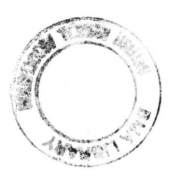

Vascular and Interventional Radiology
The Requisites

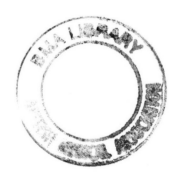

THE REQUISITES

Vascular and Interventional Radiology

Second Edition

John A. Kaufman, MD, MS, FSIR, FCIRSE
Director, Dotter Interventional Institute
Frederick S. Keller Professor of Interventional Radiology
Oregon Health & Science University Hospital
Portland, Oregon

Michael J. Lee, MSc, FRCPI, FRCR, FFR(RCSI), FSIR, EBIR
Consultant Interventional Radiologist, Beaumont Hospital
Professor of Radiology, Royal College of Surgeons in Ireland
Department of Radiology, Beaumont Hospital
Dublin, Ireland

ELSEVIER
SAUNDERS

ELSEVIER
SAUNDERS

1600 John F. Kennedy Blvd.
Ste 1800
Philadelphia, PA 19103-2899

VASCULAR AND INTERVENTIONAL RADIOLOGY:
THE REQUISITES

ISBN: 978-0-323-04584-1

Notices

Knowledge and best practice in this field are constantly changing. As new research and experience broaden our understanding, changes in research methods, professional practices, or medical treatment may become necessary.

Practitioners and researchers must always rely on their own experience and knowledge in evaluating and using any information, methods, compounds, or experiments described herein. In using such information or methods they should be mindful of their own safety and the safety of others, including parties for whom they have a professional responsibility.

With respect to any drug or pharmaceutical products identified, readers are advised to check the most current information provided (i) on procedures featured or (ii) by the manufacturer of each product to be administered, to verify the recommended dose or formula, the method and duration of administration, and contraindications. It is the responsibility of practitioners, relying on their own experience and knowledge of their patients, to make diagnoses, to determine dosages and the best treatment for each individual patient, and to take all appropriate safety precautions.

To the fullest extent of the law, neither the Publisher nor the authors, contributors, or editors, assume any liability for any injury and/or damage to persons or property as a matter of products liability, negligence or otherwise, or from any use or operation of any methods, products, instructions, or ideas contained in the material herein.

Library of Congress Cataloging-in-Publication Data
Kaufman, John A., author.
  Vascular and interventional radiology: the requisites / John A. Kaufman, Prof Michael J. Lee.—Second edition.
    p. ; cm.—(Requisites) (Requisites in radiology series)
  Includes bibliographical references and index.
  ISBN 978-0-323-04584-1 (hardcover)
  I. Lee, Michael J., author. II. Title. III. Series: Requisites series. IV. Series: Requisites in radiology.
  [DNLM: 1. Vascular Diseases—radiography. 2. Radiography, Interventional—methods. WG 500]
  RD598.67
  617.4'13059--dc23   2013009169

Senior Content Strategist: Don Scholz
Content Development Specialist: Margaret Nelson
Publishing Services Manager: Deborah Vogel
Project Manager: Brandilyn Flagg
Designer: Steve Stave

Printed in China

Last digit is the print number: 9 8 7 6 5 4 3 2 1

For our children, Nick, Claire, and Alex. You are everything to us.

John and Cathy Kaufman

For Eileen, Aoife, Ronan, Daire, and Sarah, and my parents Joe and Rose.

Michael J. Lee

Contributors

Michael D. Beland, MD
Assistant Professor
Department of Diagnostic Imaging
Alpert Medical School of Brown University;
Director of Ultrasound
Department of Diagnostic Imaging
Rhode Island Hospital
Providence, Rhode Island
Chapter 25: Image-Guided Tumor Ablation: Basic Principles

Peter J. Bromley, MD, FRCPC
Consultant Radiologist
Departments of Radiology and Surgery
Peter Lougheed Centre
Calgary, Alberta, Canada
Chapter 14: Portal and Hepatic Veins

Xavier Buy, MD
Department of Interventional Radiology
University Hospital of Strasbourg
Strasbourg, France
Chapter 24: Musculoskeletal Intervention

Colin P. Cantwell, FRCR, FFR
Consultant Interventional Radiologist
Radiology Department
St. Vincent's University Hospital
Dublin, Ireland
Chapter 26: Image-Guided Ablation of Renal Tumors
Chapter 28: Image-Guided Ablation of Liver Tumors

Damian E. Dupuy, MD, FACR
Professor of Diagnostic Imaging
Department of Diagnostic Imaging
Alpert Medical School of Brown University;
Director of Tumor Ablation
Department of Diagnostic Imaging
Rhode Island Hospital
Providence, Rhode Island
Chapter 27: Image-Guided Ablation as a Treatment Option for Thoracic Malignancies

Afshin Gangi, MD, PhD
Professor
University of Strasbourg;
Department of Interventional Radiology
Nouvel Hopital Civil (NHC)
Strasbourg, France
Chapter 24: Musculoskeletal Intervention

Debra A. Gervais, MD
Division Chief, Abdominal Imaging and Intervention
Division Chief, Pediatric Imaging
Assistant Program Director, MGH Radiology Residency
Massachusetts General Hospital and Harvard Medical School
Boston, Massachusetts
Chapter 26: Image-Guided Ablation of Renal Tumors
Chapter 28: Image-Guided Ablation of Liver Tumors

Niamh Hambly, MBBChBAO, MRCPI, FFR(RCSI)
Consultant Radiologist
Beaumont Hospital
Dublin, Ireland
Chapter 23: Image-Guided Breast Intervention

Farah G. Irani, MD
Department of Interventional Radiology
University Hospital of Strasbourg
Strasbourg, France
Chapter 24: Musculoskeletal Intervention

Alice M. Kim, MD
Clinical Instructor of Radiology
Department of Radiology
New York Hospital Queens—New York Presbyterian – Weill Cornell Medical College;
Radiologist
Department of Radiology
New York Hospital Queens
Flushing, New York
Chapter 27: Image-Guided Ablation as a Treatment Option for Thoracic Malignancies

William W. Mayo-Smith, MD, FACR
Professor of Radiology
Alpert Medical School of Brown University;
Director of CT and Body Imaging & Intervention
Department of Radiology
Rhode Island Hospital
Providence, Rhode Island
Chapter 25: Image-Guided Tumor Ablation: Basic Principles

Gary M. Nesbit, MD
Professor
Dotter Interventional Institute, Radiology, Neurosurgery, and Neurology
Oregon Health & Science University
Portland, Oregon;
Adjunct Associate Professor
Department of Radiology
University of Utah
Salt Lake City, Utah
Chapter 5: Carotid and Vertebral Arteries

Constantino S. Pena, MD
Affiliate Assistant Professor
Department of Radiology
University of South Florida College of Medicine
Tampa, Florida;
Medical Director of Vascular Imaging
Department of Interventional Radiology
Baptist Cardiac and Vascular Institute
Miami, Florida
Chapter 3: Noninvasive Vascular Imaging

Foreword

The first edition of *Vascular and Interventional Radiology: THE REQUISITES* was the tenth book in the series and shared the overall series goal of providing core material in major subspecialty areas of radiology for use by residents and fellows during their training and by practicing radiologists seeking to review or expand their knowledge. The original book achieved its goals in outstanding fashion and now it is time for the second edition, which reflects the rather remarkable strides that have been made in vascular and interventional radiology over the past several years.

As noted previously, each book in THE REQUISITES series has offered a different set of challenges. In the case of vascular and interventional radiology, a major challenge for the second edition was the need to cover many new procedures and provide outcomes information for procedures that have begun to mature. Examples from the two ends of the spectrum include the transformative development of regional delivery of targeted therapies and the growing body of knowledge about outcomes in the use of percutaneously implanted devices and stents. Drs. Kaufman and Lee have again done an outstanding job of distilling this important material and the basic concepts of vascular and interventional radiology into a text that achieves high marks for readability and accessibility.

There is no subspecialty area of radiology more vulnerable to turf battles than vascular and interventional radiology. It is imperative that radiologists continue to acquire skills in this area if the specialty is going to remain a strong provider of these services. One of the great advantages that radiologists have is their superior knowledge of imaging, which is of course the guiding hand of both diagnostic and therapeutic interventions. Drs. Kaufman and Lee have richly illustrated their book to reflect the flexibility of multi-modality imaging that is now associated with performing interventions.

In surgery morbidity is often linked to the amount of normal tissue that must be compromised in order to reach—visualize—diseased tissues. By using noninvasive imaging to achieve visualization and minimally invasive percutaneous access to treat disease, interventional radiology simply offers a better option than traditional open surgery for many conditions.

One of the major strengths of THE REQUISITES series has been the continuity of authorship from one edition to the next, allowing authors to build on their work while updating it appropriately. The current book is as fresh and relevant to today's contemporary practice of vascular and interventional radiology as its predecessor. The book also continues to be comprehensive enough to serve as both an introductory text to the subject material covered and an efficient source for review prior to examinations.

While the length and format of each volume in THE REQUISITES series are dictated by the material being covered, the principal goal of the series is to equip the reader with a text that provides the basic factual, conceptual, and interpretive material required for clinical practice. I believe residents in radiology will find that the second edition of *Vascular and Interventional Radiology: THE REQUISITES* is an excellent tool in these respects for learning the subject. Drs. Kaufman and Lee have again captured the most important material in a very user-friendly text.

In addition to residents, physicians in practice and those undertaking fellowship programs in vascular and interventional radiology will also find this book extremely useful. For seasoned practitioners and fellows alike, *Vascular and Interventional Radiology: THE REQUISITES* provides the material they need for contemporary clinical practice.

I congratulate John Kaufman and Michael Lee for another outstanding contribution to THE REQUISITES in Radiology.

James H. Thrall, MD
Radiologist-in-Chief
Department of Radiology
Massachusetts General Hospital;
Juan M. Taveras Professor of Radiology
Harvard Medical School
Boston, Massachusetts

Preface

The specialty of interventional radiology has never been, and never will be, static, boring, or easily characterized. With a unique combination of imaging, procedures, medicine, technology, and clinical variety, there is hardly a more exciting specialty. Image-guided, minimally invasive therapies are recognized by patients and other physicians as the way of the future, and interventional radiology is at the center.

The origins of this specialty lie in diagnostic imaging. In the era before cross-sectional imaging, the only nonoperative way to evaluate many pathologic conditions was to put needles into the recesses of the body, such as blood vessels, bile ducts, renal collecting systems, subarachnoid spaces, and peritoneal cavities, and then inject contrast. In 1964 in Portland, Oregon, Charles Dotter performed the first percutaneous transluminal angioplasty (see Fig. 4-1). This shifted the whole paradigm. Radiologists who performed angiography and other special diagnostic procedures began to think of themselves as interventionalists. Not only could they diagnose the disease, but they could treat it as well.

Slowly but inevitably, procedures that once required surgeons and surgical incisions have been replaced by interventionalists using percutaneous image-guided techniques. Percutaneous catheter drainage of abdominal abscesses has all but supplanted open "I & D." More recently transcatheter uterine artery embolization for symptomatic fibroids has become a major alternative to hysterectomy. With each technological innovation, the number and breadth of procedures increases. The impact of the percutaneously delivered intravascular metallic stent, particularly on the management of arterial occlusive and aneurysmal disease, has been enormous. Embolization and other procedures are now essential to the management of patients with advanced solid tumors in many organs.

Once dismissed as fringe practitioners of dangerous and unproven arts, interventional radiologists have become indispensable to the daily functioning of the medical system. Although we will never lose our imaging roots, interventional radiologists are increasingly participants in the clinical care of many different kinds of patients. Make no mistake about it; interventional radiology is here to stay.

The impact of image-guided interventions has not gone unnoticed by the rest of medicine. Early in our history, cardiologists determined that cardiac catheterization should move from radiology, where it was developed, to medicine, because that was where the heart was cared for. Interventions for arterial occlusive and aneurysmal disease have been aggressively embraced by cardiologists and vascular surgeons. It seems that everyone is now interested in image-guided interventions. What does this mean? First of all: Success! Interventional procedures are now mainstream and legitimized. Second: Excitement! There are no limits to our innovation and therapeutic horizons. Third: Change! Interventional radiologists can no longer wait for someone else to decide which procedure to order and when but must see patients in offices or clinics, render consultations, recommend a course of action, perform the procedure, and provide follow-up. Lastly: Challenge! If only for the benefit of patients, interventional radiology must mature into the core specialty for all minimally invasive practitioners, with the basic and clinical research to support the procedures and standards that ensure safe and effective care.

Volume II of THE REQUISITES provides more up-to-date information for this exciting specialty. We have endeavored to make it accessible enough for residents but detailed enough to be used by fellows and those seeking a current overview. The format is designed to allow quick reference for technical or diagnostic questions but also to provide detailed and focused information. The images have been carefully selected to be representative of current practice, with the use of cross-sectional techniques whenever possible. When the book started, the authors were colleagues at the Massachusetts General Hospital, one in the Division of Vascular Radiology (Kaufman), the other in the Division of Abdominal Imaging and Intervention (Lee). Today we are international co-conspirators, so that the book reflects a global perspective. To sum it all up, we think interventional radiology is great, this is how we do it, and we hope you enjoy this book.

John A. Kaufman, MD, MS, FSIR, FCIRSE
Michael J. Lee, MSc, FRCPI, FRCR,
FFR(RCSI), FSIR, EBIR

Acknowledgments

When James Thrall invited me to write this book, I was simultaneously ecstatic and terrified. As a junior faculty member in his department at the Massachusetts General Hospital, the invitation was an immense honor, but I had no idea how or when I would do it. After a while (well, after a few years), Jim was probably thinking the same thing. Fortunately for me, Jim has been the most patient mentor, counselor, guide, and friend that I could have ever wished for. Without his unflagging support, I could not have done this.

One of my first steps was to ask Mick Lee to collaborate on the book (read "share the pain"). Fortunately, he agreed. Mick is a superb interventionalist, great guy, and, to my chagrin, a much more efficient writer than I am. Without him the book would not be. I am proud that I can link my name with his on the cover.

Accomplishments, such as a book, mirror the people in our lives. I am a radiologist because I followed the example of someone much smarter than I, my father, Sy Kaufman. During my first year of residency, I rotated on "Specials" with Alan Greenfield and John Guben. As the cliché goes, I never looked back. In July of 1991, after my fellowship with Alan, Jim Parker, and another long-time friend Mike Bettmann, I joined the Division of Vascular Radiology at MGH. Arthur Waltman welcomed me into a dream job, a professional family, and the most formative experience of my career. Over the next 9 years I learned from an outstanding group of colleagues, including Chris Athanasoulis (whose 1982 textbook *Interventional Radiology* greatly influenced this book), Chieh-Min Fan, Mark Rieumont, Kent Yucel, and Mitch Rivitz. Above all, I worked with Stuart Geller. I have never learned so much from one person, ever. Stuart, I have tried to put all of it in here; I hope that I have it right.

In July 2000, I joined Fred Keller, Josef Rösch, Bryan Petersen, Rob Barton, Torre Andrews, Paul Lakin, Ken Kolbeck, Khashayar Farsad, Gary Nesbit, Stan Barnwell, and Dusan Pavcnik at the Dotter Institute in Portland, Oregon. Once again I found myself learning from, inspired by, and supported by superb interventionalists, innovators, and people. The majority of the images in this book are from the Dotter Institute and were created by these special colleagues

Over the years I have been fortunate to spend time with a large number of delightful fellows and residents. They don't know it, but they are the real reason for staying in academics. They have all been incredibly generous and reliable when answering my pleas for images, especially Barry Stein in Hartford, Connecticut, and Constantino ("Tino") Pena in Miami, Florida. One of my fellows from the Dotter Institute, Peter Bromley, created many excellent original line drawings in this book.

Sheri Imai-Swiggart at the Dotter Institute toiled over the images for the first edition of this book for 2 years. Special thanks to Bobby Hill for many of the CT reconstructions, including the cover, in this edition. This project has taken so long that it has outlasted several generations of Elsevier editors and production staff. Stephanie Donley, Mia Cariño, Elizabeth Corra, Hilarie Surrena, and Christy Bracken all graciously brought the first edition to life. Margaret Nelson, Sabina Borza, Stacey Fisher, Martha Limbach, and Rebecca Gaertner patiently and persistently made the second edition a reality.

An author's family sees a different side of the process. This book was time together lost, both in person and in mind. The end product has little bearing on the real stuff of family life. Yet each and every one supported and encouraged me. Cathy, my wife, learned very quickly that this book doubled her work as a parent, which she undertook with characteristic enthusiasm. She has been the co-author of my life since I was 18-years-old. My daughter Claire Kaufman and son-in-law Keith Quencer, my two favorite radiology residents in the world, were incredible proofreaders for this second edition. My two boys, Nick and Alex; mother; and in-laws all saw "the book" as yet another work-related obsession and adjusted accordingly. Even the dogs were nice about it.

Thanks to you all.

J.A.K

My journey in Interventional Radiology began in 1989 when I started a Fellowship in Abdominal Imaging and Interventional Radiology at Massachusetts General Hospital. Fresh from my radiology residency in Ireland, I was not sure what to expect. The teaching and professionalism of the staff at MGH soon dispelled my uncertainty. In particular, I would like to thank Peter Mueller, Nick Papanicolau, Steve Dawson, and Peter Hahn for imparting a wealth of wisdom and experience regarding all things interventional. As a fellow, one of the most satisfying achievements is to complete a technically difficult or challenging procedure without a staff supervisor taking over. I am sure it was difficult at times but thank you for not "taking over."

I believe that interventional radiologists should have a firm grasp of imaging to make correct therapeutic decisions for their patients. During my 6 years at MGH, I was fortunate to learn from some of the great imagers: Joe Ferucci, Jack Wittenberg, Joe Simeone, and Sanjay Saini to name but a few.

I would like to take this opportunity to especially thank Peter Mueller for his encouragement and support, both clinically and academically during my MGH years. Peter was a great mentor and continues to be a good friend.

Jim Thrall, Chairman of Radiology at MGH, allowed us the freedom to develop clinical and academic skills but also fostered leadership talents. This was accomplished with minimal fuss but occasional gentle nudging in a certain direction.

When John Kaufman asked me to co-author the first edition of this book, I was leaving MGH to take up a Chair in Radiology at the Medical School of the Royal College of Surgeons in Ireland, attached to Beaumont Hospital, Dublin (I have now been in this position for 17 years). I was delighted to accept, knowing that John is a great writer, interventionalist, and good friend. The first edition was duly completed and no sooner published when the idea of a second edition surfaced. After the many hours spent writing the first edition, the thought of a second edition took a while to flame in my mind. However, as time went by, the toil involved in writing the first edition faded and enthusiasm for the second edition increased. So here we are with the second edition. It was again a mammoth task and took much longer as John and I were both very busy with many other endeavors in the IR world. John has been President of SIR during the period of this project and I have been President of CIRSE.

I commissioned chapters from Niamh Hambly, Afshin Gangi and colleagues, Bill Mayo-Smith, Debbie Gervais, and Damian Dupuy and would like to thank them for their superb efforts. I would like to thank Sarah Taylor, Jill Kavanagh, and Gail O'Brien for their expert typing and organizational skills, and all the staff at Elsevier who have patiently reminded us over the years that these books needed to be completed. These include Stephanie Donley, Elizabeth Corra, Mia Cariño, Christy Bracken, and Hilarie Surrena for Volume I; and Margaret Nelson, Sabina Borza, Stacey Fisher, Martha Limbach, and Rebecca Gaertner for Volume II.

Finally, and most importantly, I would like to thank my wife Eileen for her unwavering support. Family, interventional radiology, and academic radiology are a difficult combination to balance. Writing a book, in addition to the latter, shifts the balance considerably. I could not have written this book without Eileen's support and understanding.

Interventional radiology is a fantastically rewarding specialty for those of us fortunate enough to practice it. I sincerely hope that Volume II of THE REQUISITES in interventional radiology contributes to the safe practice of our specialty, and I hope that it helps you, the reader, in your IR practice.

M.J.L

Contents

CHAPTER 1

Vascular Pathology

John A. Kaufman, MD, MS, FSIR, FCIRSE

THE NORMAL VASCULAR WALL	NEOPLASMS	IMPINGEMENT SYNDROMES
ATHEROSCLEROSIS	DISSECTION	ADVENTITIAL CYSTIC DISEASE
INTIMAL HYPERPLASIA	TRAUMA	MÖNCKEBERG SCLEROSIS
ANEURYSMS	VASOSPASTIC DISORDERS	THROMBOSIS
FIBROMUSCULAR DYSPLASIA	ARTERIAL EMBOLISM	
VASCULITIS	INFECTION	
HEMANGIOMAS, VASCULAR MALFORMATIONS, AND ARTERIOVENOUS FISTULAS	INHERITED DISORDERS OF THE ARTERIAL WALL	

Blood vessels are, in the simplest of terms, the plumbing of the body. Problems arise when blood flow is diminished, excessive, in the wrong direction, or when leaks occur (Table 1-1). In reality, blood vessels are complex organs within other complex organs. The degree of vascular disease that can be tolerated before symptoms occur varies with the type of blood vessel, the nature and metabolic state of the perfused organ, and the patient. Just as vascular disease can affect an organ, disease in an organ can affect its blood vessels. Often, vascular pathology can result in loss of limb, organ, or life. The ubiquitous and serious nature of vascular disease makes this a fascinating clinical area. This chapter reviews the basic types of pathology that can occur in blood vessels. The clinical presentation, diagnosis, and therapy of disease in a particular vascular bed or organ are addressed in specific chapters.

THE NORMAL VASCULAR WALL

The walls of arteries have three layers: the intima, media, and adventitia (Fig. 1-1). The intima forms the interface between the artery and the blood. Composed of endothelial cells, fibroblasts, and connective tissue, this is the site of much arterial pathology. The intima is a dynamic, hormonally active layer that responds to acute stress by release of substances such as prostaglandins and platelet activating factors. Chronic stress, such as turbulence, induces proliferation of the endothelial cells and fibroblasts. Any object in prolonged contact with the intima eventually becomes coated with a layer of new endothelial cells (neointima). In some circumstances, this proliferation results in local obstructive phenomena. The intima therefore has a central role in the natural history of vascular diseases and the outcome of vascular interventions.

The muscular media is sandwiched between and distinct from the intima and adventitia. This layer provides both structural support for the arterial wall as well as the ability to react acutely to sudden hemodynamic changes. The media is made up of well-ordered layers of elastic fibers, smooth muscle cells, and connective tissue. Smooth muscle cells are orientated in both concentric and longitudinal directions. The normal arterial media is elastic, dilating slightly with each systole and then recoiling during diastole. This is most pronounced in medium and large muscular arteries, and assists in the circulation of blood through the arterial system. In response to demands for increased blood flow the smooth muscle cells relax, resulting in enlargement of the vessel lumen (vasodilatation). Conversely, to restrict blood flow, the muscle cells contract to decrease the diameter of the lumen (vasoconstriction). With aging and certain pathologic conditions (e.g., atherosclerosis), the media loses this elasticity and responsiveness as the smooth muscle cells are replaced by fibrotic tissue or become disorganized. In fact, large atherosclerotic intimal plaques can actually invade the media. The media is also the site of expression of heritable connective tissue disorders such as Marfan syndrome and Ehlers-Danlos syndrome.

The adventitia is a tough yet filmy layer of connective tissue that forms the boundary between the artery and the surrounding structures. This layer contains collagen, fibroblasts, and some smooth muscle cells. Weaving through the interface of the adventitia and media are the small vascular channels (the vasa vasorum) that supply blood to capillaries within the adventitia and the outer third of the media. The inner part of the media and the intima receive nutrients from the blood in the vessel lumen by diffusion. The density of the vasa vasorum is highest in the thickest, most muscular portions of the arteries, such as the ascending and transverse aorta. The adventitia also contains the adrenergic nerves (nervi vascularis) that control vasoconstriction and dilatation.

Veins also have walls with three layers, similarly termed the *intima*, *media*, and *adventitia*. Venous and arterial intima and adventitia are similar in composition and function. The venous intima rarely undergoes the pathologic changes seen in arteries, unless the vein is exposed to arterial pressures, high flow rates, or foreign bodies for long periods of time. Fibrointimal hyperplasia in response to trauma, implantation of endoluminal devices, and increased flow is common. This feature of the venous intimal surface is a major determinant of the long-term outcome of many venous vascular interventions.

The medial layer of veins contains fewer smooth muscle cells than arteries, thus accounting for the relatively thinner, flaccid appearance of the walls. In addition, the connective tissue component of the venous media is less pronounced than that of arteries. As a result, veins contribute capacitance to the circulation. Blood return is facilitated by unidirectional bicuspid valves in the small to medium-sized veins that permit flow only toward the heart. Blood flow is maintained by a combination of processes, including gravity, external compression by muscle contraction, and pressure gradients created during inspiration and expiration. The smooth muscle cells of the small to medium veins can dilate and contract in response to stimuli, thus partially regulating flow.

TABLE 1-1 Clinical Manifestations of Vascular Pathology*

Manifestation	Example
Obstruction to forward flow	Arterial and venous stenoses, occlusions
Increased forward flow	Arteriovenous fistula, malformation
Increased retrograde flow	Varicose veins due to reflux through incompetent venous valves
Loss of vessel wall integrity	Aneurysm, dissection, bleeding

*These can occur alone or in any combination.

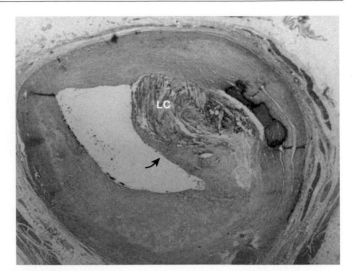

FIGURE 1-2. Atheromatous plaque. Eccentric atheroma, with thin fibrous cap *(arrow)* overlying necrotic lipid core (LC) (H&E × 50). (From Johnson DE. Anatomic aspects of vascular disease. In: Strandness ED, Breda AV, eds. *Vascular Diseases: Surgical and Interventional Therapy.* New York: Churchill Livingstone, 1994, with permission.)

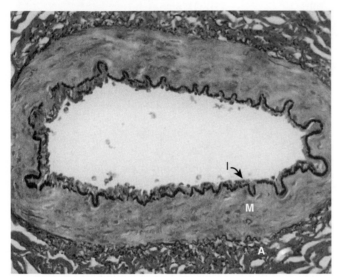

FIGURE 1-1. Photomicrograph of normal small muscular artery (VVG × 650). I, intima; M, media; A, adventitia. The wavy black line between the intima and media is the internal elastica lamina. (From Johnson DE. Anatomic aspects of vascular disease. In: Strandness ED, Breda AV, eds. *Vascular Diseases: Surgical and Interventional Therapy.* New York: Churchill Livingstone, 1994, with permission.)

Box 1-1. Risk Factors for Atherosclerosis

Genetic predisposition
Smoking
Diet
Diabetes
Chronic renal failure
Hypertension
Hyperhomocysteinemia
Advanced age
Dyslipidemia
Obesity

ATHEROSCLEROSIS

Atherosclerosis is an arterial disease that is prevalent in industrialized nations. Veins do not develop atherosclerotic lesions unless they are exposed to arterial pressures and flow over extended periods of time. The risk factors for atherosclerosis include environmental and genetic factors (Box 1-1). There are multiple theories of causation, including intimal trauma, an autoimmune response, and infection. Whatever the underlying pathogenesis, the key point is that atherosclerosis is a systemic disease, affecting arteries in all vascular beds. For example, patients presenting with peripheral arterial manifestations of atherosclerosis have risk ratios for ischemic coronary events and stroke over 10 years that are 2-6 times higher than for the general population.

The hallmark of an atherosclerotic lesion is the fibrofatty plaque, which begins as microscopic lipid deposition in areas of intimal injury. Continued injury leads to a fatty streak, an accumulation of foam cells and macrophages that is the first evidence of atherosclerosis visible with the naked eye. As the lesion progresses, the lipid content increases and a fibrotic cap forms over the surface. The cap, composed of smooth muscle cells and collagen, isolates the highly thrombogenic contents of the plaque from the blood (Fig. 1-2). If the cap is disrupted, a shower of cholesterol crystals and debris may flow downstream, producing a potentially devastating syndrome termed *cholesterol embolization.* More often, platelet aggregation leads to thrombus formation on the exposed surface of the plaque. This thrombus can embolize distally or enlarge to occlude the artery. Plaques that have little calcification and large lipid components are believed to be more prone to this complication, and have been termed *vulnerable plaque.* These lesions are often clinically asymptomatic until they rupture; they are implicated in many acute coronary and carotid artery syndromes. There is great interest in the development of imaging techniques that would identify vulnerable plaque.

Atherosclerotic lesions can be circumferential, narrowing the arterial lumen in a concentric manner (Fig. 1-3). Plaque that predominantly affects one side of the artery wall results in an eccentric lesion (Fig. 1-4). Longstanding plaque can become quite bulky, calcify, and even protrude into the arterial lumen like a coral reef.

Compromise of the arterial lumen from any cause results in restriction of flow at the site of stenosis (Fig. 1-5). Initially the velocity of flow through the stenotic area will increase, but as the lumen becomes narrower, the flow velocity eventually decreases. In general, a reduction in luminal diameter of 50% (equivalent to a 75% decrease in the area of the lumen) is required before a pressure drop across the stenosis occurs, although many other variables are important. A reduction in diameter of 75% represents a more than 90% decrease in cross-sectional area of the lumen. However, clinical symptoms occur only when the decrease in arterial flow causes end-organ ischemia or dysfunction.

There is a complex relationship between arterial occlusive disease and symptoms. The mere presence of a stenosis does not mean that a patient will have symptoms. The metabolic and

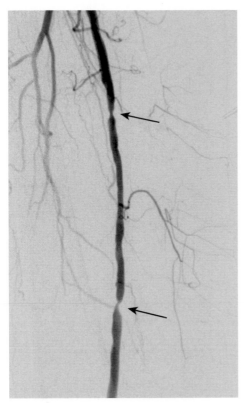

FIGURE 1-3. Angiographic appearance of concentric stenoses of the left superficial femoral artery *(arrows)*.

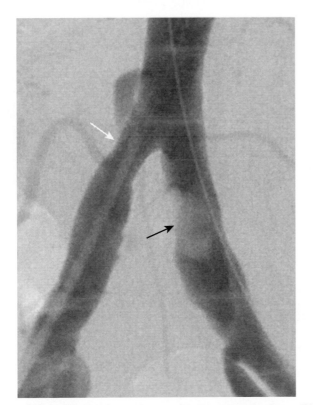

FIGURE 1-4. Angiographic appearance of bulky, eccentric plaque *(black arrow)* in the left common iliac artery. Compare this to the concentric stenosis of the right common iliac artery *(white arrow)*.

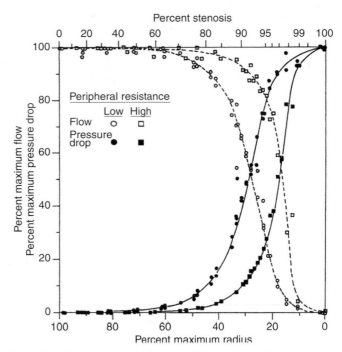

FIGURE 1-5. Relationship of pressure and flow to degree of stenosis. When peripheral resistance is high, the curves are shifted to the right. (From Sumner D. Essential hemodynamic principles. In: Rutherford RB, ed. *Vascular Surgery*, 5th ed. Philadelphia: WB Saunders, 2000, with permission.)

pathologic state of the end organ, the degree of collateralization around the stenosis, and the rapidity of onset of the reduced flow are all crucial variables. For example, the classic clinical presentation of chronic lower extremity arterial occlusive disease is ischemic muscular pain with ambulation, relieved by rest. Organs with numerous potential sources of blood supply, such as the colon, are more likely to tolerate gradual onset of occlusive disease than organs with a solitary blood supply, such as the kidney. Gradual onset of occlusion allows existing small supplementary arteries to enlarge, forming a well-developed collateral network that may compensate for most or all of the flow in the original artery (Fig. 1-6). Acute onset of stenosis or occlusion is more likely to produce symptoms, even at rest, when collateral vessels are poorly formed or cannot carry sufficient flow (Fig. 1-7).

▬ INTIMAL HYPERPLASIA

Intimal hyperplasia is not a true disease or disorder, but a complex biologic response to injury to the vessel wall (Fig. 1-8). Whenever the intimal layer of either an artery or vein is injured, fibrin deposition and platelet aggregation occurs. Macrophages and smooth muscle cells quickly migrate into the fibrin-platelet matrix, where they proliferate. Within days of the original injury, endothelial cells appear over the surface of the matrix, extending from the adjacent intact intima or by direct inoculation by circulating endothelial precursor cells. This results in formation of a neointima over the site of injury. Over approximately 12 weeks there is exuberant proliferation of smooth muscle and endothelial cells, such that some encroachment upon the vessel lumen occurs. After approximately 3 months, the entire process may slow or stop, with thinning and stabilization. For reasons that are not well understood, this process is accelerated or prolonged in some patients. The hyperplastic neointimal response can cause narrowing of the vessel lumen that is actually greater and more extensive than the original lesion.

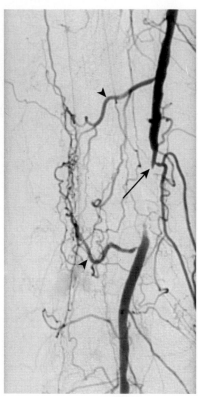

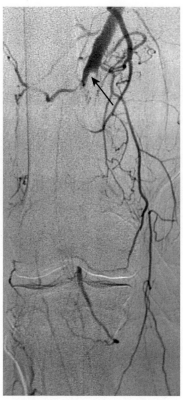

FIGURE 1-6. Hypertrophied collateral arteries around a short chronic occlusion of the distal superficial femoral artery. Digital subtraction angiogram shows enlarged muscular branches *(arrowheads)* providing flow around the occlusion with reconstitution of the above-knee popliteal artery. Note the tapered contour of the lumen at the occlusion *(arrow)*, which occurs just distal to a muscular branch.

FIGURE 1-7. Poor collateral arterial supply around an acute occlusion due to thrombosis of a popliteal artery aneurysm. Digital subtraction angiogram shows an abrupt cutoff of flow with a filling defect *(arrow)* consistent with thrombus. There is a paucity of collateral vessels and lack of reconstitution of distal vessels.

Intimal hyperplasia is the bane of vascular interventions, occurring at surgical anastomoses, angioplasty sites, and after stent deployment (Table 1-2). A number of strategies to reduce intimal hyperplasia have been proposed or are under investigation, including brachytherapy (intravascular radiation), covered stents, drug-eluting stents, freezing balloons, gene therapy, and systemic medications. No single technique has proven entirely successful. Currently, the best results are still obtained by limiting the extent of intimal injury, minimizing the use of prosthetic materials, and maximizing the final diameter of the lumen.

ANEURYSMS

Aneurysms are primarily an arterial disease, although venous aneurysms do occur. Aneurysms may be either "true" or "false," depending upon whether all three layers of the vessel wall are intact (Table 1-3 and Fig. 1-9). The etiology of the aneurysm determines the type and influences the clinical course.

True aneurysms are associated with a number of risk factors (Box 1-2). In general, focal enlargement of an artery to more than 1.5 times its normal diameter constitutes an aneurysm. The most common type of true aneurysm is degenerative. The pathogenesis of degenerative aneurysm formation is not yet fully understood, but may involve atherosclerotic, mechanical (i.e., post-stenotic dilatation), enzymatic, autoimmune, and potentially infectious mechanisms. For example, metalloproteinases are proteolytic enzymes synthesized by macrophages that are elevated in patients with abdominal aortic aneurysms. The levels drop to normal following successful repair by either surgical or endovascular techniques. Regardless of the mechanism, aneurysm formation is associated with thinning of the media and loss of smooth muscle cells, elastic fibers, and collagen.

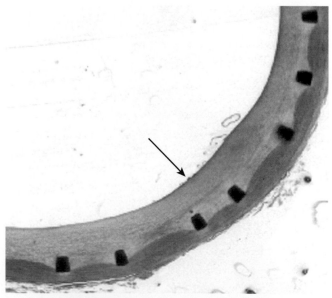

FIGURE 1-8. Intimal hyperplasia. Low-power micrograph shows thickened intima *(arrow)* lining the luminal surface of a metallic stent 6 months after placement in an external iliac artery.

Degenerative aneurysms are often multifocal, occurring in large to medium-sized arteries in numerous vascular beds in a single patient. The most common arteries in which aneurysms are found are the abdominal and thoracic aortas, the common iliac, internal iliac, common femoral, popliteal, subclavian, and visceral arteries. External iliac and extracranial carotid artery aneurysms

TABLE 1-2 Causes of Intimal Hyperplasia

Cause	Examples
Injury	Surgical anastomosis, clamps, angioplasty, excoriation of intima by any process
Foreign body	Stents, catheters
Abnormal flow	Arterialization of veins, turbulence

TABLE 1-3 True vs. False Aneurysms

Feature	True	False
Location	Expected	Often unexpected
Vessel wall	All three layers intact	Less than three layers intact
Etiology	Intrinsic abnormality	Trauma, rupture of true aneurysm, infection
Contours	Smooth	Irregular, lobulated
Calcification	Present in intima	Absent unless chronic
Rupture	Risk increases with size	Higher risk than same size true aneurysm

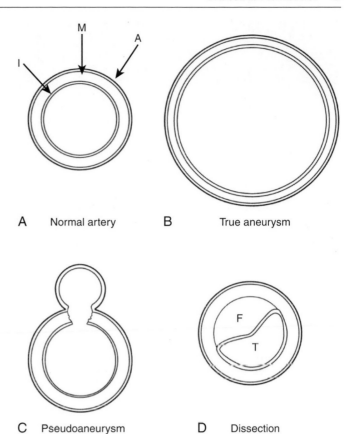

FIGURE 1-9. Diagram illustrating the differences between true aneurysms, false aneurysms, and dissections. **A,** The normal artery has three intact layers: I, intima; M, media, A, adventitia. **B,** True aneurysm. All three layers of the arterial wall remain intact, although there is thinning of the media. **C,** Pseudoaneurysm. In this drawing, there is disruption of the intima and media, with formation of a saccular aneurysm contained by the adventitia. **D,** Dissection. All three layers are essentially intact, and the artery may be normal in caliber, but the intima has separated from the media, dividing the artery into two channels (T, true lumen; F, false lumen). The false lumen may be patent or thrombosed. When patent, it is frequently larger than the true lumen. (Modified from Wojtowycz M. *Handbook of Interventional Radiology and Angiography.* St. Louis: Mosby, 1995, with permission.)

are rare. Generalized enlargement without focal aneurysm formation is termed *arteriomegaly*.

Aneurysms of large arteries most often cause symptoms by rupturing (especially the aorta, common iliac, and internal iliac arteries) (Fig. 1-10). Symptoms due to mass effect are less common but well described. Aneurysms of visceral arteries most often present clinically with rupture. Aneurysms of most other small and medium arteries (exclusive of the intracranial circulation) typically present with symptoms related to thrombosis and distal embolization (see Fig. 1-7). All aneurysms can become secondarily infected.

False aneurysms are focal enlargements of the vascular lumen due to partial or complete disruption of the arterial wall (see Fig. 1-9). The blood is contained by residual elements of the arterial wall or surrounding tissues. Also known as pseudoaneurysms (PSAs), they are more prone to rupture than similar sized true aneurysms. The cause of most PSAs encountered in clinical practice is iatrogenic, such as surgery, angiography, or percutaneous biopsies. Penetrating wounds, crush injuries, and deceleration injuries are common etiologies of PSA occurring outside of the hospital. In addition, PSA may result from contained rupture of true aneurysms or vascular infection (mycotic aneurysm).

FIBROMUSCULAR DYSPLASIA

Fibromuscular dysplasia (FMD) is a collection of fibrotic disorders of the intima, media, or adventitia of medium-sized arteries (Table 1-4). The most frequently affected arteries are the renal, extracranial internal carotid, vertebral, iliac, subclavian, and mesenteric arteries. The etiology of this nonatherosclerotic, noninflammatory abnormality is unknown, but it tends to be found in young adult female patients. The most common subtype is medial fibroplasia, in which focal weblike stenoses alternate with small aneurysms of varying sizes ("string of natural pearls"). Figure 1-11 shows the characteristic angiographic appearance. Medial fibroplasia causes symptoms by obstructing flow (webs), distal embolization (of thrombus formed in the small aneurysms), and occlusion (spontaneous dissection). Other forms of FMD result in tapered stenoses that are less characteristic in appearance, but unusual in that patients tend to be young and without evidence of atherosclerotic disease. Precise classification of the less common forms of FMD requires pathologic specimens.

Box 1-2. **Risk Factors for Arterial Aneurysms**

Age older than 60 years
Hypertension
Male
Atherosclerosis
Familial
Chronic obstructive pulmonary disease (aortic aneurysms)
Heritable disorders
• Marfan syndrome
• Ehlers-Danlos syndrome
• Loeys-Dietz syndrome
Vasculitis
Post-stenotic jet or turbulence
Repetitive trauma

FMD is frequently a bilateral and multifocal abnormality. In most cases, asymptomatic disease remains stable throughout the patient's life. Symptomatic medial fibroplasia responds well to balloon angioplasty. The experience with angioplasty in other forms of FMD is limited but favorable, although normal caliber lumens are rarely achieved.

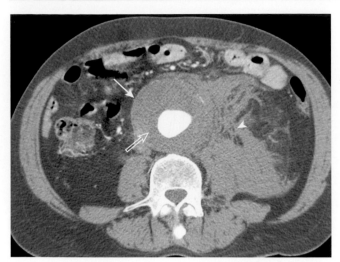

Figure 1-10. Computed tomography scan with contrast of a ruptured abdominal aortic aneurysm *(arrow)*. The lumen of the aneurysm is lined with mural thrombus *(open arrow)*. There is a hematoma in the periaortic soft tissues *(arrowhead)*.

Table 1-4 Fibromuscular Dysplasia

Type	Incidence	Predominant Features
Medial fibroplasia	85%	Alternating webs and aneurysms
Medial hyperplasia	10%	Tubular smooth stenosis
Perimedial fibroplasia	3%	Irregular, beaded stenosis
Intimal fibroplasia	1%	Focal smooth stenosis
Periarterial fibroplasia	1%	Tubular smooth stenosis

VASCULITIS

Vasculitides are inflammatory diseases of the vessel wall due to unknown causes. Inflammation due to infection is considered a mycotic process and is discussed later (see Infection). Vasculitis most commonly involves arteries, but veins can sometimes be affected. The vasculitides encountered most often in vascular imaging are those that involve large arteries (e.g., Takayasu arteritis, giant cell arteritis, and Behçet disease) and medium arteries (e.g., polyarteritis nodosa, Kawasaki disease, and Buerger disease). There are numerous types of vasculitis, most of which are associated with constitutional symptoms such as fever, arthralgia, myalgia, rash, and malaise (Table 1-5).

An elevated erythrocyte sedimentation rate (ESR) is common unless the disease has been treated or has spontaneously regressed ("burned out"). Numerous other more specific serologic markers may also be elevated, depending upon the type of vasculitis.

The diagnosis of vasculitis is usually well established before the patient is referred for imaging. The radiographic features of many of the different vasculitides overlap, such that a specific diagnosis may not be possible from the imaging studies. The diagnosis of vasculitis should be entertained whenever arterial disease such as wall thickening (especially with enhancement), bizarre-appearing stenoses, or dilations alternating with normal "skip" areas, or aneurysms, are found in unusual locations.

Takayasu arteritis is a panarteritis that involves the aorta, its major branches, and, less often, the pulmonary arteries. The cause of Takayasu arteritis is unknown, but it is presumed to be autoimmune. In the United States, the prevalence is roughly 0.5 persons per 100,000 person-years. There are no ethnic or

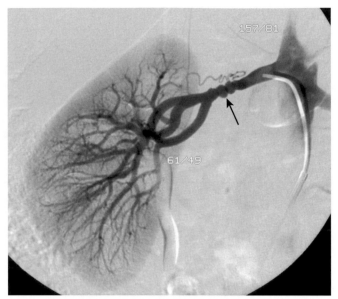

Figure 1-11. Fibromuscular dysplasia (FMD). Selective right renal artery digital subtraction angiogram in a 48-year-old woman. The irregular beaded appearance *(arrow)* and location of the abnormality in the distal main renal artery is typical of FMD of the medial fibroplasia type.

racial predilections. The typical patient is a female in her second or third decade. Granulomatous changes and lymphocytic infiltration thicken the intima and media, leading to compromise of the lumen. Chronic inflammation may also result in aneurysmal changes. There are five basic patterns of distribution of lesions, with panaortic involvement being the most common (Fig. 1-12). It is important to note that cardiac disease is present in 40% of patients, including coronary artery stenoses, aortic and mitral valvular insufficiency, and right heart failure due to pulmonary artery stenoses. A distinctive feature of active Takayasu arteritis is wall enhancement following administration of contrast on computed tomography (CT) or magnetic resonance imaging (MRI) (Fig. 1-13).

Takayasu arteritis is also known as "pulseless disease," because stenoses or occlusions of the proximal subclavian and common carotid arteries are common (Fig. 1-14; see also Fig. 9-31). Patients may present with renal hypertension due to abdominal aortic stenoses proximal to or involving the renal arteries. The stenotic lesions are usually long and smooth, although associated plaque may be present in longstanding aortic lesions of older patients. Aortic aneurysms, which are found in up to one-third of patients, rarely rupture. Treatment of uncomplicated Takayasu arteritis is with steroids.

Polyarteritis nodosa (PAN) is a systemic necrotizing vasculitis that affects primarily small and medium-sized arteries of the abdominal visceral organs, the heart, and the hands and feet. Patients are usually in their fourth or fifth decade, but may be of any age. Males are affected twice as often as females. There is a strong association between PAN and active hepatitis types B and C, as well as intravenous drug abuse, but more than 50% of patients have no known cause. Patients have constitutional, dermatologic, and neurologic manifestations, as well as abdominal pain, renal insufficiency, and spontaneous intraabdominal or retroperitoneal hemorrhage. The angiographic lesions are characteristic, with multiple small aneurysms of the renal or visceral arteries, and digital artery occlusions (Fig. 1-15). Treatment is with steroids and cyclophosphamide.

Giant cell arteritis derives its name from the presence of giant cells in the infiltrative process in all layers of the blood vessel wall. Mononuclear cells, lymphocytes, T-cells, and macrophages are more commonly present. Patients with giant cell arteritis are generally much older than those affected by Takayasu arteritis, which

TABLE 1-5 Vasculitis

Syndrome	Vasculature Affected	Imaging Findings
Takayasu arteritis ("pulseless disease")	Large: thoracic and abdominal aorta, proximal great vessels, pulmonary arteries, coronary arteries	Thickened enhancing arterial wall on CT/MRI; long aortic stenoses; long smooth non-ostial common carotid and subclavian stenoses; pulmonary artery stenosis; coronary artery stenosis; aortic aneurysm (especially ascending)
Giant cell arteritis	Large: subclavian, axillary, brachial arteries; carotid artery branches; aorta; visceral arteries (rare)	Long irregular stenoses and occlusions; aortic aneurysm/dissection
Polyarteritis nodosa	Medium and small arteries of kidney, liver, bowel, pancreas, spleen, and extremities	Micro and small aneurysms; segmental stenoses with normal skip areas; occlusions
Kawasaki disease (mucocutaneous lymph node syndrome)	Medium and small arteries	Coronary and medium-sized artery aneurysms
Buerger disease (thromboangiitis obliterans)	Medium and small arteries of the extremities; extremity veins; visceral arteries (rare)	Occlusion of all named vessels with centripetal progression and extensive per-vascular collaterals via vasa vasorum; migratory thrombophlebitis in 30%
Behçet disease	All: large and medium arteries; pulmonary arteries, systemic veins	Venous thrombosis; peripheral and aortic aneurysms; arterial thrombosis; pulmonary artery aneurysm
Radiation arteritis	All arteries	Varies with time; early thrombosis or late stenosis, with few collaterals
Systemic lupus erythematosus, scleroderma	Small arteries, usually upper extremity	Variable length tapered stenoses and occlusions, especially digital arteries
Rheumatoid arthritis and other HLA-B27 disorders	Thoracic aorta	Aortic root dilatation

CT, Computed tomography; MRI, magnetic resonance imaging.

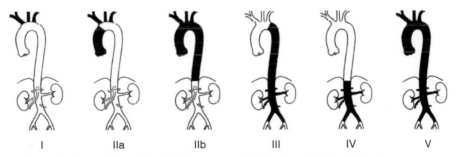

I   IIa   IIb   III   IV   V

FIGURE 1-12. Classification scheme of angiographic findings in Takayasu arteritis. The letter "C" is added when coronary artery involvement is present, and the letter "P" when pulmonary arteries are involved. (From Webb TH, Perler BA. Takayasu arteritis. In: Ernst CB, Stanley JC, eds. *Current Therapy in Vascular Surgery,* 4th ed. St. Louis: Mosby, 2001, with permission.)

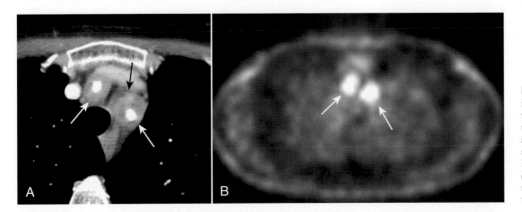

FIGURE 1-13. Takayasu arteritis involving the carotid arteries in a middle-aged woman. **A,** Contrast-enhanced computed tomography scan showing thickened arterial walls of the innominate and left subclavian arteries *(white arrows).* The left common carotid artery is occluded *(black arrow).* **B,** PET scan at same level showing activity in the thickened arterial walls *(white arrows).*

it can resemble. The classic presentation is in an older woman who suffers several weeks of fever, headaches, palpably tender temporal arteries, myalgias, and an extremely elevated ESR; also called *temporal arteritis*. Acute blindness due to involvement of the ophthalmic artery is a feared complication (40% in untreated patients). Diagnosis in these patients is most often by temporal artery biopsy.

Giant cell arteritis also causes stenoses of the extremity arteries (upper more often than lower) that manifest 8-24 weeks after onset of symptoms. The arteries involved most often are

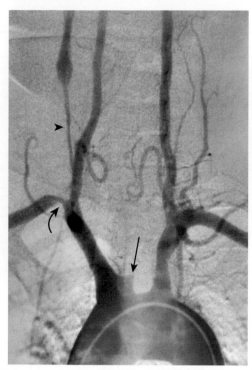

FIGURE 1-14. DSA arch aortogram showing occlusion of the left CCA *(arrow)* at the origin (bovine arch), long stenosis of the right CCA *(arrowhead)*, and stenosis of the right subclavian artery origin *(curved arrow)*.

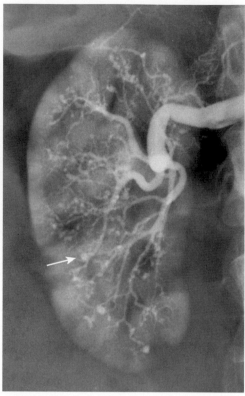

FIGURE 1-15. Polyarteritis nodosa. Angiogram of the right kidney shows numerous small peripheral aneurysms *(arrow)*. These were present in the left kidney as well.

the distal subclavian, the axillary, and the proximal brachial arteries, although a pattern very similar to Takayasu arteritis may be seen (Fig. 1-16). These patients are more likely to be referred for angiography to evaluate upper extremity ischemic symptoms. The appearance of multiple, long, irregular stenoses of these arteries is characteristic, although rarely other vasculitides, such as that associated with systemic lupus erythematosus (SLE), may produce similar lesions. Rarely, thoracic or abdominal aortic aneurysms may develop in patients with giant cell arteritis and may be the only presenting symptom. Rupture and dissection have been reported in these patients.

Buerger disease is also known as *thromboangiitis obliterans* because of the inflammatory cellular debris that occludes the vessel lumen. Even though the disease is a panarteritis, the vessel wall remains relatively intact, including the elastic lamellae. The distal small to medium arteries and veins of the lower and upper extremities are most commonly involved, usually with preservation of the proximal inflow vessels. Rarely, visceral, iliac, coronary, and pulmonary arteries can be involved. Buerger disease primarily affects male smokers younger than age 50, although female patients now comprise almost one third of all cases. This diagnosis should be suspected in any young patient presenting with small-vessel occlusive disease in the absence of diabetes. The lower extremities are almost always involved, and the upper extremities are involved in more than half of patients. A migratory thrombophlebitis, usually of the superficial veins, is seen in up to 30% of patients. The incidence of Buerger disease has decreased dramatically in the last 50 years, for reasons as yet unknown.

The angiographic appearance of Buerger disease is dramatic, with occlusion of most or all named vessels below the knee or elbow (Fig. 1-17). Because the vessel wall architecture is preserved, prominent collaterals develop in the vaso vasorum of the occluded arteries. This results in a typical "corkscrew" appearance of collaterals on angiography, quite distinct from collaterals resulting from atherosclerotic occlusions.

Behçet disease presents with recurrent oral and genital aphthous ulcers, skin lesions, ocular inflammation, arthritis, gastrointestinal

symptoms, and epididymitis. Patients are usually between 20 and 40 years of age. Males are affected more commonly than females, at a ratio of almost 2:1. Pathologically, Behçet disease is an inflammatory disorder of small blood vessels, in particular venules. The clinical vascular manifestations of Behçet disease occur in 20% of cases, with superficial venous thrombosis predominating. Aortic and pulmonary artery aneurysms, arterial occlusive disease, and central venous thrombosis occur in less than 5% of patients (Fig. 1-18).

Radiation arteritis is the result of injury to radiosensitive endothelial cells during external beam radiation for malignancy. Symptoms occur when the total radiation dose exceeds 50 Gray. The clinical presentation varies with the time interval from the radiation exposure. Thrombosis is most common within 5 years of treatment; mural fibrosis, stenosis, and occlusion with a paucity of collaterals occur between 5 and 10 years after treatment. Late manifestations include periarterial fibrosis and accelerated atherosclerosis, often in unusual distributions localized to the irradiated tissues (Fig. 1-19). New techniques for delivering radiation and careful planning limit the incidence of this complication.

Kawasaki disease, also known as *mucocutaneous lymph node syndrome*, is a rare disease of infants and children younger than 1 year. A vasculitis affects primarily small and medium-sized arteries. The most notable presenting vascular abnormality is coronary artery aneurysm, which may thrombose or rupture. Aneurysms of other arteries occur as well. This disease has been rarely reported in patients older than 9 years of age.

Systemic lupus erythematosus (SLE) and other collagen vascular diseases are usually characterized by musculoskeletal symptoms and serologic markers. Diagnosis is rarely made on the basis of angiographic findings alone. More commonly, patients with a known connective tissue disorder develop symptoms that suggest vascular involvement, such as digital ischemia and ulcerations. In these cases, angiography is performed to exclude another, correctable problem such as digital arterial emboli. The typical angiographic findings of lupus vasculitis in the hand are

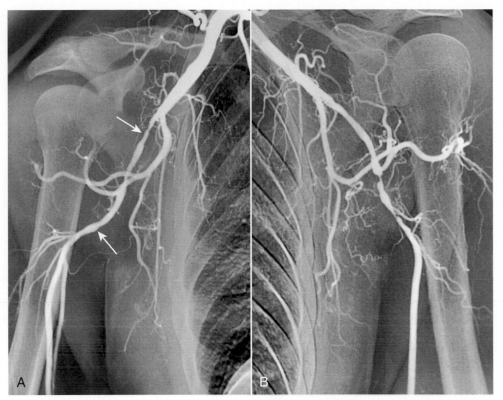

FIGURE 1-16. Giant cell arteritis in a middle-aged male with bilateral upper-extremity claudication and an elevated erythrocyte sedimentation rate. The aortic arch and subclavian arteries were normal. **A,** Digital angiogram showing irregular narrowing of the distal right axillary artery and proximal brachial arteries *(arrows)*. **B,** The same findings are present on the left. The distal arteries were normal in both arms.

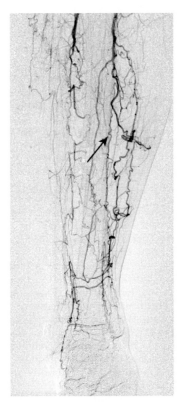

FIGURE 1-17. Buerger disease. Detailed view of digital subtraction angiogram of the calf of a 34-year-old male smoker. There are no patent named arteries. There are numerous coiled collateral arteries, including one in the vasa vasorum of the occluded posterior tibial artery *(arrow)*.

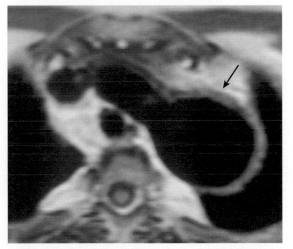

FIGURE 1-18. Behçet disease. Axial T1 weighted image of the aortic arch in a young female with a focal aneurysm of the proximal descending thoracic aorta *(arrow)*.

focal occlusions and irregular stenoses of the palmar and digital arteries (Fig. 1-20). Similar lesions may be seen in scleroderma.

Patients with rheumatoid arthritis, ankylosing spondylitis, reactive arthropathy, and psoriatic arthritis can develop ascending aortic dilatation with aortic valve insufficiency. These patients are also prone to aortic dissection.

■ HEMANGIOMAS, VASCULAR MALFORMATIONS, AND ARTERIOVENOUS FISTULAS

Precise classification of vascular lesions is important for predicting outcomes and selecting therapy, but sometimes difficult

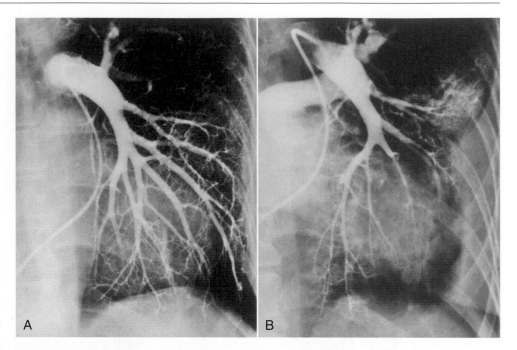

FIGURE 1-19. Radiation arteritis. **A,** Normal pulmonary angiogram of the left lung. **B,** Left pulmonary angiogram from the same patient obtained 7 years after radiation treatment for breast carcinoma shows narrowing, branch vessel occlusions and pleural thickening consistent with late radiation fibrosis.

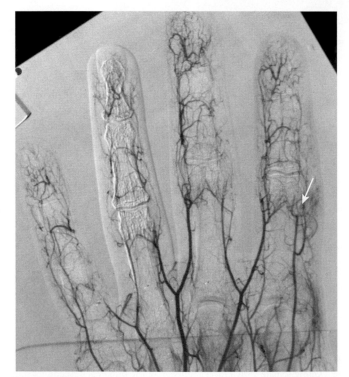

FIGURE 1-20. Systemic lupus erythematosus in a teenaged female with bilateral digital ulcers. Detail of a magnified, subtracted angiogram of the hand shows areas of digital artery narrowing with multiple occlusions *(arrow)*. There are no intraluminal filling defects or other evidence of emboli.

(Table 1-6). Infantile hemangiomas are the most common congenital vascular tumors, occurring most frequently in Caucasians (up to 10% of infants), more often in females. Infantile hemangiomas are always present at birth, 80% are solitary, and most involve the skin. These lesions are never acquired. Hemangiomas are true neoplasms but follow a benign course with a proliferative phase followed by spontaneous involution by age 9 years in most patients. When symptomatic, ulceration and compression/deformity are the most common presenting complaints. The presence of glucose transporter 1 (GLUT-1) is a tissue-specific marker.

Infantile hemangioendotheliomas are distinct from hemangiomas in that they are GLUT-1–negative, tend to be more masslike in texture, and when large can be associated with shunting, or platelet consumption and hemorrhagic complications (Kasabach-Merritt syndrome). An important association, particularly with facial infantile hemangiomas, is the PHACE (posterior fossa defects, hemangiomas, arterial anomalies, cardiac defects and aortic coarctation, and eye anomalies) syndrome. Propranolol therapy is extremely effective, more so than corticosteroids. In infants with large hepatic hemangioendotheliomas and symptomatic arteriovenous shunting, transcatheter embolization may be required (see Chapter 11, Fig. 11-36).

Cutaneous capillary malformations (slow-flow reddish-purple "port-wine" stains) are the most common vascular malformation (0.3% of the population). These are usually sporadic, often involving the face and neck. These rarely require interventional radiology procedures. Capillary malformations that have an arteriovenous component are pink-red, may have a pale halo, and can be associated with larger arteriovenous malformations and syndromes such as Parkes-Weber (venous and lymphatic malformations, cutaneous lesions, and a hypertrophic limb) and Sturge-Weber (facial cutaneous capillary malformation, ipsilateral leptomeningeal angioma, seizures, and mental deficiency).

Arteriovenous malformations (AVM) are nonproliferative high-flow congenital lesions that are usually single, can occur anywhere in the body, and comprise 36% of vascular malformations (Fig. 1-21). Approximately 60% are found in the lower limbs, 25% in the upper limbs, 12% in the pelvis and buttocks, and the remainder in other locations. These lesions are present at birth, but can remain subclinical throughout the patient's life. A characteristic feature is one or more central tangles of communicating arterioles and venules, termed the *nidus*. Arteriovenous malformations grow by recruiting additional feeding arteries and draining veins, rather than by proliferation of the component cells (Fig. 1-22). Large AVMs can cause clinically symptomatic right-to-left shunts, hypertrophy of affected extremities, and bleeding. AVMs are pulsatile, with an audible bruit, and remain distended despite elevation above the right atrium. In general, AVMs are very difficult to treat primarily with surgical resection. Careful, staged transcatheter or direct puncture embolization procedures with intravascular glues or polymers and absolute alcohol can provide remarkable control of symptoms. Complete cure is rarely achieved.

TABLE 1-6 Features of Vascular Malformations

			Lesion		
	Hemangioma	Arteriovenous Malformation	Venous Malformation	Arteriovenous Fistula	Lymphatic Malformation (Lymphangioma)
Etiology	Neoplasm	Congenital	Congenital	Acquired	Congenital
Presentation	30% at birth, remainder within 3 months	Present at birth, but may be subclinical until later	Present at birth, but may be subclinical until later	Later in life	Present at birth, but may be subclinical until later
Cellular proliferation	First year	None	None	None	None
Female-to-male ratio	2.5:1	4:1	1:1	N/A	1:1
Clinical course	Spontaneous involution by age 9 years in 95%	Growth with patient through puberty, slow growth thereafter except during pregnancy	Growth with patient through puberty, slow growth thereafter except during pregnancy	Stable or enlargement	Growth with patient.

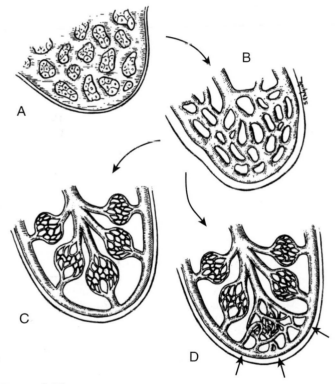

FIGURE 1-21. Diagram illustrating the development of arteriovenous malformations. **A,** Primitive mesenchyme with undifferentiated blood spaces. **B,** Primitive capillaries. **C,** Maturation of vascular bed with vascular stems leading to and from capillary beds. **D,** Local persistence of primitive capillary network results in an arteriovenous malformation *(small arrows)*. (From Rosen RJ, Riles TS. Congenital vascular malformations. In: Rutherford RB, ed. *Vascular Surgery,* 5th ed. Philadelphia: WB Saunders, 2000, with permission.)

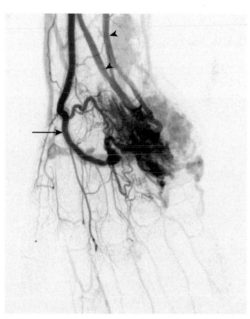

FIGURE 1-22. Arteriovenous malformation of the right hand. Selective radial artery injection *(black arrow)* shows enlarged feeding artery, an amorphous tangle of vessels in the soft tissues of the hypothenar eminence, and early venous enhancement *(arrowheads)* due to shunting. Note the weak opacification of the digital arteries due to the shunting.

Venous malformations (VM) represent 49% of congenital vascular malformations. These low-flow lesions are comprised of localized abnormal venous structures that vary in structure from spongy to varix-like, and may be isolated or communicate directly with normal veins (Fig. 1-23). Glomuvenous malformations are nodular, painful, hyperkeratotic cutaneous VMs without a deep component. The most common locations for VMs are the head and neck (40%) or the extremities (40%). The remaining 20% are truncal lesions. Large VMs can cause disfigurement, pain as a result of thrombosis or infiltration of muscle, and bleeding following minor trauma to the thin overlying skin. These lesions are soft and nonpulsatile, with no bruit, and they collapse when elevated above the right atrium. Usually single, VMs can be associated with Klippel-Trenaunay syndrome—a complex usually affecting the lower extremities, consisting of venous malformations, varicosities, cutaneous capillary malformations, limb hypertrophy, and abnormal deep venous structures. Characteristically, VMs exhibit delayed opacification (often after normal veins) and slow flow at angiography. Direct puncture venography reveals a venous space with pooling of contrast and usually drainage into normal veins. Lesions may have lymphatic as well as venous components. When readily accessible, VMs respond well to direct puncture and sclerosis with absolute alcohol or other agents.

Lymphatic malformations (LM, which represent 10% of vascular malformations, can be macrocystic (spaces > 2 cm³), microcystic, or mixed in structure (Fig. 1-24). When purely lymphatic these are soft and nonpulsatile. Venous and arterial components may be present as well. The anatomic distribution is similar to that of VMs, with approximately 45% in the head and neck, 45% in the extremities, and 10% in the trunk. Lesions can be localized

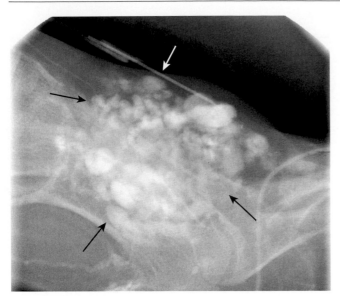

FIGURE 1-23. Venous malformation of the foot. Direct puncture venography *(white arrow)* reveals a large collection of abnormal veins in the fore-foot *(black arrows)*. This was treated with direct injection of a sclerosing agent.

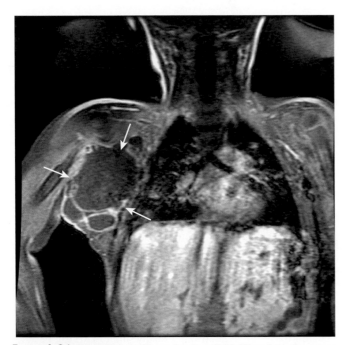

FIGURE 1-24. Lymphatic malformation in a child. T1-weighted contrast-enhanced fat saturation coronal MR image showing macrocystic lymphatic malformation in the right axilla *(arrows)*. Note the lack of central contrast enhancement and the multiple lesions.

or infiltrative, and complicated by mass effect, lymphedema, and infection. Similar to VMs these rarely involve and tend to grow as the child grows. Percutaneous treatment with direct puncture and sclerosis is an option for patients with symptomatic lesions. The agents used for sclerosis include bleomycin, doxycycline, ethanol, and OK-432 (lyophilized *Streptococcus pyogenes* exotoxin).

Arteriovenous fistulas are point-to-point communications between an artery and a vein that are almost always acquired (Fig. 1-25). The most common etiology in the hospital setting is iatrogenic following arterial catheterization or attempted central venous line placement. Small fistulas may remain asymptomatic

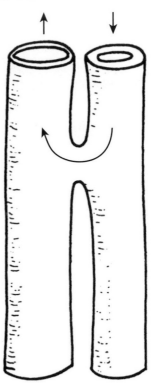

FIGURE 1-25. Schematic diagram of an arteriovenous fistula. There is a direct, point-to-point communication between the artery and vein. (From Riles TS, Rosen RJ, Jacobowitz GR. Peripheral arterial fistulae. In: Rutherford RB, ed. *Vascular Surgery,* 5th ed. Philadelphia: WB Saunders, 2000, with permission.)

or close spontaneously. Fistulas of all sizes can enlarge over time, resulting in recruitment of additional feeding arteries and draining veins. However, the actual communication always remains point-to-point. Lesions are pulsatile, with a palpable thrill and audible bruit, and the venous outflow remains distended when elevated above the right atrium. The clinical presentation can be similar to arteriovenous malformations, with symptomatic left-to-right shunts and pain. At arteriography, rapid shunting is characteristic. With chronic lesions, there is hypertrophy of the main feeding artery, but a single point of communication is characteristic. Occlusion of the point of communication using endovascular techniques or surgical ligation is curative.

MRI (including MR angiography and venography) has proven to be an excellent imaging modality for determining the nature and extent of vascular malformations. The precise relationship to superficial and deep structures can be demonstrated, as well as the dominant vascular supply. Signal characteristics of the blood in the lesion can be used to classify the lesion, and thus plan therapy (Table 1-7).

NEOPLASMS

Primary vascular neoplasms are unusual, accounting for only 2 per 100,000 cases of cancer. Neoplasms arise directly from elements in the blood vessel walls, usually the smooth muscle cells. The most common primary malignant vascular neoplasms are venous leiomyosarcomas, which involve the infrarenal IVC in 60% of patients. Lipomyosarcomas, pulmonary artery sarcomas, and aortic sarcomas can also occur. Benign lesions include lipomas and leiomyomas. These lesions are discussed later in appropriate chapters.

Secondary vascular invasion by neoplasms is much more common than primary tumors of the blood vessels. Veins, in particular the IVC, are invaded more often than arteries. Tumor invasion usually indicates malignancy, and is seen in particular

TABLE 1-7 MR and Angiographic Characteristics of Vascular Malformations*

	Hemangioma	Arteriovenous Malformation	Venous Malformation	Arteriovenous Fistula	Lymphatic Malformation (Lymphangioma)
MR appearance	Dark T1, bright T2, enhances with contrast, well-defined borders, normal arteries and veins	Dark T1 and T2, flow voids, enhances with contrast, localized or infiltrative, enlarged feeding arteries and draining veins	Intermediate T1, bright T2, absent flow voids, phleboliths/areas of thrombosis, localized or infiltrative, enhances with contrast, normal feeding arteries and draining veins	Dark T1 and T2, flow void, enlarged feeding artery and draining vein	Dark T1, bright T2, localized or infiltrative, minimal to no enhancement, normal feeding arteries and draining veins
Angiographic appearance	Normal arteries and veins, faint staining	Enlarged feeding arteries, rapid shunting to enlarged veins through multiple points of communication	Normal arteries, delayed pooling of contrast, normal draining veins, best seen with direct puncture venography	Enlarged feeding artery and draining vein with rapid shunting through single point of communication	Normal arteries and veins, hypovascular mass but may have faint rim enhancement

*Bright signal on T1 may indicate thrombosis or hemorrhage of any of these lesions.

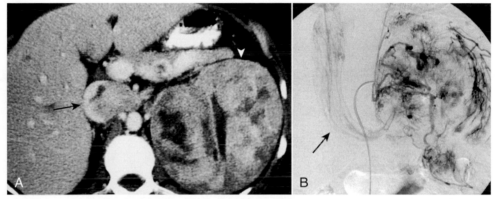

FIGURE 1-26. Adrenal carcinoma invading the inferior vena cava (IVC). **A,** Computed tomography scan with contrast shows a large heterogeneous mass in the retroperitoneum on the left *(arrowhead)*. The mass is growing through the left renal vein into the IVC. The expanded appearance of the IVC *(arrow)* with contrast around the mass is characteristic of an intraluminal process. **B,** Digital subtraction angiogram of the left inferior phrenic artery showing a large hypervascular mass with prominent neovascularity. Tumor vessels are present in the intravenous portion of the neoplasm *(arrow)*, which extends to the diaphragm.

with renal cell carcinoma, but also with hepatoma, adrenal cell carcinoma, germ cell tumors, uterine sarcoma, and thyroid carcinoma (Figs. 1-26 and 1-27). Thrombus frequently forms on the intravenous portion of the tumor, and may embolize to the lungs. Depending on the vascularity of the primary tumor, angiography may demonstrate tumor vessels in the intraluminal tumor as well as the primary mass.

The angiographic appearance of a tumor varies depending on the size of the lesion, vascular supply, and vascular architecture (see Figs. 1-26 and 1-27). Angiography is rarely performed to establish a diagnosis of malignancy, but occasionally to determine the organ of origin or extent of local invasion. An appreciation of the various appearances of malignancy on angiography is useful (Table 1-8 and Box 1-3). As a general rule, veins are subject to compression or invasion earlier than arteries. With the exception of arterial encasement or invasion, there are few signs that can conclusively distinguish a malignant from a benign mass, although the organ of origin, the size, and the number of lesions are extremely helpful clues.

Neoplasms that do not arise from the vessel wall or grow into the lumen can have distinctive (but not pathognomonic) angiographic signatures. However, many tumors, especially those with little vascularity, have very nondescript angiographic appearances (Table 1-9). In addition, the appearance of a lesion on one modality, such as CT, may not be predictive of the angiographic appearance. Lastly, the sensitivity of angiography for detection of hypovascular lesions is less than with CT and MRI.

■ DISSECTION

Dissection is a constellation of events consisting of an intimal defect, entry of blood into the medial layer, extension of blood through the media, and an intact adventitia, resulting in a second, false flow channel or lumen within the blood vessel (see Fig. 1-9). Usually, the blood cannot exit the false lumen as quickly as it enters. During diastole the false lumen remains pressurized relative to the true lumen, so that sometimes the false lumen compresses or even effaces the residual true lumen. The behavior of a dissection is unpredictable, particularly in relation to branch vessels. The dissection may extend into the branch vessel, tear the intima away from vessel ostium, or billow over the origin of the branch artery. Flow into the branch may be maintained or impaired, leading to symptomatic end-organ ischemia. Dissection is almost exclusively an arterial pathology, but has been reported in veins.

Numerous risk factors for arterial dissection range from direct trauma to inherited arterial wall abnormalities (Box 1-4). The arteries most commonly affected by spontaneous dissection are the aorta and medium-sized muscular arteries. When the media is normal, the dissection usually remains localized. In the setting of an abnormal media, such as in patients with certain heritable syndromes, the dissection may extend far from the original tear. The symptoms of dissection can be variable in severity. Pain, often described as "tearing," can occur, due to stretching of the artery and disruption of the media. Compression of the true lumen or involvement of critical branch vessels may result in distal organ ischemia. Rupture of the

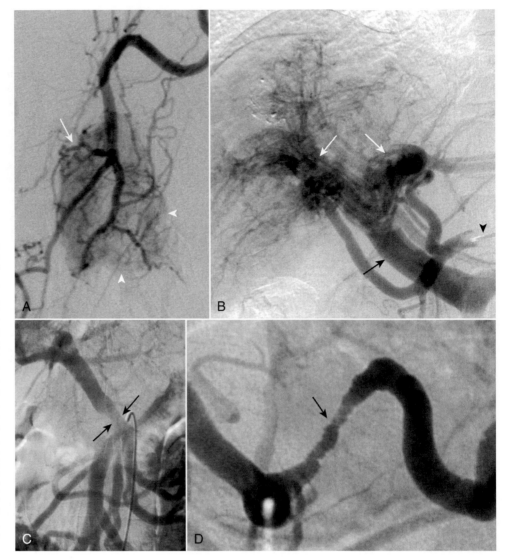

FIGURE 1-27. Varying angiographic appearances of malignancy. **A,** Tumor stain. Digital subtraction angiography of metastatic renal cell carcinoma to the left inferior pubic ramus. There is a densely staining mass *(arrowheads)* and abnormal arteries within the mass *(arrow).* **B,** Arteriovenous shunting. Arterial phase image from a patient with hepatoma invading the portal vein. Injection through a catheter in the proper hepatic artery *(arrowhead)* demonstrates classic "thread and streak" appearance of tumor in the vein *(white arrows)* and arterial-to-portal shunting *(black arrow).* **C,** Venous encasement. Portal venous phase DSA image following injection of contrast into the superior mesenteric artery (SMA) showing concentric narrowing of the portal vein *(arrows)* consistent with encasement by pancreatic head carcinoma. **D,** Arterial encasement. Arterial phase celiac artery DSA demonstrates multiple irregular areas of stenosis *(arrow)* in the splenic artery consistent with encasement by tumor in the body of the pancreas.

TABLE 1-8 Effects of Neoplasms on Adjacent Blood Vessels

Sign	Angiographic Appearance	Type of Neoplasm
Displacement	Vessel draped over mass	Benign or malignant
Compression	Smooth narrowing, no sharp angles	Benign or malignant
Encasement	Narrow vessel with sharp, variable angles	Malignant
Invasion	Jagged, irregular contour of lumen	Malignant
Intravascular	Vascularized mass in lumen	Malignant; rarely benign
Occlusion	Abrupt cutoff of normal vessel in mass	Benign or malignant

Box 1-3. Angiographic Signs of Vascular Neoplasms

Enlarged feeding arteries*
Wild, random appearing arteries in mass ("neovascularity")*
Encasement or invasion of vessel wall
Abrupt arterial occlusion*
Densely staining mass*
Rapid shunting into veins
Intravascular extension

*These signs are seen with both benign and malignant neoplasms. Location of mass and clinical history are important when interpreting the angiogram.

false lumen is a risk in the acute setting if blood pressure remains uncontrolled, or later if the false lumen becomes aneurysmal. Spontaneous thrombosis and obliteration of the false lumen can occur.

The imaging hallmark of dissection is the demonstration of blood on both sides of an intimal flap (Table 1-10 and Fig. 1-28). The true lumen is often (but by no means always) smaller and contains faster flow than the false lumen. For large vessels, such as the aorta, CTA has exquisite sensitivity and specificity for dissection, and is usually the first cross-sectional study obtained. Angiography is rarely necessary for diagnosis, but catheter-based interventions are increasingly used in these complex cases. The classification system used to describe aortic dissection is discussed in Chapter 9 (see Fig. 9-21).

TRAUMA

Blood vessels are susceptible to injury by a wide variety of mechanisms (Table 1-11). High-energy trauma may result in injury to a vessel adjacent to but not within the area of greatest soft tissue

TABLE 1-9 Angiographic Appearance of Selected Neoplasms

Neoplasm	Location	Appearance
Adenocarcinoma primary	Lung, pancreas	Hypovascular
Metastatic colon carcinoma	Liver	Hypovascular
Squamous cell carcinoma	Oropharynx, skin	Hypovascular
Gastrointestinal stromal tumor	Esophagus, bowel	Vascular
Islet cell tumor	Pancreas	Vascular
Hepatoma	Liver	Vascular
Renal cell carcinoma	Kidney	Vascular
Neuroendocrine metastases	Liver	Vascular
Melanoma metastases	Liver	Vascular
Benign leiomyoma	Uterus	Vascular
Angiomyolipoma	Kidney, adrenal	Vascular

Box 1-4. Risk Factors for Arterial Dissection

Hypertension
Atherosclerosis
Chronic obstructive pulmonary disease
Age older than 65 years
Long-term steroid use
Medial degeneration of any cause
Inherited disorder of the vascular wall (Marfan syndrome, Ehlers-Danlos syndrome)
Collagen vascular disease (rheumatoid arthritis, giant cell arteritis)
Fibromuscular dysplasia
Turner syndrome
Trauma (including iatrogenic)

injury. For example, high-power rifle bullets disperse destructive energy in a radius of millimeters to centimeters alongside their path through the soft tissues. Conversely, a knife wound creates injury only to those tissues that interact directly with the blade. However, the course of a knife blade through tissue is less predictable than that of a projectile. Consideration of the mechanism of injury is therefore important when evaluating a trauma patient for suspected vascular injury.

Traumatic vascular injuries can manifest in numerous ways (Table 1-12 and Fig. 1-29). Certain mechanisms are more likely to produce one type of injury than another, but there are no hard rules when it comes to trauma. In general, be prepared to find almost any type of injury. Common patterns of vascular injury are discussed in appropriate chapters.

A common and characteristic artifact related to power injection of contrast into normal medium and small arteries—standing waves—should not be confused with posttraumatic spasm or intimal dissection (Fig. 1-30). Usually this finding disappears on repeat injection of contrast.

VASOSPASTIC DISORDERS

Raynaud syndrome is the most common vasospastic disorder. Primary Raynaud syndrome is defined as reversible spasm of small arteries and arterioles (usually of the digits) in the absence of an underlying disorder. Secondary Raynaud syndrome is vasospasm that occurs as part of a systemic disorder such as SLE (Box 1-5). A diagnosis of primary Raynaud syndrome can only be made if symptoms are present for 2 years without an underlying

TABLE 1-10 Imaging Findings of Dissection

Modality	Findings
Computed tomography	Displacement of intimal calcification into vascular lumen; contrast on both sides of intimal flap; vascular lumen with flattened or crescentic medial contour; differential flow rates in parallel lumens within same vessel; thrombus external to intimal calcification
Magnetic resonance imaging	Contrast or flow on both sides of intimal flap; vascular lumen with flattened or crescentic medial contour; differential flow rates in parallel lumens within same vessel
Ultrasound	Flow on both sides of intimal flap; calcified flap in vessel lumen; expansion false lumen during diastole; vascular lumen with flattened or crescentic medial contour; differential flow rates in parallel lumens within same vessel
Angiography	Thick soft tissue density lateral to intimal calcification ("companion shadow"); contrast on both sides of intimal flap; differential flow rates in parallel lumens within same vessel; long spiral compression of true lumen; abrupt occlusion or unexplained absence of branch vessels

explanation. The female-to-male ratio is 4:1, with a typical age of onset in the second and third decades. Symptoms are induced by environmental factors (especially cold) in almost all patients. Patients with Raynaud syndrome experience a predictable sequence of asymmetric digital pallor or cyanosis followed by hyperemia during episodes of vasospasm. Patients with Raynaud disease rarely undergo angiography, but absence of intraluminal filling defects and reversible stenoses are useful diagnostic criteria in questionable cases (Fig. 1-31).

Ergotism is drug-induced vasospasm of small to medium-sized arteries caused by ergot alkaloids. These compounds are used to treat migraines, in the prophylaxis of deep vein thrombosis (DVT), and illicit recreation (lysergic acid diethylamide, or LSD). The incidence of vascular symptoms is less than one-hundredth of 1% of patients taking ergot alkaloids. Patients present with claudication and numbness, which can progress to tissue loss. Long smooth stenoses are seen at angiography, which reverse completely with cessation of ergot therapy (Fig. 1-32).

ARTERIAL EMBOLISM

The clinical presentation of an arterial embolus depends on the size of the embolus, the organ affected, and the presence of a collateral or alternative blood supply. A small embolus to the brain can be devastating, whereas a large embolus to a hypogastric artery can be asymptomatic when the contralateral hypogastric artery is patent. In general, emboli lodge in vessels when there is a sudden change in caliber, such as at bifurcation points and stenoses. Emboli tend to be recurrent, multiple, and unpredictable. The most common source of macroemboli is the heart (80% of all arterial emboli), and the most common etiology is atrial fibrillation (80% of cardiogenic emboli) (Box 1-6). Other etiologies include intravascular lesions such as abnormal aortic valve leaflets, exophytic aortic plaque, mural thrombus within an aortic or peripheral aneurysm, disrupted atherosclerotic plaque, and trauma (Box 1-7).

A symptomatic arterial embolus presents as an emergency when acute occlusion occurs in the absence of an established collateral blood supply. The angiographic features of emboli include abrupt occlusion with an intraluminal filling defect, lack of collateral vessels, and involvement of multiple vessels (Fig. 1-33).

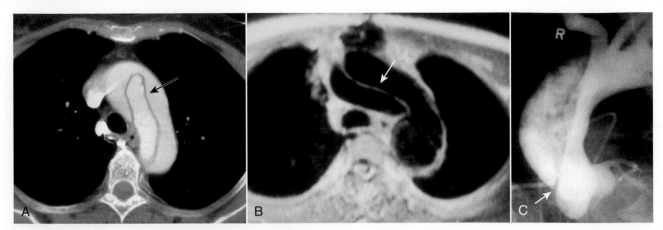

FIGURE 1-28. The appearance of aortic dissection is similar on different imaging modalities. **A,** Computed tomography scan with contrast through the aortic arch showing an intimal flap *(arrow)*. Flecks of calcium can be seen in the flap, confirming its identity as intima. **B,** Axial T1 weighted magnetic resonance image of the aortic arch from a different patient demonstrates an intimal flap *(arrow)* with a flow void on each side. The patient has undergone surgery for repair of the ascending aorta. **C,** Conventional angiogram of a patient with a dissection limited to the ascending aorta. The true lumen is compressed by the larger, less-opacified false lumen. The intimal flap *(arrow)* originates above the right coronary sinus.

TABLE 1-11 Vascular Trauma: Mechanism of Injury

Mechanism	Kinetic Energy	Example
Penetrating	High	Bullet
	Low	Knife
Blunt	High	High-speed motorvehicle accident
	Low	Surgical retractor
Stretch	High	Posterior knee dislocation
Thermal	N/A	Burn
Chemical	N/A	Intraarterial injection of absolute alcohol

N/A, Not applicable.

TABLE 1-12 Vascular Injuries

Injury	Description
Spasm	Focal smooth narrowing; resolves spontaneously, but if severe may cause thrombosis
Intramural hematoma	Focal hemorrhage into vascular wall without disruption
Intimal tear	Small intraluminal defect; usually heals with conservative management (anticoagulation); can be obstructive
Dissection	Intimal tear with creation of false lumen (frequently iatrogenic); if retrograde may heal spontaneously, but if antegrade can lead to vascular occlusion
Pseudoaneurysm	Collection of contrast due to localized disruption of vascular wall (one or more layers) with blood often contained by surrounding soft tissues; frequently associated with hematoma
Occlusion	Obstruction to flow caused by in situ thrombosis related to spasm, dissection, intimal tear, or foreign body
Transection	Circumferential disruption of vessel wall; may result in thrombosis (small vessels), pseudoaneurysm, or extravasation
Arteriovenous fistula	Direct communication between adjacent artery and vein with left-to-right shunt

Additional features that suggest emboli are occlusions in the presence of otherwise normal appearing arteries and asymmetric distribution when multiple. The anatomic distribution of emboli is determined by the source, the size of the embolus, and the flow rates. Approximately 20% emboli of cardiac origin lodge in the cerebrovascular circulation, fewer than 10% involve the visceral vessels, and the remainder lodge in the aorta and peripheral arteries (Table 1-13). When performing a diagnostic imaging study on a patient with noncardiogenic arterial embolization, it is important to evaluate the entire aorta. Recurrent embolic episodes in one limb or organ suggest an inline source close to the vascular supply of the affected anatomic region. Despite aggressive imaging with multiple modalities, a source is never found in roughly 5% of patients with arterial embolism.

Paradoxical embolism occurs when emboli of venous origin become arterial via an intracardiac (usually a patent foramen ovale) or pulmonary right-left shunt. This is believed to be an important etiology of cryptogenic embolic stroke in young patients.

Atherosclerotic microembolism (so-called cholesterol embolization) represents an important subgroup of arterial embolic disorders. Platelet aggregates, cholesterol crystals, and thrombus originating from unstable or disrupted atherosclerotic plaque embolize distally and occlude small peripheral arterioles. As a result, patients many have normal pulse examination and angiographic studies despite obvious clinical findings. Patients may present with focal areas of painful discoloration (especially in the toes, known as "blue toe syndrome"), renal failure, bowel

ischemia, and stroke (Fig. 1-34). Embolization is usually spontaneous, but can follow surgical or percutaneous manipulation of a diseased artery.

■ INFECTION

Bacterial infection of the native vessel wall can occur from several mechanisms (Table 1-14). Both arteries and veins may become infected, although venous infection is rare. Vascular bacterial infection is a mycotic process, distinct from arteritis. Patients usually present with pain related to the infected vessel, persistent bacteremia, fever, and malaise. As the infection progresses, the vessel wall is digested, resulting in a mycotic aneurysm. This is in fact a pseudoaneurysm, in that the native vessel wall no longer exists, and the inflammatory process is ongoing. Mycotic

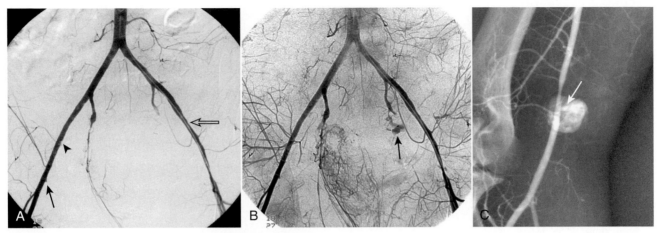

FIGURE 1-29. Angiographic findings in trauma. **A,** Digital subtraction angiogram of the pelvis in a pedestrian hit by a truck reveals numerous vascular injuries. There is occlusion of the right inferior epigastric artery *(arrow)* at its origin, as well as many hypogastric artery branches in the pelvis. Multiple small intimal flaps *(arrowhead)* are present in the right external iliac artery. There is spasm *(open arrow)* of the left external iliac artery. **B,** Later image from the same angiogram shows active extravasation *(arrow)* from the left hypogastric trunk. **C,** Brachial angiogram from a different patient following a stab wound to the arm shows a pseudoaneurysm *(arrow)*.

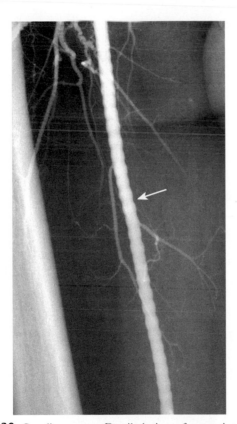

FIGURE 1-30. Standing waves. Detailed view of an angiogram of the superficial femoral artery shows a regular corrugated contour to the lumen *(arrow)*. Standing waves occur in medium to small muscular arteries during contrast injection. The exact etiology is unknown, but they are harmless and usually disappear before a second injection can be performed. This appearance should be compared to spasm (see Fig. 1-29) and fibromuscular dysplasia (see Fig. 1-11).

aneurysms tend to be located in unusual locations, and have a wild, multilobulated appearance (Fig. 1-35). Arteries containing atherosclerotic plaque, preexisting native aneurysms, or prosthetic devices are more prone to infection by hematogenous seeding and direct inoculation than are normal vessels. The organisms that are most often responsible for mycotic aneurysms are skin, oral, and enteric flora (Table 1-15). More than 50% of mycotic

Box 1-5. Causes of Secondary Raynaud Syndrome

Systemic lupus erythematosus
Scleroderma
Mixed connective tissue disorder
Rheumatoid arthritis
Sjögren syndrome
Polymyositis

aneurysms are found in the lower extremity peripheral arteries, and one third in the thoracic and abdominal aorta.

Syphilitic aortitis is a specific variant of vascular infection in which the treponeme invades the vasa vasorum of the aorta. There are relatively more vasa vasorum in the ascending than the descending thoracic aorta, and fewer still in the abdominal aorta. Syphilitic endarteritis leads to dystrophic calcification and aneurysmal dilatation during the tertiary phase of syphilis in 10% of patients. Ascending thoracic aneurysms are most common, and abdominal aortic involvement is rare. This entity is illustrated in Chapter 9 (see Fig. 9-14).

Infection of prosthetic vascular graft material may present as fever, bacteremia, wound drainage, and pain over the graft. Thrombosis of the graft material, anastomotic pseudoaneurysm, anastomotic rupture, and aortoenteric fistula can occur. Infection of autologous vein grafts is less common, but usually is localized to the surgical anastomosis. Typical organisms include skin flora for peripheral grafts with the addition of bowel flora for intraabdominal grafts. At surgery, in addition to obvious signs of sepsis, lack of incorporation of the graft material into surrounding soft tissues is highly suggestive of infection. Imaging findings include perigraft soft tissue inflammatory changes, abscess formation, perigraft and intragraft air, anastomotic pseudoaneurysms (frequently multiple), and intraluminal filling defects (Fig. 1-36). Imaging of the immediate postoperative patient can be confusing, but perigraft air should be absorbed within 2-3 weeks of surgery.

INHERITED DISORDERS OF THE ARTERIAL WALL

Marfan syndrome is an inherited disorder that results in vessel wall weakness due to abnormalities of type I collagen and fibrillin. The classic pathologic description is cystic medial necrosis.

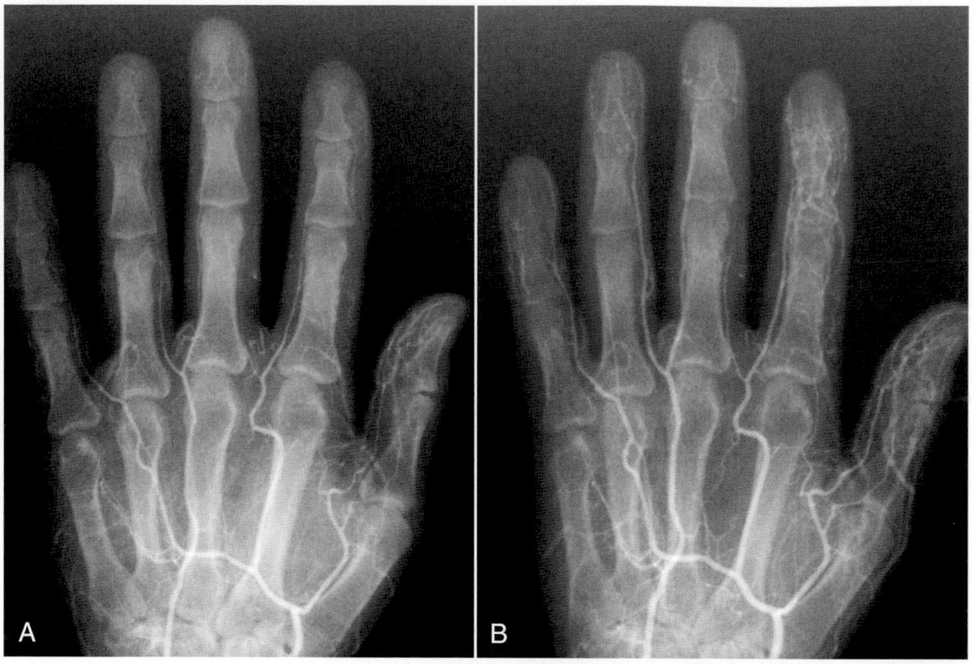

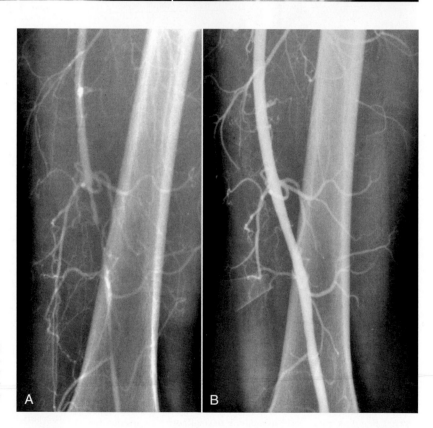

FIGURE 1-31. Angiographic demonstration of Raynaud syndrome. **A,** Hand angiogram of a patient with a long history of cold-induced blanching of the fingers and tobacco abuse. The patient was experiencing an attack during the angiogram. The arteries of the hand appear attenuated, and there is incomplete filling of the digital arteries. **B,** Following intraarterial administration of a vasodilator, there is dilatation and improved filling of the arteries, although fixed digital artery occlusions are also present.

FIGURE 1-32. Ergotism in a patient with claudication and migraine headaches. **A,** Angiogram of the left thigh demonstrates diffuse narrowing of the superficial femoral artery (SFA) and above-knee popliteal artery. **B,** Angiogram after cessation of ergot alkaloids. The SFA and popliteal artery are entirely normal.

This autosomal dominant disease has variable penetration, with no gender difference, and is found in approximately 1 per 5000 people. The clinical diagnosis is based on family history and skeletal, ocular, and cardiovascular manifestations. The classic patient is tall, thin, with long arms and fingers, pectus deformities, lens subluxation, and a family history of sudden premature death due to rupture of aortic aneurysms. Cardiovascular abnormalities occur in more than 95% of patients. The most common vascular manifestation is dilation of the ascending aorta that involves the annulus (Fig. 1-37). Aortic regurgitation and mitral valve prolapse are common. Patients with Marfan syndrome are prone to acute aortic dissection and aortic rupture.

Ehlers-Danlos syndrome is believed to occur in 1 per 5000 people. In the classic case, the patient has hyperflexible joints and elastic skin ("rubber man syndrome"). The basic defect is an abnormality in types I and III collagen. There are at least 10 subtypes, each with different genetic and clinical characteristics. Vascular complications, which are rare overall in this disease, are usually found in patients with type IV and V (vascular and vascular-like). However, 40% of patients with type IV Ehlers-Danlos syndrome develop vascular complications. Patients with type IV syndrome lack the typical joint and cutaneous laxity, so may be unaware of their diagnosis. Easy bruisability and a history of spontaneous bowel perforation, splenic rupture, or pneumothorax may

Cardiac arrhythmia (especially atrial fibrillation)
Myocardial infarction (intracavitary thrombus)
Ventricular aneurysm
Prosthetic valve
Endocarditis
Cardiomyopathy
Paradoxical embolus
Intracardiac neoplasm
Rheumatic heart disease

Box 1-7. **Noncardiac Sources of Arterial Macroemboli**

Atherosclerotic plaque
Arterial aneurysm (including aortic, subclavian, and popliteal)
Hypercoagulable states
Trauma
Foreign bodies

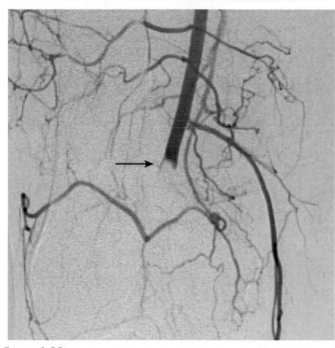

Figure 1-33. Acute arterial embolism in the above-knee popliteal artery. There is slight broadening of the contrast column and a smooth convex intraluminal filling defect *(arrow)* characteristic of an embolus. Notice that contrast outlines the top of the embolus. This appearance is similar to the acute in situ popliteal artery aneurysm thrombosis shown in Figure 1-7.

Table 1-13 Peripheral Distribution of Symptomatic Emboli of Cardiac Origin

Location	Incidence
Common femoral artery	36%
Aortic bifurcation and common iliac arteries	22%
Popliteal artery	15%
Upper extremity artery	14%
Visceral (renal and superior mesenteric arteries)	7%
Other	6%

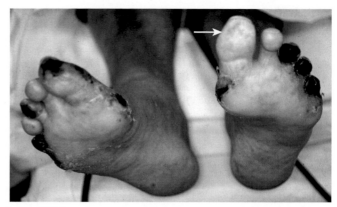

Figure 1-34. Acute and chronic atheroembolism ("blue toe syndrome") in a patient with a proximal source. Mottling consistent with acute embolism is most evident in the left great toe *(arrow)*. The gangrenous toes are typical of chronic atheroembolism.

Table 1-14 Sources of Vascular Infection

Etiology	Examples
Hematogenous	Bacteremia following dental procedure
Embolic	Septic embolus from bacterial endocarditis
Direct inoculation	Intravenous drug abuse with nonsterile technique
Contiguous spread	Aortic infection from retroperitoneal abscess

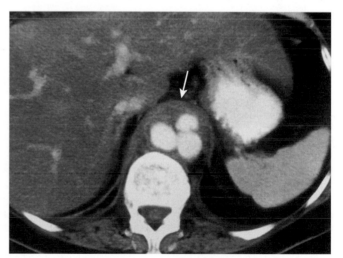

Figure 1-35. Mycotic aneurysm. Computed tomography scan with contrast at a level just proximal to the celiac artery origin in a patient with abdominal pain and *Streptococcus* species bacteremia. There is a multilobulated aneurysm with a prominent soft tissue component *(arrow)* typical of a mycotic aneurysm.

be present. Spontaneous dissection, aneurysm formation, and vessel rupture are the most common vascular symptoms (Fig. 1-38). Conventional angiography has an almost 70% major complication rate (dissection, rupture, major access-site bleeding) because of the abnormal arterial wall; it should be avoided when possible.

Loeys-Dietz syndrome is an autosomal dominant systemic disorder that has aortic aneurysms and dissection as a prominent feature. The classic triad is hypertelorism, cleft palate or bifid uvula, and arterial tortuosity and aneurysms. Patients may also have craniosynostosis, retrognathia, blue sclera, marfanoid body habitus, joint laxity, translucent skin, atrial septal defects, and developmental delay. Half of these patients will die of vascular

TABLE 1-15 Pathogens of Isolated Mycotic Aneurysms

Pathogen	Incidence
Staphylococcus aureus	30%
Salmonella species	10%
Streptococcus species	10%
Pseudomonas species	6%
Staphylococcus epidermidis	5%
Escherichia coli	3%
Klebsiella species	2%
Haemophilus influenzae	2%
Mycobacterium tuberculosis	2%
Miscellaneous	9%
Culture negative	21%

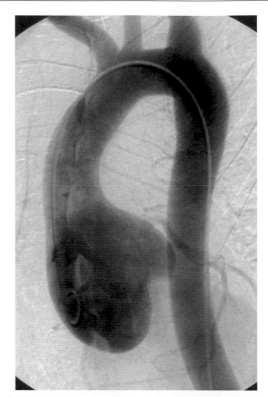

FIGURE 1-37. Marfan syndrome in an 18-year-old male. Digital subtraction angiography of the thoracic aorta in the left anterior oblique projection shows dilatation of the aortic root with loss of the sinotubular ridge.

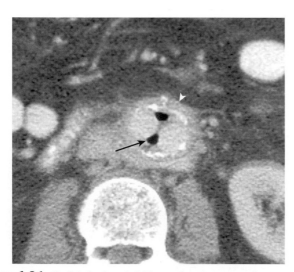

FIGURE 1-36. Graft infection. Axial image from a computed tomography scan with intravenous contrast of a patient with fever and septicemia several years after aneurysm surgery. There is gas around the limbs of the graft *(arrow)* within the old aneurysm sac. There is also enhancing soft tissue density *(arrowhead)* around the aorta.

complications (particularly rupture of ascending aortic aneurysms) before age 30 years. Aneurysms of other arteries occur in more than 50% of these patients.

IMPINGEMENT SYNDROMES

Intermittent positional external compression of a vascular structure (i.e., impingement syndrome) can be due to congenital or acquired abnormalities of form or function. These abnormalities include anomalous or hypertrophied muscles or bones, anomalous locations of vessels, and benign bony lesions such as osteochondromas. Prosthetic vascular grafts tunneled through normal muscular structures or across joints can also be subject to positional compression. Impingement syndromes are a type of repetitive trauma that results in predictable vascular lesions. In general, chronic impingement on a vein results in stenosis leading to thrombosis, whereas chronic impingement on an artery results in post-stenotic aneurysm formation with distal embolization of mural thrombus and ultimately thrombosis (Figs. 1-39 and 1-40). The two most common arterial clinical syndromes involve the subclavian artery (thoracic outlet syndrome) and the popliteal artery (popliteal artery entrapment; see Chapter 15, Figs. 15-41 to 15-43). The most

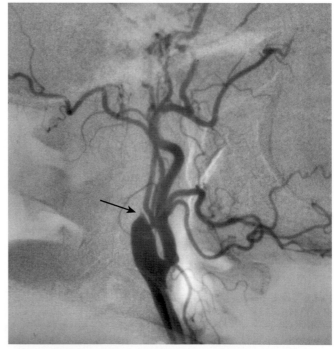

FIGURE 1-38. Ehlers-Danlos type IV in a 45-year-old woman. This carotid angiogram shows occlusion of the internal carotid artery *(arrow)* due to spontaneous dissection.

common venous syndromes involve the subclavian vein "Paget-Schroetter" or "effort thrombosis"), and the left common iliac vein (May-Thürner syndrome; see Chapter 16, Fig.16-16). These entities are discussed in later chapters. The clinical presentation of arterial and venous impingement syndromes differ (Table 1-16).

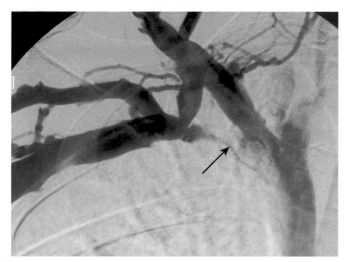

FIGURE 1-39. Subclavian venous stenosis in thoracic outlet syndrome. Right upper extremity digital subtraction venogram in a 30-year-old right-handed waiter. There is severe stenosis *(arrow)* of the right subclavian vein at the junction with the right internal jugular vein, with enlarged collateral drainage to the external jugular vein.

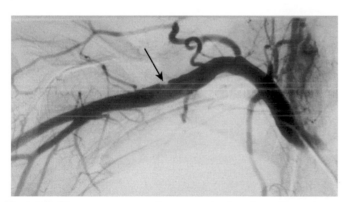

FIGURE 1-40. Subclavian artery aneurysm in thoracic outlet syndrome. Subtracted angiogram of the right subclavian artery demonstrates an aneurysm containing a small amount of mural thrombus *(arrow)*. The patient had presented with recurrent embolic episodes to the right hand. The patient has a right cervical rib (not seen on this subtraction image).

Angiographic evaluation should always include views with limbs in a position that reproduce the patient's symptoms.

ADVENTITIAL CYSTIC DISEASE

Adventitial cystic disease is a focal arterial disorder (although venous cases have been reported) in which localized accumulations of intramural fluid compress the arterial lumen. This is a disorder of young males (male-to-female ratio 5:1), that is always found near a joint, usually the knee. Adventitial cystic disease has also been reported in the external iliac, radial, ulnar, brachial, and common femoral arteries. This rare disorder results in less than 0.1% of cases of peripheral arterial occlusive disease, but should be considered in any young male presenting with claudication. The etiology is unknown, but believed to be inclusion of mucin-secreting synovial-like cells in the adventitia during fetal development. The characteristic angiographic appearance is a fixed extrinsic compression of the arterial lumen (Fig. 1-41). The only definitive treatment is surgical excision.

TABLE 1-16 Difference Between Arterial and Venous Impingement Syndromes

Feature	Venous	Arterial
Vessel abnormality	Synechia, stenosis, fibrosis	Stenosis, post-stenotic aneurysm
Clinical symptoms	Limb swelling, pain	Claudication, numbness
Complication	Thrombosis	Distal embolization, thrombosis
Treatment	Thrombolysis, angioplasty/stent, decompression	Embolectomy, thrombolysis, decompression, bypass

MÖNCKEBERG SCLEROSIS

Mönckeberg sclerosis is medial calcification of medium and small muscular arteries in association with diabetes and renal failure. Atherosclerotic calcification is different in location and distribution, occurring in intimal plaque and involving arteries of all sizes. Mönckeberg sclerosis is not an obstructive process. The circumferentially calcified vessels are readily visible on plain radiographs (Fig. 1-42).

THROMBOSIS

The formation of thrombus is a normal process, essential for maintaining life (Fig. 1-43). Two pathways are recognized, intrinsic and extrinsic, which converge when factor X is activated. The intrinsic pathway is activated by contact with platelets, whereas the extrinsic pathway is activated by contact with extravascular tissues. When a vascular injury occurs, platelets become activated when the collagen in the vessel wall is exposed. Platelets adhere to the site of injury, and initiate a process of continued platelet aggregation and fibrin formation that results in a hemostatic plug.

Derangements of thrombosis result in either hypercoagulable or hemorrhagic states. General predisposing conditions for enhanced thrombus formation have been recognized for more than 100 years. Stasis of flow, vascular injury, and a hypercoagulable state constitute *Virchow's triad,* identified by the famous 19th century German pathologist Rudolf Virchow. A clinical example is a patient with metastatic malignancy at bedrest who develops subclavian vein thrombosis after central venous line placement. A number of hypercoagulable syndromes have been identified, and new ones are realized all the time (Table 1-17).

Patients should be suspected of having a hypercoagulable condition when they present with unprovoked venous thrombosis (i.e., no obvious inciting event), thrombosis in unusual locations (sagittal sinus, portal veins, renal veins), recurrent DVT, and spontaneous arterial thrombosis in the absence of underlying stenosis or embolization. The diagnostic evaluation includes a search for an occult malignancy. Thrombotic complications following vascular interventions are more common in these patients.

In general, thrombosis itself is not the pathology, but rather the presenting symptom. Most patients will have an identifiable underlying lesion or syndrome. Treatment of patients with acute arterial or venous thrombosis is directed toward both relief of the occlusion and diagnosis of the predisposing condition.

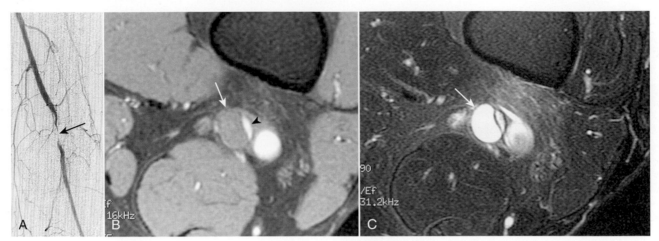

FIGURE 1-41. Adventitial cystic disease in a 55-year-old woman with left leg claudication. **A,** Digital subtraction angiogram demonstrates focal stenosis of the popliteal artery. The lumen appears compressed by a mass rather than narrowed by intraluminal plaque. **B,** Axial T1-weighted image with gadolinium and fat suppression shows an arterial lumen *(arrowhead)* compressed by a mass *(arrow)* in the wall of the artery. The adjacent popliteal vein is normal. **C,** Axial T2-weighted image at the same level shows that the mass contains fluid (bright on T2). (Case provided by Philip Rogoff, MD, and Ralph Reichle, MD, Mount Auburn Hospital, Cambridge, Mass.)

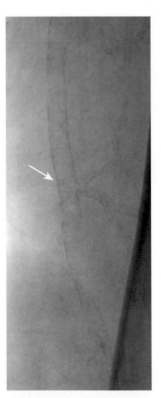

FIGURE 1-42. Mönckeberg sclerosis. Digital noncontrast image of the left thigh of a patient with diabetes and renal failure. The walls of the distal superficial femoral *(arrow)* and several muscular arteries are well visualized owing to diffuse medial calcification. The patient has a normal popliteal pulse.

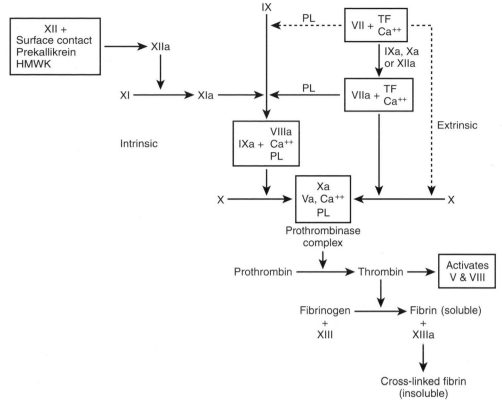

FIGURE 1-43. Two pathways of coagulation. The intrinsic pathway is initiated by surface contact, whereas the extrinsic pathway is triggered by release of tissue factor (TF). Phospholipid (PL) is found on activated platelets and endothelial membranes. HMWK, High-molecular-weight kininogen. (From Calaitges JG, Silver D. Principles of hemostasis. In: Rutherford RB, ed. *Vascular Surgery,* 5th ed. Philadelphia: WB Saunders, 2000, with permission.)

TABLE 1-17 Hypercoagulable States

Condition	Mechanism	Clinical Presentation
Heparin-induced thrombocytopenia	Type I: idiosyncratic	Transient mild decrease in platelets (remain > 100,000/mm³)
	Type II: antigenic	1%-3% population; platelets < 100,000/mm³, thrombosis, bleeding
Factor V Leiden	Resistance to inactivation of Protein C	Inherited, 3% population; venous thrombosis
Prothrombin G20210A mutation	Increased formation of prothrombin (factor II)	Inherited; venous thrombosis
Protein C deficiency	Decreased inactivation of factors Va, VIIIa	Inherited, <1% population; venous thrombosis
Protein S deficiency	Cofactor to protein C inactivation of factors Va, VIIIa; directly inhibits prothrombin activation	Acquired (pregnancy, oral contraception, HIV infection, liver disease) or hereditary; venous thrombosis
Antithrombin deficiency	Decreased inactivation of factors Xa and IXa.	Inherited, 1% patients with venous thrombosis; antithrombin levels low (type I) or normal but dysfunctional (type II)
Antiphospholipid syndrome	Exact mechanism not resolved. Elevated anticardiolipin antibodies, lupus anticoagulant	Recurrent arterial and venous thrombosis, fetal demise

▬ SUGGESTED READINGS

Abu Rahma AF, Richmond BK, Robinson PA. Etiology of peripheral arterial thromboembolism in young patients. *Am J Surg*. 1998;176:158-161.

Allaire E, Schneider F, Saucy F, et al. New insight in aetiopathogenesis of aortic diseases. *Eur J Vasc Endovasc Surg*. 2009;37:531-537.

Bergqvist D. Ehlers-Danlos type IV syndrome: a review from a vascular surgical point of view. *Eur J Surg*. 1996;162:163-170.

Bergqvist D, Björck M, Ljungman C. Popliteal venous aneurysm—a systematic review. *World J Surg*. 2006;30:273-279.

Chae EJ, Do KH, Seo JB, et al. Radiologic and clinical findings of Behçet disease: comprehensive review of multisystemic involvement. *Radiographics*. 2008; 28:e31? Epub 2008 Jul 6.

Chao CP, Walker TG, Kalva SP. Natural history and CT appearances of aortic intramural hematoma. *Radiographics*. 2009;29:791-804.

Elefteriades JA, Farkas EA. Thoracic aortic aneurysm clinically pertinent controversies and uncertainties. *J Am Coll Cardiol*. 2010;55:841-857.

Golomb BA, Dnag TT, Criqui MH. Peripheral arterial disease: morbidity and mortality implications. *Circulation*. 2006;114:688-699.

Hellmich B. Update on the management of systemic vasculitis: what did we learn in 2009? *Clin Exp Rheumatol*. 2010;28:S98-103.

Kissin EY, Merkel PA. Diagnostic imaging in Takayasu arteritis. *Curr Opin Rheumatol*. 2004;16:31-37.

Lee WK, Mossop PJ, Little AF, Fitt GJ, Vrazas JI, Hoang JK, Hennessy OF. Infected (mycotic) aneurysms: spectrum of imaging appearances and management. *Radiographics*. 2008;28:1853-1868.

Libby P, Ridker PM, Hansson GK, et al. Inflammation in atherosclerosis: from pathophysiology to practice. *J Am Coll Cardiol*. 2009;54:2129-2138.

Lopes RJ, Almeida J, Dias PJ, et al. Infectious thoracic aortitis: a literature review. *Clin Cardiol*. 2009;32:488-490.

Mattassi R, Loose DA, Vaghi M, eds. *Hemangiomas and vascular malformations*. Milan: Springer-Verlag; 2009.

Modrall JG, Sadjadi J. Early and late presentations of radiation arteritis. *Semin Vasc Surg*. 2003;16:209-214.

Norman PE, Powell JT. Site specificity of aneurysmal disease. *Circulation*. 2010;121:560-568.

Olin JW, Pierce M. Contemporary management of fibromuscular dysplasia. *Curr Opin Cardiol*. 2008;23:527-536.

Orton DF, Le Veen RF, Saigh JA, et al. Aortic prosthetic graft infections: radiologic manifestations and implications for management. *Radiographics*. 2000;20:977-993.

Piazza G, Creager MA. Thromboangiitis obliterans. *Circulation*. 2010 Apr 27;121:1858-1861.

Scolari F, Ravani P. Atheroembolic renal disease. *Lancet*. 2010;375:1650-1660.

Sidbury R. Update on vascular tumors of infancy. *Curr Opin Pediatr*. 2010;22:432-437.

Steen V, Denton CP, Pope JE, Matucci-Cerinic M. Digital ulcers: overt vascular disease in systemic sclerosis. *Rheumatology*. 2009;48(Suppl 3):iii19-iii24.

Uyeda JW, Anderson SW, Sakai O, Soto JA. CT angiography in trauma. *Radiol Clin North Am*. 2010;48:423-438.

Wojtowycz M. *Handbook of Interventional Radiology and Angiography*. St Louis: Mosby; 1995.

CHAPTER 2

Fundamentals of Angiography

John A. Kaufman, MD, MS, FSIR, FCIRSE

The development of modern angiography was enabled by one simple technique: the percutaneous introduction of devices into a blood vessel over a wire guide (Fig. 2-1). Described by Sven Ivan Seldinger in 1953, this elegant innovation (now known by Seldinger's name) eliminated the need for surgical exposure of a blood vessel before catheterization, thus allowing the transfer of angiography from the operating room to the radiology department. Virtually all vascular and many nonvascular invasive procedures are performed with Seldinger's technique.

■ PREPROCEDURE PATIENT EVALUATION AND MANAGEMENT

Knowledge empowers, and in interventional radiology it is the difference between unthinking completion of an assigned task and meaningful participation in the care of a patient. As an interventional radiologist, you should not only be skilled with a catheter, but also be a specialist in the diseases that you treat. Ideally, you will have seen the patient previously in consultation and selected which procedure to perform. The evaluation is the same in clinic or at the bedside, and begins with a review of the clinical issue. Do you understand the diagnostic questions and the information needed? Do you understand the different therapeutic options? A brief, directed history should be obtained. In particular, the symptoms or signs that precipitated the consultation are important, as this knowledge may impact the course of the subsequent examination and interpretation of the images. Other essential areas to cover in the history include prior surgical procedures (especially vascular); evidence of atherosclerotic disease (e.g., prior myocardial infarction or stroke) in "index" vascular beds; diabetes, with attention to medications; status of renal function; allergies; and known previous exposure to iodinated contrast agents. When available, office records or the patient's chart should be reviewed for similar information. Operative notes and reports from previous angiograms provide valuable information that may alter the entire approach to the procedure. Most important, personal review of noninvasive vascular studies, prior angiograms, and correlative imaging is essential before embarking upon any invasive procedure.

The immediate preprocedural physical examination is focused on the overall status of the patient and selection of a vascular access site. Introduce and identify yourself before examining the patient. The pulse examination should be conducted by the person who will perform the angiogram. A general assessment of risk for the procedure and sedation should be made. The American Society of Anesthesiologists (ASA) classification, though designed for surgical patients, is a simple way to categorize and communicate procedural risk (Table 2-1). Equally important, the patient's understanding of the procedure, ability to cooperate, current level of pain, and ability to lie on a procedure table in the position necessary for the procedure should be considered before going forward.

The strength of the pulses and the presence of peripheral aneurysm (as suggested by a broad, prominent pulse) should be recorded using a consistent system. Cellulitis, fresh surgical incisions, a large abdominal pannus, or a dense scar over the vessel all influence selection of an access site. Pulses distal to the anticipated access site must be evaluated and recorded. This baseline information is useful if an occlusive complication occurs or to determine success of a revascularization procedure. The physical examination should include both sides of the patient in case an alternate or additional access is required during the procedure. When an upper extremity approach is anticipated, blood pressures in both arms must be obtained.

Evidence of vascular disease such as trophic skin changes, hair loss, cool skin temperature, dependent rubor, delayed capillary refill, ulceration, and gangrene should be noted. Classification systems for acute and chronic ischemia have been devised, which serve to decrease ambiguity when describing a patient, have prognostic implications, and allow assessment of outcomes of interventions (see Tables 15-6 and 15-11).

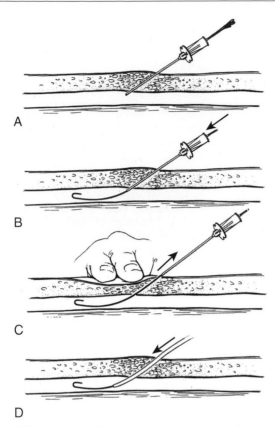

FIGURE 2-1. Seldinger technique. **A,** Percutaneous puncture of a blood vessel with a hollow needle. **B,** Introduction of an atraumatic guidewire through the needle into the blood vessel lumen. **C,** Needle is removed while guidewire remains in place. Compression over the puncture secures the guidewire and prevents bleeding. **D,** Angiographic catheter is advanced into vessel over the guidewire. (From Kadir S. *Diagnostic Angiography.* Philadelphia: WB Saunders, 1986, with permission.)

TABLE 2-1 American Society of Anesthesiologists Classification for Preoperative Risk

Class	Definition
1	A normal healthy patient
2	A patient with mild systemic disease
3	A patient with severe systemic disease
4	A patient with severe systemic disease that is a constant threat to life
5	A moribund patient who is not expected to survive without the operation
6	A declared brain-dead patient whose organs are being removed for donor purposes

From www.asahq.org/clinical/physicalstatus.htm.

Patients should be well hydrated prior to the procedure. Outpatients who will have conscious sedation should not be instructed to fast after midnight, but rather encouraged to drink clear liquids (no solid food) until 2 hours before their scheduled appointment. Medications can be taken with a sip of water. Patients for whom general anesthesia will be required should follow local anesthesiology department guidelines, usually fasting for 6 hours. Before the procedure, an intravenous infusion of (D5/0.5NS or 0.9NS) should be begun at a rate that sustains hydration (about 100 mL/hr) for adults with normal renal and cardiac function. Inpatients who will have conscious sedation should stop solid food 6 hours before the procedure, but can be given clear liquids until 2 hours before. An intravenous infusion should be established before arriving in the angiographic suite. Most hospitals have guidelines for oral intake before invasive procedures; however, these are generally not designed for patients about to receive large doses of nephrotoxic contrast.

There are no laboratory studies that are absolutely mandatory before conducting an angiogram. However, because the procedure involves making a hole in a blood vessel and administering nephrotoxic contrast material, reasonable laboratory tests in patients at risk include coagulation studies (international normalized ratio [INR] or prothrombin time (PT), activated partial thromboplastin time [aPTT]), platelet count, and serum creatinine (Cr). Routine laboratory studies can be safely omitted in young patients without known coagulation disorders or renal dysfunction.

A prolonged PT or INR is usually the result of warfarin therapy, liver disease, or poor nutritional status. Femoral arterial access is safe when the INR is 1.5 or less (or the PT less than 15 seconds). Coagulation studies should be normal for axillary, high brachial, or translumbar aortic access. Fresh frozen plasma (FFP) is used to rapidly normalize the INR or PT before a procedure. Vitamin K (phytonadione) administration for reversal of coagulopathy caused by warfarin, liver disease, or vitamin K deficiency is effective but can require a day or more to work. FFP contains normal quantities of all coagulation factors. The effect of FFP is fast but volume related; 10-20 mL per kg is usually required to normalize a coagulopathic patient (each bag contains 200-300 mL). The half-life of some of the coagulation factors in FFP is short (e.g., 3-5 hours for factor VII), so continuation of transfusion during or even after the procedure may be necessary in severely coagulopathic patients.

A prolonged aPTT is usually due to administration of unfractionated heparin (low-molecular-weight heparin does not alter the aPTT), which can be turned off when the patient arrives in the angiography suite. FFP is not indicated for reversal of heparin-induced coagulopathy. Because the half-life of heparin is roughly 60 minutes, most patients will be sufficiently reversed to allow manual compression by the end of the procedure.

Platelets have an extremely important role in hemostasis after angiographic procedures. Even in the presence of normal coagulation studies, thrombocytopenia carries a high risk of bleeding complications. Angiography is safe in patients with platelet counts greater than 50,000/mm³; venous procedures are safe when platelet counts are greater than 30,000/mm³ (assuming normal platelet function). Placement of implanted venous access ports requires platelet counts greater than 50,000/mm³. Platelet transfusion, with infusion continuing through the procedure for patients with severe consumptive thrombocytopenia, should be considered for patients with low platelet counts. Most angiographic procedures can be safely performed in patients taking platelet-inhibiting agents such as aspirin or clopidogrel. Interruption of these medications is not necessary before diagnostic angiography, and preprocedural administration of platelet inhibitors is often desirable in patients undergoing arterial interventions.

In the presence of an abnormal serum Cr, the risk of renal failure after the procedure should be weighed against the benefits of the examination. Prophylactic measures should be followed to maximize renal protection (see Contrast Agents). During the procedure, dilution of contrast in a ratio of 1:2 or even 1:1 (NS:contrast), limited use of hand injections, digital capture of fluoroscopic images, and liberal use of roadmap images to guide catheter positioning are all useful techniques to minimize contrast use.

■ BASIC SAFETY CONSIDERATIONS

Interventional radiology must be safe for patients and providers. Precautions against exposure to body fluids should be exercised

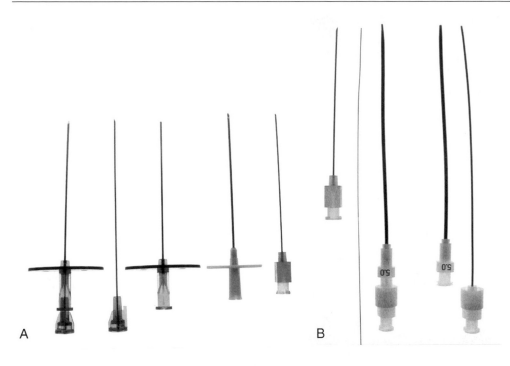

FIGURE **2-2**. Typical access needles. **A,** From left: 18-gauge Seldinger needle with hollow, sharp central stylet that extends beyond the blunt tip of the needle; stylet; Seldinger needle with stylet removed; 18-gauge sharp hollow (one-wall) needle; 21-gauge microaccess needle. **B,** Microaccess system. From left: 21-gauge needle; 0.018-inch guidewire for insertion through needle; 5-French dilator with central 3-French dilator tapered to 0.018-inch guidewire; 5-French dilator with 3-French dilator removed (accepts an 0.038-inch guidewire); 3-French dilator.

at all times, even when working with patients with no known risk factors. Consistent use of masks, face shields or other protective eyewear, sterile gloves, and impermeable gowns should be routine. Closed flush and contrast systems minimize the risk of splatter. All materials used during the case should be discarded in receptacles designed for biological waste.

Needles, scalpels, or any other sharp device used during a case should be carefully stored on the work surface in a red sharps container or removed immediately after use. Recapping is not advised. Verbal communication when handling sharps is essential. The best sharps containers contain a foam block in which the point of the sharp can be embedded. At the end of the case, it is the responsibility of the physician to dispose of the sharps in the appropriate receptacle. Puncture wounds from contaminated sharps are not only painful, but also potentially life-altering. If an accidental splash, puncture, or other exposure occurs, immediate consultation with individuals responsible for the management of occupational exposures is essential.

Radiation exposure to the patient and the staff should be kept to minimum. Use fluoroscopy only as needed. Last image hold, the ability to store and review fluoro loops, and imaging with pulse-mode fluoro (3-7.5 frames per second as compared to 15) all reduce patient and operator exposure. Prolonged fluoroscopy at high magnification with the x-ray tube in one position can cause cutaneous radiation burns to the patient. Cumulative exposure to physicians from scatter, especially when standing at the side of the patient during imaging, can be substantial. Wrap-around lead, thyroid shields, and leaded glasses should be worn. Leaded table drapes, careful coning of the beam, minimizing the air-gap between the image-intensifier and the patient, and use of boom-mounted x-ray shields are all means to decrease physician exposure to scatter. The operator's hands should never be visible on the image screen. Although it is tempting to remain at the patient's side during angiography in order to save time, this is a bad habit. Radiation badges should be worn at all times.

Many interventional radiologists report degenerative neck and back problems over time. Careful design of angiographic suites with attention to positioning of controls and monitors can reduce twisting and bending. In the future, robotically assisted or performed procedures will further decrease operator risk.

▬ TOOLS

Access Needles

All percutaneous angiographic procedures begin with an entry needle. There is great variety in vascular access needles, but all have a central channel for introduction of a guidewire (Fig. 2-2). Needles with a central sharp stylet that obturate the lumen have a blunted, atraumatic tip when the stylet is removed. The stylet allows the needle to puncture the vessel, but once removed theoretically reduces the risk of trauma. The stylet may be solid or hollow. In the latter case, blood can be visualized on the stylet hub once the vessel lumen is entered. The stylet must be removed in order to insert the guidewire. Needles with stylets are generally used only for arterial punctures. Needles without stylets have very sharp beveled tips, a quality that is useful when attempting to puncture small, mobile, or low-pressure vessels. The guidewire is introduced directly through the needle once the tip is fully within the vessel lumen. This style of needle is used for venous as well as arterial punctures.

The most common sizes for vascular access needles are 18- to 21-gauge in diameter and 2¼-5 inches in length. The lower the gauge number, the larger the diameter of the needle will be. The 18-gauge needles accommodate standard diameter guidewires. The 21-gauge needles are often packaged as part of a microaccess system that includes a small guidewire and coaxial dilators that convert the puncture to a standard-sized guidewire. These needles are designed to be highly visible under ultrasound to facilitate image-guided access. Microaccess techniques can be used for all arterial and venous punctures.

Guidewires

Guidewires are available in a wide variety of thicknesses, lengths, tip configurations, stiffnesses, coatings, and materials of construction (Fig. 2-3). In general, the guidewire thickness (always referred to in hundredths of an inch; e.g., 0.038 inch) should match the diameter of the lumen at the tip of the catheter or device that will slide over it. Guidewires that are too big will jam inside the catheter. However, if a guidewire is much smaller than the hole at the tip of the catheter or device there will be an abrupt transition or step-off that creates a gap that can trap subcutaneous tissue and cause the catheter to "stick" on the wire. The gap can

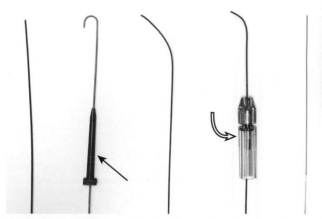

FIGURE 2-3. Common guidewires. From left: Straight 0.038-inch; J-tipped 0.038-inch with introducer device *(arrow)* to straighten guidewire during insertion into needle hub; angled high-torque 0.035-inch; angled hydrophilic-coated 0.038-inch nitinol wire with pin vise *(curved arrow)* for fine control; 0.018-inch platinum-tipped microwire.

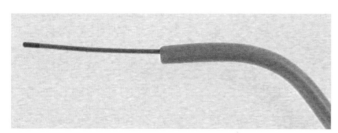

FIGURE 2-4. Catheter and guidewire mismatch. The catheter is tapered to 0.038 inch, but the guidewire is 0.018 inch in diameter. The tip of the catheter can "hang-up" on vessel wall, plaque, or the ostium of a branch vessel.

also cause the catheter tip to "hang-up" on plaque or at branch points as it is advanced along the guidewire (Fig. 2-4).

The most commonly used type of guidewire has a central stiff core around which is tightly wrapped a smaller wire, just like a coiled spring (Fig. 2-5). The outer wire is welded to the core at the back end, but not at the tip. The purpose of the coiled wrap is to decrease the area of contact between the surface of the guidewire and the tissues. Between the inner core wire and the outer wrap is a fine safety wire that runs along the length of the guidewire and is welded to the outer wrap at both ends. The safety wire prevents the wrap from unwinding. This is where the term *safety guidewire* originates. The thickness and composition of the inner core determines the degree of guidewire stiffness (Table 2-2). Flexible guidewires are important for negotiating tortuous or diseased vessels, but stiff guidewires ("working" wires) provide the most support for introducing catheters and devices. The ultimate variable-stiffness guidewire is one in which the core can be slid in and out of the spring wrap ("movable core guidewire") as needed. An important variation in guidewire design is the mandril wire, in which the springlike soft tip is limited to the tip, with the remainder of the guidewire consisting of a solid wire. This is a common construction for small-diameter guidewires, or extra rigid large-diameter guidewires.

The taper of the core at the leading end of the guidewire determines the softness or "floppiness" of the tip. The length and rate of transition of the taper defines the characteristics of the tip. Bentson guidewires, or movable core guidewires with the core retracted, have the softest tips. During diagnostic procedures, the soft end of the guidewire goes inside the patient. During interventions, the stiff back end of a guidewire can be a useful recanalization tool.

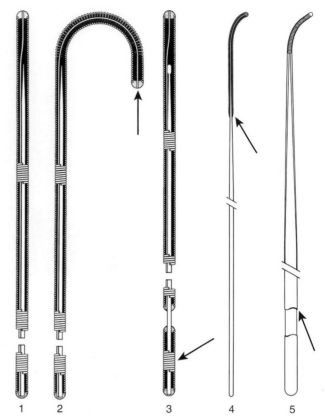

FIGURE 2-5. Basic construction of common guidewires. *1* and *2*, The straight and curved safety guidewires are basic tools. These are constructed of an outer coiled spring wrap, a central stiffening mandril welded to the outer wrap at the back end only, and a small inner safety wire *(arrow)* welded to the outer wrap at both ends. *3*, Movable core guidewire. The inner mandril slides back and forth, and can be removed entirely, using the handle at the back end of the guidewire *(arrow)*. This changes the stiffness of the wire tip. *4*, Low-profile mandril guidewire, in which the soft spring wrap is limited to one end of the guidewire *(arrow)*. The remainder of the guidewire is a plain mandril. *5*, Mandril-guidewire coated with a hydrophilic substance *(arrow)* that reduces friction and increases ability to select tortuous vessels. (Reproduced from Cook Group Incorporated, Bloomington, Ind., with permission.)

TABLE 2-2 Guidewire Stiffness

Guidewire	Stiffness
Movable core	0 (when core removed)
Standard 0.035-inch	++
Standard 0.038-inch	+++
Rosen	++++
Amplatz	+++++
Amplatz Super-Stiff	++++++
Lunderquist	+++++++

A curve in the end of the guidewire provides an additional degree of safety in diseased vessels. As the curved guidewire is advanced, the round presenting part deflects away from plaque, whereas the tip of a straight guidewire could burrow under it. A curve can be added to a straight guidewire by gently drawing the floppy tip across a firm edge (e.g., a fingernail or closed hemostat), much like curling a ribbon. In some instances, adding a curve to the body of the guidewire (especially stiff working wires) can be

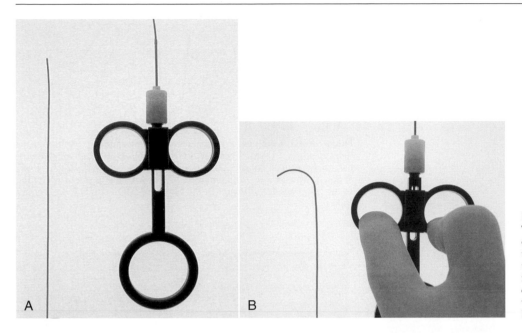

A   B

FIGURE 2-6. Tip deflecting guidewire. This wire has a stiff tip that is used to direct a catheter. **A,** The guidewire and the preattached handle. **B,** Deflection of the guidewire tip. The deflection is performed inside the catheter lumen. The catheter is then advanced off of the guidewire; the guidewire is never advanced beyond the tip of the catheter.

very useful for positioning a wire across the aortic bifurcation or in the thoracic aortic arch. Tip-deflecting guidewires allow variation in the radius of the curve while in the patient, but these guidewires have stiff tips and should never be advanced beyond the end of the catheter (Fig. 2-6).

Specialty guidewires, such as wires coated with slippery hydrophilic substances, highly torqueable guidewires, kink-resistant nitinol-based wires, and microwires are widely available. These guidewires are the difference between routine success and failure in the more challenging cases. Fine manipulation is often best with a small pin vise or other device (a "torque handle") that slides on and off of the external portion of the guidewire. Hydrophilic-coated guidewires are especially useful, because they can easily reach previously inaccessible places. This type of guidewire has a central core that is coated with an outer layer of hydrophilic material (see Fig. 2-5). These guidewires should not be inserted through access needles, because the non-radiopaque coating is easily sheared off by the metal edge at the tip of the needle when the guidewire is withdrawn. Also, unless kept moist, hydrophilic guidewires quickly become sticky. When this happens, it is difficult to advance a catheter over the guidewire. Furthermore, the entire guidewire may be pulled inadvertently out of the patient if it sticks to a gloved hand or gauze. To stabilize a hydrophilic guidewire during a catheter exchange, grip the wire with wet gauze. This allows a secure hold without drying out the guidewire.

The length of most guidewires used in routine angiography is 145-180 cm. When more guidewire is needed inside the body, or when the devices and catheters to be placed over the guidewire are long, an "exchange length" guidewire (260-300 cm) is used. This length is not used for routine cases because the length of guidewire outside the body is unwieldy and easily contaminated.

Dilators

Vessel dilators are short tapered catheters usually made of a stiffer plastic than diagnostic angiographic catheters (Fig. 2-7). The sole purpose of a dilator is to spread the soft tissues and the wall of the blood vessel to make passage of a catheter or device easier. By inserting sequentially larger dilators over a guidewire, a percutaneous access with a 21-gauge needle can be increased to almost any size. Sequential dilatation minimizes the risk of trauma to the vessel and tissues because incremental steps in size (1- to 2-French) can be accomplished with little force. The first dilator size after puncture with an 18-gauge access needle is usually 5-French.

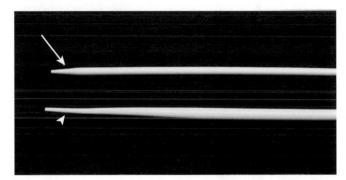

FIGURE 2-7. Vascular dilators. Standard taper *(arrow)* and longer taper *(arrowhead)* "Coons" tip. The latter is useful when more gradual dilatation is required.

Larger dilators can then be used as needed. Do not dilate an access site to more than 50% of the diameter of the artery if hemostasis with manual compression is anticipated; when the diameter of the hole in the wall approaches the diameter of the artery, the puncture becomes a partial transection.

Catheters

Angiographic catheters are made of plastic (polyurethane, polyethylene, Teflon, or nylon). The exact catheter material, construction, coatings, inner diameter, outer diameter, length, tip shape, and side-hole configuration are determined by the intended use (Fig. 2-8). Catheters for aortography are thick walled to handle large-volume, high-pressure injections, and often curled at the tip ("pigtail"), which keeps the tip of the catheter away from the vessel wall, with multiple side holes proximal to the curl such that the majority of the contrast exits the catheter in a diffuse cloud. Conversely, selective catheters are thinner walled for lower volume injections, shaped to seek branches off the main vessel, and tapered at the tip to advance smoothly into the branch vessel, with a single end hole to direct contrast in a specific direction. Precise control of the tip of the selective catheter is a top priority. Selective catheters therefore usually have fine metal or plastic strands incorporated into the wall ("braid") so that the tip is responsive to gentle rotation of the hub (Fig. 2-9).

Many different units and systems are used to describe a single catheter. The outer size is measured in French (3 French = 1 mm),

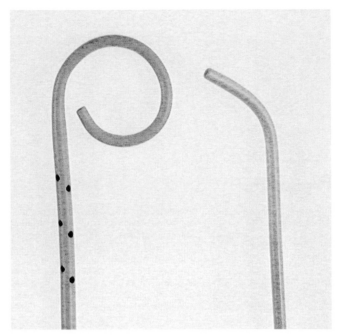

FIGURE **2-8**. Pigtail flush catheter *(left)* with multiple side holes. Selective catheter *(right)* with a single end hole.

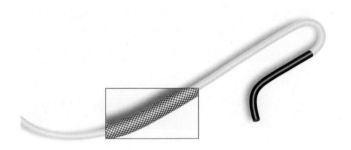

FIGURE **2-9**. Drawing illustrating the fine wire braid in the shaft of a selective catheter. The dark color at the end of the catheter is radiopaque, facilitating visualization of the catheter. (Reproduced from Cook Group Incorporated, Bloomington, Ind., with permission.)

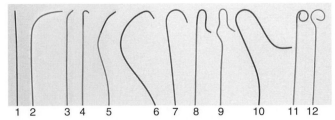

FIGURE **2-10**. Common catheter shapes. *1*, Straight. *2*, Multipurpose (hockey-stick). *3*, Davis. *4*, Binkert. *5*, Headhunter (H1). *6*, Cobra-2 (cobra-1 has a tighter curve, cobra-3 has a larger and longer curve). *7*, Rösch celiac. *8*, Sos. *9*, Mickaelson. *10*, Simmons-2 (the downgoing segment is shorter in the Simmons-1 and longer in the Simmons-3). *11*, Pigtail. *12*, Tennis racket.

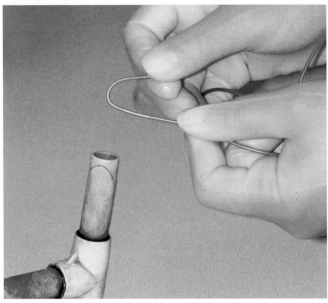

FIGURE **2-11**. Steaming a catheter. The catheter is held in steam for 30-60 seconds, then dunked in cool sterile water to "fix" the new shape.

while the diameter of the end hole (and therefore the maximum size guidewire that the catheter will accommodate) is described in hundredths of an inch. The length of the catheter is in centimeters (usually between 65 and 100 cm). The maximum flow rates are in milliliters per second (mL/sec), and maximum injection pressures are in pounds per square inch (PSI). The shape of the tip is named for either something that the catheter looks like ("pigtail," "cobra," "hockey-stick", "shepherd's crook"), the person who designed it (Simmons, Rösch, Sos, Binkert), or the intended use (celiac, left gastric, internal mammary) (Fig. 2-10). There are so many different catheters that no one department can or need stock them all. The shape of some catheters may be modified by bending into the desired configuration while heating in steam and then rapidly dunking in cool sterile water (Fig. 2-11).

Complex catheter shapes must be reformed inside the body after insertion over a guidewire. The catheter will resume its original configuration if there is sufficient space within the vessel lumen and memory in the catheter material. Some catheter shapes cannot reform spontaneously, in particular the larger recurved designs such as the Simmons. There are a number of ways to reform these catheters (Figs. 2-12 to 2-16). A recurved shape can also be created from an angled selective catheter by forming a Waltman loop (Fig. 2-17).

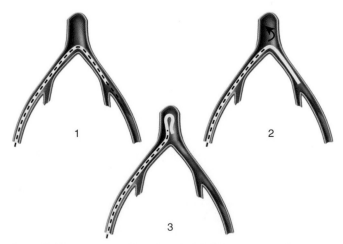

FIGURE **2-12**. Branch technique for reforming a Simmons catheter. *1*, The catheter is advanced into the branch over a guidewire *(dashed line)*. Aortic bifurcation is shown in this illustration. *2*, The guidewire is withdrawn proximal to the origin of the branch but still in the catheter. One may also remove the guidewire and reinsert the stiff end to the same point. The catheter is then simultaneously twisted and advanced. *3*, Reformed catheter.

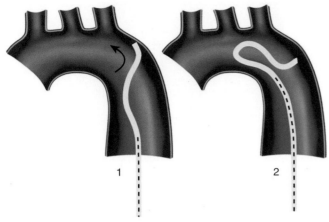

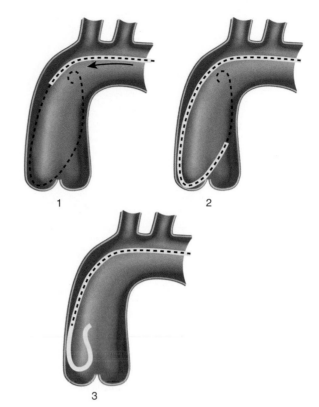

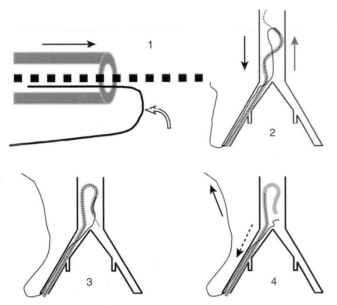

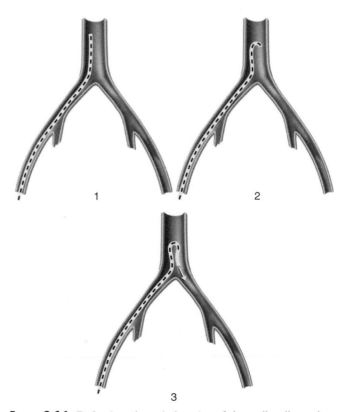

FIGURE 2-13. Aortic spin technique for reforming a Simmons catheter (works best for Simmons 1). *1*, The catheter is simultaneously twisted and advanced in the proximal descending thoracic aorta. Note the wire is withdrawn below the curved portion of the catheter. *2*, Reformed catheter.

FIGURE 2-14. Cope string technique, which easily reforms any recurved catheter. *1*, Approximately 3-4 cm of 4-0 Tevdek II (Deknatel Inc., Fall River, Mass.) suture material *(curved arrow)* has been backloaded into the catheter tip. The catheter is then loaded onto a floppy-tipped guidewire *(dashed line)* and advanced *(arrow)* into the patient. *2*, The catheter has been advanced over the guidewire into the aorta, with trailing suture material exiting the groin adjacent to the catheter. The floppy portion of the guidewire still exits the catheter, "locking" suture material in catheter tip. Suture material is pulled gently *(black arrow)* as slight forward force applied to catheter *(gray arrow)*. *3*, Simmons has been reformed. *4*, Suture is removed by first retracting the guidewire into the catheter *(dashed arrow)*, "unlocking" the suture material. Suture material can then gently be pulled out *(black arrow)*.

FIGURE 2-15. Ascending aorta technique for reforming a Simmons catheter. *1*, Floppy-tipped 3-J guidewire reflected off of the aortic valve. The catheter is advanced over the guidewire. *2*, The catheter is advanced around a bend in the guidewire. *3*, Retraction of the guidewire completes the reformation.

Straight and pigtail catheters are generally used for nonselective injections. Straight catheters should only be advanced over a guidewire; pigtail catheters can be safely advanced in normal vessels once the pigtail has reformed. Before removal of a pigtail catheter from the body, the tip is usually straightened with a guidewire. Straight catheters can be removed without a guidewire.

Selective catheters are chosen based upon the anatomy of the vessel of interest (Fig. 2-18). The technique for selecting a branch vessel with a catheter varies with the type of catheter

FIGURE 2-16. Deflecting wire technique (unsafe in small or diseased aortas). *1*, Deflecting wire is positioned near the tip of the catheter. *2*, Wire is deflected, curving the catheter as well. *3*, With the guidewire fixed, the catheter is advanced *(arrow)* to reform Simmons.

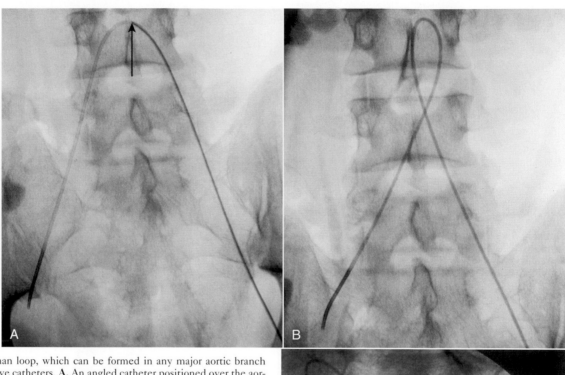

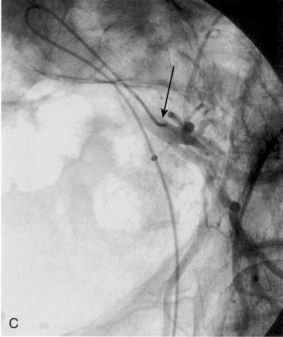

Figure 2-17. The Waltman loop, which can be formed in any major aortic branch vessel with braided selective catheters. **A,** An angled catheter positioned over the aortic bifurcation. Note the stiff end of the guidewire at the catheter apex *(arrow)*. **B,** The catheter is advanced and twisted, forming the loop. **C,** Looped catheter has been used to select the ipsilateral internal iliac artery *(arrow)*.

(Figs. 2-19 and 2-20). Aggressive probing with the catheter or guidewire, or advancing the catheter into the branch without leading with at least 1-2 cm of soft guidewire, can result in arterial dissection or perforation. The Waltman loop is particularly useful in the pelvis for selection of branches of the internal iliac artery on the same side as the arterial puncture.

Small-diameter catheters that are specially designed to fit coaxially within the lumen of a standard angiographic catheter are termed *microcatheters* (Fig. 2-21). These soft, flexible catheters are 2- to 3-French in diameter, with 0.010- to 0.027-inch inner lumens. They are designed to reach beyond standard catheters into small or tortuous vessels. The ability to reliably select these vessels without creating spasm, dissection, or thrombosis has allowed certain subspecialties (e.g., neurointerventional radiology) to flourish. To use a microcatheter, a standard angiographic catheter that accepts a 0.038- or 0.035-inch

guidewire is placed securely in a proximal position in the blood vessel. The microcatheter is then advanced in conjunction with a specially designed 0.010- to 0.018-inch selective guidewire through the standard catheter lumen. Once a superselective position has been achieved with the microcatheter, a variety of procedures can be performed such as embolization, sampling, or low-volume angiography. The resistance to flow in the small lumen prevents the use of most microcatheters for routine angiography. High-flow microcatheters can accept up to 3 mL/sec of contrast at a lower PSI than standard catheters. Contrast and flush solutions are most easily injected through these catheters with 3-mL or smaller high-pressure Luer-lock syringes.

Large guiding catheters may be used for positioning and stabilizing standard catheters and devices. These nontapered catheters have extra large lumens and a preformed simple shape

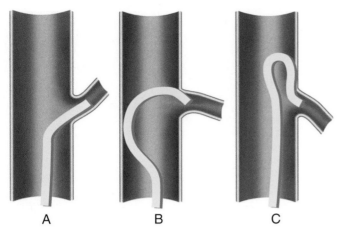

FIGURE 2-18. Choosing a selective catheter shape. **A,** Angled catheter when angle of axis of branch vessel from aortic axis is low. **B,** Curved catheter (e.g., cobra-2 or celiac) when angle of axis of branch vessel is between 60 and 120 degrees. **C,** Recurved catheter (e.g., Sos or Simmons) when angle of axis of branch vessel from aorta is great.

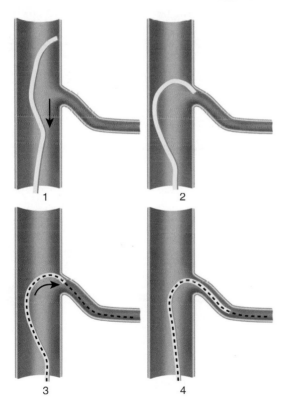

FIGURE 2-19. How to use a cobra catheter. *1,* The catheter is advanced to a position proximal to the branch over the guidewire, then pulled down *(arrow)*. *2,* The catheter tip engages the orifice of the branch. Contrast is injected gently to confirm location. *3,* Soft-tipped selective guidewire has been advanced into branch. The guidewire is held firmly and the catheter advanced *(arrow)*. *4,* Catheter in selected position.

that accepts standard sized catheters and devices (Fig. 2-22). Guiding catheters with tips can be reshaped within the patient using controls at the back end of the catheter. There are many circumstances in which standard catheters are difficult to position selectively, such as in the case of a renal artery that arises from a tortuous or aneurysmal abdominal aorta. In this situation, a larger outer catheter that can guide the standard catheter toward the renal artery and prevent it from floundering around is very helpful. Guiding catheters are usually shorter

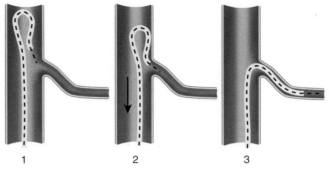

FIGURE 2-20. How to use a Simmons catheter. *1,* The catheter is positioned above the branch vessel with at least 1 cm of floppy straight guidewire beyond the catheter tip. *2,* The catheter is gently pulled down *(arrow)* until the guidewire and tip engage the orifice of the branch. *3,* Continued gentle traction results in deeper placement of catheter tip. To deselect the branch, push the catheter back into the aorta (reverse steps 1-3). To straighten the Simmons, apply continued traction after step 3.

than standard angiographic catheters, and frequently have a radiopaque band at the tip.

Be aware that guiding catheter size in French refers to the *outer,* not the *inner* diameter. The inner diameter is often described in hundredths of an inch, which must be converted to French to determine whether a standard catheter will fit (1 French = 0.012 in = 0.333 mm).

Sheaths

Most vascular interventions and many diagnostic procedures are performed through vascular access sheaths. These devices are plastic tubes of varying thickness and construction that are open at one end and capped with a hemostatic valve at the other (Fig. 2-23). The open end is not tapered, although the edges are carefully beveled to create a smooth transition to the tapered dilator that is used to introduce the sheath over a guidewire. The valve end usually has a short, flexible, and clear side arm that can be connected to a constant flush (to prevent thrombus from forming in the sheath) or an arterial pressure monitor. The valve may be a split membrane or rotating hub. The purpose of the sheath is to simplify multiple catheter exchanges through a single puncture site. When not using a sheath, it is unwise to downsize catheters during a procedure owing to the risk of bleeding around the smaller diameter catheter. Perhaps more important, devices that are irregular in contour or even nontapered can be introduced through a sheath without damaging the device or traumatizing the access vessel. Long sheaths can be used to straighten a tortuous access artery or negotiate a tortuous aorta. By convention, sheaths are described by the maximum size (in French) of the device that will fit through the sheath. Because the walls of the sheath have some thickness, the actual hole in the blood vessel is 1.5- to 2-French larger than the sheath "size." Sheaths are available in a variety of lengths, depending on the requirements of the procedure.

A useful sheath variant is the peel-away sheath (Fig. 2-24). Used frequently when inserting venous access devices, this sheath is removed by splitting lengthwise into two halves. Two wings or tabs at the hub are pulled apart to split the sheath. Some peel-away sheaths have hemostatic valves, although these are usually not as robust or efficient (particularly for air) as the valves in conventional sheaths. The sheath is introduced in standard fashion over a guidewire with a tapered plastic dilator. Once in position, the dilator is removed. The only way to achieve hemostasis with a nonvalved sheath is to block the open end with a finger or to clamp the sheath. After inserting the device or catheter through the sheath, the plastic wings are pulled in opposite directions parallel to the skin. This "breaks" the sheath into two long strips of plastic and allows complete disengagement from the catheter without having to slide it off the back end.

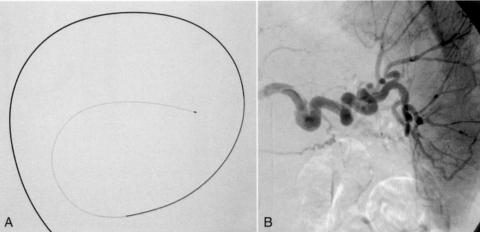

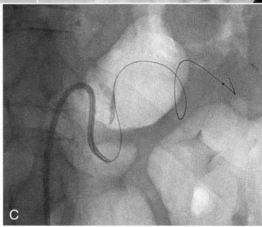

FIGURE 2-21. Use of a microcatheter. **A,** Typical microcatheter that tapers from 3-French proximally to 2.3-French at the tip. Note the radiopaque marker at the tip. **B,** Extremely tortuous splenic artery in a patient with hypersplenism. **C,** Microcatheter has been advanced over a 0.016-inch guidewire into the distal splenic artery through a 6.5-French Simmons-1 catheter.

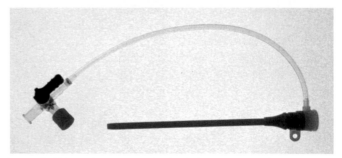

FIGURE 2-23. Typical hemostatic sheath. French size of sheaths refers to the inner diameter.

Stopcocks/Flow Switches

Controlling flow in and out of catheters once they are in the body is a priority. Stopcocks are plastic devices that allow one or more syringes to be connected to a catheter, and by turning a handle or sliding a switch, allow or block flow (Fig. 2-25). Rotating hub adaptors have one or more potential entry points for a guidewire or catheter. Hemostasis is achieved by tightening the hub by rotating it clockwise. Metal stopcocks are needed when handling oil-based contrast agents because many plastics become brittle and disintegrate when exposed to the oil.

▬ CONTRAST AGENTS

Safe and well-tolerated contrast agents are as important to angiography as the Seldinger technique. The ideal contrast agent has excellent radiopacity, mixes well with blood, is easy to use, and does not harm the patient. Iodinated contrast agents (based on benzene rings with three bound iodine atoms, termed *triiodinated*) are, as of yet, closest to ideal.

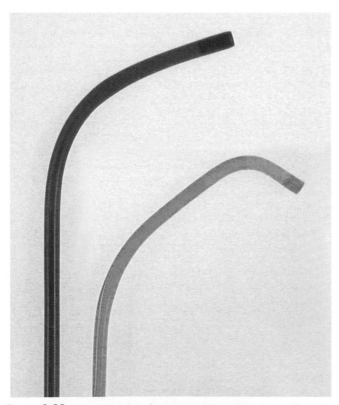

FIGURE 2-22. Two examples of nontapered large-diameter guide catheters, which can accommodate standard 5-French catheters. French size of guide catheters refers to the outer diameter.

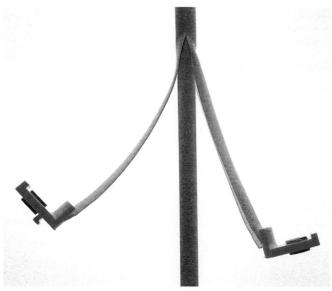

FIGURE **2-24**. Peel-away sheath. To peel the sheath away, wings are pulled in opposite directions at 90 degrees from the catheter shaft.

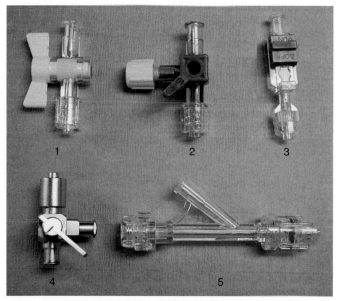

FIGURE **2-25**. Examples of flow-control devices. *1*, One-way stopcock in open position. *2*, Two-way stopcock (often called *three-way*) turned off to all lumens. *3*, Flow-switch. *4*, Metal stopcock. *5*, Rotating hub hemostatic valve (Tuohy-Borst adapter) with side arm for flushing.

There are two major classes of triiodinated contrast agents: ionic and non-ionic (Table 2-3). Ionic contrast agents are bound to a radiolucent cation, usually sodium and meglumine (N-methylglucamine), but also sometimes magnesium and calcium. This results in a highly soluble, low-viscosity, but high osmolar (two particles per iodinated ring) contrast agent. High osmolality relative to a patient's blood is believed to be a major contributing factor to adverse reactions to contrast agents. Non-ionic contrast agents have no electrical charge, so cations are not necessary. This reduces the osmolality of the contrast agent (one particle per iodinated ring), which improves the safety profile, but increases viscosity. The two major classes of contrast agents are further subdivided as either monomeric (one triiodinated benzene ring) or dimeric (two linked triiodinated benzene rings).

Adverse reactions to iodinated contrast agents are relatively common, but the majority are minor, such as nausea (Table 2-4). Most minor complications are linked to the osmolality of the contrast, so that the overall incidence is lower with non-ionic contrast

agents. Adverse reactions may be immediate (within seconds to minutes of injection) or delayed (hours to days).

The two major adverse reactions to iodinated contrast agents are anaphylaxis and renal failure. True anaphylaxis occurs shortly after contrast injection and is distinguished from a vasovagal response by tachycardia and respiratory distress (Table 2-5). The incidence of life-threatening anaphylaxis due to iodinated contrast is approximately 1 per 40,000 to 170,000, with the higher rate associated with ionic contrast. Mild reactions such as urticaria and nasal stuffiness occur more commonly (especially with ionic contrast). Contrast reactions must be treated promptly and aggressively; the most common cause of death is airway obstruction (Boxes 2-1 to 2-3). The patient with a history of prior contrast allergy should receive steroid prophylaxis beginning at least 12 hours before the procedure (unless a true emergency exists) (Box 2-4). Patients label many symptoms experienced during prior contrast injections as an "allergy," such as nausea, vagal nerve–mediated bradycardia and hypotension, or ischemic cardiac events. Whenever the precise nature of the "allergic" reaction cannot be determined from the history, steroid prophylaxis is prudent. Non-ionic contrast should be used throughout the procedure in any patient with a history of contrast allergy.

Renal failure following administration of iodinated contrast agents is more common in patients with diabetes, preexisting renal insufficiency (stage 2-5 renal failure), and multiple myeloma (Box 2-5; Table 2-6). The exact mechanism is not known, so that several different protective measures are in common use (Table 2-7). The classic presentation is an increase in creatinine 24-48 hours following exposure to contrast, peaking at 72-96 hours. Patients are usually oliguric but may become anuric. Management is usually expectant, because renal function should return to baseline in 7-14 days. However, in patients with severe preexisting renal insufficiency and diabetes, the risk of permanent dialysis after angiography may be as high as 15% despite the use of low-osmolar contrast agents and other protective measures.

Patients taking Metformin, an oral hypoglycemic agent, should be instructed to wait 48 hours after the procedure before resuming this medication. Metformin does not increase the risk of acute contrast-induced renal failure, but patients can develop fatal lactic acidosis from the drug if renal failure does occur.

Contrast is administered during angiographic procedures by hand or mechanical injection (Table 2-8). Injection by hand is useful during the initial stages of the procedure, or for low-volume and low-pressure angiograms of small vessels or through precariously situated catheters. The use of mechanical injectors is necessary for optimal contrast delivery, particularly when large volumes or high flow rates are required. In addition, there is less radiation exposure to the physician when a mechanical injector is used. Catheters are rated for both flow rates and maximum injection pressure. This information is provided on the catheter packaging. Exceeding these limits may result in bursting the catheter (usually at the hub), or premature termination of the injection by the power injector software. Careful technique is necessary when connecting a catheter to a power injector to avoid air bubbles, contamination of the catheter, or disconnection during injection (Box 2-6).

ALTERNATIVE CONTRAST AGENTS

The low but real incidence of adverse reactions to iodinated contrast agents has led to the use of alternative contrast agents in selected circumstances, particularly in patients with past histories of true anaphylactic reactions to iodinated contrast, or precarious renal function. Two alternative contrast agents have been described for patients who cannot tolerate iodinated contrast agents: carbon dioxide (CO_2) gas and gadolinium chelates.

Carbon Dioxide Gas

There is extensive experience with CO_2 gas as an angiographic contrast agent. There is no nephrotoxicity, and allergy does not

TABLE 2-3 Contrast Agents

Class of Contrast Agent	Contrast Agent	Commercial Name	Iodine (Atoms Per Molecule)	Approximate Osmolality* (300 mg I/mL Concentration)
Ionic monomer	Diatrizoate Iothalamate	Hypaque Renografin Conray	3	1500-1700
Non-ionic monomer	Iopamidol Iohexol Ioversol Ioxilan Iopromide	Isovue Omnipaque Optiray Oxilan Optivist	3	600-700
Ionic dimer	Ioxaglate	Hexabrix	6	560
Non-ionic dimer	Iodixanol	Visipaque	6	300

*mOsm/kg water.

TABLE 2-4 Contrast Reactions

Reaction	Ionic Contrast	Non-Ionic Contrast
Nausea	4.6%	1%
Vomiting	1.8%	0.4%
Itching	3.0%	0.5%
Urticaria	3.2%	0.5%
Sneezing	1.7%	0.2%
Dyspnea	0.2%	0.04%
Hypotension	0.1%	0.01%
Sialadenitis	<0.1%	<0.1%
Delayed rash	2%-3%	2%-3%
Death	1:40,000	1:170,000

TABLE 2-5 Anaphylaxis vs. Vasovagal Reaction

Feature	Anaphylaxis	Vasovagal
Blood pressure	Low	Low
Pulse	Fast	Slow
Breathing	Labored, wheezes	Normal
Skin	Flushed, urticaria	Cool, clammy

Box 2-1. Treatment of Vasovagal Reactions

Lay down patient
Elevate legs
Intravenous fluid bolus (300-500 mL normal saline)
Atropine 1 mg intravenous push (doses less than 0.5 mg
    may worsen bradycardia)

Box 2-2. Treatment of Mild Contrast Reactions

Assess airway, administer 100% oxygen
Secure intravenous access
Obtain vital signs
Benadryl 50 mg intravenously
Hydrocortisone 100-250 mg intravenously
Observe patient for 4 hours
For mild bronchospasm:
    Albuterol 0.5 mL (2.5 mg) or metaproterenol 0.3 mL
      (15 mg) in 2.5 mL normal saline, inhalation nebulizer
OR
    Epinephrine (1:1000) 0.3 mL subcutaneously or intra-
      muscularly, repeated every 20 minutes as necessary

Box 2-3. Treatment of Severe Anaphylaxis

Call a "Code"
Secure an airway (cricothyroidotomy if necessary) and
    administer 100% oxygen
Secure intravenous access
Epinephrine (1:10,000) 1 mL intravenously or via endotra-
    cheal tube
Initiate pressor support
Methylprednisolone 125 mg or hydrocortisone 500 mg
    intravenously
Aggressive fluid resuscitation with normal saline or lactated
    Ringer's solution
Admit patient to intensive care unit

Box 2-4. Suggested Preparation of Patient with Contrast Allergy

Prednisone 50 mg (oral) 13, 7, and 1 hour prior to the
    procedure (three doses) OR hydrocortisone 200 mg
    intravenously 2-3 hours prior to the procedure
Diphenhydramine (Benadryl) 50 mg (oral) 1 hour prior to
    procedure or intravenously upon arrival in angiography
    suite
H_2-blocker intravenously upon arrival in angiography suite
Alternative oral steroid regimen: prednisone 50 mg at
    12 and 2 hours before the procedure
Pediatric dosing: prednisone 0.5 mg/kg/dose, maximum
    50 mg; Benadryl 1.25 mg/kg, maximum 50 mg

exist. The gas functions as a negative contrast agent by briefly displacing the blood volume in the lumen of the vessel, resulting in decreased attenuation of the x-ray beam (Box 2-7). Dedicated CO_2 digital subtraction techniques are standard on most modern angiographic equipment (Fig. 2-26). The buoyant nature of CO_2 results in preferential filling of anterior structures. The CO_2 gas is highly soluble and excreted from the lungs.

Mechanical injectors for CO_2 are not available in the United States. All injections must therefore be performed by hand (Box 2-8). Because of the invisible nature of gases, scrupulous handling of CO_2 is necessary to prevent contamination by less soluble room air. An additional key technical aspect of CO_2 angiography is to avoid explosive delivery of gas by purging the catheter with a small volume of gas before the angiogram; otherwise tremendous pressure is generated as the gas is compressed behind the column of fluid in the catheter.

The extremely low viscosity of CO_2 is advantageous for wedged hepatic vein portography, and demonstration of subtle bleeding. CO_2 can be used for abdominal aortography, selective visceral

---

Box 2-5. **Risk Factors for Contrast-Induced Acute Renal Failure**

Underlying renal insufficiency
Diabetes mellitus
Dehydration
Nephrotoxic medications
Age >60 years
Longstanding hypertension
Cardiovascular disease
Multiple myeloma
Hyperuricemia
High-osmolar contrast
Large volume of contrast in short period of time
Recent exposure to large contrast load

TABLE 2-6 Stages of Renal Failure

Stage	Glomerular Filtration Rate (mL/min/1.73 m²)
1	>90 (normal GFR; can be present with abnormal kidneys)
2	60-89
3	30-59
4	15-29
5	<15

GFR, Glomerular filtration rate.

TABLE 2-7 Preventive Measures for Contrast-Induced Acute Renal Failure

Agent	Protocol
Hydration	1 mL/kg/hr 0.9% saline for 12 hours prior to procedure; 1 mL/kg/hr 0.9% saline for 12 hours postprocedure
Sodium bicarbonate	154 mmol/L at 3 mL/kg/hr prior to the procedure; 1 mL/kg/hr for 6 hours after the procedure
N-Acetylcysteine	1200 mg orally every 12 hours beginning 24 hours before the procedure, including one dose on morning of the angiogram, and one dose the night after the procedure. Total of 4 doses.

TABLE 2-8 Weight-Based Contrast Injection Rates

Artery	Patient Weight		
	10-20 kg	**20-50 kg**	**>50 kg**
Aorta	5-10 for 8-15*	10-20 for 20-40	20-25 for 25-50
Celiac	2-3 for 10-20	3-5 for 15-30	5-8 for 30-60
Splenic	2-3 for 10-15	3-5 for 15-20	5-8 for 20-50
Hepatic	2-3 for 5-10	3-5 for 10-15	5-8 for 15-25
Superior mesenteric artery	2-3 for 10-15	3-5 for 15-30	5-8 for 30-50
Inferior mesenteric artery	#	1-3 for 6-9	2-3 for 10-15
Renal	2-4 for 3-5	3-5 for 6-9	5-8 for 10-15
Subclavian	2-3 for 4-6	3-4 for 6-15	5-8 for 15-25
Common carotid	2-3 for 3-5	4-6 for 5-10	6-8 for 10-15
Internal carotid	1-2 for 3-5	2-4 for 5-8	4-5 for 6-10
External carotid	#	#	2-3 for 6-9
Vertebral	#	2-5 for 4-6	4-7 for 6-9

*= X-Y mL/sec for a total volume of A-B mL, for entire table.
#= hand injection.
For weights less than 10 kg, use hand injections.
Data from Heran MK, Marshalleck F, Temple M, et al. Joint quality improvement guidelines for pediatric arterial access and arteriography: from the Societies of Interventional Radiology and Pediatric Radiology. *J Vasc Interv Radiol* 2010;21:32-43.

Box 2-6. **Connecting Catheter to Power Injector**

Use sterile, clear, high-pressure Luer-lock tubing between injector and catheter
If injecting through a stopcock, be sure that it tolerates high pressures
Turn injector tubing hub counterclockwise several rotations prior to hook-up (so that potential rotational energy is not built up in tubing during attachment to catheter)
Allow backbleeding from catheter and advance contrast slowly through tubing during connection ("wet hook-up")
Make sure that connection is tight*
Withdraw contrast in tubing until blood is seen to exclude air bubbles
Advance contrast slowly to clear blood from catheter
Check catheter tip with fluoroscopy to ensure that it has remained in position after hook-up

*If the patient or injector is moved suddenly, the catheter can be pulled out of position.

Box 2-7. **Advantages of CO_2 Gas as an Angiographic Contrast Agent**

Readily available
No allergic reactions
No renal toxicity
Low viscosity
Highly soluble
No maximum total dose
Low cost

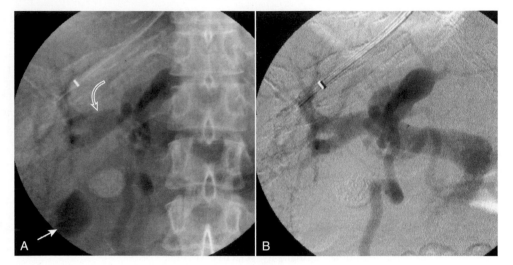

Figure 2-26. CO_2 portal venogram. **A,** Unsubtracted image from wedged hepatic venogram shows CO_2 filling portal vein *(curved arrow)*. Density of the CO_2 is the same as gas in the bowel *(straight arrow)*. **B,** Digital subtraction of the same frame. Visualization of the portal venous system is excellent.

Box 2-8. Simple Technique for Hand Injection CO_2 Angiography

60-mL Luer lock syringe containing 10 mL of flush solution, equipped with stopcock

Purge all air from syringe, so that only fluid remains

Attach to purged CO_2 source

Allow 30-40 mL of uncompressed CO_2 gas to enter syringe; use stopcock to control flow

Turn stopcock to "closed" position; disconnect from CO_2 source (closed stopcock remains on the syringe)

Keep tip of syringe pointed down

Attach to catheter while applying gentle positive pressure and opening stopcock, ensuring "wet" connection

Purge blood from catheter with small amount of CO_2 gas

Close stopcock

Compress gas with syringe plunger

Initiate digital subtraction angiography using CO_2 acquisition program

Open stopcock and vigorously inject compressed CO_2

---

injections, lower extremity runoffs, as well as most venous studies. For abdomen studies it is helpful to administer intravenous glucagon (1 mg intravenously) to decrease bowel peristalsis. CO_2 is contraindicated for angiography of the thoracic aorta, cerebral arteries, or upper extremity arteries owing to potential neurologic complications. Rarely, CO_2 gas can cause a "vapor lock" in a vessel, which obstructs blood flow and induces distal ischemia. An excessive volume of gas in the heart can obstruct the pulmonary outflow tract, with severe cardiovascular consequences.

Gadolinium Chelates

Gadolinium chelates were developed as intravenous contrast for magnetic resonance imaging. Gadolinium (Gd) has a k-edge of 50 keV, slightly higher than iodine (33 keV). This permits visualization of gadolinium with current digital subtraction angiographic equipment adjusted for a higher KVP (Fig. 2-27). The overall safety profile of these contrast agents is superior to that of iodinated contrast in normal individuals, and there is no cross-reactivity in patients with anaphylaxis to iodinated contrast. However, patients with stage 3 or higher renal insufficiency are at risk for development of nephrogenic systemic fibrosis (NSF) after injection of gadolinium agents. NSF is a debilitating, potentially fatal illness that appears to be associated with gadolinium contrast preparations that contain higher quantities of unchelated Gd (e.g., gadodiamide). Until the relationship of gadolinium to NSF is clearly understood, these contrast agents are generally only indicated in patients with normal renal function and true anaphylaxis to iodinated contrast when CO_2 is contraindicated.

Although the approved doses of most gadolinium-based agents are 0.1-0.3 mL/kg, volumes of 40-60 mL have been used for many years. Gadolinium-based contrast agents have been used in every vascular application, including carotid and coronary angiography. Gadolinium-based contrast agents are liquids, so special injection techniques or equipment is not required. Digital subtraction angiography (DSA) is necessary, in that the low gadolinium concentration in the available formulations results in relatively weak opacification of deep arteries.

▬ INTRAPROCEDURAL CARE

Sedation

Patients undergoing invasive diagnostic and therapeutic procedures tend to be nervous, apprehensive, and ill. Frequent communication with the members of the team is greatly reassuring to the patient. Small gestures, such as alerting the patient prior to any step that may be uncomfortable, can reduce anxiety and improve cooperation. Administration of intravenous sedatives (benzodiazepines) and pain medication (opioids) is frequently necessary (Table 2-9). The goal is anxiolysis or moderate ("conscious") sedation, such that the patient remains responsive with spontaneous respiration and an intact gag reflex (Table 2-10). Each facility has established requirements for training of personnel providing sedation and monitoring of these patients. As a rule, blood pressure, heart rate and rhythm, respiration rate, and oxygen saturation should be monitored and recorded at regular intervals throughout the procedure. A reliable venous access is required for administration of medications and possible resuscitation. Ready access to oxygen, suction, and defibrillation equipment is necessary.

Antibiotic Prophylaxis

Angiograms are sterile procedures. Hair at the puncture site should be shaved immediately prior to the procedure using an electric razor. The skin over the access site should be prepared according to institutional guidelines for open procedures. Prepackaged single-use sponge-sticks containing a skin-prep solution (e.g., a mixture of 2% chlorhexidine and 70% isopropyl alcohol) simplify and standardize this process. The patient is then covered with sterile drapes so that only the puncture site is accessible. Personnel directly involved in performing the procedure should wear sterile gloves and gown, as well as a hat, mask, and splatter shield. Other personnel can wear scrub clothes, hat, and mask.

Antibiotic prophylaxis is not necessary for the majority of patients undergoing diagnostic angiography. Rare exceptions

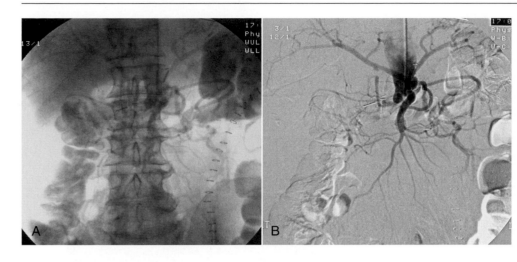

FIGURE 2-27. Gadolinium digital subtraction angiogram. **A,** Unsubtracted image from aortic injection in a patient with infrarenal aortic occlusion shows weak vascular opacification. **B,** Digital subtraction of the same frame. There is excellent opacification of the visceral vessels.

TABLE 2-9 Medications for Conscious Sedation

Medication	Type	IV Dose*	Duration	Antagonist
Midazolam	Benzodiazepine	0.5-1 mg[†]	30 min	Flumazenil
Diazepam	Benzodiazepine	1-3 mg[†]	6-10 hr	Flumazenil
Flumazenil	Benzodiazepine antagonist	0.1-0.2 mg[†]	45 min	None
Fentanyl	Opioid	25-50 µg[†]	30-60 min	Naloxone
Morphine	Opioid	1-3 mg[†]	3-4 hr	Naloxone
Naloxone	Opioid antagonist	0.1-0.2 mg[†]	45 min	None
Odansetron	Antiemetic	4 mg[‡]	4-8 hr	None
Promethazine	Antiemetic	6.25-12.5 mg[‡]	4-8 hr	None

*IV, intravenous dose.
[†]Repeated as necessary until desired affect achieved.
[‡]Repeated × 1 if necessary.

TABLE 2-10 Sedation/Analgesia Levels

Level	Description
Minimal sedation (anxiolysis)	Normal response to verbal commands, normal ventilation and cardiovascular function
Moderate sedation ("conscious" sedation)	Depressed consciousness with purposeful response to verbal commands, adequate spontaneous respiration, normal cardiovascular function
Deep sedation	Depressed consciousness, repeated or painful stimulus required for purposeful response, ability to maintain airway and ventilation may be impaired
Anesthesia	Loss of consciousness, ventilatory function often impaired, cardiovascular function may be impaired

TABLE 2-11 Medications for Hypertensive Crisis

Medication	Initial Dose	Titration Schedule	Duration
Labetalol*	20-80 mg bolus	5-10 min up to 300 mg	3-6 hr
Hydralazine	5 mg bolus	Repeat up to 20 mg	3-6 hr
Fenoldopam	0.1-3 µg/kg/min	15 min to desired blood pressure	30 min
Nitroprusside[†]	0.5-10 µg/kg/min	5-10 min to desired blood pressure	1-3 min
Phentolamine[‡]	5-10 mg bolus	5-15 min to desired blood pressure	3-10 min

*May not be effective in patients receiving α and β antagonists.
[†]Avoid in patients with increased central nervous system pressures.
[‡]Adrenergic crisis in patients with pheochromocytoma.

include asplenic and severely neutropenic patients. Patients with prosthetic heart valves or other indications for endocarditis prophylaxis do not require antibiotics before angiography. When indicated, antibiotics appropriate for skin flora should be used, such as cephazolin 1 g, clindamycin 300 mg, or vancomycin 500 mg.

Blood Pressure Control

Anxious or uncomfortable patients may develop elevated blood pressures before or during the procedure. A systolic blood pressure less than 170 mm Hg is desirable to avoid cardiac ischemia in older patients and to facilitate hemostasis at the end of the procedure. In most cases, the blood pressure returns to normal once adequate sedation and pain control is achieved. When immediate reduction of blood pressure is indicated, or if patients do not respond to sedation, pharmacologic intervention is warranted (Table 2-11). When pheochromocytoma is suspected as the cause of the hypertensive crisis, the drug of choice is phentolamine, a nonselective α-adrenergic blocker.

Carcinoid Crisis

Patients with metastatic carcinoid tumor to the liver should receive octreotide (a somatostatin analog) 500 µg intravenously (infused over 20 minutes) or subcutaneously before diagnostic angiography, particularly when selective hepatic angiography or an intervention will be performed. Symptoms of carcinoid crisis include sudden onset of flushing, hypertension or hypotension, tachycardia, arrhythmias, bronchospasm, abdominal pain, and diarrhea. The cornerstone of treatment is intravenous octreotide in boluses of 250-500 µg over several minutes, repeated as necessary, followed by a continuous infusion of 100-200 µg/hr. Fluid resuscitation, corticosteroids, and antihypertensive medications may also be necessary. If untreated, carcinoid crisis can be fatal.

Anticoagulation

Anticoagulation during diagnostic peripheral angiography is rarely necessary in adults unless the catheter impedes flow in a diseased or small vessel. Some physicians routinely administer heparin to patients during selective carotid angiography for occlusive disease. The typical adult dose is a 3000-5000 U intravenous bolus, followed by 1000 U each hour. The effect of the heparin can be monitored by measuring an activated clotting time (ACT), with a target of greater than 250 seconds. Heparin can be reversed with Protamine, administered as a slow intravenous bolus. The usual dose is 10 mg of Protamine for every 1000 U of unfractionated heparin presumed to be still active. Protamine does not reverse low-molecular-weight heparin.

Pediatric Patients

Angiography in pediatric patients requires several modifications of standard techniques. General anesthesia is recommended for any prepubescent child, and for immature adolescents. Pediatric patients weighing less than 15 kg should be routinely anticoagulated with heparin (75-100 U/kg) because the risk of catheter-induced arterial spasm and thrombosis is as high as 10% in patients younger than 1 year of age. The common femoral artery access is preferred. Microaccess needles, ultrasound guidance for access, local anesthetic with 1% lidocaine (following weight-based dosing guidelines of 5 mg/kg without epinephrine, 7 mg/kg with epinephrine), and smaller catheter systems (3- or 4-French) should be used. Temperature control during long procedures is an important concern in infants. Non-ionic contrast should always be used, with a total contrast usage not exceeding 5 mL/kg during short procedures in infants and toddlers. Hand injection of contrast is recommended for infants weighing less than 10 kg because this allows the angiographer to adjust the injection during filming. Weight-based injection rates are listed in Table 2-8. The volume of flush and test injections should be limited to 2-3 mL in small children to avoid volume overload. All children with meningomyeloceles should be assumed to be allergic to latex.

■ THE ARTERIAL PUNCTURE

General Considerations

The patient should be positioned on the angiographic table in such a way as to provide the easiest, most direct access to the puncture site. Patient comfort during procedures is extremely important, but the physician's ability to access the artery, manipulate the catheter, observe the puncture site, and use the table controls during the procedure are paramount. Also, be sure that all tools are nearby before beginning, so that time is not wasted during the procedure looking for something that is needed routinely. Most departments have a standardized sterile angiographic table setup that contains the basic components necessary to begin an angiogram.

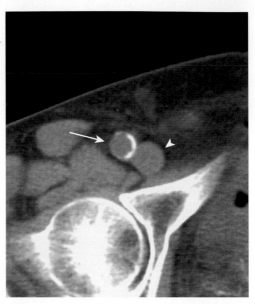

FIGURE 2-28. Axial computed tomography scan without contrast at the level of the femoral head showing the relationship of the common femoral artery (CFA) *(arrow)* and common femoral vein (CFV) *(arrowhead)* within the femoral sheath. The femoral nerve (lateral to the CFA) is not seen on this image. Note the proximity of the CFA to the skin and the calcified medial plaque.

There are a few general guidelines for selecting an arterial access (Box 2-9). The area of interest should be accessible from the artery through which the catheter is introduced. The access artery must be large enough to accommodate diagnostic devices. There should not be any critical or fragile organs interposed between the skin and the artery to be accessed. The puncture should be over bone when possible so that the vessel can be compressed against something hard at the end of the procedure. The vessel to be punctured should be as normal as possible; bad arteries have bad complications. Lastly, the overlying skin should be free of infection, fresh surgical incisions, or any other unpalatable features.

Common Femoral Artery

The common femoral artery (CFA) is the most frequent access site for angiography. The CFA pulse is readily palpated in most patients, large enough to accommodate standard angiographic devices, and easy to compress against the underlying femoral head. Furthermore, the CFA is contained within the anatomic femoral sheath, which helps to limit peripuncture bleeding (Fig. 2-28).

The majority of CFA punctures are retrograde (against arterial blood flow) as opposed to antegrade (in the direction of arterial blood flow). An abdominal pannus in obese patients can be retracted with tape in order to expose the inguinal region for retrograde access. Antegrade punctures can be difficult or impossible in these patients due to the pannus. Regardless of the approach, the CFA should be accessed over the middle or lower third of the femoral head to facilitate compression at the termination of the procedure. The artery is first localized by palpation of the pulse. The course of the artery under the skin and the point

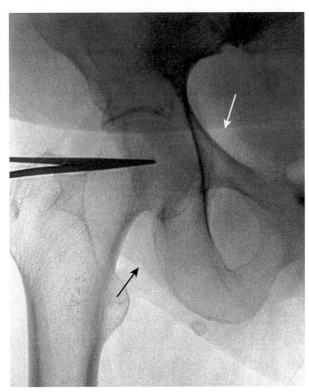

FIGURE 2-29. Common femoral artery (CFA) puncture in a large individual. After identifying the CFA pulse, a blunt metallic instrument is used for fluoroscopic localization of the desired site of entry into the vessel. The skin nick will be made a few centimeters distal to this point. Note the relationship of the large pannus *(white arrow)* and inguinal fold *(black arrow)* to the puncture site.

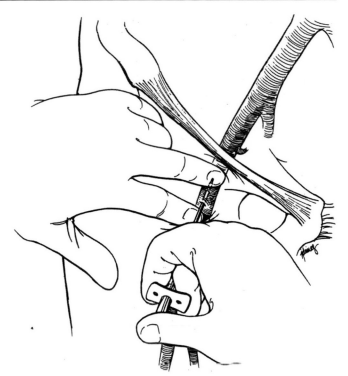

FIGURE 2-30. Technique for localizing the arterial pulse during puncture. (From Kadir S. *Diagnostic Angiography*. Philadelphia: WB Saunders, 1986, with permission.)

of maximum impulse are determined. In large or older patients, the inguinal crease cannot be relied upon to localize the common femoral artery, because it may shift downward over the superficial femoral artery. A blunt metal instrument can be placed on the skin at the anticipated point of access and fluoroscoped to determine its relationship to the femoral head (Fig. 2-29). The skin incision should be 1-2 cm below the intended entry into the artery (for antegrade punctures, make the skin incision the same distance above) to allow a 45-degree angle between the needle and the artery during access. The skin is anesthetized with 1%-2% lidocaine (buffered with 1 mL of 8.4% sodium bicarbonate per 10 mL anesthetic) injected as a superficial wheal and in the underlying deep tissues. Aspiration before injecting in the deep tissues helps avoid intravascular lidocaine. Using the tip of a pointed (#11) scalpel blade, a 3- to 5-mm incision is made in the skin along a natural skin line. The skin incision and a subcutaneous tract are then dilated by gently spreading a straight surgical snap. The purpose of creating this tract is to facilitate catheter insertion during the procedure and egress of blood in the event of bleeding.

The access needle is held firmly by the hub in one hand while the skin incision is straddled by the tips of the second and third fingers (either one above and one below, or one on each side) of the other hand (Fig. 2-30). The pulse should be palpable at all times during the puncture with these fingers. The needle is advanced slowly through the incision at a 45-degree angle to the artery until pulsations can be felt transmitted through the needle. The needle is then thrust forward until the underlying bone is encountered. If the needle has a stylet, this is then removed. The periosteum can be anesthetized with an additional 1 mL of lidocaine injected through the puncture needle (be sure that blood cannot be aspirated before injecting). The hub of the needle is grasped with the thumb and index finger from each hand

on either side; the hub is depressed a few degrees toward the patient's thigh and then slowly withdrawn until blood spurts out of the hub. A slight "pop" is frequently felt just as the needle tip enters the lumen of the artery. The flow of blood should be pulsatile and vigorous. When the flow does not correlate with the quality of the pulse, the needle tip may be partially intramural ("side-walled"), under a plaque, in a vein, or in the orifice of a small branch vessel.

With one hand the needle is held steady while an atraumatic guidewire (such as a 3-J long taper or a Bentson wire) is introduced through the hub. There should be absolutely no resistance to advancement of the guidewire—stop immediately if there is any resistance (Fig. 2-31). The tip of the needle may be only partially in the artery, or directing the guidewire against the wall or under a plaque. Sometimes it is necessary to gently retract the needle to reposition the tip into the center of the vessel. When the guidewire will not advance freely, the tip should be inspected fluoroscopically while the angle of the needle is changed slightly to align with the long axis of the artery. The guidewire is then gently readvanced, with continuous fluoroscopic monitoring. When moving the needle hub slightly does not correct the problem, remove the guidewire to check for good blood return through the needle. A small injection of contrast may help identify the problem, but only do this if there is easy blood return. Otherwise, the injection may be into the wall of the artery and create an obstructing dissection.

During antegrade access, keep in mind that the superficial femoral artery (SFA) origin is medial and anterior to the profunda femoris artery (PFA) origin. With a 45-degree entry angle, the guidewire is often directed posteriorly into the PFA. Depressing the needle hub close to the skin as the guidewire is advanced elevates the tip of the needle and directs the guidewire toward the SFA. A floppy-tipped 3-J guidewire may self-select the SFA as the origin during an antegrade access because this vessel is usually larger than the PFA.

Guidewires should be advanced with slow, deliberate motions. Rapid, forceful introduction of a guidewire risks dissection,

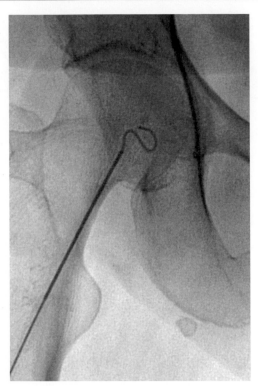

FIGURE 2-31. The operator felt resistance while inserting the guidewire and stopped to obtain this image. The guidewire could be extravascular, subintimal, or coiling against an obstruction. The key is to stop, look, withdraw the guidewire, and readjust the needle.

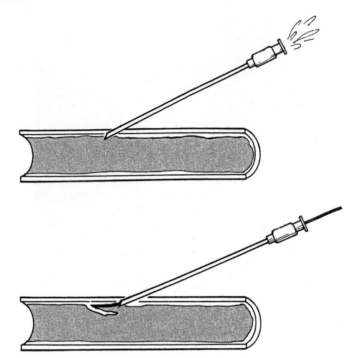

FIGURE 2-32. Potential mechanism of vessel wall injury during single-wall puncture. *Top:* Good blood return is obtained although the needle is only partially in the lumen. *Bottom:* Guidewire passes into the subintimal plane. (From Kim D, Orron DE. *Peripheral Vascular Imaging and Intervention.* St. Louis: Mosby, 1992, with permission.)

kinking, or other problems. A guidewire that forms a "J" or seems to move freely is usually intravascular. A guidewire that spirals or crumples as it advances may have encountered an obstruction, dissected the wall of the artery, or become extravascular (see Fig. 2-31). When this occurs, the guidewire should be pulled back until it assumes a normal shape and then gently readvanced. If the guidewire hangs up on the edge of the needle, remove everything as a single unit. Compress for a few minutes, check that the pulse is still good, and then repeat the access.

Arterial punctures are characterized as double-walled (as described earlier) or single-walled. In a single-wall puncture, the needle is advanced a few millimeters after the tip touches the artery, just through the anterior wall of the vessel. This creates only one hole in the artery, which is plugged with the catheter throughout the procedure, thus theoretically decreasing the chance of a bleeding complication. Single-wall punctures based on palpation are more difficult than the standard double-wall technique. If the needle tip only partially enters the lumen, there will be good blood return but the guidewire can pass into the subintimal layer as it exits the needle (Fig. 2-32). The use of ultrasound guidance and the 21-gauge echo-tip needle commonly found in microaccess kits makes single-wall puncture much easier and safer than by manual palpation with 18-gauge needles. Fluoroscopic location of the femoral head is still strongly recommended when using ultrasound.

Puncturing the nonpalpable artery (owing to an obstruction, low blood pressure, or patient obesity) can be frustrating. Puncture under ultrasound guidance is an excellent technique in this situation, eliminating all guesswork. When ultrasound is not readily available, fluoroscopic evaluation of the groin may reveal calcification in the CFA. Calcified vessels can be punctured with direct fluoroscopic guidance. Another strategy is to opacify the vessel with contrast from a catheter placed through a different access site, but this should be used only if two catheters are needed, such as prior to a bilateral iliac artery intervention. Blind puncture over the medial third of the femoral head may yield

success, but is least productive. If the femoral vein is entered during any of these attempts, a guidewire can be inserted. This is then used as a guide to direct the needle lateral toward the adjacent CFA during fluoroscopy.

Puncture of the postoperative groin requires knowledge of the type and age of the surgery, particularly when a vascular anastomosis is present. Most angiographers prefer to wait 6 weeks before puncture of a recently operated groin, because the area can be very tender, and there is a small concern about damaging the vascular suture line. In reality, the artery or graft can be punctured immediately if necessary. Antibiotics are not necessary when puncturing a synthetic graft. An important potential pitfall exists when a graft has been anastomosed to the top of the CFA, such as in an aortofemoral bypass. During percutaneous access it can be difficult to negotiate out of the native CFA into the more anterior graft (Fig. 2-33). In addition, scarring in the groin may make it difficult to introduce catheters. Overdilation of the tract by one French size larger than the catheter and a stiff guidewire may be required to introduce even a 5-French catheter.

Complications from CFA punctures are related primarily to vascular trauma and deficient hemostasis (Table 2-12). Attention to detail and a gentle touch help avoid most intraprocedural complications. Brute force is rarely needed and a frequent precursor to an adverse outcome in the vascular system. Dissections that occur during retrograde puncture are frequently subclinical, in that antegrade blood flow tends to compress the false lumen (Fig. 2-34). Thrombosis is unusual unless a tight stenosis is present; anticoagulation with heparin during the procedure is warranted in this situation.

The riskiest part of the procedure is after the catheter has been removed, when arterial bleeding may occur. Patients who received heparin during the procedure should have an ACT checked before compression. Protamine sulfate (10 mg/1000 U heparin still active) can be given intravenously over 10-15 minutes to correct prolonged ACTs. Patients with an abnormal INR (>1.5) or PT (>15 seconds) can be given 2 units of fresh frozen

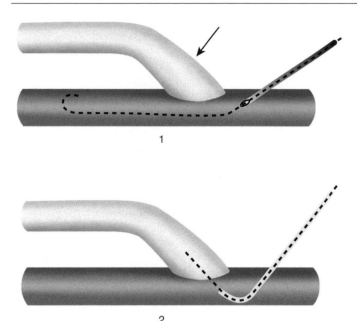

FIGURE **2-33**. Puncture of the groin after aortofemoral bypass. *1*, The guidewire is directed into the native vessel by the access needle. Note the anterior relationship of the graft *(arrow)* to the native artery. *2*, A short, angled catheter is used to redirect the guidewire into the graft.

TABLE 2-12 Complications of Common Femoral Artery Puncture

Complication	Acceptable Incidence
Hematoma (requiring transfusion, surgery, or delayed discharge)	<0.5%
Occlusion	<0.2%
Pseudoaneurysm	<0.2%
Arteriovenous fistula	<0.2%

Data from Singh H, Cardella JF, Cole PE, et al. Quality improvement guidelines for diagnostic arteriography. *J Vasc Interv Radiol* 2002;13:1-6.

plasma during the compression. Before removing the catheter, the tips of the second through fourth fingers are placed so that the third finger is over the estimated arterial entry site (which may be above or below the skin nick). This provides proximal and distal control of the artery as well as the puncture site. The person performing the compression must know the location of the catheter entry site in the artery relative to the skin nick and the quality of the pulse prior to the procedure. The pulse should be identified with certainty before the catheter is removed. The catheter is removed as pressure is applied. Occlusive pressure is maintained for 1-2 minutes, after which it is reduced slightly to allow some blood flow (usually this results in a palpable thrill or slight pulse under the fingertips). The occlusive time should be limited to 1 minute when compressing a graft, in that the likelihood of thrombosis is higher than with a native vessel. Pressure is gradually reduced over 15 minutes. If bleeding resumes, occlusive pressure is reapplied and the 15-minute clock restarted. If an obvious hematoma begins to form during compression, the pressure may be inadequate or may be applied in the wrong place. Patients with heavily calcified vessels, with systolic blood pressure greater than 160 mm Hg, or who are systemically anticoagulated are at greater risk of bleeding and may require prolonged compressions. A sandbag should never be used to augment compression

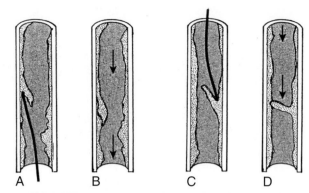

FIGURE **2-34**. Different outcomes of retrograde and antegrade iatrogenic dissections. Arrows indicate direction of flow. **A** and **B,** Retrograde dissections tend to be compressed by antegrade flow. **C** and **D,** Antegrade dissections tend to be exacerbated and enlarged by antegrade flow. (From Kim D, Orron DE. *Peripheral Vascular Imaging and Intervention.* St. Louis: Mosby, 1992, with permission.)

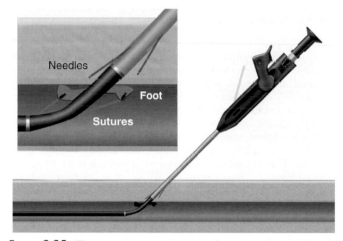

FIGURE **2-35**. There are numerous strategies for remote closure of arterial puncture sites. Shown is a suture-based device. (From Abbott Laboratories Incorporated, Abbott Park, Ill, with permission.)

because it cannot apply sufficient point pressure to control the artery, and it hides the development of a hematoma. Patients who undergo manual compression of the puncture should remain in bed with the leg immobilized for 6 hours. The head of the bed may be elevated to 30 degrees.

Vascular Closure Devices

There are several alternatives to manual compression of arteries that may allow the patient to ambulate sooner and reduce the risk of bleeding in anticoagulated, thrombocytopenic, or uncooperative patients (Fig. 2-35). Device-mediated vascular closure strategies include a patch inside the lumen, remote suturing of the vessel, placement of a metal clip on the outer surface of the artery, and deposition of a hemostatic plug or procoagulant gel on the artery. All of these devices require training for proper use. Operators should put on new sterile gloves and the access site should be re-prepped with antiseptic solution. Additional injection of subcutaneous local anesthetic should be considered, especially when the procedure has been long. For some devices an ipsilateral anterior oblique angiogram is required to locate the actual entry into the artery in relation to the inguinal ligament proximally and the CFA bifurcation distally. Closure devices require additional manual compression after deployment in 5%-10% of patients, although outright failures are uncommon (Fig. 2-36). Closure devices should not be used if there is any

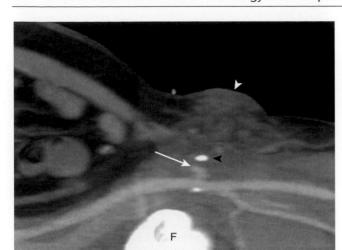

FIGURE 2-36. Failed closure device. Sagittal reconstruction of a computed tomography scan showing that the metal clip *(black arrowhead)* has come away from the artery. A small, irregular pseudoaneurysm arises from the common femoral artery puncture site *(arrow)* beneath the clip. The patient had a visible hematoma *(white arrowhead)*. There is posterior calcification in the artery at the puncture site. F, Femoral head.

question of contamination of the access site. Complications are rare, but include pseudoaneurysm, arterial injury, arterial occlusion, and infection. A dense fibrotic reaction in the soft tissues may be associated with some closure devices. All closure devices incur an added expense to the procedure, but patients can ambulate after 1 hour.

Another closure strategy is to hold a pad impregnated with a prothrombotic agent over the access site during manual compression. This avoids leaving any sort of foreign material in the patient. Several of the agents used are derived from military wound management applications. Compression times are shortened as is the required bedrest, without direct manipulation of the artery. Mechanical external compression devices can substitute or augment manual compression.

"Preclose" Technique

When large vascular access is anticipated (10 French and larger), a suture-mediated closure device can be partially deployed before insertion of the large sheath (see Fig. 2-35). The sutures are not tied until the end of the procedure when the large device is removed. This allows percutaneous management of arterial access for sheaths as large as 24-French inner diameter (the outer diameter is close to 28 French) (Box 2-10).

Axillary or High Brachial Artery

The upper extremity approach to arterial access is an alternative to the common femoral artery in patients with occluded femoral arteries, groin conditions that preclude safe access, when antegrade approach to visceral vessels is desirable, or when an upper extremity intervention is anticipated (Fig. 2-37). This approach is a secondary access because it introduces a small (0.5%) risk of stroke (related to the catheter crossing the origins of one or more great vessels) and peripheral upper extremity nerve injury due to nerve compression by a hematoma in the medial brachial fascial compartment. Furthermore, the upper extremity arteries tend to be smaller and more prone to spasm than the CFA, which limits the size of devices that can be introduced. In general, the axillary artery can accommodate up to a 7-French sheath without difficulty. Patients with uncorrected coagulopathy, uncontrolled hypertension, and morbid obesity are at higher risk for a hematoma. In addition, because the hand must be placed over and behind the patient's head for the duration of the angiogram, individuals with severe arthritis or other shoulder pathology may

---

Box 2-10. "Preclose" Technique for Large-Diameter Arterial Access

Access artery should be good quality, at least as big as desired sheath
Puncture artery with ultrasound guidance; avoid side wall, branch-vessel entry
Limited angiogram of access artery to confirm suitable entry
Deploy 6-French Perclose ProGlide* (1 suture) or 10-French ProStar XL* (2 suture)
Partially remove Perclose device
Secure sutures with metal snap(s)
Reinsert guidewire (angled hydrophilic) through orifice on Perclose catheter
Remove Perclose device over guidewire
Insert second Perclose device and deploy at 45 degrees to first device
Partially remove Perclose device, secure sutures, and reinsert guidewire.
Remove Perclose device over the guidewire, insert large sheath
At end of procedure, reinsert sheath dilator
Attach knot pushers to sutures
First operator removes sheath slowly over hydrophilic wire
As dilator appears, second operator pushes knots down, alternating sides
With sheath removed but guidewire still in place, assess for hemostasis
If uncontrolled bleeding, reinsert sheath over guidewire, proceed to open repair
If minimal or no bleeding, remove guidewire, complete Perclose
For final sheath size less than 14 French, consider a single 6-French "preclose."

*Abbott Laboratories, Abbott Park, Ill.

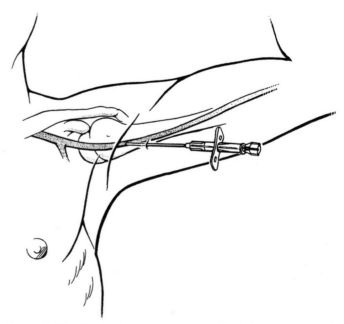

FIGURE 2-37. High brachial artery puncture of the left arm. The artery is entered lateral to the pectoral fold. (From Kadir S. *Diagnostic Angiography*. Philadelphia: WB Saunders, 1986, with permission.)

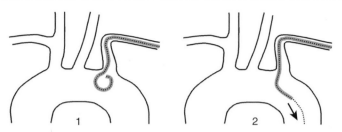

FIGURE 2-38. Technique to direct a pigtail catheter into the descending thoracic aorta from the left axillary approach. *1*, In the left anterior oblique (LAO) projection, the pigtail catheter is positioned at the origin of the left subclavian artery, oriented toward the descending thoracic aorta. A cobra or other curved selective catheter can also be used. *2*, The guidewire *(dashed line)* is advanced, opening the pigtail, which directs the wire into the descending thoracic aorta. The catheter is then advanced over the guidewire *(arrow).*

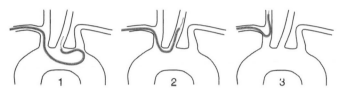

FIGURE 2-39. Selective catheterization of arch vessels from the right axillary approach. *1*, Simmons 1 or 2 catheter in the distal aortic arch *(dashed line* represents soft-tipped guidewire). *2*, Simmons catheter gently pulled into the left common carotid artery. *3*, Simmons catheter pulled into the right common carotid artery.

not be able to tolerate an upper extremity approach. The overall incidence of complications with axillary and high brachial artery punctures is believed to be higher than with CFA puncture, primarily because of an increased incidence of neurologic, hemorrhagic, and occlusive incidents.

For procedures involving imaging of the abdominal aorta or the lower extremities, the left arm should be used if possible so that the catheter crosses only one cerebral artery (the left vertebral artery) (Fig. 2-38). When imaging the ascending thoracic aorta or selecting the cerebral vessels from an axillary approach, the right arm provides the best access (Fig. 2-39). Before the procedure, the upper extremity pulses should be palpated and the blood pressures in both arms compared. A blood pressure differential of more than 10-20 mm Hg suggests the presence of a proximal stenosis on the lower side, and puncture should be performed in the opposite arm.

The patient is positioned on the angiographic table so that the arm is abducted 90 degrees with the elbow flexed and the hand placed under the back of the head. A pulse oximeter placed on a finger on the side of the puncture helps monitor perfusion of the extremity during the case. The axillary artery is palpated in the axilla and as it crosses the lateral edge of the pectoralis major muscle to become the brachial artery. The preferred site of arterial puncture is actually the high brachial artery as it lies against the humerus, because this site is easier to compress than the true axillary artery. The skin overlying the artery is anesthetized, but little deep anesthesia is used to avoid an inadvertent nerve block (a confusing situation because nerve compression is a potential complication of the procedure). The arterial puncture is performed with a 21-gauge microaccess needle using ultrasound guidance or manual palpation. The sharp microaccess needle facilitates puncture of the mobile brachial and axillary arteries. When using palpation to access the artery, remember that in the upper extremity the humerus is superior as well as posterior to the artery (not directly posterior like the femoral head in relation to the CFA). The needle tip should be angled slightly toward the patient's head in order to hit the artery. A good guidewire

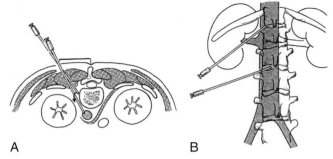

FIGURE 2-40. Translumbar puncture of the abdominal aorta. **A,** Cross-sectional diagram demonstrates anterior redirection of the needle away from the vertebral body toward the aorta. **B,** The two sites for puncture of the aorta are at the T12-L1 interspace (high) and the L2-L3 interspace (low). (From Kim D, Orron DE. *Peripheral Vascular Imaging and Intervention.* St. Louis: Mosby, 1992, with permission.)

for axillary or brachial access is a floppy 3-J to prevent accidental selection of the vertebral artery and other branch vessels.

After the catheter is removed and manual compression completed, the arm should be immobilized in a sling for 6 hours with the back of the patient's bed elevated at least 30 degrees. Patients who have had brachial or axillary artery punctures require periodic neurologic examinations during the 6-hour recovery period. Hematoma formation in the neurovascular sheath can occur without visible evidence of bleeding and can result in compression of adjacent nerves. Nurses should be instructed to check grip and sensation in the hand along with vital signs and inspection of the puncture site. Weakness, paresthesias, or sensory changes in the hand following upper extremity arterial puncture requires urgent evaluation for possible surgical decompression of the hematoma.

Translumbar Aorta

The translumbar approach to the aorta (TLA) seems like a crude and dangerous approach to angiography, but is actually a simple and safe access. The aorta is a large structure with a constant position, and the puncture is guided fluoroscopically using bony landmarks, allowing reliable access in most cases. The main disadvantages of direct aortic puncture are that selective angiography is more difficult, anticoagulation is contraindicated, and the patient must remain in the prone position for the examination. This access is therefore usually restricted to procedures that involve only aortic injections in patients who can lie on their stomachs for 1-2 hours.

The chief complication of translumbar aortography is retroperitoneal hematoma. Virtually all patients will have a small self-contained psoas hematoma (up to ½ unit of blood) after the procedure, but fewer than 1% require treatment. Very rarely the pleural space may be crossed, resulting in a hemopneumothorax. Visceral artery injury caused by the needle has also been reported. Contraindications to TLA puncture include uncontrolled hypertension and coagulopathy, known juxta- or supra-renal aortic aneurysm, a severely scoliotic spine, and dense circumferential aortic calcification.

The two types of TLA puncture for a diagnostic procedure are high (entry at the inferior endplate of the T12 vertebral body) and low (entry at the inferior endplate of L3) (Fig. 2-40). The high approach is most commonly used, because the low puncture is impossible in patients with infrarenal aortic occlusion (i.e., the typical TLA patient) and avoided in the presence of an untreated infrarenal abdominal aortic aneurysm. With the patient prone, the T12 vertebral body, as well as the iliac crest, are localized. The skin is anesthetized at a point roughly midway from the spinous process to the flank and several centimeters below the 12th rib. A skin entry site midway between the iliac crest and the 12th rib is used for a low TLA. If the skin incision is too medial, the needle will be blocked by a transverse process or vertebral body. An access too lateral may result in puncture of the kidney or inability to reach all the way to the aorta with the needle. Deep anesthesia can be administered with a 20-gauge spinal needle. Needles designed for TLA are usually 18-gauge, long, and may be preloaded coaxial dilators. The needle is advanced medially and cephalad toward the inferior endplate of T12. If the vertebral body is encountered, the needle is withdrawn several centimeters, the angle changed, and the needle readvanced. Passing through the psoas muscle fascia may be uncomfortable for the patient. Deflection of aortic calcification by the needle may be visible or a transmitted aortic pulsation felt. To enter the aorta, the needle is firmly advanced forward a centimeter (but not across the midline). The stylet is removed, confirming blood return before introduction of a guidewire. A 0.038-inch guidewire should be used to prevent kinking in the retroperitoneal tissues during catheter exchanges. Insertion of a long 5-French sheath allows catheter exchanges if necessary. Reversal of direction of the catheter can be accomplished by pulling a pigtail catheter or Simmons-1 catheter to the edge of the sheath to direct a floppy guidewire into the distal abdominal aorta.

With TLA, there is no compression. At the end of the procedure, patients are rolled onto their back on a stretcher, and the sheath or catheter is simply pulled out. Patients commonly experience a mild backache from the retroperitoneal hematoma, but otherwise should be asymptomatic. Blood pressure and vital signs should be checked frequently for several hours. Patients may ambulate after 4-6 hours of bedrest.

Unusual Arterial Access

Almost any artery in the body can be accessed percutaneously, but this is not always safe. A few unusual approaches should be kept in mind for special circumstances. The radial artery can accommodate up to 6-French sheaths and long catheters that can be passed in a retrograde direction into the central arterial structures. This is a favored arterial access for cardiac catheterization and interventions, but with long devices can also be used for lower extremity arterial procedures. The overall complication rate is low, and bedrest is not required after compression. Patients should have a normal or near normal perfusion of the hand with the Allen test (compression of both arteries of the wrist followed by sequential release of the ulnar then radial arteries with inspection of the pattern of hand reperfusion); radial artery occlusion occurs in a small percentage of patients. The left hand is preferred to the right for abdominal and lower extremity angiography. Anticoagulation during the procedure is recommended.

The popliteal artery can be accessed in the popliteal space using ultrasound guidance. The usual indication for this access is an intervention, such as angioplasty of a superficial femoral artery origin stenosis or embolization of a distal foot lesion. Popliteal artery access is rarely necessary for diagnostic procedures. With the patient in the prone position, the popliteal artery is punctured with a microaccess needle and ultrasound guidance in a retrograde or antegrade direction as determined by the type of procedure. The popliteal vein, which lies superficial to the artery when the patient is in the prone position, should be avoided. Tibial arteries can be accessed in the distal leg or foot for retrograde lower extremity interventions, but only small catheters (3-4 French) can be used.

▬ THE VENOUS PUNCTURE

Percutaneous puncture of deep venous structures differs from arterial access in that the veins cannot be palpated. Superficial anatomy, relationship to palpable arterial or bony structures, or imaging with ultrasound or fluoroscopy are the major localization techniques. With the exception of femoral vein punctures, it is worthwhile to take advantage of image guidance techniques for most venous punctures.

Veins and the venous system are forgiving, in that the ambient intraluminal pressure is low or even negative, and the walls of the vessels are generally soft and pliable. Large catheters and devices are readily accommodated through most percutaneous central venous punctures with satisfactory hemostasis at the end of the procedure. In comparison to arterial punctures, the primary complications associated with deep venous punctures are thrombosis, injury to adjacent arteries or organs (e.g., the lung), and rarely air embolism (Table 2-13). Clinically important hematomas or bleeding are rare, although they can occur in coagulopathic patients, especially in the presence of a central obstruction or other situations with high venous pressures.

Common Femoral Vein

The common femoral vein (CFV) is most often accessed over the femoral head, above the junction with the deep (profunda) femoral vein and the saphenous vein (see Fig. 2-28). This segment of vein is analogous to the CFA in that it is relatively large, constant in position, and contained within the fascia of the femoral sheath. The vein lies medial and deep to the palpable arterial pulse. To access the CFV without ultrasound, first localize the CFA, then anesthetize the skin just medial to the arterial pulse. The skin incision is usually lower than would be used for arterial puncture, in that the goal is to enter the vein over the lower third of the femoral head. A sharp open needle without a stylet is used, and suction is applied to the hub as the needle is advanced. Blood is aspirated when the needle enters the vessel. Continuous localization of the arterial pulse with fingers of one while advancing the needle with the other hand prevents arterial puncture. If the underlying femoral head is reached without seeing a blood return, slowly withdraw the needle while maintaining suction. Remove the fingers from over the femoral pulse during this step because these may compress the adjacent vein. Vary the angle of the needle slightly with each pass if no blood return is obtained; the more lateral the trajectory, the greater the risk of arterial puncture. The femoral vein can be accessed in both the antegrade (toward the head) or retrograde (toward the foot) direction depending on the goal of the procedure. Difficult punctures can be performed with ultrasound guidance. Most femoral venous punctures for diagnostic procedures require only 5-10 minutes of compression. Interventional procedures with large sheaths in anticoagulated patients may require longer compression times. Postprocedure bedrest with the leg immobile for 3-4 hours is adequate for hemostasis.

TABLE 2-13 Complications of Central Venous Punctures

Complication	Acceptable Incidence
Pneumothorax*	1%-3%
Hemothorax*	1%
Air embolism*	1%
Hematoma	1%-3%
Perforation of vein	0.5%-1%
Thrombosis of puncture site (symptomatic)	4%
Arterial injury	<1%

*Jugular and thoracic veins only.
Data from Dariushnia SR, Wallace MJ, Siddiqi NH, et al. Quality improvement guidelines for central venous access. *J Vasc Interv Radiol* 2010;21:976-981.

Internal Jugular Vein

The internal jugular vein (IJV) is a valuable access for many diagnostic and interventional procedures (Fig. 2-41). The right IJV is the optimal site for insertion of dialysis catheters. The traditional approach to IJV puncture is based upon anatomic landmarks, with access from a posterior, middle, or anterior approach. Access with ultrasound guidance is the preferred method by interventional radiologists, because it is quick, safe, and reliable. Puncture of the carotid artery and pneumothorax, the major complications of blind IJV puncture, can be almost eliminated by using ultrasound guidance.

The IJVs should be checked with ultrasound for location relative to the carotid arteries, compressibility, and change in size with respiration and cardiac cycle (indicating central patency) before preparing the skin. Note the depth of the vein for future reference during the puncture. The patient should be placed in Trendelenburg position or with the legs elevated on pillows to increase central venous pressure and dilate the IJVs. Microaccess needles are ideal for ultrasound-guided IJV puncture.

The access site for an IJV puncture for diagnostic and interventional procedures is in the midportion of the neck. For tunneled venous access devices, a low posterior access is preferred. The right IJV is the easiest approach for diagnostic or interventional venous procedures involving the thorax or abdomen in that it provides straight-line access to the superior vena cava (SVC). The needle is advanced under ultrasound guidance until it enters the vein or until blood can be aspirated (Fig. 2-42). Aspiration of air may indicate transgression of the pleural cavity or (more typically) that the syringe is not attached firmly to the needle. The needle position and the status of the ipsilateral lung can be checked with fluoroscopy if there is any question. The guidewire should pass easily to the right atrium, and in many patients into the inferior vena cava (IVC). If accidental carotid puncture is suspected for any reason, either pull out everything, or insert the

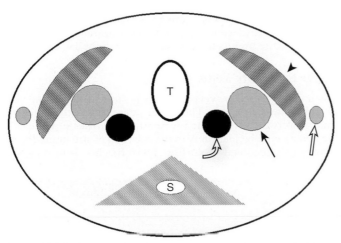

FIGURE **2-41**. Cross-sectional vascular anatomy of the neck. *Straight arrow* = internal jugular vein. *Curved arrow* = common carotid artery. *Arrowhead* = sternocleidomastoid muscle. *Open straight arrow* = external jugular vein. T = trachea. S = spine.

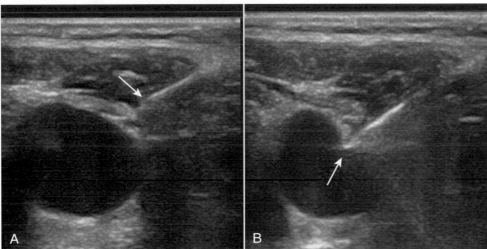

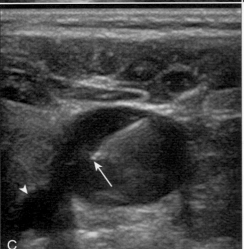

FIGURE **2-42**. Ultrasound-guided puncture of the internal jugular vein (IJV) at the base of the neck. The needle tip should be visualized at all times. **A,** Axial view of the IJV showing the microaccess needle *(arrow)* in the sternocleidomastoid muscle. **B,** The needle tip *(arrow)* is tenting the IJV just before entering it. **C,** The needle *(arrow)* in the vein. Note the proximity to the common carotid artery *(arrowhead)*.

3-French inner dilator from the microaccess kit over the 0.018-inch guidewire and inject a small amount of contrast (without any air bubbles!).

Percutaneous access via the IJVs has a low overall complication rate (see Table 2-13). Puncture-related thrombosis is less likely in the IJVs than with most other venous access sites. However, a unique and potentially lethal risk of IJV access (as well as subclavian vein access) is the introduction of air (air embolism) through an open catheter, dilator, or sheath (particularly the peel-away type) into the systemic circulation if the patient takes a breath at the wrong moment. A small amount of air introduced into the central venous system is harmless, but a large amount (20-30 mL) can create an obstruction in the pulmonary outflow tract. To minimize the risk of air embolism, the patient should be instructed to perform Valsalva maneuver or hum whenever a needle, catheter, or sheath is open to room air. Placing the patient in Trendelenburg position also helps to decrease the risk of air embolism.

If an air embolism occurs during a procedure, first check the patient's vital signs for a drop in blood pressure or oxygen saturation (Box 2-11). The patient may complain of chest pain. A patient in stable condition can be observed for several minutes until the air is absorbed. The air can sometimes be seen outlining the pulmonary valve with fluoroscopy. A patient whose condition is unstable should be turned left side down to trap the air in the capacious right atrium. In severe cases, a catheter may be introduced into the right atrium to attempt to aspirate the air.

Jugular vein punctures can be compressed with the back of the patient's bed elevated. The patient should be instructed to perform Valsalva maneuver during catheter removal, and occlusive pressure should be applied as the catheter is removed. Air embolism through the subcutaneous tract can occur. The duration of compression is usually only 5-10 minutes. After the procedure, the patient should be on bedrest with the head of the bed upright for 1-2 hours.

Subclavian Vein

Percutaneous access to the subclavian vein has traditionally been based on superficial landmarks, similar to the IJV puncture. When this approach is used, access is achieved in 90%-95% of attempts, but pneumothorax and subclavian artery puncture occur in 3%-5%. With image-guided puncture, these complications are reduced to less than 1% combined, with an almost 100% success rate.

The safest place to access the subclavian vein is where it crosses over the anterior aspect of the first rib, lateral to the clavicle (Fig. 2-43). The vein should not be accessed under the clavicle, particularly when placing long-term central venous catheters, because this may lead to compression and fracture of the catheter ("pinch-off syndrome;" see Fig. 7-29) between the clavicle and the 1st rib. The subclavian vein is inferior and anterior to the artery over the 1st rib, and the presence of underlying bone minimizes the risk of pneumothorax during puncture. Lateral to the 1st rib the vessel becomes the axillary vein, which is best accessed over the anterior portion of the 2nd rib for the same reasons listed.

Puncture of the subclavian vein can be guided with ultrasound or fluoroscopy. The disadvantage of ultrasound is that the structures below the vein (rib and lung) may be difficult to visualize, and patency of the central veins cannot be assessed. The technique is virtually identical to that used for the IJVs. The advantage of ultrasound guidance is that contrast is not necessary, and exposure to radiation for both the operator and the patient is minimized. For a fluoroscopically guided puncture, a limited upper extremity venogram can be performed by injecting 10-20 mL of contrast material through a vein in the hand or forearm. This allows precise localization of the subclavian vein as it crosses the ribs and confirms patency of the central venous system before beginning the procedure. Puncture can then be performed with carefully coned-down fluoroscopy over the needle tip. A microaccess needle is advanced under direct visualization until blood is aspirated or the tip hits the anterior surface of the 1st rib.

Upper Extremity Veins

When upper extremity venous access is desired, the basilic vein should be the first target. The basilic vein is larger than the brachial veins (which are frequently multiple), and lies superficial to the nerves and brachial artery in the segment of arm immediately above the antecubital fossa (Fig. 2-44). Brachial vein puncture

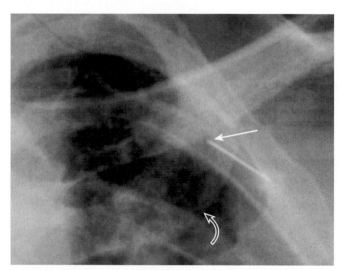

FIGURE 2-43. Puncture of the subclavian vein over the 1st rib. The vein was localized with contrast injection during the puncture. The tip of the needle *(arrow)* could be visualized over the 1st rib *(curved arrow)* the entire time during the puncture.

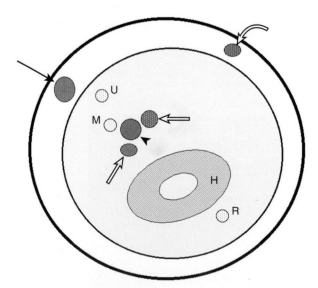

FIGURE 2-44. Cross-sectional anatomy of the upper arm proximal to the antecubital fossa. *Straight arrow* = basilic vein. *Curved arrow* = cephalic vein. *Open straight arrows* = brachial veins. *Arrowhead* = brachial artery. U = ulnar nerve. M = median nerve. R = radial nerve. H = humerus.

Box 2-11. Management of Central Venous Air Embolism

Control source (clamp, compress, or plug)
Turn patient to left lateral decubitus position
Administer 100% oxygen
Aspirate air from heart with catheter

has the risk (albeit low) of injury to the adjacent artery or nerves. The cephalic vein can be punctured without fear of damage to surrounding structures, but this vessel is small and subject to spasm. The basilic vein is readily accessed with either ultrasound or venographic guidance.

Inferior Vena Cava

Translumbar Access

Direct puncture of the IVC is used primarily for placement of long-term central venous access devices (see Fig. 7-25). Diagnostic procedures can almost always be performed from a peripheral approach. This puncture is similar in technique and materials to a low TLA (discussed earlier), with the difference being that the approach is from the right rather than the left (unless a left-sided IVC is present).

Previous studies such as computed tomography (CT) scans should be reviewed before the procedure to determine IVC anatomy, particularly in a patient with an abdominal aortic aneurysm or retroperitoneal mass. When first performing this procedure, it may be helpful to insert a small pigtail catheter into the IVC from a femoral approach to localize the cava during puncture.

The patient is placed either prone or in the left lateral decubitus position, with a small towel roll under the left flank to straighten the spine. A translumbar aortography needle/sheath system or a long 18-gauge needle (e.g., Hawkins needle) is inserted at a point approximately 10 cm to the right of the spinous process just above the right iliac crest. The needle is advanced at approximately a 45-degree angle cephalad from the skin entry toward the top of the L3 vertebral body until the vertebral body is encountered. The needle is then withdrawn and angled more anteriorly, so that it passes just anterior to the vertebral body. The stylet is removed, and the needle withdrawn until blood can be aspirated. A pigtail catheter placed previously in the inferior cava from another access is an excellent target for puncture.

Entry by the needle into an arterial structure should not cause alarm unless the patient is coagulopathic. After trans-lumbar puncture of the IVC, patients should be observed with the same postprocedure protocol used for TLA punctures. Many patients note transient pain radiating to the right leg during the procedure. When the pain is severe the needle should be reinserted from a more lateral position to avoid the psoas muscle.

Transhepatic Access

This approach is indicated only when the thoracic veins and the infrarenal IVC are occluded. As with the translumbar puncture of the IVC, this technique is most often used for an intervention rather than a diagnostic procedure (see Fig. 7-25). Review of previous imaging is essential to determine hepatic anatomy and exclude dilated bile ducts, cysts, hemangiomas, or tumors along the access route. The right upper abdomen should be fluoroscoped to select a puncture site in the anterior axillary line that avoids transpleural, or at least transpulmonary, placement of the catheter. Ultrasound is useful to identify the hepatic and portal veins. A long 21-gauge microaccess needle is advanced in a horizontal course through the liver toward the vertebral column. The needle should not be advanced beyond the midportion of the vertebral body. Aspiration of blood during withdrawal of the needle signifies entry into a vascular structure. Contrast should be injected to identify the vessel. Either a hepatic vein or the IVC can be used for access.

Other Venous Access

The median antecubital vein can be punctured under direct vision, but it is frequently thrombosed or already in use in hospitalized patients. The external jugular (EJ) veins are similarly easy to access, and are a useful alternative when the IJV is occluded. The EJ vein enters the subclavian vein at an angle that is easily negotiated with catheters and guidewires. Popliteal, saphenous, and tibial veins can be used as access for lower extremity venous interventions. Puncture of these veins requires ultrasound guidance. Lastly, an enlarged collateral vein may provide access to the central circulation in patients with occlusion of the more typical access sites.

ANGIOGRAPHIC "DO'S AND DON'TS"

Never underestimate the amount of damage that can be done with a needle, guidewire, or catheter (Table 2-14). When performing an invasive vascular procedure, there are several general guidelines that should be followed to ensure that the examination is performed safely and completely. One of the most important technical points is safe catheter flush technique (Box 2-12). This simple procedure maintains catheter patency and avoids potential embolic complications from injection of air bubbles or thrombus that can form in the catheter (Fig. 2-45).

Guidewires must be wiped with a moist nonfraying gauze or Telfa pad between exchanges or when removed from a catheter. Platelets, fibrin, and thrombus can form on guidewires. Even a thin film of material on a guidewire can make it sticky and cause substantial resistance when advancing a catheter. Similarly, catheters should be flushed with heparinized saline and wiped clean when first brought on to the sterile field and whenever removed from a patient. Many physicians keep guidewires and catheters in a basin of sterile heparinized saline when not in use.

During an arterial procedure it is essential to watch with fluoroscopy any time that a catheter or guidewire is moved, particularly when advancing. Very experienced operators may deviate from this when introducing a soft-tipped guidewire into a large

TABLE 2-14 Catheter-Induced Complications

Complication	Acceptable Incidence
Distal emboli	<0.5%
Arterial dissection/subintimal passage	<0.5%
Subintimal injection of contrast	<0.5%

Data from Singh H, Cardella JF, Cole PE, et al. Quality improvement guidelines for diagnostic arteriography. *J Vasc Interv Radiol* 2002;13:1-6.

BOX 2-12. Angiographic Catheter Flush Technique

Open stopcock on catheter if present
Aspirate catheter (approximately 5 mL of blood) with 20-mL syringe
For end-hole catheters, apply mild to moderate suction
For multiple side-hole catheters, aspirate vigorously to empty catheter tip distal to side holes
If no blood return, do one of the following while aspirating until blood returns:
  • Turn catheter slightly (tip may be against wall of vessel)
  • Retract catheter (tip may be subintimal or wedged)
Attach 20-mL syringe containing 5-10 mL heparinized saline (6000 U/1000 mL) to catheter
Hold syringe tip down and tap several times to dislodge any bubbles in tip
Withdraw plunger until a puff of blood is seen in syringe
Inject flush solution:
  • For end-hole catheters, inject with mild to moderate force
  • For multiple side-hole catheters, inject forcibly to ensure flush reaches catheter tip
Close stopcock if present while injecting

normal vessel. New or inexperienced physicians should visually monitor all catheter or guidewire manipulations.

Always aspirate blood before injecting anything through a catheter. Never inject when blood cannot be aspirated; the catheter tip may be subintimal, wedged in a tiny branch, or occluded. Withdraw the catheter while applying negative pressure with a syringe until vigorous blood return is obtained; then inject. When aspiration is still not possible, the catheter, or less likely the artery, may be thrombosed. An attempt to aspirate with a 60-mL syringe may clear the thrombus. Never simply flush the catheter or ream out the thrombus with a guidewire in an artery, although this is sometimes acceptable in a vein. As a last resort, the hub of the occluded catheter can be cut and a sheath advanced over the catheter as if it was a dilator. The occluded catheter can then be removed while preserving the access.

Frequently the tip of a guidewire may advance beyond the field of view of the image intensifier. This is a common situation when exchanging catheters or selecting a branch vessel. Vascular perforations can occur if the guidewire selects a small branch vessel. In the thoracic aorta, the guidewire can dislodge plaque, resulting in a stroke or transient ischemic attack. Always think about where the tip of the guidewire *might* be, even when it is not visible.

Diseased or delicate vessels can be easily traumatized by catheters and guidewires. In particular, patients on long-term high-dose steroids are prone to catheter-induced dissection. Straight or angled catheters should be advanced over a guidewire, whereas pigtail or recurved catheters can be safely advanced alone once they have reformed. Select diseased or delicate vessels with at least 1 cm of a soft guidewire protruding from the tip of the catheter. A soft guidewire will become very stiff if only a millimeter or two protrudes from the catheter.

A common dilemma during selective angiography is distinguishing arterial dissection from arterial spasm. Both are caused by manipulation of guidewires and catheters, and avoided by using soft and small devices such as microguidewires and catheters. Spasm reverses with injection of a vasodilator (intraarterial nitroglycerin, 100-200 μg in adults, 1-3 μg/kg in children), followed by repeat contrast injection 2-3 minutes later (Fig. 2-46). If the new stenosis persists and is flow-limiting, the patients should be heparinized. Many limited branch-artery dissections heal spontaneously with time. For extensive or obstructive dissections in critical arteries, a course of low-molecular-weight heparin and aspirin 80 mg daily for 2-4 weeks should be considered. Alternatively, a stent can be placed to restore flow in the true lumen.

Listen to the patient: if something hurts, stop and figure out why. Often, reassurance is all that is necessary, but sometimes a complication or other adverse outcome can be avoided. When something won't go, don't just push harder; try a different catheter or guidewire.

Changing one variable at a time helps determine the primary limiting factor. When advancing the catheter shaft through an access site, make sure the tip advances appropriately inside the patient. If the tip does not seem to move a distance equal to the amount that is going into the patient, stop and fluoroscope the entire catheter: the catheter may be coiling in the subcutaneous tissues or buckling somewhere inside the patient (Fig. 2-47).

Always test inject through a catheter before a power injection after positioning or repositioning. This ensures that the catheter is in the proper position and that the tip is free within the lumen rather than against the wall or subintimal, and it may lead to a modification in the injection rate. Major complications can be created by large subintimal injections of contrast. Catheters should not remain connected to the power injector for more than 1-2 minutes without flushing, because thrombus will form in the tip.

Study symptomatic lesions first, particularly in the cerebral circulation. Image inflow, the lesion, and outflow. If an adverse event occurs, such as a contrast reaction or equipment failure, useful information will still have been collected. In addition, have a low threshold for intraprocedural heparin. A groin hematoma is more acceptable than an ischemic complication.

Severely tortuous vessels are a common finding during diagnostic angiography in older patients. These can be difficult or impossible to negotiate safely with standard catheters and guidewires. A useful technique is to cross these vessels with a soft guidewire, followed by a hydrophilic catheter. Exchange for a stiffer guidewire through the hydrophilic catheter enables introduction of additional catheters or devices. However, the stiff guidewire can cause distortion and "accordioning" of the artery. The vessel usually returns to normal after the stiff devices are removed (Fig. 2-48). Long sheaths that reach beyond the area of tortuosity can be extremely helpful in this situation.

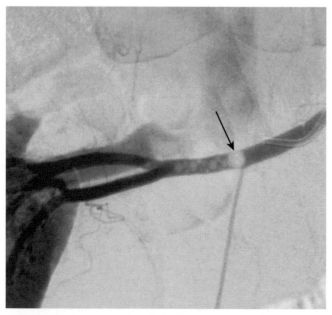

FIGURE 2-45. Importance of careful flush technique. Air bubbles *(arrow)* in an accessory renal artery during hand injection of contrast. These were easily aspirated.

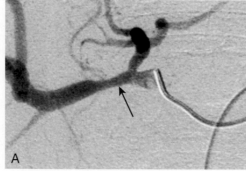 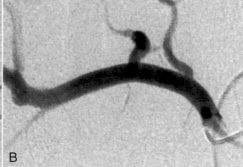

FIGURE 2-46. Catheter-induced vasospasm. **A,** Proper hepatic angiogram through a 5-French catheter shows focal, smooth, concentric narrowing *(arrow)* consistent with spasm. This was not present on the celiac angiogram obtained earlier. **B,** After withdrawing the catheter slightly and injecting 200 μg of nitroglycerin into the artery, the spasm has resolved.

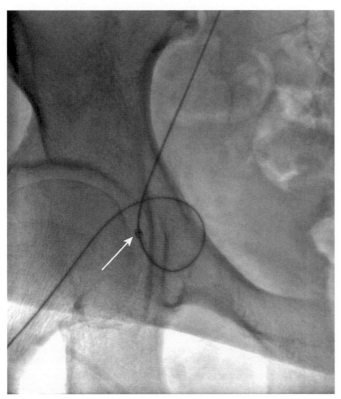

FIGURE 2-47. Coiling *(arrow)* of a 5-French sheath and guidewire in the soft tissues in an obese patient with a very scarred groin. The patient was so large that the operator could not feel the sheath buckling in the soft tissues. After predilating with a 7-French dilator, a fresh 5-French sheath was easily inserted.

Occasionally a vessel cannot be found in its usual location. A common example is failure to visualize the right hepatic artery during injection of the celiac artery. In this situation, there are several considerations, including anomalous origin of the vessel from another location (e.g., the right hepatic artery from the superior mesenteric artery in the example described), occlusion by disease or other causes, congenital absence of the vessel, or surgical absence of the organ that the vessel used to supply. When the origin of a vessel cannot be selected with a catheter but the vessel is known to be present, a tight origin stenosis may be present, or the wrong catheter shape may be employed. A moment's pause to reflect on the cause of the problem usually identifies a simple solution.

Rarely, a catheter will form a true knot during extensive manipulation. This is usually the result of a combination of inattention and difficult anatomy. Knots may sometimes be undone by advancing a stiff guidewire through the catheter, forcing the catheter to unwind. Alternatively, a second catheter inserted from another access may be needed to "untie" the knot (Fig. 2-49). Small knots can be extracted through an appropriate sized sheath, but arteriotomy may be required.

IMAGING

A key element of angiography is the recording of the contrast injection (i.e., imaging). Simple observation with fluoroscopy is not sufficient (no recorded images = no diagnosis). There are two basic modes of recording angiographic images, film-screen and digital angiography. Film-screen imaging is now archaic and rarely used in current angiographic facilities. All new equipment is based on digital imaging.

Digital Subtraction Angiography

The original digital subtraction angiography (DSA) technique was rapid peripheral venous injection of contrast with acquisition of digitally subtracted images timed to record arterial passage of the bolus (IVDSA). This was an unsatisfactory application of a

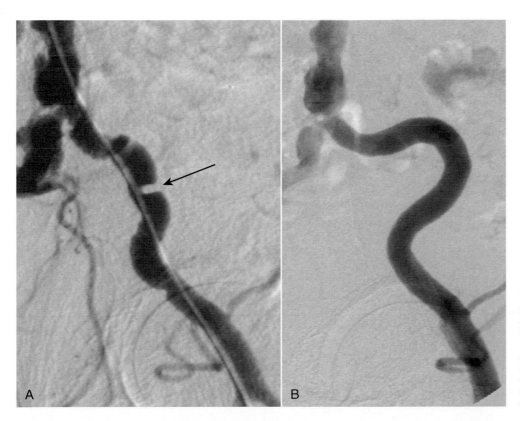

FIGURE 2-48. Accordion effect. **A,** Multiple eccentric, irregular stenoses *(arrow)* noted in the left external iliac artery during a pelvic angiogram with a stiff guidewire in place. **B,** Retrograde injection of the same vessel with the guidewire removed reveals a normal but tortuous artery. The apparent stenoses were caused when the artery was straightened and shortened by the guidewire.

brilliant innovation, owing to unpredictable variations in cardiac output, poor resolution of the weakly opacified arteries, inability to selectively inject arteries, and motion artifacts. Direct intraarterial injection of contrast, as used with film-screen angiography, rapidly supplanted IVDSA.

Digital angiography currently has lower resolution than the older film-screen images, but provides extremely rapid acquisition of images and processing (the subtraction is performed instantaneously and displayed on a monitor), and the ability to manipulate the image appearance online to compensate for poor vascular opacification. Most current angiographic units utilize at least a 1024-pixel matrix with a flat panel detector technology. The interchange between fluoroscopic and angiographic modes is electronic and almost instantaneous rather than mechanical and slow. Images can be viewed in either subtracted or unsubtracted (raw) format (Fig. 2-50). Filming can be as rapid as 30 frames per second with some units, with continuous acquisition while moving the angiographic table (bolus chase) or the tube (rotational

angiography). An extremely useful feature of DSA is "road mapping," in which an angiographic image is acquired and superimposed over a live fluoroscopic image. This allows negotiation of complex anatomy or occlusions with greater confidence. Newer units with flat-panel detectors can reconstruct three-dimensional models or CT-like axial images from rotational angiographic data, a very useful tool for evaluating complex anatomy or during some interventions (Fig. 2-51). With DSA, lower concentrations of contrast can be used (30%-50% less iodine than with film-screen angiography), without altering the injection rates. The exquisite sensitivity of DSA allows use of alternative negative contrast agents such as CO_2 for angiography (see Figs. 2-26 and 2-27).

The limitations of DSA, in addition to lower resolution, include subtraction artifacts from involuntary motion such as bowel peristalsis, respiration, and cardiac pulsation. There is a tendency to "shoot first and ask questions later" (i.e., collect lots of images and views quickly with only superficial review of the results on a monitor during the procedure).

Procedural Issues

The angiographer should determine patient positioning and filming rates for each injection. Patient positioning has been loosely standardized for most types of angiograms based on anatomy and the empiricism that two different views of the same vascular structure are necessary for evaluation of most pathologic processes ("one view = no view"; Fig. 2-52).

Similarly, contrast injection and filming rates are determined for different studies based upon expected flow rates and pathology. Suggestions for tube angulation, patient positioning, contrast injection rates, and filming rates for specific studies are in later chapters. Variations in positioning, injection rates, and filming are frequently necessary to suit an individual patient, in that flow may be slower or faster than anticipated, or the pathology may be visible only on delayed images. In general, film faster during the contrast injection (arterial phase) and then slow down to follow the capillary and venous phases. Large vascular spaces such as aortic aneurysms need longer injections of large volumes of contrast (not faster injection rates) to be adequately opacified; large

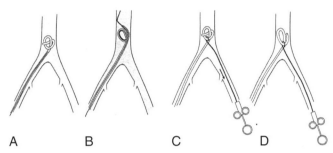

FIGURE 2-49. The knotted catheter. **A,** An extra-stiff hydrophilic guidewire is advanced to the knot. **B,** The knot is forced open as progressively stiffer portions of the guidewire exit the catheter. This technique is successful in the majority of instances. **C,** Alternatively, the knot can be teased open with downward traction from the opposite iliac access. A selective catheter is insinuated through the knot. Shown is a deflecting guidewire, which would be activated inside the selective catheter. **D,** The knot opens as traction is applied. (From Kim D, Orron DE. *Peripheral Vascular Imaging and Intervention.* St. Louis: Mosby, 1992, with permission.)

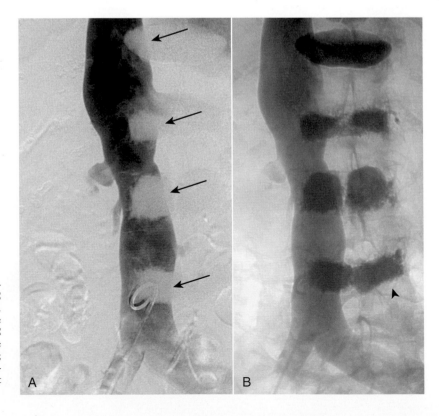

FIGURE 2-50. Digital subtraction angiography. **A,** Subtracted image from an inferior vena cavogram. The IVC contrast appears very dense compared to the background. There appear to be multiple filling defects *(arrows)* in the IVC. **B,** The same image, viewed unsubtracted. The IVC contrast is less dense relative to the background, but the explanation for the apparent filling defects is revealed; radiopaque intravertebral cement *(arrowhead)* from multiple vertebroplasties created subtraction artifacts that looked like filling defects in image **A.**

vascular beds (e.g., the lower extremities) need long injections at a lower rate to ensure complete opacification, and rapidly flowing blood may require both high flow rates and large volumes (e.g., a thoracic aortogram in a young hyperdynamic patient).

Image intensifiers with large fields of view are desirable for most applications. Electronic magnification, careful coning of images, and application of filters enhance image quality. During prolonged procedures, pulse-mode fluoroscopy can reduce patient and operator exposure, as well as prevent tube overheating. The standard pulse rate for fluoroscopy is 15 pulses per second. With experience and during simple procedures, pulse rates as low as 3 pulses per second can be used. The image intensifier should always be as close to the patient as possible to minimize scatter and improve image quality.

■ INTRAVASCULAR ULTRASOUND

Intravascular ultrasound (IVUS) is a technology that combines features of both invasive and noninvasive imaging. Although ultrasound is generally considered noninvasive, this is true only as long as the probe is outside of the body. By placing a probe on the end of a catheter (usually 3- to 9-French in diameter), direct imaging of the vascular lumen becomes possible by inserting the catheter over a guidewire (Fig. 2-53). A hemostatic sheath is necessary to allow safe introduction of the IVUS probe.

Instead of looking from outside in, IVUS looks from inside out (Fig. 2-54). This technique is useful as an adjunct to conventional angiography to evaluate intraluminal processes such as dissections, or vessel wall abnormalities such as eccentric stenoses that are difficult to visualize on an angiogram. Precise luminal measurements can be obtained, as well as localization of stenoses. This may be particularly useful during a complex intervention. The quality of the arterial wall can also be assessed for subtle changes of atherosclerosis. Reconstruction of two- and three-dimensional models from IVUS data is very useful for measurements, understanding anatomy, and interventions. The limitations of the technique are the expense of the additional equipment, the potential need for a second access, the inability to look forward with the catheter (most designs can image only in the axial or sagittal planes), and the small field of view when compared to external probes.

■ POSTPROCEDURE CARE

The care of the patient after an angiogram is equal in importance to the procedure itself. Patients should be observed in a supervised setting for a length of time befitting the procedure and the sedation. For example, following a translumbar aortogram, a patient is kept on bedrest for 4-6 hours, whereas a patient may be discharged immediately following an arm venogram through

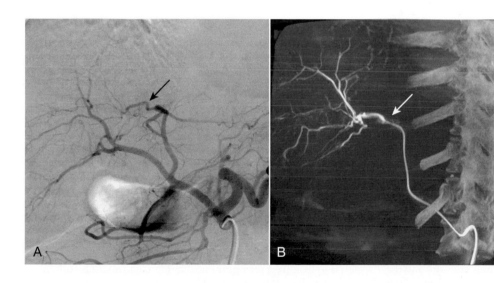

FIGURE 2-51. Postprocessed rotational digital subtraction angiogram using a flat-panel image intensifier. **A,** Celiac artery injection. Note the medial branch *(arrow)* of the left hepatic artery to segment 4 of the liver. **B,** Maximum intensity projection (MIP) image of a rotational angiogram obtained during superselective angiography of the segment 4 branch. A 3-French microcatheter has been advanced into the left hepatic artery branch *(arrow)* from the 5-French catheter in the celiac artery. Dilute contrast was injected through the microcatheter as the x-ray tube and flat-panel image-intensifier rotated around the patient.

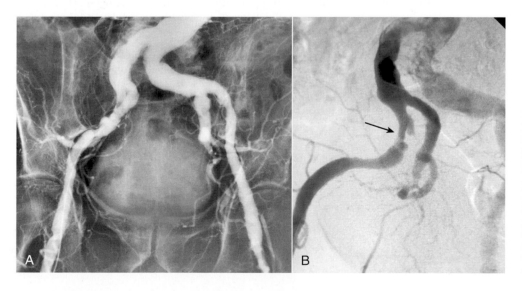

FIGURE 2-52. Evaluation of most vascular structures requires imaging in at least two views. **A,** Screen-film pelvic angiogram (note the standard white-on-black display) in the anteroposterior projection. There is no obvious lesion on the right, but the patient had a slightly diminished right femoral pulse. **B,** Digital subtraction view (note the black-on-white display) of the right external iliac artery in the right posterior oblique projection. An eccentric stenosis *(arrow)* is now readily visible. The internal iliac artery origin is also clearly seen in this view.

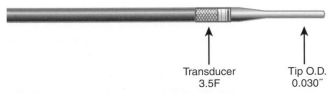

Transducer
3.5F

Tip O.D.
0.030″

FIGURE 2-53. Intravascular ultrasound probe (3.5-French, 20-MHz). The catheter can be inserted over a 0.018-inch guidewire. (Image courtesy of Volcano Corporation, San Diego, Calif.)

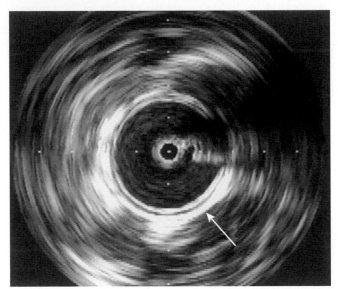

FIGURE 2-54. Normal intravascular ultrasound (IVUS) images of the popliteal artery. A 6-French probe (12.5-MHz) is visible in the center of the vessel. The echogenic intima, hypoechoic media, and echogenic adventitia are clearly visualized *(arrow)*.

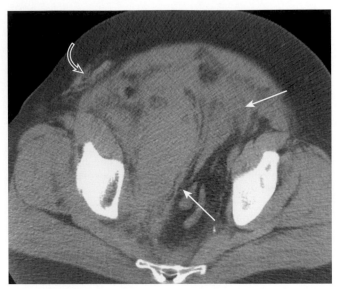

FIGURE 2-55. Hematomas following angiography. Noncontrast computed tomography scan of patient who developed hypotension following a percutaneous procedure. There is a small subcutaneous hematoma *(curved arrow)* and a massive retroperitoneal hematoma *(arrows)* in the pelvis. At surgery the arterial puncture was noted to be in the external iliac artery above the inguinal ligament.

a peripheral intravenous catheter performed without sedation. Patients may resume their previous diet as soon as they are awake enough to eat safely, but intravenous hydration with an appropriate solution should be continued until oral intake is satisfactory. Patients with severely compromised renal function should be hydrated for 12 hours following the procedure.

When discharging an outpatient after an arterial procedure, check and record the pulse and status of the puncture site and the distal pulses. Be sure that the patient is tolerating food by mouth and has urinated at least once. Give the patient clear instructions regarding activity for the next 24 hours, what to look for that might indicate a complication (cold extremity, painful puncture site, obvious hematoma or bleeding, or absence of urination for 24 hours), and what to do if the patient suspects a complication.

When called to evaluate a patient for a suspected puncture site complication after an angiogram, be sure to bring a pair of gloves and some sterile gauze. Ischemic complications are rare, but manifest as diminished or absent pulses, rest pain, pallor, or loss of nerve function. Knowledge of the patient's preprocedural examination and the angiographic findings are important to determine whether the pulse abnormality is new. The differential diagnosis includes thrombosis of a preexisting critical stenosis, puncture site thrombosis or dissection, and distal embolization of thrombus or plaque. Rarely, a catheter may fragment and embolize distally. Management includes heparinization, emergent angiography with possible thrombolysis or stent placement, or surgical thrombectomy.

Hemorrhagic complications include overt bleeding or hematoma formation. The patient's blood pressure and pulse should be checked immediately while inspecting the puncture site.

If the patient is hypotensive, a bolus of 300-500 mL of crystalloid (NS or lactated Ringer's solution) should be administered, and blood obtained for a stat complete blood count, coagulation studies, and blood bank sample. The initial treatment of overt bleeding or hematoma formation are identical: compression. It can be difficult to locate a pulse in the midst of a large hematoma; application of continuous firm pressure can displace the hematoma sufficiently to uncover the pulse. Knowledge of the type of puncture is essential so that pressure can be applied in the appropriate place. For example, the arterial entry site for an antegrade femoral angiogram is distal to the skin incision, not proximal. While compressing, reiterate to the patient that the extremity must be kept still. After 15 minutes, reinspect the puncture site. Be prepared to compress for an additional 15 minutes if necessary. If bleeding persists after repeat compression, consider checking the patient's coagulation studies and platelet count if not already done. A noncontrast CT scan of the abdomen and pelvis to look for a retroperitoneal hematoma should be obtained when a patient develops unexplained hypotension, abdominal or back pain, or a drop in hematocrit after an angiogram (Fig. 2-55). A large bleed following an angiogram is a risk factor for pseudoaneurysm formation (see Fig. 2-36).

Patients experience mild to moderate discomfort at the puncture site for several days, followed by 10-14 days of slight tenderness. A small area of focal induration may develop related to resolution of subcutaneous blood. Ecchymosis is common and can track into the ipsilateral thigh and perineum. Patients should be instructed to return if there is increased pain, swelling, or bleeding at the puncture site.

▬ SUGGESTED READINGS

Angle JF, Nemcek AA, Cohen AM, et al. Quality improvement guidelines for preventing wrong site, wrong procedure, and wrong person errors: application of the Joint Commission "universal protocol for preventing wrong site, wrong procedure, wrong person surgery" to the practice of interventional radiology. *J Vasc Interv Radiol.* 2008;19:1145-1151.

Barret BJ, Parfrey PS. Preventing nephropathy induced by contrast medium. *N Engl J Med.* 2006;354:379-386.

Bechara CF, Annambhotia S, Lin PH. Access site management with vascular closure devices for percutaneous transarterial procedures. *J Vasc Surg.* 2010;52:1682-1696.

Brockow K. Immediate and delayed reactions to radiocontrast media: is there an allergic mechanism? *Immunol Allergy Clin North Am.* 2009;29:453-468.

Brueck M, Bandorski D, Kramer W, et al. A randomized comparison of transradial versus transfemoral approach for coronary angiography and angioplasty. *J Am Coll Cardiol Cardiovasc Interv.* 2009;2:1047-1054.

Chan D, Downing D, Keough CE, et al. Joint practice guideline for sterile technique during vascular and interventional radiology procedures. *J Vasc Interv Radiol.* 2012;23:715-724.

Dariushnia SR, Wallace MJ, Siddiqi NH, et al. Quality improvement guidelines for central venous access. *J Vasc Interv Radiol.* 2010;21:976-981.

Das R, Ahmed K, Athanasiou T, Morgan RA, Belli AM. Arterial closure devices versus manual compression for femoral haemostasis in interventional radiological procedures: a systematic review and meta-analysis. *Cardiovasc Intervent Radiol.* 2011;34:723-738.

Hawkins IF, Cho KJ, Caridi JG. Carbon dioxide in angiography to reduce the risk of contrast-induced nephropathy. *Radiol Clin North Am.* 2009;47:813-825.

Heran MK, Marshalleck F, Temple M, et al. Joint quality improvement guidelines for pediatric arterial access and arteriography: from the Societies of Interventional Radiology and Pediatric Radiology J. *Vasc Interv Radiol.* 2010;21:32-43.

Kadir S. *Diagnostic Angiography.* Philadelphia: WB Saunders; 1986.

Kandarpa K, Machan L. *Handbook of Interventional Radiologic Procedures.* 4th ed. Philadelphia: Wolters Kluwer; 2011.

Kerns SR, Hawkins IF. Carbon dioxide digital subtraction angiography: expanding applications and technical evolution. *Am J Roentgenol.* 1995;164:735-741.

Kim D, Orron DE. *Peripheral Vascular Imaging and Intervention.* St. Louis: Mosby-Yearbook; 1992.

Leiner T, Kucharczyk W. NSF prevention in clinical practice: summary of recommendations and guidelines in the United States, Canada, and Europe. *J Magn Reson Imaging.* 2009,30.1357-1363.

Levitin A. Intravascular ultrasound. *Tech Vasc Interv Radiol.* 2001;4:66-74.

Miller DL, Vano E, Bartal G, et al. Occupational radiation protection in interventional radiology: a joint guideline of the Cardiovascular and Interventional Radiology Society of Europe and the Society of Interventional Radiology. *J Vasc Interv Radiol.* 2010;21:607-615.

Mistretta CA, Crummy AB. Diagnosis of cardiovascular disease by digital subtraction angiography. *Science.* 1981;214:761-765.

Segal AJ, Bush WH Jr. Avoidable errors in dealing with anaphylactoid reactions to iodinated contrast media. Invest Radiol. 2011;46:147-51.

Seldinger SI. Catheter replacement of the needle in percutaneous arteriography. *Acta Radiologica.* 1953;39:368-376.

Singh H, Cardella JF, Cole PE, et al. Quality improvement guidelines for diagnostic arteriography. *J Vasc Interv Radiol.* 2002;13:1-6.

Solomon R, Werner C, Mann D, et al. Effects of saline, mannitol, and furosemide to prevent acute decreases in renal function induced by radiocontrast agents. *N Engl J Med.* 1994;331:1416-1420.

Spies JB, Bakal CR, Burke DR, et al. Standards for diagnostic arteriography in adults. *J Vasc Interv Radiol.* 1993;4:385-395.

Spinosa DJ, Kaufmann JA, Hartwell GD. Gadolinium chelates in angiography and interventional radiology: a useful alternative to iodinated contrast media for angiography. *Radiology.* 2002;223:319-327.

Stecker MS, Balter S, Towbin RB, et al. Guidelines for patient radiation dose management. *J Vasc Interv Radiol.* 2009;20:S263-S273.

Trerotola SO, Kuhlman JE, Fishman EK. Bleeding complications of femoral catheterization: CT evaluation. *Radiology.* 1990;174:37-40.

Valji K. *Vascular and Interventional Radiology.* 2nd ed. Philadelphia: WB Saunders; 2006.

Weisbord SD, Palevsky PM. Strategies for the prevention of contrast-induced acute kidney injury. *Curr Opin Nephrol Hypertens.* 2010;19:539-549.

CHAPTER 3

Noninvasive Vascular Imaging

John A. Kaufman, MD, MS, FSIR, FCIRSE, and Constantino S. Pena, MD

ULTRASOUND
  Grayscale Ultrasound
  Doppler Ultrasound
  Color Doppler
  Power Doppler

Ultrasound Contrast Agents

**MAGNETIC RESONANCE IMAGING
AND MAGNETIC RESONANCE
ANGIOGRAPHY**

**COMPUTED TOMOGRAPHY AND
COMPUTED TOMOGRAPHY
ANGIOGRAPHY**

POSTPROCESSING

Diagnostic imaging of patients with vascular disease is most often performed with ultrasound (US), computed tomography (CT), or magnetic resonance imaging (MRI). The purpose of this chapter is to provide an understanding of the basic principles of each of the noninvasive modalities.

ULTRASOUND

Grayscale Ultrasound

Much of the evaluation of blood vessels with ultrasound can be accomplished with conventional grayscale imaging. A transducer that emits high-frequency sound waves (usually 2-7 MHz) is held to the skin using a coupling gel to eliminate the air gap between the transducer and the skin. The sound waves are reflected to variable degrees by the internal structures. A computer measures the time that it takes for the sound waves to return to the transducer and then creates an image. Sound waves that are reflected by a tissue, such as the wall of a blood vessel, are visible as echoic structures. Sound waves that are transmitted by structures, such as the fluid-filled lumen of a blood vessel, have no echoes (anechoic). Grayscale ultrasound is a powerful tool for defining the morphology of blood vessels, but it has distinct limitations. Air, bone, and metal are so highly reflective that sound waves cannot penetrate to visualize underlying tissues. The two areas of the body where this is most problematic are the chest (air in the lungs) and the head (bone in the skull). Another limitation of grayscale ultrasound is that it does not image blood flow. The presence of a vascular disease may be suspected on the basis of the grayscale appearance of the vessel wall, such as a large echogenic plaque in an artery, visualization of wall pulsatile motion, echogenic material in the vessel lumen, or inability to compress the vessel. Fortunately, a very basic principle of ultrasound, Doppler shift, can be used to indirectly measure the velocity of flow.

Doppler Ultrasound

When a sound wave is reflected from a stationary object, the frequency of the returning wave is the same as that of the initial wave. The frequency of a wave that is reflected from an object moving toward the sound source is higher in proportion to the speed of that object. Conversely, the frequency of a wave reflected from an object moving away from the sound source is lower in proportion to the velocity of the object. This is why the tone of a siren drops noticeably lower as an ambulance drives by. The audible difference between the two frequencies is termed the "Doppler shift." This same phenomenon can be applied to flowing blood during an ultrasound examination using the sound waves emitted from and reflected back to the transducer.

Most diagnostic ultrasound equipment utilizes a thin beam of pulsed ultrasound (known as *pulsed-wave Doppler*) because this allows precise spatial localization of the measured velocity within the tissues. Continuous-wave Doppler (e.g., the small handheld units used to detect arterial pulses) measures all flow within the emitted beam, such that overlapping structures are easily confused.

Review of the Doppler equation helps to understand the strengths and limitations of this technique. The simplified equation is as follows:

$$\text{Doppler shift}$$
$$= (F_r - F_t)$$
$$= 2 \times F_t \times V \times \cos \theta \times (1/c)$$

where F_r is the frequency of the reflected sound, F_t is the frequency of the transmitted sound, V is the velocity of flow, θ is the angle of the ultrasound beam with respect to the long axis of the vessel lumen, and c is the speed of sound in soft tissues. The velocity of flow is useful for detection of disease, so the equation can be rearranged as:

$$V(\text{cm/s})$$
$$= F_d \times (1/F_t) \times (c/2) \times (1/\cos \theta),$$

where F_d is the Doppler shift. Notice that the calculated velocity is directly proportional to the Doppler shift, but inversely proportional to cos θ (the angle of the ultrasound beam to the direction of flow). This last fact explains why the best angles for measurement of velocity are less than 60 degrees. Below a θ of 60 degrees the value of $1/\cos \theta$ changes at a relatively leisurely rate. At a θ greater than 60 degrees the changes in the value of $1/\cos \theta$ are large with only incremental changes in θ. This leads to magnification of errors during the velocity calculation, rendering the results unreliable.

Velocity of flow is most commonly displayed as a tracing on a scale determined by the operator. By convention, flow toward the transducer is displayed above the baseline, and flow away from the transducer is displayed below. The characteristics of the tracing are determined by the type of vessel, the organ which it supplies, and the presence of disease states. Arterial flow varies with the cardiac cycle, with a rapid rise to peak velocity during systole, and gradual decrease in velocity during diastole. Shortly after flow peaks, the aortic valve closes, creating a small secondary peak in flow termed the dicrotic notch. Blood flow in high-resistance structures, such as the leg muscles, is triphasic with a brief period of retrograde flow during diastole (Fig. 3-1). Blood flow in low-resistance structures,

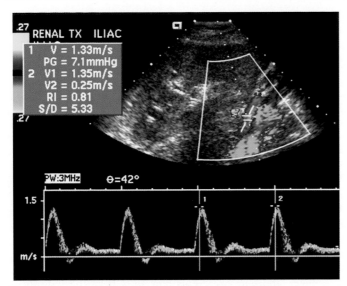

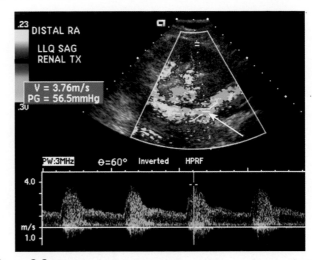

FIGURE 3-1. The normal Doppler waveform in high-resistance arteries is triphasic: fast antegrade flow during systole, reversed briefly at the beginning of diastole, then antegrade at a lower velocity. An external iliac artery tracing is shown.

FIGURE 3-3. Doppler tracing from a patient with transplant renal artery stenosis shows increased velocity and broadening of the waveform in the region of greatest arterial narrowing *(arrow)*.

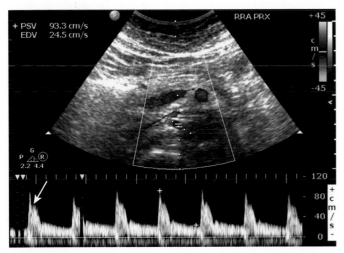

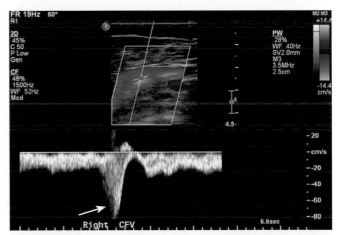

FIGURE 3-2. The normal Doppler waveform in a low-resistance visceral artery is biphasic: fast antegrade flow during systole with slower antegrade flow during diastole. Flow is never reversed in normal visceral arteries. A renal artery tracing is shown *(arrow on dicrotic notch)*.

FIGURE 3-4. Doppler waveform in a normal common femoral vein shows gentle respiratory variation in flow. A sharp increase in flow *(arrow)* occurs with manual compression of the calf.

such as visceral organs, remains antegrade throughout diastole (Fig. 3-2). With occlusive disease the velocity of flow in the stenosis rises and the Doppler tracing thickens (termed *spectral broadening*) as the range of velocities present increases (Fig. 3-3). As the stenosis progresses in severity, the velocity may decrease and the waveform becomes dampened or disappears altogether.

Blood flow in veins characteristically has a lower velocity than in arteries, with a less pulsatile Doppler waveform (Fig. 3-4). The velocity and pulsation vary depending on the proximity of the vein to the heart, the health of the heart, and the volume status of the patient. Phasic changes in velocity with respiration also occurs, with substantial increases in flow during inspiration and dampened flow during expiration. With forced expiration (the Valsalva maneuver) flow may be completely arrested (Fig. 3-5). In general, the more distant the vein is from the central circulation, the slower and more constant the flow.

Two vascular abnormalities with distinct Doppler signatures that are important to angiographers are arteriovenous fistula

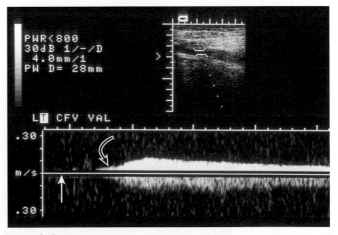

FIGURE 3-5. During Valsalva maneuver there is cessation of flow *(straight arrow)* in the common femoral vein. With relaxation, flow resumes *(curved arrow)*.

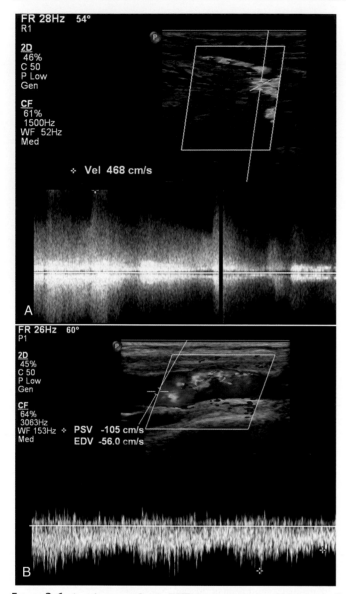

FR 28Hz 54°
R1

2D
46%
C 50
P Low
Gen

CF
61%
1500Hz
WF 52Hz
Med

❖ Vel 468 cm/s

A

FR 26Hz 60°
P1

2D
45%
C 50
P Low
Gen

CF
64%
3063Hz
WF 153Hz ❖ PSV −105 cm/s
Med   EDV −56.0 cm/s

B

FIGURE 3-6. Arteriovenous fistula (AVF) between the brachial artery and vein after attempted peripherally inserted central catheter line placement. A, Doppler waveform in the fistula shows greatly accelerated velocities with extreme spectral broadening. B, Doppler waveform from the vein central to the AVF shows a pulsatile venous waveform consistent with arterialized venous flow.

(AVF) and arterial pseudoaneurysm (PSA). Both lesions can occur following percutaneous vascular procedures. An AVF is a direct communication between an artery and a vein (see Fig. 1-25). The Doppler characteristics are accentuated diastolic flow (i.e., a low-resistance pattern) in the artery proximal to the AVF, a jet of extremely high-velocity flow through the point of communication, and an arterialized waveform in the vein central to the fistula (Fig. 3-6). A PSA is a focal disruption of at least one layer of the arterial wall communicating with a blood-filled space that is usually contained by the adjacent soft tissues (see Fig. 1-9). The Doppler characteristics are a jet of high-velocity flow through the neck that may reverse during diastole ("to-and-fro") with swirling flow in the pseudoaneurysm (Fig. 3-7).

Color Doppler

The Doppler shift can be assigned colors that reflect both the relative direction and velocity of the flow. All flow within a specified area of a fan beam is assigned a color, with red and blue being the most conventional. Red usually indicates flow toward the transducer, and blue represents flow away from the transducer. The color of the flow is determined by how the operator holds the transducer; one should never try to identify a vessel based on color alone. The color image is superimposed upon a grayscale image to provide anatomic definition, and many ultrasound machines also allow simultaneous display of a pulsed-wave tracing.

With color-flow Doppler, very fast flow is usually displayed as white or yellow. This helps localize areas of stenosis or other pathologies such as an AVF or neck of a PSA by visualization of the accelerated flow. Subsequently, precise velocity measurements in the area of abnormality are obtained with pulsed-wave Doppler. The appearance of turbulent flow is exemplified by the color pattern found inside an arterial PSA, in which the color changes from red to blue as the blood swirls around in the cavity. Color imaging can also be very useful when evaluating intraluminal processes, such as partially occlusive thrombus.

Power Doppler

Power Doppler is an important modification of color-flow techniques. With standard color-flow imaging, the color is linked to the Doppler shift. Power Doppler uses the overall energy in the Doppler signal to assign color, without regard for the magnitude of the phase shift (velocity) or direction. Since the majority of the signal is created by moving red blood cells, this technique is more sensitive to flow than standard color imaging. Although this is useful when evaluating areas of slow flow or small structures, other movement such as transmitted pulsations or vibrations will also be more apparent on the images.

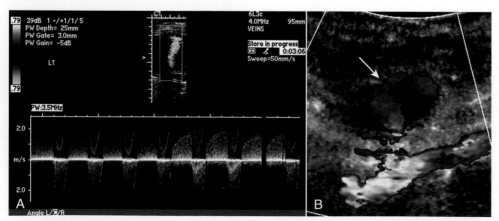

FIGURE 3-7. Arterial pseudoaneurysm (PSA). A, Doppler waveform in the neck of an iatrogenic popliteal artery PSA shows high velocity to-and-fro flow. B, Color-flow image of an iatrogenic common femoral artery PSA (arrow) shows swirling turbulent flow in the aneurysm ("yin-yang" sign).

Ultrasound imaging has several limitations, some of which are related to the physics of the technique, and some to the person performing the examination. The greatest limitation is that ultrasound is reflected by bone and air-tissue interfaces. Structures surrounded by or consisting primarily of these components can be difficult or impossible to image. A second limitation is that imaging occurs in a single plane determined by the person holding the transducer. Complex nonlinear structures must be evaluated in a piecemeal fashion, with intense concentration upon the part of the examiner in order to perform a complete study. The application of three-dimensional (3-D) image reconstruction software to ultrasound will facilitate these examinations.

Doppler imaging has several key weaknesses, including unreliable velocity calculations when the angle of insonation is greater than 60 degrees, as described earlier. Very slow flow is difficult to detect, particularly in deep vessels, which may lead to the false conclusion that a vessel is occluded, a potentially serious error when evaluating the carotid arteries. On the other hand, extremely fast flow may exceed the ability of a particular ultrasound machine to measure or display the velocity, but this is rarely an important problem in patient management.

Color-flow Doppler imaging does not display velocity as accurately as the waveform. The severity of a stenosis is inferred from the visualized color changes. Selection of an inappropriate color scale may result in overestimation or underestimation of the degree of stenosis. Furthermore, because color-encoding is determined by the operator, the identity of a vessel cannot be assumed from the color of the flow.

Ultrasound Contrast Agents

Intravascular contrast agents for ultrasound are 3-5 micron microspheres of encapsulated gas that reflect sound. The bubbles oscillate in the ultrasound beam, so that imaging at high power disrupts the shells. The microbubbles remain intravascular such that tissue enhancement does not occur as with computed tomography (CT) and magnetic resonance (MR) contrast agents. The gas is absorbed over approximately 5 minutes. The most common applications for ultrasound contrast agents are in the detection and characterization of solid organ lesions. The use of ultrasound contrast for vascular imaging is less common, but has been described in the follow-up of abdominal aortic endografts. Contrast reactions are rare, with true anaphylaxis reported in 0.014% of administrations.

▬ MAGNETIC RESONANCE IMAGING AND MAGNETIC RESONANCE ANGIOGRAPHY

Magnetic resonance imaging (MRI) is based upon the detection of radiofrequency signals emitted by protons within a powerful magnetic field. Protons in the tissue being imaged align their axes with the strong magnetic field in the MR scanner (longitudinal magnetization). Application of an additional radiofrequency pulse to the protons tips the spins out of alignment with the magnetic field in a plane perpendicular to the magnetic field (transverse magnetization). The natural tendency of the protons is to realign themselves with the magnetic field (relaxation), which creates a detectable signal (echo). Images are created from the signals emitted during longitudinal (T1) or transverse (T2) relaxation of the spins. In general, images based on short echo times are T1-weighted while those based on long echo times are T2-weighted.

The MR signal characteristics of tissues can be complex. Normal fat, muscle, tendon, solid organs, and fluids have different signal intensities on T1- and T2-weighted images. These signal characteristics can change with the presence of pathology or bleeding, or following administration of a contrast agent. In general, fast-flowing blood is usually black, because it moves out of the image before any signal can be collected (Fig. 3-8). The signal characteristics of static blood (thrombus) are variable but specific with respect to the pulse sequence and the age of the

thrombus. After administration of contrast, blood and organs usually become bright on most sequences. Inflammatory changes in the wall of a blood vessel enhance. However, bone and air always appear dark. The inability to visualize vascular calcification is an important limitation of MRI when applied to vascular pathology. Nevertheless, conventional MR images can be invaluable in the evaluation of vascular diseases and are included in most vascular studies except lower extremity runoffs.

Magnetic resonance angiography (MRA) is the application of MR techniques to the imaging of flowing blood (Box 3-1). First described in 1985, there are now numerous strategies for imaging flow in a magnetic field (Table 3-1). Each technique relies upon a different aspect of MRI to visualize blood flow. Time-of-flight (TOF) and phase-contrast (PC) sequences are both non–contrast-enhanced techniques that image flowing protons and are susceptible to signal loss due to turbulence, slow flow, and rapid changes in velocity, which are conditions that frequently exist in diseased blood vessels (Figs. 3-9 and 3-10). These techniques are used for either slice-by-slice (two-dimensional, or 2-D) or volume (3-D) acquisitions. In general, 2-D imaging provides excellent vascular signal at the expense of image resolution, whereas 3-D imaging provides better resolution (thinner slices) but is susceptible to signal loss as volumes increase in size. 3-D acquisitions are now performed in an interleaving technique to maintain image signal. Both TOF and PC

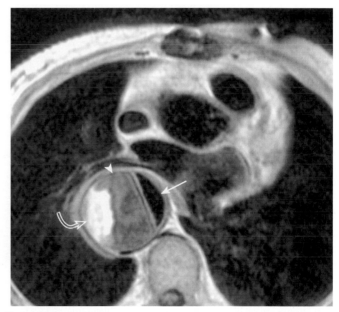

FIGURE 3-8. Axial T1-weighted image of chronic aortic dissection. Fast flow in the true lumen is black *(straight arrow)*, slow flow in the false lumen is gray *(arrowhead)*, and chronic mural thrombus in the false lumen is bright *(curved arrow)*.

Box 3-1. Magnetic Resonance Angiography Advantages

No loss of vascular signal with gadolinium MRA
Large field of view
Single breath-hold acquisition
Bones invisible
Multiple station lower extremity runoffs
Time-resolved imaging
Allergic reactions to contrast rare
Noncontrast techniques in renal failure
No exposure to ionizing radiation

TABLE 3-1 Magnetic Resonance Imaging Techniques

Technique	Basic Principle	Blood/Background Signal
Black blood	No signal from rapidly flowing blood; normal signal from surrounding tissues	Dark/bright
Time-of-flight	Signal from fresh protons in flowing blood visible against suppressed signal from background tissues; slowly moving blood may lose signal; venous/arterial selection by saturation of opposite inflow; time-consuming and limited anatomic coverage for volume imaging	Bright/dark
Phase-contrast	Measurement of phase shift of spinning proton at two time points as it moves through magnetic field; provides directional and velocity information; stationary protons have no phase shift; volume imaging time-consuming and limited anatomic coverage	Bright/dark
ECG-gated 3-D partial-Fourier fast spin echo	Subtraction of systolic from diastolic images to visualize arterial flow; arterial flow is dark and venous flow bright on systolic T2 image, whereas both artery and venous blood are bright on diastolic images; subtraction creates angiographic image; requires several minutes and susceptible to motion artifacts	Bright/dark
Balanced steady-state free precession*	Gradient echo sequences that use the ratio of T2 to T1 relaxation times to depict bright blood; saturation bands are necessary to suppress unwanted vascular signal; can be used with arterial spin labeling (ASL) in which protons are preexcited before entering the imaging field of view; imaging with ASL relies on rapid directional flow	Bright/dark
Gadolinium-enhanced	Signal from intravascular contrast agent (no saturation); timing critical, especially to separate arteries and veins; background signal present but minimal; quick volume imaging of large body areas; use in patients with renal dysfunction limited	Bright/dark

*Other versions include fast imaging employing steady-state acquisition, true fast imaging with steady-state precession, and balanced fast filed echo.

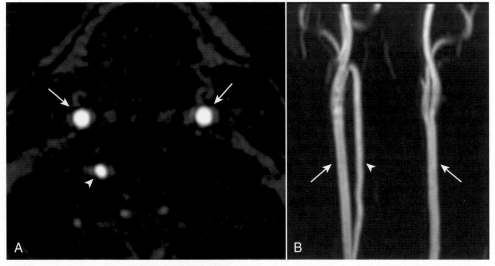

FIGURE 3-9. Time-of-flight (TOF) magnetic resonance angiography (MRA) of the carotid arteries. TOF MRA is based upon saturation of signal from background tissues and detection of signal from "fresh" spins in blood flowing into the slice or volume. **A,** Axial 2-D TOF image of the neck. The complete study consists of many more contiguous images, collected individually and sequentially. The common carotid *(arrows)* and right vertebral *(arrowhead)* arteries are visible as white structures. The signal from the background tissues is suppressed. The venous signal is eliminated by a saturation band that is positioned superior to and moves with each slice. Note the absence of visualization of the left vertebral artery. The artery may be occluded, severely stenotic with such slow flow that signal is suppressed along with the background tissues, or have reversed flow that is saturated along with the venous flow. **B,** Maximum intensity projection (MIP) of a portion of the same 2-D TOF MRA provides an angiographic view of arteries. Only the brightest pixels are displayed on the 2-D MIP image. Note again the absence of signal in the left vertebral artery (see Fig. 3-11). *Arrows* = carotid arteries; *arrowhead* = right vertebral artery.

imaging decreased in importance following the introduction of gadolinium-enhanced 3-D MRA by Prince in 1993.

Gadolinium-enhanced MRA sequences directly image the intravascular contrast agent, with minimal signal from flow-related enhancement leading to minimal degradation from abnormal flow patterns. The gadolinium contrast agent is injected rapidly through a peripheral vein, with image acquisition timed to occur as the contrast enters the arterial circulation in the region of interest. Imaging with this technique can be accomplished in a single breath-hold, encompassing large fields of view. Images are acquired before the injection of the contrast agent and can serve as a mask to subtract background signal and increase the conspicuity of the contrast agent (Fig. 3-11). Although 3-D volumes are routinely used, there is no loss of signal due to saturation effects as experienced with noncontrast techniques. Peripheral lower extremity MRA sequences routinely are performed in overlapping stations (Fig. 3-12). Newer acquisition techniques such as parallel imaging have allowed for faster and higher resolution images. Time-resolved imaging permits rapid repetitive acquisitions of a single anatomic region, so that four-dimensional evaluation of the blood flow is possible (Fig. 3-13).

There are fewer adverse reactions to gadolinium contrast agents than with iodinated contrast, and gadolinium appears to have little clinical nephrotoxicity. The recognition of rare complication

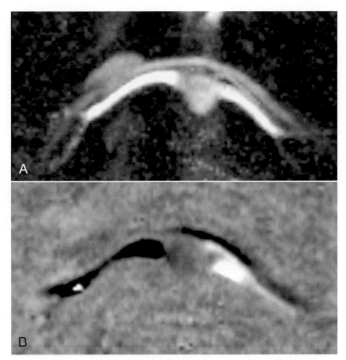

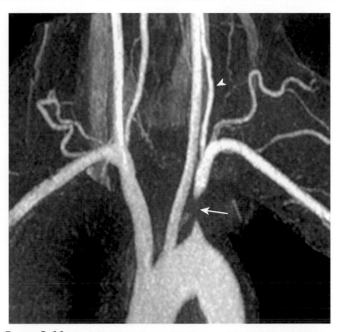

FIGURE **3-11**. Gadolinium-enhanced 3-D magnetic resonance angiography (MRA). Coronal oblique maximum intensity projection image of a gadolinium-enhanced 3-D MRA of the same patient as in Figure 3-9 shows that the left vertebral artery is patent *(arrowhead)* with reversed flow due to a left subclavian artery origin occlusion *(arrow)*. The signal loss in the left vertebral artery on the 2-D time-of-flight study was due to saturation of reversed flow. Note the smooth vessel contours and ability to image flow in all directions in this 3-D acquisition.

FIGURE **3-10**. Phase-contrast (PC) magnetic resonance angiography of the renal arteries. PC MRA is based upon measurement of phase shifts of protons moving through the magnetic field. Stationary protons have no phase shift, resulting in absence of signal from background tissues. The velocity encoding (VENC) for this study was 40 cm/sec. This parameter is selected by the operator in PC MRA to purposely maximize signal from flow at a specific velocity. **A,** Axial maximum intensity projection of a 3-D PC MRA of normal renal arteries. Flow in every direction is depicted as white and there is no background signal. Note the renal veins anterior to the arterial structures. A small accessory renal artery is visible on the left between the left renal artery and vein. **B,** Single slice from the same study encoded for directional flow (right to left). Flow in the left renal arteries is white, and flow in the left renal vein is black. Note that flow in the right renal artery, which is in the same direction as flow in the left renal vein, is also black. Little signal is seen in the aorta, because the predominant direction of flow is superior to inferior. PC images are very sensitive to turbulent flow.

of gadolinium contrast agents, nephrogenic systemic fibrosis (see Chapter 2) has resulted in renewed interest in noncontrast MRA (Fig. 3-14).

MRI techniques are subject to a number of limitations (Box 3-2). Patients with most cardiac pacemakers, defibrillators, intraocular or intraaural metallic foreign bodies, or claustrophobia cannot be imaged. Ferromagnetic objects in or adjacent to blood vessels can create susceptibility artifacts that result in signal loss (Fig. 3-15). Highly concentrated gadolinium shortens T2, such that too much gadolinium results in signal loss in vessels and surrounding susceptibility artifacts (Fig. 3-16). Heavy circumferential intimal calcification in medium or small arteries may also result in susceptibility artifacts and apparent stenoses on MRA sequences. Specialized MR-compatible equipment is required for hemodynamic monitoring of unstable patients; lethal complications can occur when metallic objects are sucked into the bore while a patient is being scanned. Uncooperative or demented patients who are not able to hold still during image acquisition can render a study useless.

▬ COMPUTED TOMOGRAPHY AND COMPUTED TOMOGRAPHY ANGIOGRAPHY

The development of helical CT scanners revitalized the vascular applications of this imaging modality. Conventional scanners imaged one slice at a time, with the table in a stationary position.

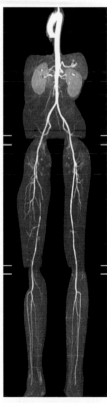

FIGURE **3-12**. Gadolinium-enhanced 3-D magnetic resonance angiography of the aorta and bilateral lower extremity arteries in a patient with peripheral arterial disease. The study was acquired in the coronal plane with overlapping slabs, a moving scanning table, and a single injection of gadolinium. The study is displayed as a combined maximum intensity projection image.

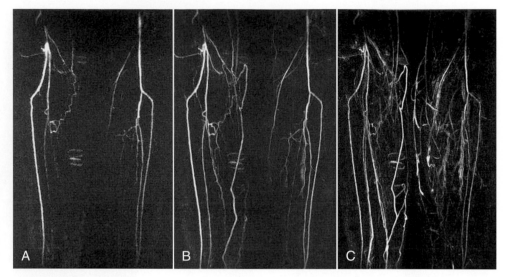

Figure 3-13. Time-resolved gadolinium-enhanced imaging of the tibial arteries in a patient with peripheral arterial disease, displayed as maximum intensity projection images. **A,** Early arterial phase. **B,** Midarterial phase with some early venous opacification, particularly in the medial superficial veins of the right calf. **C,** Late phase with more extensive venous opacification bilaterally as the arteries become less prominent.

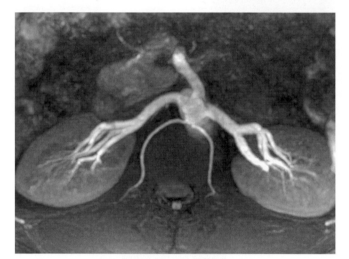

Figure 3-14. Renal magnetic resonance angiography obtained without contrast using an IFIR (enhance inflow inversion recovery), a FIESTA-based (fast imaging employing steady-state acquisition) sequence. Shown is an axial thick multiplanar reformation. (Courtesy of Barry Stein, MD, Hartford, Conn.)

Although conventional CT was recognized as an excellent modality for visualizing blood vessel morphology, imaging was too slow to be used for angiographic studies. Helical (or spiral) CT scanners image continuously as the patient is moved rapidly through the gantry. Slip-ring technology in the CT scan gantry allows continuous rotation of the x-ray tube, without the need to stop and "rewind" between slices. Data are acquired in a volume, as with 3-D MRA, rather than as individual slices. The scan time is dramatically reduced compared to conventional CT, so that a bolus of contrast can be tracked as it opacifies a vascular bed.

The initial helical scanners were equipped with a single row of detector elements. Multidetector row technology (MDCT) and dual energy scanning have further decreased imaging times, with improved image quality. Whole body scanning in less than 5 seconds is now feasible. Multiple interweaving helices are acquired at the same time, allowing reduced scan times, reduced volumes of contrast, reduced motion and pulsatility artifacts, and improved spatial resolution. Slice thickness is determined by the thickness of the detector elements rather than beam collimation, and may be substantially less than 1 mm. Some flat-panel rotational diagnostic angiographic units are equipped with CT

Box 3-2. Magnetic Resonance Angiography Limitations

Timing critical for single-pass gadolinium MRA
Risk of nephrogenic systemic fibrosis with some gadolinium agents in renal failure
Overestimates stenosis
Signal loss due to metal artifact
Signal loss due to heavy calcification in small vessels
Degradation of study due to patient motion
Contraindicated in patients with certain implants
Special nonmagnetic monitoring/respiratory equipment required
Limited availability of imaging equipment

reconstruction algorithms but at reduced image quality compared to dedicated CT units (see Fig. 2-51).

CT images are reconstructed initially as axial images. The decrease in collimation and scanning times afforded by MDCT has resulted in ballooning of the total number of images acquired per study. It is not unusual to have more than 1000 images in each examination. Image review on a digital workstation (PACS) is essential.

Important information can be obtained about the vascular system without the use of intravenous contrast. Most CT scans for vascular pathology should begin with a noncontrast scan. The size of the blood vessel and the degree of vascular calcification can be easily assessed on noncontrast CT (Fig. 3-17). Acute extravascular blood appears dense on noncontrast CT, so that the diagnosis of acute hemorrhage from vascular injury or rupture does not require intravenous contrast. Synthetic graft materials are usually high-density on non-contrast scans, but often obscured by contrast-enhanced blood.

The basic principle of CT angiography (CTA) is a carefully timed helical acquisition during the rapid peripheral infusion of iodinated contrast. Determination of correct timing is usually performed with automated techniques (Fig. 3-18), test boluses, or "best guess" based upon empirical delays. The latter method is least reliable in older patients or those with cardiac disease. The region of interest determines the parameters used for the scan. In general, CTA is less complicated and faster than MRA. When creating study protocols, keep in mind that the thinner the collimation or greater the pitch, the lower the ratio of signal to noise in the image.

CTA is entirely dependent upon imaging when the vessels are of increased intravascular density due to the contrast agent.

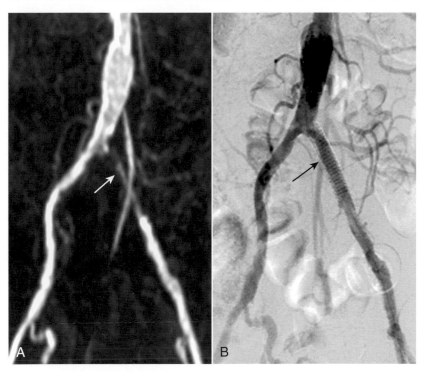

FIGURE 3-15. Signal loss due to metallic susceptibility artifact from an arterial stent. **A,** Coronal maximum intensity projection of a gadolinium-enhanced 3-D magnetic resonance angiography of the pelvis. There is apparent diffuse stenosis in the left common iliac artery *(arrow)*. **B,** Digital subtraction angiography of the distal abdominal aorta and pelvis demonstrates a stent in the left common iliac artery *(arrow)* that has mild proximal in-stent restenosis but is otherwise patent.

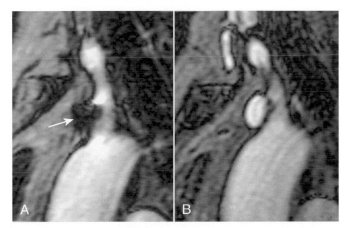

FIGURE 3-16. Signal loss due to concentrated gadolinium. **A,** Single slice from a gadolinium-enhanced 3-D magnetic resonance angiography of the aortic arch obtained during injection of contrast through a left upper extremity vein. There is a signal void in the left brachiocephalic vein *(arrow)* with surrounding susceptibility artifact causing an apparent bulky eccentric stenosis of the adjacent brachiocephalic artery. **B,** Single slice (same location) from the same study obtained 30 seconds after the first image. The concentration of gadolinium in the left upper extremity veins has decreased. The left brachiocephalic vein is normal and the brachiocephalic artery stenosis is less impressive.

Information from background tissues is not suppressed as it is in MRA. Three factors are considered when choosing a contrast protocol for CTA: injection rate, total volume, and concentration of iodine. Visualization of small vessels improves as the concentration of iodine in the blood increases. Most CTA studies utilize injection rates of 3-5 mL/sec for a total volume of 70-150 mL. One of the major advantages of CTA is that the source images are conventional axial slices with intense vascular opacification (see Fig. 3-17). All of the information that one would normally expect regarding the vascular wall and perivascular structures on a CT scan is still present on the source images. This allows more

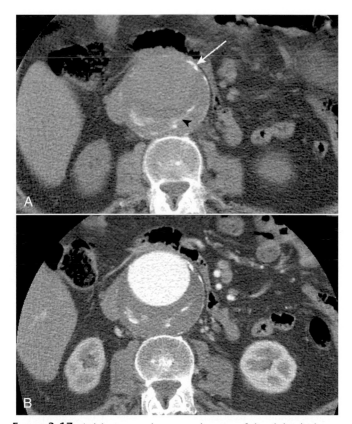

FIGURE 3-17. Axial computed tomography scan of the abdominal aorta from a helical acquisition. **A,** Image without contrast of an abdominal aortic aneurysm. The wall of the aneurysm is identified by the calcification in the intimal layer *(arrow)*. The patency of the aneurysm cannot be determined from this image, but mural thrombus containing calcium *(arrowhead)* is present. **B,** Contrast-enhanced image at a similar level shows the aortic lumen. The mural thrombus is lower in density than the blood. Without the precontrast study the calcified areas in the thrombus could be misinterpreted as contrast.

FIGURE **3-18**. Timing is critical for computed tomography angiography (CTA), as well as for contrast-enhanced magnetic resonance angiography. **A,** There are many techniques for optimizing image acquisition during peak vascular opacification. Shown is the curve of measured Hounsfield units in the proximal descending thoracic aorta *(inset)*. When a threshold value of 150 HU was reached, the scan was automatically initiated. **B,** Oblique 3-D volume rendering of the CTA obtained in this manner. The image is windowed to show the blood vessels against the bony skeleton. The patient had treatment of a thoracoabdominal aneurysm with surgical bypasses to the celiac, superior mesenteric artery, and right renal artery from the left common iliac artery *(arrow)* and placement of endografts *(arrowhead)* from the thoracic aorta to the infrarenal abdominal aorta. This is termed a *debranching* procedure.

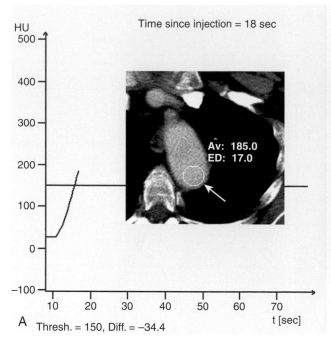

Time since injection = 18 sec

Av: 185.0
ED: 17.0

A Thresh. = 150, Diff. = −34.4

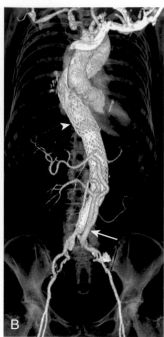

B

Box 3-3. **Computed Tomography Angiography Advantages**

Large field of view
Vascular enhancement by contrast
Rapid scan time allowing extensive longitudinal coverage (whole-body scan)
Limited number of variables to manipulate
Valuable information in source images
Scanners readily available
Conventional monitoring/respiratory equipment usable

Box 3-4. **Computed Tomography Angiography Limitations**

Timing critical
Overestimates degree of stenosis, especially in calcified vessels
Metal and bone obscure vascular structures
Signal-to-noise ratio poor in large patients
Nephrotoxic contrast material
Study degradation by patient motion
Exposure to ionizing radiation

---

comprehensive evaluation of the vascular structures than with MRA (Box 3-3). Although metal can create streak artifacts that degrade images, carefully windowed thin-slice CTA data can be used to evaluate intravascular stents (Fig. 3-19).

CTA has certain important limitations (Box 3-4). Patients with contrast allergies or renal failure, as well as those with contraindications to ionizing radiation (e.g., patients in the first trimester of pregnancy), may not be candidates for elective studies. As the number of slices and scans increases, the absorbed radiation dose to the patient increases. When CTA is used repeatedly to follow pathology, the accumulated dose can be substantial. Low-dose protocols, especially for children, and carefully tailored scans can reduce this exposure. Larger patients are hard to image even with high doses.

Small, heavily calcified vessels are difficult to evaluate, because bulky intimal calcium can be indistinguishable from the opacified vessel lumen. Concentrated contrast can cause streak artifacts that mimic pathology or obscure detail. Pulsatile vessels (particularly the ascending aorta) can be similarly difficult to image owing to motion artifacts, although this is less of a problem with ECG-gated MDCT scanners (Fig. 3-20). Uncooperative patients introduce motion or respiratory artifacts that seriously degrade the final images.

POSTPROCESSING

In order to view data from MRA and CTA studies as angiograms, postprocessing of source digital data is necessary. This crucial step occurs after the study has been completed, and frequently after the patient has been removed from the scanner. A number of postprocessing options are available, ranging from simple reformatting of data into different planes (i.e., coronal slices from axially acquired data), to 3-D renderings that permit an endoscopic viewpoint of the vascular lumen (Table 3-2 and Fig. 3-21; see also Figs. 3-11, 3-12, and 3-18). Excellent postprocessed images can only be created from excellent original data.

The source data for MRA and CTA are composed of discrete elements termed *voxels*. Each voxel has only one numerical value, determined by the measured density or signal from the structures in the voxel. If a voxel contains two structures with differing values, it will be assigned a value that is an average of both. There is no way to retrospectively separate these two structures with current postprocessing techniques. For this reason, small cube-shaped (isotropic) voxels are most desirable to maximize image detail and facilitate postprocessing. If an image is constructed of large rectangular voxels, small objects may get "lost" (partial volume averaging), particularly when viewed from a perspective perpendicular to the long axis of the voxel. The regions of an image in which this becomes most apparent are curved edges or borders of structures. However, the smaller the voxel, the greater the impact of background noise.

Postprocessing is the sophisticated manipulation of voxels in order to enhance or emphasize important features of an image. With the exception of reformatting, angiographic postprocessing results in loss of data as nonvascular voxels are rendered

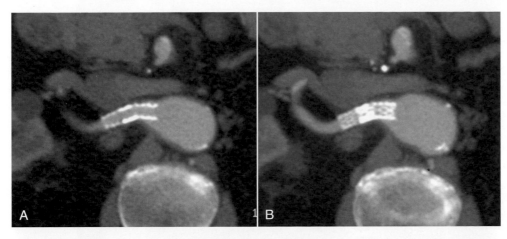

FIGURE 3-19. CTA can be used to evaluate metal stents. **A,** Single axial slice from a contrast-enhanced CT through the right renal artery origin showing patent stents, but the renal artery distal to the stents is not well seen. **B,** Summation (thick slab) of several slices from the same dataset as in A shows the two overlapping stents. More of the main renal artery is visualized, but now it is not possible to assess for stenosis within the stents.

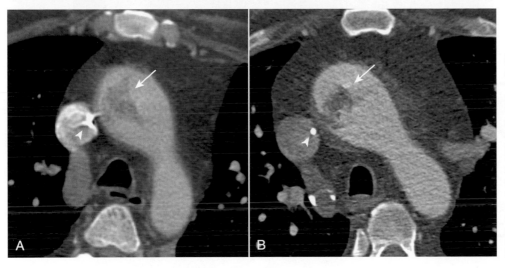

FIGURE 3-20. Nongated and gated CTA of the thoracic aorta in a patient presenting with recurrent embolic strokes. **A,** Nongated CTA. Source axial image shows a filling defect in the ascending thoracic aorta *(arrow)*. Note the motion artifact *(arrowhead)* from the catheter in the superior vena cava (SVC). The edges of the aorta are blurred. **B,** ECG-gated CTA. The intraluminal filling defect *(arrow)* is not only crisply defined, but the attachment to the wall of the aorta is clearly seen. There is no motion artifact from the SVC catheter *(arrowhead)*, and the walls of the aorta appear sharp. This patient had a mural aortic thrombus secondary to a hypercoagulable condition.

TABLE 3-2 Postprocessing Techniques

Technique	Basic Principle	Strengths	Weaknesses
Reformat	Allows display of all data in volume in user-defined 2-D planes, including curved	Quick; no loss of data; can display complex anatomy	Overlap of structures can be confusing, 2-D display only
Maximum intensity projection	Displays brightest voxels in user-defined 2-D planes; discards background information	Quick; bright vessels	Threshold for display may result in loss of critical information; 2-D display only
Volume rendering	Displays voxels as a virtual 3-dimensional volume; objects selected by setting threshold, opacity values	3-D-like rendition of selected voxel values while retaining complete data set	Threshold for model may render critical voxels transparent
Endoscopic	Displays tubular structures without intraluminal contents with 3-D appearance	Allows viewer to enter and travel through lumen of blood vessel	Intraluminal perspective only

transparent or discarded. The remaining voxels are then manipulated to enhance the appearance of the final images, often by adding or further subtracting data as needed.

A few generalizations can be made regarding postprocessing techniques. Basic reformatting algorithms are integrated into many PACS workstations. Most sophisticated postprocessing is performed on fast independent workstations equipped with proprietary software. Datasets must be heavily edited with excision of unwanted portions of the images in order to produce satisfactory 3-D models. This requires some understanding of vascular anatomy and pathology. In addition, the source data must have excellent contrast between vascular structures and background tissues. For these reasons, all 3-D models must be viewed with some skepticism and correlated to the axial images, because important information can be omitted at several stages during creation of the final images (Box 3-5).

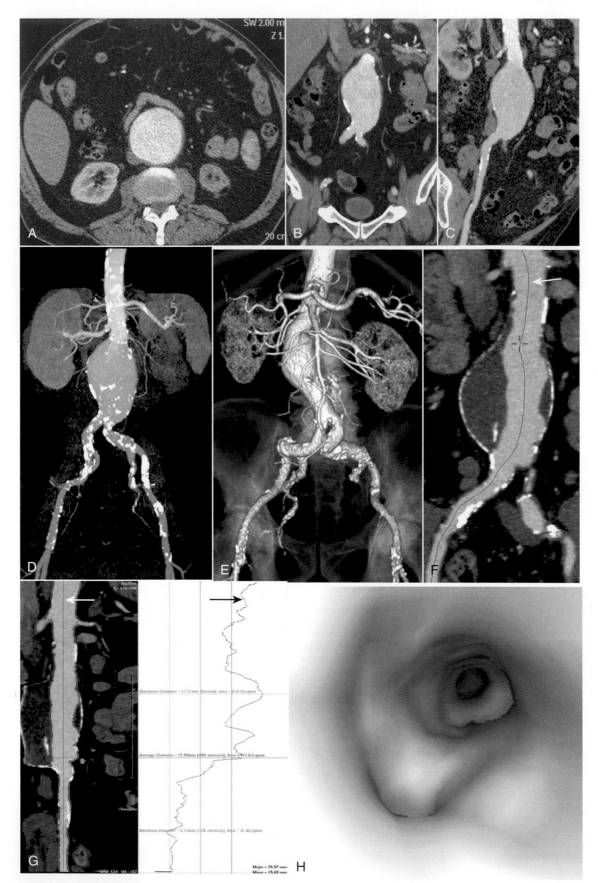

Figure 3-21. Image postprocessing is crucial to magnetic resonance angiography (MRA) and computed tomography angiography (CTA). **A,** Axial source CTA image of a patient with abdominal aortic aneurysm (AAA). **B,** Coronal multiplanar reformat (MPR) image of the same data set. This thin image shows only a slice of the aneurysm. Note that all of the source image data are preserved. **C,** Curved MPR image using same data set showing the aneurysm and right iliac arteries. This is also a thin image, so that the left iliac arteries, which are out of plane, are not visualized. Note the decrease in contrast density within the aneurysm relative to the suprarenal aorta. Flow in the AAA is slower and more turbulent. **D,** Thick coronal maximum intensity projection (MIP) image of the same data set. The brightest pixels are summated so that the arteries are displayed in a single image, but there is loss of much of the source image data. **E,** Volume rendering of a CTA of a different patient with an AAA showing the 3-D representation of the vascular data. **F,** Coronal reformat of a CTA of another patient with an abdominal aortic aneurysm. A centerline *(arrow)* has been drawn in the lumen. **G,** Using the centerline from **F** *(white arrow)*, a coronal reformatted image has been rendered in which the lumen is straightened (i.e., the axial plane of the lumen is now always at a 90-degree angle to the centerline). This allows measurement of true diameters at all points *(black arrow)*. **H,** Endoscopic image from another aortic CTA showing the origin of a branch vessel.

Box 3-5. Postprocessing Hints

Learn how to do it yourself
Always review source data for any questionable finding
There is no magic: bad source data yield bad postprocessed images

■ SUGGESTED READINGS

Chavhan GB, Parra DA, Mann A, Navarro OM. Normal Doppler spectral waveforms of major pediatric vessels: specific patterns. *Radiographics.* 2008;28:691-706.

Chrysochou C, Buckley DL, Dark P, Cowie A, Kalra PA. Gadolinium-enhanced magnetic resonance imaging for renovascular disease and nephrogenic systemic fibrosis: critical review of the literature and UK experience. *J Magn Reson Imaging.* 2009;29:887-894.

Fleischmann D, Kamaya A. Optimal vascular and parenchymal contrast enhancement: the current state of the art. *Radiol Clin North Am.* 2009;47:13-26.

Gerhard-Herman M, Gardin JM, Jaff M, et al. Guidelines for noninvasive vascular laboratory testing: a report from the American Society of Echocardiography and the Society for Vascular Medicine and Biology. *Vasc Med.* 2006;11:183-200.

Griffin M, Grist TM, François CJ. Dynamic four-dimensional MR angiography of the chest and abdomen. *Magn Reson Imaging Clin N Am.* 2009 Feb;17(1):77-90.

Kumamaru KK, Hoppel BE, Mather RT, Rybicki FJ. CT angiography: current technology and clinical use. *Radiol Clin North Am.* 2010;48:213-235.

Meaney JF, Goyen M. Recent advances in contrast-enhanced magnetic resonance angiography. *Eur Radiol.* 2007;17(Suppl 2):B2-B6.

Miyazaki M, Lee VS. Nonenhanced MR angiography. *Radiology.* 2008;248:20-43.

Prince MR, Yucel EK, Kaufman JA, et al. Dynamic gadolinium-enhanced three-dimensional abdominal MR arteriography. *J Magn Reson Imaging.* 1993;3:877-881.

Roditi G, Maki JH, Oliveira G, Michaely HJ. Renovascular imaging in the NSF era. *J Magn Reson Imaging.* 2009;30:1323-1334.

Rose SC, Nelson TR. Ultrasonographic modalities to assess vascular anatomy and disease. *J Vasc Interv Radiol.* 2004;15:25-38.

Scoutt LM, Zawin ML, Taylor KJ. Doppler US: II. Clinical applications. *Radiology.* 1990;174:309-319.

Strandness DE. *Duplex Scanning of Vascular Disorders.* 3rd ed. Philadelphia: Lippincott Williams & Wilkins; 2002.

Taylor KJ, Holland S. Doppler US: I. Basic principles, instrumentation, and pitfalls. *Radiology.* 1990;174:297-307.

Wedeen VJ, Meuli RA, Edelman RR, et al. Projective imaging of pulsatile flow with magnetic resonance. *Science.* 1985;230:946-968.

Wilson GJ, Maki JH. Non-contrast-enhanced MR imaging of renal artery stenosis at 1.5 tesla. *Magn Reson Imaging Clin N Am.* 2009;17:13-27.

Wilson SR, Burns PN. Microbubble-enhanced US in body imaging: what role? *Radiology.* 2010;257:24-39.

Wood MM, Romine LE, Lee YK, Richman KM, O'Boyle MK, Paz DA, Chu PK, Pretorius DH. Spectral Doppler signature waveforms in ultrasonography: a review of normal and abnormal waveforms. *Ultrasound Q.* 2010;26:83-99.

Zhang H, Maki JH, Prince MR. 3D contrast-enhanced MR angiography. *J Magn Reson Imaging.* 2007;25:13-25.

CHAPTER 4

Vascular Interventions

John A. Kaufman, MD, MS, FSIR, FCIRSE

Percutaneous vascular interventions can be grouped into those that improve or occlude the lumen and those that implant or remove things. The fundamentals of each of these interventions are the same across most of the vascular system. This chapter describes the basic principles of how to perform vascular interventions. The results of specific interventions are discussed in the appropriate anatomic chapters.

The history of percutaneous catheter-based vascular interventions mirrors the development of interventional radiology as a specialty. Diagnostic angiography was originally just one of the several imaging technologies (albeit the most invasive) used by radiologists to obtain diagnostic images for other physicians. At the end of the procedure, the catheter was removed and the patient went for surgery or medical treatment by someone else. In 1964, Charles Dotter dilated an above-knee popliteal artery stenosis using progressively larger catheters, thus performing the first percutaneous transluminal angioplasty (Fig. 4-1). Surgery was avoided, and a new paradigm was born: arterial disease diagnosed by catheters could be treated by catheters. The milestones in vascular intervention are listed in Table 4-1.

When the first image-guided peripheral arterial intervention was performed by a radiologist, medicine was transformed. Percutaneous vascular interventions are now widely accepted and performed by a wide range of physicians. Interventional radiology has grown to include the clinical management of patients undergoing image-guided therapy and focused areas of disease-specific practice such as oncology and peripheral vascular disease.

IMPROVING THE LUMEN

Fundamentals

Abnormalities of the blood vessel lumen, whether resulting in a lumen that is too small (stenosis) or too big (aneurysm), are readily treated with percutaneous techniques. We will first focus on stenotic or occluded blood vessels. A variety of strategies have been devised to restore patency of both arteries and veins, but all have certain elements in common (Box 4-1). This section focuses on these fundamentals, with specific interventions discussed in subsequent sections. Interventions should be performed only after a complete diagnostic evaluation in appropriately symptomatic patients. The lesion responsible for the symptoms should be identified and characterized, and both the inflow and outflow evaluated. Lesion morphology is very important in guiding intervention and predicting outcome (Fig. 4-2). For example, short concentric noncalcified atherosclerotic lesions usually respond well to simple angioplasty, whereas long, calcified occlusions may be impossible to cross or dilate. Careful review of the appearance of the lesion, sometimes in several obliquities, may be necessary.

Once the decision to intervene is made, a vascular sheath should be inserted. If a large sheath will be required, consider partially deploying a suture-mediated closure device before the sheath is inserted (see Box 2-10). Medications commonly used during interventions should be prepared in advance (Table 4-2). The patient should be anticoagulated with unfractionated heparin or bivalirudin just before or immediately after crossing the lesion.

Crossing the lesion is essential to completing a revascularization procedure. Stenoses are crossed with an atraumatic torqueable selective guidewire, often directed by a selective catheter (Box 4-2). The use of digital "roadmap" fluoroscopy is extremely helpful, especially for complex and long lesions. Once the guidewire is across the lesion, the catheter is advanced over the guidewire, and the guidewire removed. Aspiration of blood followed by gentle injection of contrast confirms that the lumen has been reached on the other side. Static flow indicates either occlusion of the stenosis by the catheter or subintimal injection (Fig. 4-3). Distinguishing between the two is essential; filling of normal caliber lumen and branches indicates successful crossing of the lesion, whereas focal pooling of contrast or tracking around a central unopacified lumen indicates a subintimal location. A pressure gradient can be measured at this time if necessary.

Crossing an occlusion is more difficult than crossing a stenosis. The longer and more calcified the occlusion, the less probable the successful negotiation from one side to the other. There are two basic approaches: intraluminal and intentional subintimal. With intraluminal revascularization, the obliterated vascular lumen is recanalized. The procedure begins with injection of contrast close to the site of occlusion. This may unveil a tapered lumen that will direct the wire through the occlusion. Often, a smooth fibrotic cap adjacent to the last collateral around the lesion is present. To gain access to the occluded lumen, an angled or straight catheter is advanced up to the cap and a guidewire is then used to probe for a "soft spot." The choice of initial guidewire varies with the operator, the vessel, and the anatomy, but often a straight hydrophilic guidewire stays within the lumen once it gets through the cap. When the initial attempts to cross the occlusion fail, different shaped catheters and guidewires with gradually increased stiffness are used. Mechanical devices that burrow, vibrate, drill, or melt their way through the obliterated lumen are available (Fig. 4-4). If all else fails, the back end of a hydrophilic guidewire can

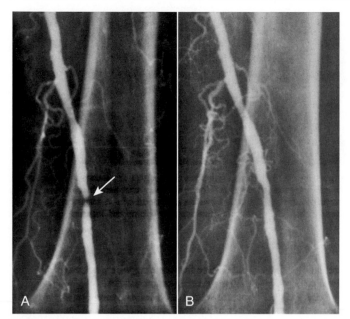

FIGURE 4-1. The first percutaneous angioplasty, 1964. **A,** Focal stenosis in the popliteal artery *(arrow)*. **B,** Using progressively larger coaxial catheters, the lesion was dilated. The patient's rest pain resolved and toe ulcers healed.

TABLE 4-1 Milestones in Vascular Intervention

Innovation	Year	Innovator
Embolization	1960	Luessenhop
Transvascular biopsy	1962	Sakakibara
Percutaneous angioplasty	1964	Dotter
Percutaneous foreign body retrieval	1964	Thomas
Percutaneous stent	1969	Dotter
Intraarterial thrombolysis	1974	Dotter
Stent-graft	1986	Balko

Box 4-1. Basic Steps in Recanalization Procedures

Patient history and physical examination
Diagnose lesion
Administer ancillary drugs (especially heparin)
Cross lesion with selective catheter and guidewire
Confirm intraluminal position distal to lesion
Exchange for working guidewire
Perform intervention
Document result
Schedule and perform follow-up

---

be used to puncture the cap, but this risks puncture of the artery wall as well.

Subintimal revascularization is an intentional dissection in the media around the occluded lumen and intimal disease. The proposed benefits of this approach are the absence of atheromatous disease in the media and the ability to recanalize extremely long distances, such as groin to ankle. An angled catheter is used to direct a guidewire (usually angled hydrophilic) into the subintimal space above the obstruction (Fig. 4-5). A loop of guidewire is formed in the subintimal space and used to dissect

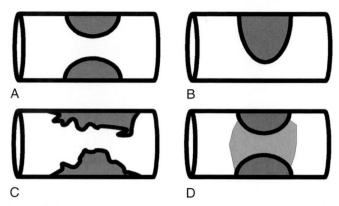

FIGURE 4-2. Drawings of basic lesion morphologies. Any of these lesions may be soft or heavily calcified. **A,** Concentric stenosis. This is an optimal lesion for intervention, especially angioplasty alone. **B,** Eccentric stenosis. This lesion is difficult to treat with angioplasty alone because the normal wall opposing the lesion will stretch and recoil with balloon inflation. **C,** Irregular stenosis. This lesion may be more difficult to cross due to the irregularity of the surface. **D,** Occlusion. If this occlusion is due to fresh thrombus within the lesion, consider thrombolysis or mechanical thrombectomy before treating the underlying stenosis.

TABLE 4-2 Drugs Commonly Used During Revascularization Procedures

Medication	Dose	Purpose
Heparin (1000 U/mL)	3000-7000 units IA	Prevent thrombus formation
Bivalirudin	0.75 mg/kg bolus, 1.75 mg/kg/hr infusion	Prevent thrombus formation
Nitroglycerin (100 µg/mL)	200-250 µg aliquots IA	Prevent/treat local spasm
Adenosine diphosphate receptor antagonists		Platelet inhibition
Clopidogrel	300 mg PO loading dose 2-3 hr before procedure, then 75 mg daily for 1-3 mo	
Aspirin	325 mg PO	Platelet inhibition
Glycoprotein IIb/IIIa antagonists	12-24 hr infusion IV	Prevent platelet aggregation
Abciximab	0.25 mg/kg bolus, then 0.125 µg/kg/min (max. 10 mg/min)	
Eptifibatide	180 µg/kg bolus, then 0.5 µg/kg/min	
Tirofiban	0.4 µg/kg/min for 30 min, then 0.1 µg/kg/min	

IA, Intraarterial; IV, intravenous; PO, by mouth.

Box 4-2. Crossing the Lesion

Be sure of lesion morphology
Choose optimal obliquity
Use "roadmap" fluoroscopy
Start slowly and gently
Use atraumatic tools
Redirect rather than push harder
Spiral or "barber pole" trajectory of guidewire frequently indicates subintimal location

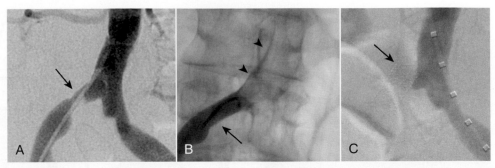

Figure 4-3. The importance of confirming an intraluminal location after crossing a stenosis. **A,** Pelvic angiogram showing a tight stenosis *(arrow)* of the proximal right common iliac artery. Guidewire access across the lesion was lost briefly after this angiogram. The lesion was recrossed, but a test injection was not performed before stenting. **B,** Retrograde injection of contrast after stent placement *(arrow)* shows an occlusion of the common iliac artery proximal to the stent and subintimal contrast *(arrowheads)* outlining the infrarenal aorta. **C,** Aortogram showing the subintimal location of the stent *(arrow)* and right common iliac artery occlusion.

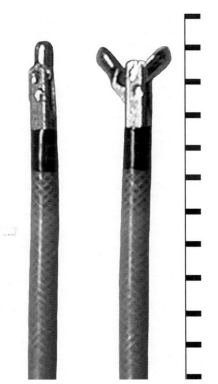

Figure 4-4. Device used for intravascular blunt dissection through firm arterial occlusions. The device is pushed when closed against the occlusion, and then opened to create a channel. *Left*, device in closed position. *Right*, opened device. The scale on the right is in millimeters. (Courtesy Frontrunner, Cordis Corp, Warren, N.J.)

around the lesion. The guidewire spontaneously reenters the true lumen distally at the interface of the plaque and normal intima in approximately two thirds of the procedures. This may occur well distal to the actual obstruction. When spontaneous reentry does not occur, specialized devices can puncture back into the lumen (Fig. 4-6). At centers experienced with the technique, failure to successfully reenter the true lumen is reported in about 10% of cases.

After confirming successful navigation across the lesion by aspirating blood or injecting contrast, a working guidewire is advanced through the catheter to provide stability for the intervention. In general, relatively stiff guidewires are used that allow devices to be advanced into position without losing access across the lesion. These are available in a range of lengths and diameters, including as small as 0.010-inch diameter. Hydrophilic coated guidewires

are usually not a good choice for working wires, because they easily slip out of place during catheter exchanges.

Accurate device sizing (e.g., for balloons, stents, or stent-grafts) requires consideration of several factors (Box 4-3). Oversizing of device diameters by 5%-10% greater than the diameter of the normal lumen is the general rule. Very tight or calcified lesions may require progressive dilation with sequentially larger balloons. The final desired diameter of a blood vessel is determined from an adjacent normal segment of vessel, the same vessel on the other side of the body in the case of bilateral structures or the known average size of the vessel (i.e., "rule of thumb" technique) (Fig. 4-7). When measuring directly from images, it is helpful to calibrate to a known internal standard such as a marker catheter or guidewire, but this method is not always accurate. Many digital units include electronic measuring software. Intravascular ultrasound can be used to obtain direct measurements. The vessel and the type of lesion also impact sizing, in that veins are usually more compliant, whereas heavily calcified arteries may fracture when overdilated.

The length of the device should be sufficient to treat the diseased area, with minimal trauma to adjacent normal or slightly diseased vessels. When the area of disease to be treated extends up to or across a bifurcation into a smaller diameter vessel, the device should be sized or delivered in a manner that avoids trauma to the smaller or normal vessel. (See Balloon Angioplasty.)

The optimal clinical outcome of revascularization procedures is durable improvement of the patient's symptoms. Because the clinical outcome cannot always be measured during a procedure, most interventionalists use technical endpoints such as a residual luminal stenosis of less than 20% or reduction of the pressure gradient across the lesion to a predetermined level. Pressure gradients across lesions are a very useful means of deciding when to perform and when to stop a procedure. Reliance upon angiographic appearance as the sole indication for intervention leads to treating the image not the patient. Pressures are measured intravascularly, both proximal and distal to the lesion (Table 4-3). The most accurate systems obtain simultaneous pressures using two end-hole catheters or an end-hole catheter and a sheath (Fig. 4-8). A quick approach is to withdraw a catheter through the lesion while continuously recording pressures, but the patient's baseline pressure could change during this process. In many instances a catheter must be through the lesion of interest in order to obtain a distal pressure, such as in the renal artery. If the lesion is tight, the catheter itself accentuates the severity of the gradient by partially obstructing the lumen. Specialized pressure-sensing guidewires may be useful in these cases, but in general most interventionalists believe that any symptomatic lesion tight enough to be partially obstructed by an angiographic catheter requires treatment. When in doubt, injection of 200-300 µg of nitroglycerin or another vasodilator through a catheter distal to the lesion may

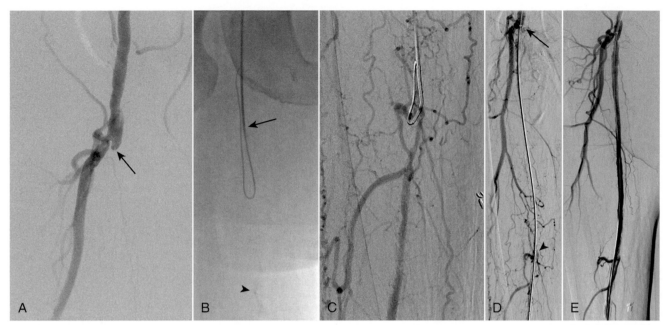

FIGURE **4-5**. Subintimal recanalization of a chronically occluded superficial femoral artery (SFA). **A,** Anterior oblique angiogram of the right common femoral artery (CFA) showing a smooth, chronic appearing occlusion of the SFA *(arrow)*. **B,** Loop of guidewire in the subintimal space, supported by a 5-French catheter *(arrow)*. Intimal calcification *(arrowhead)* can be seen more distal in the SFA. **C,** The subintimal wire and catheter in the distal SFA, just before reentry into the true lumen. Contrast was injected from a sheath in the CFA. **D,** Angiogram of the SFA through the sheath in the CFA *(arrow)* after reentry into the true lumen *(arrowhead)* showing the length of the occlusion. **E,** Angiogram after angioplasty of the entire SFA. The SFA was subsequently stented with self-expanding bare metal stents.

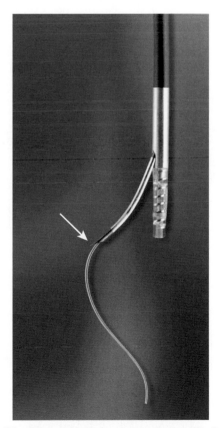

FIGURE **4-6**. The Outback Catheter reentry device. The hollow curved needle *(arrow)* is used to puncture from one lumen to the other, through which a guidewire can be advanced into the newly entered lumen. (Courtesy Cordis Corp., Warren, N.J., modified with permission.)

Box 4-3. Factors to Consider When Sizing Balloons, Stents, and Stent-Grafts

DELIVERY SYSTEM CHARACTERISTICS
Catheter size
Sheath size
Flexibility of device

LESION CHARACTERISTICS
Type of vessel
Type of lesion
Initial lumen diameter
Diameter of vessel over length of lesion
Desired final diameter
Length of vessel to be treated

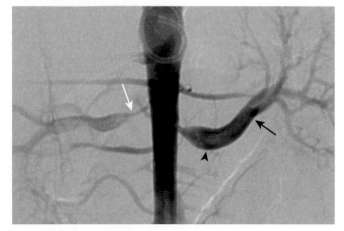

FIGURE **4-7**. Poststenotic dilation *(black arrowhead)* due to left renal artery stenosis in a 5-year-old with neurofibromatosis. The distal left renal artery approaches the normal diameter *(black arrow)*. The right renal artery stenosis *(white arrow)* is so tight that the remainder of the right renal artery (also with post-stenotic dilation) is barely opacified. The infrarenal aorta is slightly narrowed as well.

induce hyperemia and unmask a gradient. Technical success and clinical success do not always coincide; pushing an intervention to an extreme to obtain an ideal image or perfect gradient risks harming the patient (see Fig. 4-8).

The guidewire should remain across the lesion until success has been documented. When appropriate, the status of the vessels distal to or proximal to the intervention should be reevalu-

TABLE 4-3 Acceptable Postintervention Pressure Gradients (mm Hg)*

Anatomic Region	Parameter	At Rest	Augmented[†]
Arterial	Systolic	≤10	≤15
Venous	Mean	≤5	NA
TIPS[‡]	Mean	≤12	NA

*Patient supine.
[†]Following injection of 200-300 µg of nitroglycerin or 15-25 mg tolazoline distal to lesion.
[‡]Transjugular intrahepatic portosystemic shunt, portal to inferior vena cava gradient for patient with variceal bleeding. For ascites, a 50% decrease from the initial gradient is preferable.

ated as well. Clinical follow-up tailored to the intervention should be performed by the interventional radiologist.

Procedural complications associated with opening of blood vessels are related to the patient's general status, the difficulty of the procedure, the size and type of the device, the underlying condition of the vessels, and the intensity of anticoagulation (Box 4-4). Older patients with acute illnesses, diffuse vascular disease, and concurrent major illnesses are most likely to experience a complication. Large complex devices have more complications than small simple devices.

Failure (i.e., return of symptoms) of revascularization procedures occurs for different reasons at different times (Table 4-4). Most early failures are due to technical issues such as an occlusive dissection adjacent to the intervention site that impedes flow, elastic recoil of a fibrotic lesion, or perhaps a missed lesion that continues to impair flow. Hypercoagulable syndromes, episodes of hypotension, or other low-flow states can result in acute thrombosis at arterial or venous intervention sites at any time. After approximately 3 months, and up to 1 year from the intervention, intimal hyperplasia is the main cause of failure. The degree of intimal hyperplasia that occurs after an intervention is dependent upon the biology of the vessel and the extent of the trauma to the endothelium (see Fig. 1-8). In general, the more extensive the area that is treated, the higher the likelihood that intimal

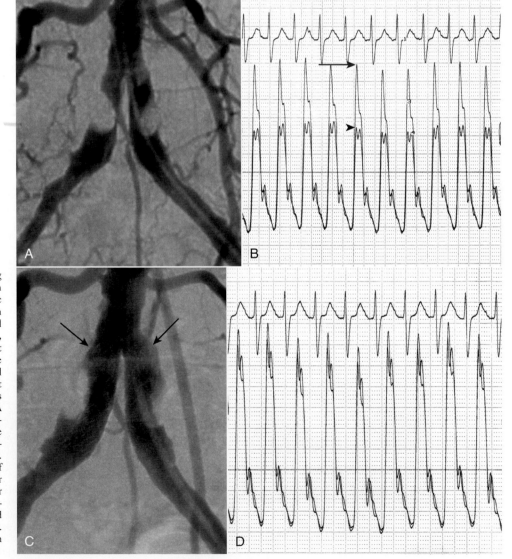

FIGURE 4-8. Pressure gradients during an intervention. **A,** Pelvic angiogram showing eccentric bilateral common iliac artery (CIA) stenoses, right worse than left. These were heavily calcified, and the patient was a high surgical risk. **B,** Simultaneous pressures reveal a gradient (44 mm Hg) between a catheter in the aorta and a catheter in the left external iliac artery (EIA). A 57 mm Hg gradient was present on the right. *Arrow* shows aortic pressure; *arrowhead* shows left EIA pressure. **C,** Pelvic angiogram after placement of bilateral balloon-expandable CIA stents *(arrows)*. Note that the eccentric plaque is still present on both sides. The patient had notable pain (7 out of 10) with balloon inflation, so the operator did not try to dilate the stents further for fear of rupturing an artery. **D,** Final pressure measurements show superimposed aortic and left EIA pressure tracings. There was also no residual gradient on the right.

hyperplasia will be a problem. Restenosis occurs in or adjacent to the original lesion. Drug-eluting balloons, drug-eluting stents, and stent-grafts show promise for improved long-term clinical success rates in various vascular applications. There is evidence suggesting that antiplatelet and statin therapies may reduce restenosis rates following peripheral arterial interventions. After 1 year, failure of a revascularization procedure is more likely to be due to progression of the original disease in the inflow or outflow vessels. Factors such as smoking, diet, hyperlipidemia, and homocysteinemia contribute to late failure of arterial interventions.

Balloon Angioplasty

The primary mechanism of arterial balloon angioplasty is controlled fracture of the obstructing plaque (Fig. 4-9). This results in formation of fissures in the plaque itself, and tearing of the edges of the plaque away from the adjacent normal intima. With proper oversizing of the balloon, the muscular media is stretched as well. Plaque is not remodeled, redistributed, or vaporized by the balloon. Distal embolization of microscopic and, occasionally, macroscopic debris does occur but is usually asymptomatic. Visualization of "cracks" or small dissections in lesions following angioplasty is a normal finding at angiography (Fig. 4-10). Over time these areas may remodel and the lumen resume a more normal appearance. Venous lesions, which are usually fibrotic, are primarily stretched during angioplasty.

Andreas Gruentzig performed the first successful balloon angioplasty in 1977. Since then, the technology of balloons has become very complex, but in practical terms it can be divided into compliant and noncompliant devices (Fig. 4-11). Compliant balloons are constructed from material that continues to stretch as pressure is applied, allowing the balloon to expand until the

point of rupture. Compliant balloons conform to the vessel walls rather than dilate. This type of balloon is most commonly used to temporarily occlude flow or sweep away thrombus during a balloon thrombectomy.

Noncompliant balloons reach a nominal predetermined diameter during inflation and remain close to that diameter as pressure is increased to the bursting point (many of these balloons actually increase slightly in diameter as pressure increases). During inflation, a waist is visualized in the balloon at the site of maximal stenosis (Fig. 4-12). Continued inflation of the balloon ultimately obliterates the waist, often suddenly. Noncompliant balloons are desirable for angioplasty; otherwise the balloon expands on either side of the waist without dilating the stenosis. Very high pressure noncompliant balloons (up to 30 atm) are used in venous and nonvascular applications, whereas lower pressure balloons are used in arterial lesions. However, some lesions cannot be dilated no matter how much pressure is applied. In this situation, balloon rupture may occur. Burst pressures are included on the packaging of all balloons.

The balloon material and construction determine the burst pressure. A balloon that ruptures before the lesion is fully dilated is of little value, but a balloon that is so strong that the vessel ruptures first is potentially dangerous. Balloons are designed to split longitudinally to minimize damage to the vessel wall and facilitate removal (Fig. 4-13).

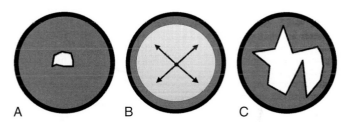

FIGURE 4-9. Schematic of the mechanism of angioplasty. **A,** Concentric stenosis with a small residual lumen. **B,** An appropriately sized angioplasty balloon is inflated *(arrows)* in the lumen. **C,** Fracturing, fissuring, and subintimal dissection of the plaque greatly increase the cross-sectional area of the lumen.

Box 4-4. Complications of Revascularization Procedures

Vessel spasm
Intimal dissection
Occlusion of branch vessels
Thrombosis
Embolization
 • Atheromatous plaque
 • Thrombus
 • Cholesterol
Vessel rupture
Access site hemorrhage
Remote hemorrhage

TABLE 4-4 Causes of Failure of Arterial Recanalization Procedures

Etiology	0-30 days	30-60 days	3-12 months	>12 months
Occlusive dissection	×			
Elastic recoil	×			
Thrombosis	×			
Inadequate dilation	×	×		
Missed lesion	×	×	×	
Intimal hyperplasia			×	
Progressive atherosclerosis				×
Kinked or crushed stent	×	×	×	×

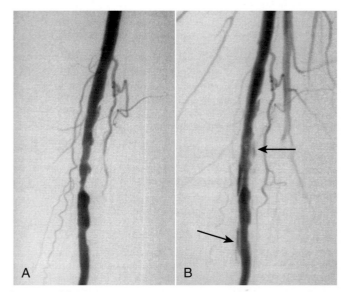

FIGURE 4-10. Normal angiographic appearance of an artery following angioplasty. **A,** Diseased segment of superficial femoral artery. **B,** After angioplasty with a 5-mm balloon, there is fissuring *(arrows)* of the plaque. This is a normal post-angioplasty appearance and requires no further intervention unless it is flow-limiting.

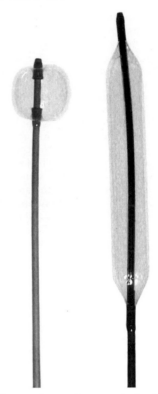

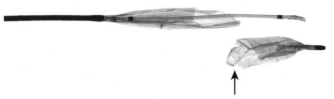

FIGURE 4-13. Danger of transverse rather than longitudinal balloon rupture. This balloon split circumferentially. The distal portion *(arrow)* detached from the catheter in the vascular system during attempted extraction because the balloon membrane mushroomed and jammed against the tip of the sheath.

TABLE 4-5 Typical Angioplasty Balloon Sizes*

Vessel†	Balloon Diameter (mm)	Balloon Length (cm)
Internal carotid artery (cervical)	5-6	2-4
Subclavian artery	6-7	2-4
Abdominal aorta	10-16	2-4
Superior mesenteric/celiac artery	6-7	2-4
Renal artery	5-6	2-4
Common iliac artery	8-10	2-4
External iliac artery	6-7	2-4
Superficial femoral artery	5-6	2-20
Popliteal artery	4-5	2-6
Tibial artery	2-4	2-20
Pedal artery	1.5-2	2-15
Superior vena cava	10-18	4-6
Subclavian/brachiocephalic vein	8-16	4-6
Brachial/basilic veins	6-10	2-4
Iliac veins	8-16	4-6

*These sizes serve as a rough guide; measurements from reliable imaging should always be used when possible for selection of balloon dimensions.
†There is a greater range of diameters for veins.

FIGURE 4-11. Balloon catheters. Latex occlusion balloon *(left);* 8-mm diameter angioplasty balloon on a 5-French shaft *(right).* The occlusion balloon is compliant and responds to increased pressure by enlarging. The angioplasty balloon is relatively noncompliant and reaches a fixed diameter and shape. Increased pressure may slightly increase the diameter, but primarily makes the balloon firmer. Note the short sloping "shoulders" at each end of the angioplasty balloon.

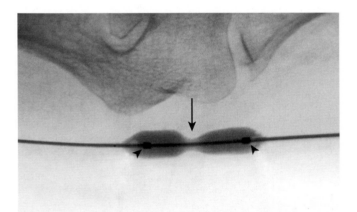

FIGURE 4-12. Typical appearance of a waist *(arrow)* in a balloon during an angioplasty (in this case dilation of a fibrotic venous lesion). Note the radiopaque markers *(arrowheads)* on the balloon catheter that help in positioning the device. Disappearance of the waist is suggestive of successful angioplasty.

> ### *Box 4-5.* Angioplasty Tips
>
> Size balloon conservatively
> Give heparin or other anticoagulant before crossing lesion
> Center balloon on the lesion
> Stabilize balloon at sheath during inflation
> Use dilute contrast for inflation
> Inflate with 10-mL Luer-lock syringe by hand or insufflation device
> Slow, steady inflation
> Deflate with 20-mL syringe
> Counterclockwise rotation during removal from sheath
> Maintain guidewire access across lesion until completely finished

---

Balloon diameters range from a millimeters to more than 4 cm, and lengths range from less than 1 cm to more than 20 cm. The vascular bed and lesion length influence the balloon choice (Table 4-5). When in doubt, undersize. An initially undersized balloon rarely causes a complication, and a larger balloon can always be used if the result is unsatisfactory. The reverse is not true for an initially oversized balloon. Because of the physics of balloons (tension = pressure × radius), the larger the balloon, the lower the necessary inflation pressure.

The balloon material is not radiopaque. To aid in positioning of the balloon, metallic rings are placed on the catheter at both ends of the balloon (see Fig. 4-12, Box 4-5). Dilute contrast (1 part contrast to 2-3 parts flush solution) is used for inflation to allow visualization of the balloon–lesion interaction and facilitate rapid deflation. Centering the balloon on the lesion maximizes stability during inflation and force transmitted to the lesion. During inflation, the ends of the balloon inflate first, so-called "dog-boning," followed by "popping" the waist (see Fig. 4-12). Soft lesions

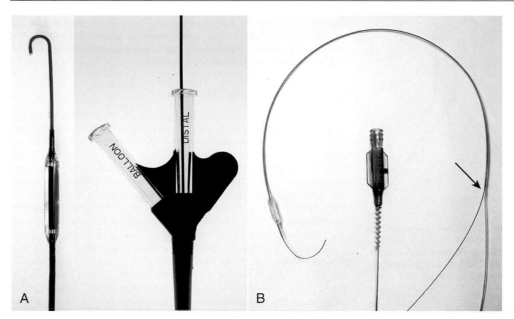

FIGURE **4-14**. Interventional devices can be either over-the-wire or rapid exchange. **A,** The distal and proximal ends of an over-the-wire angioplasty balloon. Note the separate access points for the guidewire ("Distal") and balloon lumens at the hub. A guidewire is in place. **B,** The distal and proximal ends of a rapid exchange angioplasty balloon. The guidewire exits the catheter *(arrow)* near the balloon end, so only a small portion of this 150 cm long catheter travels over the guidewire. The single access at the hub is only for the balloon.

dilate with relatively little pressure. Calcified or fibrotic lesions may require substantial pressure and may never fully dilate. Inflation should be gradual, in that rapid, explosive dilation results in greater trauma to the adjacent normal vessel. In the hands of most humans, a 10-mL Luer-lock syringe can maximally generate 10-12 atm, which is sufficient to dilate the majority of arterial lesions. A mechanical inflation device or a smaller syringe (5 or 3 mL) can be used to generate the higher pressures sometimes needed for fibrotic or venous lesions. Balloons are kept inflated for 20-120 seconds depending on the lesion, the vessel, and the degree of anticoagulation. The patient should be asked about discomfort during inflation. Total lack of sensation on the patient's part implies an undersized balloon (provided there is normal vascular innervation). Mild pressure or pain indicates stretching of the adventitia and a properly oversized balloon. Intense, severe, or sharp pain suggests overdilation with possible dissection or rupture of the blood vessel. To minimize trauma, balloons should not be moved back and forth through the lesion while inflated. Short balloons have a tendency squirt out of a lesion during inflation (similar to pinching a wet watermelon seed). This can be prevented by stabilizing the balloon shaft at the diaphragm of the sheath and using a longer balloon. Deflation of the balloon with a 20-mL syringe is quicker and more complete than with a 10-mL syringe. Rapid deflation is desirable to restore flow as quickly as possible.

Angioplasty balloons are mounted on angiographic catheters, usually with two lumens: one for a guidewire and one for balloon inflation/deflation. The back end of the standard over-the-wire balloon catheter usually has two separate Luer-lock hubs, one for the central guidewire lumen and one for balloon inflation. Balloons mounted on 3- or 4-French catheters have the smallest overall insertion profiles, require 0.018 inch or smaller guidewires, and can be inserted through 4- or 5-French sheaths. Rapid exchange balloon catheters have two lumens in the distal portion of the catheter, with the shorter guidewire lumen exiting the side of the catheter (Fig. 4-14). The balloon lumen continues for the entire length of the catheter, ending in single Luer hub. This allows for lower catheter profiles and insertion of a long catheter over a standard length guidewire, because the majority of the catheter slides alongside the guidewire, not over it.

When removing a balloon through a sheath, resistance may be encountered because the deflated balloon does not return to its original low profile. Continued aspiration and counterclockwise rotation as the catheter is withdrawn into the sheath rewraps the balloon around the shaft and facilitates removal.

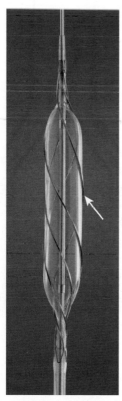

FIGURE **4-15**. Scoring balloon for controlled plaque disruption during angioplasty. The metallic elements *(arrow)* are pushed against the plaque during balloon inflation. (Courtesy AngioScore Inc., Freemont, Calif., modified with permission.)

Several enhanced angioplasty balloons are available. Cutting and sculpting balloons use small longitudinal blades on the balloon surface or a metallic cage on the outside of the balloon to create controlled splitting rather than random plaque fractures (Fig. 4-15). This may enable successful angioplasty of tough, fibrotic lesions. Cryoplasty, in which liquid nitrogen is used to inflate a specially designed balloon, results in apoptosis of smooth muscle cells in the media. Angioplasty balloons are increasingly used to deliver drugs or gene therapy vectors directly to lesions.

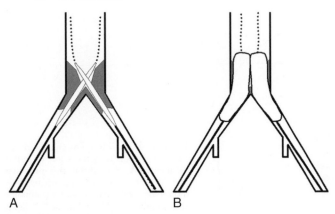

Figure 4-16. Schematic of kissing balloons. **A,** Balloon dilation of a lesion that extends from a larger vessel (the aorta) into two smaller branches (the common iliac arteries). Each balloon is sized for the common iliac artery lesion, not the aortic lesion. **B,** The balloons are inflated simultaneously, individually dilating the common iliac arteries and dilating the aorta as a pair.

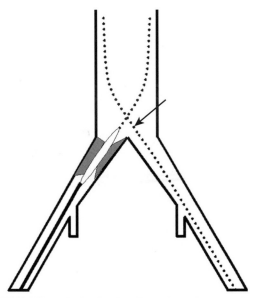

Figure 4-17. When a lesion involves the ostium of one vessel at a bifurcation, a safety wire *(arrow)* should be placed in the normal vessel during the intervention to preserve access in case a dissection extends across the bifurcation. Alternatively, a smaller balloon can be inflated simultaneously in the normal vessel.

Angioplasty of lesions that involve or are close to a vascular bifurcation can be challenging because of the size discrepancy of the lumens proximal and distal to the branch point. Simultaneous inflation of two balloons across the branch point, each sized to the diameter of the vessel distal to the branch, prevents complications at the vessel origins (Fig. 4-16). This is known as the "kissing balloon" technique and is also used with stent deployment. In some cases the lesion in the branch is close to, but does not involve, the vessel origin. Rather than insert a second balloon, a "safety wire" in the uninvolved vessel can be used to preserve access in case a complication (e.g., origin dissection) occurs (Fig. 4-17).

Specific complication rates for angioplasty of each anatomic area will be found in later chapters. One of the most potentially devastating generic complications is vascular rupture (Fig. 4-18). Patients complain of severe pain persisting after deflation of the balloon, which may be accompanied by hypotension and tachycardia. Immediate reinflation of the balloon across or proximal to the lesion is a life-saving maneuver (Box 4-6). Prolonged balloon inflation, reversal of anticoagulation, stent-graft placement, or urgent surgical repair (see later) may be required to stop the bleeding. The risk of vessel rupture during revascularization procedures, however, is much less than 1%.

Embolic Protection Devices

Particulate embolization likely occurs with all revascularization procedures, but it is clinically silent in most cases. In some vascular beds, such as the kidneys, the manifestations of particulate embolization may be subtle, such as a blunted or paradoxical clinical response to the intervention. The risk of clinically apparent embolization is highest with interventions in diseased arteries. Embolization of plaque elements is termed "cholesterol" embolization (Box 4-7). This can occur as chunks of plaque (macroembolization) or cholesterol crystals (microembolization). Macroembolization results in acute occlusion of branch arteries with acute ischemia. Cholesterol crystals are mobilized during procedures by unroofing lipid-rich plaques and can continue to shower for days to weeks. Crystalline emboli lodged in arterioles are not angiographically visible, cause localized ischemia, and incite a painful inflammatory reaction in addition to the occlusion that can ultimately lead to tissue ischemia and necrosis (see Fig. 1-34). The overall incidence of cholesterol embolization is less than 1%, with patients with extensive atheromatous disease or friable plaques at greatest risk. Amputation, permanent renal failure, bowel ischemia, stroke, and death are all potential outcomes of cholesterol embolization.

Protection devices have been developed to minimize the risk of particulate embolization (Fig. 4-19). The clinical drivers for these devices were originally coronary saphenous vein bypass and carotid artery interventions, but application to renal and other peripheral arterial interventions are being evaluated. There are three basic types: distal filters, distal occlusion balloons, and proximal occlusion balloons with or without flow reversal. Filter and distal occlusion balloons are advanced through the lesion on a guidewire before the intervention and then must be recovered afterward. The filtration devices have pore sizes from 80 to about 200 μm and permit continued antegrade flow of blood during the procedure unless a large volume of debris is collected. One limitation of filters is that small debris can pass through the filter. Distal occlusion balloons prevent all emboli while inflated, but do not allow any antegrade flow during the procedure and rely on complete aspiration of debris to prevent emboli after deflation. Proximal occlusion devices also prevent antegrade flow, but usually rely on reversal of flow rather than aspiration to remove debris. The efficacy of these devices in peripheral interventions is under evaluation.

Stents

Stents provide an intravascular scaffold for the vessel lumen. The mechanism of action of stents is very different from angioplasty, in that the plaque and vessel wall are literally pushed aside by the stent to enlarge the lumen (Figs. 4-8 and 4-20). Many different stents are available, but not all are approved for vascular use in the United States (Figs. 4-21 and 4-22). Many stents are approved and labeled as biliary or tracheal stents. The off-label use of stents in blood vessels is ubiquitous but not officially promoted by manufacturers.

The metal used to make the stent as well as the manufacturing technique have a major impact on the clinical performance of the device (Table 4-6). The typical metals used are stainless steel (iron and chromium), nitinol (nickel and titanium), and Elgiloy (cobalt, chromium, nickel, and molybdenum). The latter two metals are not ferromagnetic and therefore do not cause artifacts on magnetic resonance imaging. Stents are categorized as either *balloon-expandable* (deployed by inflating an angioplasty balloon) or *self-expanding* (deployed by releasing a constraining

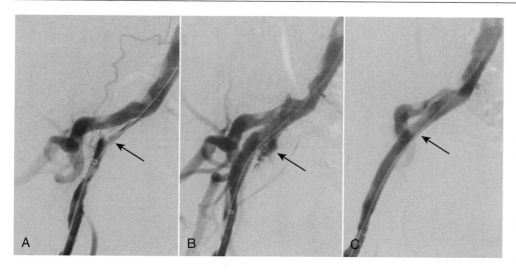

FIGURE **4-18**. External iliac artery (EIA) rupture during stent placement. **A,** DSA of the right EIA *(arrow)* before stent placement showing a diffusely diseased artery. **B,** After placement of a balloon-expandable bare metal stent, the patient complained of pain in the right groin. There is extravasation of contrast *(arrow)* from the EIA. **C,** DSA after placement of a covered stent *(arrow)* within the bare stent and extending distally shows that the extravasation has resolved. The patient's pain resolved as well.

Box 4-6. Arterial Rupture During Angioplasty/Stent Placement

SYMPTOMS
Severe pain during balloon inflation, persists after balloon deflation
Hypotension
Tachycardia

MANAGEMENT
Maintain access across lesion with guidewire!
Check vital signs
If stable blood pressure/pulse, inject contrast and localize extravasation
If hemodynamically unstable, reinflated balloon across or proximal to lesion
Fluid resuscitation
Percutaneous stent-graft or surgical repair

Box 4-7. Cholesterol Embolization

CLINICAL FINDINGS
Livido reticularis
Blue toe syndrome
Bowel/renal ischemia
Transient ischemic attack/stroke (ascending and arch aortic source)

LABORATORY FINDINGS
Progressive renal failure
Eosinophilia (urine and serum)

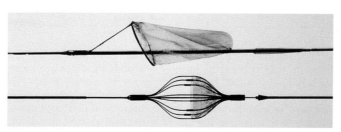

FIGURE **4-19**. Distal embolic protection devices based on microporous filters, both on 0.014-inch wires. (*Top,* MicroFilterWire EZ, Boston Scientific, Natick, Mass. *Bottom,* Angioguard XP, Cordis Corp, Warren, N.J.)

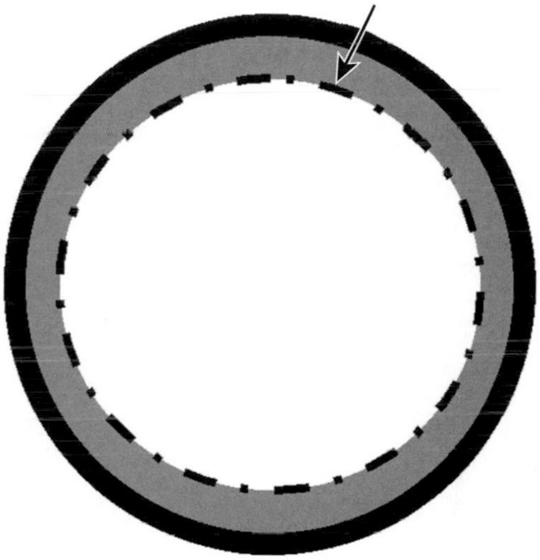

FIGURE **4-20**. Schematic representation of a deployed stent *(arrow).* Compare with the postangioplasty lumen depicted in Figure 4-9.

mechanism). Stents are further categorized as *closed* or *open-celled.* Open-celled stents are the most flexible, but can "shingle" or "fish scale" when deployed in tight curves or over irregular lesions. Most stents are manufactured from small diameter tubes of metal that are cut in a proprietary pattern with a laser to create an expandable device, with the type depending on the properties of the metal. Self-expanding stents may also be made from wire woven or sewn together. Nitinol has thermal memory, so that it is soft and flexible at room temperature but becomes rigid and resumes a predetermined shape and size at body temperature. This property is useful for self-expanding intravascular devices.

Stent design greatly influences clinical use. Balloon-expandable stents are deployed by applying force from within (usually with an angioplasty balloon), and they resist vessel wall elastic recoil. However, they will not reexpand spontaneously if the resistance is temporarily overcome (i.e., the stent remains collapsed). Self-expanding stents attempt to reach a predetermined diameter unless continuously and externally constrained. Although not as resistant to elastic recoil as balloon-expandable stents, self-expanding stents reexpand spontaneously if compressed. This is desirable in superficial locations, such as the cervical carotid artery and superficial femoral artery.

Drug-eluting or releasing stents are a class of devices that combine the mechanical properties of a stent with the ability to locally

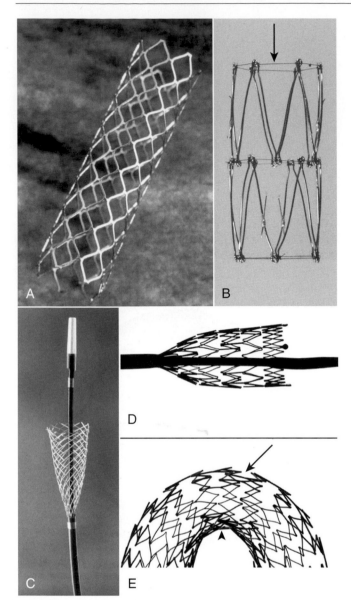

FIGURE **4-21**. Examples of metallic stents. **A,** Balloon-expandable stent. **B,** Self-expanding Gianturco-Rösch stainless steel Z-stents. Note sutures *(arrow)* constraining stents. **C,** Self-expanding woven stainless steel Wall-stent **D,** Self-expanding laser-cut nitinol Zilver stent. **E,** Open-cell self-expanding stent in a tight curve to accentuate the opening of cells on the outer curve *(arrow)* and compression of stent elements ("shingling") on the inner curve *(arrowhead)*. (**A,** Courtesy Cordis Corp., Warren, N.J.; **B** and **D,** courtesy Cook Group, Bloomington, Ind.; **C,** courtesy Boston Scientific, Natick, Mass.)

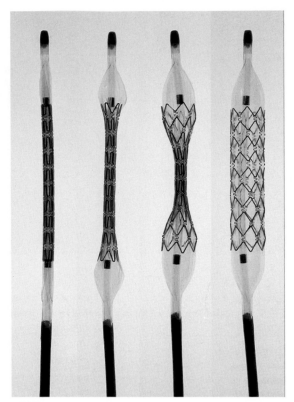

FIGURE **4-22**. Stages of balloon-expandable stent deployment, from left to right. The stent expands first at both ends; the central portion opens last (compare to the angioplasty balloon in a stenosis in Fig. 4-12). Note slight decrease in overall length of the stent with full expansion compared to the markers on the balloon catheter. (Courtesy Genesis, Cordis Corp, Warren, N.J.)

TABLE 4-6 Stent Features

Feature	Variables
Metal	Stainless steel, nitinol, Elgiloy, tantalum, platinum
Construction	Laser-cut, welded, woven, wire spring, sutured
Deployment	Balloon-expanded, elastic recoil, thermal memory
Precision of deployment	Stent design, deployment technique
Hoop strength	Stent design, type of metal
Flexibility	Stent design, construction, type of metal
Radiopacity	Type of metal, coatings, markers
Sizes	Diameter and length before and after deployment
Drug eluting	For example, paclitaxel heparin, dexamethasone
Delivery system	French size, flexibility, guidewire requirements
Regulatory status	Government approval for vascular and nonvascular use

deliver drugs to prevent restenosis. There are several strategies for bonding drugs to stents, including applying polymer coatings on the surface or microscopic "wells" in the stent metal. These devices were used initially in coronary arteries but are now being applied in the peripheral arteries. Using polymer and metal stents that dissolve over time is another approach to reducing restenosis.

The indications for stent placement depend on patient- and lesion-specific factors as well as the preference of the operator (Box 4-8). In practice, the tendency is to place a stent as the first intervention without trying to optimize the result of angioplasty ("primary stenting"). Although expensive (stents can cost more than $1000 each), a good initial result is obtained quickly and with greater certainty. Nevertheless, in many instances it is wise to attempt angioplasty first, reserving stents for failed or recurrent lesions. This is especially true in heavily calcified lesions that

may not respond to angioplasty, let alone stent placement. The long-term results of stents in most anatomic locations are better than angioplasty alone, but sometimes not by a great amount. In certain conditions, such as fibromuscular dysplasia, stents do not seem to offer any advantage over angioplasty, and therefore should probably be reserved to salvage failed angioplasty. Stents should not be placed at sites of anticipated surgical anastomoses, because the presence of the device may complicate surgery or render it impossible. Anticoagulation (e.g., heparin or bivalirudin bolus)

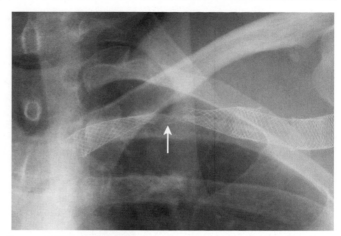

FIGURE 4-23. Fracture of a Wallstent *(arrow)* placed in the subclavian vein for venous thoracic outlet syndrome without first rib resection. Chronic compression between the clavicle and first rib has destroyed the metallic stent.

TABLE 4-7 Complications Unique to Stent Placement

Complication	Etiology	Prevention
Stent loose on balloon during delivery	Loose crimp	Tight crimp, correct balloon size, slight positive pressure in balloon after mounting
Stent embolization after deployment	Undersized stent	Oversize stent 5%-10% in diameter
Stent will not expand lesion	Nondilatable or fibrotic lesion	Test with angioplasty balloon before deploying stent; use stent with high hoop strength
Stent kinks in lesion after deployment	Angled vessel	Use flexible self-expanding stent

should be used during stent placement. A 1- to 3-month course of antiplatelet therapy (aspirin, clopidogrel, or both) is often prescribed following stent placement although efficacy in preventing restenosis in peripheral arteries has not been studied thoroughly.

The techniques for stent placement vary depending upon the device, but certain broad principles can be followed. Delivery over a guidewire is essential to maintain access through the stent after deployment. Predilation of very tight lesions with an angioplasty balloon ensures that the lesion is stretchable (i.e., can be treated with a stent), and makes positioning the device easier. However, primary stent placement reduces overall manipulation of the lesion with potentially fewer distal embolic complications. All stents should be long enough to cover the lesion, with minimal extension into normal areas of the vessel.

Balloon-expandable stents deploy from both ends toward the middle (see Fig. 4-22). These stents are sized in the same manner as angioplasty balloons, up to 5%-10% greater in diameter than the measured normal lumen. Balloon-expandable stents shorten slightly during expansion in proportion to the final diameter. This shortening can be dramatic if the stent is markedly overdilated. When mounting a stent on a balloon by hand, careful crimping in a radial fashion (not twisting) is necessary to prevent dislodgment of the balloon during delivery. The stent should not be longer than the working surface of the balloon (i.e., the distance between the radiopaque marker bands on the catheter shaft inside the balloon). When placing a balloon-expandable stent, it may be necessary to first advance a long sheath or guiding catheter across the lesion so that the stent can be positioned without catching on plaque. Premounted balloon-expandable stents with smooth polished edges that are firmly situated on a balloon can often be "bare-backed" through lesions that are not too tight or irregular. Small-diameter stents mounted on small-shafted balloons are surprisingly flexible and can negotiate tortuous vessels.

Self-expanding stents typically deploy from distal to proximal relative to the operator. The unconstrained diameter of the stent should be 10%-20% larger than the normal diameter of the target vessel because fixation depends on secure apposition of the stent to the vessel wall. Self-expanding stents are usually constrained by an outer sleeve or membrane (see Fig. 4-21). These devices do not necessarily require the protection of a long sheath or guiding catheter to advance through a lesion, but predilation of the lesion is useful. Radiopacity of the stent is crucial to aid in correct

placement and complete expansion. Most nitinol-based stents have highly radiopaque markers at the ends. Laser-cut nitinol-based stents have the least shortening during delivery, but are not reconstrainable like some woven stents. However, woven stents may shorten markedly because they are made small in diameter for insertion by being stretched out on the delivery catheter. Laser-cut self-expanding nitinol stents cannot be dilated beyond their resting maximum diameter. Woven stents have some capability to be dilated beyond their nominal resting diameter, but will shorten.

In general, a stent cannot do anything that an inflated balloon cannot (see Fig. 4-8). In other words, if the lesion cannot be dilated with a balloon, then a stent will not provide any additional benefit. When the primary abnormality is chronic extrinsic compression of the lumen by an extravascular structure, placement of a stent without first relieving the compression may result in stent fracture (Fig. 4-23).

Stent placement originally had a higher overall complication rate than angioplasty alone owing to the larger size of the first devices and more complex delivery. Complication rates have decreased dramatically as experience has increased and devices refined. In most cases the complication rates are probably lower than aggressive angioplasty, in that acceptable results are easily obtained with a stent whereas multiple balloon inflations would have been required in the past. The types of procedural complications are largely the same as for angioplasty. However, there are several that are unique to stent placement (Table 4-7). Early thrombosis of fully deployed stents is unusual unless runoff or inflow is compromised (see Fig. 4-3). Stent fracture can result when there is repetitive compression, torsion, or flexion of a

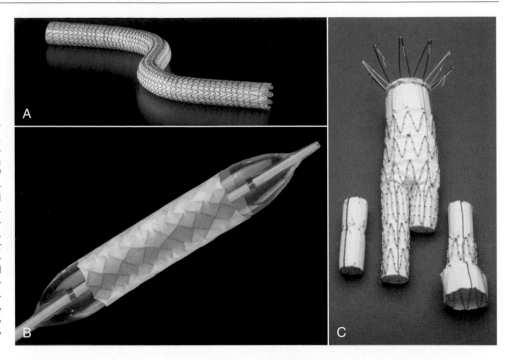

FIGURE 4-24. Examples of commercially available stent-grafts, fully expanded. These are delivered constrained on a catheter and expand within the vessel once released. **A,** The self-expanding GORE® VIABAHN® Endoprosthesis. The stent-graft is constructed from nitinol metal and expanded polytetrafluoroethylene (PTFE). **B,** The balloon-expandable iCAST stainless steel stent encapsulated in PTFE film. **C,** The Zenith bifurcated stent-graft for abdominal aortic aneurysms. The stent-graft is constructed from stainless steel and woven polyester. The modular components are assembled within the patient. (**A,** Image © 2009 W. L. Gore & Associates, Inc.; **B,** courtesy of Atrium Medical, Hudson, N.H.; **C,** Courtesy Cook Inc., Bloomington, Ind.)

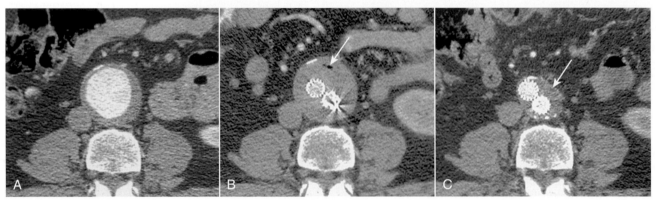

FIGURE 4-25. Stent-graft exclusion of an abdominal aortic aneurysm. **A,** Computed tomography (CT) scan before bifurcated stent-graft placement shows a patent aneurysm. **B,** CT scan at the same level 24 hours after stent-graft insertion. The lumen of the aneurysm is thrombosed. Note the air bubble *(arrow)* in the excluded aneurysm sac, a common early finding. **C,** CT scan 1 year later shows dramatic decrease in the diameter of the aneurysm *(arrow)*.

device (see Fig. 4-23). Fractures are thought to be associated with restenosis. Infection is rare but usually results in pseudoaneurysm formation around the stent.

Stent-Grafts

A stent-graft is a device constructed from a stent and a fabric that is inserted from a remote access using catheter techniques and image guidance. The stent anchors the graft in the blood vessel lumen and in most cases also provides structural support for the graft material. The graft material provides a conduit for blood flow. The first clinically successful stent-grafts were handmade by physicians by combining available stents and surgical vascular grafts. There are now a variety of specially designed and commercially manufactured stent-grafts (Fig. 4-24). These devices employ a range of metals, designs, and graft materials. Nitinol, stainless steel, and Elgiloy are commonly used to make the stents. The stents may be rigid or flexible, continuous or interrupted, and located inside, outside, or in a sandwich of graft material. The graft material may be synthetic, such as woven polyester or expanded polytetrafluoroethylene, or biological.

The function of a stent-graft varies with the application. In occlusive disease the stent-graft not only props the vessel open but also forms a physical barrier between the diseased intima and the lumen. When used to treat an aneurysm, the stent-graft provides a new flow channel and excludes the sac of the aneurysm from the circulation (Fig. 4-25). In the treatment of vascular injuries such as an acute arteriovenous fistula or pseudoaneurysm, the stent-graft seals over the hole in the wall of the vessel. In each of these cases, the basic principle is diversion of blood flow through the stent-graft. Therefore, in order to function, the stent-graft must fully appose the inner walls of the vessel at the attachment sites. Otherwise, blood will leak between the stent-graft and the intimal surface. This is a fundamental difference between stent-grafts and surgical grafts, which are sewn to the vessel wall.

The indications for stent-grafts are evolving as new devices and data become available (Box 4-9). Stent-grafts are considered a standard treatment for arterial aneurysms, particularly of the abdominal and thoracic aorta. The results of the transjugular intrahepatic portosystemic shunt procedure have been improved dramatically by stent-grafts. Recanalization of arterial occlusions, kissing common iliac artery stents, and long segment superficial femoral arterial disease are some of the peripheral arterial applications of stent-grafts.

The technique of stent-graft delivery is determined by the design of the stent, the graft material, and the size of the

CIA, Common iliac artery; SFA, superficial femoral artery.

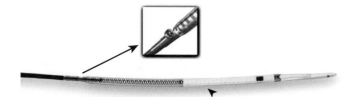

FIGURE **4-27**. Atherectomy device. Box shows the cutting blade. The strips of atheroma are collected in the long chamber *(arrowhead)* distal to the cutting orifice. (SilverHawk, courtesy of eV3 Endovascular, Plymouth, Minn.)

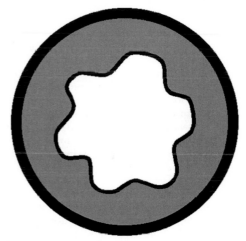

FIGURE **4-26**. Schematic representation of lesion following a debulking procedure. Compare with Figures 4-9 and 4-20.

delivery system. The very first clinical stent-grafts were based on balloon-expandable stents. Most devices are now self-expanding, although postplacement "tacking" with a balloon is common. In addition, gentle inflation of a balloon along the length of the device may be necessary to "iron" the graft material. Each device has its own specific delivery procedure. The size of the delivery system is determined by the amount of metal in the stent and the thickness of the graft material.

Intimal hyperplasia at the ends of the stent-graft remains a problem when used to treat occlusive disease. Thrombosis of stent-grafts is a risk when placed in small-diameter arteries or when there is slow flow. Strut fracture, dislodgment, kinking, or shifting of the stent-graft have been reported as late complications in treatment of large aneurysms. Infection is rare but often manifested by pseudoaneurysm formation at the ends of the stent-graft.

Debulking Atheroma

Angioplasty, stents, and stent-grafts increase the size of the vessel lumen by actions that do not change the volume of preexisting disease. An alternative approach is to debulk the obstruction by removing the plaque (Fig. 4-26). This is the basic principle of surgical endarterectomy, in which the vessel is incised and the plaque cored out. Doing the same thing with a catheter is challenging, as a large plaque cannot be easily removed in one piece. A variety

of devices have been invented that bite, bore, or blast the plaque using cutting blades, drills, and lasers (Fig. 4-27). Drills and lasers create a channel no larger than the diameter of the device itself, so that an additional intervention is almost always required. The long-term outcomes of these devices are difficult to separate from the subsequent angioplasty or stent placements. Cutting atherectomy catheters can be directed to remove sufficient volumes of plaque so that other interventions may not be necessary. Fibrotic lesions, lesions in anatomic areas not suitable for stent placement, or instances in which recovered material would be useful for pathologic diagnosis are some of the uses of tissue-extracting technologies. Atherectomy of long lesions in large vessels can be time-consuming. Heavily calcified lesions and severely tortuous arteries are difficult to treat.

Pharmacologic Thrombolysis

Thrombosis of a blood vessel rarely occurs in the absence of one or more of the following: an endothelial abnormality, a systemic abnormality of coagulation, or low flow (the "Virchow's triad"). Acute thrombosis is therefore the expression of one or more underlying problems. The goals of the interventional treatment of thrombosis are to relieve the acute obstruction and unmask the underlying etiology (Fig. 4-28).

The human body has an endogenous mechanism for lysis of thrombus (Fig. 4-29). The surgical approach to thrombus management is to open the vessel and pull or flush out the clot. Interventionalists employ both pharmacologic and mechanical tools when dealing with thrombus. This section discusses the pharmacologic approach, termed *thrombolysis*.

The native thrombolytic system can be enhanced by the administration of drugs that ultimately activate plasminogen. Although peripheral infusion of these drugs can accomplish this to some extent, catheter-directed drug delivery into the thrombus is the core principle of the interventional radiology approach to thrombolysis (like angioplasty, also an innovation of Charles Dotter). The thrombolytic infusion is performed over many hours and up to several days.

Streptokinase, derived from streptococcal bacteria, was the first thrombolytic drug available (Table 4-8). Streptokinase forms complexes with free plasminogen, and later plasmin, that in turn convert plasminogen to plasmin. Although inexpensive, streptokinase works slowly, so infusion times are long. Up to 14% of patients have allergic reactions because of sensitivity to streptococci. Urokinase was the second thrombolytic to become widely available. Urokinase is a non-antigenic substance produced by human renal tissue. A direct plasminogen activator with little fibrin specificity, thrombolysis with urokinase is faster (24-48 hr) than streptokinase and has fewer bleeding complications. Direct tissue plasminogen activators became popular for peripheral interventions in the late 1990s when urokinase was removed from the market for several years. These had previously been used primarily in coronary arteries. Recombinant tissue plasminogen activator alteplase (t-PA) and a derivative—reteplase (r-PA)—both have increased activity in the presence of fibrin (t-PA greater than r-PA). Theoretically this makes these agents

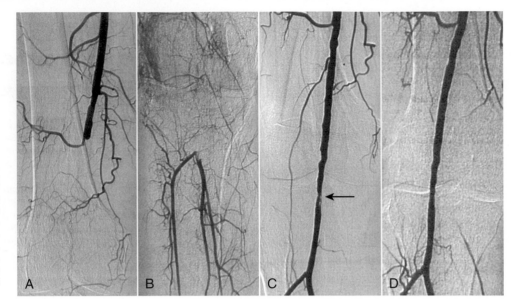

Figure 4-28. Thrombolysis of popliteal artery thrombosis. **A,** Popliteal artery occlusion in a patient with sudden increase in calf claudication. **B,** There is reconstitution of the tibial arteries. **C,** Following overnight thrombolysis, there is complete clearing of thrombus, which reveals a focal stenosis *(arrow)*. **D,** The lesion was dilated with a 5-mm balloon. (Case courtesy of Thomas Burdick, MD, Seattle, Wash.)

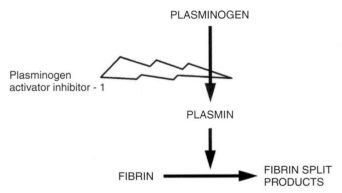

Figure 4-29. The final steps in the lytic pathway.

more thrombus-specific than urokinase or streptokinase. The duration of thrombolytic therapy with tissue plasminogen activators is usually short, in the range of 12-36 hours. Many additional agents have been studied, but few have reached clinical practice. The dosages of each agent vary based on the vascular bed, the volume of thrombus, and the method of delivery.

All thrombolytic agents ultimately result in dissolution and fragmentation of thrombus. The fresher the thrombus, the faster and more complete the thrombolysis. Chronic organized thrombus that has become fibrotic and endothelialized is less likely to be successfully thrombolysed. Inability to cross the thrombus with a guidewire is a rough predictor of unsuccessful thrombolysis. Mechanical disruption of the thrombus accelerates thrombolysis by exposing a larger surface area to the agent, leading to enhanced local activation of plasminogen.

Thrombolytic agents do not prevent formation of new thrombus or platelet aggregation. The smaller the vessel and the slower the flow, the more important it is that the patient be anticoagulated during the procedure. However, bleeding complications increase with anticoagulation. The dose of heparin varies with the thrombolytic agent. When urokinase is used, patients are fully heparinized to an activated partial thromboplastin time (aPTT) of 1.5 times normal. Smaller doses of heparin, such as 500 U/hr, are often used with t-PA and r-PA to offset the higher rate of bleeding complications with these agents.

The indications for catheter-directed thrombolysis in most vascular beds are acute or subacute thrombosis resulting in clinical symptoms that require urgent resolution (Box 4-10). There are

a few notable exceptions. Thrombosed dialysis grafts cause no immediate symptoms but require treatment. Occasionally a brief course of thrombolysis before angioplasty or stenting is employed when fresh thrombus is suspected in a chronic lesion.

Success of a thrombolytic procedure can be defined as technical, hemodynamic, or clinical. Technical success is restoration of prograde blood flow with less than 5% residual thrombus. Hemodynamic success is the return of the patient to the preocclusive vascular status. Clinical success is the relief of acute symptoms with return to baseline functional level. In peripheral arterial thrombolysis, amputation rates at 1 year are also an important measure of success.

The established contraindications to thrombolysis are generally related to bleeding in undesirable locations or the complications of revascularization of already dead tissue (Box 4-11). Thrombolytic drugs cannot distinguish between "good" thrombus, such as at an arterial access site, and "bad" thrombus in a stenosis. Already bleeding patients bleed more during thrombolysis. In addition, preexisting lesions (e.g., vascular brain metastases) that already have a tendency to bleed spontaneously are more likely to bleed during thrombolysis. Limbs or organs that are irreversibly ischemic should not undergo thrombolysis, because reperfusion of dead tissue may lead to severe metabolic disturbances *(reperfusion syndrome)*. Furthermore, vessels opened during thrombolysis that have no runoff do not stay open. Lastly, an uncooperative patient cannot undergo this procedure.

The two basic techniques for pharmacologic thrombolysis are drip infusion and pulse-spray. The essential feature of a drip infusion is to span the entire length of the thrombus with a catheter (Box 4-12). Most catheters are designed with multiple side-holes between two radio-opaque makers to facilitate positioning. The catheter(s) should be positioned so that the most proximal sidehole is just above the top of the thrombus, otherwise the distal clot will thrombolyse leaving an obstructing proximal plug (Fig. 4-30). Dosage is controversial, with passionate advocates for all regimens, but in general complications are fewer and results satisfactory using modest doses. Drip infusions usually require 12-48 hours depending on the drug (shorter with tissue plasminogen activators, longer with urokinase), so patients must be monitored in a controlled setting. In most hospitals, this is in an intensive care unit. When concurrent anticoagulation is used the aPTT should be followed during treatment. Daily hematocrit and serum creatinine should also be obtained. Fibrinogen levels and fibrin split products have little correlation with outcomes.

TABLE **4-8** Thrombolytic Agents

Agent	Trade Name	Description	Half-Life	Mechanism of Action
Streptokinase (SK)	Streptase	Derived from group-C β-hemolytic streptococci	20 min	Indirect; SK-plasminogen and plasmin complexes activate plasminogen; no fibrin specificity
Urokinase (UK)	Abbokinase	Derived from fetal kidney cells	14 min	Direct; no fibrin specificity
Recombinant urokinase	r-UK	Recombinant double-chain analogue of UK	7 min	Direct: no fibrin specificity
Recombinant pro-urokinase or single-chain UK-type plasminogen activator	Saruplase	Recombinant single-chain precursor of UK	7 min	Direct; fibrin-specific
Alteplase	Activase	Recombinant tissue plasminogen activator (527-unit amino acid chain)	5 min	Direct; moderate fibrin specificity
Reteplase	Retavase	Recombinant mutein of tissue plasminogen activator (355-unit amino acid chain)	15 min	Direct; low-fibrin specificity
TNK-tissue plasminogen activator	Tenecteplase	Modified recombinant mutein of tissue plasminogen activator	20 min	Direct; high-fibrin specificity; only agent resistant to inactivation by plasminogen activator inhibitor-1

Box 4-10. Vascular Indications for Thrombolysis

Arterial occlusions with viable extremity or organ*
Thrombotic occlusion of dialysis graft*
Conversion of thrombotic occlusion to stenosis before angioplasty or stent
Acute thrombotic stroke (anterior circulation < 6 hr; posterior circulation 12-24 hr)
Extensive deep venous thrombosis*
Massive pulmonary embolism*
Central venous access catheter malfunction

*<14 days old, but exceptions may be made in specific cases.

Box 4-11. Contraindications to Thrombolysis

Irreversible limb or organ ischemia
Active hemorrhage
Recent major surgery
Recent intraocular surgery/bleeding
Craniotomy within 2 months
Brain tumor (primary or metastatic)
Stroke within 6 months
History of spontaneous intracranial hemorrhage
Uncooperative or demented patient

Box 4-12. Catheter-Directed Thrombolysis

Position catheter system across entire length of thrombus
  • 5-French multiple side-hole catheter ± coaxial 3-French catheter
  • One side hole should be just proximal to top of thrombus
Infuse thrombolytic agent through each catheter
Dosage (empirical total hourly doses)*
  • Alteplase (rt-PA): 0.5-1 mg/hr
  • Reteplase (r-PA): 0.5-1 U/hr
  • Urokinase: 100,000 U/hr
Infuse with high-pressure mechanical pumps
Concurrent heparin and platelet inhibitor therapy (lower doses with tissue plasminogen activators)
Secure catheter at insertion site
Periodic neurologic checks
Frequent monitoring of access site for bleeding
Strict bedrest with access limb immobilized
Frequent monitoring of limb for changes in vascular examination
Foley catheter in bladder
Minimize blood draws; no arterial punctures

*Risk of bleeding complication increases as dose and duration of therapy increase.

Pulse-spray thrombolysis (a form of pharmacomechanical thrombolysis) also uses a catheter with multiple small side holes or slits at the distal end of the catheter (Box 4-13). Small aliquots of concentrated thrombolytic drug are forcibly injected through the catheter at short intervals, creating quick bursts of high-velocity fluid jets (Fig. 4-31). The jets disrupt thrombus as well as deliver the drug, resulting in a faster lysis time, frequently 1-2 hours. The patient remains in the angiography suite for the duration of the procedure. A mechanical injector is available in some countries, but this is usually done by hand in North America.

Thrombolysis with urokinase, t-PA, or r-PA has an 80%-90% technical success rate for recent occlusions in most applications. Success rates decrease with increase in the age of the occlusion and vary among different vascular beds and types of lesions. Clinical success in peripheral arterial occlusions, defined as limb salvage, is approximately 70% at 1 year. The results with streptokinase were less favorable and required longer infusions.

The majority of complications of thrombolysis procedures are hemorrhagic, involving the access site (Table 4-9). Careful technique during arterial puncture, the use of vascular sheaths, immobilization of the limb on the side of access, and gentle anticoagulation minimize this problem. Central nervous system bleeding occurs in 0.5%-2% of cases, with apparent higher risk with r-UK, t-PA, and r-PA. The risk of central nervous system bleeding seems to persist for at least 12-24 hours following termination of therapy. Distal embolization of fragments of thrombus occurs in up to 20% of peripheral arterial thrombolysis procedures as flow is restored. Patients complain of sudden acute worsening of ischemic symptoms just when things seemed to be getting better. Known as the "darkness before the dawn," this situation resolves in almost all cases within an hour or two with continued therapy as the embolized thrombus lyses. Persistence of symptoms requires return to the angiography suite or surgical thrombectomy.

Mechanical Thrombectomy

Catheter-based mechanical devices can pulverize and/or remove thrombus without the use of a thrombolytic agent. These devices use impellers, fluid jets, brushes, baskets, lasers, and ultrasound to break thrombus into fragments small enough to be aspirated through a catheter or released into the circulation (Fig. 4-32). The goal of all of these devices is rapid restoration of blood flow by rapid reduction of the volume of thrombus.

Mechanical thrombectomy devices vary in sheath requirements and their ability to be advanced over a guidewire. These devices can be used to declot surgical dialysis access or bypasses, as well as native arteries or veins. Fresh thrombus responds best, particularly within small-diameter surgical grafts. A common limitation is an inability to completely clear thrombus in large-diameter vessels such as the inferior vena cava. However, when used appropriately, excellent results can be obtained. One area in which these devices are particularly useful is in the treatment of massive pulmonary embolism, when fragmentation of the embolus frequently results in major improvement in pulmonary arterial flow.

A very simple mechanical approach to removal of fresh thrombus that uses readily available equipment is suction thrombectomy. For this procedure, a sheath should always be used at the access site. A nontapered catheter large enough to accommodate the thrombus and still fit inside the vessel is advanced into the thrombus over a smaller tapered catheter. The inner catheter is removed, and an empty 60-mL syringe is attached

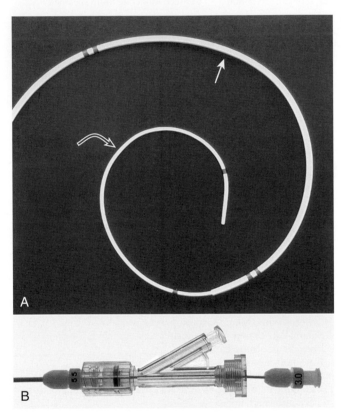

FIGURE 4-30. Example of coaxial catheter infusion system for thrombolysis infusion. **A,** The outer 5.5-French catheter (*straight arrow*) has multiple side holes between the paired radiopaque marker bands. The 3-French inner coaxial catheter *(curved arrow)* with multiple side holes between the single marker bands. **B,** Close-up of the Y-adapter that allows simultaneous infusion through both catheters.

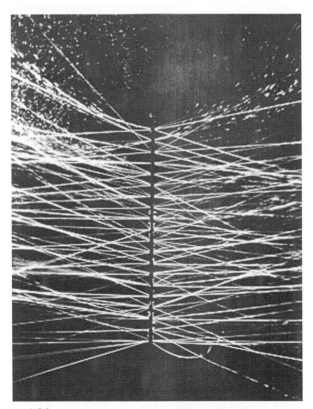

FIGURE 4-31. Photograph of multiple fluid jets exiting from a pulse-spray catheter (Courtesy Angiodynamics Inc., Queensbury, N.Y.)

Box 4-13. Manual Pulse-Spray Pharmacomechanical Thrombolysis

Position catheter across thrombus

t-PA: 2-10 mg in 10 mL (± heparin; may precipitate); inject 0.5 mL every 30-90 seconds

r-PA: 2-10 U in 10 mL (± heparin); inject 0.5 mL every 30-90 seconds

Urokinase: 250,000 U in 9-mL sterile water plus 5000 U heparin (1 mL); inject 0.2-0.3 mL every 30-90 seconds

Concurrent heparin/platelet inhibitor therapy (lower doses with tissue plasminogen activators)

Immobilize catheters at insertion site

Frequent monitoring of access site for bleeding

Frequent monitoring of limb for changes in vascular examination

---

TABLE 4-9 Complication Rates with Peripheral Arterial Thrombolysis*

Complication	Streptokinase	Urokinase	t-PA and Derivatives
Access-site bleeding			
Minor[†]	20%-40%	20%-40%	20%-40%
Major[‡]	10%-20%	5%	5%-15%
Intracranial bleed	0.5%	0.5%	0.5%-3%
Distal embolization	15%	15%	15%
Failed procedure	30%-40%	5%-10%	5%-10%

*Complication rates are generalizations based on highly inhomogeneous (and sometimes suspect) data and vary greatly with the dose of lytic agent, age of occlusion, length of therapy, and concurrent anticoagulation.
[†]Almost all patients develop a small access-site hematoma.
[‡]Requires transfusion or operative therapy.

to the nontapered catheter. A vigorous, continuous suction is then applied to the catheter as it as advanced into, and then withdrawn through, the thrombus (Fig. 4-33). Suction is applied without interruption until the catheter is removed completely from the sheath, otherwise thrombus may dislodge from the catheter and embolize. This quick technique is particularly useful for management of acute intraprocedural thrombus in medium to small-diameter vessels or for removal of embolized atheromatous debris.

The complications of mechanical thrombectomy are somewhat device-dependent and include embolization, hemolysis, and volume overload. Unusual problems such as device fracture can result from improper or prolonged use. In general, these are very safe devices when used appropriately.

Pharmacomechanical Thrombolysis

The simultaneous use of a device that disrupts thrombus with a thrombolytic agent is termed *pharmacomechanical* thrombolysis. This promising approach seeks to take advantage of the best of both thrombolysis and mechanical thrombectomy. Any device that breaks up thrombus can be combined with a thrombolytic agent to decrease overall treatment times and improve efficacy. For example, the AngioJet catheter (MEDRAD, Warrendale, PA.) can be set to deliver the thrombolytic into the clot under pressure. After a short dwell time, the lysed thrombus is aspirated using the usual operating mode for the device (Power Pulse Spray) (Box 4-14). Some mechanical devices are specifically designed to be used in combination with a thrombolytic agent (Fig. 4-34). The fundamental concepts are fragmentation of the thrombus to expose more surface area to the thrombolytic agent and triggering additive endogenous lytic pathways. An alternative to mechanical thrombus disruption is the local delivery of high-frequency low-power ultrasound from within the infusion catheter along with the agent to accelerate catheter-directed thrombolysis (EKOS Corp, Bethell, Wash.).

The results of pharmacomechanical thrombolytic techniques are promising, with rapid restoration of flow and often reduced overall doses of thrombolytic agents. In approximately 30%-40% of patients, additional catheter-directed thrombolysis is required to "clean up" residual thrombus, especially when large volumes of thrombus are treated with mechanical devices.

Vasodilating Drugs

Vascular spasm can restrict blood flow to the point of occlusion in the absence of an underlying structural lesion. Spasm can be

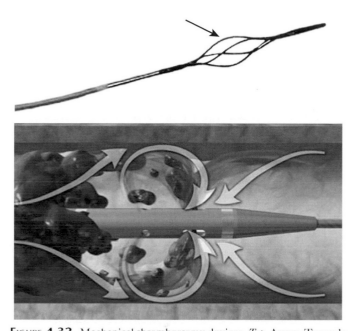

FIGURE 4-32. Mechanical thrombectomy devices. *Top,* Arrow–Trerotola PTD device (Arrow International, Reading, PA.). Battery-powered motor-driven rotating basket *(arrow)* pulverizes thrombus that can be aspirated from a sheath. *Bottom,* drawing of AngioJet catheter. Heparinized saline is forcefully injected through the proximal ports to fragment thrombus, which is continuously aspirated through the distal ports. (*Top,* Courtesy Scott Trerotola, MD; *bottom,* courtesy MEDRAD Inc., Warrendale, PA.)

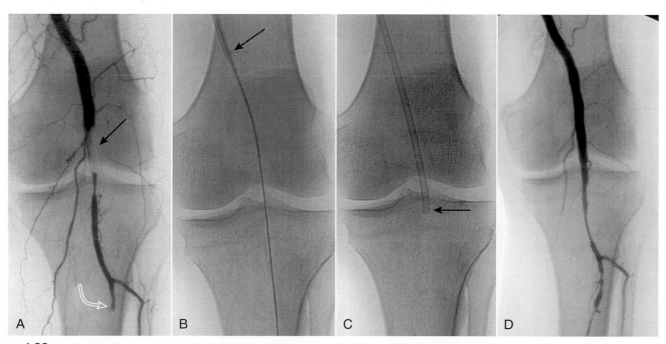

FIGURE 4-33. Aspiration thrombectomy. **A,** Emboli in the popliteal artery *(straight arrow)* and tibioperoneal trunk *(curved arrow)*. **B,** After crossing the lesions with a guidewire, an 8-French nontapered guiding catheter *(arrow)* was advanced over a 5-French catheter beyond both emboli. **C,** The guidewire and inner catheter were removed. Suction was applied to the guiding catheter *(arrow)* with a 60-mL syringe as it was withdrawn. **D,** Postaspiration run shows patent vessels, although there is now some spasm in the distal popliteal artery.

Box 4-14. Power Pulse Spray Pharmacomechanical Thrombolysis

Mix 25 mg t-PA (25U r-PA) in 100 mL saline
Set to "Power Pulse Spray"
Position catheter across thrombosis
Deliver thrombolytic agent over entire length of thrombus
Withdraw at 0.5 cm/pulse, distal-to-proximal relative to access site
Wait 20 minutes
Replace thrombolytic with 500 mL NS with 2500 U heparin
Set to "AngioJet"
Reposition catheter across thrombosis
Withdraw catheter 2-3 mm/sec during activation

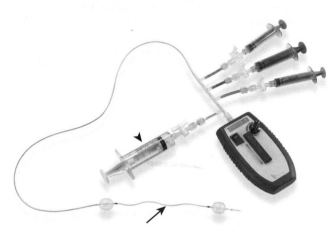

FIGURE 4-34. Pharmacomechanical thrombectomy device. The two occlusion balloons isolate the vascular segment to be treated. A thrombolytic agent is injected into the isolated blood vessel, and the sinusoidal catheter *(arrow)* is rotated using a battery-powered motor. After the thrombus is lysed, the vascular segment can be aspirated *(arrowhead)* before lowering the occlusion balloons. (Courtesy Trellis Covidien, Mansfield, Mass. COVIDIEN, COVIDIEN with logo are U.S. and/or internationally registered trademarks of Covidien AG. Other brands are trademarks of a Covidien company. © 2009 Achille Bigliardi Photography, used by permission.)

caused by external trauma to the vessel, guidewire manipulation in the vessel lumen, shock, hypothermia, or the use of vasoconstrictor drugs (see Fig. 2-46). Vasoactive drugs can be used intraarterially to reverse or reduce vasospasm (Table 4-10). When induced by a guidewire or catheter, removal of the offending device frequently allows the spasm to resolve. The most useful drug for acute intraprocedural spasm is nitroglycerin, which can be given every 5-10 minutes until the spasm improves or the blood pressure drops. When more prolonged therapy is required, an infusion of papaverine may be used. In cases of severe procedure-related spasm that does not resolve quickly, heparin should be given to prevent thrombosis.

DECREASING BLOOD FLOW THROUGH VESSELS

Fundamentals

Partial or complete occlusion of blood flow using catheter-based techniques is desirable to treat many conditions, including holes in blood vessels, tumors (both benign and malignant), abnormal communications between blood vessels, and abnormal blood vessels in abnormal locations. Although the pathologies are varied, the basics of the procedures are the same. The essential considerations are the underlying lesion, the clinical problem that needs

TABLE 4-10 Vasodilating Agents

Drug*	Dose	Half-life	Mechanism of Action
Nitroglycerin	100-250 μg bolus IA (100 μg/mL)	4-6 min	Direct vasodilator (metabolized to nitric oxide)
Papaverine	30-60 mg/h infusion IA (1 mg/mL NS)	30-120 min	Direct smooth muscle relaxant (inhibits cyclic nucleotide phosphodiesterase)
Verapamil	2.5 mg bolus IV 1-2 mg bolus IA	2-5 hr	Calcium-channel blocker

*Both nitroglycerin and verapamil can be repeated as blood pressure permits.
IA, Intraarterial; IV, intravenous;

TABLE 4-11 Planning an Occlusion Procedure

Category	Considerations
Goal of procedure	Decrease flow; complete occlusion; deliver drug; kill organ
Level of occlusion	Proximal; distal; capillary
Precision of delivery	Exact; flow-directed; regional
Delivery system	Microcatheters; diagnostic catheters; direct puncture
Vascular anatomy	Access vessels; major blood supply; accessory/collateral vessels
Adjacent structures	Risks of nontarget organ embolization, compartment syndrome

to be addressed, the feasibility of a percutaneous approach to the lesion, the ability to accomplish what is required, and the management plans for the patient after the procedure.

The lesions most amenable to treatment with percutaneous vascular occlusion techniques are those that involve or are supplied by blood vessels. Avascular lesions usually cannot be treated effectively through an intravascular route.

A clear understanding of the clinical problem is essential (Table 4-11). The rapidity with which the occlusion must be achieved, the occlusive technique, and the tolerance for complications can be very different depending on the goals of the procedure. For example, both life-threatening hemorrhage from pelvic fracture and symptomatic uterine fibroids can be treated with transcatheter pelvic embolization, but the approach to each procedure is very different.

In order to perform the procedure, it is necessary to gain access to the lesion and to deliver an effective device or drug. Access can be accomplished through a blood vessel or by direct puncture. Very tortuous vessels can be successfully negotiated with specialized microcatheters (see Fig. 2-21). However, an effective occlusive agent may be impossible to deliver through such a small catheter. Careful review of imaging studies and performance of a complete diagnostic angiogram (when the clinical situation allows) assist in formulation of a successful strategy. A crucial step in this process is consideration of potential collateral or accessory blood supply to a lesion, because failure to identify these vessels may result in a failed procedure (Fig. 4-35).

The management plan for the patient after embolization has great bearing on the details of the occlusion procedure. For example, embolizing an organ that will subsequently be removed surgically is approached differently than an organ that must remain

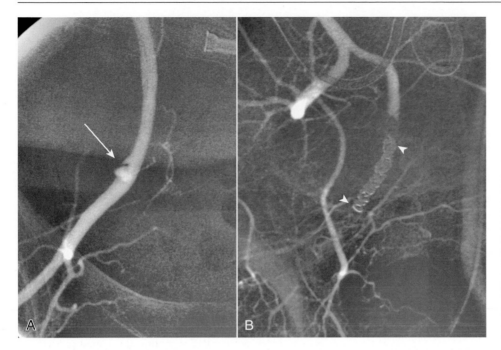

FIGURE 4-35. Embolization of an inferior gluteal artery to treat a pseudoaneurysm following transgluteal abscess drainage. Coils were used in this case. **A,** Digital angiogram showing the pseudoaneurysm *(arrow)* of the inferior gluteal artery. **B,** Coils have been densely packed on both sides of the pseudoaneurysm *(arrowheads)* to block antegrade perfusion from the hypogastric artery and retrograde perfusion from collaterals to the distal inferior gluteal artery from the superior gluteal and profunda femoris arteries. Simply embolizing the inferior gluteal artery proximal to the pseudoaneurysm would have resulted in inadequate treatment.

TABLE 4-12 Techniques and Tools for Vascular Occlusion

Technique	Sample Tools
Intraluminal obstruction	Steel coils, plug, particles
Delivery of chemotherapeutic agent	Lipiodol, drug-eluting beads
Vasoconstriction	Vasopressin drip
Sclerosis of lumen	Dehydrated ethanol, sodium tetradecyl sulfate
Sealing hole in vessel wall: Intraluminal approach	Stent-graft
Extraluminal	Ultrasound-guided compression; thrombin injection into pseudoaneurysm

in place and functional. In the former, total infarction is acceptable, but in the latter it would be undesirable.

A variety of tools and techniques can be used to slow flow or occlude blood vessels (Table 4-12). Matching the tools and techniques to the clinical situation is frequently a matter of judgment, experience, and device availability.

Embolization

There are a large number of embolic agents, with varying physical properties, methods of delivery, and permanence (Table 4-13). Selection of an embolic agent depends on the clinical factors and the technical aspects of the procedure. There are a few basic rules for embolization procedures that, when followed, lead to a successful procedure with minimal complications (Box 4-15).

Proximal vessel occlusion is useful when a single vessel supplies the target area, a quick result is necessary, or preservation of distal collateral vessels is desirable. Large agents such as coils or plugs are ideal for this situation. Distal occlusion has a higher chance of tissue infarction. Liquid agents penetrate more deeply than solid agents. Detachable coils and plugs are the most precise embolic agents, in that they can be repositioned or removed if placement is unsatisfactory. Lastly, secure placement of large embolic agents in areas of narrowing prevents distal migration.

Coils

Embolization coils are available in a variety of sizes, lengths, shapes, and materials (Fig. 4-36). Coils are lengths of coil-spring wire (usually stainless steel or platinum) that may be preformed into any number of shapes. Wire diameters range from 0.010 to 0.052 inches. Tufts of synthetic fibers may be attached to the coil to promote platelet aggregation and thrombosis. Some coils are coated with a polymer that swells when exposed to liquids (Fig. 4-37). Coils occlude vessels by physically obstructing the lumen. Packaging for coils usually is labeled with the diameter of the wire, the length of the coil wire, and the diameter when reformed. Careful attention to the labeling is necessary to avoid inserting inappropriately sized devices (Fig. 4-38). Coils are supplied straightened in a metal or plastic tube, either free or attached to a delivery wire. The loading tube must be placed firmly into the hub of the catheter, and the coil advanced into the catheter (Box 4-16). The diameter of the coil wire should always closely match the inner diameter of the delivery catheter; otherwise the coil may begin to reform and jam in the catheter. Coils can be advanced through the catheter with a floppy-tipped guidewire or coil pusher that matches the inner diameter of the catheter. Gentle but firm forward pressure on the catheter may be necessary during the final stages of coil delivery to prevent excessive "bucking" of the catheter tip or improper placement. Alternatively, when catheter position is secure, coils may be injected using 1-3 mL Luer-lock syringes. Detachable coils remain connected to the pusher wire until an electric current is applied to break a bond or until a mechanical technique is used to release the coil. These are particularly useful in procedures when precise placement is critical. Another specialty coil is the "liquid coil," an extremely limp length of nonfibered platinum coil that, when injected through a microcatheter, piles up in the target vessel like soft-serve ice cream.

A single coil rarely occludes a vessel because it usually does not completely obstruct the lumen, and platelet aggregation on the fibers may take time. This is especially true in large, high-flow vessels. In these cases it is useful to place a few stiff coils first that can serve as a framework (or "nest") in which softer coils can be packed. Soft coils can be swept away by high flow even when properly sized. Another strategy to use in this situation is to "anchor" the coil by starting the deployment in a small branch vessel and then retracting the catheter into the larger lumen for the majority of the coil deployment. The occlusive effect of

TABLE **4-13** Embolic Agents

Agent	Properties	Durability	Vessel Size	Delivery
Coils	Solid; obstructs flow	Permanent	Large, medium, small	Push or inject through catheter; some detachable
Plugs	Solid; obstructs flow	Permanent	Large, medium	Detachable from catheter
Particles (flakes or spheres)	Solid; obstructs flow	Permanent	Small	Injected
Gelfoam gelatin sponge	Solid; obstructs flow	4-6 weeks	Medium to small	Injected; pushed
Autologous clot	Solid; obstructs flow	4-7 days	Medium	Injected
Glues and polymers:	Liquid turns to solid; obstructs flow	Permanent	Determined by vessel lumen	Injected
Lipiodol (iodized oil)	Liquid; obstructs flow	Varies	Small to capillary	Injected
Thrombin	Liquid; induces thrombosis	Varies	Large to capillary	Injected
Sotradecol	Liquid; sclerosant	Permanent	Medium to capillary	Injected
Ethanol (95% ETOH)	Liquid; tissue destruction	Permanent	Large to capillary	Injected

---

Box 4-15. Embolization Rules

Have a plan
Be sure of the pathology and anatomy
Maintain stable, secure catheter position
Embolize antegrade (with flow) when possible
Use coaxial microcatheters for small vessels
If image quality is poor, do not embolize
Embolize to a predetermined endpoint
Avoid "just one more for good luck"; it is frequently one too many
Document results: always check for collateral reconstitution distal to occlusion
Consider prophylactic antibiotics (primarily solid organ embolization)

---

fibered coils can be enhanced by soaking the coil in a thrombin solution before delivery.

Vascular Plugs

Vascular plugs create rapid occlusion of vessels with a limited number of devices. Larger devices can be repositioned or removed before deployment. The most widely used plugs are made from a fine nitinol metallic mesh that assumes a preformed shape when unconstrained but that can be elongated to fit through a catheter (Fig. 4-39). The larger plugs are detachable, allowing repositioning or removal before final deployment. This is very useful when working in large, high-flow vessels, because the stability of the embolic device can be determined before it is released. Large plugs are delivered through guide catheters. Smaller plugs can be pushed through regular angiographic catheters, but may not be detachable or repositionable. The dense mesh does not instantly obstruct flow, but serves as a scaffold for rapid thrombus formation that completes the occlusion, usually within 5-10 minutes. Covered plugs are less commonly available, but occlusion times are more rapid than with mesh plugs.

Polyvinyl Alcohol (Ivalon)

Ivalon, one of the oldest particulate embolic materials, is inexpensive, inert, and permanent (Fig. 4-40). The particles are injected through a catheter and carried to the site of embolization by the arterial flow (Box 4-17). Correct sizing of the Ivalon is critical to prevent blockage of the delivery catheter and to achieve the desired embolization. Ivalon is supplied dry or in suspension in vials or syringes as irregular or spherically shaped particles in sizes from 50 to 1200 μm in diameter. Spherical Ivalon is more uniform in size than irregular particles, and compresses 20%-30% in catheters and blood vessels. Irregular particles are more likely to clump and occlude proximally, whereas spheres are more likely to occlude distally. The particles are not visible radiographically, so they are usually mixed with contrast before injection. Adding albumin to the suspension helps prevent clumping of irregular particles. The particles are delivered by gentle injection with 1- to 3-mL syringes using a pulsing motion during fluoroscopy. Embolic endpoints are determined by the quality of flow in the vessel. As the embolization approaches completion, flow becomes slower. Forceful injection of particles or contrast during the procedure may result in reflux out of the target vessel into another vessel.

Microspheres

Numerous spherical embolic agents are available made from acrylics, hydrogels, resins, polymers, glass, and, as noted earlier, Ivalon (Table 4-14). Some of these agents have the added capability of controlled delivery of a therapeutic agent in addition to obstructing flow. Spheres are uniformly shaped, flow-directed, solid embolic agents (Fig. 4-41). Most spheres can be compressed approximately 20%-30% in diameter, a feature that requires consideration when selecting a size. The spheres range in diameter from 40 to 1200 μm and are available dry or suspended in solution. The range of sizes included in each container varies by manufacturer and can be as little as 0 μm and as great as 300 μm. The spheres are not radiopaque and therefore are usually suspended in contrast before injection. The ratios of contrast to spheres for even suspension vary by manufacturer; the instructions for use should be consulted before performing the procedure. Some spheres increase in size when hydrated (see Table 4-14)

Spheres that can bind positively charged ions to their surface or absorb drugs can be used to deliver therapeutic agents. Mixing spheres with the drugs is done a few hours before the embolization procedure to ensure maximum uptake of the agent. Both mechanisms permit a controlled delivery of drug after embolization (drug-eluting beads).

The uniform shape and compressibility of spheres results in less clumping than with irregular Ivalon particles. This makes delivery of relatively large particles through microcatheters possible. However, overcompression of the spheres can result in fractures and biodegradation over time.

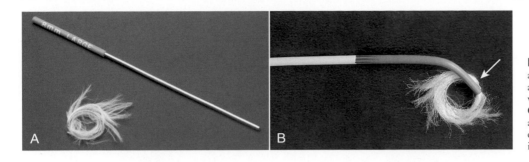

FIGURE 4-36. Embolization coils. **A,** Coils are supplied preloaded in tubes. Shown is a standard Gianturco stainless steel coil with polyester fibers (Courtesy Cook Group, Bloomington, Ind.). **B,** Delivery of a coil through a catheter *(arrow).* The coil can be pushed with a soft guidewire, or injected.

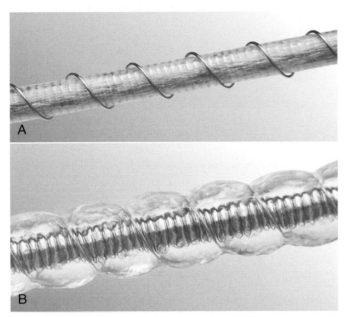

FIGURE 4-37. Coil coated with a hydrogel that swells upon contact with blood. **A,** Coil in dry state. **B,** Coil after hydration. This process requires approximately 20 minutes to complete in the body. (Courtesy MicroVention Inc., Tustin, Calif.)

Radioembolization

Yttrium-90 loaded glass or resin microspheres are used for embolization of primary and metastatic hepatic arterial lesions. Yttrium-90 is a powerful β-emitter with a short penetration (just centimeters) and a half-life of 64.2 hours. The isotope degrades to zirconium-90. There are two available preparations, both approximately 20-30 μm in diameter but different in composition and activity (see Table 4-14). Radioactive spheres require special shipping, handling protocols, certification for operators, and administration techniques. The planning for a radioembolization differs substantially from other embolizations, because each dose must be estimated and then ordered well in advance for each patient. Use of these agents is described in Chapter 11.

Gelfoam

Gelfoam (gelatin sponge) was one of the earliest embolics and remains among the most versatile. This substance is compressible and absorbed over a period of 4-6 weeks. Gelfoam is supplied in small sterile bricks or a fine (approximately 50-μm) powder (Fig. 4-42). The brick can be cut to the size needed to occlude the vessel of interest, compressed to fit through a catheter, and then injected into the vessel where it will expand to a larger size than when dry (Box 4-18). The size of the piece can range from several millimeters wide and a centimeter long (a Gelfoam "torpedo") for occluding a single vessel to a slurry of fine particles

(Gelfoam "snowstorm") for embolizing an entire vascular bed. The pieces can be suspended in contrast before injection to aid in fluoroscopic visualization (Fig. 4-43). Gelfoam can also be soaked in thrombin or a sclerosing agent before injection. As with all particulates, overly forceful injection can result in reflux of the Gelfoam into a nontarget vessel. Gelfoam pieces are useful any time that temporary occlusion is desired. In addition, Gelfoam torpedoes can be used in combination with coil embolization: after initial placement of a few coils, Gelfoam pieces are injected and lodge in the coils to complete the occlusion. Afterward, coils can be placed to finalize the embolization (the "Gelfoam sandwich").

Gelfoam powder frequently results in permanent occlusion owing to the small size of the particles. The level of occlusion is so distal that tissue necrosis can occur.

Autologous Clot

Rarely used except when very temporary (hours to days) occlusion is desired, autologous clot was actually one of the first solid embolic agents. Pieces of thrombus formed from the patient's blood are injected in a similar fashion as Gelfoam torpedoes.

Glues and Polymers

Liquid embolic materials that can be injected through a small catheter and then solidify to occlude a larger space are very useful flow-directed agents (Fig. 4-44). These agents flow into complex vascular structures and then solidify (Fig. 4-45). This is of particular value in treatment of arteriovenous malformations, in which a central nidus with multiple feeding arteries and draining veins can be effectively treated. Cyanoacrylate glues and derivatives "set" upon contact with ionic solutions such as blood or saline. The time required for the glue to set can be adjusted by mixing with varying amounts of iodized oil (Box 4-19). In addition, the oil opacifies the otherwise radiolucent glue. Meticulous technique is required to prevent solidification in the catheter; the catheter must be flushed with a glucose solution prior to injection of glue. The injection of the glue cannot be interrupted, as it will solidify and obstruct the catheter tip. These are very quick procedures as the glue sets within seconds. For this reason, there is very little opportunity to modify the injection once begun. When the injection is complete the catheter must be rapidly withdrawn to avoid cementing it in place.

Ethylene vinyl alcohol copolymer (EVOH, Onyx, eV3 Inc, Plymouth, Minn.) is a biocompatible agent that is opacified with tantalum and dissolved in dimethyl sulfoxide (DMSO) (Fig. 4-46). Upon contact with an aqueous solution it precipitates into a spongy mass. The precipitation is much slower and more controlled than glue polymerization. Delivery is through specialized microcatheters that are not dissolved by DMSO (Box 4-20). The catheter is first purged with saline and then filled with DMSO. Multiple vials of EVOH can be delivered through the same catheter, because the agent flows like molten lava (without the heat) into the space being embolized, gradually filling it. Different viscosities are available; thinner viscosity is better for deeper penetration into smaller vessels. The delivery can be paused to allow some areas to set and redirect the subsequent

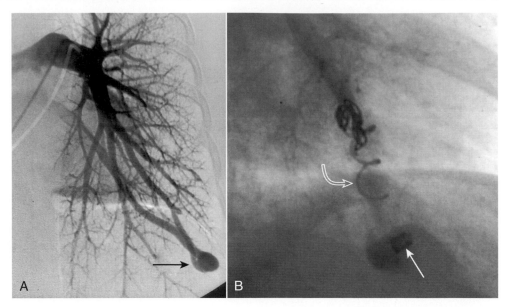

FIGURE 4-38. Improper coil selection. **A,** Pulmonary arteriovenous malformation *(arrow)*. **B,** One coil was too small and embolized into the malformation *(straight arrow)*. This could have resulted in systemic arterial embolization. Another coil was too big, and could not adequately reform in the feeding pulmonary artery *(curved arrow)*.

Box 4-16. **Coil Tips**

Read labels carefully: be sure of coil dimensions before inserting into the patient

Final diameter of coil should be 20%-30% larger than target vessel

Match diameter of coil wire to catheter lumen; smaller coils will jam in the catheter

Push coils with the guidewire/pusher that matches catheter lumen; otherwise the pusher will jam alongside the coil in the catheter

Gentle forward pressure on the catheter helps coil to "pack"

Coils can be injected with 1-3 mL Luer-lock syringes

Platinum coils are softer and easier to see than steel coils

Avoid sharp angles or redundancy in the delivery catheter

Flush gently after coil placement or contrast injections

EVOH elsewhere. Unlike glue, there is no urgency to the delivery. Embolization of large lesions can take time, so reduced fluoroscopic pulse rates should be used because the injection must be monitored continuously. Patients may feel the DMSO as a deep ache. The EVOH mass is less adhesive to the catheter than glue, but can still trap the catheter. Patients emit a characteristic odor of rotten eggs and garlic for several days after the procedure (the DMSO), so warn the family in advance.

Iodized Oil

An inert iodinated oil and one of the oldest radiographic contrast agents, Lipiodol (Guerbet, Roissy CDG, France) obstructs small vessels owing to its high viscosity relative to blood. In addition, hepatomas have a specific affinity for iodinated oil (Fig. 4-47). Supplied in 10-mL vials, it is frequently used to create an emulsion with chemotherapy for embolization of hepatic tumors. Delivery is by gentle injection. Lipiodol is readily visible during injection, which facilitates a controlled delivery. This material should not be used in high-flow tumors with large arteriovenous shunts without previous particulate embolization to control the shunt.

Lipiodol is also used to opacify or modify other liquid embolic agents (see Glues and Polymers above, and see Other Liquid Sclerosants below).

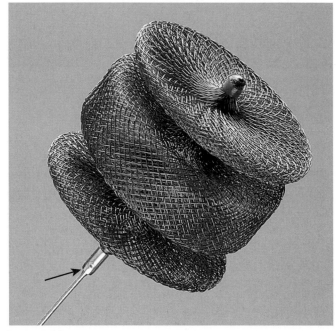

FIGURE 4-39. A vascular plug. Shown is the Amplatzer II plug. The three lobes increase the surface area of the plug to promote occlusion. Note the delivery wire *(arrow)*, which remains attached to the plug until released with a counterclockwise rotation. (Modified image courtesy of AGA Medical, Plymouth, Minn.)

Chemoembolization

Chemotherapeutic agents can be delivered directly into an organ or tumor through an artery to treat certain tumors (particularly primary and metastatic hepatic lesions). When combined with an embolic agent, this is termed *chemoembolization*. A wide variety of chemotherapeutic agents are used, depending on the tumor and the institutional experience. In general, vascular and hypervascular tumors respond best to chemoembolization. The chemotherapy is usually mixed with contrast to allow visualization and an embolic agent to slow flow and trap the drugs in the organ of interest. Iodized oil and/or particles such as spheres, irregular Ivalon, or Gelfoam are used as the embolic agent (see Fig. 4-47). Drug-eluting beads (see Microspheres above) can provide a controlled and sustained release of the chemotherapeutic agent rather than a single large dose. The goal of chemoembolization is to deliver the chemotherapy, not permanently occlude the major access vessels, because multiple treatments are frequently required. Chemoembolization can be performed alone or in conjunction with other therapies such as radiofrequency ablation, external beam radiation, or surgical excision. This procedure is described in more detail in Chapter 14.

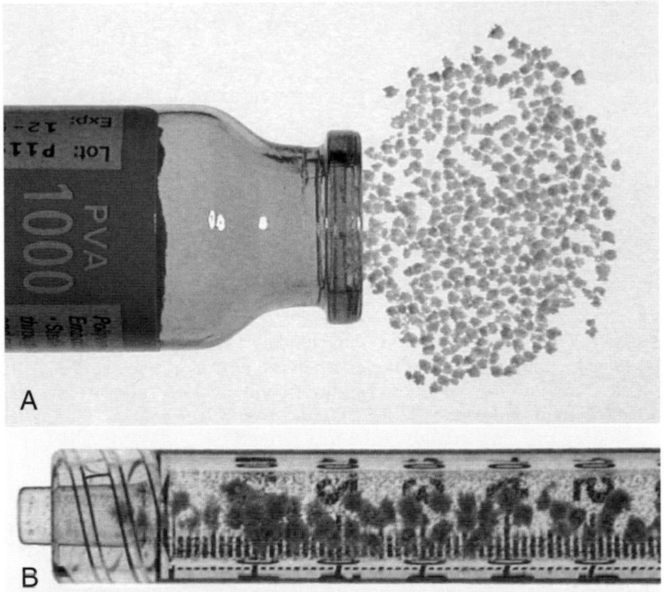

Thrombin

Topical thrombin is a potent agent that causes vascular obstruction by rapidly inducing thrombosis when injected intravascularly (Fig. 4-48). Approved by the FDA only for topical use, it is used intravascularly to treat aneurysms or induce thrombosis during stubborn embolization cases. Thrombin powder is reconstituted in saline and injected slowly in aliquots of 500-1000 units. When contrast is not added to make the solution radiopaque, or injection is performed with ultrasound monitoring, extreme care must be taken to prevent reflux into the systemic circulation. Following catheter injection of thrombin, the catheter should be flushed gently to evacuate any residual thrombin. Lesions with rapid washout, such as high-flow arteriovenous malformations or fistulas, should not be treated with thrombin. Entire limbs or vascular beds may occlude if too much thrombin refluxes or washes out into nontarget vessels. Thrombosis is initiated instantly upon injection, but may take several minutes to complete. Gentle injections of contrast can help determine the progress of the thrombosis without refluxing residual thrombin or fresh thrombus out of the target artery.

Endovascular Ablation

Destructive obliteration of the vascular lumen effectively eliminates blood flow. In some cases, the destruction may extend beyond the endothelial cell layer of the blood vessel to the media or even the surrounding tissues. The level of destruction desired depends on the goal of the procedure. The next three sections describe different endovascular ablation techniques.

Absolute Ethanol

Dehydrated alcohol (98% ethanol, absolute ETOH) is a powerful agent that produces intravascular thrombosis, vessel wall sclerosis, and cell death in perfused tissue. Absolute ETOH does not simply cause occlusion of flow, but ablates tissue as well. This quality is an advantage when treating certain types of vascular malformations or tumors. Supplied in glass vials, ETOH is injected slowly in small volumes sufficient to fill the vessel or vascular bed to be obliterated. Large volumes can result in systemic ETOH toxicity. The pain associated with ETOH embolization can be so severe that general anesthesia may be required for treatment of superficial vascular malformations. Control of flow is essential when

FIGURE 4-40. Polyvinyl alcohol particles. **A,** These particles are very large (up to 1000 μm in diameter). **B,** Particles suspended n a 1-mL syringe: a 2:1 mixture of contrast and 5% albumin.

Box 4-17. Ivalon Tips

Mix particles in clean small bowl with 2:1 mixture of contrast and 5% albumin (irregular particles only)

Inject using 1-mL or 3-mL Luer-lock syringes

Use 700 μm or smaller particles through microcatheters

Flush catheter with 1- to 3-mL after each syringe of Ivalon

Blocked catheters can be cleared by flushing with 1-mL Luer-lock syringe

Inject Ivalon using fluoroscopic guidance ("roadmapping" if available)

Embolize until stasis or reflux is visible along the catheter

---

TABLE 4-14 Embolic Spheres

Trade Name	Composition	Active features	Company
LC Bead	PVA hydrogel microsphere	Drug delivery* (marketed as DC Beads outside the United States)	Biocompatibles, Oxford, Conn.
Contour SE	Spherical PVA	No	Boston Scientific, Natick, Mass.
Embozene	Hydrogel core, Polyzene-F coating	No	CeloNova BioSciences, Peachtree City, Ga.
Embospheres	Trisacryl cross-linked with gelatin	No	BioSphere Medical/Merit Medical, South Jordan, Utah
Quadraspheres	PVA-sodium acrylate copolymer	Drug delivery* (expand 400% with hydration)	BioSphere Medical/Merit Medical, South Jordan, Utah
Bead Block	Acrylamido PVA macropolymer	No	Biocompatibles, Oxford, Conn.
TheraSphere	Glass loaded with yttrium-90 isotope	Beta emitter, 2500 Bq/bead	Nordion, Ottawa, Ontario
SirSpheres	Resin loaded with yttrium-90 isotope	Beta emitter, 50 Bq/bead	Sirtex Medical, Wilmington, Mass.

*Off-label use as of March 2013.
Bq, Becquerel; PVA, polyvinyl alcohol.

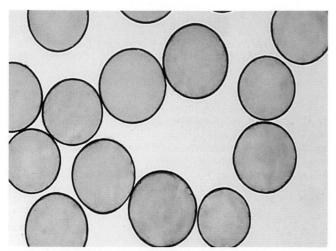

FIGURE **4-41**. Microspheres for embolization. Note the uniform shape. (Courtesy BioSphere Medical/Merit Medical, South Jordan, Utah.)

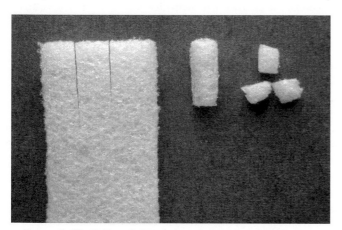

FIGURE **4-42**. Gelfoam brick cut into "torpedo" and small cubes.

Box 4-18. Gelfoam Tips

Cut dry brick with scalpel or scissors
Place piece(s) in syringe
Soak with contrast in syringe
Long "torpedoes" can be delivered individually with 1-mL syringes
Multiple small cubes can be injected with 3- to 5-mL syringe
Smaller pieces are necessary for microcatheters
Flush catheter with 1-mL syringe after each Gelfoam syringe
Gelfoam stuck in syringe can be cleared with 1-mL syringe

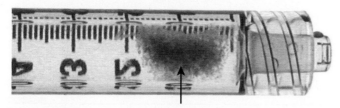

FIGURE **4-43**. Gelfoam "torpedo" *(arrow)* suspended in a 1-mL Luer-lock syringe.

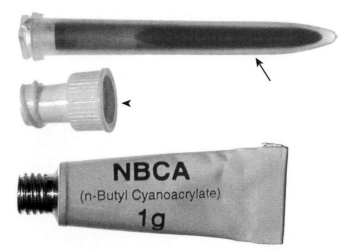

FIGURE **4-44**. Tube of N-butyl cyanoacrylate and a vial of tantalum powder *(arrow)*. The powder can be mixed in the glue to enhance radiopacity, but the iodized oil used to modify the polymerization time usually provides adequate radiopacity. The white adapter *(arrowhead)* is used when transferring the glue from the tube to a syringe.

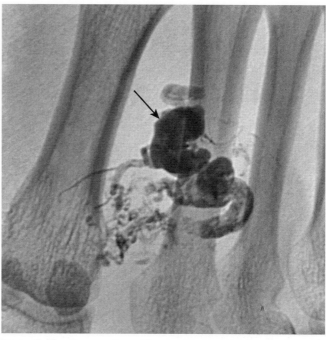

FIGURE **4-45**. Glue cast *(arrow)* in an arteriovenous malformation of the foot. The glue is visible because of the iodized oil.

Box 4-19. Glue Tips

Use a coaxial microcatheter system
Angiogram through microcatheter at 1 frame/sec to estimate rate of flow in lesion
Mix oil and glue in a ratio to obtain an appropriate "set" time
Flush catheter with 5% dextrose solution before introducing glue
Inject glue with 1- to 5-mL syringe
Once glue begins to set, inject until no forward flow
Immediately retract microcatheter to avoid glue "tail" on catheter
Aspirate microcatheter while removing from patient
Use new microcatheter for each glue injection

using absolute ETOH, because rapid washout causes dilution and limits contact with the vessel wall, or results in destruction of downstream tissues (Box 4-21). For this reason, control of flow with balloon occlusion catheters or compression is frequently employed when ETOH is used in arteries so that the alcohol can dwell in the target vessel for several minutes. Balloon occlusion catheters also prevent reflux into proximal nontarget organs. The specific gravity of ethanol is lower than that of blood, so anterior structures are particularly at risk when reflux occurs in arteries. When sclerosing venous structures, obstruction of outflow veins can be used to trap the ETOH in the treated segments. Absolute ETOH may be mixed with Lipiodol (usually in a ratio of 3-9:1 ETOH:Lipiodol) for embolization of some tumors.

Other Liquid Sclerosants

A wide variety of liquid sclerosants are used for treating primarily venous structures, including hypertonic saline, glycerine, bromated iodine, ethanolamine, sodium tetradecyl sulfate (Sotradecol), and polidocanol (Asclera in the United States, Aethoxysklerol in Europe). The agent used for any particular procedure depends on the experience of the operator, local regulations, cost, and availability. Superficial varicose veins are the most commonly sclerosed veins, and sodium tetradecyl sulfate and polidocanol are thought to be the most widely used agents.

Sodium tetradecyl sulfate and polidocanol are detergents that denature proteins in cell walls, resulting in cell death, inflammation, and eventual obliteration of the vascular lumen. The location of action is the vascular endothelial cell. Commonly used to treat superficial lower extremity venous varicosities, this agent can also be used for venous malformations. Supplied as a liquid, sodium tetradecyl sulfate is available in 1%-3% solution, and polidocanol in 0.5%-1% solution. These agents are injected slowly into the target vessel in 1- to 2-mL aliquots. For use in small veins, the solution is diluted lower than 1%. Alternatively, a foam can be created by mixing 1 part sclerosant with 3-5 parts room air and cycling the mixture rapidly between two syringes connected by a 3-way stopcock (the Tessari technique) (Fig. 4-49). The microbubbles expand the total volume and potential surface area of the injected sclerosant, allowing more extensive contact with the endothelium. The air content renders foam very conspicuous with ultrasound, which can be used to guide deep injections. Foam can also be created with small amounts of iodized oil, with or without room air/CO_2, which allows visualization of the mixture under fluoroscopy (Fig. 4-50). These agents should not be used in high-flow lesions, or when reflux into nontarget vessels is likely. In some situations, a balloon occlusion catheter can be used to control inflow or outflow. Extravasation can cause damage to adjacent tissues (e.g., skin ulceration), especially with higher concentrations of sodium tetradecyl sulfate, but is uncommon when dilute concentration doses are used. Polidocanol has been associated with a lower incidence of anaphylaxis than sodium tetradecyl sulfate. This is

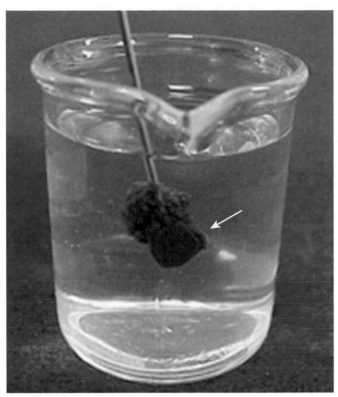

FIGURE **4-46**. Slow polymerization of ethylene vinyl alcohol copolymer (EVOH, Onyx, eV3 Inc., Plymouth, Minn.) as it is extruded from a catheter into saline *(arrow)*. The outer shell hardens but inside remains liquid. As more Onyx is injected, the liquid breaks through the shell like lava, allowing a controlled delivery. (Modified image courtesy of eV3 Inc., Plymouth, Minn.)

Box 4-20. Onyx Tips*

Start agitating bottles at beginning of case
Use dimethyl sulfoxide (DMSO)-compatible microcatheter
Position catheter in lesion at optimal starting point
Select Onyx viscosity base on flow rates in lesion, depth of penetration
Flush microcatheter with saline
Load microcatheter with DMSO
Inject Onyx slowly; allow "bead" to form at catheter tip
Follow injection with "roadmap" fluoroscopy
Pause to allow embolic to "set" if reflux
Reposition (withdraw) catheter as needed to redirect flow
Change viscosity as needed to control flow
Aspirate on catheter when withdrawing

*Ethylene vinyl alcohol copolymer (Onyx), eV3 Inc, Plymouth, Minn.

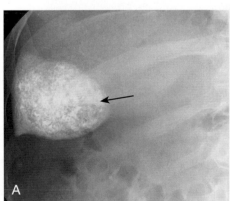
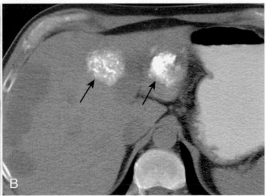

FIGURE **4-47**. Oil-based chemoembolization of hepatoma. **A,** Dense staining and iodized oil uptake in a right lobe hepatoma *(arrow)* following chemoembolization. **B,** Noncontrast computed tomography scan from another patient with multifocal hepatoma following chemoembolization shows oil uptake in several tumors *(arrows)*.

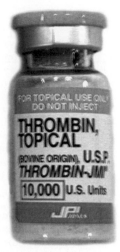

FIGURE 4-48. Topical thrombin is supplied in powdered form and must be reconstituted before injection. This agent is not FDA approved for intravascular injection but is commonly used in this fashion.

Box 4-21. Ethanol Tips

Use only 98% ethanol
For renal angiomyolipoma, mix 3-9:1 ETOH/iodized oil
General anesthesia for superficial vascular lesions
Use 3- to 5-mL syringes
Test injection with contrast to determine volume, rate of injection
Consider balloon occlusion catheter in arteries to control inflow, reflux
Consider compression, occlusion of outflow for venous lesions
Inject slowly
Use "roadmap" imaging if feasible
Inject volume of alcohol sufficient to fill target lesion
Wait 5-10 minutes
Aspirate residual alcohol (especially before deflating occlusion balloons)
Confirm occlusion with gentle injection of contrast

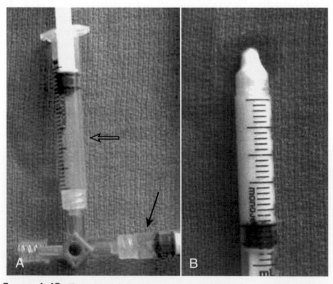

FIGURE 4-49. Foaming of detergent sclerosant (in this case sodium tetradecyl sulfate). The ratio of room air or CO_2 gas to sclerosant is 4-5:1. **A,** Syringe set-up before foaming. Room air *(open arrow)* will be mixed with liquid sclerosant *(solid arrow)*. **B,** After cycling 30 times rapidly from syringe to syringe, a uniform foam that will last for a few minutes is obtained.

---

further reduced by avoiding any contact of the agents with latex, including using nonlatex gloves for the procedure.

Endoluminal Thermal Ablation

Thermal ablation of the vessel lumen is used most often for treatment of greater and lesser saphenous veins in patients with symptomatic venous insufficiency. The heat destroys the endothelium, denatures proteins in the vessel wall, and induces wall edema, all of which lead to obliteration of the lumen during healing. Surrounding tissues are protected by the limited penetration of the heat as well as infiltration of the perivenous tissues with a dilute local anesthetic solution. The two most commonly used heat sources are lasers and radiofrequency probes. Lasers work primarily by boiling the blood adjacent to the tip of the probe, although some wavelengths are thought to selectively destroy the vascular endothelium. Radiofrequency probes heat the vessel wall by either direct contact or boiling the blood along the probe. These technologies could potentially also be applied to other endothelial lined tubular structures, such as ureters and bile ducts. The venous procedures are discussed in more detail in Chapter 16.

Vasoconstricting Drugs

Blood flow can be diminished without obstructing an artery by inducing vasoconstriction. This is a particularly useful strategy when the goal is to temporarily decrease the pressure or volume of blood reaching a specific area. A common example is gastrointestinal bleeding from sigmoid colon diverticulosis, in which preservation of flow is desired to prevent bowel infarction, but decreased flow is necessary to allow the natural hemostatic mechanism to work. Vasoconstricting agents have little value in the venous system.

In the past, the most commonly used agent was vasopressin for gastrointestinal bleeding (Box 4-22). Although rarely needed today, this remains occasionally a useful alternative to embolization. Vasopressin causes smooth muscle contraction in the

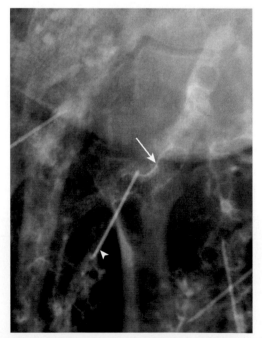

FIGURE 4-50. Spot film obtained during treatment of a large foot venous malformation with sodium tetradecyl sulfate foam created with addition of a small quantity of iodized oil. The oily contrast outlines the foam filling one of the venous spaces *(arrow)*. Injection was through direct puncture with a needle *(arrowhead)*. Other needles can be seen already in place around the foot.

peripheral arteries and water retention by the kidneys. The indication for intraarterial use is intestinal bleeding. Because of the potential for systemic vasoconstriction, patients with symptomatic coronary artery disease should not be treated with vasopressin. The initial dose is 0.2 U/min, with a maximum dose of 0.4 U/min. Patients frequently have abdominal cramping with initiation of therapy due to enhanced peristalsis, and pass old clot per rectum. This should not be confused with either intestinal ischemia or recurrent bleeding.

Epinephrine can be used for arterial injection to cause transient vasoconstriction, but should not be used for continuous infusions. There are few applications for this drug, but at one time it was useful in the angiographic diagnosis of tumors. On occasion it is still used to decrease renal arterial flow to allow satisfactory renal venography. For this application a mixture of 2 μg/mL is prepared by diluting 1 mL of 1:1000 epinephrine in 500 mL of 5% dextrose or saline. Injection of 8-10 μg into the renal artery immediately before the retrograde renal venogram decreases flow sufficiently to allow reflux into the intrarenal venules. Smaller doses (5-6 μg) can be used in diagnosis of renal and hepatic tumors. Normal arteries vasoconstrict in response to epinephrine, but tumor arteries do not, making it easier to see vascular renal or hepatic malignancies at angiography.

Treatment of Arterial Access Pseudoaneurysms

Pseudoaneurysms at the site of an arterial puncture occur in less than 5% of cases. Large catheter size, anticoagulation, calcified arteries, hypertension, puncture of the superficial femoral rather than the common femoral artery, and obesity are contributing risk factors. On physical examination, patients may have a pulsatile hematoma at the puncture site, frequently with a bruit. A discrete pulsatile mass may or may not be present. Color-flow ultrasound allows rapid diagnosis (see Fig. 3-7). Many pseudoaneurysms resolve spontaneously, particularly when small in size and in the absence of anticoagulation. However, rupture and infection can occur. The conventional treatment of pseudoaneurysms is surgical repair.

There are two basic image-guided therapies for femoral artery pseudo-aneurysms. Ultrasound-guided compression of the neck of the pseudoaneurysm is successful in approximately 80% of attempts. This procedure requires careful identification of the neck of the pseudoaneurysm and the ability to compress this neck without obliterating the lumen of the underlying normal vessel. This can be a very uncomfortable procedure for the patient, particularly those with fresh pseudoaneurysms and large hematomas. Compression for 20-30 minutes may be required. Complications with this procedure are rare, but distal embolization or thrombosis can occur. The rate of recurrence of the pseudoaneurysm is less than 5%.

As an alternative to compression therapy, direct percutaneous injection of the pseudoaneurysm with thrombin using ultrasound guidance results in rapid thrombosis of the pseudoaneurysm. A discrete neck should be identified by ultrasound, and the presence of an arteriovenous fistula excluded. Meticulous sterile technique is essential for the entire procedure, including the skin preparation. A small diameter needle (21-gauge) is advanced into the center of the pseudoaneurysm using ultrasound guidance. The thrombin is prepared in a concentration of 1000 U/mL. Small aliquots of thrombin (500-1000 U) are injected gently through the needle using a 1-mL syringe. Thrombosis of the pseudoaneurysm is usually instantaneous, but a small additional injection may be required. Reflux of thrombin into the systemic circulation can result in arterial thrombosis distal to the pseudoaneurysm. Careful positioning of the needle away from the pseudoaneurysm neck and gentle injection of small volumes of thrombin help avoid this complication. Recurrence of the pseudoaneurysm occurs in fewer than 5% of cases.

▬ IMPLANTING DEVICES

The insertion of intravascular devices for purposes other than increasing or decreasing blood flow has become an important part of vascular and interventional radiology. The two devices most commonly inserted (other than vascular stents) are central venous access catheters and vena cava filters. These subjects are covered in detail in Chapters 7 and 13.

▬ TAKING THINGS OUT OF BLOOD VESSELS

Intravascular Foreign Body Retrieval

Certain criteria must be satisfied for a successful retrieval (Box 4-23). The most important consideration is whether the object needs to be retrieved. This judgment is often based on individual opinion rather than scientific fact, but it should always be considered. The most common "lost" objects are central venous catheter fragments, which are also the easiest objects to retrieve because they are flexible and narrow, have well-defined ends, and are usually lodged in a capacious low-pressure vessel. Retrieval of objects from the arterial system differs from retrieval from the venous system in that the clinical presentation may be obstruction of flow, prompting a more urgent procedure. Objects lost in veins tend to move centrally, whereas objects lost in arteries move peripherally. A wide spectrum of objects have been retrieved from the vascular system, including embolization coils, pacemaker wires, stents, stent-grafts, vena cava filters, bullets, and fragments of angiographic catheters.

Devices used for retrieval are listed in Table 4-15. The most ubiquitous and simple device is the snare (Figs. 4-51 and 4-52,

---

Box 4-22. Vasopressin (Pitressin)

Localize bleeding source with arteriography
Place catheter in proximal superior or inferior mesenteric artery
Infusion dosage:
- Infuse 0.2 U/min for 30 minutes, then reassess with angiography
- If still bleeding, increase to 0.3 or 0.4 U/min for 30 minutes; repeat angiogram; if still bleeding, pursue different therapy

When bleeding is controlled, secure catheter
Infuse at successful dose for 12-24 hours
Monitor serum sodium, serial hematocrit
For rebleeding during therapy:
- Check that patient is still getting drug
- Check that catheter is not dislodged (inject contrast at bedside with portable abdominal film)
- Increase to maximum dose (0.4 U/min)

When completed, Taper to normal saline over 12 hours
Leave catheter in place for 6 hours after Pitressin is stopped before removal (in case of re-bleeding)

Box 4-23. Intravascular Foreign Body Retrieval

Is it necessary to remove foreign body (what is risk of just leaving it)?
Is it really intravascular?
Is it accessible from a peripheral access?
Can it be moved (i.e., is not sewn, stapled, glued, or otherwise permanently attached to blood vessel)?
Can it be moved without endangering patient?
Does size of object permit removal from a peripheral location?

Box 4-24). Other devices include wire baskets that can engage an object in a similar manner, grasping cones, special forceps that actually grasp an object, multistranded "mops" that can be used to entangle a coil, and large nontapered catheters than can be used to aspirate a small object.

When a catheter fragment is positioned so that neither end is free, retrieval is still possible with a snare if one end can be dislodged. Pigtail or recurved catheters can be used to hook the central portion of the fragment. Applying traction can pull an end of the fragment free. A deflecting guidewire advanced to the end of the catheter (but not beyond) may be needed to provide extra stiffness when the fragment cannot be easily

TABLE 4-15 Retrieval Devices

Device	Mechanism
Snare	Encircles
Basket	Encircles
Forceps	Pincer
Aspiration catheter	Suction
Balloon	Dislodgment

repositioned. Another strategy is to use a recurved catheter to pass a guidewire over the fragment. The guidewire can then be snared from below, forming a closed loop that can dislodge even the most stubborn objects (Fig. 4-53).

Rarely, an object gets away from the operator during a procedure but is still on the guidewire. This is the ideal situation for snare retrieval. A typical example is a stent that becomes dislodged from an angioplasty balloon but remains on the guidewire in the vessel (Fig. 4-54). The loop of a snare can be placed over the back end of the guidewire and advanced to the stent using the guidewire as a monorail. The loop is then carefully advanced over the stent without pushing it off of the guidewire. Once engaged, the loop is closed over the stent and guidewire, and retrieved through a large-caliber sheath or guide catheter. Great care should be taken to keep the stent on the guidewire at all times, as retrieval of a free-floating stent can be extremely difficult.

In some circumstances it may possible to engage a large object, but not remove it percutaneously. In this situation the object can

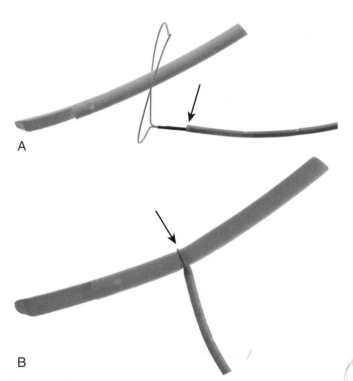

FIGURE 4-52. How a snare works. **A,** Snare is looped around one end of the catheter fragment. Note that this snare forms at a right-angle to the guiding catheter *(arrow)*. **B,** The snare is locked down on the fragment *(arrow)* by advancing the guiding catheter to close the loop.

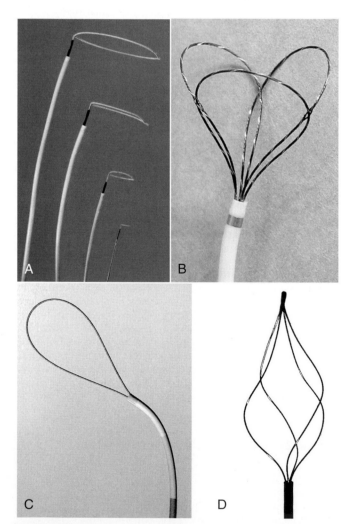

FIGURE 4-51. Different snare retrieval devices. **A,** Amplatz gooseneck snares. **B,** EnSnare. **C,** Snare formed by looping a guidewire through a catheter. **D,** Basket. (**A,** Courtesy eV3 Inc., Plymouth, Minn., with permission; **B,** courtesy Merit Medical Systems Inc., South Jordan, Utah).

Box 4-24. Using a Snare

Select loop diameter equal to or slightly larger than lumen in which object is located

Insert sheath large enough to accommodate snare and object

Engage object with snare (selective catheter very useful to direct snare)

Advance catheter over snare to close loop and lock object

Apply firm, continuous traction on snare wire from this point on ("death grip")

Using continuous fluoroscopic monitoring, withdraw snare, catheter, and object as single unit

Release death grip only when object and snare are outside of body

be repositioned in a peripheral location, where a simple cut-down can be performed. This is usually preferable to a major operation.

Transvascular Biopsy

Transvascular biopsy of masses or organs is a valuable technique when conventional percutaneous biopsy has a high risk of hemorrhagic complication, or the only access is through a blood vessel. The basic premise of transvascular biopsy is that any potential bleeding from the biopsy site will be into a blood vessel. The most common indication is suspected liver parenchymal disease in patients with coagulopathy or ascites, although transvascular

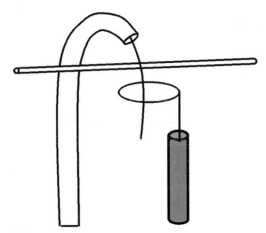

FIGURE 4-53. When the ends of an object are not free, a snare can be formed around the object. A wire is passed over the object and snared. The snare and the wire are brought out through the same sheath, forming a loop around the object. A guiding catheter can be advanced over both ends of the wire to the object, completing the snare.

renal biopsy is becoming more common (Table 4-16). Focal liver and renal masses are, in general, more successfully biopsied in a conventional manner using a cross-sectional imaging modality such as computed tomography, ultrasound, or magnetic resonance imaging. Some vascular tumors present as entirely intraluminal masses, particularly venous and arterial sarcomas. These lesions are ideal for transvascular biopsy.

The access route is determined by the organ or vessel that is involved. For liver and kidney biopsies, a transvenous route from a jugular access is preferred, because the hepatic and renal veins are easy to catheterize from this approach, stiff devices track well to the target organ, and hemostasis at the venipuncture site is readily achieved with compression. The appropriate laboratory tests and specimen solutions should be determined in advance for each type of specimen.

Dedicated transvascular biopsy kits use automated cutting needles to obtain a core of tissue (e.g., Quick Core 18-gauge needle from Cook Group) (Fig. 4-55). These are primarily designed for liver or renal biopsy through a 7-French sheath and a curved inner metal cannula. A modified needle with a shorter intraparenchymal excursion is available for renal biopsies. Other biopsy tools include biting clamshell forceps, similar to devices used during endoscopy. Guiding catheters are helpful to position these devices adjacent to the mass. Occasionally, an atherectomy device can be used to obtain shavings from an intravascular mass (see Fig. 4-27).

The overall complication rate of transvascular liver and renal biopsy is less than 6%, with the majority being hemorrhagic. This tends to occur when the liver or renal capsule is inadvertently transgressed during the biopsy. Death from intraabdominal bleeding is a particular risk in coagulopathic patients, especially when combined with ascites. Patients should be observed for several hours after a biopsy in a monitored setting. When hemorrhage is suspected, a noncontrast computed tomography scan should be obtained, and angiography with intent to embolize considered early.

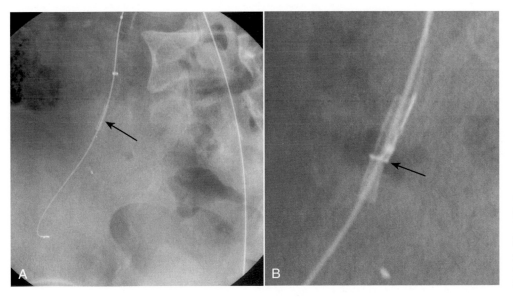

FIGURE 4-54. Snaring a stent that is free on a guidewire. **A,** A stent *(arrow)* has become dislodged from the balloon during an intervention on a transplant renal artery. The stent remains on the guidewire. **B,** A snare *(arrow)* has been passed over the guidewire and used to capture the stent.

TABLE 4-16 Indications for Transvascular Biopsy

Organ	Indications
Liver	Coagulopathy; ascites; failed percutaneous attempt
Renal	Coagulopathy; failed percutaneous attempt
Intravascular masses	Only available access route

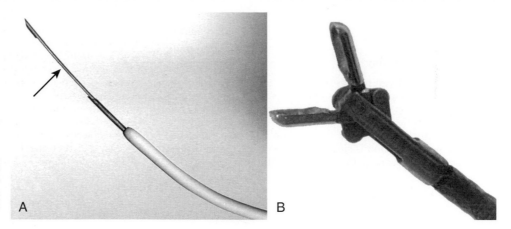

Figure 4-55. Intravascular biopsy devices. **A,** Close-up of cutting needle *(arrow)* used for transjugular liver biopsy. The needle extends beyond the curved 7-French guiding catheter. **B,** Close-up of clam-shell biopsy forceps in the open position.

Suggested Readings

Angle JF, Siddiqi NH, Wallace MJ, et al. Quality improvement guidelines for percutaneous transcatheter embolization: Society of Interventional Radiology Standards of Practice Committee. *J Vasc Interv Radiol*. 2010;21:1479-1486.

Balko A, Piasecki GJ, Shah DM, et al. Transfemoral placement of intraluminal polyurethane prosthesis for abdominal aortic aneurysm. *J Surg Res*. 1986;40: 305-309.

Block PC, Myler RK, Stertzer S, et al. Morphology after transluminal angioplasty in human beings. *N Engl J Med*. 1981;305:382-385.

Brown BD, Cardella JF, Sacks D, et al. Quality improvement guidelines for transhepatic arterial chemoembolization, embolization, and chemotherapeutic infusion for hepatic malignancy. *J Vasc Interv Radiol*. 2006;17:225-232.

Cluzel P, Martinez F, Bellin MF, et al. Transjugular versus percutaneous renal biopsy for the diagnosis of parenchymal disease: comparison of sampling effectiveness and complications. *Radiology*. 2000;215:689-693.

Das TS. Excimer laser-assisted angioplasty for infrainguinal artery disease. *J Endovasc Ther*. 2009;16(Suppl 2):98-104.

Diehm NA, Hoppe H, Do DD. Drug eluting balloons. *Tech Vasc Interv Radiol*. 2010;13:59-63.

Dindyal S, Kyriakides C. A review of cilostazol, a phosphodiesterase inhibitor, and its role in preventing both coronary and peripheral arterial restenosis following endovascular therapy. *Recent Pat Cardiovasc Drug Discov*. 2009;4:6-14.

Dotter CT. Transluminally-placed coilspring endarterial tube grafts: long-term patency in canine popliteal artery. *Invest Radiol*. 1969;4:329-332.

Dotter CT, Judkins MP. Transluminal treatment of arteriosclerotic obstruction: description of a new technic and a preliminary report of its application. *Circulation*. 1964;30:654.

Dotter CT, Rösch J, Seaman AJ. Selective clot lysis with low dose streptokinase. *Radiology*. 1974;111:31.

Drooz AT, Lewis CA, Allen TE, et al. Quality improvement guidelines for percutaneous transcatheter embolization. *J Vasc Interv Radiol*. 1997;8:889-895.

Fisher RG, Ferreyro R. Evaluation of current techniques for nonsurgical removal of intravascular iatrogenic foreign bodies. *AJR*. 1978;130:541-548.

Katzen BT, Kaplan JO, Dake MD. Developing an interventional radiology practice in a community hospital: the interventional radiologist as an equal partner in patient care. *Radiology*. 1989;170(3 Pt 2):955-958.

Kinney TB, Rose SC. Intraarterial pressure measurements during angiographic evaluation of peripheral vascular disease: techniques, interpretation, applications, and limitations. *AJR Am J Roentgenol*. 1996;166:277-284.

Luessenhop AJ, Spence WT. Artificial embolization of cerebral arteries. *JAMA*. 1960;172:1153.

Mammen T, Keshava SN, Eapen CE, et al. Transjugular liver biopsy: a retrospective analysis of 601 cases. *J Vasc Interv Radiol*. 2008;19:351-358.

Met R, Van Lienden KP, Koelemay MJ, et al. Subintimal angioplasty for peripheral arterial occlusive disease: a systematic review. *Cardiovasc Intervent Radiol*. 2008;31:687-697.

Misra S, Gyamlani G, Swaminathan S, et al. Safety and diagnostic yield of transjugular renal biopsy. *J Vasc Interv Radiol*. 2008;19:546-551.

Ouriel K, Gray B, Clair DG, et al. Complications associated with the use of urokinase and recombinant tissue plasminogen activator for catheter-directed peripheral arterial and venous thrombolysis. *J Vasc Interv Radiol*. 2000;11:295-298.

Patel N, Sacks D, Patel RG, et al. SCVIR reporting standards for the treatment of acute limb ischemia with the use of transluminal removal of arterial thrombus. *J Vasc Interv Radiol*. 2001; 2:559-570.

Reekers JA, Bolia A. Percutaneous intentional extraluminal (subintimal) recanalization: how to do it yourself. *Eur J Radiol*. 1998;28:192-198.

Robertson I, Kessel DO, Berridge DC. Fibrinolytic agents for peripheral arterial occlusion. *Cochrane Database Syst Rev*. 2010 Mar 17;(3):CD001099.

Sakakibara S, Kono S. Endomyocardial biopsy. *Jpn Heart J*. 1962;3:537.

Schwarzwälder U, Zeller T. Debulking procedures: potential device specific indications. *Tech Vasc Interv Radiol*. 2010;13:43-53.

Spies JB, Bakal CW, Burke DR, et al. Angioplasty Standard of Practice. *J Vasc Interv Radiol*. 2003;14:S219-S221.

Thomas J, Sinclair-Smith B, Bloomfield D, et al. Nonsurgical retrieval of a broken segment of steel spring guide from the right atrium and inferior vena cava. *Circulation*. 1964;30:106.

Tsetis D, Morgan R, Belli AM. Cutting balloons for the treatment of vascular stenoses. *Eur Radiol*. 2006;16:1675-1683.

Venkatesan AM, Kundu S, Sacks D, et al. Practice guideline for adult antibiotic prophylaxis during vascular and interventional radiology procedures thrombolysis in the management of lower limb peripheral arterial occlusion—a consensus document. *J Vasc Interv Radiol*. 2010;21:1611-1630.

Working Party on Thrombolysis in the Management of Limb Ischemia. Thrombolysis in the management of lower limb peripheral arterial occlusion—a consensus document. *J Vasc Interv Radiol*. 2003;14:S337-S349.

CHAPTER 5

Carotid and Vertebral Arteries

John A. Kaufman, MD, MS, FSIR, FCIRSE, and Gary M. Nesbit, MD

ANATOMY	FIBROMUSCULAR DYSPLASIA	EPISTAXIS
KEY COLLATERAL PATHWAYS	VASCULITIS	CAROTID BODY TUMORS
IMAGING	SPONTANEOUS CAROTID AND VERTEBRAL DISSECTION	HEAD AND NECK MALIGNANCY
ATHEROSCLEROTIC OCCLUSIVE DISEASE	TRAUMA	STROKE THERAPY

The organ at risk from carotid and vertebral artery disease is the brain. Central nervous system ischemia can be severely debilitating and even lethal. Vascular imaging has a major role in the diagnosis of all aspects of cerebrovascular disease. Catheter-based interventions are frequently utilized in the therapy of occlusive disease and acute stroke. This chapter focuses primarily on diagnosis and catheter-based interventions in the extracranial carotid and vertebral arteries, but also includes stroke treatment.

ANATOMY

The right common carotid artery (CCA) arises from the brachiocephalic artery, while the left CCA usually originates directly from the aortic arch (Fig. 5-1). The common carotid arteries ascend through the mediastinum and lie posterior and medial to the internal jugular veins in the neck (see Fig. 2-41). Typical internal diameters of the CCA are 6-8 mm. The CCA bifurcates into the external carotid artery (ECA) and internal carotid artery (ICA) in the upper neck, typically at the upper edge of the thyroid cartilage (between the third and fifth cervical vertebrae). The ICA arises posterolateral to the ECA in approximately 90% of individuals; a medial origin is present in the remaining 10%. The ICA and ECA are normally the only branches of the CCA, small cervical branches directly from the CCA are extremely rare (Fig. 5-2).

The ECA supplies the structures of the neck, face, and scalp (Fig. 5-3). The ECA branches that supply the midline structures of the face frequently anastomose with one another. Many memorable (but unprintable) mnemonics have been devised for the branches of the ECA.

The ICA is usually a branchless vessel until it reaches the base of the skull (Fig. 5-4). The internal diameter of this vessel ranges from 4 to 6 mm. Rarely, persistent embryonic branches to the basilar artery from the cervical ICA may be encountered at the C1-C2 (persistent hypoglossal artery) and C2-C3 (proatlantal intersegmental artery) levels. At the skull base the internal carotid artery enters the serpentine carotid canal within the petrous bone, traveling medial and anterior toward the cavernous sinus. Small branches can communicate from this portion of the ICA with the internal maxillary artery. The ICA exits the petrous canal into the cavernous sinus. An anomalous branch from the cavernous ICA to the basilar artery, the persistent trigeminal artery, is found in 0.5% of patients (Fig. 5-5). Typically, the ophthalmic artery is the first major branch of the distal ICA, arising just above the cavernous sinus. The posterior communicating and anterior choroidal arteries arise from the ICA within the subarachnoid space just before the bifurcation into anterior and middle cerebral arteries.

The vertebral arteries arise from the proximal subclavian arteries in almost 95% of patients, traveling in a posterior and medial direction toward the skull (Fig. 5-6). In 5% of patients the left vertebral artery arises directly from the aortic arch. The diameter of the cervical vertebral artery is 3-5 mm. The left vertebral artery is equal to or larger than the right in 75% of individuals. Unlike the CCA and ICA, the cervical portion of the vertebral artery has many small unnamed muscular branches. The vertebral arteries lie within a series of bony rings formed by the transverse processes of C6 or C5 to C1, before looping posteriorly into the spinal canal between the skull base and C1 (see Fig. 5-4). The segment from the artery origin to where it enters the lowest transverse process is termed *V1*; the section within the transverse processes up to C2 is *V2*; the section between C2 and the spinal canal is *V3*; the final section *(V4)* travels medially through foramen magnum to the basilar artery. Within the skull the vertebral arteries are subarachnoid and give rise to the posterior inferior cerebellar arteries before joining to form the basilar artery. The basilar artery, which runs along the posterior surface of the clivus, terminates by branching into the posterior cerebral arteries. Numerous small branches to the pons, as well as the paired anterior inferior and superior cerebellar arteries, arise from the basilar artery before it bifurcates.

The majority of anatomic variations of the CCA, ICA, and vertebral arteries occur at vessel origins (Table 5-1). These anomalies are related to the development of the thoracic arch (see Chapter 9).

KEY COLLATERAL PATHWAYS

There are two levels of cerebrovascular collaterals: extracranial and intracranial. The ECA is an important source of collateral blood supply to both the ipsilateral and contralateral ICA. In the setting of a proximal ICA occlusion, retrograde flow in the ophthalmic artery can reconstitute the intracranial portion of the distal ICA, thus supplying the brain (Fig. 5-7). With occlusion of a CCA, collateral flow from the contralateral ECA and the ipsilateral vertebral artery can reconstitute the cervical ICA (Fig. 5-8). Rarely, the superficial temporal and middle meningeal arteries can provide collateral supply through the skull to leptomeningeal arteries on the surface of the brain.

In the neck, the vertebral artery is an additional potential source of collateral blood supply to the carotid arteries. Muscular branches of the vertebral artery communicate with the occipital branch of the ECA, which can then reconstitute the ICA. Conversely, the ECA can provide collateral blood supply to the distal cervical vertebral artery through the same pathway. The distal cervical vertebral artery can be reconstituted by muscular arteries of the neck such as the ascending cervical artery.

Within the skull the anterior (carotid) and posterior (vertebral) circulations communicate through a vascular ring, the circle of Willis, located at the base of the brain (Fig. 5-9). This network potentially allows perfusion of the entire brain via any one of four vessels that supply the head. Similarly, the circle of Willis serves as a potential collateral pathway to the upper extremities. The circle of Willis is incomplete or contains hypoplastic elements in more than 50% of individuals. One or both posterior communicating arteries are absent in up to a third of patients. A hypoplastic

or absent A1 segment of the anterior cerebral artery is found in approximately 15%. The posterior cerebral artery arises directly from the ICA in up to 20%. These variants can occur in isolation or in conjunction with other circle anomalies.

IMAGING

The most widely used imaging tool for the extracranial cerebral circulation is ultrasound with pulsed Doppler and duplex color flow. Grayscale imaging with a 4- to 7.5-MHz linear array transducer is sufficient in most patients to identify the CCA, ICA, ECA, and

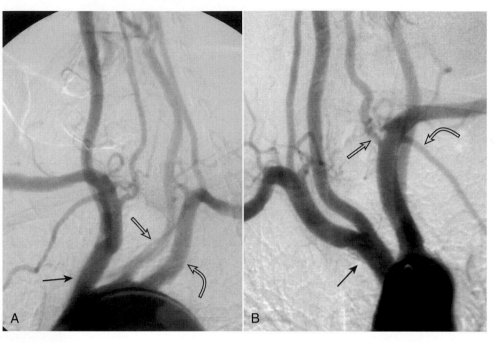

FIGURE 5-1. Normal great vessel origin anatomy. **A,** Digital subtraction (DSA) arch aortogram in the left anterior oblique projection. The brachiocephalic *(solid arrow)*, left common carotid *(open arrow)*, and left subclavian artery *(curved arrow)* origins are best visualized in this obliquity. The bifurcation of the brachiocephalic artery into the right subclavian and common carotid artery origins is obscured in this projection. **B,** DSA arch in the right anterior oblique projection allows evaluation of the bifurcation of the brachiocephalic artery *(solid arrow)* into the right subclavian and common carotid arteries. The left vertebral *(open arrow)* and internal mammary *(curved arrows)* artery origins are seen best in this projection.

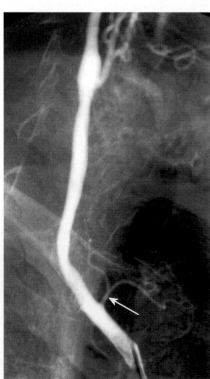

FIGURE 5-2. Branches from the common carotid artery (CCA) are very rare. An artery to the thyroid gland *(arrow)* arises from the right CCA in this patient.

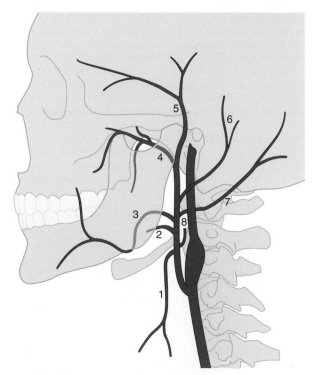

FIGURE 5-3. Line drawing of the external carotid artery branches. *1,* Superior thyroidal artery. *2,* Lingual artery. *3,* Facial artery. *4,* Internal maxillary artery. *5,* Superficial temporal artery. *6,* Posterior auricular artery. *7,* Occipital artery. *8,* Ascending pharyngeal artery.

areas of plaque. Grayscale imaging alone does not perform well in the determination of the degree of stenosis, because hypoechoic "soft" plaque may be indistinguishable from the residual lumen, and calcification in the anterior wall of the vessel can reflect the ultrasound beam so that the lumen cannot be visualized. Sometimes it can be difficult to distinguish the ICA from the ECA. Doppler interrogation of flow improves identification of the vessels and quantification of stenoses. The normal CCA, ICA, and ECA have distinctive Doppler waveforms (Fig. 5-10). The CCA, ICA, and vertebral artery have low-resistance waveforms, whereas the ECA has a high-resistance waveform. Color flow is helpful in localizing vessels and selecting the best place to measure velocities in a stenosis.

The intracranial arteries cannot be directly visualized with current ultrasound units owing to the reflective properties of the skull. Transcranial Doppler (TCD) uses low-frequency (2-MHz) pulsed-wave Doppler to evaluate the intracranial arteries. The low-frequency sound waves can penetrate the thinner portions of the skull. The arteries of the circle of Willis can be evaluated through the temporal bone, the ophthalmic artery through the orbit, and the vertebral artery through the foramen magnum. Direction of flow and alterations in flow velocity and waveforms can be used to infer the presence of occlusive disease.

A number of potential pitfalls exist with carotid ultrasound. The quality of the study is dependent upon a skilled and knowledgeable sonographer. The great vessel origins cannot be reliably imaged. A complete study may not be possible in a patient with a high carotid artery bifurcation situated behind the ramus of the mandible. Lastly, the cervical vertebral arteries are difficult to image in their entirety with ultrasound owing to the surrounding bony vertebra, although direction of flow can be readily determined.

The cervical vessels are excellent subjects for magnetic resonance angiography (MRA). Imaging should cover from the arch to the circle of Willis (intracranial MRA requires dedicated imaging sequences). Two-dimensional (2-D) and three-dimensional (3-D) time-of-flight (TOF) MRA with a superior saturation band were the first clinically useful techniques developed for imaging the cervical arteries. The superior saturation band eliminates jugular venous flow, but also masks reversed flow in a vertebral artery. Calcification of lesions does not impair the ability of MRA to image the carotid arteries, but the degree of stenosis is routinely overestimated. The 3-D techniques provide higher resolution than 2-D, but the area imaged is much smaller. The great vessel origins cannot be adequately evaluated with TOF, and flow in kinked or tortuous carotid arteries loses signal due to saturation. Lastly, very slow flow distal to a severe stenosis may become completely saturated and produce no signal, so that the vessel appears occluded.

Dynamic gadolinium-enhanced 3-D sequences overcome many of the limitations of TOF carotid MRA. Rapid acquisitions during breath-holding are necessary to avoid enhancement of the adjacent jugular veins. However, stenosis, tortuosity, and slow flow do not impair gadolinium-enhanced 3-D carotid MRA. The absence of signal loss from turbulence allows more accurate grading of stenoses. A larger field of view may be used than with TOF MRA, so that diagnostic images can be obtained from origin of the great vessels to the carotid siphon (Fig. 5-11). Dedicated separate sequences should be used to image the circle of Willis and the intracranial circulation. When coupled with anatomic and perfusion/diffusion brain imaging, MR with MRA has the potential to provide complete cerebrovascular evaluation.

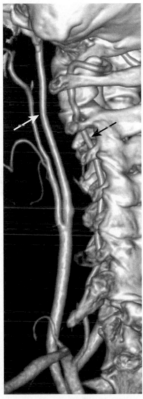

FIGURE 5-4. Internal carotid artery (ICA) anatomy shown on volume rendering of computed tomography angiogram. The cervical ICA *(white arrow)* is a branchless vessel. Note the course of the vertebral artery *(black arrow).*

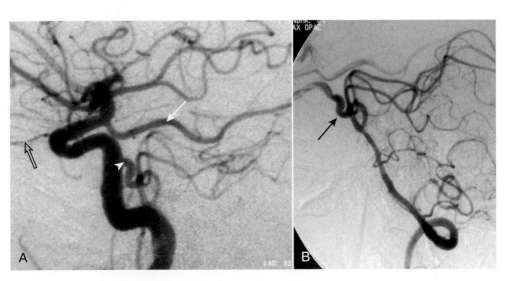

FIGURE 5-5. Anomalous branches of the internal carotid artery (ICA). **A,** Lateral view of the cavernous ICA. Two anomalous branches are present: a posterior cerebral artery *(arrow)* arising exclusively from the ICA (termed a *fetal origin,* found in 20% of patients, bilateral in 8%), and a persistent trigeminal artery *(arrowhead).* The ophthalmic artery *(open arrow)* is a normal branch of the cavernous ICA. **B,** Lateral view of vertebral artery injection in the same patient confirms the identity of the trigeminal artery *(arrow)* anastomosing with the basilar artery.

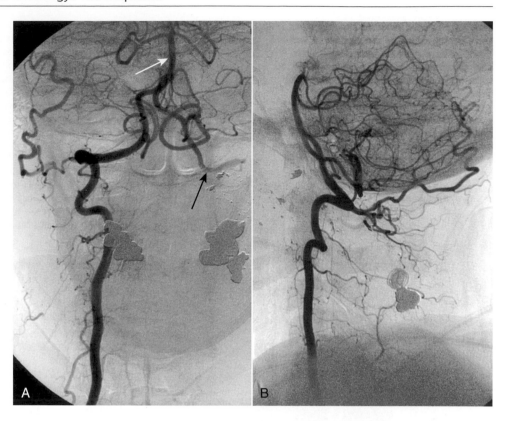

FIGURE 5-6. Vertebral artery anatomy. **A,** Anteroposterior view of right vertebral artery injection in a patient with traumatic occlusion of the V2 segment of the left vertebral artery *(black arrow)*. The vertebral arteries join to form the basilar artery *(white arrow)*. **B,** Lateral view from the same injection.

TABLE 5-1 Anatomic Variants of the Carotid and Vertebral Arteries

Variant	Incidence
Left common carotid artery from brachiocephalic artery ("bovine arch")	22%
Left vertebral artery directly from aortic arch	5%
Combined left common carotid and left subclavian artery origin	1%
Aberrant right subclavian artery (last branch from aortic arch)	1%
Persistent trigeminal artery	0.5%
Persistent hypoglossal artery	0.03%
Congenital absence of the internal carotid artery	0.01%

Limitations of all forms of carotid MRA include signal loss due to presence of metal (e.g., stents or adjacent surgical clips), motion artifacts (e.g., when swallowing or yodeling during the study), and spatial image resolution.

Computed tomography angiography (CTA) is also used extensively to image the cervical carotid and vertebral arteries (see Fig. 5-4). Rapid bolus injection of iodinated contrast with a short delay is necessary to avoid venous enhancement. Imaging should be inclusive from the arch through the brain. Thin slices and careful postprocessing allows accurate evaluation of stenoses, dissections, and aneurysmal disease. Slow flow in a vessel distal to a pinpoint lesion can be reliably detected with CTA, although reversed flow cannot be distinguished from flow in the normal direction. The degree of vascular calcification is readily apparent, but metal in the teeth or cervical spine can create limiting streak artifacts. Major advantages of CTA are that image acquisition times are short (and includes the brain), the adjacent soft tissues can be evaluated as well, and CT scanners are readily available.

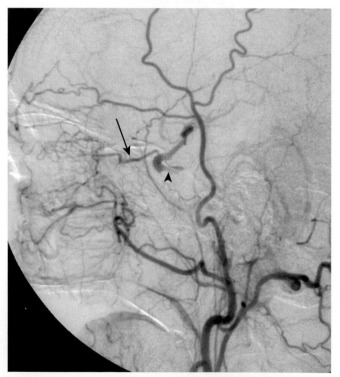

FIGURE 5-7. Lateral view (anterior is to left of image) showing reconstitution of the cavernous portion of the ipsilateral internal carotid artery (ICA) *(arrowhead)* from retrograde flow in the ophthalmic artery *(arrow)* in a patient with occlusion of the cervical ICA.

Imaging of atherosclerotic plaque is of great interest in the cervical carotid, in that plaque composition as well as degree of stenosis influences the risk of stroke. Plaques with a lipid core greater than 25%, a thin overlying fibrous cap, or intraplaque hemorrhage are associated with an increased stroke risk ("vulnerable plaque").

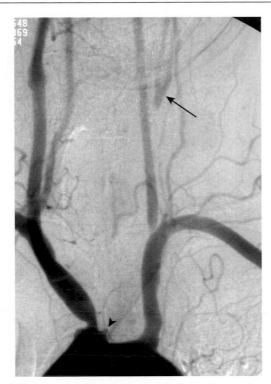

FIGURE 5-8. Reconstitution of the cervical internal carotid artery from retrograde flow in the external carotid artery branches. Left anterior oblique arch aortogram in a patient with left common carotid artery (CCA) origin occlusion *(arrowhead)* and innominate artery stenosis. The left CCA bifurcation *(arrow)* appears to be "floating" in the neck.

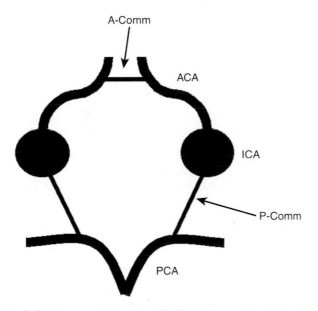

FIGURE 5-9. Diagram of the circle of Willis. A-Comm, Anterior communicating artery; ACA, A1 segment of the anterior cerebral artery; ICA, internal carotid artery; P-Comm, posterior communicating artery; PCA, posterior cerebral artery arising from the bifurcation of the basilar artery.

Plaque imaging is not yet mainstream, but several techniques appear promising. These include high-resolution magnetic resonance imaging (MRI) that can identify plaque components and internal hemorrhage, as well as positron-emission tomography (PET) CT or MRI in which increased metabolic activity is associated with vulnerable plaque. Characterization of the plaque components may become an essential part of carotid imaging for atherosclerotic disease.

Catheter angiography of the extracranial carotid and vertebral arteries is the standard against which other imaging modalities have been validated. Although infrequently used for diagnosis, this modality remains important for resolving diagnostic dilemmas and for interventions. The study should begin with a flush aortic injection through a 5-French pigtail catheter positioned so that the side holes are in the transverse portion of the aortic arch. Filming should be rapid (4-6 frames per second) in the left anterior oblique (LAO) projection (the exact degree depends on patient anatomy, but is usually about 45 degrees). This obliquity opens up the arch to show the origins of the brachiocephalic, left common carotid, and left subclavian vessels to best advantage. If there is a question about the right common carotid or subclavian artery origin, a second injection in the right anterior oblique (RAO) projection should be obtained (see Fig. 5-1). The common carotid arteries can be selected with 5-French catheters, usually with an H-1, Davis, or Berenstein-type shape. When the great vessels arise from the arch at a steep angle, a Simmons shape (S1 for the left CCA and S2 for the right CCA) may be necessary. A short segment (1-2 cm) of soft guidewire (e.g., Bentson) should protrude from the tip of the catheter during selection of the vessel to minimize the risk of trauma. Selection of the ICA and ECA can be accomplished with the same catheters and a hydrophilic-coated or a Bentson guidewire. Carotid injections should be viewed in two planes, usually anteroposterior (AP) and lateral (Table 5-2). Imaging in an anterior oblique view may be necessary to profile ICA and ECA origins.

Vertebral arteries are selected with the same catheter shapes used for the CCA. An H-1, Davis, or Berenstein catheter is advanced into the subclavian artery, rotated so that the tip points superiorly, and gently withdrawn with intermittent puffs of contrast until the vertebral artery orifice is engaged. Careful selection of the vertebral artery is then performed with a hydrophilic or Bentson guidewire. When selection of the vertebral artery is difficult, a subclavian artery angiogram with the ipsilateral brachial artery outflow temporarily occluded with a blood pressure cuff inflated to suprasystolic pressures will opacify the vertebral artery. Vertebral artery angiograms should be performed in at least two planes (AP and lateral) (see Fig. 5-6).

In the unusual situation of performing selective carotid angiography from the upper extremity approach, the preferred access is in the right arm. A Simmons 1 catheter (see Fig. 2-39) can be used to select both carotid arteries. Selection of the right CCA from a left arm access can be challenging and usually requires a Simmons 2 catheter.

Extreme care is necessary when manipulating or flushing any catheter in the aortic arch or cerebral vessels, because small thrombi or air bubbles create huge problems in this vascular bed. Double flush all catheters in these locations every 90 seconds. Many angiographers administer a bolus of 3000-5000 U of heparin during diagnostic studies after obtaining vascular access. The overall risk of permanent stroke during cerebral angiography is about 0.5% with current techniques and equipment. Reversible ischemic events occur in as many as 2% of patients. In patients with ongoing transient ischemic attacks (TIAs), the neurologic complication rates are slightly higher.

ATHEROSCLEROTIC OCCLUSIVE DISEASE

The most common pathologic condition in the extracranial carotid and vertebral arteries is occlusive atherosclerotic disease. About 7% of adults older than 65 years of age have asymptomatic narrowing of cervical carotid arteries of 50% or more due to atherosclerosis. More than 90% of carotid artery stenoses are localized to the bifurcation of the CCA or the proximal ICA (Fig. 5-12). Origin stenoses of the common carotid artery are present in fewer than 5% of patients with concurrent disease at the CCA bifurcation (see Fig. 5-8). Similarly, occlusive disease in the distal ICA is found in 5% of patients with ICA bifurcation disease. Stenoses

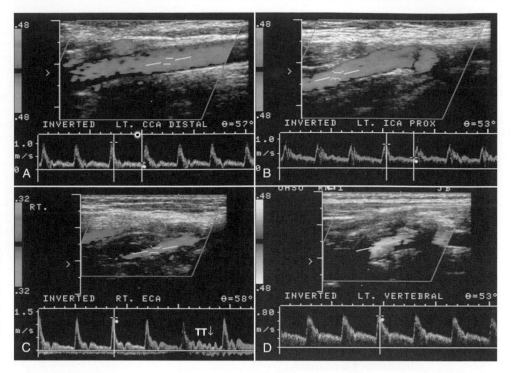

FIGURE 5-10. Normal Doppler waveforms and flow velocities in the cervical carotid and vertebral arteries. **A,** Common carotid artery (CCA). The waveform is low resistance. **B,** Internal carotid artery. The waveform is noticeably more low resistance than the CCA. **C,** External carotid artery. Note the high-resistance waveform. TT = tapping over temporal artery; used to confirm the identity of the artery being imaged. **D,** Vertebral artery. The waveform is low resistance.

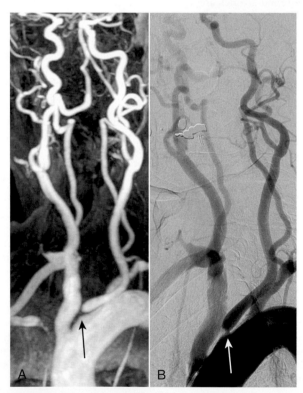

FIGURE 5-11. Three-dimensional gadolinium-enhanced magnetic resonance angiogram of the carotid arteries. **A,** Anterior maximum intensity projection shows from the great vessel origins to the circle of Willis. Loss of signal at the origin of the common carotid artery (CCA) suggests a tight stenosis *(arrow).* **B,** Left anterior oblique digital subtraction angiogram of the aortic arch confirms that there is a stenosis of the left CCA origin *(arrow).*

of the cervical vertebral arteries are found in approximately one third of patients with ICA stenosis, but are rarely symptomatic.

The risk to patients from carotid atherosclerosis is stroke, with about 15% of all strokes thought to be due to debris or thrombus from carotid plaque (Boxes 5-1 and 5-2). Asymptomatic stenosis of the internal carotid artery of less than 75% has only a 1% yearly

risk of stroke, which increases to 2%-5% for tighter lesions. Symptomatic lesions (i.e., those causing reversible episodes of cerebral ischemia, or TIAs) have stroke rates approaching 35% over 5 years. The characteristics of the carotid plaque influence the risk of stroke, with softer, more vulnerable plaques having a higher risk.

The most widely accepted criteria of carotid stenosis on MRA, CTA, and catheter angiography uses the ratio of the diameter of the lumen at the point of maximal stenosis to the diameter of the lumen in the closest normal nontapered segment of cervical internal carotid artery (the NASCET technique: North American Symptomatic Carotid Endarterectomy Trial) (Fig. 5-13). The estimated or true maximal diameter of the ICA bulb or CCA is less accurate and should not be used. A method to calibrate measurements during angiography is to place a radiopaque object with a known diameter on the ipsilateral neck as a reference (especially for sizing stents and balloons).

The mechanism of stroke due to carotid disease is predominantly embolic, either from thrombus or platelet aggregates that form within a lesion, or debris released when an unstable plaque ruptures into the vessel lumen. Irregularities of the plaque surface that look like pits are termed *ulcers* and may have a higher propensity for causing stroke (see Fig. 5-12). Acute carotid occlusion or extreme carotid stenosis can result in ipsilateral stroke when the intracranial collateral circulation is insufficient or thrombus embolizes from the ICA, but cases with adequate collateral perfusion may remain clinically silent.

Patients with carotid stenosis may present with symptoms of transient cerebral or retinal ischemia, presumably due to small emboli that spontaneously lyse or fragment. A TIA is manifested clinically by a neurologic or visual abnormality that usually reverses completely within minutes, but may last up to 24 hours. The risk of a stroke increases 10-fold in patients experiencing TIAs, but only one third of patients with carotid distribution TIAs have moderate or severe carotid artery disease. In other words, plaque composition and degree of stenosis influences risk, and cardiac and aortic sources of emboli are common.

Vertebral and basilar artery occlusive disease has a different clinical presentation than ICA stenosis. The neurologic territory at risk involves the brainstem, cerebellum, and posterior

TABLE 5-2 Injection Rates for Carotid and Vertebral Angiography

Location	Injection Rate	Total Volume	Projections	Filming Rate	Duration
Arch	20-25 mL/sec	30-50 mL	LAO, RAO	4-6 sec	10 sec
CCA	7-9 mL/sec	11-12 mL	AP, Lat, AO	2-4 sec	15 sec
ECA	2-4 mL/sec	4-6 mL	AP, Lat	2-4 sec	15 sec
ICA	6-7 mL/sec	8-9 mL	AP, Lat, AO	2-4 sec	20 sec
Vertebral	3-5 mL/sec	5-7 mL	AP, Lat	2-4 sec	15 sec

AO, Anterior oblique; AP, anteroposterior; CCA, common carotid artery; ECA, external carotid artery; ICA, internal carotid artery; Lat, lateral; LAO, left anterior oblique; RAO, right anterior oblique.

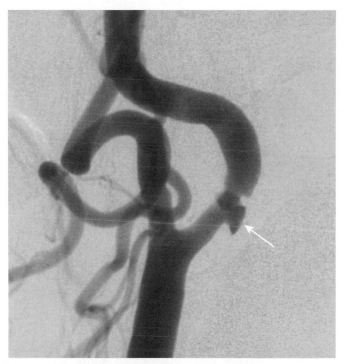

FIGURE 5-12. Digital subtraction angiogram in the anterior oblique projection showing a stenotic proximal internal carotid artery with an ulcer *(arrow)*. The clinical importance of this angiographic appearance is not certain, but would be suspicious as a source of emboli in a patient with recurrent transient ischemic attacks.

Box 5-1. Risk Factors for Stroke

Smoking
Hypertension
Diabetes
Elevated cholesterol
Male sex
Advanced age
African-American or Asian
Family history

Box 5-2. Clinical Features of Anterior Circulation Stroke

Hemiplegia
Hemiparesis
Aphasia, dominant hemisphere
Neglect, nondominant hemisphere
Gaze deviation toward affected hemisphere

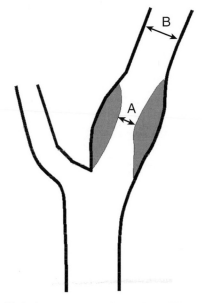

FIGURE 5-13. Technique to measure internal carotid artery (ICA) stenosis. The diameter of the lumen in the most narrow portion is divided by the diameter of the most normal appearing adjacent cervical ICA. The degree of stenosis is $[(B - A)/B] \times 100$.

cerebral lobes. Occlusive disease of the posterior circulation results in a complex of symptoms referred to as *vertebrobasilar syndrome* (Box 5-3). Asymptomatic moderate to severe vertebral artery stenoses result in stroke in about 5% of patients. Patients with TIAs related to posterior circulation lesions have a risk of subsequent stroke of about 22% within 90 days. The anatomic distribution of symptomatic lesions is predominantly at or near the vertebral artery origin (V1 and V2), with about 8% occurring in the basilar artery. Occlusive lesions of the subclavian artery origin cause retrograde flow in the ipsilateral vertebral artery which results in vertebrobasilar syndrome in 25% of patients (see Fig. 3-11).

When carotid occlusive disease is suspected, the first imaging examination for the majority of patients is grayscale and Doppler ultrasound (Fig. 5-14). Velocity measurements proximal, within, and distal to the area of stenosis allow accurate determination of the degree of stenosis (Table 5-3). The flow through an area of stenosis is at first accelerated and remains so until the lumen becomes severely narrowed. Flow then decreases and may be barely detectable by ultrasound. Doppler waveforms distal to the stenosis broaden with first loss in amplitude and ultimately loss of pulsatility. The generally accepted sensitivity and specificity of ultrasound for clinically significant carotid stenosis are each greater than 90%.

The presence of severe disease or occlusion in one ICA may result in ultrasound overestimation of the degree of stenosis in the other ICA owing to normal compensatory increased flow.

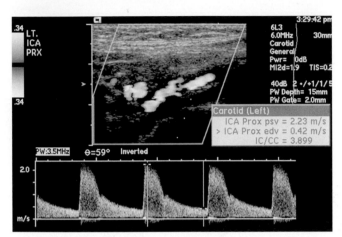

FIGURE 5-14. Ultrasound of carotid stenosis. Spectral broadening and elevated velocities in a patient with left internal carotid artery stenosis.

TABLE 5-3 Ultrasound Evaluation of Internal Carotid Artery Stenosis

Stenosis	PSV (cm/s)	Plaque (%)	EDV (cm/s)	VICA/VCCA
<50%	<120-139	<50	<40	<2
50%-69%	140-230	≥50	40-100	2-4
>70%*	>230	>50	>100	>4

EDV, End diastolic velocity in lesion; plaque, visible plaque reducing diameter of lumen; PSV, peak systolic velocity in lesion; VICA/VCCA, ratio of internal carotid artery PSV to the PSV of the middle/distal common carotid artery.

*For asymptomatic patients, consider using PSV, EDV, and VICA/VCCA to increase positive predictive value.

Data from AbuRahma AF, Srivastava M, Stone PA, et al. Critical appraisal of the Carotid Duplex Consensus criteria in the diagnosis of carotid artery stenosis. *J Vasc Surg.* 2011;53:53-60.

A pinpoint residual ICA lumen with very slow distal flow may be indistinguishable from a total occlusion by ultrasound. This distinction is important because the management is different (see later).

Contrast-enhanced MRA has a sensitivity of greater than 90% and a specificity of greater than 90% for the detection of hemodynamically significant (>50% reduction in luminal diameter) carotid stenosis (Fig. 5-15). However, as a rule, the degree of stenosis is overestimated by MRA, particularly on 2-D TOF sequences. Precise determination of the degree of stenosis requires high-resolution gadolinium-enhanced 3-D sequences. The vertebral arteries are reliably imaged with MRA techniques. The origins at the subclavian arteries or arch can be seen best with gadolinium enhanced 3-D sequences, although motion artifact can degrade images.

The sensitivity and specificity of CTA for detection of carotid stenoses are reportedly slightly less than MRA, but are also greater than 90% each (Fig. 5-16). The vertebral arteries can be evaluated for patency, but direction of flow cannot be determined.

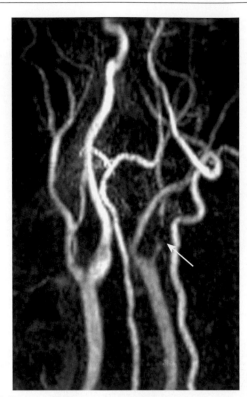

FIGURE 5-15. Magnetic resonance angiogram (MRA) of internal carotid artery (ICA) stenosis. Oblique maximum intensity projection of a 3-D gadolinium-enhanced MRA of the neck demonstrates a tight left ICA origin stenosis *(arrow)* with weak opacification of the distal artery.

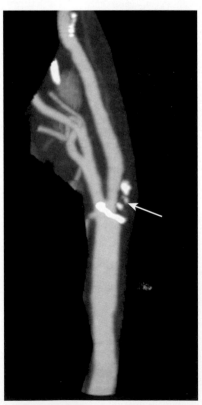

FIGURE 5-16. Sagittal reformat of a computed tomography angiogram showing calcified internal carotid artery origin stenosis *(arrow)*. (Courtesy Larry Tanenbaum, MD, Edison Imaging, N.J.)

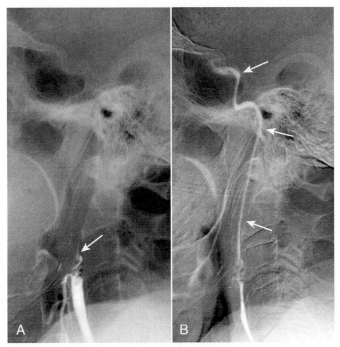

FIGURE 5-17. String sign. **A,** Early lateral film from selective common carotid artery injection shows filling of a few external carotid artery branches and what appears to be an internal carotid artery (ICA) occlusion *(arrow).* **B,** Later image from the same injection shows layering of contrast and slow prograde flow in a patent ICA *(arrows)* beyond a severe origin stenosis. Delayed filming is necessary to detect a string sign.

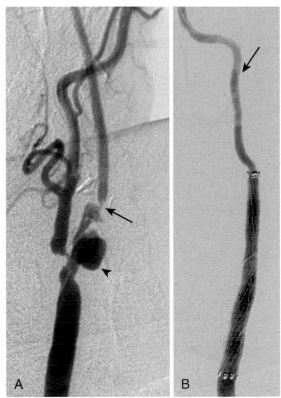

FIGURE 5-18. Focal severe internal carotid artery (ICA) restenosis after carotid endarterectomy associated with aneurysmal dilation at the endarterectomy site. The patient has had several operations on this artery and reoperation is considered high risk. **A,** Oblique digital subtraction angiography shows the stenosis at the distal end of the endarterectomy *(arrow)* and focal dilation *(arrowhead)* presumed to be a patch pseudoaneurysm. Surgical clips are present in the soft tissues near the ICA stenosis. Note the severe stenosis of the external carotid artery origin and the mild narrowing of the distal common carotid artery. **B,** Angiogram after placement of a stent-graft. The stenosis is resolved, the pseudoaneurysm excluded (as well as the external carotid artery). A distal protection device *(arrow)* was used.

Heavily calcified plaque, streak artifact from dental amalgam, and vascular tortuosity can make image interpretation difficult.

Selective common carotid angiography remains widely accepted as a reliable technique for evaluation of ICA stenosis. However, owing to the cost, patient inconvenience, and small risk of stroke, routine use of angiography for diagnosis alone is uncommon. The current indications for catheter angiography include discordant results of noninvasive imaging modalities, technically inadequate noninvasive studies, suspected concurrent great vessel origin or intracranial ICA occlusive disease, and differentiation of severe stenosis from occlusion of the ICA. In the later case, delayed filming in the lateral plane should be obtained in order to detect a "string sign" (Fig. 5-17).

There continues to be great debate over intervention for ICA stenosis. The debate is framed by the morbidity and mortality associated with the intervention versus the risk associated with medical management. Medical management, surgical technique, and catheter-based interventions have all improved rapidly, making comparisons at one point in time difficult to extrapolate to current clinical practice. Furthermore, randomized prospective controlled trials necessarily study homogeneous patient populations that do not reflect the variety of daily practice. Nevertheless, the intervention that is still used as a benchmark is surgical carotid endarterectomy (CEA), which has a reported operative stroke rate of 2%-3%, mortality of less than 1%, cranial nerve injury in 1%-2%, and a symptomatic restenosis rate of 1%-2% (Fig. 5-18). The adoption of surgical patch angioplasty rather than eversion endarterectomy has further decreased restenosis rates.

A number of prospective studies comparing CEA with medical therapy profoundly influenced the management and subsequent investigation of this disease. The North American Symptomatic Carotid Endarterectomy Trial (NASCET) and the European Carotid Surgery Trial (ECST), both reported in the 1990s, were randomized comparisons of optimal medical therapy (of that time) and combined CEA and medical therapy in patients with symptomatic carotid stenosis. For patients with 70%-99% stenoses, the

cumulative risks of any ipsilateral stroke at 2 years were 26% and 32% (NASCET and ECST, respectively) in the medical patients and 9% and 16% (NASCET and ECST, respectively) in the surgical patients. In the NASCET trial, the risk for a major or fatal ipsilateral stroke was 13.1% for medical patients versus 2.5% for surgical patients. The risk reduction for symptomatic patients with 50%-70% stenoses was less pronounced, but still significant.

Asymptomatic patients were studied in the Asymptomatic Carotid Atherosclerosis Study (ACAS), the Veterans Affairs Cooperative Study Group, and the Asymptomatic Carotid Surgery Trial. In these studies, asymptomatic men and women with 60% or greater stenoses of the ICA were randomized to either CEA and medical therapy or medical therapy alone. The risk of stroke or death within 30 days of surgery was up to 3.3% in the CEA group, significantly higher than the first 30 days of medical therapy. However, over time, CEA patients fared better. In the ACAS trial the aggregate risk of stroke at 5 years was 5.1% for the surgical group and 11% for medical therapy. These studies established 60% diameter reduction of the ICA as the threshold for intervention in patients with asymptomatic stenoses.

Carotid artery stenting (CAS) is undergoing intensive investigation as an alternative to CEA. The studies have evolved as techniques and devices have matured, skills improved, and target patient populations changed. For example, in the Carotid and Vertebral Artery Transluminal Angioplasty Study (CAVATAS), only high-risk surgical patients were included, distal protection was not available, and stents were not used in all patients. However, this study did show that, when used, stents reduced the risk of procedural stroke compared to angioplasty alone. In the Stenting and Angioplasty with Protection in Patients at Risk for Endarterectomy study (SAPPHIRE), distal protection and dedicated stents were used in all patients. The majority of patients had asymptomatic carotid stenosis. There was an initial advantage of CAS over CEA, with 1-year risk of stroke or death at 1.9% versus 5.3%, respectively. At 3 years, the two treatments became equivalent.

The Stent-protected Percutaneous Angioplasty of the Carotid vs. Endarterectomy (SPACE) trial studied symptomatic patients with greater than 50% stenosis. Distal protection devices were used in only 27% of CAS cases. This study demonstrated no difference in ipsilateral stroke that persisted through 2 years. Another study, the Endarterectomy vs. Angioplasty in Patients with Symptomatic Severe Carotid Stenosis (EVA-3S) was stopped early due to safety concerns related to high stroke rates in CAS patients. Distal protection was initially not mandated in the study, and operators with limited experience were allowed to participate.

The International Carotid Stenting Study (ICSS) and the Carotid Revascularization Endarterectomy vs. Stenting Trial (CREST) are the two largest studies of CAS. Asymptomatic and symptomatic patients were included. The ICSS trial allowed a variety of stents and distal protection was used in 72% of patients. At 120 days, the incidence of stroke, death, or procedural myocardial infarction (MI) was 8.5% and 5.2% for CAS and CEA, respectively, a significant difference. The CREST trial was not only larger, but had a strict credentialing process for investigators and uniformity in the stent and protection device (with 96% application). The primary endpoint was any periprocedural stroke, MI, death, or postprocedural ipsilateral stroke for up to 4 years. At 2.5 years, there was no significant difference (7.2% and 6.8% for CAS and CEA, respectively), but there were more strokes in the CAS group and more MIs in the CEA group during the first 30 days whether analyzed in aggregate or by symptom status. Interestingly, the rate of stroke and death in the CAS patients at 30 days for both symptomatic (6%) and asymptomatic patients (2.5%) were equivalent to those reported for CEA in the ACAS and NASCET trials.

The indications for carotid stenting are in flux, and local talent has great influence on which procedure to perform. Assuming the availability of both skilled interventionalists and surgeons, for symptomatic patients younger than 70 years with low surgical risk, CAS and CEA are equivalent in terms of overall outcomes, with the tradeoff between increased stroke in CAS and increased MI and cranial nerve injury in CEA. In patients younger than 60 years, the stroke outcomes with CAS may be better than with CEA. Symptomatic patients at high surgical risk are good candidates for CAS, but age older than 80 years increases CAS risk substantially. Asymptomatic patients are more challenging to triage, but CAS should be considered in patients with greater than 70% stenosis and high surgical risk.

Carotid stenting should be performed within the context of adequate training in the technique, competence in cerebral angiography (performance and interpretation), and access to specialty stroke-related support. Meticulous technique is essential during carotid stent procedures (one small air bubble can ruin everything). A standardized catheter and sheath flush protocol should be in place, with careful debubbling of all pressure infusion setups for sheaths. Patients at increased risk of procedural complication with CAS include those with poor access (i.e., tortuous or diseased iliac arteries, thoracic aorta, or carotid arteries), heavily calcified lesions, age older than 80 years, and multiple or tandem lesions, especially those involving the carotid siphon.

A very important component of the procedure is the use of a cerebral embolic protection apparatus. The two basic approaches to cerebral protection are distal ICA filters or occlusion, or flow reversal in the ICA (Fig. 5-19 and see Fig. 4-19). Distal devices require crossing the lesion in order to position the

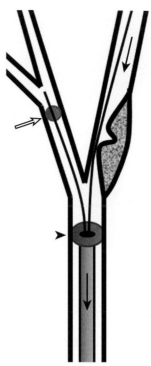

FIGURE 5-19. Schematic of flow reversal apparatus deployed for a carotid intervention. The proximal balloon *(arrowhead)* on the large guide catheter occludes flow in the common carotid artery, and the distal balloon *(open arrow)* occludes flow in the external carotid artery. This results in reversal of flow in the internal carotid artery that is aspirated through the guide catheter *(solid arrows)*. During an intervention on the ICA stenosis, this prevents distal embolization of debris.

protection system but allow continued antegrade cerebral perfusion, whereas flow reversal systems require an intact circle of Willis and positioning of occlusion balloons in the CCA and ECA to control inflow. Distal protection devices can induce spasm in the ICA, which resolves with removal of the device. Each patient and lesion should be evaluated for suitability for the available devices, because no single device can be used for every patient or lesion.

The patient undergoing carotid artery stenting should be pretreated with dual antiplatelet medication such as clopidogrel and aspirin, and anticoagulated during the procedure with heparin. A 6- or 7-French guiding catheter in the carotid artery is necessary to provide a stable working platform. The lesion is carefully crossed, a protection device deployed, the lesion predilated with an undersized balloon using short inflation times, a self-expanding stent deployed with or without postdilation, angiographic confirmation of a satisfactory result, and then removal of the protection device (Fig. 5-20). Dedicated balloon and stent systems that use 0.014- to 0.018-inch guidewires are often used. Typical angioplasty balloon diameters are 4-6 mm for the ICA. Self-expanding stents are preferred in this region, because it is subject to rotation and external compression, which could crush a balloon-expandable stent. Perhaps more important, self-expanding stents conform better to the anatomy, which can involve disparate diameter vessels and tortuosity. Stent placement across the origin of the ECA is frequently necessary to adequately treat ICA-origin stenoses and is well tolerated. Stretching of the carotid bulb during the procedure can trigger a reflex bradycardia or asystole, so atropine 1 mg should be available or given intravenously before balloon inflation, and a transvenous or transcutaneous pacemaker should be close at hand. Persistent hypotension for 12-24 hours can also occur, such that close hemodynamic monitoring overnight is required. The goal of stenting is to increase flow across the lesion, not make it equal or better than new. This is a vascular bed in which the old adage "the enemy of good is better" applies.

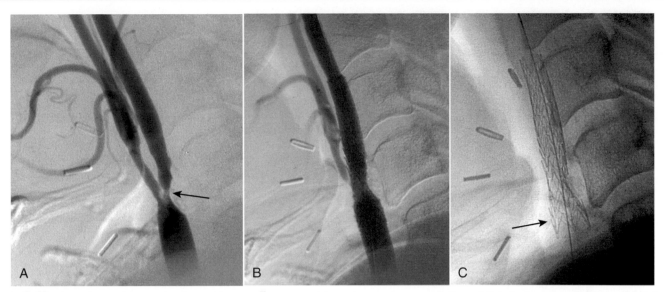

FIGURE 5-20. Carotid stenosis treated with metallic stent in a patient with previous neck surgery. **A,** Lateral digital subtraction angiogram (DSA) showing stenosis of the common carotid artery (CCA) bifurcation extending into the internal carotid artery (ICA) *(arrow)* and external carotid artery (ECA). **B,** Lateral DSA after placement of a self-expanding stent. The ICA is widely patent, but the ECA does not fill as well as before. **C,** Unsubtracted lateral image showing that the stent extends from the distal CCA *(arrow)* into the ICA. This placement is intentional in order to treat the full length of the stenosis. Note that the guidewire remains in place across the stent until the very end of the procedure.

Patients can be followed with duplex ultrasound or angiography. The restenosis rate (>70%) is approximately 3%-6% over 4 years, with a similar incidence of stent fractures.

The endovascular treatment of symptomatic vertebral artery atherosclerotic stenosis depends on the location of the lesion. Balloon-expandable stent placement in origin lesions produces relief of symptoms, with a restenosis rate of approximately 10% at 1 year, and subsequent stroke is less than 2%. The restenosis rate may be reduced with the use of drug-eluting stents.

FIBROMUSCULAR DYSPLASIA

The ICA is the second most common site of fibromuscular dysplasia (FMD), with the renal arteries being the first. Overall, FMD of the ICA is found in just under 1% of patients undergoing carotid arteriography, with the typical location at the level of C2-C1. Vertebral FMD is much less common. There are a number of forms of FMD (see Table 1-4), but 85% of cases are of the medial fibroplasia type, which has a distinctive "string of pearls" appearance. FMD is localized to the cervical portion of the ICA distal to the bulb in 90% of cases. This process can also involve the vertebral artery (10%-40%). Lesions are bilateral in up to two thirds of patients. Approximately 20% of patients with carotid FMD also have intracranial aneurysms (Fig. 5-21).

The presence of FMD in the carotid or vertebral circulation is frequently an asymptomatic incidental finding on physical examination (an audible bruit) or imaging studies. Progression to symptomatic FMD is very rare. Patients may complain of symptoms that are difficult to attribute directly to the FMD, such as headache, a swishing sound in the ears, and dizziness. However, patients can present with more significant symptoms of TIAs, presumably due to embolization of small thrombi that form in the aneurysmal "pearls." Other sources of emboli, such as the heart and atherosclerotic ICA stenosis, should be excluded before attributing these symptoms to FMD. Subarachnoid hemorrhage due to associated intracranial aneurysms can occur. Spontaneous ICA or vertebral artery dissection can be due to underlying FMD, although establishing the diagnosis after the dissection has occurred can be difficult unless FMD can be found in a nondissected cerebral artery.

The most sensitive imaging modality for detecting FMD is conventional angiography. Subtle FMD can be difficult or

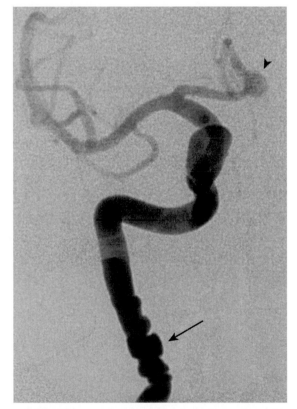

FIGURE 5-21. Fibromuscular dysplasia of the internal carotid artery (ICA). Digital subtraction angiogram of the right ICA showing a beaded appearance *(arrow)* of the distal cervical ICA typical of medial fibroplasia. Note the anterior circulation intracranial aneurysm *(arrowhead)*.

impossible to visualize with ultrasound, MRA, and CTA because image resolution is too low. A flow disturbance or area of stenosis may be detected by ultrasound, but the full extent of the FMD in the cervical ICA cannot be determined with this modality.

Intervention in carotid FMD is warranted in symptomatic patients (e.g., TIA without another source) or when a critical stenosis is present. Surgical resection of the abnormal segment

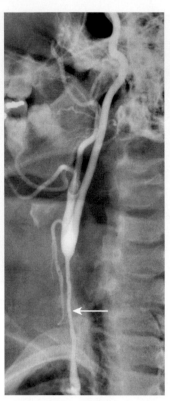

Figure 5-22. Takayasu arteritis involving the carotid arteries in a young woman. Selective right common carotid artery angiogram showing the long, smooth stenosis *(arrow)* that spares the bifurcation, internal carotid artery, and external carotid artery (see Fig. 1-14).

may be possible if the FMD is low enough and limited in extent. However, medial fibroplasia is ideally suited for angioplasty (and stents when necessary), because distal lesions can be treated. Results in small series of patients undergoing ICA angioplasty for FMD have been excellent and durable.

VASCULITIS

Vasculitides involving the carotid and vertebral arteries are rare in North America, but much more common in portions of Asia and South America. Long, smooth stenoses are characteristic, although irregular lesions or a "sausage link" appearance may be present. Concurrent atherosclerosis can be seen in older patients or with radiation vasculitis.

The best known vasculitis that affects the carotid arteries is Takayasu arteritis. This granulomatous disease can involve the CCA, great vessel origins, subclavian arteries, thoracic and abdominal aorta, coronary arteries, visceral arteries, and pulmonary arteries (Fig. 5-22; see Figs. 1-12 and 9-31). Patients usually present with signs of a systemic illness such as fever and malaise, but may have vascular occlusion as their only symptom. However, TIA and stroke can occur. The typical patient is a young woman aged 20-40 years (female-to-male ratio 9:1), although the disease has been reported in males, children, and septuagenarians as well. Angiographically, long smooth stenoses of the common carotid and subclavian arteries are characteristic. A thickened, enhancing arterial wall can be seen with ultrasound, CT, MRI, and PET (see Fig. 1-13). Angioplasty and stenting of severe stenoses due to Takayasu arteritis during the inactive or "burned out" phase is successful.

Giant cell arteritis is the most common primary vasculitis, affecting large and medium arteries in 2-20/100,000 persons older than age 50 years. Involvement of branches of the ECA is common, with anterior ischemic neuropathy being a particular risk. Headache and jaw claudication are typical symptoms, and stroke

has been reported in 1%-3% of patients. Angiography is rarely performed for the diagnosis of GCA in the carotids. Temporal artery ultrasound and large artery PET, CT, and MRI scans are useful for diagnosis, but temporal artery biopsy is usually performed.

Radiation vasculitis occurs months to years following external beam therapy. The typical appearance is diffuse stenosis that can look very much like atherosclerosis with intimal calcification and focal irregularity. The distribution of the lesions is the key to the diagnosis, because they are localized to the radiation portal and involve many vessels. Patients may present with acute stroke or chronic ischemic symptoms. Intervention is difficult in that the vessels do not respond well to angioplasty, and the surgical field is challenging owing to the location of the lesions and scarring.

SPONTANEOUS CAROTID AND VERTEBRAL DISSECTION

Spontaneous (i.e., in the absence of trauma) dissection of the CCA, ICA, or vertebral arteries is the most common cause of stroke in young patients. The incidence of spontaneous carotid dissection is 2.6/100,000, and the incidence of vertebral dissection is 1-1.5/100,000. There are numerous etiologies, including FMD, hypertension, and underlying arterial wall abnormalities (Box 5-4; see Fig. 1-38). Patients tend to be in their third to fifth decade, but dissection can occur in any age group. The presenting symptoms can be misleading and result in delay in diagnosis. Ipsilateral headache is characteristic, but incomplete Horner syndrome, cranial nerve dysfunction (VII, IX, X, and XII), and focal cerebral ischemic events due to reduced flow or emboli also occur (Box 5-5). The neurologic findings may be delayed by hours, days, and even months.

CT, MRI, and ultrasound are particularly useful for diagnosis of carotid and vertebral dissection. The intimal flap or a compressed true lumen may be visualized (Fig. 5-23). Slow flow or a thrombosed false lumen may appear bright on both T1- and T2-weighted MRI, depending on velocity of flow or the age of the thrombus. Compression or long tapered occlusion of the lumen is characteristic on angiography. Focal pseudoaneurysms can occur if the dissection penetrates into the subadventitia. Dissection of the ICA may extend into the cavernous portion of the artery, and 10% of vertebral artery dissections extend intracranially.

At least 85% of patients can be successfully managed with long-term anticoagulation. Identification and, if possible, modification of underlying risk factors is a crucial aspect of treatment. However, in most patients, no etiology can be found. Patients

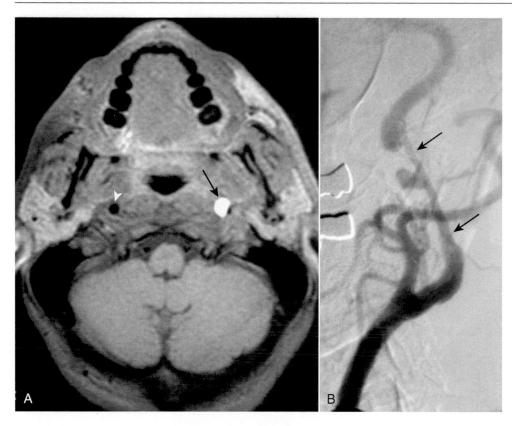

FIGURE 5-23. Spontaneous carotid dissection. **A**, Axial T1-weighted magnetic resonance image showing the true lumen of the left internal carotid artery (ICA) lumen compressed by a false lumen that has bright signal *(arrow)* consistent with thrombus or slow flow. The right ICA *(arrowhead)* is normal. **B**, Digital subtraction angiogram in the same patient showing the compressed true lumen of the left ICA *(arrows)*. The false lumen does not fill.

who experience ongoing ischemic events, progressive neurologic symptoms, or enlarging pseudoaneurysms, or who have contraindication to anticoagulation can be treated with self-expanding stent placement in the true lumen. Pseudoaneurysms may require coil embolization as well. Distal protection is rarely indicated in these procedures. Following stent placement the patients should be maintained on antiplatelet therapy if possible. Permanent occlusion of the pseudoaneurysm is achieved in 90% of cases. The long-term restenosis and occlusion rates (1%-3% total in the carotid, 12% in the vertebral arteries) are low.

▬ TRAUMA

Traumatic lesions to the extracranial cervical vessels can be caused by any mechanism, but they are most commonly related to penetrating, blunt, hyperextension, and blast injuries. Common associations include cervical fractures and dislocations, and airway and esophageal trauma. Injury can occur to both the arteries and the veins, particularly the internal jugular vein. Clinical presentation varies with the type and mechanism of trauma, and severity of other injuries. The full spectrum of vascular injuries may be present, ranging from spasm to transection with active extravasation.

Penetrating neck injuries result in vascular injury in up to 25% of patients and have an overall mortality rate of approximately 5%. The neck is divided into three vascular zones (Table 5-4). Zones 3 and 1 injuries are extremely difficult to approach surgically (the mandible obstructs access to zone 3, and thoracotomy is required for control of arteries in zone 1). Vascular injuries in zone 1 have a 12% mortality rate. Stable patients with suspected vascular injury in these zones usually undergo CT scan and sometimes angiography. Injuries to zone 2 are not only more common (60%-70%), but are readily accessible for physical examination and surgery (Fig. 5-24). Stable patients may undergo exploratory surgery, CT, ultrasound examination, serial physical examinations, or angiography depending on the local standard of care.

The majority of major vascular injuries in the neck due to penetrating wounds involve the carotid arteries, although the

TABLE 5-4 Vascular Zones in Penetrating Neck Trauma

Zone	Definition
1	Below cricoid cartilage to clavicles
2	Cricoid cartilage to mandibular angle
3	Above angle of mandible to skull base

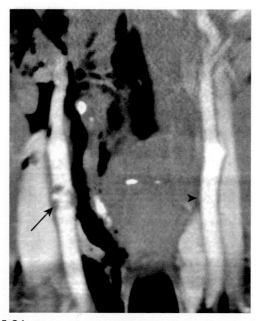

FIGURE 5-24. Right common carotid artery (CCA) dissection *(arrow)* in zone 2 following blunt trauma to the neck. Compare to the normal left CCA *(arrowhead)*. There is extensive soft tissue emphysema consistent with either esophageal or tracheal injury.

vertebral arteries are injured in up to 4% of patients (Fig. 5-25). Branches of the external carotid artery may be involved as well as the major veins. Angiography for trauma of the cervical vessels should therefore always include delayed images that visualize the veins.

Arterial injury from a direct blow, the shoulder strap of seat belts, and strangulation is found in fewer than 2% of all blunt trauma cases. However, TIA or stroke occurs in more than 40% of patients with arterial injury in some series. Autopsy studies of injuries have shown intimal and medial tears in 64%, adventitial contusions in 70%, and multiartery involvement in 39%. The most common location for traumatic dissection is the cervical ICA, extending into the skull base. Vertebral artery dissection

may be found in as many as 20% of patients (Fig. 5-26). Symptoms develop in up to two thirds of patients within the first 24 hours, but only 10% have focal neurologic findings on initial presentation. Symptoms may develop weeks to months following injury. The etiology of the delayed symptoms is believed to be emboli originating from the dissection rather than compromise of ICA flow. A high level of suspicion is necessary to diagnose these lesions. Ultrasound, MRI/MRA, CT, and angiography are all used for evaluation of suspected carotid injury in blunt trauma.

Intervention in carotid and vertebral injury is determined by the type of injury, symptoms, accessibility of the vessel, and overall status of the patient. Spasm, intimal tears, and nonocclusive dissection are managed with anticoagulation or antiplatelet

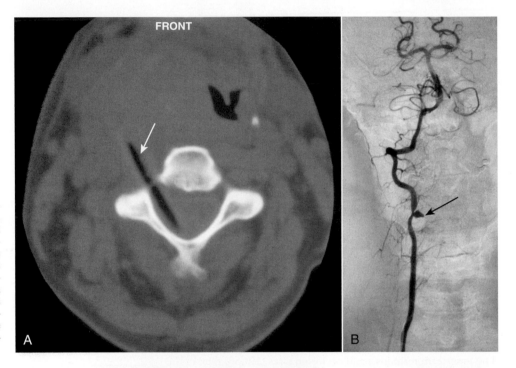

FIGURE 5-25. Vertebral artery pseudoaneurysm due to penetrating injury. **A,** Computed tomography scan of the neck showing a wood splinter through the neural foramina *(arrow)*. There is a large hematoma in the neck that displaces the airway. **B,** Selective right vertebral angiogram after removal of the splinter shows a small pseudoaneurysm *(arrow)*. This was treated by balloon occlusion of the vertebral artery proximal and distal to the lesion after ensuring that the left vertebral artery was normal.

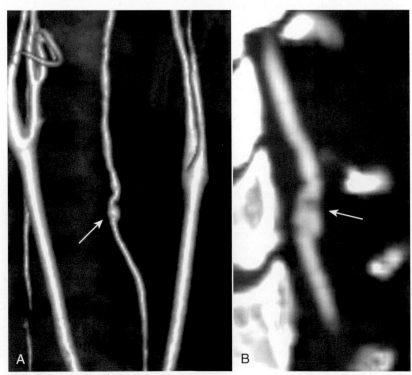

FIGURE 5-26. Vertebral artery dissection following motor vehicle accident. **A,** Volume rendering of cervical computed tomography angiogram shows focal irregular enlargement of the left vertebral artery *(arrow)*. **B,** Coronal reformation through the same area shows the intimal irregularity within the artery.

therapy alone when feasible. Stent or stent-graft placement may be considered for substantial zone 1 and 3 injuries to reduce the risk of stroke or bleeding. Long-term antiplatelet therapy is necessary to decrease the rate of stent occlusion, which has been high in some early series. Endovascular occlusion of surgically inaccessible transected vessels can be performed with coils, plugs, or other devices. These procedures are usually tolerated well in patients with intact intracranial collateral pathways.

EPISTAXIS

Nosebleeds are common and usually due to a source in the anterior portion of the nose. These bleeds usually stop spontaneously, or can be readily visualized and treated with local measures. Posterior epistaxis occurs in a more inaccessible region and is much more difficult to control. In addition, bleeding in this location is more frequent in older patients with multiple medical problems. Uncommon etiologies include tumors, penetrating trauma, and carotid artery laceration in the siphon due to fractures of the skull base. Up to 25% of patients with Osler-Weber-Rendu disease have frequent bleeding from nasopharyngeal telangiectases.

The initial management of severe posterior epistaxis is resuscitation (including blood products), correction of coagulopathies, intravenous vasoconstrictors, and application of direct pressure to the area with nasal packing. The latter is extremely uncomfortable and fails in roughly 25% of cases. The arterial supply to the posterior nasal cavity is primarily from the internal maxillary artery. Surgical ligation or clipping of the internal maxillary artery has a 10%-30% failure rate. Endoscopic cautery has similar rates of success and rebleeding.

Selective catheterization of the internal maxillary artery and embolization with particles and Gelfoam successfully controls bleeding in 75%-95% of cases (Fig. 5-27). Extravasation is rarely seen at angiography. Patients should be counseled on the risks of pain and stroke related to nontarget organ embolization. Bilateral embolization should be performed to prevent reconstitution of the distal internal maxillary branches from the opposite side. Collateral supply to the posterior nasopharynx from sources such as the facial artery should be evaluated when internal maxillary artery embolization is insufficient. Epistaxis due to rupture of the ICA in the siphon is managed with proximal and distal balloon occlusion of the ICA.

CAROTID BODY TUMORS

The carotid body comprises neural tissue located in the adventitia of the posterior medial CCA bifurcation. The carotid body is a chemoreceptor that is responsive to hypoxia, hypercapnia, and acidosis, producing an increased respiratory and heart rate, tidal volume, blood pressure, and circulating catecholamines.

Tumors of the carotid body are rare; 5% are bilateral (unless familial, in which bilateral lesions are found in one third), about 5% are endocrinologically active, and up to 50% are malignant (although metastases are present in fewer than 5%). The typical presentation is a painless neck mass at the angle of the mandible. Carotid body tumors are highly vascular, receiving arterial blood supply from the ECA in the majority of cases. Splaying of the CCA bifurcation by a vascular mass is a characteristic finding on imaging studies (Fig. 5-28). Large lesions can encase the ICA and ECA.

The treatment of carotid body tumors is surgical excision because of the progressive growth and malignant potential of these masses. Preoperative embolization reduces blood loss. Selective catheterization of supplying arterial branches and embolization with small-diameter particles is performed shortly before surgery.

HEAD AND NECK MALIGNANCY

Primary tumors of the carotid arteries are exceedingly rare, but secondary involvement by head and neck tumors is a well-known phenomenon. Arterial encasement and invasion of the CCA, ICA, or ECA occurs in at least 5% of patients with squamous cell carcinomas. Rarely, stent placement is required to relieve symptomatic CCA or ICA compression by an unresectable tumor. Massive arterial bleeding ("carotid blow-out") may occur due to direct tumor invasion, infection, tumor necrosis, iatrogenic injury, or radiation necrosis. Endovascular treatment of bleeding with endograft placement or embolization (including carotid artery occlusion) is temporarily life-saving (Fig. 5-29).

STROKE THERAPY

Approximately 800,000 strokes occur each year in the United States, of which 600,000 are first time events, with a 30-day mortality of 17%. An ischemic or thromboembolic etiology is responsible for almost 85% of strokes. The underlying etiology of stroke is extracranial carotid artery disease in 15%, a cardiac source in 20%, intracranial disease in 20%, emboli from aortic plaque in 20%, and unknown in about 25%. Approximately 15% of strokes are hemorrhagic in nature, due to hypertensive vasculopathy, ruptured cerebral aneurysms or arteriovenous malformations, and hematologic disorders. The estimated total cost of the care of patients with stroke approached $80 billion in 2010.

The aggressive early treatment of stroke with the aim to reverse the neurologic injury is a relatively recent phenomenon. A number of randomized trials beginning in the 1990s established that intravenous thrombolytics resulted in improved long-term outcomes (by a factor of 4 to 5) but an increased risk of intracranial hemorrhage compared to conservative management. As a result,

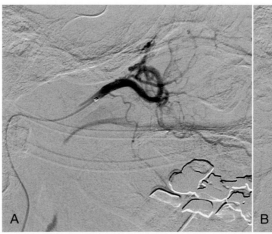
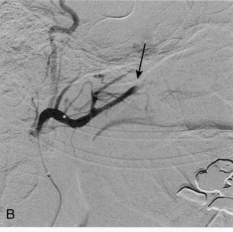

FIGURE 5-27. Embolization of the internal maxillary artery in a patient with epistaxis unresponsive to conservative treatment. **A,** Lateral digital subtraction angiogram with selective injection into internal maxillary artery. **B,** Selective internal maxillary artery injection following embolization with Ivalon particles. There is stasis of flow *(arrow)*. The contralateral internal maxillary artery was subsequently embolized.

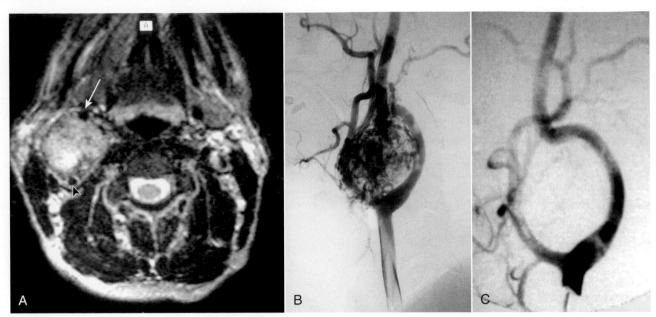

FIGURE 5-28. Carotid body tumor. **A,** T2-weighted magnetic resonance image showing the tumor splaying the internal carotid artery (ICA) *(arrowhead)* and external carotid artery *(arrow).* **B,** Lateral common carotid artery digital subtraction angiogram showing a hypervascular mass splaying the ICA and ECA. **C,** Following embolization, the mass is devascularized. The patient then underwent uncomplicated surgical resection.

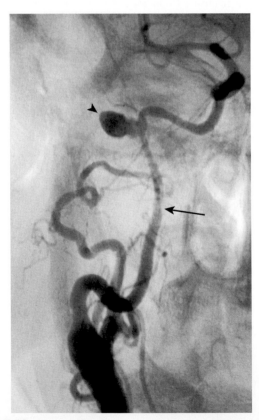

FIGURE 5-29. Massive intermittent posterior pharyngeal bleeding in a patient with inoperable squamous cell carcinoma who has been treated with radiation. Unsubtracted angiogram in the anterior projection showing a diffusely narrowing cervical internal carotid artery (ICA) *(arrow)* and a pseudoaneurysm *(arrowhead).* This was treated with balloon occlusion of the ICA proximal and distal to the lesion. Prior to the balloon occlusion, an injection in the left common carotid artery (CCA) was performed while compressing the right CCA to confirm that the right anterior and middle cerebral arteries would fill from the left ICA. The patient tolerated the balloon occlusion without complication.

intravenous thrombolysis became an accepted option if initiated within 4.5 hours of onset of symptoms for patients younger than 80 years of age (Box 5-6). The recommended dose is 0.9 mg/kg recombinant tissue plasminogen activator (maximum dose 90 mg) over 60 minutes with 10% of the dose given as a bolus over 1 minute.

The direct delivery of thrombolytic agents into the occlusion improves overall recanalization rates and clinical outcomes. With intravenous infusion, recanalization of occlusions occurs in less than 50% of patients. Large vessel (ICA) thrombosis in particular and about two thirds of proximal middle cerebral occlusions do not respond well to the intravenous approach. Direct intraarterial administration of thrombolytic agents increases the recanalization rates to more than 60%, with the best results with soft thrombus. The intracranial hemorrhage rate is approximately 10%. In addition, the treatment window can be extended to 6 hours, but the best results remain in patients treated early.

Some strokes are caused by organized emboli that are resistant to thrombolysis, whether it is intravenous or intraarterial. In addition, the ability to rapidly restore flow, potentially without the use of thrombolytics, may expand the indications for acute stroke treatment. Mechanical approaches have been developed that can be used instead of or with thrombolytics. The basic strategies are to pull out the clot with a retrieval device, aspirate the clot, accelerate thrombolysis with low-frequency ultrasound, or to compress the thrombus with angioplasty and possibly a stent. Employed in isolation, each of these techniques have recanalization rates that approach 60% with symptomatic intracranial hemorrhage rates that are similar to intraarterial thrombolysis. The superiority of one particular technique has not been established. However, when used in combination with thrombolysis, the overall recanalization rates increase to greater than 75% with no increased risk of symptomatic hemorrhage. Aggressive multimodal therapies for stroke have become established as options in the treatment of patients with acute stroke.

When managing the acute stroke patient, "time is brain." The faster blood flow is restored, the better the recovery, with intervention within the first 90 minutes being optimal. The best setting for stroke treatment is within an organized stroke center with trained personnel prepared to rapidly and consistently triage, image, and treat patients. When the expertise and tools are

Box 5-6. AHA/ASA Indications for Intravenous Thrombolysis in Acute Stroke

Stroke within 3 hr:

- Diagnosis of ischemic stroke causing measurable neurologic deficit
- Neurologic signs should not be clearing spontaneously
- Neurologic signs should not be minor and isolated
- Caution should be exercised in treating a patient with major deficits
- Symptoms of stroke should not be suggestive of subarachnoid hemorrhage
- Onset of symptoms less than 3 hours before beginning treatment
- No head trauma or prior stroke in previous 3 months
- No myocardial infarction in the previous 3 months
- No gastrointestinal or urinary tract hemorrhage in previous 21 days
- No major surgery in the previous 14 days
- No arterial puncture at a noncompressible site in the previous 7 days
- No history of previous intracranial hemorrhage
- Blood pressure not elevated (systolic < 185 mm Hg; diastolic > 110 mm Hg)
- No evidence of active bleeding or acute trauma (fracture) on examination
- Not taking an oral anticoagulant or, if so, INR ≤ 1.7
- If receiving heparin in previous 48 hours, aPTT must be in normal range
- Platelet count ≥ 100,000 mm^3
- Blood glucose concentration ≥ 50 mg/dL (2.7 mmol/L)
- No seizure with postictal residual neurologic impairments
- Computed tomography does not show a multilobar infarction (hypodensity greater than one-third cerebral hemisphere)
- Patient or family members understand the potential risks and benefits of treatment

Stroke within 3-4.5 hours: All of the above plus:

- Age ≤ 80 years
- NIHSS ≤ 25
- Does not have history of both stroke and diabetes

aPTT, Activated partial thromboplastin time INR, international normalized ratio; NIHSS, NIH Stroke Scale, see Table 5-6.
Adapted from Adams HP, del Zoppo GJ, Alberts MJ, et al. Guidelines for the early management of adults with ischemic stroke. *Stroke.* 2007;38:1655-1711; del Zoppo GJ, Saver JL, Jauch EC, et al. Expansion of the time window for the treatment of acute ischemic stroke with intravenous tissue plasminogen activator. *Stroke.* 2009;40:2945-2948.

available, this intervention should be considered for any patient with an acute stroke.

The most important initial step in the process is to determine the onset of symptoms, because completed strokes do not benefit from invasive therapy and may have worse outcomes with intervention. This assessment is usually performed by a dedicated stroke team mobilized when the patient is first evaluated either in the field or hospital. Standardized systems for scaling the severity of the deficit should be used (Tables 5-5 and 5-6). Once a stroke is confirmed clinically and the time of onset established, the patient is imaged with MRI or CT. In addition to excluding a hemorrhagic stroke, advanced MRI and CT imaging techniques can help distinguish areas of irreversible ischemia from the ischemic penumbra. Blood pressure control is important, with a target of less than 180 mm Hg systolic and 100 mm Hg diastolic.

The emergent revascularization procedure begins with a rapid diagnostic angiographic evaluation of the cerebral circulation to determine the arterial anatomy, location of the occlusion, presence of concomitant arterial disease, and status of collateral pathways (Fig. 5-30). In general, acute anterior circulation strokes are due to emboli, while posterior circulation strokes are more likely to be caused by local thrombosis of underlying stenosis. The majority of emboli to the anterior circulation lodge in the middle cerebral artery (MCA). The risk of procedural bleeding increases with the duration of occlusion of the lenticulostriate arteries arising from the horizontal portion of the MCA (M1 segment). All glucose-containing fluids are banned from the procedure. The patient should be heparinized with a low systemic dose, such as a 2000 U bolus. Using a guiding catheter in the ICA, a coaxial superselective catheter is advanced into the thrombus. The dosage and type of thrombolytic agent is currently in flux, but when using recombinant tissue plasminogen activator, the usual maximal intra-arterial dose is 22 mg (2 mg intrathrombotic bolus followed by 20 mg infusion over 2 hours). Catheters that also deliver low-frequency ultrasound to the artery at the site of occlusion can accelerate thrombolysis times. Intravenous and intraarterial administration of thrombolytic agents can be combined.

Any restoration of antegrade flow is a hopeful angiographic sign. In particular, obtaining TICI 2b or 3 flow is associated with a good prognosis (Table 5-7). Repositioning of the microcatheter may be necessary during the procedure to thrombolyse small distal emboli that result from dissolution of the original obstruction. Thrombolysis should be stopped and heparin reversed immediately if an intracranial bleed is suspected. Following successful thrombolysis of an ICA territory thrombosis, heparin is stopped within 4 hours and the patient is usually managed with aspirin alone. The patient is carefully followed for clinical or imaging signs of stroke or bleed. In the posterior circulation, thrombolysis frequently reveals an underlying stenosis which may require angioplasty and/or stent placement if flow remains marginal.

TABLE 5-5 Glasgow Coma Scale

	1	2	3	4	5	6
Eyes	Does not open eyes	Opens eyes in response to painful stimuli	Opens eyes in response to voice	Opens eyes spontaneously	N/A	N/A
Verbal	Makes no sounds	Incomprehensible sounds	Utters inappropriate words	Confused, disoriented	Oriented, converses normally	N/A
Motor	Makes no movements	Extension to painful stimuli *(decerebrate response)*	Abnormal flexion to painful stimuli *(decorticate response)*	Flexion / Withdrawal to painful stimuli	Localizes painful stimuli	Obeys commands

Modified from Teasdale G, Jennett B. Assessment of coma and impaired consciousness: a practical scale. *Lancet.* 1974;304:81-84.

TABLE 5-6 NIH Stroke Scale

Tested Item	Title	Responses and Scores
1A	Level of consciousness	0—alert 1—drowsy 2—obtunded 3—coma/unresponsive
1B	Orientation questions (2)	0—answers both correctly 1—answers one correctly 2—answers neither correctly
1C	Response to commands (2)	0—performs both tasks correctly 1—performs one task correctly 2—performs neither
2	Gaze	0—normal horizontal movements 1—partial gaze palsy 2—complete gaze palsy
3	Visual fields	0—no visual field defect 1—partial hemianopia 2—complete hemianopia 3—bilateral hemianopia
4	Facial movement	0—normal 1—minor facial weakness 2—partial facial weakness 3—complete unilateral palsy
5	Motor function (arm) a, left b, right	0—no drift 1—drift before 5 seconds 2—falls before 10 seconds 3—no effort against gravity 4—no movement
6	Motor function (leg) a, left b, right	0—no drift 1—drift before 5 seconds 2—falls before 10 seconds 3—no effort against gravity 4—no movement
7	Limb ataxia	0—no ataxia 1—ataxia in 1 limb 2—ataxia in 2 limbs
8	Sensory	0—no sensory loss 1—mild sensory loss 2—severe sensory loss
9	Language	0—normal 1—mild aphasia 2—severe aphasia 3—mute or global aphasia
10	Articulation	0—normal 1—mild dysarthria 2—severe dysarthria
11	Extinction or inattention	0—absent 1—mild (loss 1 sensory modality) 2—severe (loss 2 modalities)

Adapted from Adams HP, del Zoppo GJ, Alberts MJ, et al. AHA/ASA guidelines for the early management of adults with ischemic stroke. *Stroke.* 2007;38:1655-1711.

A number of mechanical devices for retrieval of thrombus or emboli are now available and are often the initial choice for rapid restoration of flow. There are typically two components to these devices, a sheath with an occlusion balloon and the retrieval device (Fig. 5-31). The combined use of a mechanical device and thrombolytics has the highest revascularization rates, although large-scale randomized studies of clinical outcomes have not been performed.

Innovation in the treatment of stroke is continuing. Developing therapies include transcranial ultrasound disruption of thrombolytic-bearing microbubbles that locally disrupt the thrombus, and the use of adjunctive neuroprotective medications or cooling. Some of these innovations may allow pre-hospital treatment of stroke in the future.

TABLE 5-7 Modified Thrombolysis in Cerebral Infarction (TICI) Anterior Cerebral Artery (ACA) Distal Perfusion Score

0	No perfusion
1	Perfusion past the initial obstruction but limited to distal branch filling with little or slow distal perfusion
2A	Perfusion < 50% of the vascular distribution of the occluded artery
2B	Perfusion ≥ 50% of the vascular distribution of the occluded artery
3	Full perfusion with filling of all distal branches

Adapted from Tomsick T, Broderick J, Carrozella J, et al. Revascularization results in the Interventional Management of Stroke II Trial. *AJNR Am J Neuroradiol.* 2008;29:582-587.

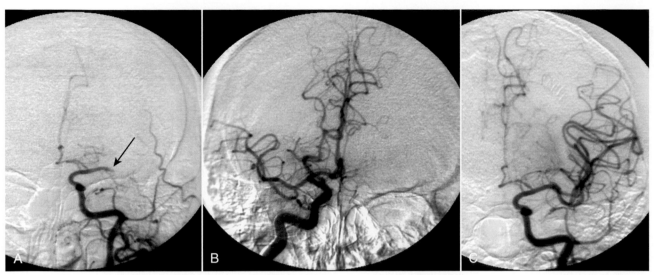

FIGURE 5-30. Thrombolysis in a patient presenting with acute onset of left hemispheric ischemia of 3 hours' duration. An emergent head computed tomography scan was negative for extravascular blood or edema. **A,** Digital subtraction angiography (DSA) image from left internal carotid artery (ICA) injection (anteroposterior projection) showing no filling of the middle cerebral artery branches *(arrow)*. **B,** DSA image from injection in the right ICA shows normal vessels. There is filling of the left anterior cerebral artery from the right through a patent anterior communicating artery. **C,** Following thrombolysis with urokinase (700,000 U) through a microcatheter in the middle cerebral artery, the vessel is patent. The patient experienced a full neurologic recovery.

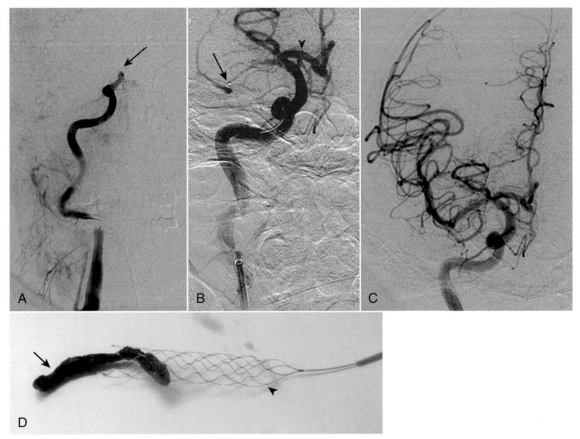

FIGURE 5-31. Stroke therapy with a clot retrieval device (the Solitaire retrievable stent, eV3, Plymouth, Minn.) **A,** Carotid angiogram showing abrupt occlusion of the right cavernous internal carotid artery (ICA) *(arrow)*. **B,** Angiogram after first pass with the stent shows that the right anterior cerebral artery is now patent *(arrowhead)*. The stent has been positioned in the occluded middle cerebral artery *(arrow)*. **C,** Completion angiogram showing excellent reperfusion of the right anterior and middle cerebral arteries. **D,** The thrombus *(arrow)* removed from the middle cerebral artery, trapped in the retrievable stent *(arrowhead)*.

■ SUGGESTED READINGS

AbuRahma AF, Srivastava M, Stone PA, et al. Critical appraisal of the Carotid Duplex Consensus criteria in the diagnosis of carotid artery stenosis. *J Vasc Surg.* 2011;53:53-59.

Adams HP, del Zoppo GJ, Alberts MJ, et al. AHA/ASA guidelines for the early management of adults with ischemic stroke. *Stroke.* 2007;38:1655-1711.

Begelman SM, Olin JW. Nonatherosclerotic arterial disease of the extracranial cerebrovasculature. *Semin Vasc Surg.* 2000;13:153-164.

Brott TG, Halperin JL, Abbara S, et al. ASA/ACCF/AHA/AANN/AANS/ACR/ ASNR/CNS/SAIP/SCAI/SIR/SNIS/SVM/SVS guideline on the management of patients with extracranial carotid and vertebral artery disease: Executive summary. *J Am Coll Cardiol.* 2011;57:1002-1044.

Brywczynski JJ, Barrett TW, Lyon JA, Cotton BA. Management of penetrating neck injury in the emergency department: a structured literature review. *Emerg Med J.* 2008;25:711-715.

Clevert DA, Sommer WH, Zengel P, et al. Imaging of carotid arterial diseases with contrast-enhanced ultrasound (CEUS). *Eur J Radiol.* 2011;80:68-76.

Executive Committee for the Asymptomatic Carotid Atherosclerosis (ACAS) Study. Endarterectomy for asymptomatic carotid artery stenosis. *JAMA.* 1995;273:1421-1428.

Furlan A, Higashida R, Wechsler L, et al. Intra-arterial prourokinase for acute ischemic stroke. The PROACT II study: a randomized controlled trial. Prolyse in Acute Cerebral Thromboembolism. *JAMA.* 1999;282:2003-2011.

Gonzalez-Gay MA, Martinez-Dubois C, Agudo M, et al. Giant cell arteritis: epidemiology, diagnosis, and management. *Curr Rheumatol Rep.* 2010;12: 436-442.

Goodney PP, Nolan BW, Eldrup-Jorgensen J, et al. Restenosis after carotid endarterectomy in a multicenter regional registry. *J Vasc Surg.* 2010;52: 897-904.

Gupta R, Tayal AH, Levy EI, et al. Intra-arterial thrombolysis or stent placement during endovascular treatment for acute ischemic stroke leads to the highest recanalization rate: Results of a multi-center retrospective study. *Neurosurgery.* 2011;68:1618-1622.

Hatano T, Tsukahara T, Miyakoshi A, et al. Stent placement for atherosclerotic stenosis of the vertebral artery ostium: angiographic and clinical outcomes in 117 consecutive patients. *Neurosurgery.* 2011;68:108-116.

Lanzino G, Tallarita T, Rabinstein AA. Internal carotid artery stenosis: natural history and management. *Semin Neurol.* 2010;30:518-527.

Mason JC. Takayasu arteritis--advances in diagnosis and management. *Nat Rev Rheumatol.* 2010;6:406-415.

Menke J. Diagnostic accuracy of contrast-enhanced MR angiography in severe carotid stenosis: meta-analysis with metaregression of different techniques. *Eur Radiol.* 2009;19:2204-2216.

Molina CA. Reperfusion therapies for acute ischemic stroke: current pharmacological and mechanical approaches. *Stroke.* 2011;42:S16-S19.

Moulakakis KG, Mylonas S, Avgerinos E, Kotsis T, Liapis CD. An update of the role of endovascular repair in blunt carotid artery trauma. *Eur J Vasc Endovasc Surg.* 2010;40:312-319.

Morrissey DD, Andersen PE, Nesbit GM, et al. Endovascular management of hemorrhage in patients with head and neck cancer. *Arch Otolaryngol Head Neck Surg.* 1997;123:15-19.

North American Symptomatic Carotid Endarterectomy Trial (NASCET) Collaborators. Beneficial effect of carotid endarterectomy in symptomatic patients with high-grade carotid stenosis. *N Engl J Med.* 1991;325:445-453.

Olin JW, Sealove BA. Diagnosis, management, and future developments of fibromuscular dysplasia. *J Vasc Surg.* 2011;53:826-836.

O'Rourke K, Berge E, Walsh CD, Kelly PJ. Percutaneous vascular interventions for acute ischaemic stroke. *Cochrane Database Syst Rev.* 2010 Oct; 6(10):CD007574.

Perkins WJ, Lanzino G, Brott TG. Carotid stenting vs endarterectomy: new results in perspective. *Mayo Clin Proc.* 2010;85:1101-1108.

Provenzale JM, Sarikaya B. Comparison of test performance characteristics of MRI, MR angiography, and CT angiography in the diagnosis of carotid and vertebral artery dissection: a review of the medical literature. *AJR Am J Roentgenol.* 2009;193:1167-1174.

Rossi CM, Di Comite G. The clinical spectrum of the neurological involvement in vasculitides. *J Neurol Sci.* 2009;285:13-21.

Schievink WI. Spontaneous dissection of the carotid and vertebral arteries. *N Engl J Med.* 2001;344:898-906.

Schlosser RJ. Clinical practice. Epistaxis. *N Engl J Med.* 2009;360:784-789.

Schroeder JW, Baskaran V, Aygun N. Imaging of traumatic arterial injuries in the neck with an emphasis on CTA. *Emerg Radiol.* 2010;17:109-122.

Tomsick T, Broderick J, Carrozzella J, et al. Revascularization results in the Interventional Management of Stroke II Trial. *AJNR.* 2008;29:582-587.

U-King-Im JM, Young V, Gillard JH. Carotid-artery imaging in the diagnosis and management of patients at risk of stroke. *Lancet Neurol.* 2009;8:569-580.

van den Berg R. Imaging and management of head and neck paragangliomas. *Eur Radiol.* 2005;15:1310-1318.

Wardlaw JM, Chappell FM, Best JJ, et al. Non-invasive imaging compared with intra-arterial angiography in the diagnosis of symptomatic carotid stenosis: a meta-analysis. *Lancet.* 2006;367:1503-1512.

Willems PW, Farb RI, Agid R. Endovascular treatment of epistaxis. *Am J Neuroradiol.* 2009;30:1637-1645.

CHAPTER 6

Upper Extremity Arteries

John A. Kaufman, MD, MS, FSIR, FCIRSE

NORMAL AND VARIANT ANATOMY	**CHRONIC ISCHEMIA**	**VASCULITIS**
KEY COLLATERAL PATHWAYS	**ACUTE ISCHEMIA**	**TRAUMA**
IMAGING	**THORACIC OUTLET SYNDROME**	**FIBROMUSCULAR DYSPLASIA**
VASOSPASTIC DISORDERS	**ANEURYSMS**	**PRIMARY HYPERPARATHYROIDISM**

Arterial disease is diagnosed less often in the upper than in the lower extremities, but unusual pathologies such as vasculitis, entrapment syndromes, and trauma are more common. This makes upper extremity arterial diagnosis challenging and intervention interesting.

NORMAL AND VARIANT ANATOMY

The arterial blood supply of the upper extremities begins with the subclavian artery on the left and the brachiocephalic (also known as the innominate) artery on the right. The left subclavian artery arises directly from the aorta, while on the right the brachiocephalic artery bifurcates into the right common carotid and subclavian arteries (see Fig. 5-1). The subclavian arteries are defined as the segment of vessel between the aortic arch or brachiocephalic artery bifurcation and the lateral border of the first rib. The subclavian artery exits the thoracic cavity between the anterior and middle scalene muscles, and then passes between the clavicle and first rib (Fig. 6-1). The typical diameter of the subclavian artery is 7-10 mm. The subclavian arteries provide blood to the upper chest, the arms, and the central nervous system (through the vertebral artery).

The internal mammary arteries are constant vessels that arise from the anterior inferior aspect of the subclavian arteries just opposite or slightly distal to the vertebral arteries. These vessels course anteriorly and medially along the inner surface of the chest wall. The internal mammary arteries are important potential sources of collateral blood supply in cases of thoracic or abdominal aortic obstruction (via the anterior anastomoses with the intercostal arteries in the former, and the inferior epigastric arteries in the latter). The internal mammary arteries can provide collateral supply to bronchial arteries as well.

The other named branches of the subclavian arteries are highly variable in origin, but relatively constant in presence. The vertebral arteries arise from the superoposterior surface of the subclavian arteries and are discussed in Chapter 5. The thyrocervical trunk arises just distal to the internal mammary arteries from the superior surface of the subclavian artery, often lateral to the vertebral artery. This vessel is subject to enormous variability, but is typically the origin of the inferior thyroidal, superficial cervical, and suprascapular arteries. Only slightly more than 50% of individuals have this classic anatomy. Independent origins of one or more of these vessels from the subclavian artery are common. The next major branch of the subclavian artery is the costocervical trunk, which gives rise to the deep cervical, supreme intercostal (highest thoracic), and occasionally the anterior spinal (radiculomedullary) arteries (Fig. 6-2). The supreme intercostal artery contributes to the blood supply of the first through third ribs. This anatomy is found in approximately 80% of individuals, with the most common variants being independent origins of the two branches.

The axillary artery begins at the lateral margin of the first rib, extending to the lateral margin of the teres major muscle tendon. Thus a portion of the axillary artery is located quite medial to the anatomic axilla. The branches of the axillary artery are highly variable in origin. These are the superior thoracic artery (to the anterior portions of the first through third intercostal spaces); the lateral thoracic artery (to the lateral chest, with a prominent mammary branch in women); the thoracoacromial artery (with branches to the clavicle, the acromion, and deltoid); the subscapular artery, which gives rise to the thoracodorsal artery (supplying the musculature along the lateral margin of the scapula); and the scapular circumflex artery (supplying the muscles of the back deep to the scapula). The last branch of the axillary artery is the circumflex humeral artery, which supplies the humeral head and the surrounding soft tissues. All of the axillary and subclavian artery branches (exclusive of the vertebral artery) have potential anastomoses with each other that become evident in the presence of occlusive disease or vascular tumors. Of great importance, the radial, ulnar, and median nerves lie in close proximity to the axillary artery. Contained in a sheath of connective tissue along with the artery, these neural structures are at risk for compression by even a small amount of bleeding within the sheath after axillary artery punctures.

The brachial artery begins lateral to the teres major muscle tendon (see Fig. 6-1). Variants of the brachial artery proper are uncommon, but include a small accessory branch to the radial artery (persistent superficial brachial artery, 1%-2%) and duplication (0.1%). The profunda brachialis artery is usually the first major branch of this vessel, traveling with the ulnar nerve in a posterolateral course around the humerus (Fig. 6-3). This vessel supplies the muscular structures of the posterior aspect of the upper arm, as well as collateral supply around the elbow. There are many unnamed muscular branches of this artery, but those that anastomose to muscular branches distal to the elbow joint are termed *collateral vessels*. These variable vessels are named after the forearm vessel to which they collateralize (e.g., ulnar collateral artery).

The terminal branches of the brachial artery are the radial, ulnar, and interosseous arteries (Fig. 6-4). Anomalous high origins of the radial or ulnar artery from the brachial or axillary arteries are present in 15% and 3% of patients, respectively. These variants are potential sources of confusion during upper extremity angiography if the catheter is unknowingly placed distal to an anomalously high origin (Fig. 6-5). The forearm arteries supply the adjacent muscles and (usually only the radial and ulnar arteries) continue into the hand. The interosseous artery divides into an anterior and posterior branch. In fewer than 2% of individuals, the interosseous artery may continue into the hand as the median artery (Fig. 6-6).

The classic arterial anatomy of the hand is comprised of two complete palmar arcades, both of which receive contributions

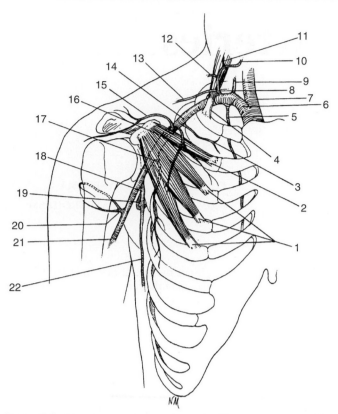

FIGURE 6-1. Line drawing of subclavian and axillary artery anatomy. The clavicle is not shown. *1*, Pectoralis minor muscle. *2*, Pectoral branch of the thoracoacromial artery. *3*, Superior thoracic artery. *4*, Anterior scalene muscle. *5*, Internal mammary artery. *6*, Subclavian artery. *7*, Right common carotid artery. *8*, Thyrocervical trunk. *9*, Vertebral artery. *10*, Inferior thyroid artery. *11*, Ascending cervical artery. *12*, Superficial cervical artery. *13*, Suprascapular artery. *14*, Axillary artery. *15*, Acromial branch of the thoracoacromial artery. *16*, Thoracoacromial artery. *17*, Lateral thoracic artery. *18*, Subscapular artery. *19*, Circumflex scapular artery. *20*, Circumflex humeral artery. *21*, Brachial artery. *22*, Thoracodorsal artery. (From Kadir S. *Atlas of Normal and Variant Anatomy.* Philadelphia: WB Saunders, 1991, with permission.)

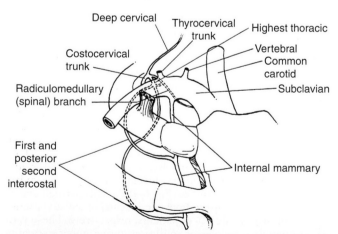

FIGURE 6-2. Line drawing of costocervical trunk anatomy. (From Kadir S. *Atlas of Normal and Variant Anatomy.* Philadelphia: WB Saunders, 1991, with permission.)

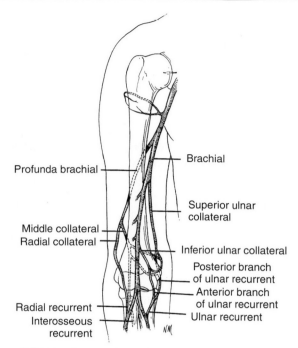

FIGURE 6-3. Line drawing of normal brachial artery anatomy. (From Kadir S. *Atlas of Normal and Variant Anatomy.* Philadelphia: WB Saunders, 1991, with permission.)

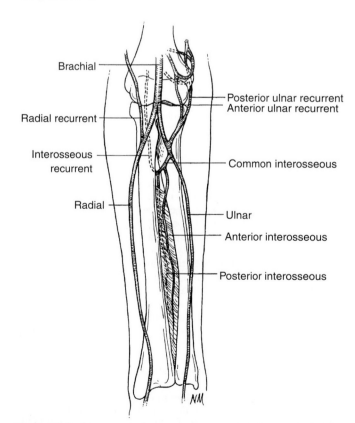

FIGURE 6-4. Line drawing of normal forearm arterial anatomy. (From Kadir S. *Atlas of Normal and Variant Anatomy.* Philadelphia: WB Saunders, 1991, with permission.)

from the radial and the ulnar arteries (Fig. 6-7). The more proximal arcade, the deep palmar arch, is primarily supplied by the radial artery. The more distal arcade, the superficial palmar arch, is supplied primarily by the ulnar artery. Variations of this anatomy are so prevalent that the classic anatomy of two

complete interconnected arcades is present in fewer than 50% of patients (Table 6-1). These variants are the rule rather than the exception.

The blood supply to the fingers is derived from the paired palmar metacarpal and common palmar digital arteries that originate

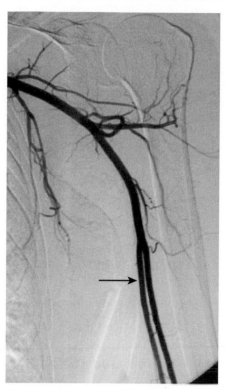

FIGURE 6-5. Proximal origin of the radial artery. Digital subtraction angiogram (DSA) of the left upper arm with injection in the subclavian artery showing a large branch *(arrow)* arising from the proximal brachial artery and continuing toward the hand. This proved to be the radial artery on distal images.

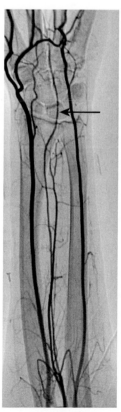

FIGURE 6-6. Median artery. Digital subtraction angiogram of the forearm with the hand in the anatomic position. The interosseous artery continues across the wrist as the median artery *(arrow)*.

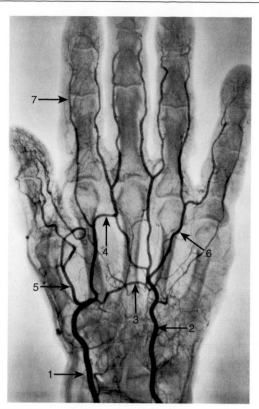

FIGURE 6-7. Subtracted angiogram of the hand in a 54-year-old male smoker. There are distal occlusions of the proper palmar digital arteries, and the palmar metacarpal arteries are not visualized. *1*, Radial artery. *2*, Ulnar artery. *3*, Deep palmar arch. *4*, Superficial palmar arch. *5*, Princeps pollicis artery. *6*, Common palmar digital artery. *7*, Proper palmar digital artery.

TABLE 6-1 Variant Arterial Anatomy of the Hand

Variant	Approximate Incidence
Incomplete superficial arch	55%
Ulnar artery supplies entire incomplete superficial arch	13%
Superficial arch from median and ulnar arteries	4%
Superficial arch from radial, median, and ulnar arteries	1%
Independent radial, median, and ulnar arteries (no arch)	1%
Incomplete deep arch	5%

from the deep and superficial palmar arches, respectively. These arteries join at the interdigital webspace to form the paired proper palmar digital arteries of the fingers. The radial artery is usually the dominant blood supply to the thumb and the second digit, while the ulnar artery supplies the fourth and fifth digits. The third digit may be supplied by either artery. The dominant blood supply to the fingers varies with the arch anatomy.

KEY COLLATERAL PATHWAYS

The potential collateral routes around a subclavian artery origin stenosis or occlusion are numerous, in that they include all of the branches of the subclavian and axillary artery. One pattern, subclavian steal, describes retrograde flow in the ipsilateral vertebral

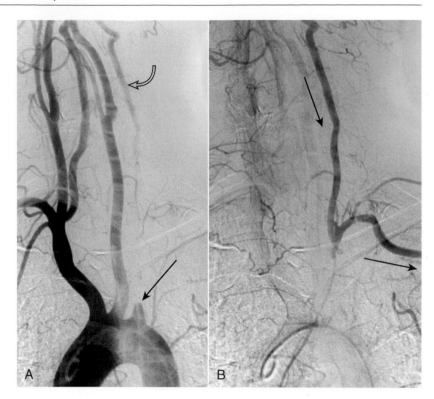

FIGURE 6-8. Subclavian steal. **A,** Digital subtraction angiogram of the arch in the left anterior oblique projection. There is occlusion of the left subclavian artery origin *(straight arrow).* Faint retrograde opacification of the left vertebral artery is present *(curved arrow).* **B,** Later image from the same injection showing retrograde flow in the left vertebral artery reconstituting the left subclavian artery. Arrows indicate direction of blood flow.

Box 6-1. Symptoms of Subclavian Steal

Vertebrobasilar insufficiency
Dizziness
Drop attack
Ataxia
Vertigo
Syncope
Exercise-induced upper extremity ischemia
Hemispheric transient ischemic attack

---

artery (Fig. 6-8; see Fig. 3-11). Subclavian steal is associated with arm pain or central neurologic symptoms in a third of patients. Symptoms may be exacerbated with use of the arm (Box 6-1). Bilateral subclavian steal is uncommon.

Steal physiology can affect other vessels in the upper extremity. Proximal occlusion of the brachiocephalic artery origin can result in retrograde flow down the right common carotid artery as well as the right vertebral artery. Reversal of flow can occur in smaller subclavian artery branches such as the thyrocervical trunk and the internal mammary artery. In patients with cardiac bypass surgery based on an internal mammary artery, proximal subclavian stenosis can cause a steal phenomenon involving the internal mammary artery that presents as angina (Fig. 6-9).

Axillary artery occlusion is usually well tolerated because of the rich potential collateral pathways around the scapula and humerus. Frequently, the subscapular artery assumes a dominant role in reconstituting the distal axillary artery. In addition, the intercostal arteries can provide collateral blood supply to the upper extremity through anastomoses with the vessels of the chest wall, such as the lateral thoracic artery. Occlusion of the distal brachial artery results in collateral supply from the profunda brachialis artery high in the arm and around the elbow through the radial and ulnar collateral arteries to radial and ulnar recurrent arteries.

Occlusion of either the radial or ulnar artery is well tolerated by the fingers as long as one or both arches are intact. When the deep and superficial arches are incomplete or absent, acute occlusion of a forearm artery may result in severe digital ischemia. Over time, collateral supply can develop from the opposite forearm vessel or the interosseous artery.

IMAGING

Ultrasound examination of the upper extremity arteries distal to the clavicle is relatively straightforward. Standard duplex color-flow ultrasound techniques can be used for the peripheral vessels. A high-resistance triphasic waveform is normal in the upper extremity except in the fingers, which are biphasic. Pulse volume recordings of the fingers can be used to assess digital perfusion (Fig. 6-10). The superficial location of these vessels facilitates visualization with ultrasound. Medial to the clavicle, the vessels dive deep into the mediastinum, beyond the reach of surface probes. To fully evaluate the subclavian artery origins and brachiocephalic artery, a transesophageal probe is needed. However, even with this technique the origins of the arteries may not be completely visualized.

Computed tomography angiography (CTA) of the upper extremity vessels is an excellent modality for evaluation of the axillosubclavian arteries, especially within the mediastinum. CTA requires the patient to breath-hold, with a short delay after injection of contrast. As a general rule, a noncontrast scan should be obtained before contrast injection. Thick collimation is appropriate for the noncontrast scan. Thinner effective collimation (sub 1 cm) should be used for the contrast-enhanced scan. The area of coverage should include the proximal neck to the hand for complete upper extremity studies. A very important technical consideration is the route of administration of contrast. Contrast injected into an upper extremity vein remains extremely dense on CT scan before it reaches the central circulation. This causes streak artifacts that degrade image quality, particularly across the great vessel origins. The arm opposite the side of interest should therefore be used for contrast administration. The vessels can be evaluated using simple postprocessing techniques such as reformatting.

The upper extremity arteries are well suited for evaluation with magnetic resonance angiographic (MRA) techniques. Gadolinium-enhanced three-dimensional (3-D) acquisitions provide

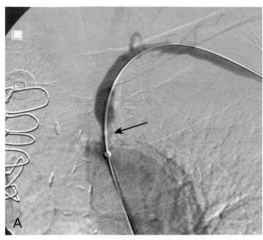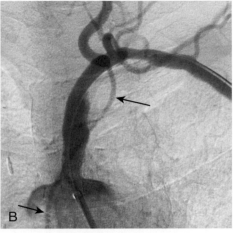

FIGURE 6-9. Symptomatic left internal mammary artery (LIMA) steal in a patient in whom recurrent angina developed several years after coronary artery revascularization with the LIMA. A coronary angiogram showed retrograde flow in a patent LIMA away from the heart. **A,** Selective left subclavian artery digital subtraction angiogram shows absent filling of both the LIMA and the vertebral artery. The origin of the subclavian artery is stenotic *(arrow)*. **B,** Following stent placement in the subclavian artery origin, there is antegrade flow in the LIMA *(arrows)* as well as the vertebral artery. The patient's angina resolved.

excellent images of the arch and proximal portions of the upper extremity arteries (Fig. 6-11). Acquisitions oriented in the coronal plane can include both the arch and the upper extremity vessels to the shoulder. An important pitfall is signal loss due to susceptibility artifact from adjacent veins caused by undiluted gadolinium injected in an upper extremity vein (see Fig. 3-17). As with CTA of the upper extremities, contrast should be injected into the extremity opposite the side of clinical interest. Imaging arteries of the arm and hand can be accomplished with either contrast-enhanced or noncontrast acquisitions. Small coils can be used to maximize image detail (Fig. 6-12).

Angiographic studies are usually performed from a femoral arterial approach, but retrograde access from axillary, brachial, or radial arteries can be used. Documentation of the upper extremity pulses (axillary, brachial, radial, and ulnar arteries) in both arms, the carotid pulses, and bilateral brachial artery blood pressure measurements should be confirmed before inserting a catheter, even when the problem is unilateral. Subclavian artery aneurysms may be palpable as a pulsatile mass in the supraclavicular fossa, although a tortuous but normal-caliber artery may feel similar.

The complete angiographic study of the upper extremity involves visualization of all arteries from the aortic arch to the tips of the fingers. Anything less risks missing important pathology. Exceptions to this rule should be made only after careful analysis of the clinical scenario and of the patient. For each injection it is essential to ensure that there is satisfactory overlap of coverage with the preceding injection so that the extremity is imaged in its entirety.

An arch aortogram in the left anterior oblique (LAO) projection will profile the origins of the great vessels (see Fig. 6-8). To open the brachiocephalic artery bifurcation, filming in the right anterior oblique (RAO) projection is necessary (see Fig. 5-1). The pigtail catheter should be positioned in the ascending aorta just proximal to the brachiocephalic artery origin. Specific injection and exposure rates are listed in Table 6-2. To select the subclavian arteries, the pigtail catheter is exchanged for a 5-French 100-cm length catheter with a gentle angle at the tip, such as Davis or H-1 (see Fig. 2-10). Arteries that arise from the arch at an acute angle can be selected with a Simmons-2 (right subclavian) or Simmons-1 (left subclavian). With the tube angled to show the arch in an LAO projection, the catheter is positioned in the aorta proximal to the great vessel origins. The catheter is then turned so that the tip points toward the head and is slowly withdrawn until it pops up into a great vessel origin. Leading with 1 cm of soft guidewire (e.g., Bentson) minimizes the risk of vessel trauma. In older patients there is frequently enough calcification at the ostia of the great vessels to provide a fluoroscopic landmark. A gentle test of contrast (no air bubbles!) can be used to identify the vessel. The subclavian artery can be selected using almost any atraumatic guidewire,

such as a 3-J long taper or an angled hydrophilic guidewire. If the guidewire passes into the neck toward the head, it may be in a vertebral artery or, on the right, in the common carotid artery. When selecting the right subclavian artery, remember that the origin is usually posterior to the right common carotid artery (see Fig. 5-1).

The subclavian and axillary arteries can usually be included on one image with the catheter tip positioned just beyond the origin of the vertebral artery. Non-ionic contrast should be used to minimize patient discomfort during the examination. An angled hydrophilic guidewire can then be used to select a more peripheral location. The brachial artery should be imaged with the catheter in the proximal axillary artery in order to avoid causing spasm or missing a high origin of a radial or ulnar artery. Once these anomalies have been excluded, the catheter can be positioned in the mid or distal brachial artery for angiography of the forearm or hand. The hand should be in anatomic position (palm up and hand flat on the table) for forearm angiography (see Fig. 6-6). Otherwise it can be extremely difficult to identify vessels in the forearm or hand. Selective angiography of the individual forearm arteries is best performed with small high-flow microcatheters, because these vessels are subject to spasm when manipulated.

The hand can be maintained in anatomic position (palm up) or placed completely flat with the fingers spread slightly for the hand angiogram (see Fig. 6-7). Since the digital arteries are small and numerous, magnification views and vasodilation are frequently necessary to obtain the best images. Vasodilation of the arteries of the hand can be induced by wrapping the hand in warm towels or having the patient hold a warm pack during the initial parts of the examination. Another effective method is reactive hyperemia with the blood pressure cuff on the upper arm. Intraarterial injection of a vasodilating agent (such as 200 μg of nitroglycerin) through the catheter just before injection of contrast can also be used (see Fig. 6-10). There are few radiographic images more distinctive and beautiful than high-quality magnification arteriograms of the human hand.

VASOSPASTIC DISORDERS

Raynaud phenomenon (primary or secondary) is the most common cause of symptomatic upper extremity ischemia (see Box 1-5). More prevalent in cold climates, the classic presentation is onset of a white digit or digits in response to cold exposure, followed by transition to blue, then red. The duration of the attack may be up to 1 hour. Patients with Raynaud phenomenon usually have a normal baseline physical examination. Although rarely performed, angiography demonstrates reversible vasospasm (induced by cold and ameliorated by heat or vasodilators) (see Fig. 1-31). Patients with secondary Raynaud phenomenon (i.e., associated connective tissue disorders, atherosclerosis, and history of repetitive trauma) may have underlying fixed small vessel arterial obstruction.

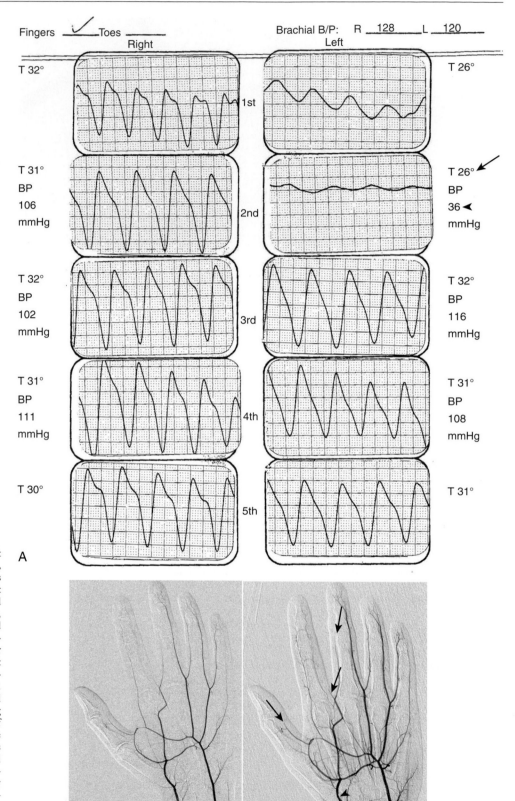

Fingers ✓ Toes ____
Right

Brachial B/P: R ___128___ L ___120___
Left

FIGURE 6-10. Acute ischemia of left first and second digits due to emboli. **A,** Noninvasive evaluation of the fingers shows dampened waveforms in the left digits 1 and 2 (compare with normal biphasic waveform in the other fingers), with decreased temperature *(arrow)* and pressure *(arrowhead)*. Note that the finger pressures are normally slightly lower than the brachial artery pressure. **B,** Left hand digital subtraction angiogram without hand warming or a vasodilator. There is poor opacification of the digital arteries. **C,** Repeat study after warming the hand and intraarterial injection of 200 µg of nitroglycerin just prior to the angiogram. The arterial opacification is improved, and occlusions of the digital arteries are evident *(arrows)* with a subtle irregularity of the distal radial artery *(arrowhead)* at the base of the first metacarpal suggestive of mural thrombus. The patient gave a history of repeated trauma to this area.

The differential diagnosis of the fixed purple digit is broad, including acrocyanosis, frostbite, insect or snake bite, antiphospholipid antibody syndrome, and cholesterol embolization. In each of these cases, the lack of improvement with warming is a distinguishing characteristic to differentiate from primary or secondary Raynaud syndrome.

■ CHRONIC ISCHEMIA

Symptomatic chronic ischemia of the upper extremities can be divided into small (hand) or large (wrist to arch) vessel etiologies (Boxes 6-2 and 6-3). Atherosclerotic occlusive disease is the cause of approximately 5% of all cases of clinically evident upper limb

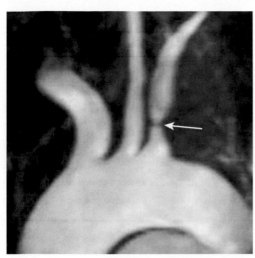

FIGURE 6-11. Gadolinium-enhanced three-dimensional magnetic resonance angiogram viewed in the left anterior oblique projection showing a focal proximal left subclavian artery stenosis *(arrow)*. (Courtesy of Barry Stein, MD, Hartford Hospital, Hartford, Conn.)

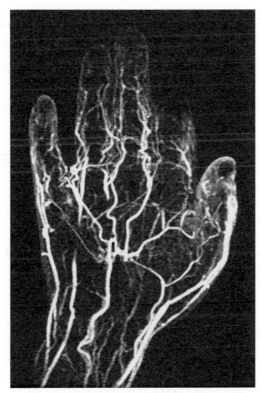

FIGURE 6-12. Late image from gadolinium-enhanced time-resolved contrast imaging magnetic resonance angiogram of the hand in a patient with second digit ischemia due to a small embolus. The image spatial resolution is not sufficient to permit evaluation of the peripheral digital arteries, and there is venous filling on this late image, but the abnormal perfusion of the second digit is evident.

ischemia. The muscle mass of the upper body is smaller than in the lower limbs and is used less vigorously (perhaps if we walked on all fours symptomatic upper extremity arterial disease would be more common). In addition, the collateral pathways are numerous and well developed at multiple levels. The most frequent etiology of chronic large vessel upper extremity occlusive disease is atherosclerosis. The risk factors for atherosclerotic disease of the upper extremity arteries are the same as everywhere else in the body. Patients are usually older, with other manifestations of

atherosclerosis. Cramping or a tight feeling in the upper arm and forearm muscles with activity due to proximal arterial occlusive disease is considered true arm claudication. Rest pain and tissue loss are rare. When ulcerations occur, the fingers are usually most affected (Fig. 6-13).

On physical examination, diminished pulses or a lower blood pressure in an arm may indicate the presence of proximal occlusive disease. The Allen test (compression of both the radial and ulnar artery to prevent blood flow to the hand followed by sequential release of the arteries and inspection of pattern of reperfusion) is a simple measure that gauges both the relative contributions of the radial and ulnar arteries to the hand and the degree of collateralization between the deep and superficial arches.

Atherosclerotic occlusive disease can occur anywhere in the upper extremity arteries, but is most often manifested clinically when it is located at the subclavian artery origins (see Figs. 6-8 and 6-9). The left subclavian artery is affected more often than the brachiocephalic artery or the right subclavian artery. Obstruction at the ostia of the left subclavian artery is the result of aortic plaque, a feature that impacts on the types and outcomes of interventions. Ostial stenosis of the right subclavian artery may also involve the right common carotid artery origin. Subclavian artery occlusive disease proximal to the vertebral artery frequently results in subclavian steal physiology (see Key Collateral Pathways and Fig. 6-8).

Atherosclerotic digital arterial occlusive disease is more prevalent than it is symptomatic. Abnormal digital arteries are often found in smokers, patients with renal failure, diabetics, and individuals who perform heavy manual work. Symptoms may be precipitated by creation of a proximal surgical dialysis access which effectively "steals" arterial blood from the hand or after placement of a radial arterial catheter in a patient with an occluded ulnar artery (see Fig. 7-31).

The subclavian artery origins are difficult to visualize with ultrasound, but abnormal waveforms and flow velocities in accessible portions of the vessel infer a proximal lesion. The vertebral arteries are easily interrogated, as are the extremity arteries distal to the clavicle. Detailed ultrasound evaluation of the intrinsic small vessels of the hand can be challenging, but digital pressures and waveforms provide useful information about hand and digital perfusion (see Fig. 6-10).

CTA and contrast-enhanced MRA are excellent modalities for evaluation of the occlusive disease of the subclavian artery origins. Retrograde flow in the vertebral artery due to a proximal subclavian stenosis is indistinguishable from antegrade flow on CTA and conventional contrast-enhanced MRA. Noncontrast two-dimensional time-of-flight phase contrast images or time-resolved contrast imaging (TRICKS) of the vertebral artery can provide information about directional flow. Neither CTA nor MRA is suitable for routine vascular imaging of the hand owing to limited resolution and small size of the vessels (see Fig. 6-12).

Conventional angiography remains the definitive imaging modality for evaluation of symptomatic chronic upper extremity ischemia. Arch aortography should always precede selective angiography. Magnification angiography is usually necessary to adequately evaluate the hand vessels.

Surgical access to the subclavian artery origins requires a thoracotomy. This permits direct transaortic endarterectomy or bypass with a graft arising from the ascending aorta. Alternatively, bypass from a more accessible inflow source such as either common carotid artery or the contralateral axillary artery is less rigorous for the patient and usually performed if the anatomy permits. In extreme situations, a common femoral to axillary artery bypass can be used. Thoracic sympathectomy may delay or prevent amputation in patients with intractable digital ischemia due to fixed occlusive disease.

The most frequent percutaneous intervention in chronic upper extremity arterial occlusive disease is stent placement in

TABLE 6-2 Upper Extremity Angiography

Vessel	Catheter	Position	Projection*	Injection†
Great vessel origins	Pigtail	Ascending aorta	LAO	20/30
Right subclavian origin	Pigtail	Ascending aorta	RAO	20/30
Right subclavian origin	H-1, Davis‡	Brachiocephalic	RAO	5-8/12-16
Subclavian	H-1, Davis, Simmons-1 or -2	Proximal subclavian	AP	6-8/12-16
Axillary	H-1, Davis	Distal subclavian	AP	5-8/10-16
Brachial	H-1, Davis	Distal subclavian	AP	5-8/10-16
Forearm	H-1, Davis	Mid-brachial	AP, hand in anatomic position	5-8/10-16
Hand	H-1, Davis	Mid-brachial	AP, hand in anatomic position§	5-6/20-30

*Imaging obliquity.
†Rate per second/total volume.
‡H-1, Headhunter 1; Davis, Davis A1.
§Flow augmentation with warming of hand with heat lamp or by holding hot pack during examination; inject vasodilator (nitroglycerin, 200 µg in 10-mL table flush) immediately before contrast; reactive hyperemia (2-3 minutes).
AP, Anteroposterior projection; LAO, left anterior oblique; RAO, right anterior oblique.

Box 6-2. Causes of Chronic Upper Extremity Ischemia: Small Vessel

Raynaud syndrome/disease
Atherosclerosis
Connective tissue disease
Vibration injury
Buerger disease
Hypercoagulable syndromes
Frostbite
Chronic renal failure
Diabetes
Recurrent embolization
Acrocyanosis

Box 6-3. Causes of Chronic Upper Extremity Ischemia: Large Vessel

Atherosclerosis
Trauma
Recurrent embolization
Thoracic outlet syndrome
Steal (dialysis fistula or graft)
Vasculitis
• Giant cell arteritis
• Takayasu arteritis
• Radiation arteritis
• Buerger disease
Fibromuscular dysplasia

---

the subclavian and brachiocephalic artery origins (see Fig. 6-9). This procedure can be performed from either a femoral, brachial, or (for the brachiocephalic artery) even carotid artery access. The relationship of the stenosis to the origin of cerebral branches and the status of the other cerebral arteries are key considerations when planning the procedure. Occlusion of a vertebral artery origin by a dissection flap during subclavian artery angioplasty, although rare, could result in a stroke in a patient with poor intracranial collateral circulation. Common balloon sizes range from 6 to 10 mm in diameter in the subclavian and

innominate arteries. Balloon-expandable stent placement is almost always necessary when the lesion involves the arterial ostium. Careful stent positioning is required in this location to avoid compression of the orifice of the common carotid artery on the right or protruding too far into the aorta on the left. Self-expanding stents can be used in more peripheral locations. However, stents should be avoided in the segment of the subclavian artery between the clavicle and the first rib, because they can be crushed by the bony structures. The technical success rate of subclavian and innominate artery angioplasty and stent placement is greater than 95%, with a complication rate (stroke and distal embolization) of less than 1%. There is relatively little information on the long-term patency of these procedures, but available results suggest excellent outcomes.

ACUTE ISCHEMIA

Acute upper extremity ischemia usually presents with digital and hand symptoms. Mild ischemia may result in simply a cold finger or hand with delayed capillary refill, whereas severe ischemia produces a cadaveric extremity.

The pulse examination provides clues as to the level of occlusion. Always examine both upper extremities, in that bilateral findings suggest an embolic etiology. When a patient presents with ischemia localized to the fingers, the distribution of affected fingers suggests the arteries involved (first and second digits, radial artery; third, radial or ulnar arteries; fourth and fifth, ulnar artery).

The patient's history may provide clues about the etiology of the ischemia and directs subsequent imaging. The most common cause of acute ischemia is an embolus of cardiac origin (Boxes 6-4 and 6-5). These patients report acute onset of severe symptoms in association with a known or newly discovered cardiac arrhythmia or structural abnormality (e.g., dilatative cardiomyopathy). Recurrent emboli in the same arm implicate a source within that extremity, such as a subclavian aneurysm (see Thoracic Outlet Syndrome). Other etiologies are trauma (including iatrogenic), aortic dissection, thrombosis of an existing lesion, severe vasospasm, and in situ thrombosis due to a hypercoagulable syndrome.

Acute hand ischemia due to steal following surgical creation of a proximal dialysis access occurs in 5%-10% of patients. The symptoms occur immediately in two thirds of cases and are delayed in one third. Patients at risk are older diabetics and smokers with preexisting but asymptomatic occlusive disease of the forearm and digital arteries. When the arteriovenous communication is created,

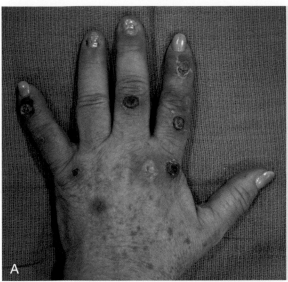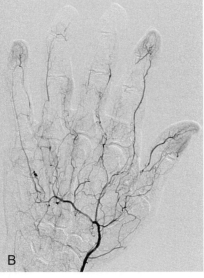

FIGURE 6-13. A 56-year-old woman with chronic renal failure in whom hand pain and ulceration developed over several months. **A,** Multiple ischemic ulcers on the hand distally. **B,** Digital subtraction angiogram of the hand, with warming, shows occlusion of the ulnar artery and diffuse small artery occlusive disease involving all of the digits.

BOX 6-4. Causes of Acute Upper Extremity Ischemia

Embolus
Trauma
Brachial, radial artery catheterization
Hypercoagulable syndrome
Aortic dissection
Steal (dialysis fistula or graft)
Vasospasm
Compartment syndrome

BOX 6-5. Sources of Upper Extremity Emboli

Heart
  • Left ventricle
  • Left atrium
  • Aortic valve
Upper extremity artery aneurysm (subclavian, axillary, ulnar)
Atherosclerotic plaque
Ascending aortic aneurysm
Subclavian and axillary artery fibromuscular dysplasia
Iatrogenic
  • Dialysis access declotting
  • Cardiac surgery
Paradoxical

TABLE 6-3 Location of Upper Extremity Emboli

Location	Incidence
Brachial artery	60%
Axillary artery	23%
Subclavian artery	12%
Forearm and digital arteries	5%

---

a pressure drop distal to the fistula and even reversal of flow in the distal radial artery (after a Brescia Cimino fistula) can result in neurologic injury, pain, and eventually ulceration and even gangrene.

When patients present with acute upper extremity ischemia, physical examination and history alone may be sufficient to plan management. For example, a patient with acute hand ischemia, a bounding pulse that terminates abruptly in the antecubital brachial artery, and an arrhythmia likely has a brachial artery embolus and should proceed to embolectomy (Table 6-3). When indicated, imaging of acute upper extremity ischemia is best accomplished with angiography, because everything between the aortic valve and the fingertips can be visualized (Fig. 6-14). Noninvasive imaging modalities do not yet provide sufficient anatomic coverage and resolution of detail. Furthermore, diagnostic angiography can be converted to an interventional procedure at a moment's notice. Magnification views of the fingers

may be essential to distinguish between embolic occlusion (intraluminal filing defects) and other causes (Fig. 6-15). Injection of a vasodilator may improve visualization of digital arteries, and resolve ischemia related to severe vasospasm (see Fig. 6-10). The subclavian artery should be carefully inspected for the presence of a subtle aneurysm or an ulcerated plaque. The finding of small emboli in proximal branch vessels supports the diagnosis of embolus. Although rare, aneurysms can occur at any point beyond the subclavian artery. The findings of a focal aneurysm or occlusion of the ulnar artery in the base of the hand is suggestive of hypothenar hammer syndrome (see Trauma). When hand ischemia occurs in the presence of a dialysis graft or fistula, injections with temporary occlusion of the venous outflow (usually by manual compression) are necessary to assess the hand arteries (see Fig. 7-31).

Patients with critical ischemia should undergo surgical thromboembolectomy. This can be very difficult when the small vessels of the hand are involved. In these cases, proximal surgical thromboembolectomy can be combined with intraoperative local distal injection of a thrombolytic agent.

Percutaneous intervention for acute upper extremity ischemia is performed less often than for lower extremity acute ischemia because the condition is not as common and the neighboring vascular bed at risk (the central nervous system) is less forgiving. The upper extremity must be viable in order to consider percutaneous intervention. Thrombolysis, either pharmacologic, pharmacomechanical, or mechanical may be helpful when extensive thrombus is present, particularly in the small vessels of the hand. These procedures can be performed from either the femoral artery or brachial artery (antegrade or retrograde) approach, depending on the location and extent of the thrombus (Fig. 6-16). Treatment of proximal subclavian artery thrombus risks vertebral artery embolization and stroke during the procedure. When treatment in the forearm arteries is necessary, a microcatheter or coronary artery thrombectomy device is required due to the small size of the arteries and the propensity to develop spasm. For very distal thrombosis, good results with thrombolysis are frequently obtained with the catheter positioned in the distal brachial artery to perfuse the entire forearm and hand. A microcatheter should be used when delivering thrombolytics directly into the hand.

When a femoral artery approach is used, anticoagulation with heparin is important to prevent pericatheter thrombus formation in the subclavian artery and subsequent vertebral artery embolization. Published experience with upper extremity thrombolysis suggests that overall results are promising with few complications in properly selected patients.

When the source of distal embolization is a focal atherosclerotic lesion in the subclavian or axillary artery, this may be treated with dilation and stent placement (Fig. 6-17). A self-expanding stent should be used because it will not remain crushed if accidently compressed. Stenting the subclavian artery between the clavicle and first rib should be avoided (unless the first rib has been removed) because the repeated external compression in this location will fracture any stent.

There are several operative approaches to the management of steal syndrome due to surgical dialysis access. Ligation of the fistula or graft results in loss of the dialysis access. Banding of the fistula or revision of the arterial anastomosis can decrease the degree of shunting while preserving dialysis access. Ligation of the artery distal to the fistula with placement of an arterial jump graft from proximal to distal around the fistula, termed the *DRIL procedure* (distal revascularization with interval ligation), also preserves the access (Fig. 6-18). Occasionally, coil occlusion of the radial artery distal to the arterial anastomosis of a Brescia-Cimino (radial artery to cephalic vein at the wrist) fistula is used to eliminate steal from

the fingers through the palmar arches. The ulnar arterial supply to the fingers must be confirmed before this intervention.

▰ THORACIC OUTLET SYNDROME

Symptomatic extrinsic compression of the neurovascular structures of the upper extremity as they exit the bony thorax is termed *thoracic outlet syndrome*. Neurologic symptoms are by far the most common manifestation, accounting for 90% of cases. Neurogenic thoracic outlet syndrome is most often found in women (female-to-male ratio 4:1) between the ages of 20 and 50 years. Symptomatic arterial thoracic outlet syndrome is unusual, comprising roughly 1% of cases. The usual patient with arterial thoracic outlet syndrome is a young, athletic male. Patients may present with hand numbness, tingling, or coolness with activities that require arm abduction, and diminished extremity pulses. Acute embolic events to the forearm and hand occur in up to 40% of patients (due to clot formation in poststenotic subclavian artery aneurysms), and may be the initial presenting symptom. Combined neurologic and vascular symptoms may be present.

The physical examination is usually unremarkable, but a pulsatile mass may be present in the supraclavicular fossa with diminished distal pulses (Fig. 6-19). Several evocative maneuvers have been advocated for detection of arterial thoracic outlet syndrome, such as the Adson maneuver (caudal traction on the arm, head turned toward the arm, and inspiration) and 90-degree abduction and external rotation. However, compression of the subclavian artery resulting in diminished distal pulses is very common (at least 50%) in normal subjects (try it on yourself).

There are three locations at which thoracic outlet syndrome can occur: the scalene triangle, the costoclavicular space, and

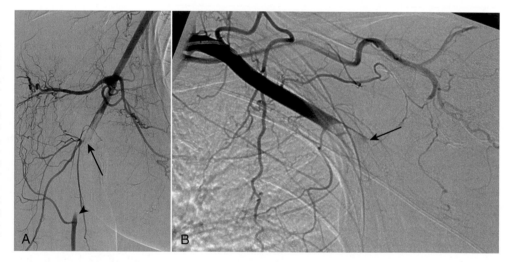

FIGURE 6-14. A 53-year-old man with bilateral upper extremity paradoxical emboli. The patient presented with acute bilateral upper extremity ischemia with a known diagnosis of bilateral pulmonary embolism. The complete study included arch aortogram and bilateral selective upper extremity angiograms from the arch to the hands. **A,** Digital subtraction angiogram (DSA) of selective right axillary artery injection showing embolic occlusion of the proximal brachial artery *(arrow)* with distal reconstitution *(arrowhead)* via collaterals from the circumflex humeral artery. **B,** DSA of selective left axillary artery injection showing embolic occlusion *(arrow)* of the distal axillary artery.

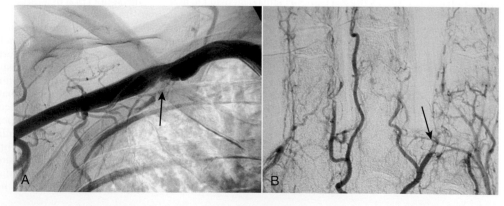

FIGURE 6-15. Patient with acute and chronic right hand digital ischemia. The underlying diagnosis is arterial thoracic outlet syndrome. **A,** Subclavian artery digital subtraction angiogram (DSA) showing slight aneurysmal dilation and mural irregularity (thrombus) where the artery crosses between the clavicle and first rib *(arrow)*. **B,** Magnification DSA of the right hand showing multiple digital artery occlusions and an intraluminal filling defect *(arrow)* consistent with an embolus.

the subpectoral space. The most common site of arterial compression is the scalene triangle (often associated with an anomalous or accessory rib), followed by the costoclavicular space. Compression of arterial structures in the subpectoral space is extremely rare. Arterial compression may be due to hypertrophy of normal structures or anomalous muscular, ligamentous, or bony structures. Repetitive crushing of the artery with arm

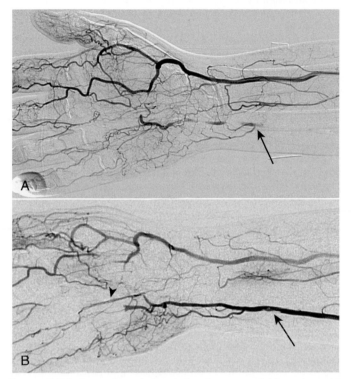

FIGURE 6-16. Acute finger ischemia in a hypercoagulable patient with prior episodes of ischemia. **A,** Digital subtraction angiogram (DSA) of the forearm and proximal hand showing occlusion of the ulnar artery with distal reconstitution *(arrow)* from radial and interosseus artery collaterals. **B,** DSA after infusion of tissue plasminogen activator into the ulnar artery for 48 hours (using antegrade brachial artery approach). The ulnar artery is patent with a small amount of residual thrombus *(arrow)*. There has been only slight improvement in the hand, because most of the occlusions are chronic *(arrowhead* on palmar digital artery showing intraluminal webs consistent with chronic thrombosis).

motion results in development of a focal narrowing and poststenotic dilation. Thrombus may form in these dilated or aneurysmal segments, with subsequent distal embolization (see Figs. 1-40 and 6-15).

Imaging of thoracic outlet syndrome must include both the inside and the outside of the lumen. The structures outside the lumen are imaged to determine the cause of the compression. The arterial lumen is imaged to confirm the compression and diagnose a complication of the syndrome such as distal embolization. Imaging should begin with a simple chest radiograph, which may reveal a cervical rib or other bony anomaly. Cross-sectional imaging of the upper thorax with CT/CTA or MR/MRA is useful for evaluating both the artery and the surrounding soft tissues. Postprocessing of the CTA or MRA may be needed to identify the cause of the aneurysm (Fig. 6-20). The goals of angiography in these patients are to evaluate the subclavian artery for stenosis, aneurysmal change, the presence of thrombus, and to detect distal emboli. A complete angiographic examination from the aortic arch to the hand is necessary. Subclavian aneurysms in thoracic outlet syndrome can be subtle, so comparison with the opposite side is useful. Injections with the arm in neutral position, and one with the arm in a position that elicits symptoms, have been considered essential in the past. As noted, evocative maneuvers can induce arterial compression in half of normal patients and should be interpreted with caution (Fig. 6-21). In positive cases, both subclavian arteries should be studied.

Definitive therapy requires surgical decompression of the thoracic outlet, resection of the aneurysm, and placement of a bypass graft. Patients who present with distal emboli may first undergo thrombolysis. Exclusion of the aneurysm can also be accomplished with a stent-graft, but prior decompression of the extrinsic structures is necessary.

ANEURYSMS

Upper extremity arterial aneurysms are unusual, representing fewer than 2% of all peripheral aneurysms. There are numerous etiologies of upper extremity aneurysms, several of which are discussed in other sections of this chapter (Box 6-6). Degenerative aneurysms are uncommon, but usually involve the proximal or intrathoracic portion of the subclavian artery. These aneurysms are associated with atherosclerosis and aortic, contralateral subclavian, or visceral artery aneurysms in up to 50% of patients. Older men are most often affected. Aneurysms of the extrathoracic subclavian and proximal axillary artery are typically due to thoracic outlet syndrome, and more distal aneurysms are often

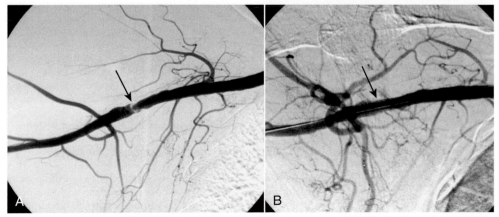

FIGURE 6-17. Ulcerated plaque in the axillary artery causing acute and chronic digital artery atheroembolization in a 58-year-old woman with vasculopathy presenting with finger gangrene, ulcerations, and superimposed acute digital ischemia. The brachial pulse was diminished. **A,** Irregular, weblike stenosis of the axillary artery *(arrow)*. The arterial inflow was normal. **B,** The stenosis was treated with primary stent placement *(arrow)* using a self-expanding nitinol stent (8 mm × 20 mm), followed by angioplasty to 7 mm. A self-expanding stent was used because of the peripheral location of the lesion. The patient had immediate relief of her hand pain with improved perfusion and subsequent healing of her digital ulcerations.

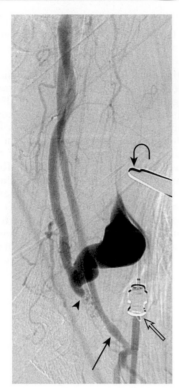

FIGURE 6-18. Distal revascularization with interval ligation (DRIL) for hand ischemia in a patient with a large brachial artery to cephalic vein fistula. The brachial artery has been ligated distal to the fistula *(arrowhead)*, and a vein bypass *(arrow)* placed from the proximal to distal brachial artery around the fistula. The image was created by compressing the venous outflow *(curved arrow)*, with access directly into the cephalic vein *(open arrow)*.

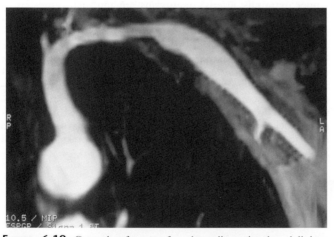

FIGURE 6-19. Coronal reformat of a three-dimensional gadolinium-enhanced magnetic resonance angiogram showing an aneurysm of the distal subclavian and axillary arteries in a woman who presented with a cervical rib and pulsatile supraclavicular mass. The distal pulses were normal. The aneurysm and rib were resected without additional imaging.

traumatic in origin. A detailed history and careful imaging are essential to determine the nature of the aneurysm.

Central (intrathoracic) aneurysms can present with pain, compression of adjacent structures such as veins and nerves (including hoarseness when the right recurrent laryngeal nerve is involved), distal thromboembolism, and rupture. Extrathoracic subclavian and more distal aneurysms present with distal embolization and thrombosis.

Aberrant right subclavian arteries (arising as the last branch of the arch) occur in 1% of individuals. The origin of this artery is frequently patulous, termed a *diverticulum of Kommerell.* When the diameter exceeds 2 cm, it is considered an aneurysm. In 80% of patients, the aberrant subclavian artery lies posterior to the esophagus, in 15% between the esophagus and trachea, and anterior to both in 5%. Aneurysms of this artery can compress and obstruct the esophagus resulting in difficulty swallowing (dysphagia lusoria). These aneurysms appear to be at high risk of rupture and are usually surgically resected when diagnosed (Fig. 6-22). Although extremely rare, the same pathology can be found in an aberrant left subclavian artery in patients with right-sided aortic arches.

Imaging with ultrasound, CTA, and MRA is frequently sufficient to detect an upper extremity aneurysm and differentiate it from a tortuous but otherwise normal artery. CTA and MRA can often provide definitive evaluation of aneurysms of the intrathoracic subclavian artery. Etiologies of intrathoracic subclavian aneurysms other than degeneration should be carefully excluded, particularly trauma and chronic dissection. Angiography may not be necessary unless the relationship of the aneurysm to cerebral artery origins or the aorta cannot be determined.

Therapy of upper extremity aneurysms is determined by the etiology, size, and location. The majority of aneurysms are treated surgically with excision and bypass, although stent-grafts are increasingly used.

VASCULITIS

The arteries of the upper extremity can be affected by any of the arteritides (Box 6-7). The typical patient is younger than would be expected for atherosclerotic disease and usually has constitutional symptoms. Patients may present with intermittent or fixed ischemic symptoms, ranging from diminished upper extremity pulses to digital ulceration. A frequent association is Raynaud syndrome.

Imaging of vasculitides that have a more central distribution, such as Takayasu arteritis, can be initiated with cross-sectional techniques such as CT or MR imaging. Wall thickening that enhances with contrast, central stenoses, and central aneurysms suggest a vasculitis. When there is digital involvement, angiography is necessary to differentiate between embolic, atherosclerotic, and inflammatory diseases.

The location of the vascular abnormality is somewhat helpful in classifying the vasculitis, although in this situation the destiny of all rules (to be broken) is often fulfilled. Proximal stenoses and occlusions (brachiocephalic and subclavian arteries) strongly suggest Takayasu arteritis (see Fig. 1-14). Subclavian, axillary, and proximal brachial artery occlusions suggest giant cell arteritis (see Fig. 1-16). These occlusions are usually well collateralized, with preservation of the distal runoff to the forearm and hand. The patient history is equally important in determining the etiology of the lesion. For example, radiation treatments that included the extremity in the therapy portal may result in radiation vasculitis.

Buerger disease (thromboangiitis obliterans) affects the upper extremities in more than two thirds of patients with this disorder. Occlusion of named arteries and hypertrophy of small perineural vessels and vasa vasorum are characteristic (Fig. 6-23). In addition to tobacco abuse, frequent use of marijuana also appears to be a risk factor.

The angiographic appearance of systemic lupus erythematosus (SLE), scleroderma, rheumatoid arthritis, and many other connective tissue disorders is similar (see Fig. 1-20). In general there are multiple occlusions of the medium to small arteries of the hand, particularly in the digits, with poor collateralization. The occlusions are usually tapered, although there may be intimal irregularity and abrupt changes in caliber of the patent vessels. The absence of intraluminal filling defects is a key diagnostic feature. The arteries of the upper arm and forearm are usually spared, although axillary occlusion has been reported in SLE. The presence of multiple small aneurysms is typical of polyarteritis nodosa (PAN), but atypical with other vasculitides.

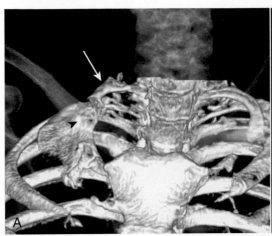
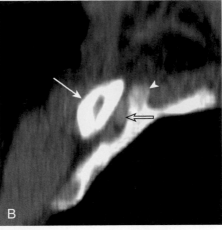

FIGURE **6-20**. Right-handed male electrician with right hand pain when he works with his hands over his head. **A,** Three-dimensional surface rendering from a chest computed tomography scan shows a hypoplastic first right rib *(arrow)*, which articulates with an exostosis *(arrowhead)* arising from a hypertrophied second rib. **B,** Sagittal reconstruction shows the subclavian artery *(open arrow)* compressed between the clavicle *(white arrow)* and the exostosis *(arrowhead)*.

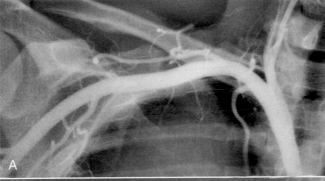
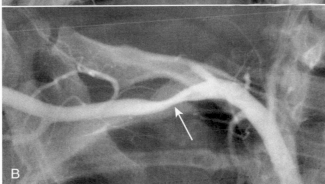

FIGURE **6-21**. Evocative maneuvers in a patient with suspected arterial thoracic outlet syndrome. **A,** The subclavian artery appears normal in neutral position. **B,** With the arm abducted 90 degrees, there is compression of the subclavian artery *(arrow)*. Care in interpretation of this result in the absence of a subclavian artery aneurysm is necessary because this same finding can be induced in asymptomatic individuals.

Box 6-6. Etiologies of Upper Extremity Aneurysms

TRUE
Thoracic outlet syndrome
Chronic dissection (originating in aorta)
Degenerative
Marfan syndrome
Vasculitis

FALSE
Trauma
Iatrogenic
Infection
Ehlers-Danlos syndrome
Behçet disease

TRAUMA

The upper limb is involved in approximately 40% of all cases of extremity penetrating trauma. The likelihood of an arterial injury that requires intervention is 40%-50% when hard clinical findings are present (Box 6-8). Angiography is the optimal imaging modality, as it can be both diagnostic and therapeutic. The diagnostic angiographic examination in trauma patients is focused on the injured limb segment. The full range of vascular injuries may be found, including spasm, intimal tear, pseudoaneurysm, extravasation, occlusion, and arteriovenous fistula (Fig. 6-24). Branch vessel pseudoaneurysms and arteriovenous fistulas can be easily treated by transcatheter embolization. Similar injuries to the subclavian and axillary arteries can be effectively managed with stent-grafts.

In the absence of hard clinical signs, a major vascular injury is unlikely, and patients are managed conservatively with observation and clinical follow-up. Vascular ultrasound has been used to confirm absence of vascular injury when clinical suspicion is low but is probably unnecessary. Shotgun wounds are an exception, in that the large area of soft tissue trauma and the multiple pellets makes physical examination difficult and less reliable. These patients should undergo angiography despite the absence of hard clinical signs. Penetrating injury to the chest in the vicinity of the intrathoracic portions of subclavian artery (zone 1, see Table 5-4) is also considered differently, in that physical examination of these vessels is impossible, and surgical repair requires a thoracotomy. CTA or angiography is warranted if vascular injury is suspected, even in the absence of objective evidence of vascular injury.

Stretch as a mechanism of injury is somewhat unique to the upper extremities, particularly the axillosubclavian arteries (Fig. 6-25). This occurs when there is sudden extreme traction on the arm, such as when trying to stop a fall from a tree by grabbing a branch, or dislocation. The artery is stretched along its long axis, resulting in intimal tears and disruption of the media. Small branch arteries may be sheared away. Secondary thrombosis with distal embolization may complicate the injury. Concomitant neurologic injury occurs in over 40% of traction injuries to the arm owing to avulsion of the brachial plexus nerve roots. The combination of neurologic and vascular injury can be devastating, with poor long-term functional results. Chronic forceful stretching, such as in baseball pitchers, may result in localized arterial dissection or thrombosis.

Iatrogenic injuries to the upper extremity arteries occur most often during central venous access procedures or placement of an arterial line for hemodynamic monitoring. When central lines are placed using blind bedside techniques, the incidence of inadvertent arterial puncture may be as high as 2%. The arteries most commonly injured are the subclavian and carotid, although other branch vessels such as the internal mammary artery and thyrocervical trunk can be involved (Fig. 6-26). In

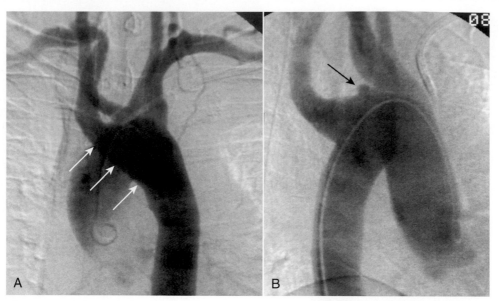

FIGURE 6-22. Ruptured aneurysm of aberrant right subclavian artery in a 49-year-old hypertensive woman presenting with acute chest pain and transient hypotension. **A,** Digital subtraction angiogram (DSA) of the aorta in the anteroposterior projection shows the origin of the aberrant right subclavian artery *(arrows)* projected posterior to the arch. **B,** DSA of the aorta in the right anterior oblique projection showing the aneurysmal origin of the aberrant right subclavian artery and a contained rupture *(arrow)*. (Case courtesy of Drs. John Thomas, San Antonio, Texas, and Charles Trinh, Houston, Texas.)

Box 6-7. Vasculitides Affecting the Upper Extremities

Digital
- Systemic lupus erythematosus
- Scleroderma
- Rheumatoid
- Buerger disease
- Polyarteritis nodosa

Forearm
- Buerger disease

Axillary artery
- Giant cell
- Systemic lupus erythematosus (rare)

Subclavian artery
- Takayasu arteritis
- Behçet disease

Box 6-8. Clinical Signs of Vascular Injury

HARD
Active arterial hemorrhage
Thrill or bruit
Expanding hematoma
Extremity ischemia
Pulse deficit

SOFT
Adjacent fracture
Adjacent nerve injury
Stable hematoma
Delayed or decreased capillary refill
History of hypotension or bleeding
Extensive soft tissue injury

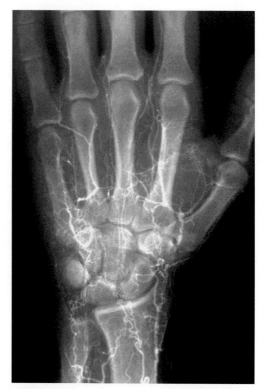

FIGURE 6-23. Upper extremity Buerger disease in a 33-year-old male heavy smoker. Angiogram of the hand shows widespread arterial occlusions with numerous corkscrew collaterals.

the most instances, the arterial puncture is of no consequence. Arterial dissection can result from attempts to cannulate the artery with a guidewire or large central venous access device. Pseudoaneurysms and arteriovenous fistulas are more likely to occur in patients with coagulation disorders. Sudden widening of the mediastinum or hemo-pneumothorax after placement of a central line should suggest an unrecognized arterial injury. Further evaluation may be attempted with ultrasound (if the suspected location of the injury is peripheral), or contrast-enhanced CT. Angiography is both definitive and possibly therapeutic. Keep in mind that during bedside attempts to place central venous catheters nobody really knows how deep or far the needle went.

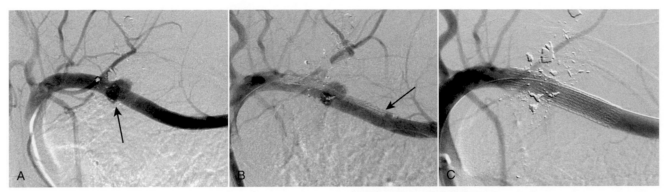

FIGURE 6-24. Left subclavian pseudoaneurysm following a gunshot wound. **A,** Selective left subclavian digital subtraction angiogram (DSA) showing a pseudoaneurysm *(arrow).* **B,** DSA showing the position of the endograft *(arrow)* before deployment. **C,** DSA after endograft deployment showing exclusion of the pseudoaneurysm.

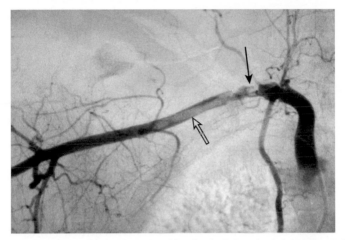

FIGURE 6-25. Subtracted angiogram showing intimal irregularity *(arrow)* and intraluminal thrombosis *(open arrow)* of the subclavian and axillary arteries in a patient who had diminished right upper extremity pulses and a brachial plexus injury after falling from a tree. The patient tried to grab a branch half way down.

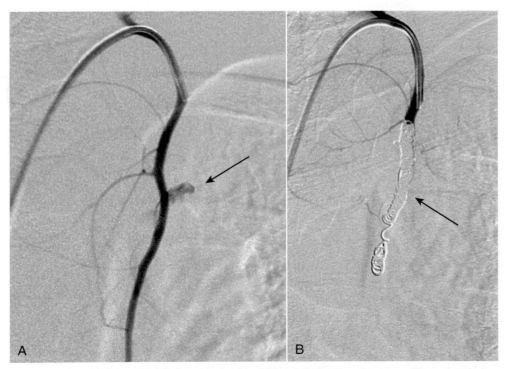

FIGURE 6-26. Internal mammary artery injury caused during attempted bedside subclavian line placement. The patient had an expanding chest wall hematoma. **A,** Selective left internal mammary artery digital subtraction angiogram (DSA) showing extravasation *(arrow).* **B,** Control DSA after coil embolization *(arrow).* Note that the coils were placed from distal to proximal across the injury to prevent retrograde perfusion from intercostals and inferior epigastric arteries.

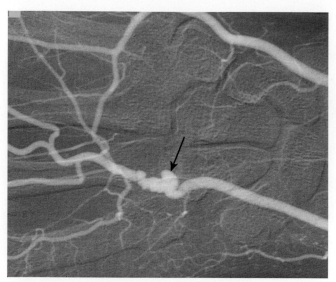

FIGURE 6-27. Hand angiogram in a 37-year-old male mechanic presenting with recurrent episodes of digital ischemia. There is irregularity and enlargement of the ulnar artery *(arrow)* in the region of the hamate bone. This is characteristic of hypothenar hammer syndrome.

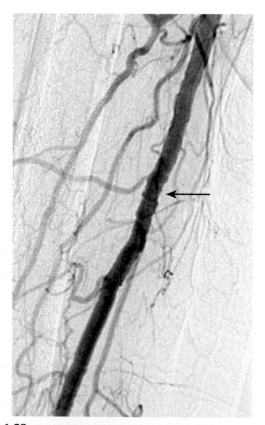

FIGURE 6-28. Angiogram of the right brachial artery showing the typical beaded appearance of medial fibroplasia *(arrow)*.

The brachial artery can be injured by blunt trauma to the inside of the upper arm such as might occur with chronic improper use of crutches. Aneurysmal degeneration of the artery leads to thrombus formation with local occlusion or distal embolization. Stretch injury, thrombosis, and transection can occur in association with dislocations and fractures. Extravasation from disrupted branch arteries can be managed with embolization in most instances (see Fig. 6-26).

Box 6-9. Primary Hyperparathyroidism

Incidence 4-6 per 100,000
Female-to-male ratio 3:2
Fifth and sixth decades
Single adenomas in 80%
Multiple adenomas in 15%
Ectopic adenomas 1%
Parathyroid carcinoma 1%
Usually sporadic, but associated with multiple endocrine neoplasia syndromes

Chronic trauma to the base of the hand, such as occurs when the "butt" of the hand is used as a hammer, can result in intimal injury and aneurysm formation in the ulnar artery as it crosses the base of the metacarpals (Fig. 6-27). An underlying intrinsic abnormality of the ulnar artery, such as fibromuscular dysplasia, has been proposed as a contributing factor. Symptoms occur when the aneurysms or intimal irregularities thrombose or become a source of digital emboli, characteristically to the third through fifth fingers. This complex is termed *hypothenar hammer syndrome.* Angiography remains the best imaging modality for this entity, although ultrasound may be used to determine the size of the aneurysm. Digital artery emboli with an ulnar artery aneurysm or focal ulnar occlusion at the hypothenar eminence are diagnostic findings.

Self-administered drugs injected directly into an upper extremity artery can result in pseudoaneurysms, arteriovenous fistulas, dissections, and thrombosis. Acute hand and digital ischemia may complicate the local arterial injury. Mycotic pseudoaneurysms are prevalent in this patient population.

FIBROMUSCULAR DYSPLASIA

Fibromuscular dysplasia (FMD) may affect any medium-sized artery in the body. As a group, the subclavian, axillary, and brachial arteries are the fifth most common location for this process (Fig. 6-28). Ulnar and radial artery involvement has also been reported. Patients are usually asymptomatic, but may present with distal embolization. The diagnosis is usually not suspected before imaging, but angiography is required for confirmation. Both upper extremities should be studied, in that FMD is frequently bilateral. Angioplasty of symptomatic lesions is safe and effective.

PRIMARY HYPERPARATHYROIDISM

Hyperparathyroidism can be divided into three forms. Primary hyperparathyroidism is due to independent secretion of parathyroid hormone (PTH) by an adenoma in the gland (Box 6-9). Secondary hyperparathyroidism is due to stimulation of PTH by hypocalcemia. The tertiary form is due to autonomous hypersecretion of PTH due to chronic hypocalcemia or chronic renal failure. Vascular imaging and intervention has a role in the diagnosis and treatment of primary hyperparathyroidism.

There are normally four parathyroid glands, each residing posterior to the poles of the thyroid. Ectopic parathyroid glands can occur in the neck and mediastinum. The blood supply to normally situated glands is from the inferior and superior thyroidal arteries. Rarely, a small branch may arise directly from the aortic arch (thyroid ima).

Imaging of patients with suspected primary hyperparathyroidism is usually with neck ultrasound, CT, MRI, and technetium-99m sestamibi scans. Angiography or venous sampling is not indicated in patients when first diagnosed with primary hyperparathyroidism. Neck exploration, inspection of all four parathyroid glands, and resection of the abnormal gland is curative

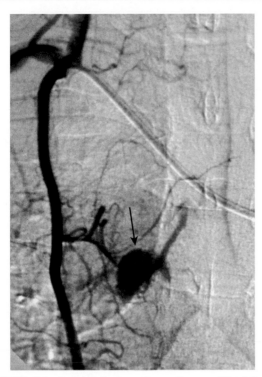

FIGURE 6-29. Selective digital subtraction angiogram of the right internal mammary artery in a patient with persistent hyperparathyroidism after neck exploration. There is a densely staining, well-circumscribed right paratracheal mass *(arrow)*. This proved to be an adenoma in an ectopic parathyroid gland.

in 90%-95% of cases. Those that continue to manifest primary hyperparathyroidism should undergo angiography followed by venous sampling (discussed in Chapter 7).

When undergoing an angiographic search for an ectopic parathyroid gland, selective injection of the thyrocervical trunk, the internal mammary arteries, and external carotid or superior thyroidal arteries should be performed (Fig. 6-29). Parathyroid adenomas appear as densely staining masses on angiography. Angiographic localization is successful in 60%-70%. An aortic arch injection in the LAO projection is necessary to identify a thyroid IMA artery.

Wedged injection of hypertonic contrast or absolute alcohol into a parathyroid adenoma results in cure in 60%-70% of patients, but most reoccur within 5 years. This can be a valuable therapy in those rare patients who have failed repeated surgical exploration.

▬▬ SUGGESTED READINGS

Angle JF, Matsumoto AH, McGraw JK, et al. Percutaneous angioplasty and stenting of left subclavian artery stenosis in patients with left internal mammary-coronary bypass grafts: clinical experience and long-term follow-up. *Vasc Endovasc Surg.* 2003;37:89-97.

Brown PJ, Zirwas MJ, English 3rd JC. The purple digit: an algorithmic approach to diagnosis. *Am J Clin Dermatol.* 2010;11:103-116.

Carrafiello G, Laganà D, Mangini M, et al. Percutaneous treatment of traumatic upper-extremity arterial injuries: a single-center experience. *J Vasc Interv Radiol.* 2011;22:34-39.

Cejna M, Salomonowitz E, Wohlschlager H, et al. rt-PA thrombolysis in acute thromboembolic upper-extremity arterial occlusion. *Cardiovasc Intervent Radiol.* 2001;24:218-223.

Chemelli AP, Wiedermann F, Klocker J, et al. Endovascular management of inadvertent subclavian artery catheterization during subclavian vein cannulation. *J Vasc Interv Radiol.* 2010;21:470-476.

Criado E, Berguer R, Greenfield L. The spectrum of arterial compression at the thoracic outlet. *J Vasc Surg.* 2010;52:406-411.

Doherty GM, Doppman JL, Miller DL, et al. Results of a multidisciplinary strategy for management of mediastinal parathyroid adenoma as a cause of persistent primary hyperparathyroidism. *Ann Surg.* 1992;215:101-106.

Duwayri YM, Emery VB, Driskill MR, et al. Positional compression of the axillary artery causing upper extremity thrombosis and embolism in the elite overhead throwing athlete. *J Vasc Surg.* 2011;53:1329-1340.

Ferris BL, Taylor LM, Oyama K, et al. Hypothenar hammer syndrome: proposed etiology. *J Vasc Surg.* 2000;31:104-113.

Gonzalez-Gay MA, Martinez-Dubois C, et al. Giant cell arteritis: epidemiology, diagnosis, and management. *Curr Rheumatol Rep.* 2010;12:436-442.

Hwang HY, Kim JH, Lee W, et al. Left subclavian artery stenosis in coronary artery bypass: prevalence and revascularization strategies. *Ann Thorac Surg.* 2010;89:1146-1150.

Kawarada O, Yokoi Y, Higashimori A. Angioplasty of ulnar or radial arteries to treat critical hand ischemia: use of 3- and 4-French systems. *Catheter Cardiovasc Interv.* 2010;76:345-350.

Kopp R, Wizgall I, Kreuzer E, et al. Surgical and endovascular treatment of symptomatic aberrant right subclavian artery (arteria lusoria). *Vascular.* 2007;15:84-91.

Labropoulos N, Nandivada P, Bekelis K. Prevalence and impact of the subclavian steal syndrome. *Ann Surg.* 2010;252:166-170.

Landry GJ, Edwards JM, McLafferty RB, et al. Long-term outcome of Raynaud's syndrome in a prospectively analyzed patient cohort. *J Vasc Surg.* 1996;23:76-85.

Licht PB, Balezantis T, Wolff B, et al. Long-term outcome following thromboembolectomy in the upper extremity. *Eur J Vasc Endovasc Surg.* 2004;28:508-512.

Malik J, Tuka V, Kasalova Z, et al. Understanding the dialysis access steal syndrome. A review of the etiologies, diagnosis, prevention and treatment strategies. *J Vasc Access.* 2008;9:155-166.

Matsumura JS, Rizvi AZ, Society for Vascular Surgery. Left subclavian artery revascularization: Society for Vascular Surgery Practice Guidelines. *J Vasc Surg.* 2010;52(Suppl 4):65S-70S.

McCready RA, Bryant MA, Divelbiss JL. Combined thenar and hypothenar hammer syndromes: case report and review of the literature. *J Vasc Surg.* 2008;48:741-744.

Mills Sr JL. Buerger's disease in the 21st century: diagnosis, clinical features, and therapy. *Semin Vasc Surg.* 2003;16:179-189.

Mosley JG. Arterial problems in athletes. *Br J Surg.* 2003;90:1461-1469.

Ouriel K. Noninvasive diagnosis of upper extremity vascular disease. *Semin Vasc Surg.* 1998;11:54-59.

Rice RD, Armstrong PJ. Brachial artery fibromuscular dysplasia. *Ann Vasc Surg.* 2010;24:255:e1-4.

Rose SC. Noninvasive vascular laboratory for evaluation of peripheral arterial occlusive disease: III. Clinical applications: nonatherosclerotic lower extremity arterial conditions and upper extremity arterial disease. *J Vasc Interv Radiol.* 2001;12:11-18.

Saemi AM, Johnson JM, Morris CS. Treatment of bilateral hand frostbite using transcatheter arterial thrombolysis after papaverine infusion. *Cardiovasc Intervent Radiol.* 2009;32:1280-1283.

Sanders RJ, Hammond SL, Rao NM. Diagnosis of thoracic outlet syndrome. *J Vasc Surg.* 2007;46:601-604.

Stepansky F, Hecht EM, Rivera R, et al. Dynamic MR angiography of upper extremity vascular disease: pictorial review. *Radiographics.* 2008;28:e28.

Stone PA, Srivastiva M, Campbell JE, Mousa AY. Diagnosis and treatment of subclavian artery occlusive disease. *Expert Rev Cardiovasc Ther.* 2010;8:1275-1282.

Suding PN, Wilson SE. Strategies for management of ischemic steal syndrome. *Semin Vasc Surg.* 2007;20:184-188.

Vierhout BP, Zeebregts CJ, van den Dungen JJ, Reijnen MM. Changing profiles of diagnostic and treatment options in subclavian artery aneurysms. *Eur J Vasc Endovasc Surg.* 2010;40:27-34.

Willmann JK, Wildermuth S. Multidetector-row CT angiography of upper and lower-extremity peripheral arteries. *Eur Radiol.* 2005;15(Suppl 4):D3-D9.

Winterer JT, Ghanem N, Roth M, et al. Diagnosis of the hypothenar hammer syndrome by high-resolution contrast-enhanced MR angiography. *Eur Radiol.* 2002;12:2457-2462.

CHAPTER 7

Upper Extremity, Neck, and Central Thoracic Veins

John A. Kaufman, MD, MS, FSIR, FCIRSE

The veins of the neck, arms, and chest are visited frequently by interventional radiologists. Placement of long-term central venous access catheters is a common yet essential procedure. The upper extremity veins are of critical importance for dialysis patients, whether they are managed with venous catheters or surgically created access. Upper extremity and central venous occlusions can cause severe symptoms, and are best managed with catheter-based techniques. In many interventional practices, procedures involving the veins of the upper body comprise a large portion of patients treated.

ANATOMY

Veins of the Neck

The internal jugular veins (IJV) are the largest veins of the head and neck. These valveless veins begin at the sigmoid fossa of the skull and anastomose with the subclavian veins at the base of the neck, behind the proximal head of the clavicle. There is almost always a valve in the IJV at this junction. Within the middle and lower neck the IJV lies within the carotid sheath anterior and slightly lateral to the carotid artery and beneath the sternocleidomastoid muscle (see Fig. 2-41). One IJV tends to be larger or "dominant" in most patients, usually the right. Important tributaries of the IJVs include the inferior petrosal sinuses (venous blood from the pituitary) at the jugular foramen, and the superior and middle thyroidal veins in the neck (Fig. 7-1). The inferior thyroidal vein is usually a single structure that drains vertically into the left brachiocephalic vein.

The external jugular veins (EJVs) are much smaller in size than their internal counterparts (see Fig. 7-1). The EJVs drain soft tissue structures of the face, scalp, and neck. Superficial in location, these veins are frequently visible as they pass over the upper sternocleidomastoid muscle and travel in an oblique course toward the supraclavicular fossa. The EJVs enter the subclavian veins just lateral to the IJVs. Additional drainage of the head and neck is provided by the vertebral veins, which also drain into the subclavian veins.

Key Collateral Pathways

Obstruction of one IJV results in drainage through the opposite vein. Obstruction of both IJVs is usually well tolerated due to the numerous potential collateral drainage pathways. These include the external jugular, vertebral, inferior thyroidal, and muscular veins of the neck.

Veins of the Upper Extremities

The veins of the upper extremities are divided into superficial and deep systems. From the hand to the shoulder, the superficial veins are the major drainage pathway. At the shoulder the deep veins become the primary drainage route. This is different from the venous anatomy of the lower extremities, where the deep veins are the dominant drainage throughout.

The superficial veins of the forearm are the cephalic along the anterior radial edge, the basilic along the posterior ulnar edge, and the median along the anterior aspect in the midline (Fig. 7-2). At the antecubital fossa just below the elbow joint, the cephalic vein sends a branch, the median cubital vein, obliquely across to join the basilic vein, which swings anteriorly in the upper third of the forearm to meet this branch. The median vein of the forearm drains into the median cubital vein.

In the upper arm, the cephalic vein lies in the groove between the biceps and brachialis muscles. At the shoulder, the cephalic vein passes between the pectoralis and deltoid muscles, diving over the medial edge of the pectoralis minor muscle to join the deeper axillary vein. There are no critical arterial or neural structures near the cephalic vein. The basilic vein ascends along the medial border of the biceps muscle, superficial to the brachial fascia, accompanied by only a few small superficial nerves. The brachial artery, veins, and associated major nerves lurk below the brachial fascia. At the junction of the distal and middle thirds of the upper arm, the basilic vein pierces the brachial fascia to join the deep (brachial) veins. The basilic vein becomes confluent with the brachial veins at the lower border of the teres major muscle to form the axillary vein. The basilic vein is easily identified in the upper arm as the largest single, most superficial medial draining vein.

The deep veins of the arm are small paired structures that parallel their associated namesake arteries (Fig. 7-3). Predictably, the deep veins of the forearm are the ulnar, interosseous, and radial veins. These drain into the paired brachial veins at the level of the antecubital fossa. In the upper arm, the brachial veins are closely related to the brachial artery and the median and radial nerves. At the lateral border of the teres major muscle, the brachial veins fuse with the basilic vein to form the axillary vein. Up until this point, the deep veins are smaller in size than the superficial veins. However, from the axillary vein centrally the deep veins assume dominance. The axillary vein lies slightly inferior and anterior to the axillary artery. At the lateral edge of the first rib, the axillary vein becomes the subclavian vein. This vein passes between the first rib and the clavicle to combine with the IJV at the thoracic inlet to form the brachiocephalic veins. Of all the upper extremity veins, only the subclavian vein is consistently valveless.

Key Collateral Pathways

The venous drainage of the upper extremities is rich with potential collateral pathways. Because of the multiplicity of veins in the arm, occlusion of a basilic or brachial vein is usually well tolerated.

Occlusion of an axillary or subclavian vein results in collateral flow through muscular and superficial veins about the shoulder, scapula, and chest wall. Dilated subcutaneous veins over the upper chest and shoulder are frequently visible in patients with occluded central veins. Potential decompressive pathways include the ipsilateral IJV, the ipsilateral intercostal veins, and the contralateral jugular or subclavian veins (Fig. 7-4).

Central Thoracic Veins

Blood from the upper extremities and the head returns to the heart through the brachiocephalic (or innominate) veins and the

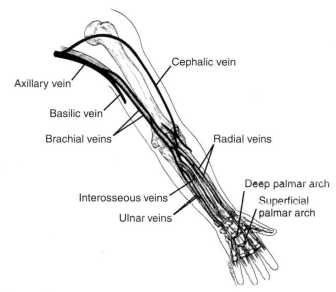

FIGURE 7-3. Drawing of the deep upper extremity veins. (From Lundell C, Kadir S. Superior vena cava and thoracic veins. In: Kadir S, ed. *Atlas of Normal and Angiographic Anatomy*. Philadelphia: WB Saunders, 1991, with permission.)

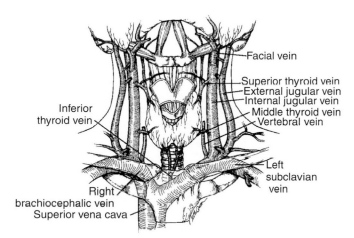

FIGURE 7-1. Drawing of the venous anatomy of the neck. (From Lundell C, Kadir S. Superior vena cava and thoracic veins. In: Kadir S, ed. *Atlas of Normal and Angiographic Anatomy*. Philadelphia: WB Saunders, 1991, with permission.)

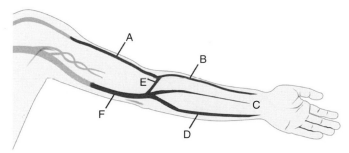

FIGURE 7-2. Drawing of the superficial veins of the arm. **A,** Cephalic vein in upper arm. **B,** Cephalic vein in forearm. **C,** Median vein of forearm. **D,** Basilic vein in forearm. **E,** Median cubital vein. **F,** Basilic vein in upper arm.

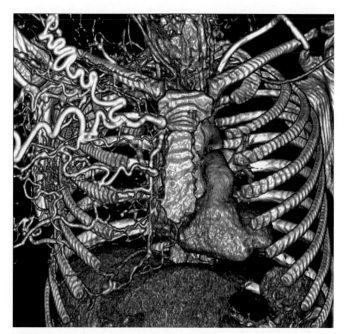

FIGURE 7-4. Subclavian vein occlusion. Volume rendering of a direct right upper extremity computed tomography venogram in a dialysis patient with longstanding subclavian vein occlusion due to repeated line placements shows drainage via large right chest wall collaterals. The beaded appearance of the bones is an imaging artifact. (Courtesy Constantino S. Pena, MD, Miami, Fla.)

superior vena cava (SVC) (Fig. 7-5). The right brachiocephalic vein is a short (2- to 3-cm) structure that has a vertical trajectory into the SVC. The left brachiocephalic vein, fully 2-3 times longer than the right, crosses from the left side of the mediastinum anterior to the great vessels to join the right brachiocephalic vein. This defines the origin of the SVC. Important tributaries of the brachiocephalic vein include the internal mammary, vertebral, pericardiophrenic, and the first intercostal veins. On the left, the inferior thyroidal vein drains into the superior aspect of the midpoint of the brachiocephalic vein.

The left brachiocephalic vein crosses the midline to join the right in more than 99% of normal individuals. In less than 1% of patients without congenital heart disease, the left brachiocephalic vein does not anastomose with the right but drains into the coronary sinus through a second, left-sided SVC (Fig. 7-6). This anomaly is observed in 4%-5% of patients with congenital heart disease.

The SVC is generally 6-8 cm in length, and up to 2 cm in diameter. The main tributaries of the SVC are the brachiocephalic veins and the azygos vein. The SVC generally enters the pericardium below the orifice of the azygos vein. In more than 99% of individuals, this vessel is single, right-sided, and drains into the right atrium.

The azygos and hemiazygos veins are posterior mediastinal structures that originate at the L1-L2 level (Fig. 7-7). The azygos vein ascends anterior to the thoracic spine to the right of the midline, while the hemiazygos vein lies slightly to the left of the midline anterior to the spine. Both veins receive blood from ascending lumbar, intercostal, subcostal, esophageal, and bronchial veins. The hemiazygos vein crosses anterior to the spine at the level of the T8 vertebral body to join the azygos vein. The azygos vein continues cephalad to the level of the T4 vertebral body, where it passes anteriorly over the right hilum to empty into the SVC. The accessory hemiazygos vein is a small, left-sided tributary of either the azygos or hemiazygos vein that drains the upper (through T8) intercostal veins. This vein will sometimes empty anteriorly and superiorly into the left brachiocephalic vein, in which case it can be visualized along the lateral border of the proximal descending thoracic aorta.

Key Collateral Pathways

Occlusion of a brachiocephalic vein results in obstruction of flow from both the ipsilateral arm and neck. Facial swelling on the side of the occlusion is rare as long as the contralateral IJV is patent. The venous blood from the arm may drain across the back, chest, and neck via deep and superficial collaterals to the opposite jugular, subclavian, and brachiocephalic veins. The superficial chest wall veins such as internal mammary and intercostal veins may also serve as collateral drainage pathways. These veins drain into the azygos vein on the right and hemiazygos vein on the left, or may continue down the abdominal wall to the inferior epigastric veins. Pericardial and phrenic veins may also be recruited as collateral drainage pathways.

The level of occlusion of the SVC determines which collateral pathway will be dominant. When occlusion is above the azygos vein, the collateral drainage involves primarily the chest wall and intercostal veins, emptying into the azygos system. The direction of flow within the azygos veins remains toward the SVC. Some drainage through the pericardial and abdominal wall veins

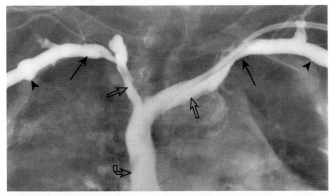

FIGURE 7-5. Central venogram obtained by simultaneous injection of both upper extremities. The patient has bilateral indwelling subclavian vein catheters. Axillary vein *(arrowheads)*, subclavian vein *(arrows)*, brachiocephalic veins *(open arrows)*, superior vena cava *(curved arrow)*.

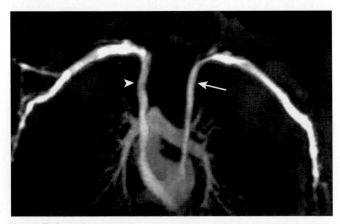

FIGURE 7-6. Persistent left superior vena cava (SVC). Coronal maximum intensity projection of bilateral upper extremity direct magnetic resonance venography in a patient with a persistent left SVC *(arrow)* showing the normal course of the right SVC *(arrowhead)*. Both drain to the right atrium, with the left SVC entering through the coronary sinus. (Courtesy Constantino S. Pena, MD, Miami, Fla.)

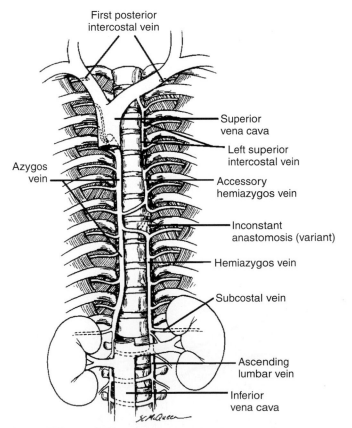

FIGURE 7-7. Drawing of the azygos veins. (From Lundell C, Kadir S. Superior vena cava and thoracic veins. In: Kadir S, ed. *Atlas of Normal and Angiographic Anatomy.* Philadelphia: WB Saunders, 1991, with permission.)

may be present as well. When the occlusion is localized below the azygos vein, flow reverses in this vein with drainage into the inferior vena cava (IVC) (Fig. 7-8). Chest wall and pericardial collaterals may also develop. Occlusion of the SVC above and below the azygos veins results in azygos and hemiazygos drainage into the IVC, as well as extensive chest wall and pericardial collateral veins.

▰ IMAGING

The superficial veins of the neck and upper extremity can be readily imaged with ultrasound. When evaluating a patient for upper extremity central venous thrombosis, the neck as well as the upper extremity veins should be studied, because the jugular veins are frequently involved. Gray scale imaging with compression and Doppler with color flow can provide information about venous patency and direction of flow (Fig. 7-9). The central veins such as the brachiocephalic veins and SVC cannot be directly imaged satisfactorily with external ultrasound transducers owing to the surrounding bone and lung. The patency of the central vessels can be inferred by studying subclavian vein and IJV Doppler waveforms at rest and in response to respiration and Valsalva maneuver. However, the impact of central stenoses on flow in the more peripheral veins has not been carefully worked out and may be masked by a well-developed collateral network. If, for some reason, ultrasound examination of the intrathoracic veins is strongly desired, then a transesophageal study is required.

Contrast-enhanced computed tomography (CT) is an excellent modality for evaluation of the jugular, proximal subclavian, brachiocephalic, and central veins, as well as the surrounding structures. The veins from the forearm to the axilla are difficult to image with CT. The advantages of this modality are the ability to map out collateral pathways, such as superficial chest wall veins in SVC obstruction, as well as revealing extrinsic causes of venous obstruction. Injection of contrast into the upper extremity

opposite the side of interest followed by a saline "chaser" for indirect CT venography can limit streak artifact from dense contrast. A delayed scan after the initial contrast injection is often useful to obtain opacification of all veins. Direct CT venography is performed with dilute contrast injected into the arm of interest during image acquisition. For all CT venography, careful postprocessing is useful when tracing collateral pathways and determining the etiology of extrinsic compression.

Magnetic resonance venography (MRV) is an excellent cross-sectional modality for evaluating the upper extremity, neck, and central veins (Fig. 7-10). Suppression of signal from background structures results in images that are easy to view, in comparison to CT in which bone and other tissues can obscure the veins. The most robust techniques involve gadolinium-enhanced acquisitions, preferably with subtraction of the enhanced arteries. The side of injection of contrast is not an issue with this technique, except that concentrated gadolinium may result in signal loss due to dominance of T2 shortening effects (see Fig. 3-16). This is easily solved by sequential acquisitions over several minutes, during which time the gadolinium becomes diluted. Conventional two-dimensional time-of-flight (2-D TOF) techniques have also been used with great success, although multiple acquisitions with careful orientation of the slices and saturation bands are necessary to image all of the veins (e.g., axial slices with inferior saturation for the jugular veins and SVC, but sagittal slices with medial saturation slabs for the brachiocephalic and subclavian veins). MRV of the veins of the forearms can be used for planning surgical dialysis access, but ultrasound and conventional venography are more readily available.

Although MRV is excellent for visualizing the vein lumen, the surrounding structures are not well seen. At a minimum, conventional anatomic T1-weighted images are necessary to evaluate the adjacent soft tissues.

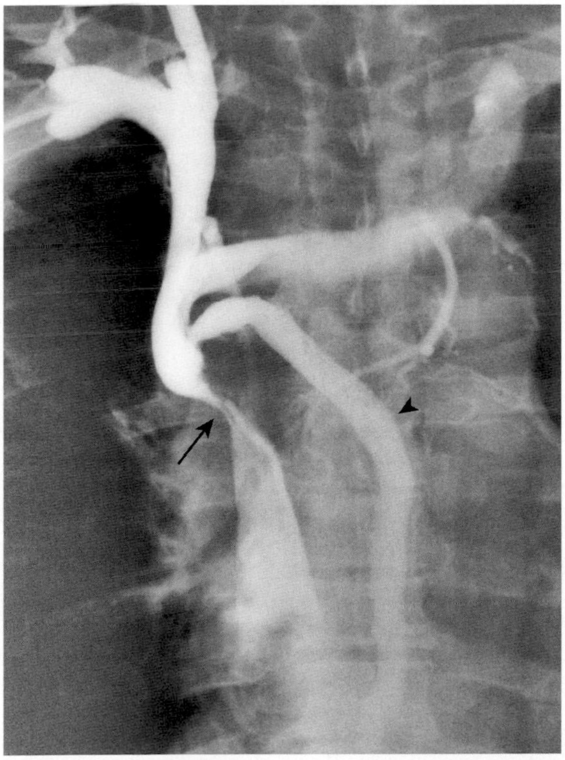

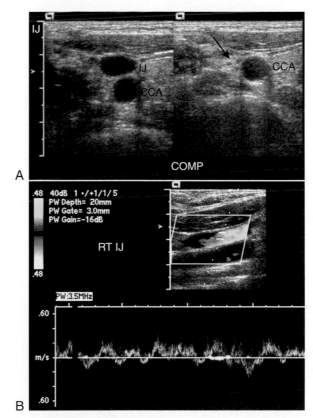

FIGURE 7-8. Collateral pathways in superior vena cava (SVC) obstruction. Venogram showing severe stenosis of the central SVC *(arrow)* with collateral drainage via the azygos vein *(arrowhead)*.

FIGURE 7-9. Ultrasound of jugular veins. **A,** Gray scale image showing normal, compressible internal jugular vein (IJ). CCA, Common carotid artery; Comp, compression Arrow, compressed IJ vein. **B,** Normal IJV Doppler waveform.

Arm venography is a simple, quick procedure for evaluation of the upper extremity and central veins. The IJVs are not routinely studied with this technique. For arm venography, an 18- to 20-gauge intravenous (IV) line should be started in a hand or forearm vein. When using existing IV access, test it first to ensure that it is patent and in a vein. Injection of the antecubital vein or upper arm cephalic vein may fail to opacify the basilic, brachial, and proximal axillary veins. Two or three 20-mL syringes of dilute contrast (20%-30% iodine) are injected by hand. Carbon dioxide gas is an excellent alternative contrast agent, except in patients with dialysis access grafts or fistulas. A tourniquet at the axilla enhances filling of deep and superficial veins. The hand should be in anatomic position (palm up) with the arm slightly abducted. In large patients, compression by the chest wall soft tissues can cause pseudostenosis of the veins in the medial aspect of the upper arm (Fig. 7-11). Both spot films and digital subtraction images are satisfactory for the arm veins. Digital subtraction is usually required to adequately visualize the brachiocephalic veins

and SVC. Unopacified inflow from other central veins should not be mistaken for thrombus or other filling defects. Bilateral injections can be performed to evaluate central processes (see Fig. 7-5). One of the major advantages of conventional arm venography is that there is an option to proceed directly to an intervention if an amenable abnormality is found.

■ UPPER EXTREMITY VENOUS THROMBOSIS

Acute thrombosis of a single peripheral upper extremity vein rarely results in arm swelling, but patients may have pain and tenderness over the involved vein. A common etiology is intravenous injection of medication or illicit drugs. The treatment is oral antiinflammatory agents and local measures such as heat packs. Thrombosis of central veins such as the axillary, subclavian, or brachiocephalic veins may result in swelling and cyanosis of the arm, especially when the limb is dependent. Frequently, patients report the first symptom as a ring or wristwatch feeling tight. Acute thrombosis may also be locally painful, possibly due to the expansion of the vein by thrombus or tense edema of the extremity. When the jugular vein is involved patients may complain of neck stiffness, tenderness, or a sense of swelling of the face on the affected side. Facial swelling is rarely a symptom of unilateral (or even bilateral) jugular vein thrombosis in a patient with patent central veins. Phlegmasia (alba or cerulea dolens) is also extremely rare in the upper extremity. Pulmonary embolization from the upper extremity is thought to occur in up to 15%-30% of cases, but is often asymptomatic.

Chronic occlusion of the small superficial upper extremity veins produces a hard, cordlike structure, but is usually otherwise innocuous. Chronic central thrombosis is suggested by the presence of well-developed superficial chest wall collateral veins. Patients may complain of arm swelling, particularly with use of the limb, but many are asymptomatic.

Central venous catheterization is the most common underlying etiology of upper extremity and jugular thrombosis (Box 7-1). Reported rates of pericatheter thrombus range from 3% to 60% with chronic indwelling subclavian venous catheters, although fewer (5%-10%) are symptomatic (Fig. 7-12). Many factors influence the incidence of this complication in specific patient populations, such as catheter size, location, and the presence of an underlying hypercoagulable state. There are no pharmacologic measures that have been shown conclusively to prevent acute catheter-related upper extremity venous thrombosis. Heparin or antibiotic impregnated catheters are promising technologies. Late thrombosis due to venous stenosis from catheter-related intimal injury can present at a time remote from the venous catheterization. Pacemaker wires are associated with an incidence of occlusive thrombosis of approximately 10% (Fig. 7-13).

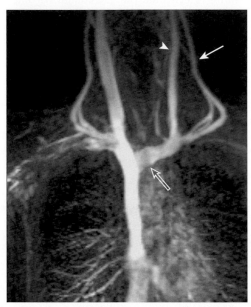

FIGURE 7-10. Gadolinium-enhanced 3-D magnetic resonance venogram of normal neck and central veins. The deep and superficial neck veins (*arrowhead* on left IJV, *solid arrow* on left EJV) are well visualized. An impression *(open arrow)* from the brachiocephalic artery can be seen on the left brachiocephalic vein. The heart and subclavian veins are not included in this restricted maximum-intensity projection. (Courtesy Barry Stein, MD, Hartford Hospital, Hartford, Conn.)

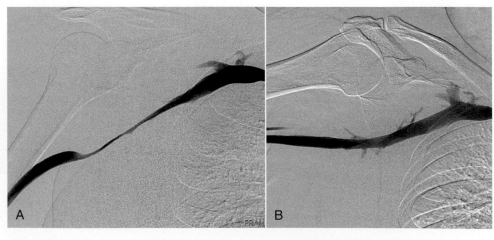

FIGURE 7-11. Axillary vein pseudolesion due to compression by chest wall soft tissues in an obese patient. **A,** Digital subtraction venogram of the right upper extremity with the arm at the patient's side. There appears to be a long stenosis of the axillary vein. Note the copious soft tissues of the chest. **B,** Venographic image of the same patient with the arm abducted. The stenosis has resolved.

Imaging findings of acute venous thrombosis are similar across most imaging modalities, although each has additional specific findings (Boxes 7-2 and 7-3). Patients should be initially evaluated with ultrasound, although the ability of this modality to image the central veins is limited. CT or MR allows diagnosis of thrombus, determination of the extent of obstruction, and identification of contributing pathologic processes in the adjacent soft tissues. Venography is not necessary unless the diagnosis is uncertain or an intervention is contemplated. Chronic venous thrombosis has a different appearance than acute venous thrombosis, but both can and often do coexist (Box 7-4).

The volume of thrombus encountered in the upper and central veins is less than that in the lower extremities because the upper venous bed is less capacious. When thrombosis occurs in the setting of a chronic underlying stenosis, the symptoms are caused by obstruction of the collateral veins by retrograde propagation of thrombus, not occlusion of the stenosis. Often, a little thrombus causes a lot of symptoms in the central thoracic veins. These features make catheter-based interventions an excellent choice for these patients.

The management of upper extremity central venous thrombosis depends on the chronicity, underlying cause, and clinical

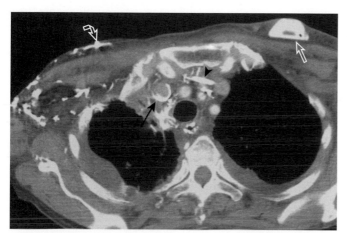

FIGURE 7-12. Axial computed tomography scan with injection through the right arm showing thrombus in the right brachiocephalic vein *(straight arrow)* and extensive chest wall collaterals *(curved arrow)*. The patient has a left chest port *(open arrow)* with a catheter *(arrowhead)* visible in the unopacified left brachiocephalic vein.

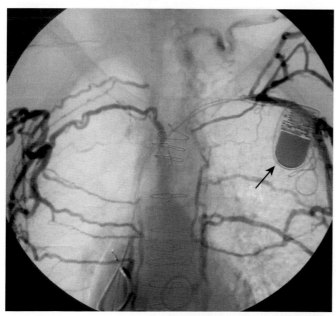

FIGURE 7-13. Digital venogram showing central venous occlusions in a patient with a left-sided pacemaker *(arrow)* and previous right subclavian catheters.

scenario. Acute thrombosis associated with a central line may be managed with simple local measures such as arm elevation, a compression sleeve, or full anticoagulation. Thrombosis in patients without central lines is managed with anticoagulation when possible, and a workup to identify an inciting cause such as venous stenosis. Evaluation for a prothrombotic state is important when the thrombosis is unprovoked. Patients with severe or persistent symptoms despite anticoagulation should be evaluated for catheter-based treatment of the thrombosis. Early clinical improvement is often dramatic with catheter-based treatments, although an advantage in the long-term outcome compared to anticoagulation remains ambiguous.

Pharmacomechanical thrombolysis of acute upper extremity venous thrombosis relieves symptoms and may unmask the underlying etiology. The goal is to open as many collaterals as possible in addition to the in-line venous drainage. Ultrasound or venographically guided puncture of the ipsilateral basilic vein (when patent) with a microaccess needle allows a direct approach to subclavian thrombosis. Femoral or jugular vein access may be used as well. When using an antegrade upper arm access, a sheath should be placed as an additional infusion site for the thrombolytic agent or heparin. The area of thrombosis should be crossed with a selective guidewire and catheter. Often the ease of crossing provides important clues about the age of the thrombus and predicts the overall success of the procedure, with fresh soft thrombus responding better than hard chronic organized clot.

Pharmacologic thrombolysis is accomplished by placing a multi-side-holed infusion catheter across the thrombus. Infusions should be continued for 12-24 hours at a minimum. Concurrent anticoagulation with low doses of heparin, ideally through an IV peripheral to the thrombus, should be administered. Success rates are high with acute thrombus.

Pharmacomechanical and mechanical thrombectomy result in rapid restoration of flow through the occluded segment, with complete treatment possible in a single session. However, subsequent overnight infusion to treat residual thrombus may be needed. The same access techniques and sites are used as for pharmacologic thrombolysis, but use of a sheath is mandatory. These methods are the preferred first option for many interventionalists.

When a venous stenosis is unmasked after the thrombus is cleared, angioplasty should be performed unless thoracic outlet syndrome is the underlying etiology (see later). The availability of noncompliant high-pressure balloons is essential, in that these lesions tend to be fibrotic and elastic. Prolonged inflations, often several minutes, and inflation devices that permit controlled application of high pressures are used. Patients are uncomfortable during these inflations. Angioplasty can also be helpful to disrupt residual thrombus. Do not be afraid to push a little thrombus out of the vein with the inflated balloon, especially when it is saturated with a thrombolytic agent.

The need for stents depends on the angioplasty results and the quantity of venous flow. Patients without a dialysis fistula peripheral to the obstruction (i.e., low flow) respond well to even modest angioplasty results and restored patency of collateral veins. Stent placement is more often necessary to relieve symptoms when there is high flow in the vein. Self-expanding stents are commonly used, especially in the brachiocephalic veins. Stenting across jugular or brachiocephalic vein orifices could impede future venous access and should be avoided. Stents placed in the subclavian vein beneath the clavicle are at risk for fracture due to compression (see Fig. 4-23). Large stents are needed for most central veins, often 14 mm in diameter. Patients require long-term anticoagulation following successful thrombolysis/thrombectomy whether or not stents are used.

In rare cases, patients with acute upper extremity thrombosis may have documented symptomatic pulmonary embolism and a contraindication to anticoagulation. Placement of an SVC filter may be necessary (Fig. 7-14).

Chronic occlusions require treatment only if symptomatic or the vein is needed as a conduit for another procedure. These lesions can be densely fibrotic and difficult to cross with guidewires. Catheters on both sides of the occlusion are extremely helpful, in that the precise length of the occlusion is known and a target clearly identified. Aggressive measures, such as probing with the back end of a stiff hydrophilic guidewire or even a TIPS needle (see Chapter 14) may ultimately be required. Stents are almost always necessary, but the restenosis rate approaches 45% at 1 year. Covered stents (usually with ePTFE material) are increasingly used in this setting with promising early results.

THORACIC OUTLET SYNDROME

Venous thoracic outlet syndrome usually first presents with acute thrombosis (Box 7-5). Also known as *Paget Schroetter* or *effort*

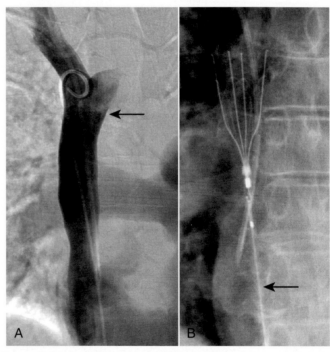

FIGURE 7-14. Superior vena cava (SVC) filter in a patient with massive upper extremity thrombosis, pulmonary embolism, and contraindication to anticoagulation. **A,** Venogram performed from a femoral approach showing the right and left brachiocephalic veins and the SVC. The arrow indicates the intended location for the base of the filter. A triple-lumen catheter is present in the SVC, which was left in place for the procedure. **B,** A Gunther Tulip filter (Cook Group, Bloomington, Ind.) before final release with the feet just below the confluence of the brachiocephalic veins and the apex pointed toward the right atrium. This was a jugular access filter placed from a femoral access *(arrow)* to ensure proper orientation of the device.

Box 7-5. Venous Thoracic Outlet Syndrome

Locations
- Thoracic outlet
- Pectoralis minor muscle
- Subacromial space

Male:female = 2:1
Second through fifth decade
Right > left
Bilateral thrombosis in 6%
Combined venous thrombosis and neurogenic thoracic outlet syndrome in 10%

thrombosis syndromes, this diagnosis should be suspected in any young, healthy (especially athletic) patient presenting with unexplained acute subclavian vein thrombosis. About 5% of all cases of acute upper extremity venous thrombosis are due to thoracic outlet syndrome. Extrinsic compression of the subclavian or axillary vein by a cervical rib, bony exostosis, anomalous ligament or muscle, or hypertrophied scalene muscles (exercise can be dangerous) results in intimal hyperplasia, fibrosis, and stenosis (see Fig. 1-39). Collaterals develop that compensate for the obstruction and prevent symptoms, although many patients give a history of arm swelling and heaviness when questioned. Thrombosis isolated to the residual lumen is usually accompanied by minimal or mild symptoms. Propagation of thrombus into the collateral veins causes acute obstruction of venous outflow. Patients frequently report onset of symptoms after vigorous upper body activity, such as painting a ceiling. Pulmonary embolus from upper extremity thrombosis due to thoracic outlet syndrome is unusual, in that the underlying pathology is a fixed venous obstruction. The long-term natural history is not well known, but estimates of chronic disability due to swelling and discomfort range from 10% to 60%.

In patients with acute symptoms and suspected thoracic outlet syndrome, the chest radiograph should be reviewed for anomalous cervical ribs. The presence of thrombus can be confirmed with ultrasound or venography. MRI or CT, either acutely or after treatment, is helpful to evaluate for anomalous muscles or ligaments.

When thoracic outlet syndrome is suspected in the absence of acute symptoms, the same imaging studies should be obtained. Venography should be performed with the arm positioned to reproduce the patient's symptoms. Using the Adson maneuver, the shoulder is depressed with the arm at the side and the patient's head turned toward the shoulder. When thoracic outlet syndrome is found or suspected, bilateral subclavian venograms should be obtained. However, be wary because subclavian vein compression with extreme abduction of the arm can be induced in half the population (Fig. 7-15).

Thoracic outlet syndrome is initially managed with heparinization and catheter-based treatment of the thrombus, usually from an ipsilateral upper extremity approach (Fig. 7-16). This quickly

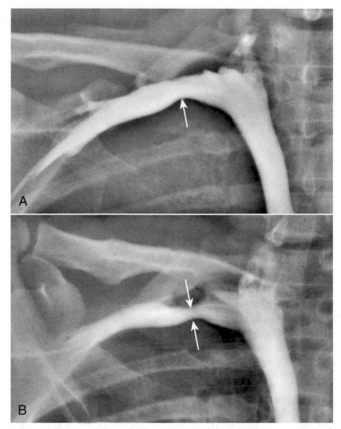

Figure 7-15. Compression of the subclavian vein in a normal individual. **A,** Venogram with the arm in neutral position shows minimal inferior indentation *(arrow)* of the subclavian vein. Note the absence of collateral veins. **B,** Venogram with the arm abducted shows partial compression of the subclavian vein *(arrows)*. Again note the absence of collateral veins.

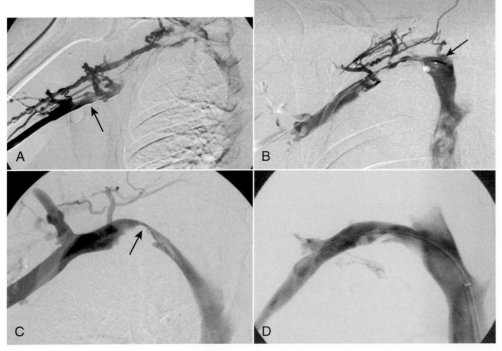

Figure 7-16. Upper extremity venous thrombosis in a young athlete. **A,** Right upper extremity venogram in a healthy young male with acute arm swelling. There is obstruction at the level of the axillary vein. Note the intraluminal filling defect characteristic of thrombus *(arrow)* and the drainage through collateral veins. **B,** Venogram after 4 hours of thrombolysis shows multi-side-hole catheter positioned across the thrombus with the tip *(arrow)* in the right brachiocephalic vein. **C,** After 24 hours of catheter-directed thrombolysis, a focal, bulky stenosis *(arrow)* is present at the junction of the subclavian and internal jugular vein. **D,** Venogram following first rib resection with subsequent angioplasty (12-mm diameter balloon) shows minimal residual stenosis.

Box 7-6. Causes of Superior Vena Cava Syndrome

Malignancy
- Bronchogenic carcinoma
- Lymphoma
- Small-cell carcinoma
- Mediastinal metastases

Central venous catheter
Trauma
Mediastinal hematoma
Mediastinal fibrosis
Sarcoid
Radiation
Thoracic aortic aneurysm
Anastomotic stenosis (heart-lung transplant)

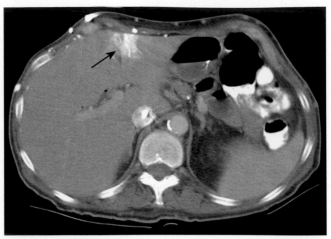

FIGURE 7-17. Characteristic enhancement of segment IV *(arrow)* of the liver by chest and mediastinal collateral veins in a patient with superior vena cava syndrome following injection of contrast in an upper extremity vein. Note the numerous collateral veins in the abdominal wall.

reduces arm swelling and allows delineation of the underlying venous lesion. The cause of the extrinsic compression must also be determined, because the second step in treatment is decompression of the thoracic outlet. An obvious stenosis in the subclavian vein is usually present. This responds poorly to angioplasty or stents because the problem is the extrinsic compression. Surgical decompression is performed before any additional interventions. Repeat venography is performed after surgical decompression, with angioplasty of residual stenoses. Stents should be used only when stenoses are both recurrent and severely symptomatic. The unknown long-term patency and the young age of most of these patients should caution against routine stent use. Stents should not be placed without surgical decompression of the thoracic outlet, or the stent may be crushed or fractured (see Fig. 4-23).

▬ SUPERIOR VENA CAVA SYNDROME

Abrupt occlusion of the SVC results in a characteristic syndrome of facial and upper extremity edema, superficial venous distention, and cyanosis. These patients are usually extremely uncomfortable, especially when lying flat. Acute SVC syndrome is considered a medical emergency. Chronic occlusion or stenosis may be asymptomatic or cause moderate facial edema or pressure that improves when the patient is upright. The level of obstruction is important, because occlusion below the azygos vein may be well tolerated if the azygos drainage is robust (see Fig. 7-8). Obstruction of the SVC can be due to intrinsic or extrinsic causes (Box 7-6). The most common etiology (>80%) is compression by thoracic malignancy, usually originating in the lung. Patients with SVC syndrome caused by malignancy have less than 50% survival at 6 months.

Although SVC syndrome is a clinical diagnosis, imaging is necessary for confirmation and planning therapy. The most expeditious imaging modality is contrast-enhanced CT, which allows evaluation of venous patency and the surrounding tissues (see Fig. 7-12). Injection of contrast into the upper extremity with filling of abdominal wall collateral veins suggests central stenosis or occlusion (Fig. 7-17). Opacification of the more central veins may be delayed, so a second scan after 60-90 seconds may be necessary to avoid overestimating the extent of occlusion. The lower neck should be included in the imaged area so that jugular vein patency can be assessed. Gadolinium-enhanced MR venography is also very useful in the evaluation of suspected SVC syndrome. Upper extremity venography with simultaneous injection of contrast into both arms defines the status of the veins, but does not provide information about the extravascular structures (see Fig. 7-13).

Symptomatic chronic SVC stenosis should be managed by angioplasty first, with stents reserved for recurrent or recalcitrant lesions (Fig. 7-18). Identification of the underlying etiology is essential to provide proper treatment. Thrombosis of a chronic lesion is usually amenable to thrombolysis/pharmacomechanical

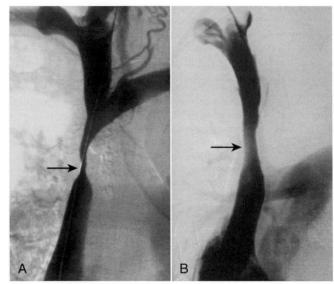

FIGURE 7-18. Superior vena cava (SVC) syndrome due to mediastinal fibrosis in a patient with histoplasmosis exposure. **A,** Contrast venogram performed by injection from the right internal jugular vein showing severe SVC stenosis *(arrow)* and reflux into the left brachiocephalic vein. **B,** Contrast venogram following stent placement *(arrow)* dilated to 10 mm, at which point the patient complained of chest pain. Note absence of reflux into other mediastinal veins.

thrombectomy (PMT). Indwelling long-term central venous access catheters are a common cause of benign stenoses, and can be repositioned into a jugular or subclavian vein during placement of an SVC stent. Stents can be placed over pacemaker wires when necessary. Balloon and stent diameters range from 8 to 16 mm, but must be tailored to the patient and the underlying pathology. Reestablishment of inline drainage from one jugular vein to the right atrium is usually sufficient to relieve head and neck symptoms acutely. Extension of stents into the right atrium may induce arrhythmia and should be avoided.

Recanalization of an occluded SVC is frequently successful when combined IJV and femoral venous approaches are used. Access through the right IJV provides a short, straight path to the right atrium and is preferred. A second catheter placed in the residual patent SVC below the obstruction from a femoral approach can be used to guide recanalization. Care must be taken

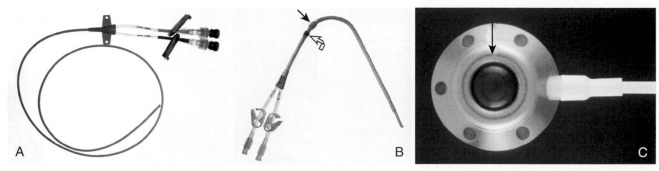

FIGURE 7-19. Typical long-term central venous access devices. **A,** Peripherally inserted central catheter (PICC), double lumen. Catheter may be silicone or polyurethane, usually 3-6 French, single or double lumen, valved or nonvalved. There is no cuff for tissue ingrowth. **B,** Tunneled catheter (in this case for dialysis). Tunneled catheters may be silicone or polyurethane, up to 16 French or larger, have up to three lumens, and be valved or nonvalved. Tunneled catheters are characterized by the presence of a cuff for tissue ingrowth *(straight arrow)* that stabilizes the catheter after 3-4 weeks. The catheter shown here also has a silver-impregnated cuff *(curved arrow)* to reduce tunnel infections. **C,** Port for subcutaneous implantation. A silicone membrane *(arrow)* for access with a noncoring needle is characteristic. Ports may be metal or plastic, single or double lumen, with a range of sizes suitable for arm or chest placement. Catheters are silicone or polyurethane, usually 5-8 French in diameter.

TABLE 7-1 Types of Central Venous Access Devices

Device	Duration	Uses
Nontunneled central catheter	7-14 days	Resuscitation; acute dialysis; stem cell harvest
Nontunneled PICC	1-12 weeks	Antibiotics; TPN
Tunneled catheter	>1 month	Chemotherapy; TPN; dialysis; plasmapheresis
Implantable port	>3 months	Chemotherapy; chronic transfusion; chronic blood tests

PICC, Peripherally inserted central catheter; TPN, total parenteral nutrition.

not to perforate the SVC below the azygos vein, because this portion is frequently intrapericardial and may result in hemopericardium with tamponade. Stent placement is almost always required in these patients. Surgical bypass of the SVC is reported to have 60%-70% patency rates at 1 year, but is rarely performed.

Acute SVC syndrome due to malignancy can be treated with external radiation and steroids. This treatment can rapidly shrink some mediastinal tumors. Nevertheless, interventional radiology has much to offer these patients, particularly when there is a large thrombus burden or an intrinsic lesion within the SVC. Thrombolysis/PMT restores patency and reveals the underlying lesion, but use of thrombolytic agents is not possible in patients with brain or pericardial metastases. Mechanical thrombectomy can partially restore flow without the use of thrombolytic agents, but stent placement is almost always necessary. Stents can be placed despite incomplete clearing of thrombus because the objective is to relieve the extrinsic compression, not maximize clearing of thrombus. Some operators treat this lesion primarily with stents without first treating the thrombus. Flexible, self-expanding stents are ideal for extensive reconstructions. After crossing the thrombosed SVC, the self-expanding stent can be deployed and then postdilated. This minimizes the risk of massive pulmonary embolization. The relief of symptoms can be so dramatic that the patient feels improved before the end of the case. The goal of this procedure is palliation rather than an angiographically elegant result.

CENTRAL VENOUS ACCESS

One of the most common vascular interventional procedures currently performed is placement of long-term central venous access devices. This simple procedure is also one of the most

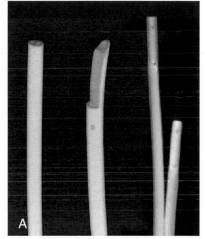
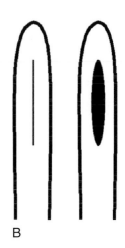

FIGURE 7-20. Catheter tips. **A,** From left to right, nontapered dual-lumen; staggered-tip dual-lumen; split catheter. **B,** Schematic of mechanism of action of a Groshong valve-tipped catheter. The end of the catheter is sealed, and flow is through a slit in the side near the tip. *Left:* Resting closed state. *Right:* With aspiration or injection the slit opens to allow flow.

important in terms of overall patient care and is most likely the manner in which much of the general patient population will be exposed to interventional radiology. A large variety of venous access devices are available (Fig. 7-19 and Table 7-1). Devices that are designed for high-pressure, high-volume injections used in CT and MRI are identified as CT-compatible. Drug-coated catheters that reduce the risk of infection, thrombosis, or both, are an exciting advance. There are several basic configurations of catheter tips, including open and valved (Fig. 7-20). Valves can also be incorporated into the hub of the catheter. Valved catheters are useful for patients with heparin allergies, because the flush solution can be sterile saline. However, current valves prevent high flow rates, so dialysis and plasmapheresis catheters are open-ended. Specific flush solutions for various devices vary greatly by hospital, with higher concentrations usually required for dialysis catheters.

Image-guided placement of long-term venous access devices is safe, cost-effective, and efficacious. Selection of an appropriate device requires familiarity with the access device, an understanding of the patient's access needs, and knowledge of the patient's venous anatomy. Many patients have specific requests regarding location of devices that should be taken into consideration.

TABLE 7-2 Suggested Coagulation Parameters for Central Venous Access Procedures

	INR (seconds)	aPTT (seconds)	Platelets/mL
Nontunneled	<2	<50	≥15,000
Tunneled	≤1.5*	<50	≥30,000
Port	Normal	Normal	≥30,000†

*Infusion of fresh frozen plasma during the procedure should be considered when these levels are exceeded.
†Infusion of platelets during the procedure is recommended.
Note: Patients in renal failure or on platelet-inhibiting medications may still bleed despite normal or near normal platelet counts.
aPTT, Activated partial thromboplastin time; INR, international normalized ratio.

TABLE 7-3 Preferred Veins (in Order) for Long-Term Central Access

Device	Vein
PICC line*	Basilic, cephalic,† brachial‡ veins
Dialysis	RIJ, REJ, LIJ, LEJ; avoid LSCV, RSCV
Nondialysis tunneled	RIJ, LIJ, RSCV, LSCV
Implantable ports	RIJ, LIJ, RSCV, LSCV

*Should not be placed in arm in patients with renal failure. Use neck veins.
†More subject to spasm; angle in shoulder can be difficult to negotiate.
‡Close to brachial artery and to radial and median nerves.
LEJ, Left external jugular vein; LIJ, left internal jugular vein; LSCV, left subclavian vein; REJ, right external jugular vein; RIJ, right internal jugular vein; RSCV, right subclavian vein.

Basic Principles of Device Implantation

There are a few guidelines to follow during device insertion that are applicable to all venous access devices. Suggested coagulation parameters are listed in Table 7-2. The right IJV is the preferred access because it is large, close to the skin, and provides a short, straight route to the SVC. This vein should be used whenever possible for dialysis catheters or in renal failure patients to avoid compromise of subclavian veins and the left brachiocephalic vein, which are important for the success of upper arm surgical dialysis access (grafts and fistulas) (Table 7-3). Techniques for puncture of internal jugular, subclavian, and upper extremity veins are described in Chapter 2. The one potential procedural complication that can result in immediate death is massive air embolism through large peel-away sheaths during catheter insertion. Specific measures to avoid and manage this complication are described in Chapter 2 (Venous Access, Internal Jugular Vein, and Box 2-11). In addition, tunneled catheters should be flushed, clamped, and capped before insertion into the patient to prevent inadvertent aspiration of air through an open catheter.

The tip of a long-term central venous access device should lie in the high right atrium (Fig. 7-21). Catheter tips that end in the SVC or brachiocephalic vein have a higher incidence of catheter malfunction due to formation of fibrin sheaths, as well as catheter-related central venous stenosis and thrombosis (Fig. 7-22). The etiology of stenotic complications are not known with certainty, but are probably related to trauma to the endothelium by the catheter tip and the injected medications. Catheter tips in the high right atrium are rarely in contact with endothelium. During positioning of the catheter in a supine patient, it is important to note that chest wall tissues may drop and the mediastinum lengthen when the patient stands or sits upright. Catheters withdraw a few centimeters when this

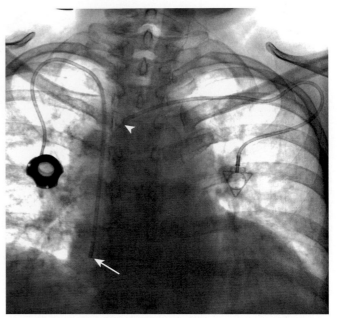

FIGURE 7-21. Chest radiograph after insertion of a new single-lumen right chest port through the right internal jugular vein to replace a malfunctioning left chest port (inserted through the left subclavian vein). The catheter tip of the new port is in the high right atrium *(arrow)*. The left port was placed without imaging guidance; the tip ends in the brachiocephalic vein *(arrowhead)*. This port was removed.

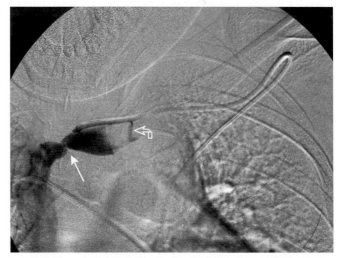

FIGURE 7-22. Consequences of catheter malpositioning. The tip of this chest port has withdrawn into the left brachiocephalic vein. A stenosis *(straight arrow)* has developed central to the catheter tip. A fibrin sheath has formed around the catheter tip, so that blood could not be aspirated. Contrast injected through the catheter tracks underneath the fibrin sheath, entering the vessel lumen through gaps in the fibrin *(curved arrow)*.

happens (Fig. 7-23). To compensate for this natural pull-back, the catheter tip should be placed a few centimeters deeper into the atrium than the intended final location, especially in patients with loose chest wall tissues. Most conventional catheters can be trimmed to length by the operator after determining the amount of catheter needed to reach a desired central location. Special use catheters, such as for dialysis, have staggered tip configurations that should not be altered.

When placing tunneled catheters or ports, infected or irradiated skin should be avoided. An appropriate thickness of skin

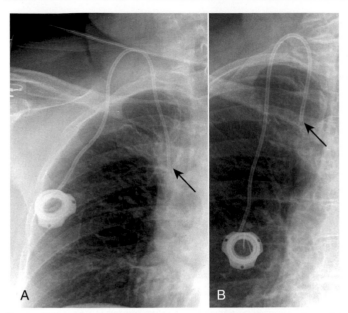

FIGURE 7-23. Positional change in catheter tip location in patient with abundant, loose chest wall tissues. A, Chest radiograph with patient in semiupright position immediately after port placement (without imaging guidance). This catheter, placed without imaging guidance, is just barely in the superior vena cava. B, Same patient in upright position several weeks later. The port is located lower on the chest wall, and the catheter tip has withdrawn to a less central position *(arrow)*.

Box 7-7. Peripherally Inserted Central Catheter Line Placement

Surgical arm prep
Basilic or cephalic vein preferred
Ultrasound or arm venogram to confirm venous anatomy/ patency
Access vein with micropuncture needle
Advance wire to superior vena cava
Determine appropriate intravascular length of catheter; tip should be in high right atrium
Insert peel-away sheath
Advance catheter through sheath
Secure to skin

Box 7-8. Placement of Tunneled Catheters

Confirm patency of access vein
Surgical prep skin
±Prophylactic antibiotics
Surgical scrub operator hands
Image-guided access; micropuncture needle
Determine appropriate intravascular length with guidewire; tip should be in high right atrium
Tunnel catheter to puncture site; tunnel on chest wall should have gentle curve to access site
Insert catheter through peel-away sheath: Valsalva, Trendelenburg position to prevent air embolism during catheter insertion
Close venous access site
Secure catheter to skin

Box 7-9. Port Placement

Confirm patency of access site
Surgical prep skin
Prophylactic antibiotics
Surgical scrub operator hands
Image-guided access; micropuncture needle
Insert catheter through peel-away sheath: Valsalva, Trendelenburg position to prevent air embolism
Position catheter tip in high right atrium
Create pocket
Tunnel catheter retrograde into pocket
Trim catheter, assemble port, flush
Place port in pocket, secure with 3-0 absorbable sutures
Close skin in layers: 3-0 absorbable suture deep layer; 4-0 or 5-0 absorbable suture subcuticular skin
Close venous access site
Access port, confirm correct function, flush

Box 7-10. Alternative Access Routes for Long-Term Central Venous Access

Recanalization of occluded central vein
Translumbar inferior vena cava (IVC)
Collateral vein
Femoral vein
Direct brachiocephalic vein
Transhepatic IVC

---

and subcutaneous tissue over the device is 5-10 mm. Otherwise, erosion may occur, particularly in oncology patients who may lose substantial amounts of weight during their illness. Conversely, ports should not be placed too deeply, as they become difficult to access. In women, it is always wise to avoid placing the port in breast tissue as access is uncomfortable and inconvenient, and scarring will be created that could confuse the mammographer.

The use of prophylactic antibiotics during device insertion varies from one institution to another. One dose of an antibiotic that provides coverage for *Staphylococcus aureus*, such as cefazolin or vancomycin, can be given immediately before the procedure. Catheters coated with bacteriocidal or bacteriostatic drugs can reduce the incidence of late infections, as does meticulous catheter care. Tunneled or implanted devices should not be placed into patients with sepsis or who have been febrile within the previous 48 hours.

Each type of device has certain unique aspects of the insertion procedure (Boxes 7-7 to 7-9). Generally, it is best not to tunnel or create pockets until venous access has been obtained. Tunneling tools are used to pull catheters through subcutaneous tunnels

without damaging the catheter tips. The majority of implantation procedures can be performed with local anesthetic and light conscious sedation.

Patients with occlusion of conventional access sites represent particular challenges. Image-guided placement of central venous access devices may be life-saving in these patients (Box 7-10). The first consideration is whether recanalization of an already occluded vein is possible (Fig. 7-24). This preserves future alternative access sites, without risking a new occlusion. Standard recanalization techniques can be used to allow positioning of a catheter to a central location. Stent placement is not necessary unless the occlusion was symptomatic. When recanalization is not possible, consider alternative access techniques, including translumbar to the IVC, transhepatic to the IVC, common femoral vein, direct suprasternal puncture of a brachiocephalic vein, and through collaterals (Fig. 7-25). These puncture techniques

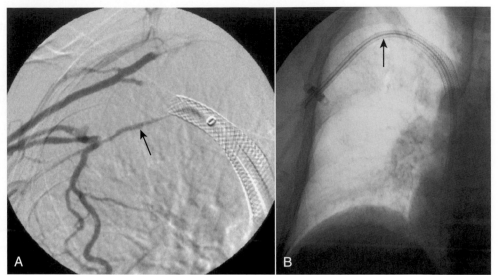

Figure 7-24. Recanalization of the right subclavian vein in a chronic dialysis patient with occlusion of both internal jugular veins and the left brachiocephalic vein. **A,** Digital subtraction venogram showing a severely stenotic right subclavian vein *(arrow)* and stent. The vein was dilated with a 6-mm angioplasty balloon from a femoral vein access, and then punctured lateral to the stent with a micropuncture needle. **B,** Final radiograph showing a 16-French dialysis catheter *(arrow)* inserted through the subclavian vein and stent.

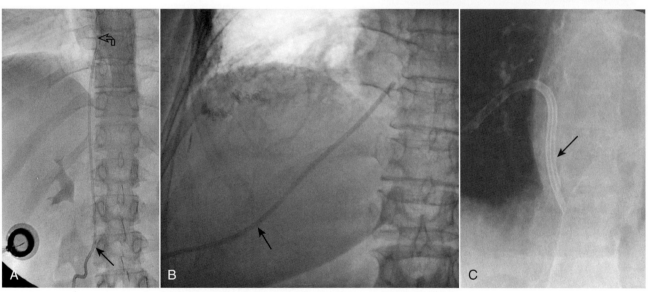

Figure 7-25. Alternative access sites for long-term central venous catheter placement. **A,** Translumbar placement of a port through the inferior vena cava (IVC) in a patient with superior vena cava (SVC) occlusion. The catheter enters the IVC at the level of the L3 vertebral body *(straight arrow)*. The tip is in the right atrium *(curved arrow)*. **B,** Transhepatic placement of a tunneled catheter *(arrow)* through the middle hepatic vein. The patient had occlusion of the infrarenal IVC as well as the SVC. **C,** Direct right atrial catheter *(arrow)* inserted surgically in a patient with thrombosis of all central veins.

are described in Chapter 2. The greatest experience has been accumulated with translumbar IVC catheters, with a less than 5% rate of caval thrombosis. Although once discouraged, femoral venous access is becoming more accepted. In all cases, the tip of the catheter should be positioned in the right atrium to maximize the functional life of the device. In extreme cases, direct surgical placement into the right atrium is possible.

Complications of Venous Access Devices

Procedural complications of central venous catheter placement are related primarily to the venous access, such as injury to adjacent structures (lung or artery), and air embolism (Table 7-4). Meticulous technique, ultrasound image-guided venous puncture (with visualization of the needle tip at all times), image-guided catheter insertion, and use of valved peel-away sheaths minimize some of these complications.

Excessive oozing around a tunneled catheter, especially in dialysis patients, can be managed first with application of gentle

pressure. Prothrombotic pads or powders (e.g., thrombin) can be applied as well. When oozing seems to be coming from the skin edges, injection of 1%-2% lidocaine with epinephrine around the entry site induces vasoconstriction and permits hemostasis. When patients continue to bleed excessively, a coagulation profile should be obtained.

Catheter malfunction, venous thrombosis, and infection are the most common late complications. Careful device selection, placement, and education of the patient and staff using the device can minimize late complications.

Catheter malfunction, defined as suboptimal infusion or aspiration of blood, is the most common problem encountered after catheter placement. This is usually due to fibrin deposition in or around the tip of the catheter, but may also be caused by venous thrombosis, catheter malpositioning, catheter kinking, or catheter fracture (Fig. 7-26). Any patient that complains of pain during injection through a catheter should be evaluated promptly with physical examination of the access looking for evidence of extravasation or infection, chest radiograph to assess for device position and integrity,

TABLE **7-4** Complications of Central Venous Catheters

Complication	Incidence
Insertion procedure	
Pneumothorax	<2%
Air embolism	<2%
Arterial puncture	1%
Failure to insert catheter	<1%
Catheter malposition	<1%
Indwelling catheter	
Catheter malfunction	10%-20%*
Symptomatic venous thrombosis	5%-15%†
Infection	5%-10%
Catheter fracture	<1%

*Most catheter malfunctions are transitory.
†Varies by access site, catheter size, and patient factors. Highest for large subclavian catheters in patients with cancer.
Data from Lewis CA, Allen TE, Burke DR, et al. Quality improvement guidelines for central venous access. The Standards of Practice Committee of the Society of Cardiovascular & Interventional Radiology. *J Vasc Interv Radiol.* 1997;8:475–479.

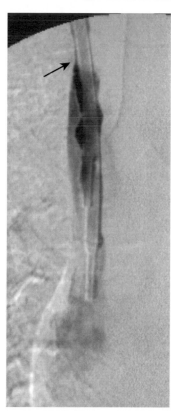

FIGURE 7-26. Typical appearance of fibrin sheath on a split-tip dialysis catheter. Injection through the proximal lumen shows contrast collecting around the catheter and tracking retrograde *(arrow)* before it enters the vessel lumen.

and injection of contrast through the catheter to assess for device integrity and patency. In most patients, a fibrin sheath obstructing the catheter tip is responsible for inability to aspirate. A simple algorithm involving administration of thrombolytic agents, catheter replacement with sheath disruption, or percutaneous mechanical stripping of the fibrin from the catheter maintains most access (Fig. 7-27 and Box 7-11). Poorly functioning tunneled catheters that have no outward signs of infection can usually be replaced over a

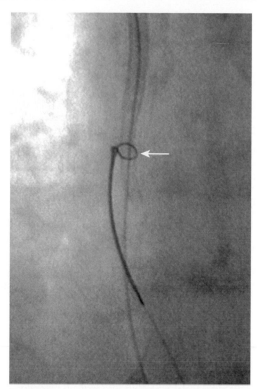

FIGURE 7-27. A snare can be used to pull a fibrin sheath off a catheter. A guidewire through the catheter was used to guide the snare (inserted from a femoral access) over the catheter. The snare was tightened to the point where it would slide down the catheter with moderate force, stripping off the fibrin. In this image, the snare *(arrow)* is almost at the tip of the catheter.

Box 7-11. Management of the Malfunctioning Catheter

Check catheter position on chest radiograph
Fill catheter with small dose thrombolytic agent (e.g., tPA 1-2 mg, urokinase 5000 U)
Check catheter function after 30-60 minutes
If no change, repeat dose of thrombolytic agent
Check catheter function after 30-60 minutes
If no change, obtain contrast study of catheter:
- For extensive fibrin sheath, infuse thrombolytic agent for 4-8 hours (e.g., tPA 1 mg/hr, urokinase 50,000 U/hr). Should this fail, consider stripping with snare, or catheter exchange over a guidewire. Angioplasty balloon may be used to disrupt sheath
- For central venous thrombosis, infuse thrombolytic agent through catheter for 8-12 hours
- For catheter malpositioning, reposition catheter tip or replace. Tip must be in high right atrium at end of procedure

tPA, Tissue plasminogen activator.

guidewire through the original tunnel. When the cause of catheter malfunction is central venous thrombosis, thrombolysis through the catheter followed by anticoagulation may restore function.

There are no proven preventative measures for catheter malfunction, but new strategies such as low-molecular-weight heparin, weekly catheter flushes with a thrombolytic agent, or drug-coated catheters may reduce this problem.

Catheters that have migrated into unsatisfactory locations can be repositioned with percutaneous techniques, but frequently return to the poor position (Fig. 7-28 and Box 7-12). If catheter

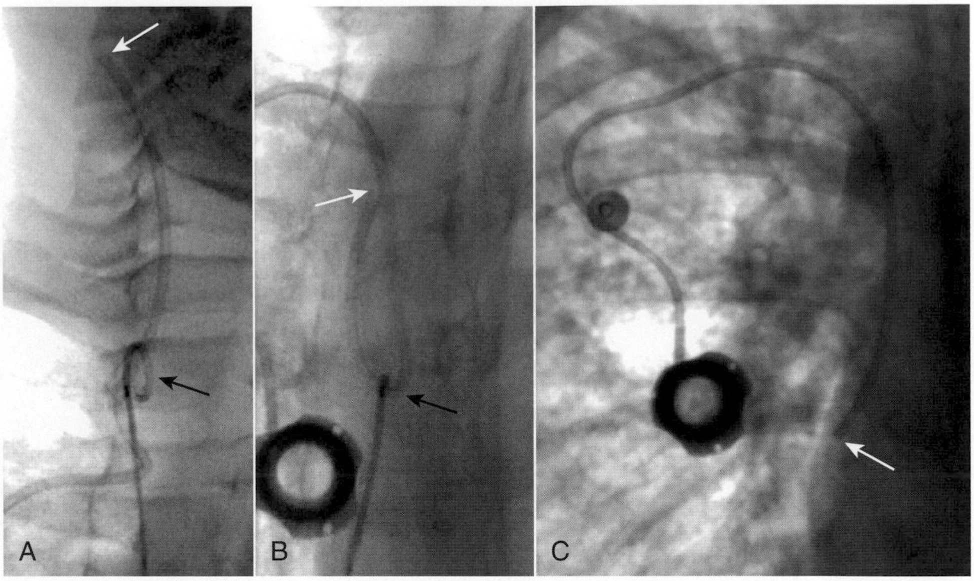

FIGURE 7-28. Catheter repositioning. **A,** Digital image showing single-lumen chest port catheter that has flipped into the right internal jugular vein *(white arrow)*. A pigtail catheter placed from a femoral approach has engaged the port catheter *(black arrow)*. A deflecting wire is used inside the pigtail catheter to provide rigidity. **B,** As the pigtail catheter is withdrawn *(black arrow)*, the port catheter *(white arrow)* is pulled back into the superior vena cava. **C,** The port catheter tip *(white arrow)* is in proper central position.

Box 7-12. Techniques for Repositioning Catheters

All catheters
- Snare end of catheter, pull into central location
- Engage catheter body with recurved or pigtail catheter, pull into central location
- Use deflecting wire in working catheter to increase rigidity
- Form snare loop around body of catheter, pull into central location (see Fig. 4-53)

Additional option for externalized catheters
- Advance guidewire through catheter, withdraw catheter until wire can be used to select central location, re-advance catheter over guidewire
- Strict aseptic technique must be maintained

---

migration occurs again, revision or replacement of the catheter is usually necessary.

Thrombosis of the access vein may be asymptomatic, but can cause pain at the insertion site and limb swelling if an arm vein has been used. Catheter-related central venous thrombosis can rarely be a source of symptomatic pulmonary emboli. In most cases the catheter is still fully functional unless the thrombus extends centrally to the catheter tip. Whenever possible, the catheter should be left in place while the thrombosis is treated with anticoagulation, unless the patient no longer requires venous access.

Catheter fracture is extremely rare owing to the durability of silicone and polyurethane. When fracture occurs it is frequently due to unusual stress upon the catheter. "Pinch-off" syndrome, in which a catheter is compressed between bony or ligamentous structures, predisposes to catheter fracture (Fig. 7-29). This occurs most often with blind subclavian vein puncture when the catheter enters the vein under the clavicle from an inferior approach. The extravascular portion of the catheter is subject to compression and shearing between the first rib and the clavicle.

Infection of a venous access device is a vexing issue as it complicates patient management and can cause life-threatening sepsis. Drug-coated catheters have great promise to reduce this complication, but fastidious aseptic technique during placement and subsequent use will always be necessary. Infections may manifest as unexplained fever, rigors with injection, positive blood cultures, purulence at the tunnel or port pocket, and sepsis. When patients with catheters have a fever, the catheter is often presumed to be the culprit without proof. This can lead to repeated catheter removals and insertions. Culturing the catheter tip may provide an answer, but usually the patient is already on antibiotics. Removal is rarely an emergency procedure unless the patient is neutropenic or septic. Whenever feasible, the patient should be afebrile for 48 hours with negative blood cultures after removal of an infected device before reinsertion of new access.

Device Removal

Removal of venous access devices is part of the responsibility of insertion. Catheters containing concentrated heparin, such as dialysis catheters, should be aspirated before manipulation to avoid inadvertent injection of a large bolus of anticoagulant. Patients with central venous catheters should be placed flat in the supine position for the removal procedure. Nontunneled catheters can be removed by compressing over the skin entry site and gently pulling the catheter. Tunneled catheters that have been in place for less than 2 weeks can often be removed in a similar fashion. The cuffs of tunneled catheters that have been in place for more than 2 weeks have usually become incorporated into the soft tissues unless the tunnel is infected. The cuff should be identified and the area around it infiltrated with local anesthetic. When the cuff is close to the skin exit site, a blunt instrument can be used to free the cuff. Occasionally a small incision directly over the cuff is necessary. Overaggressive traction can cause catheter fracture in the tunnel. If this happens, pressure should be applied over the tunnel immediately to prevent air embolism or excessive blood loss. Using local anesthetic, a small incision should be made over the cuff and the catheter freed. After catheter removal, pressure should be held over the exit site for 5 minutes. The skin exit site can be closed with a Steri-Strip or simply covered with a small sterile dressing. The device should be inspected to ensure that it has been removed in one piece.

To remove a noninfected port, the area around the device (including the pocket) is extensively infiltrated with local anesthetic. Try to use the scar from the insertion for the new incision. Dissect down to the catheter and place a clamp on it. At this point, it is wise to pull the catheter out of the venous system before trying to free the port. Then, dissect back to the device using the catheter stem as a guide. Once the pocket has been entered, fibrotic bands that have formed through suture holes on the port are broken, freeing the device. The pocket should be closed in layers unless infection is suspected. Infected pockets should be packed with sterile gauze with daily changes, allowing healing by secondary intention.

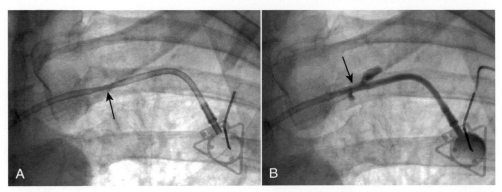

FIGURE 7-29. "Pinch-off" syndrome. **A,** Compression *(arrow)* of an 8-French catheter between the clavicle and the first rib. This port was placed using surface landmarks for venous access. Note that the port, suitable for power injection, has the letters "CT" faintly visible straddling the catheter stem. **B,** Digital spot film obtained during a catheter check. The patient had pain under the clavicle with injection in the port. Extravasation of contrast *(arrow)* from a fracture in the catheter is visible. Ultimately this will lead to catheter transection with central embolization of the distal fragment. The catheter was removed and a new port was placed through the right internal jugular vein.

■ PERMANENT DIALYSIS ACCESS

Approximately 230,000 patients are on permanent hemodialysis in the United States. Goals for optimized care of these patients have been formulated by the National Kidney Foundation (NKF) and disseminated as the Dialysis Outcomes Quality Initiative (DOQI) guidelines. This is a living public document that can be accessed electronically through the NKF website. A major goal of the document is improvement of the outcomes of dialysis access.

Venous catheters do not provide reliable long-term access owing to infection and malfunction rates. Permanent access for dialysis is usually accomplished by surgical creation of an arteriovenous fistula (AVF) or interposition of a short bridge of synthetic vascular graft material between an artery and vein in a superficial location (Box 7-13 and Fig. 7-30). Whenever possible, a fistula is preferred over a graft. The anastomoses are usually end-to-side for both fistulas and bridge grafts to preserve the continuity of the native vessels. Grafts are typically polytetrafluoroethylene or Dacron material, 6-8 mm in diameter and 6-12 cm in length in the forearm.

The most common immediate complications after creation of surgical dialysis access are thrombosis or inadequate flow rates. The causes include technical error, preexisting venous outflow obstruction, and unrecognized arterial inflow disease. Surgical thrombectomy and revision is the appropriate treatment for an access that fails shortly after creation, although venography may be useful to delineate venous anatomy.

Fistulas have a superior longevity in comparison to bridge grafts (85% vs. 50% patency at 2 years), but require several months for the veins to enlarge sufficiently ("mature") to accommodate the large needles and flow rates used during dialysis. As many as 30% of fistulas fail to mature or thrombose acutely. Ultrasound, conventional venography, and MR venography can be useful to evaluate the upper extremity veins before creation of the fistula.

The normal fistula should have a continuous thrill at the anastomosis; a thrill only during systole indicates a stenosis, as does a localized thrill elsewhere in the venous outflow. However, a low-pitched bruit in the outflow vein is normal. A very pulsatile fistula indicates a more central stenosis; the normal fistula is usually not pulsatile, or only slightly. A stenosis can sometimes be localized by a palpable step-off in a pulsatile arm vein.

Once established, fistulas can maintain patency with flow rates as low as 80 mL/min. Late failures occur most often due to venous outflow stenosis or, less often, anastomotic stenoses. Stenosis at the arterial-venous anastomosis occurs in fewer than 4% of patients. Venous stenoses occur most commonly located in the juxtaanastomotic and runoff vein, although up to one third may have a central venous stenosis. Once a stenosis has occurred,

---

Box 7-13. Surgical Dialysis Access

ARTERIOVENOUS FISTULA
Radial artery to cephalic vein at wrist
Brachial artery to antecubital, cephalic, or transposed basilic vein in forearm or upper arm

BRIDGE GRAFTS
Forearm
- Radial artery to antecubital, basilic, or brachial vein straight/curved
- Brachial artery to antecubital, basilic, or brachial vein loop

Upper arm
- Brachial artery to brachial or axillary vein straight/curved
- Axillary artery to axillary vein loop

Leg
- Femoral artery to saphenous or femoral vein loop

Chest
- Axillary artery to contralateral axillary vein (necklace)

---

recurrence is common, and up to 70% may require additional intervention within 6 months.

Bridge grafts can be accessed sooner after creation than fistulas, and may be advantageous in certain patients (e.g., those with limited usable veins or obesity) but have higher failure rates due to development of stenoses at the venous anastomosis and in the outflow veins. When a graft fails, arterial anastomotic stenoses are found in 1%-2%, venous anastomotic stenoses in 60%, and outflow or central venous stenoses in 28%. Up to one fifth of acute graft failures can be due to infection. Bridge grafts require higher flow rates than AVFs (450 mL/min or more) to maintain patency. Repeated punctures can lead to pseudoaneurysm formation in the grafts.

The normal dialysis graft should have a thrill at the arterial anastomosis and be only slightly pulsatile. A bruit should be audible throughout the graft. The bruit becomes high-pitched in the presence of a stenosis.

Both fistulas and bridge grafts are accessed for dialysis by inserting one large-bore needle in the vein or graft close to the arterial anastomosis and another in a more central location in the same vein or graft. Blood is withdrawn from the first (termed *arterial*) needle and returned through the second (termed *venous*) needle. Assuming that the needles are in good position, inability to aspirate blood at a satisfactory flow rate may indicate an inflow problem such as stenosis at the arterial anastomosis or, less

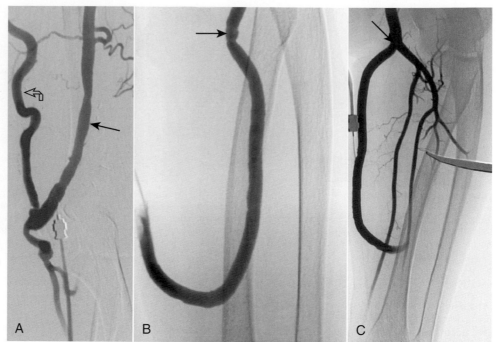

FIGURE 7-30. Permanent surgical dialysis access. **A,** Arm fistula: brachial artery to cephalic vein. The venous outflow was compressed with a clamp during contrast injection, allowing visualization of the vein *(straight arrow)* and inflow artery *(curved arrow)*. **B,** Forearm bridge graft. Injection of contrast without occlusion of venous outflow shows the venous anastomosis *(arrow)*. **C,** Contrast injection in the same graft with compression of the outflow with a clamp shows the arterial anastomosis *(arrow)* and a portion of the arterial inflow.

TABLE 7-5 Surgical Dialysis Access Parameters

Parameter	Value
Maximum flow rate bridge graft	800 mL/min
Maximum flow rate forearm fistula	300 mL/min
Maximum flow rate upper arm fistula	1000 mL/min
Indicators of venous outflow stenosis (grafts):	
Intraaccess flow measurements	<600 mL/min or decreased by 25%
Venous pressure* at flow rate of 200 mL/min	>125 mm Hg
Ratio of venous to systemic arterial pressure†	>0.4
Decrease in (K × t)/V‡	>0.2

*Pressure measured in dialysis needle returning blood to patient during dialysis.
†Baseline venous pressure in dialysis access compared to ipsilateral upper arm cuff pressure.
‡K = clearance of urea, t = dialysis time, and V = estimated patient body water. This measure has no units. Target Kt/V = 1.2 or greater for patients undergoing dialysis three times per week.

often, a stenosis in the native artery proximal to the access. Low pressures in both the arterial and venous needles have the same implication. When excessive pressure is required to return blood through the venous needle or when clearance of metabolites is very slow, a venous outflow lesion may be present (Table 7-5).

Distinguishing between the arterial and venous anastomoses in a loop graft can sometimes be difficult on physical exam when the thrill is absent and the anastomoses are in close proximity. Interrogation with ultrasound or compression over the midpoint of the graft reveals direction of flow, with the arterial anastomosis located on the side that remains pulsatile.

A swollen arm and dilated chest wall veins suggests a central venous stenosis. Graft infection or arm cellulitis should be considered when the arm is hot and erythematous and the patient febrile. Infection is more common with grafts than fistulas. Other complications include pseudoaneurysm formation and steal syndrome (see Chapter 6, Acute Ischemia) (Fig. 7-31).

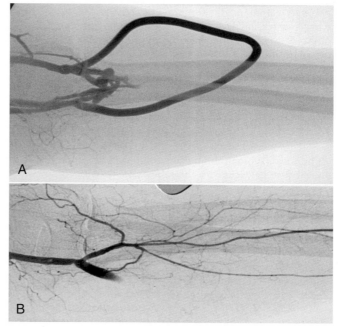

FIGURE 7-31. Patient with hand ischemia developing several months after placement of a bridge graft. Symptoms are worse during dialysis. **A,** Angiogram showing a patent bridge graft, but no visible distal runoff. **B,** Angiogram with compression of the venous outflow shows opacification of forearm arteries.

Imaging of a patent dialysis access is indicated when flow rates are unsatisfactory, physical examination suggests decreased flow (e.g., loss of a palpable thrill), or the patient develops upper extremity swelling or hand ischemia (Table 7-6). Duplex color-flow ultrasound can be used to evaluate the access and upper extremity veins for stenosis, but it is limited in ability to visualize the central veins. Imaging with CTA/CTV or MRA/MRV (especially noncontrast techniques) is used in some centers, because these visualize both the arterial and venous structures.

TABLE 7-6 Venography of Surgical Dialysis Access

Indication	Technique	Imaging Goals
Access planning	Venogram from dorsum of hand	Document patency of upper extremity veins from forearm to right atrium
Malfunctioning but patent dialysis access	Venogram from access; include view of arterial anastomosis	Localize and correct stenotic lesions in inflow and outflow from arterial anastomosis to right atrium
Thrombosed dialysis access	5-French catheter from access into patent outflow veins; injection in access after declotting	Before declotting, document absence of thrombus in outflow veins; following declotting, identify and correct stenotic lesions in access or at anastomoses
Upper extremity swelling with patent dialysis access	Venogram from access	Localize and correct obstruction of outflow from upper extremity veins to right atrium
Upper extremity ischemia with patent dialysis access	5-French catheter retrograde from access to aortic arch, or from femoral arterial access	Aortic arch injection to show subclavian artery origin, selective injection upper extremity arteries, and injection with obstruction of venous outflow to visualize arteries distal to access

Conventional venography allows both diagnosis and intervention during the same procedure (see Fig. 7-30). Either an 18-gauge intravenous catheter or a 4- or 5-French microaccess set can be used for access. The skin should be prepped and draped for sterile access, and the arm abducted and supported on an arm board. To visualize the arm, either the angiographic table or the C-arm may have to be swiveled out of normal position. As an alternative, the patient can lie across a stretcher with head, upper back and arm on the angiographic table. The access is often directly into the dialysis fistula or graft, oriented toward the venous anastomosis (or outflow in the case of a fistula) unless an arterial inflow lesion is suspected. For fistulas, some interventionalists advocate obtaining access in the brachial artery proximal to the fistula because venous spasm at the puncture site can sometimes occur and is difficult to distinguish from stenosis. Non-ionic contrast is injected by hand (using extension tubing so that the radiologist can stand behind a lead shield) and filmed with digital subtraction angiography technique. Images from the arterial anastomosis to the right atrium should be obtained with careful overlap of each field of view. The arterial anastomosis is visualized by injection with obstruction of the venous outflow by external compression (a clamp or blood pressure cuff) or an angioplasty balloon in the outflow, which allows contrast to reflux into the artery. The hand or arm should be rotated to improve visualization of the anastomosis. Patients do not need immediate dialysis following venography unless volume status is tenuous.

Angioplasty and Stents

The diagnostic examination can be converted to an intervention by exchanging the 18-gauge catheter or microaccess dilator for a 5- or 6-French sheath over a 0.035-inch guidewire. When the lesion is located in a direction opposite to that of the initial access, a second puncture in an appropriate direction is made. The patient should be anticoagulated with 3000–5000 U heparin. Stenosis of the venous anastomosis of a loop graft is dilated with a 6- to 8-mm diameter high-pressure balloon, depending on the known diameter of the graft (Fig. 7-32). Lesions in outflow veins can be dilated with appropriate diameter high-pressure balloons. Multiple, slow, and prolonged (5 minutes or more) inflations may be required to prevent elastic recoil. Often a very thin but stubborn waist in the balloon is visualized (see Fig. 4-12). Patients may experience considerable pain during angioplasty of venous lesions. Pain that persists after balloon deflation may signify rupture of the vein. Inflow lesions in the forearm arteries can be angioplastied with 0.035- or 0.018-inch based systems as appropriate.

Lesions that do not respond to angioplasty can be treated with a cutting or scoring balloons, metallic stents, short stent-grafts, or surgical revision (when accessible). Cutting balloons are used

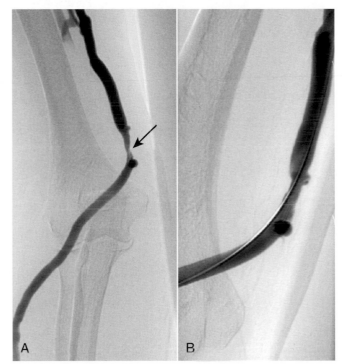

FIGURE 7-32. Angioplasty of a venous anastomotic stenosis. **A,** Digital angiogram showing stenosis *(arrow)* at the anastomosis with the basilic vein. **B,** Postangioplasty venogram showing improved caliber of the lumen. The thrill returned in the graft, and the patient resumed successful dialysis.

for lesions that resist angioplasty, and stents and stent-grafts are used for lesions that recoil. Angioplasty should always be tried first, with stents reserved for inadequate acute results or recurrent lesions in the outflow veins (Fig. 7-33). Stenting under the clavicle should be avoided because stent fractures will occur. Dedicated stent-grafts improve patency of venous anastomotic stenoses in dialysis loop grafts and may have some advantage in central veins as well (Fig 7-34). Arterial inflow lesions that cannot be dilated are usually managed with surgical revision. The endpoints of these procedures are return to successful dialysis, restoration of a palpable thrill, improved intragraft flow rates, or a venous to brachial artery pressure ratio less than 0.4.

Removal of the sheaths can be safely performed while the patient is still anticoagulated. Gentle compression or a cerclage suture can be used to obtain hemostasis (Fig. 7-35). The suture should be removed before the patient is discharged home.

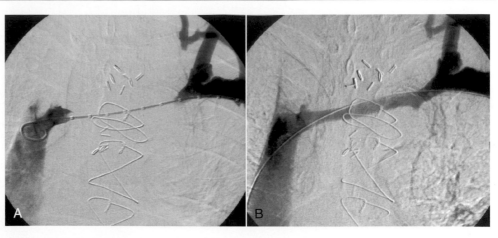

FIGURE 7-33. Patient with a left forearm dialysis fistula and high venous pressures at dialysis. The fistula and veins in the arm were normal, but the brachiocephalic vein was occluded. **A,** Image showing a measuring catheter across the brachiocephalic vein to determine the length of the occlusion. This aids in selection of a stent. **B,** Digital subtraction venogram after placement of a self-expanding stent due to unsatisfactory result with angioplasty alone.

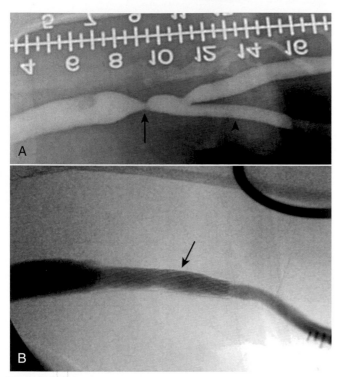

FIGURE 7-34. Endograft placement in a venous anastomotic stenosis of a dialysis loop graft. **A,** Pretreatment image with stenosis at venous anastomosis *(arrow)* of loop graft *(arrowhead).* **B,** Image from 6-month follow-up study showing a widely patent endograft *(arrow,* Flair endograft, Bard Peripheral Vascular, Tempe, Ariz.). (Courtesy Ziv Haskal, MD, Baltimore, MD.)

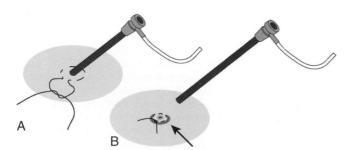

FIGURE 7-35. Cerclage or "purse-string" suture for removal of sheaths following dialysis intervention. **A,** A monofilament nylon suture has been placed in the skin around the sheath and a half-hitch thrown. **B,** As the sheath is removed the purse-string is tightened *(arrow)* to obtain hemostasis.

TABLE 7-7 Outcomes of Central Venous Angioplasty/Stents in Dialysis Access

Outcome	Percent
Technical success angioplasty	90
Technical success stents	95
Primary patency venous angioplasty at 6 months	65
Primary patency venous angioplasty at 12 months	30
Primary patency bare stents at 12 months	30

Satisfactory dialysis can be achieved after intervention for stenotic (not thrombosed) access in 90%-95% of patients. Stenoses at the bridge-graft venous anastomoses recur within 6 months after angioplasty in at least 50% of patients, but this is reduced to 23% after placement of a dedicated stent-graft. The results of angioplasty and stents in venous outflow veins approach 60% primary patency at 6 months, but there is no demonstrable advantage to bare metal stents over successful angioplasty (Table 7-7).

The acute complications of angioplasty and stent placement in dialysis access include thrombosis, dissection, and rupture (Fig. 7-36). Acute thrombosis responds well to pharmacologic or mechanical thrombectomy (see next section). Dissection of a vessel can sometimes be managed by prolonged balloon inflation to tack down the flap (with aggressive anticoagulation to prevent thrombosis of the entire access). When this fails, stent placement is usually curative. Rupture of a vessel in the arm can sometimes be treated successfully with 10-15 minutes of manual compression or prolonged balloon inflation across the site of rupture. The vein remains patent while extravasation ceases. When this technique fails, placement of a bare metal stent across the defect in the vessel wall can stop extravasation, possibly by eliminating any outflow obstruction. Stent-grafts can also be used, particularly for central ruptures.

Management of the Thrombosed Dialysis Access

Acute thrombosis of a mature dialysis access requires urgent, but not emergent intervention. Patients in need of immediate dialysis can be managed with placement of a short-term nontunneled dialysis catheter. The two basic approaches for declotting a dialysis access are (1) surgical cutdown with extraction of the thrombus with a small balloon catheter and (2) percutaneous methods. The superiority of one technique over another has not been established, although surgical declotting is greatly enhanced when combined with venographic evaluation of the runoff and central veins. Percutaneous declotting can be accomplished

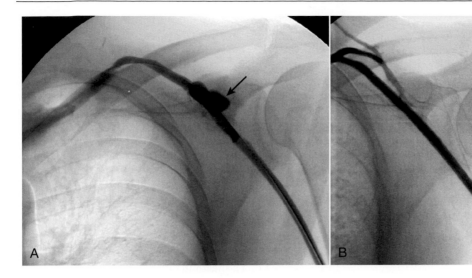

Figure 7-36. Vein rupture during angioplasty of stenotic venous outflow in a dialysis patient. **A**, Venogram after angioplasty shows vein rupture and a pseudoaneurysm *(arrow)*. Reversal of heparin, prolonged balloon inflations across the rupture, and manual compression failed, and an expanding hematoma developed. **B**, Venogram after placement of a stent-graft across the rupture site.

with pharmacologic thrombolysis, mechanical thrombolysis, or a combination of both techniques. In all cases, identification of an underlying lesion that predisposed to thrombosis is of paramount importance. Regardless of the technique used to restore patency, thrombosis is associated with a 50%-70% rate of irreversible failure of the access within 1 year.

The NKF DOQI guidelines have established overall target outcomes for graft declotting of 85% acute success (ability to use graft for dialysis), 40% primary patency at 6 months for percutaneous techniques, and 40% primary patency at 12 months for surgical thrombectomy.

General principles are common to all percutaneous declotting techniques (both pharmacologic and mechanical) (Box 7-14). First, bridge grafts are easier to declot than fistulas because the anatomy is straightforward and the thrombus is usually limited to the graft, between the arterial and venous anastomoses. The anatomy of dialysis fistulas is less predictable, and the presence of multiple side branches may complicate the declotting procedure. Second, grafts and fistulas almost always thrombose due to a stenotic lesion; the goal of the declotting procedure is to find and treat this lesion. Third, there is always a hard plug of white thrombus (platelets and fibrin) at the arterial anastomosis, whereas thrombus in the access and at the venous end is soft and red (full of red blood cells). Fourth, when puncturing a clotted dialysis access dark blood or no blood may be aspirated. A small, very low-pressure injection of contrast can be used to document correct position of the needle. A large or forceful injection should be avoided, as this may cause reflux of thrombus into the arterial circulation. Fifth, the venous system central to the dialysis access must be patent before embarking on a declotting procedure. This can be easily determined by advancing a short 5-French catheter centrally from the clotted access while injecting contrast until patent veins are found. Finally, declotting procedures should not be performed in patients with suspected graft infection, severely limited cardiac reserve (as small asymptomatic pulmonary emboli are common during the procedure), or known central right-to-left shunts (due to the risk of paradoxical embolism).

Pharmacologic Thrombolysis

There are many techniques described for pharmacologic thrombolysis of dialysis access, but the two most popular are "pulse-spray" and "lyse-and-wait" (see Box 4-13.) These two techniques are preferred because they are the quickest. The pulse-spray technique, originally described by Bookstein, is a pharmacomechanical process in which a specially designed 5-French multi-side-hole catheter is inserted into the thrombosed portion of the dialysis access through a 5- or 6-French

Box 7-14. Common Principles of Dialysis Declot Procedures

Do not perform procedure in patients with
- Known central right-to-left shunts
- Limited pulmonary reserve
- Severe pulmonary hypertension or right heart failure
- Dialysis access infection
- Emergent need for immediate dialysis

Determine type of access from history or records
Localize all anastomoses
Examine access for pulse, thrill, aneurysm, and evidence of infection
Use sterile technique
Anticoagulate patient with 3000-5000 U heparin during procedure
Use low-pressure injections in clotted access
Avoid CO_2 gas as contrast agent
Document patency of central veins before attempting to declot
Identify and correct stenotic lesions after declotting
Keep your hands out of the x-ray beam
Use careful radiation protection measures

sheath and small aliquots of a thrombolytic agent are forcefully injected using a 1-mL Luer-lock syringe (see Fig. 4-31). The jets of fluid exiting the side holes act to fragment the thrombus, while the thrombolytic agent induces fibrinolysis. Two catheters are used, inserted in a criss-cross orientation to treat the entire access (Fig. 7-37). The catheters cross at the midpoint of the access. Injection of small amounts of contrast during the process is used to assess progress. Once satisfactory lysis has been achieved (the definition of this varies, but generally indicates substantial reduction of the volume of thrombus), the venous anastomosis is angioplastied, usually with a balloon sized to the bridge graft. This relieves any potential outflow obstruction. The arterial anastomosis is cleared by pulling the plug into the access with a balloon. This is accomplished by advancing the deflated angioplasty or thrombectomy balloon through the arterial anastomosis over a guidewire, and then withdrawing the gently inflated balloon into the access. Any arterial inflow obstruction can then be angioplastied.

The "lyse-and-wait" technique, described by Cynamon, varies from the pulse-spray in that the thrombolytic agent is introduced into the thrombus approximately 15-30 minutes before the

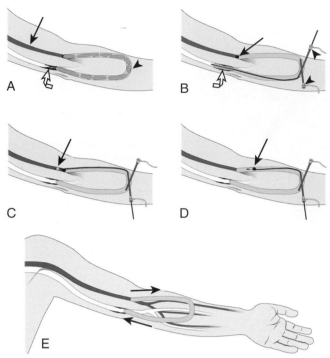

FIGURE 7-37. Basic elements of restoring flow in a thrombosed bridge graft. **A,** Thrombosis of a synthetic dialysis graft from the brachial artery to basilic vein. (*Arrow*, brachial artery; *curved arrow*, basilic vein with intimal hyperplasia at anastomosis; *arrowhead*, thrombosed graft). **B,** Sheaths have been placed (*arrowheads*) to allow access to both the arterial and venous anastomoses; a diagnostic venogram was performed through a 5-French catheter advanced beyond the venous anastomosis to confirm patent outflow veins, and the thrombus in the graft was then thrombolysed. At this point, an angioplasty balloon is used to dilate the region of the venous anastomosis (*curved arrow*), opening the outflow. Note the platelet plug (*straight arrow*) obstructing flow through the arterial anastomosis. **C,** A Fogarty-type balloon (*arrow*) is advanced past the platelet plug and gently inflated in the brachial artery. **D,** As the balloon is withdrawn into the graft, the plug (*arrow*) is pulled with it, restoring inflow. **E,** The graft is patent. Arrows show the direction of flow.

procedure is initiated (Box 7-15). The thrombolytic agent is mixed to a total volume of 7-10 mL. The graft or fistula is accessed with a small catheter as close to the arterial anastomosis as possible pointing toward the venous outflow. The arterial anastomosis and venous anastomosis of bridge grafts should be compressed while the thrombolytic agent is slowly injected. This prevents reflux of thrombus into the arterial supply as well as traps the lytic agent in the dialysis access. The catheter is then capped for 15-30 minutes (longer with urokinase, shorter with tPA, rPA, or other newer thrombolytic drugs). A small amount of contrast is then injected to determine the extent of thrombolysis. Typically, the thrombolysis within the bridge graft or fistula is complete with the exception of the arterial plug and venous anastomosis. The catheter is then exchanged over a guidewire for a 5- or 6-French sheath for intervention on the venous outflow. A second sheath is inserted in the direction of the arterial anastomosis for dislodgment of the arterial plug.

Pharmacologic thrombolysis techniques are successful in restoring patency of bridge grafts in more than 90% of patients. Intervention is almost universally required, usually for an outflow lesion. Rethrombosis occurs within 6 months in more than 50% of bridge grafts and 30% of fistulas.

Percutaneous Mechanical Thrombectomy

There are a number of mechanical thrombectomy devices available (see Fig. 4-32 and Table 7-8). Each is based upon a different mechanical principle, with the common goal of fragmenting

---

BOX 7-15. "Lyse and Wait" Technique for Dialysis Access Declot

Insert access in direction of venous outflow close to arterial anastomosis
Compress arterial and venous anastomosis (bridge graft)
Compress arterial anastomosis and distal extent of palpable thrombosed vein (fistula)
Inject thrombolytic agent slowly:
- Urokinase 250,000 U plus 5000 U heparin (total volume 6 mL)
- tPA 5 mg (total volume 5 mL)
- rtPA 5 U plus 5000 U heparin (total volume 6 mL)
Wait for:
- 30-60 minutes urokinase
- 15-30 minutes tPA, rtPA
Exchange intravenous catheter for 5- to 6-French sheath
Angioplasty venous outflow stenosis
Insert 5- to 6-French sheath in direction toward arterial anastomosis
Dislodge arterial plug

TABLE 7-8 Mechanical Thrombectomy Device Principles

Principle	Examples
Fragmentation	Rotating baskets; brushes; vortex
Venturi effect	Saline jets directed into catheters
Aspiration	Reciprocating clot spoon

---

the thrombus into pieces small enough that they can be either released into the systemic circulation or removed through the device. The purpose of these devices is to rapidly declot the graft without the need for a thrombolytic agent. The arterial and venous anastomoses are still managed with balloons in the same way as during pharmacologic thrombolysis. Patients should be adequately heparinized during the procedure to prevent rethrombosis before outflow and inflow are restored.

Mechanical thrombectomy devices are inserted into the thrombosed graft following the same principles as thrombolysis catheters. The status of the central venous outflow is documented at the beginning of the procedure prior to initiating thrombectomy. The sheath requirements for each device should be carefully checked to ensure compatibility. Some devices can be utilized over a guidewire, whereas others do not have this capability. Not all devices are approved for use in native vessels, so the anatomy of the graft should be well understood before inserting the device. The duration of activation of the device must be carefully monitored, because the mechanical elements may fracture with prolonged use or cause clinically significant hemolysis. Overall procedural times are shorter with mechanical rather than pharmacologic thrombolysis. The success rates and outcomes of mechanical thrombectomy in bridge grafts are similar to pharmacologic thrombolysis.

Percutaneous Pharmacomechanical Thrombectomy

Augmentation of thrombolysis with high-frequency ultrasound, mechanical agitation of the thrombus, or powered injection of lytic agent followed by aspiration have all been applied to thrombosed dialysis access (see Fig. 4-34). The ultrasound-assisted techniques use specialized transducer wires that are inserted through an infusion catheter. The ultrasound improves penetration of the lytic agent into the thrombus as well as degrades

TABLE 7-9 Procedural Complications of Percutaneous Declotting Procedures

Complication	Incidence
Immediate thrombosis	5%
Vein rupture (usually peripheral)	2%
Arterial embolization	2%
Pseudoaneurysm (immediate and delayed)	1%
Infection	<1%

Data from Aruny JE, Lewis CA, Cardella JF, et al. Quality improvement guidelines for percutaneous management of the thrombosed or dysfunctional dialysis access. Standards of Practice Committee of the Society of Cardiovascular & Interventional Radiology. *J Vasc Interv Radiol.* 1999;10:491-498.

fibrin. All of the techniques have been successful in rapid declotting of thrombosed dialysis access.

Complications of Dialysis Access Declotting Procedures

Complications of thrombolysis, mechanical, and pharmacomechanical declotting procedures are similar (Table 7-9). Arterial embolization due to reflux of thrombus can be successfully managed with percutaneous methods, such as withdrawing the embolus into the dialysis access with a Fogarty balloon or thrombolysis, but surgical embolectomy may be necessary (Fig. 7-38). Lethal complications are rare, but can occur, usually due to pulmonary embolization in patients with limited pulmonary arterial reserve.

▬ CHRONIC CEREBROSPINAL VENOUS INSUFFICIENCY

Multiple sclerosis (MS) is a chronic neurologic disorder characterized by chronic inflammation, demyelination, and gliosis. This is a heterogeneous disease that typically affects young adults, with a prevalence of 1 case per 1000 in the United States. Rates of diagnosis vary by geography. MS can be relapsing or progressive, and may have autoimmune, inflammatory, genetic, and environmental factors. Women are affected almost twice as often as men. Recently, a vascular component related to insufficient venous drainage of central nervous venous system (chronic cerebrospinal venous insufficiency, or CCSVI) leading to perivenular inflammation has been proposed. This hypothesis was based on the observation that stenoses of the jugular and azygous veins are prevalent in patients with MS. Treatment with angioplasty and/or stenting of the internal jugular and azygous veins is being performed to treat this condition with encouraging reports of early responses (Fig. 7-39). This treatment is best offered in the setting of multidisciplinary care and management of MS patients. Prospective controlled trials are needed to confirm short- and long-term results.

▬ PRIMARY HYPERPARATHYROIDISM

The clinical features of hyperparathyroidism are discussed in Chapter 6 (see Box 6-9). Venous sampling is indicated in patients with persistent primary hyperparathyroidism following neck exploration. Venous sampling is usually performed following unsuccessful localization by angiography.

The technique of venous sampling ideally involves selection of the superior, middle, and inferior thyroid, thymic, and vertebral veins, as well as a peripheral vein. However, many of the thyroidal veins may have been ligated during surgery, and the anatomy is highly variable. Samples from multiple levels in the brachiocephalic vein, IJV, and SVC are generally easier to obtain and allow lateralization of the adenoma. An angled 5-French catheter with

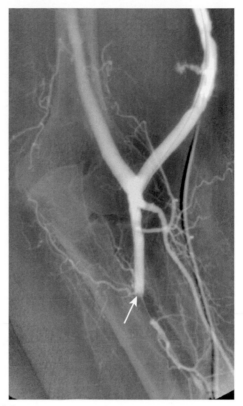

FIGURE 7-38. Brachial artery embolus *(arrow)* during declotting of a dialysis graft. The embolus was successfully treated with catheter-directed thrombolysis.

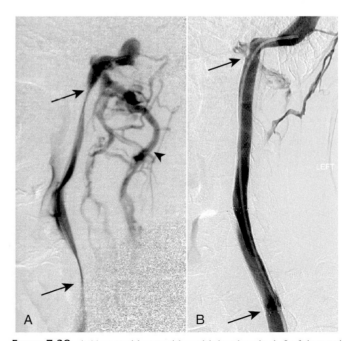

FIGURE 7-39. A 44-year-old man with multiple sclerosis. **A,** Left internal jugular venogram in a steep left anterior oblique projection shows diffuse stenosis of the internal jugular vein (IJV) *(arrows)* with drainage through cervical collateral veins *(arrowhead).* The right IJV had a similar appearance. Both veins were treated with angioplasty followed by self-expanding stent placement. **B,** One year later the left IJV stents are widely patent stents *(arrows)* with absence of collateral drainage. The right IJV stents were also patent.

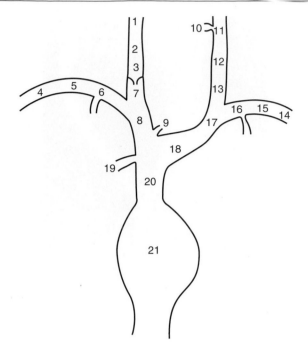

Figure 7-40. Diagram of the venous samples obtained in a patient with failed surgical localization of a parathyroid adenoma. Precise labeling and recording of sampling locations is critical.

an added side hole at the tip, such as a Davis, can be used with an angled 0.038-inch hydrophilic guidewire to select these veins. Crossing the valve at the junction of the IJV and subclavian vein can be difficult. Having the patient inhale, turn the head, or shrug can open the valve. Test injection of contrast confirms the identity of the vein before sampling. Careful labeling and recording of each sample is critical (Fig. 7-40). Samples are analyzed for parathyroid hormone.

Venous sampling is successful in lateralizing an adenoma in approximately 80% of cases. A ratio of at least 2:1 compared to a peripheral vein sample is considered diagnostic.

▬ Suggested Readings

Augustine MM, Bravo PE, Zeiger MA. Surgical treatment of primary hyperparathyroidism. *Endocr Pract.* 2011;17:S75-S82.

Bent CL, Sahni VA, Matson MB. The radiological management of the thrombosed arteriovenous dialysis fistula. *Clin Radiol.* 2011;66:1-12.

Czihal M, Hoffmann U. Upper extremity deep venous thrombosis. *Vascular Medicine.* 2011;16:191-202.

Cynamon J, Lakritz P, Wahl S, et al. Hemodialysis graft declotting: description of the "lyse and wait" technique. *J Vasc Interv Radiol.* 1997;8:925-929.

Dale JD, Dolmatch BL, Duch JM, et al. Expanded polytetrafluoroethylene-covered stent treatment of angioplasty-related extravasation during hemodialysis access intervention: technical and 180-day patency. *J Vasc Interv Radiol.* 2010;21:322-326.

Demondion X, Herbinet P, Van Sint Jan S, et al. Imaging assessment of thoracic outlet syndrome. *Radiographics.* 2006;26:1735-1750.

Dwyer A. Surface-treated catheters–a review. *Semin Dial.* 2008;21:542-546.

Ferral H, Bjarnason H, Wholey M, et al. Recanalization of occluded veins to provide access for central catheter placement. *J Vasc Interv Radiol.* 1996;7:681-685.

Ganeshan A, Hon LQ, Warakaulle DR, et al. Superior vena caval stenting for SVC obstruction: current status. *Eur J Radiol.* 2009;71:343-349.

Gray RJ, Sacks D, Martin LG, et al. Reporting standards for percutaneous interventions in dialysis access. Technology Assessment Committee. *J Vasc Interv Radiol.* 1999;10:1405-1415.

Hamilton HC, Foxcroft DR. Central venous access sites for the prevention of venous thrombosis, stenosis and infection in patients requiring long-term intravenous therapy. *Cochrane Database Syst Rev.* 2007;CD004084.

Haskal ZJ, Trerotola S, Dolmatch B, et al. Stent graft versus balloon angioplasty for failing dialysis-access grafts. *N Engl J Med.* 2010;362:494-503.

Illig KA, Doyle AJ. A comprehensive review of Paget-Schroetter syndrome. *J Vasc Surg.* 2010;51:1538-1547.

Kaufman JA, Kazanjian SA, Rivitz SM, et al. Long-term central venous catheterization in patients with limited access. *Am J Roentgenol.* 1996;167:1327-1333.

Kundu S. Review of central venous disease in hemodialysis patients. *J Vasc Interv Radiol.* 2010;21:963-968.

Kundu S, Modabber M, You JM, et al. Use of PTFE stent grafts for hemodialysis-related central venous occlusions: intermediate-term results. *Cardiovasc Intervent Radiol.* 2011;34:949-957.

Laissy JP, Fernandez P, Karila-Cohen P, et al. Upper limb vein anatomy before hemodialysis fistula creation: cross-sectional anatomy using MR venography. *Eur Radiol.* 2003;13:256-261.

Lau TN, Kinney TB. Direct US-guided puncture of the innominate veins for central venous access. *J Vasc Interv Radiol.* 2001;12:641-645.

Lewis CA, Allen TE, Burke DR, et al. Quality improvement guidelines for central venous access. The Standards of Practice Committee of the Society of Cardiovascular & Interventional Radiology. *J Vasc Interv Radiol.* 2003;14:S231-S235.

Lundell C, Kadir S. Upper extremity veins. In: Kadir S, ed. *Atlas of Normal and Angiographic Anatomy.* Philadelphia: WB Saunders; 1991.

Lundell C, Kadir S. Superior vena cava and thoracic veins. In: Kadir S, ed. *Atlas of Normal and Angiographic Anatomy.* Philadelphia: WB Saunders; 1991.

Seehofer D, Steinmüller T, Rayes N, et al. Parathyroid hormone venous sampling before reoperative surgery in renal hyperparathyroidism: comparison with noninvasive localization procedures and review of the literature. *Arch Surg.* 2004;139:1331-1338.

Sheth S, Ebert MD, Fishman EK. Superior vena cava obstruction evaluation with MDCT. *AJR.* 2010;194:336-346.

Silberzweig JE, Sacks D, Khorsandi AS, et al. Reporting standards for central venous access. *J Vasc Interv Radiol.* 2000;11:391-400.

Vedantham S, Benenati JF, Kundu S, et al. Interventional endovascular management of chronic cerebrospinal venous insufficiency in patients with multiple sclerosis: a position statement by the Society of Interventional Radiology, endorsed by the Canadian Interventional Radiology Association. *J Vasc Interv Radiol.* 2010;21:1335-1337.

Vesely TM. Central venous catheter tip position: a continuing controversy. *J Vasc Interv Radiol.* 2003;14:527-534.

Vo JN, Hoffer FA, Shaw DW. Techniques in vascular and interventional radiology: pediatric central venous access. *Tech Vasc Interv Radiol.* 2010;13:250-257.

Watkinson AF, Yeow TN, Fraser C. Endovascular stenting to treat obstruction of the superior vena cava. *Br Med J.* 2008;336:1434-1437.

Yurkovic A, Cohen RD, Mantell MP, et al. Outcomes of thrombectomy procedures performed in hemodialysis grafts with early failure. *J Vasc Interv Radiol.* 2011;22:317-324.

CHAPTER 8

Pulmonary Circulation

John A. Kaufman, MD, MS, FSIR, FCIRSE

The lungs receive blood from both ventricles—the entire volume of the right heart and also a small fraction of blood from the left heart (via the bronchial arteries). Functionally, the lungs have two roles: oxygenation of venous blood and filtration of the systemic venous blood. Pulmonary vascular pathology, imaging, and intervention frequently have a clinical impact that extends far beyond the lungs.

ANATOMY

The pulmonary arterial blood undergoes oxygenation and filtration in the lung. The pulmonary arterial vascular circuit is comprised of the pulmonary arteries, the alveolar capillary network, and the pulmonary veins. Systemic venous blood exits the heart from the right ventricle through the main pulmonary artery, an anterior and intrapericardial structure. After a distance of approximately 3-5 cm, the main pulmonary artery bifurcates into right and left main pulmonary arteries. The right main pulmonary artery crosses the mediastinum to the right hilum posterior to the ascending aorta and superior vena cava (SVC) and anterior to the carina and the esophagus (Fig. 8-1). Within the right hemithorax the artery branches first into upper and lower trunks, and then into segmental vessels that roughly follow the bronchial segments. Beyond this point pulmonary artery anatomy becomes extremely variable. Common variants of the right pulmonary artery include an accessory branch to the posterior segment of the upper lobe from the lower trunk, and two arteries to the middle lobe.

The left pulmonary artery courses superiorly and posteriorly toward the left hilum (see Fig. 8-1). In this location the artery is anterior to the descending thoracic aorta and closely approximated to the undersurface of the arch. At the hilum the left pulmonary artery gives off its first branches to the upper lobe. These are usually multiple individual or paired arteries. A single common upper lobe trunk is seen in fewer than 20% of individuals. The lingula is usually supplied next, from the descending portion of the left pulmonary artery before it divides into the lower lobe vessels. As with the right pulmonary artery, the lower lobe left pulmonary arterial branches approximate the segmental bronchial anatomy, but are highly variable.

The pulmonary arteries are elastic vessels that contain only small amounts of smooth muscle cells down to the level of fifth-order branches. Conversely, the pulmonary arterioles are very muscular. Because of the elastic nature of the pulmonary arteries and the extensive capillary network, the capacity of this vascular bed is enormous. Normal main pulmonary artery pressures are approximately 22/8 mm Hg, with a mean of 13 mm Hg.

The diameter of the individual pulmonary capillaries averages 8-9 μm. The capillary bed is vast (almost 90 m²), which permits efficient and rapid gas exchange at the alveolar level.

This bed also performs another important function—filtration of solid waste from the venous blood before it reaches the left side of the heart and the systemic arteries. The small size but immense number of capillaries allows filtration of large quantities of particulate material without compromising gas exchange or blood flow. Active intrinsic thrombolytic and phagocytic systems in the lung rapidly dispose of normal physiologic debris. There are also anastomoses to the systemic (bronchial) arteries at the capillary level, although in normal individuals these have no clinical importance.

Oxygenated blood is returned to the left atrium by the pulmonary veins (Fig. 8-2). Typically, one upper and two lower veins are formed from coalescence of the segmental veins in each lung. The right pulmonary veins lie inferior to the pulmonary artery and posterior to the SVC. The right middle lobe usually drains into the upper vein, but may empty directly into the left atrium. On the left, the pulmonary veins also lie inferior to the pulmonary artery, and anterior to the descending thoracic aorta. The lingular veins drain with the upper lobe segments. Anomalous venous drainage to the SVC, systemic thoracic veins, or coronary sinus may be found in association with congenital heart disease, pulmonary sequestration, or as an isolated occurrence (Fig. 8-3).

At any point in time, 30% of pulmonary blood is in the arteries, 20% is in the capillaries, and 50% is in the veins. In the supine position the blood volume is relatively evenly distributed between the upper and lower lobes. When upright, the lower lobes are preferentially perfused.

The bronchial arteries, branches of the thoracic aorta, provide blood supply to the airways. Bronchial arteries are normally small vessels that are highly variable in number, but the most common pattern (45%) is two on the left and one on the right. The right bronchial artery arises from a common intercostal trunk in over 70% of individuals, but only 5% of left bronchial arteries have a common origin with an intercostal artery. One quarter of individuals will have single bronchial arteries bilaterally, whereas 30% will have four or more. Right and left bronchial arteries have a common origin in about 40% of individuals (Figs. 8-4 and 8-5). Bronchial arteries usually are located on the anterolateral surface of the thoracic aorta just below the ligamentum arteriosum at the level of the T3-T4 vertebral bodies. Variant sites of origin include the inner surface of the aortic arch (15%), internal mammary, brachiocephalic, inferior thyroidal, and subclavian arteries. Bronchial arteries (especially those on the right) have communication with the anterior spinal artery in 10% of patients. Anastomoses may also be present with the coronary arteries. The venous drainage of the bronchi is through both the systemic veins of the thorax and the pulmonary veins.

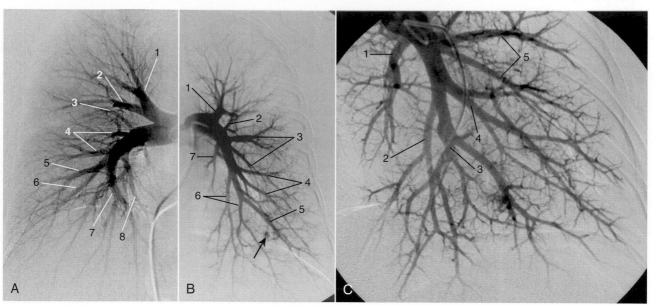

Figure 8-1. Pulmonary artery anatomy as seen on bilateral selective digital subtraction pulmonary angiograms. **A,** Right pulmonary angiogram: *1,* Apical posterior branch right upper lobe (RUL). *2,* Anterior branch RUL. *3,* Superior branch right lower lobe (RLL). *4,* Middle lobe branches. *5,* Lateral basal branch RLL. *6,* Anterior basal branch RLL. *7,* Posterior basal branch RLL. *8,* Medial basal branch RLL. **B,** Left pulmonary artery: *1,* Apical posterior branch left upper lobe (LUL). *2,* Anterior branch LUL. *3,* Lingular branches. *4,* Anteromedial branches left lower lobe (LLL). *5,* Lateral branch LLL. *6,* Posterior branch(es) LLL. *7,* Superior branch LLL. *Arrow,* small pulmonary arteriovenous fistula. **C,** Left posterior oblique magnification selective left pulmonary angiogram. The basal vessels are displayed to best advantage in this view. *1,* Superior branch LLL. *2,* Posterior branch LLL. *3,* Lateral branch LLL. *4,* Anteromedial branch LLL. *5,* Lingular branches.

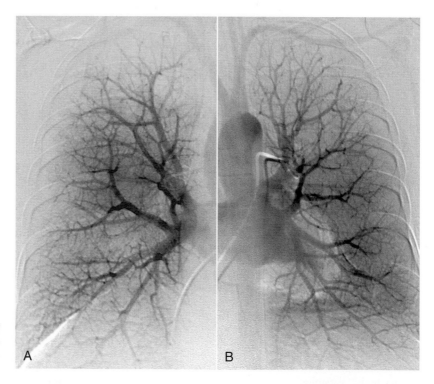

Figure 8-2. Pulmonary veins seen on the late phase of selective digital subtraction pulmonary angiograms. Note the opacification of the thoracic aorta on both studies. **A,** Right pulmonary veins. **B,** Left pulmonary veins.

▬ KEY COLLATERAL PATHWAYS

Pulmonary arteries are considered end arteries, in that few normal intrapulmonary anastomoses exist. Acute proximal occlusion of a normal pulmonary artery segment usually results in distal infarction of the subtended lung parenchyma. Congenital proximal pulmonary artery obstruction is relieved by flow through a patent ductus arteriosus, as well as the bronchial arteries and other mediastinal arteries. In adults with longstanding acquired pulmonary artery occlusions, reconstitution of peripheral pulmonary arteries by small distal intrapulmonary collaterals can occur. The bronchial arteries can provide collateral supply to both the lung parenchyma and the pulmonary arteries (Fig. 8-6). Almost every artery that supplies the thorax (including the diaphragm) can potentially provide collateral supply to the pulmonary arteries. When systemic arteries provide substantial collateral flow to the pulmonary arteries, a measurable left-to-right shunt may develop.

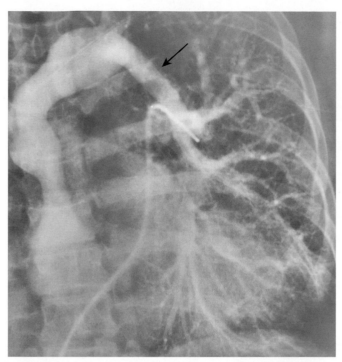

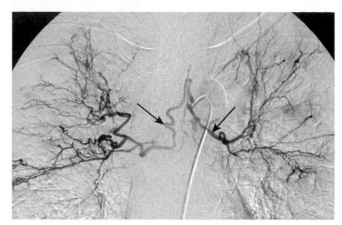

FIGURE 8-5. Digital subtraction angiogram (DSA) showing conjoint origin of hypertrophied right and left bronchial arteries *(arrows)* in a patient with cystic fibrosis (compare to the size of the bronchial arteries in Fig. 8-4).

Bronchial arteries and the lung parenchyma have multiple potential sources of collateral supply (Box 8-1). These usually develop in response to increased arterial flow demands in the lung tissues from chronic pulmonary infections, granulomatous diseases, and tumors, as well as in congenital or acquired pulmonary artery obstruction (Fig. 8-7). Knowledge of these collateral pathways becomes important during interventions for bronchial artery bleeding. Successful occlusion of the bronchial arteries may fail to control bleeding in patients with well-developed collaterals.

◾ IMAGING

Pulmonary Circulation

The optimum imaging modality for the pulmonary vasculature depends on the clinical question, the vessels of interest, available technology, and available technique. Multidetector computed tomography angiography (CTA) is the most widely used imaging technique; it is readily available, fast, and accurate, and it provides comprehensive imaging. Scans performed to evaluate for pulmonary artery embolism follow a different protocol than those to evaluated bronchial arteries. The scan direction (diaphragm to apex for pulmonary embolism, apex to diaphragm for systemic arteries) varies depending on the clinical question and the number of detectors (Fig. 8-8). When possible a peripheral intravenous catheter is used. Injection of contrast through a vein in the right upper extremity minimizes artifact from dense contrast in the left brachiocephalic vein. Power injection of 80-120 mL of contrast at 3-5 mL/sec is crucial to obtain satisfactory images. A scan delay of approximately 20-25 seconds is often used. Prospective cardiac triggering improves image quality but is not routinely used. Streak artifact from contrast in the SVC can interfere with evaluation of the main right pulmonary artery. Delayed scans are useful when evaluating central veins and vascular masses.

Careful postprocessing on an independent workstation facilitates inspection of the pulmonary vasculature. One of the great advantages of pulmonary CTA is the vast amount of additional information about the lung parenchyma, mediastinal structures, and thoracic arteries that can be acquired by simply viewing the same data at different window levels. Patients with suspected pulmonary arterial pathology often have alternate thoracic disease processes that account for or contribute to their symptoms.

Pulmonary arterial magnetic resonance angiography (MRA) usually requires contrast enhancement with gadolinium to obtain satisfactory images (Fig. 8-9). The surrounding aerated

FIGURE 8-3. Partial anomalous venous return of the left lung demonstrated on late image from screen film selective left pulmonary angiogram. The pulmonary vein *(arrow)* draining the left upper lobe and lingula empties directly into the left brachiocephalic vein and then returns to the heart. A pigtail catheter can be seen in the left main pulmonary artery.

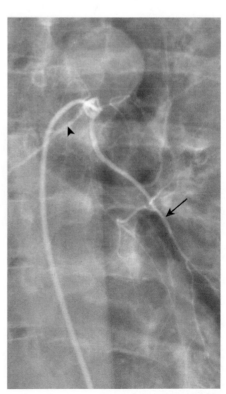

FIGURE 8-4. Selective left bronchial artery injection showing a normal-caliber vessel *(arrow)*. In this patient, a right bronchial artery branch *(arrowhead)* arises with the left.

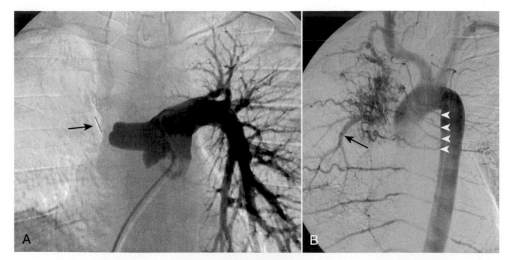

FIGURE 8-6. Systemic to pulmonary artery collateralization due to iatrogenic pulmonary artery occlusion following right upper lobectomy for chronic inflammation. **A,** Main pulmonary angiogram showing occlusion of the right pulmonary artery. Note the surgical clip in the right hilum *(arrow)*. **B,** Aortogram showing numerous bronchial and intercostal arteries *(arrowheads)* supplying hypervascular lung tissue and reconstituting the pulmonary artery *(arrow)*.

Box 8-1. Sources of Potential Collateral Supply to Bronchial Arteries

Intercostal arteries
Branches of the subclavian artery
- Thyrocervical trunk
- Internal mammary artery
- Lateral thoracic artery
- Long thoracic artery

Phrenic arteries
Coronary arteries

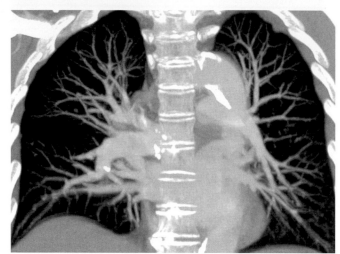

FIGURE 8-8. Pulmonary computed tomography angiogram (128 detector row, 1.5-mm slice thickness, 0.75 mm intervals) displayed as thick coronal maximum intensity projections to demonstrate the level of detail that can be obtained. Interpretation of this study requires review of the individual axial slices.

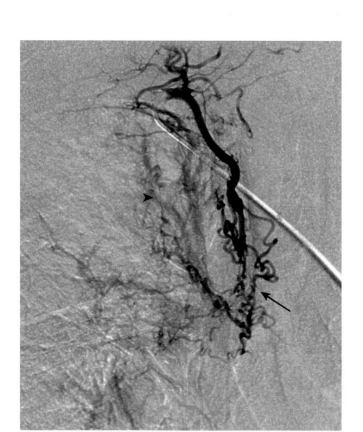

FIGURE 8-7. Collateral supply to the bronchial circulation in a patient with cystic fibrosis and four prior bronchial artery embolizations. Selective right thyrocervical trunk digital subtraction angiogram showing multiple collaterals *(arrow)* to the right upper lobe bronchial arteries. There is shunting into pulmonary artery branches *(arrowhead)*, a common finding in patients with chronic inflammatory diseases leading to bronchial artery hypertrophy.

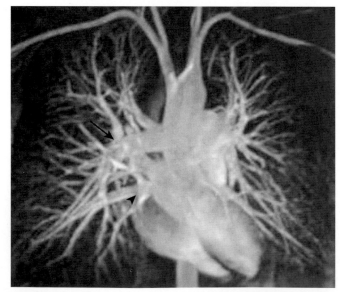

FIGURE 8-9. Pulmonary artery magnetic resonance angiogram using gadolinium-enhanced three-dimensional acquisition displayed as a coronal maximum intensity projection. The pulmonary artery *(arrow)* and veins *(arrowhead)* are visualized, as is the thoracic aorta. (Courtesy Barry Stein, MD, Hartford Hospital, Hartford, Conn.)

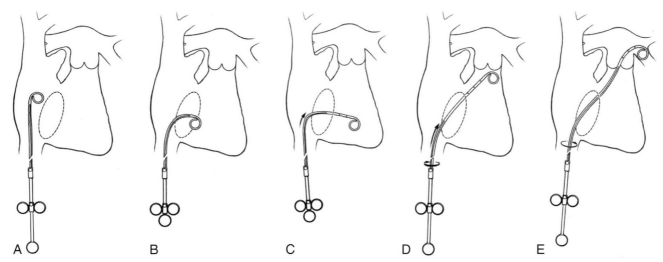

A   B   C   D   E

FIGURE 8-10. Deflecting wire technique for selective catheterization of the pulmonary arteries. Note that the wire never exits the catheter. **A,** The deflecting wire is positioned in the catheter just below the pigtail. **B,** The wire is deflected, directing the catheter toward the tricuspid valve. **C,** The catheter is advanced off the wire into the right ventricle. **D,** The deflection is released and the catheter is advanced through the pulmonary valve while being rotated counterclockwise. **E,** The deflecting wire can be used to direct the catheter from the left to the right pulmonary artery by deflecting and rotating the catheter in a clockwise direction. (Adapted from Kadir S. Pulmonary angiography. In: Kadir S, ed. *Diagnostic Angiography.* Philadelphia: WB Saunders, 1986, with permission.)

lung and cardiac motion limits conventional spin-echo images to evaluation of the central pulmonary arteries. The intrinsic black-blood nature of these images is useful for depiction of central vascular tumors or thrombi. Acquisition times for conventional time-of-flight (TOF) angiographic techniques are too long, and signal loss from in-plane flow is problematic. The most promising techniques are breath-hold fast three-dimensional (3-D) gradient echo time-resolved sequences with bolus injection of gadolinium. Ultra-fast scanners can image the contrast bolus at each step in the pulmonary circuit. Very powerful and fast gradients are required to obtain the extremely short echo times used for time-resolved pulmonary MRA. Limitations of pulmonary MRA are the lack of discrimination of small peripheral vessels with current technology, limited availability, and long duration of the scans compared to CTA.

Catheter angiography remains an extremely important though seldom used diagnostic tool for imaging the peripheral pulmonary arterial circulation. More often, pulmonary angiography is performed as part of an intervention. Selective pulmonary arteriography with a pigtail catheter and low-osmolar contrast agents is more invasive than either CTA or MRA, but safe and definitive in experienced hands.

The patient's electrocardiogram should be reviewed before pulmonary angiography to evaluate for left bundle branch block. If present, temporary pacing (either external or internal) should be in place before a catheter is introduced into the right heart because transient right bundle branch block can be caused by catheter manipulation. In patients with preexisting left bundle branch, this will result in complete heart block.

Contraindications to pulmonary angiography are severe pulmonary hypertension with an end-diastolic right ventricular pressure of 20 mm Hg or more, unstable ventricular arrhythmias, and untreatable severe contrast allergy.

Pulmonary angiography can be performed from either the femoral (most commonly) or jugular venous approach. Nonselective injection of contrast into the vena cava, right atrium, or main pulmonary artery usually does not provide satisfactory visualization of the peripheral pulmonary vessels and requires very large volumes of contrast. Selective pulmonary angiography is safer and provides the best images. Large pigtail catheters (6- or 7-French) that can tolerate high flow rates without whipping in the artery or unwinding are used. The catheter is advanced to the right atrium and then

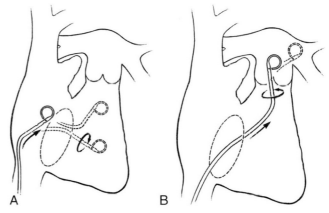

A   B

FIGURE 8-11. Grollman catheter technique. **A,** A pigtail catheter with a secondary curve is advanced across the tricuspid valve. **B,** Using a rotary motion, the catheter is advanced through the pulmonary valve. (Adapted from Kadir S. Pulmonary angiography. In: Kadir S, ed. *Diagnostic Angiography.* Philadelphia: WB Saunders, 1986, with permission.)

through the heart selectively into a right or left pulmonary artery. Several techniques can be used to catheterize the pulmonary arteries, including the use of a deflecting wire to direct a standard pigtail catheter through the valves or the manipulation of a pre-shaped catheter (Figs. 8-10 and 8-11). Ventricular arrhythmias are common because the catheter is manipulated through the right ventricle, but they are almost always self-limited. When elevated right ventricular pressures are suspected, a pressure measurement should be obtained in this location. A pressure measurement should always be obtained in the pulmonary artery before contrast injection. Careful and frequent flushing of the catheter prevents thrombus formation in the lumen, which, if injected into the lung during the study, mimics small emboli originating from peripheral veins. In patients with pulmonary arteriovenous fistulas or malformations, small thrombi or air bubbles could result in a stroke. The main concern related to contrast injection in the pulmonary artery is causing acute right heart failure due to increase afterload. Normal contrast injection rates are 25-30 mL/sec for 2 seconds (see Fig. 8-1). Patients with chronic pulmonary artery hypertension are

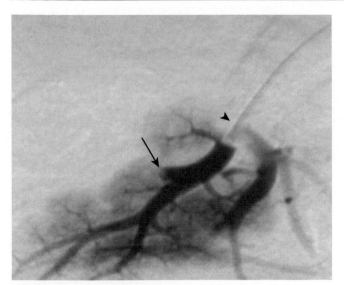

FIGURE 8-12. Balloon occlusion catheter *(arrowhead)* in the right lateral basal segmental artery demonstrating a small embolus *(arrow)*.

<table>
</table>

Box 8-2. Risk Factors for Pulmonary Angiography

Complete left bundle branch block
Severe uncompensated right heart failure
Severe pulmonary hypertension
Acute myocardial infarction
Pulmonary edema
History of anaphylaxis to iodinated contrast

Box 8-3. Sources of Acute Thrombotic Pulmonary Emboli

Lower extremity deep venous thrombosis
Pelvic vein thrombosis
Gonadal vein thrombosis (postpartum)
Renal vein thrombosis
Upper extremity central vein thrombosis
Vascular invasion by malignancy (renal cell carcinoma, adrenal carcinoma, hepatoma)

often well compensated and may not require alteration in contrast injection parameters. In patients with uncompensated pulmonary hypertension, the rate and volume of contrast should be reduced to avoid acute right heart failure, sometimes to less than half of the volumes described. There are no generally agreed upon or validated guidelines for contrast reduction; observation of a small test dose (8-10 mL) of contrast injected by hand can be very helpful. Brisk flow, even in the setting of extremely elevated pressures, indicates adequate right ventricular function and the ability to tolerate normal injection rates. Slow flow and delayed washout of test contrast in the pulmonary arteries in the setting of a normal or elevated heart rate suggests a severely impaired right ventricle, and contrast volumes should be reduced appropriately.

The choice of imaging projection depends on the clinical question, but usually an anteroposterior (AP) view of the entire lung and a posterior oblique magnification view of the lung base with the catheter advanced beyond the upper lobe branches is sufficient for pulmonary embolism studies (see Fig. 8-1). When basilar lung segments are atelectatic, the anterior oblique view may provide the best view of the lower lobe pulmonary arteries. Rapid filming (at least four frames per second) is necessary. Imaging should be continued into the venous phase to evaluate the pulmonary veins (see Figs. 8-2 and 8-3). Diluting contrast containing more than 30% iodine by one third with saline reduces burnout against aerated lung in some digital subtraction angiograph systems. In rare instances, a balloon occlusion catheter may be necessary to isolate a pulmonary artery segment to image a peripheral embolus or high-flow abnormality (Fig. 8-12).

There is a lot of lore about the proper way to remove a pigtail catheter from the pulmonary artery. The theoretical concern is that the catheter will become entangled in valve elements and will either tear them or become trapped. The most conservative approach is to open the pigtail with a soft-tipped guidewire in the pulmonary artery before removing it. Gentle withdrawal of the closed pigtail while observing under fluoroscopy works well. The pigtail frequently opens while exiting through the tricuspid valve, with no sequelae. Do not spin the pigtail, especially if it seems to get stuck, because it may indeed become entangled valve chordae. Either push it back into the heart or insert a soft straight guidewire to open the pig.

Overall complication rates of pulmonary angiography are less than 3%, with the majority related to access site issues or contrast-induced nephropathy. The mortality rate is less than 1% when the procedure is performed for suspected thromboembolic disease, with death occurring more commonly in critically ill

patients with acute right heart strain, pulmonary hypertension, or elevated cardiac troponins due to the thromboembolic event (Box 8-2).

Right ventricular overload is avoided by reduction of contrast rate and volume in patients with acutely elevated pulmonary artery pressures. Once induced, right ventricular decompensation is difficult to reverse.

Bronchial Arteries

Bronchial artery angiography is usually performed as part of an embolization procedure for hemoptysis. Fortunately, the normally small bronchial arteries are typically hypertrophied in these patients. A digital subtraction aortogram in the AP projection with a pigtail catheter positioned in the transverse arch and injection of full-strength contrast at 20-30 mL/sec for 2 seconds allows rapid identification of the enlarged and tortuous bronchial arteries (see Fig. 8-6). The arteries can then be selected with 5-French catheters using a variety of shapes, such as Cobra 2, Simmons 1, and Shepherd's crook. Gentle hand injection of small volumes of contrast (3-10 mL) is usually sufficient unless massive collaterals have developed. Branches to intercostal arteries, the esophagus, and the spinal cord may be seen. When more selective catheterization is required, a microcatheter can be advanced into the bronchial artery. In patients with chronic pulmonary inflammatory processes, multiple selective injections looking for sources of potential collaterals, such as the internal mammary and other subclavian artery branches, may be necessary to map out the entire bronchial arterial supply (see Fig. 8-7).

The most feared complication of diagnostic bronchial arteriography is paraplegia due to transverse myelitis. The exact mechanism is unknown, but it is exceedingly rare (much less than 1%) with current catheters and contrast agents. However, all patients must be advised of this potential complication before bronchial angiography.

▪ ACUTE PULMONARY EMBOLISM

Acute thrombotic pulmonary embolism (PE) occurs when thrombus that has formed in the systemic veins breaks free and is carried by the venous return to the heart and, ultimately, the lungs (Box 8-3). In situ formation of thrombus in the pulmonary arteries is rare and usually related to a surgical procedure, proximal obstruction, or pulmonary artery tumor. The actual incidence of PE is not known but is suspected to be more than 600,000 cases

TABLE 8-1 Prognosis of Pulmonary Embolism

Risk Level	Mortality	Clinical Findings
High	15%	Systolic BP ≤ 90 mm Hg or ≥ 40 mm Hg decrease for ≥ 15 minutes
Intermediate	3%-15%	Hemodynamic stability with impaired RV function*
Low	1%	Hemodynamic stability and normal RV function

BP, Blood pressure; RV, right ventricle.
*Function assessed by imaging or electrocardiogram criteria; elevated cardiac troponins; clinical symptoms. Risk increases with severity of RV dysfunction.

per year in the United States. Untreated, it is thought that the mortality rate of acute PE is 30%.

The clinical effects and prognosis of PE are dependent upon the following factors: degree and level of obstruction; baseline conditions of the pulmonary vasculature and lung parenchyma; and the status of the heart (Table 8-1). Healthy patients with normal lungs and hearts can tolerate massive pulmonary emboli, whereas older patients with end-stage pulmonary diseases may succumb to relatively small emboli. In general, large emboli lodge in the central pulmonary arteries and present with cardiopulmonary collapse, elevated right heart pressures, and hypoxia with evidence of poor oxygen exchange (the so-called "death embolus") (Fig. 8-13). Small emboli lodge in peripheral pulmonary arteries and cause infarcts, which result in pleuritic chest pain and tachypnea but stable hemodynamic parameters and normal oxygenation (Fig. 8-14). Subsegmental emboli tend to be multiple, bilateral, and in the lower lobes.

Lower extremity deep vein thrombosis (DVT) is present in up to 75% of patients with documented PE, but is often asymptomatic. Conversely, 50% of patients with symptomatic DVT have abnormal ventilation/perfusion (V̇/Q̇) scans that are consistent with PE, despite the lack of pulmonary symptoms.

The clinical diagnosis of PE remains elusive, with several models proposed that incorporate symptoms, clinical parameters, and history to arrive at a probability of PE. The D-dimer test provides additional information when negative in patients with a low to moderate probability of PE. However, no scoring system has proven sufficient to obviate imaging evaluation.

Suspicion of acute PE is the most common indication for imaging the pulmonary vasculature. Plain radiographs are useful only to identify alternate explanations for the patient's pulmonary symptoms and as a correlate for other studies. Peripheral wedge-shaped infiltrates can be seen in pulmonary infarcts, but emboli by themselves are not visible.

The V̇/Q̇ scan was once commonly used in the evaluation of patients with suspected PE and still retains some utility. Unlike other imaging tests, the V̇/Q̇ scan compares pulmonary perfusion with pulmonary ventilation. Ventilation of nonperfused areas of lung that are normal on chest radiograph allows a presumptive diagnosis of pulmonary artery obstruction. Conversely, PE does not explain perfusion of areas of nonventilated lung. This modality was validated in a landmark multicenter trial (Prospective Investigation of Pulmonary Embolism Diagnosis, or PIOPED) that comprised 933 patients and compared V̇/Q̇ to pulmonary angiography. The PIOPED II trial, which compared pulmonary CTA, CT venography of the pelvis and lower extremities, V̇/Q̇ scan, and compression venous ultrasound of the lower extremities suggested that perfusion scans can be interpreted without the ventilation component in patients with normal chest radiographs with an accuracy equivalent to pulmonary CTA. Uncooperative patients with obvious chest radiograph abnormalities are poor candidates for V̇/Q̇ scans because perfusion abnormalities may result from pneumonia, atelectasis, and other nonembolic causes.

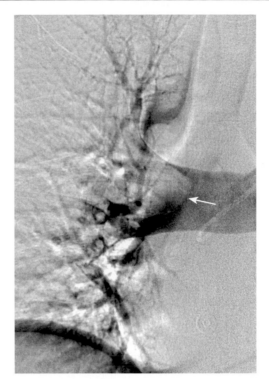

FIGURE 8-13. Digital subtraction angiogram showing a massive embolus *(arrow)* occluding the right upper and lower pulmonary arteries. The patient presented with sudden, transient hypotension.

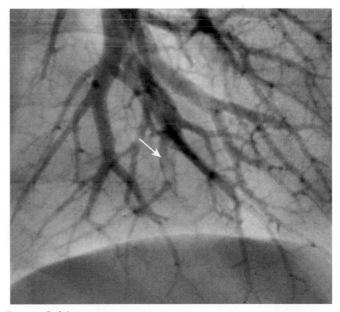

FIGURE 8-14. Subsegmental pulmonary embolus *(arrow)* shown on magnification angiogram of the left lung base. The patient presented with pleuritic chest pain.

Refer to *Nuclear Medicine: The Requisites* for a complete description of V̇/Q̇ scan interpretation (Box 8-4). In summary, the results of V̇/Q̇ scans are expressed in terms of probability of pulmonary embolism. High probability scans have sensitivity of 77% for detection of PE, and low probability or normal scans have a specificity of 98% (no PE). However, a definitive diagnosis or exclusion of PE based on V̇/Q̇ scanning alone is possible in about 50% of patients. For this reason, a number of strategies have been proposed to enhance the diagnosis of PE using V̇/Q̇ scans, including combining the results with lower extremity venous ultrasound and clinical probability scores.

Direct imaging of the pulmonary arteries remains a fundamental approach to the diagnosis of PE. All vascular imaging modalities (CTA, MRA, and conventional angiography) base the diagnosis of PE on the same criteria: visualization of an intraluminal filling defect, which is defined as an unopacified object in the vessel lumen surrounded by contrast-enhanced blood. This finding is not exclusive to PE and must be interpreted in the context of the patient's history, because postoperative changes and pulmonary artery tumors may also produce intraluminal filling defects. Acute emboli fill the lumen of the artery, have smooth contours, and

are most common at bifurcation points in the pulmonary artery (Fig. 8-15; see Figs. 8-13 and 8-14). Subacute or partially lysed emboli appear contracted, with slightly irregular contours (see Fig. 8-15). All other "signs" of PE are secondary and can possibly be explained by nonembolic etiologies (Box 8-5). When undertaking imaging for PE, plan to make a definitive diagnosis; the answer should be either "positive" or "negative."

Multidetector CTA is the imaging modality used most often for patients with suspected acute PE. The PIOPED II trial provided validation of this imaging modality, with a sensitivity of 83% and specificity of 96%. Emboli appear as nonenhancing intraluminal filling defects (see Fig. 8-15). The age of the thrombus may be inferred from the appearance (see later), but acute and chronic PE can be present in the same patient. Straightening of the intracardiac intraventricular septum, dilation of the right ventricle, and reflux of contrast into the inferior vena cava (IVC) and hepatic veins in the presence of acute PE are suggestive of right ventricular strain. Areas of decreased perfusion on lung windows imply pulmonary artery obstruction, but cannot be used to diagnose PE in the absence of an intraluminal filling defect. False-positive diagnoses can result from volume averaging of extrapulmonary structures, particularly peribronchial lymph nodes at bifurcation points. Atelectasis, tumors, and infiltrates can make interpretation of studies difficult. As emboli become smaller in size and number, and more peripheral, sensitivity and specificity decrease. This limitation is counteracted by increasing numbers of detectors and faster scan times. A major advantage of CTA is the vast amount of information that is acquired about the other intrathoracic structures, which sometimes leads to the alternate and correct diagnosis.

Box 8-4. Modified PIOPED Criteria

NORMAL
No perfusion defects

LOW PROBABILITY: <20%
Any perfusion defect with a substantially larger radiographic abnormality
Matched ventilation and perfusion defects with a normal chest radiograph
Nonsegmental perfusion defects (e.g., cardiomegaly, aortic aneurysm, hilar mass, mediastinal mass, elevated diaphragm, small pleural effusion with blunting of costophrenic angle)
Small subsegmental perfusion defects

MEDIUM PROBABILITY: 20%-80%
One moderate mismatched segmental defect with a normal radiograph
One large and one moderate mismatched segmental defect with a normal radiograph
Difficult to categorize as high or low probability
Not meeting the stated criteria for high or low probability

HIGH PROBABILITY: >80%
Two or more large mismatched segmental defects without a radiographic abnormality (or the perfusion defect is substantially larger than the radiographic abnormality)
Any combination of mismatched defects equivalent to the above (two moderate defects = one large defect)

PIOPED, Prospective investigation of pulmonary embolism diagnosis

---

Box 8-5. Imaging Criteria for Diagnosis of Pulmonary Embolism

ABSOLUTE
Intraluminal filling defect

SECONDARY
Abrupt cutoff of pulmonary artery
Abrupt transition artery diameter without branch
Unexplained absence of pulmonary artery branch(es)
Oligemia of lung parenchyma
Slow flow in pulmonary artery segment
Absent venous drainage of lung segment

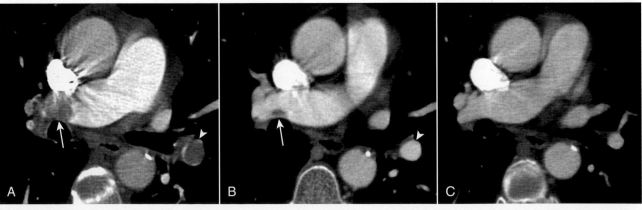

FIGURE 8-15. Bilateral pulmonary emboli on computed tomography angiogram (CTA), appearance over time with treatment. **A,** Axial image from pulmonary CTA showing large right *(arrow)* and left *(arrowhead)* emboli. Note the rim of contrast visible around the left lower lobe embolus *(arrowhead)*. There is streak artifact from contrast in the superior vena cava. The patient, who was hemodynamically stable, was treated with systemic anticoagulation. **B,** Repeat CTA 14 days later. On the right, a small amount of residual thrombus is present *(arrow)*. The left lower lobe pulmonary artery is patent *(arrowhead)*. **C,** Follow-up CTA 1 year later shows no evidence of the emboli.

After acquiring the pulmonary arterial images, a venous phase scan through the pelvis and legs (CT venography [CTV]) may detect DVT. The clinical value of this additional scan when the CTA is positive for PE is uncertain but may direct further therapy. In patients with negative CTA for PE, DVT was detected in 8% in the PIOPED II trial, leading to a recommendation to perform both studies. The addition of CTV improved the diagnostic performance of CTA for PE in patients with negative or inconclusive studies, but increased radiation and cost. Because very few diagnosed DVTs have been isolated to the pelvis, lower extremity venous duplex ultrasound is an alternative to CTV in these patients.

Gadolinium-enhanced MRA has performed well in the diagnosis of proximal and central PE, and was the subject of the PIOPED III trial. Although the sensitivity was 78% and the specificity 99% in this trial, clinical application remains limited due to longer scan times and more complex imaging protocols. Emboli are seen as intraluminal filling defects. Fast gadolinium-enhanced 3-D gradient echo acquisitions can be acquired in a single breath-hold with most equipment. As more MR scanners become available, use of MRA for diagnosis of acute PE may increase.

Pulmonary angiography is rarely required in the diagnosis of acute PE. Conventional angiography is indicated when CTA has been inconclusive or a catheter-based intervention for PE is anticipated. When performed properly, it is a safe examination, even in very ill patients. As with both CTA and MRA, the definitive diagnosis of PE is made by finding an intraluminal filling defect in the pulmonary artery (see Figs. 8-12 through 8-14). The most common location for emboli to lodge is at bifurcation points, so these areas should be inspected carefully. Overlap of pulmonary arteries may obscure or mimic PE, so a second view in a different projection is frequently obtained. When peripheral emboli are suspected, magnification views (sometimes in multiple obliquities) may be necessary (see Fig. 8-14). A filling defect due to an embolus is constant on several images. Inflow of unopacified blood can mimic an embolus on a single image, but is easily identified on serial images by its changing morphology (Fig. 8-16). Secondary signs of PE are helpful but do not substitute for a filling defect. Injection of a sufficient volume of contrast and rapid filming are the keys to obtaining diagnostic pulmonary angiograms. However, contrast volumes and rates must be adjusted based on pulmonary artery pressures and qualitative assessment of flow.

The lung of interest should be studied first, based on either clinical symptoms or other imaging tests. The right lung may be studied first when there is no obvious choice, as it is harder to catheterize than the left. When the diagnosis is made on the first angiogram, obtain at least one view of the opposite lung unless contraindicated by the patient's condition. A small number of patients will be suspected of having recurrent PE during initiation of therapy, and baseline studies will be helpful during interpretation of repeat studies.

The conventional treatment of acute PE has two objectives: (1) to permit or enhance resolution of emboli and thrombus by the intrinsic thrombolytic pathways and (2) to reduce the risk of additional emboli by preventing new thrombus formation and allowing stabilization of existing venous thrombus. Both objectives are usually successfully accomplished with anticoagulation. Patients may be treated with unfractionated heparin followed by warfarin or low-molecular-weight heparin compounds. The recommended duration of anticoagulation varies depending on the clinical scenario, but should be at least 6 months in most patients. The American College of Chest Physicians (ACCP) evidence-based guidelines for anticoagulation are widely used and are updated regularly.

Symptomatic recurrent PE occurs in almost 5% of patients during the initial phase of anticoagulation, usually during the first 2 weeks of therapy. Mortality from PE is directly related to recurrent PE and varies with the degree of thrombus burden and right heart dysfunction. The ability of normal lung to lyse thrombus is remarkable (see Fig. 8-15). Fewer than 3% of patients treated with anticoagulation develop symptomatic chronic pulmonary arterial hypertension due to obstruction of flow.

Patients with massive PE and cardiac compromise are candidates for acute relief of central pulmonary artery obstruction. Surgical pulmonary thromboembolectomy is the traditional approach, with an operative mortality rate of 5%-8% and excellent 10-year survival results. Systemic thrombolysis has been studied extensively, but mostly in patients with intermediate risk PE, with inconclusive results. In patients with massive PE, there are few studies but there does appear to be a survival benefit and this is an accepted therapy. Dosing varies by agent (Table 8-2). Systemic thrombolysis has a 25% risk for bleeding complications overall, with an approximately 2%-3% risk of intracranial hemorrhage.

Percutaneous catheter-directed techniques are an increasingly popular alternative to systemic thrombolysis and surgical thromboembolectomy in patients with massive PE. The outcomes are similar to those of surgery, with clinical success reported in approximately 91% of patients. A critical variable in this success is the timing of intervention; the more profound the right ventricular dysfunction, the worse the outcome. A variety of percutaneous thrombectomy devices have been used, as has fragmentation by a rotating a pigtail catheter and angioplasty balloon. A long guiding catheter in the pulmonary artery is necessary with most mechanical devices to provide stability. Pharmacomechanical thrombolysis accelerates the fragmentation of the thrombus, relieving outflow obstruction of the right ventricle and improving survival (Fig. 8-17). In these procedures, mechanical techniques are often combined with doses of a thrombolytic agent (such as

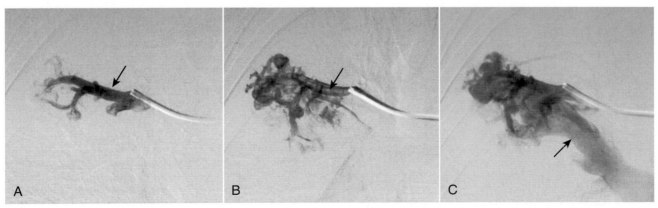

FIGURE 8-16. Inflow of unopacified blood simulating a filling defect. **A,** Selective right upper lobe pulmonary angiogram in a patient with a complex pulmonary arteriovenous malformation (AVM). The feeding artery *(arrow)* is completely opacified with contrast. **B,** The next frame shows unopacified blood in the center of the feeding artery *(arrow),* surrounded by slower moving contrast-enhanced blood along the walls of the vessel, causing the appearance of a filling defect. Note the numerous communicating branches with the AVM. **C,** A few frames later (during diastole) the feeding artery is again completely opacified. A single draining vein is visible *(arrow).*

5-10 mg tPA) delivered into the thrombus. Subsequent catheter infusion of a thrombolytic agent directly into the pulmonary arteries can be continued using standard catheters or ultrasound assisted devices. When delivered centrally, lower doses of thrombolytic are required than for systemic therapy. Thrombolytic agents should be used sparingly in patients with recent major surgery, hemorrhagic stroke, or contraindications to anticoagulation. Emergency surgical pulmonary thromboembolectomy should be considered when percutaneous intervention is not readily available or a significant chronic component of thrombus is suspected.

When anticoagulation is not feasible or an additional PE would be life-threatening, interruption of the inferior vena cava (IVC) with a filter is indicated (see Chapter 13).

CHRONIC PULMONARY EMBOLISM

Although the lungs are capable of absorbing relatively large acute embolic loads, repeat embolization over a long period is one of the causes of chronic pulmonary arterial hypertension. The pathophysiology is a combination of macrovascular obstruction, chronic vasoconstriction, and a small vessel arteriopathy of the media and intima. Partial recanalization of emboli results in luminal compromise by weblike stenoses, linear strands of organized intraluminal thrombus, and mural thrombus. The organized thrombus is firm, rubbery, and forms a cast of the pulmonary vasculature. As the available pulmonary artery vascular bed decreases, pulmonary artery pressure increases, the main pulmonary arteries and right ventricle become enlarged, and gas exchange is compromised. Ultimately, right heart failure ensues. Clinically significant chronic PE is estimated to occur in only 2%-4% of patients following acute PE.

The diagnosis of chronic PE is frequently arrived at during evaluation for other more common disorders such as pulmonary hypertension or fibrosis. Patients with chronic PE frequently have no history of prior documented PE or DVT. Symptoms include dyspnea on exertion, pulmonary artery hypertension, and right heart failure, as well as nondescript complaints such as fatigue and failure to thrive. Acute PE can coexist with chronic PE.

The approach to imaging patients with suspected chronic PE is somewhat different from imaging acute PE. Patients are usually stable, although sometimes very ill. Accurate determination of the extent of pulmonary artery involvement is crucial for planning therapy. Emergent imaging is rarely necessary.

As with acute PE, the plain radiograph is rarely useful in the diagnosis of chronic PE other than to possibly provide alternative diagnoses. Enlarged central pulmonary arteries, absence or "pruned" appearance of peripheral pulmonary artery branches, and wedge-shaped peripheral infarcts have all been reported in chronic PE.

The findings on $\dot{V}/\dot{Q}$ scan for chronic PE are the same as in acute PE (Table 8-3). Nevertheless, the study is useful in that a normal examination excludes chronic PE as an explanation for dyspnea, pulmonary artery hypertension, and right heart failure. In order to develop these symptoms, a large quantity of the pulmonary vasculature must be obstructed.

CTA is an excellent modality for evaluation of suspected chronic PE. The typical findings include mural thrombus in the pulmonary arteries, stenoses, central pulmonary artery enlargement, and parenchymal abnormalities such as a mosaic pattern

TABLE 8-2 Thrombolytic Dosing for Pulmonary Emboli

Drug	Systemic Dose	Catheter-Directed Infusion
tPA	100 mg over 2 hr, or 0.6 mg/kg over 15 min	1-2 mg/hr over 12-24 hr
rtPA	10 U × 2, 30 min apart	1 U/hr for 12-24 hr
TNK	30-50 mg over 5-10 sec*	1 mg/hr for 12-24 hr
UK	4400 IU/kg over 10 min, then 4400/kg/hr for 12-24 hr	100,000-200,000 IU/hr over 12-24 hr

IU, International units; tPA, tissue plasminogen activator; rtPA, recombinant tPA; TNK, tenecteplase.
*Tenecteplase dosing: 30 mg for < 60 kg, then increase 5 mg every 10 kg to maximum 50 mg.

TABLE 8-3 Findings in Chronic Pulmonary Embolism

Finding	$\dot{V}/\dot{Q}$	CTA	MRA	Angio
Perfusion/ventilation mismatch	+*	N/A	N/A	N/A
Mural thrombus	N/A	+	+	-
Enlarged central PA	N/A	+	+	+
PA stenoses/webs	N/A	+	+	+
PA hypertension	N/A	+	+	+†
Proximal PA occlusions	N/A	+	+	+
Peripheral PA occlusions	N/A	-	-	+

*Also found in acute pulmonary embolism.
†Direct measurement.
N/A, Not applicable; PA, pulmonary artery.

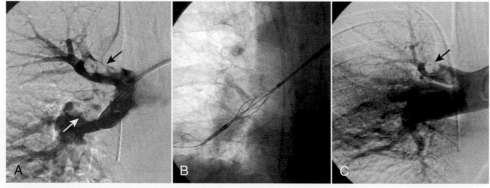

FIGURE 8-17. Catheter-directed therapy of acute massive pulmonary embolism. **A,** Selective right pulmonary artery angiogram showing large lower *(white arrow)* and upper *(black arrow)* lobe pulmonary emboli in a patient with hemodynamic compromise. **B,** Spot film of a percutaneous thrombectomy device (PTD) in the right lower lobe pulmonary artery. The patient also received 6 mg of alteplase directly into the pulmonary artery before activation of the device. **C,** Right pulmonary angiogram after catheter-directed treatment shows improvement in the right lower lobe perfusion and residual thrombus *(arrow)* in the upper lobe (not treated with the PTD due to the small size of the artery). The patient was hemodynamically improved. An important component of this procedure not shown was placement of an inferior vena cava filter.

and peripheral nodules (Fig. 8-18). Small peripheral areas of obstruction may be missed. MRA provides similar information about the vasculature, but is not as useful for the pulmonary parenchyma.

The angiographic findings of chronic PE are listed in Table 8-3. Angiography allows direct determination of right heart and pulmonary artery pressures. Subtle intimal irregularities, stenoses, occlusions, and a "pruned" or branchless appearance of the pulmonary artery are all typical of chronic PE (see Fig. 8-18). Remnants of recanalized emboli can be seen as linear filling defects, termed *synechia*. An important limitation of angiography is the inability to characterize the extent of mural thrombus in the pulmonary artery.

Surgical removal of the chronic thrombus (pulmonary thromboendarterectomy) is the accepted treatment and has excellent results. The rubbery thrombus is shelled out of the pulmonary arteries. Often the pulmonary arteries distal to the chronic obstruction are normal compared to the patent vessels that are subject to chronic pulmonary artery hypertension. Patients require cardiopulmonary bypass and have an operative mortality of approximately 5%. Currently, there are no effective percutaneous techniques for removing chronic pulmonary thrombus. Stent placement to relieve stenoses caused by chronic thrombus in nonoperative candidates has been described.

An important aspect of the treatment of chronic PE is based on preventing further emboli from occurring. Long-term anticoagulation prevents development of new peripheral sources of thrombus that may embolize. Many of these patients are candidates for IVC filters.

PULMONARY ARTERY STENOSIS

There are multiple causes of pulmonary artery stenoses in adults (Table 8-4). In children, pulmonary artery stenosis may be associated with congenital heart defects such as tetralogy of Fallot, atrial and ventricular septal defects, rubella syndrome, and Williams syndrome.

The etiology of pulmonary stenosis may be suggested by the appearance (Table 8-5). Stenoses that are focal and smooth with obtuse angles imply extrinsic compression by masses (Fig. 8-19). Diffuse smooth stenoses are more likely to be due to congenital abnormalities of the pulmonary artery or vasculitis (Fig. 8-20; see also Fig. 1-19). Stenoses that are irregular with acute angles or obvious webs imply an intrinsic lesion such as chronic PE (see Fig. 8-18). Other important factors are the patient's age, associated conditions, and past history. Plain radiographs may reveal calcified lymph nodes, pulmonary fibrosis, or masses. Conventional CT and magnetic resonance imaging of the chest are extremely useful for evaluation of the mediastinal and hilar structures, as well as

the lung parenchyma. CTA and MRA accurately depict central pulmonary artery stenosis. Pulmonary angiography is necessary to diagnose small vessel stenoses, as cross-sectional imaging lacks the required resolution.

Therapy is determined by the severity of the symptoms and the underlying etiology of the lesion. Stenoses due to chronic PE may be amenable to thromboendarterectomy. Focal proximal lesions respond to placement of a balloon-expandable stent.

PULMONARY VASCULAR MALFORMATIONS

The most common pulmonary vascular malformations are congenital pulmonary artery to venous communications. Broadly termed *pulmonary arteriovenous malformations* (AVM), many are simple artery to vein connections and therefore more like an arteriovenous fistula (AVF) (Fig. 8-21; see also Figs. 8-16 and 4-38). Patients with cirrhosis can develop multiple symptomatic fistulas at the lung base (hepatopulmonary syndrome). Rarely, congenital systemic artery to pulmonary artery fistulas or malformations can occur (Fig. 8-22).

In patients with abnormal pulmonary artery to vein communications, blood is shunted directly from the right heart to the left without benefiting from two major functions of the pulmonary capillary bed: oxygenation and filtration. Patients with pulmonary arteriovenous lesions may present with symptoms of hypoxia due to shunting, high-output cardiac failure, or, more seriously, paradoxical embolization. Dyspnea and hypoxia due to shunting that

TABLE 8-4 Causes of Pulmonary Artery Stenoses in Adults

Etiology	Central	Peripheral
Chronic pulmonary embolism	+	+
Vasculitis		
Takayasu arteritis	+	+
Radiation	+	+
Chronic inflammation	+	+
Tumor	+	+
Congenital rubella	+	−
Adenopathy	+	−
Fibrosing mediastinitis	+	−
Aortic aneurysm	+	−
Prior surgery	+	−

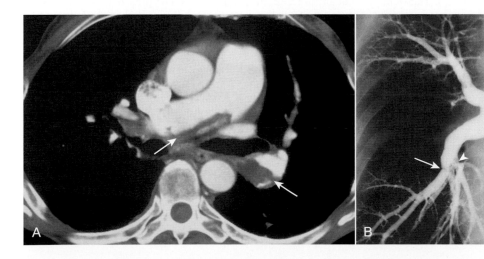

FIGURE 8-18. Chronic pulmonary embolism (PE). **A,** Contrast-enhanced computed tomography scan in a patient with chronic PE showing mural thrombus *(arrows)* lining the left and right pulmonary arteries. (Compare with the acute PE in Figs. 18-15 and 18-17) **B,** Selective right pulmonary angiogram from a different patient with chronic PE showing webs *(arrow)*, partially recanalized occlusions *(arrowhead)*, and diminished parenchymal vascularity. (Courtesy David Levin, MD, and Thomas Kinney, MD, UCSD Department of Radiology, San Diego, Calif.)

TABLE 8-5 Anatomic Location of Pulmonary Artery Stenosis

Etiology	Extrinsic	Intrinsic
Chronic pulmonary embolism	−	+
Vasculitis		
Takayasu arteritis	−	+
Radiation	−	+
Congenital rubella	−	+
Post lung transplant	−	+
Williams syndrome	−	+
Chronic inflammation	+	−
Tumor	+	−
Adenopathy	+	−
Fibrosing mediastinitis	+	−
Aortic aneurysm	+	−

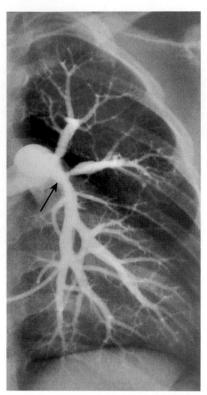

FIGURE 8-20. Selective left pulmonary artery angiogram in a child with congenital rubella infection showing pulmonary artery stenoses *(arrow)*.

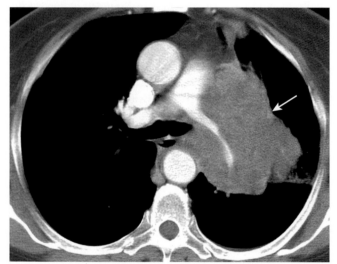

FIGURE 8-19. Contrast-enhanced computed tomography scan of a patient with a large lung carcinoma *(arrow)* encasing and compressing the right pulmonary artery.

are worse with standing is typical in patients with large lower lobe lesions (platypnea and orthodeoxia, respectively). Transient ischemic attacks, strokes, brain abscesses, and peripheral arterial emboli may occur. The risk of paradoxical embolus increases with the number of malformations and the size of the feeding arteries. A rare complication is acute hemorrhage, either intrapulmonary or intrapleural, particularly in pregnant women.

Pulmonary vascular malformations occur sporadically (30%) or as part of a diagnosable autosomal dominant disorder (70%) known as either hereditary hemorrhagic telangiectasia (HHT) or Osler-Weber-Rendu disease. In addition to pulmonary lesions, almost all patients with HHT have recurrent epistaxis, 75% have skin telangiectasias, 33% have liver involvement by AVM, up to 20% have brain or spine AVMs, and about 15% have gastrointestinal bleeding. There are at least four types of HHT, each related to a specific chromosomal abnormality. Type 1 (chromosome 9) has the highest association with pulmonary artery lesions (30%), whereas only 3% of patients with type 2 (chromosome 12) have lung abnormalities. Patients with type 4 have an increased incidence of juvenile polyposis.

The overall incidence of HHT varies from 1 per 40,000 in parts of England to 1 per 200 in certain Caribbean populations. Pulmonary lesions are multiple in 35%-58% of patients and bilateral in 40%, occurring predominantly in the lower lobes. Simple AVMs (supply from one artery) occur in 80%, and complex AVMs (supply from multiple arteries) in 20%. A new diagnosis of HHT should prompt two actions: (1) a search for pulmonary lesions in the patient and (2) a search for HHT in the patient's relatives.

Identification of intrapulmonary shunting is a useful parameter in the diagnosis and postintervention follow-up. Contrast echocardiography (with agitated saline) is highly sensitive with higher degrees of shunting correlating well with the presence of pulmonary vascular malformations. A right to left shunt is suggested when contrast is visualized in the left atrium within four cardiac beats of its appearance in the right atrium.

Pulmonary lesions appear on chest radiographs as smooth, round, or lobulated mass lesions and are frequently initially thought to represent solid tumors. The presence of large vessels extending from the mass to the hilum is highly suggestive of an AVM. A normal chest radiograph does not exclude the presence of pulmonary vascular lesions.

Thin-section CT scans are the preferred imaging for evaluation of suspected pulmonary lesions in HHT patients. The sensitivity and specificity of thin-section CT for pulmonary AVMs are each approximately 80% (see Fig. 8-21). Tiny AVMs that may have a lower risk for paradoxical shunting can be missed. Thin-section noncontrast scans, as well as CTA, allow accurate planning for therapy. Contrast-enhanced 3-D MRA can also be used for evaluation of these patients. With both CT and MRA, great care (using inline filters) must be observed during insertion of the peripheral intravenous catheter and injection of contrast to avoid introduction of particulate debris or air bubbles.

Pulmonary angiography for pulmonary AVM is performed to confirm the diagnosis before embolotherapy. Angiographic technique must be fastidious. Intravenous lines should be free of air bubbles and have particulate filters. Heparinization with

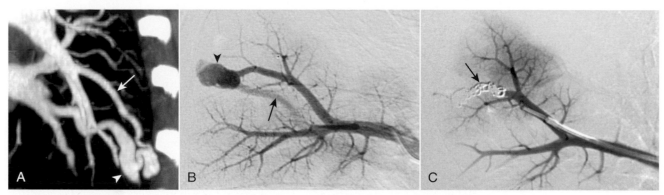

FIGURE 8-21. Pulmonary arteriovenous malformations (PAVM) in patients with hereditary hemorrhagic telangiectasia syndrome. **A,** Coronal thick multiplanar reformation (MPR) of pulmonary computed tomography angiogram showing a simple left lower lobe PAVM. A small aneurysm is seen just before the artery joins the vein. *(Arrow,* feeding artery; *arrowhead,* draining vein.) **B,** Selective right upper lobe pulmonary artery digital subtraction angiogram shows a PAVM *(arrowhead)* with a single enlarged feeding artery and early filling of a draining pulmonary vein *(arrow)* in a different patient than in **A.** Note again the typical aneurysm at the point of arteriovenous communication. **C,** Same patient as in **B.** Angiogram after successful coil occlusion *(arrow)* of the feeding artery.

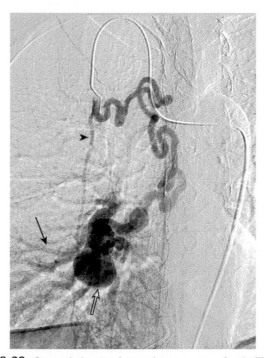

FIGURE 8-22. Congenital systemic to pulmonary artery fistula. The catheter is in the right internal mammary artery. An enlarged mediastinal artery fills an aneurysm *(open arrow)* just before joining the right lower lobe pulmonary artery *(black arrow).* The normal internal mammary artery *(arrowhead)* can be seen distal to the artery supplying the fistula. The patient was asymptomatic, but the aneurysm was increasing in size.

a bolus of 3000-5000 U after introduction of the catheter provides a measure of security against thrombus formation in or around the catheter. All catheter and guidewire manipulations should be conducted in a manner that prevents air from entering the catheter, such as submersion of the catheter hub in a saline-filled bowl during wire exchanges. Frequent catheter flushing with bubble-free flush solution is a critical point of technique.

Patients with pulmonary lesions are generally young and nervous about their diagnosis, factors that result in a hyperdynamic state. Pulmonary angiography in this population may require higher flow rates (30-35 mL/sec for 2 seconds) than the typical older patient with thromboembolic disease. Complete

angiography with multiple views of both lungs should be obtained to identify all pulmonary vascular lesions. Small AVMs may be missed at CT, and detection at angiography is important when planning long-term follow-up. AVMs are identifiable by one or more large feeding arteries and a large draining vein that opacifies before the remainder of the pulmonary veins. The actual arteriovenous communication is frequently saccular or aneurysmal in appearance.

The therapy of the majority of simple and complex pulmonary AVMs is embolization. In the past, only AVMs with feeding pulmonary arteries that were 3 mm or greater in diameter were embolized, because these were thought to be the lesions most likely to permit paradoxical emboli. More recent practice has been to embolize any AVM that can be catheterized, because even small lesions can lead to stroke. The intended site of occlusion is the feeding artery, not the actual fistula or the outflow vein. Long guiding catheters are used to stabilize the system in the pulmonary artery (see Fig. 8-21). After selection of the feeding artery, hand injection of contrast in multiple views may be necessary to define the anatomy. The guiding catheter is then advanced as close to the actual shunt as possible. Occlusion of the feeding artery can be accomplished with coils or detachable plugs. The choice of the embolic agent depends on the dimensions of the artery to be occluded, the ability to deliver the embolic device to the target location, and operator preference. The occluding devices should have a diameter at least 20% larger than the target vessel to avoid becoming paradoxical emboli themselves (see Fig. 4-38). The first coil or plug should be relatively large and placed close to the shunt in the feeding artery. A technique for secure placement of the first coil is to anchor the first centimeter or two in a small side branch of the feeding artery near the fistula. As the coil is deployed, the delivery catheter is backed into the feeding artery so that that majority of the coil is delivered in this location. Additional coils or plugs more closely sized to the artery are then deposited until there is no longer filling of the shunt.

Complications of embolization are rare, but include systemic embolization of a coil (<1%), air embolus to the right coronary artery (<1%), and stroke. Many patients have transient pleural pain and fever following embolization. Recanalization after embolization occurs in up to 20% of patients. Combined with the slow progressive enlargement of small AVMs over time, this mandates lifelong follow-up for patients.

▬ PULMONARY SEQUESTRATION

Pulmonary sequestration is a portion of lung that either has no connection to the bronchi or pulmonary arteries, or derives its major blood supply from an aberrant systemic artery (Fig. 8-23).

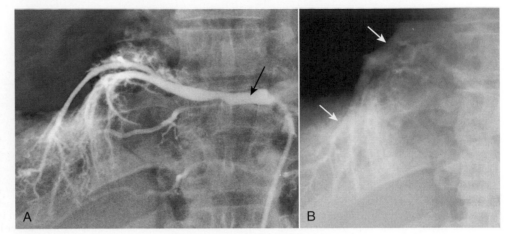

Figure 8-23. Angiographic findings of intralobar pulmonary sequestration. **A,** Selective injection of an anomalous large artery *(arrow)* arising from the distal thoracic aorta opacifies a portion of right lower lobe lung parenchyma. **B,** Later image from the same injection shows filling of pulmonary veins *(arrows)*.

When present, this artery typically originates from the distal descending thoracic or the upper abdominal aorta. Sequestrations are either contained within the pleura of the normal lung (intralobar) or have their own separate pleura (extralobar). Intralobar sequestrations drain to the pulmonary veins, are usually found in adults, and are more common than extralobar sequestration. Extralobar sequestration is found in children, is less common than the intralobar variety, and drains to the systemic veins. Both types of sequestration occur more commonly at the left lung base. Bilateral sequestration is rare. Patients may be asymptomatic but commonly present with hemoptysis, recurrent infection, or chest pain.

Sequestration appears as a mass lesion on chest radiographs. Chest CT may reveal a mass, a cystic lesion, or a cavitation. Pulmonary CTA is an excellent modality for evaluating suspected pulmonary sequestration. Angiography is occasionally required to conclusively demonstrate the blood supply to the abnormal lung tissue. Pulmonary angiography, aortography, and selective injection of the aberrant arterial supply should be performed. Although the traditional therapy of sequestration is surgical resection, embolization alone has been reported with success. Coil embolization of the feeding arteries results in infarction of the sequestration in approximately 75% of patients. In neonates, embolization can be performed via the umbilical artery.

◼ PULMONARY ARTERY TUMORS

Primary malignant pulmonary artery tumors are rare, accounting for fewer than 1% of thoracic tumors. These are usually sarcomatous lesions, arising from elements of the pulmonary artery (Box 8-6). The tumors commonly occur in a central location, but can be multifocal. Pulmonary artery invasion by adjacent tumor can also occur with bronchogenic carcinoma, germ-cell tumors, and other mediastinal malignancies. The prognosis of primary and secondary pulmonary artery tumors is poor.

Patients may be asymptomatic when the mass is nonobstructive or slowly enlarging. These lesions may be identified incidentally during evaluation of suspected thoracic malignancy or pulmonary embolism. More often, patients have several months of nonspecific complaints such as cough and progressive dyspnea. Large central masses may obstruct the main pulmonary artery outflow, resulting in hypoxia, syncope, and right heart failure.

The CT and MR findings of a primary pulmonary artery tumor are an intraluminal mass that may partially or completely obstruct the lumen that often has some enhancement and may demonstrate uptake on positron emission tomography (PET) scan (Fig. 8-24). Enhancement is a critical distinguishing feature between a mass and a chronic bland embolus, which does not enhance but which can be mildly PET avid. Secondary involvement of the pulmonary arteries by a primary mediastinal or lung

---

Box 8-6. Primary Pulmonary Artery Tumors

Rhabdomyosarcoma
Angiosarcoma
Malignant fibrous histiocytoma
Malignant mesenchymoma
Fibrosarcoma
Myxosarcoma
Liposarcoma
Chondrosarcoma
Osteosarcoma
Spindle cell
Undifferentiated

---

tumor is usually easily determined based on cross-sectional imaging findings. Angiography demonstrates intraluminal filling defects, frequently with a lobulated contour. Intravascular biopsy can be performed to obtain a tissue diagnosis before surgery (see Fig. 8-24).

Treatment is with surgery, systemic chemotherapy, and radiation. Mean survival is about 3 years for patients undergoing combined therapy. Stent placement to relieve obstructive symptoms can be beneficial as palliative therapy.

◼ PULMONARY ARTERY ANEURYSMS AND PSEUDOANEURYSMS

There are numerous etiologies of pulmonary artery aneurysms and pseudoaneurysms (PSA) (Box 8-7). The clinical presentation and course vary with the etiology. The risk of rupture probably increases with size, but clear guidelines for intervention have not been formulated. Acute dissection can occur in aneurysmal pulmonary arteries in patients with chronic pulmonary artery hypertension.

Aneurysms are often identified incidentally during evaluation of unrelated thoracic diseases (Fig. 8-25). The presence of a large draining vein suggests AVM as the etiology (see Fig. 8-21). Location of the aneurysm (central vs. peripheral), the presence of calcification, and multiplicity can be clues to the underlying cause. Hemoptysis is a typical acute presenting symptom, particularly with PSAs and mycotic aneurysms. When the infectious etiology is tuberculosis, the lesion is termed a *Rasmussen aneurysm*.

The most commonly encountered pulmonary artery PSAs are iatrogenic, usually related to flow-directed balloon-tipped catheters placed for hemodynamic monitoring in acutely ill patients (Fig. 8-26). Although the balloons are made from compliant materials, inflation in a small pulmonary artery branch can lead to rupture of the vessel and a PSA. Alternatively, the catheter itself

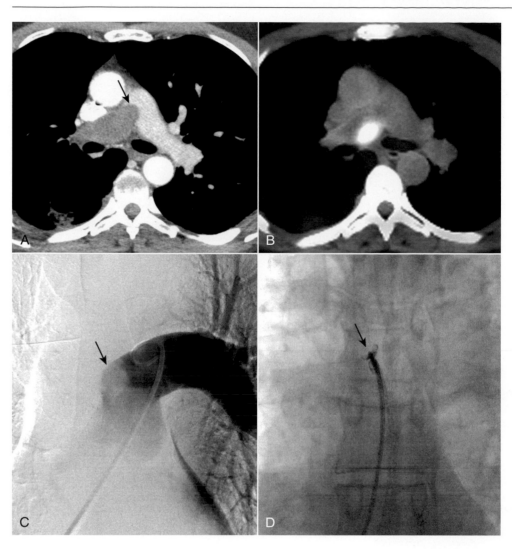

FIGURE 8-24. Pulmonary artery sarcoma (spindle cell). **A,** Axial computed tomography image after administration of contrast shows a mass obstructing and expanding the right pulmonary artery and extending into the main pulmonary artery *(arrow).* **B,** Fusion positron emission tomography image shows intensive activity in the posterior portion of the mass. **C,** Pulmonary angiogram shows obstruction of the right pulmonary artery with a bulky filling defect *(arrow)* protruding from the right pulmonary artery consistent with a tumor. **D,** An intravascular biopsy of the mass was performed with grasping forceps *(arrow).*

Box 8-7. Pulmonary Artery Aneurysms

TRUE
Chronic pulmonary hypertension
Pulmonic valve stenosis
Behçet disease
Takayasu arteritis
Congenital
Hughes Stovin syndrome
Marfan syndrome
Arteriovenous malformation

FALSE
Infection
• Endocarditis
• Septic emboli
• Necrotizing pneumonia
• Tuberculosis
Trauma
• Penetrating
• Deceleration
• Swan-Ganz catheter perforation

---

may perforate the wall of the artery. The estimated incidence is as high as 1 in 1600 insertions. Acute hemoptysis is the typical presentation, occurring at the presumed time of arterial injury. Hemoptysis may be massive, life-threatening, and recurrent. Pulmonary artery hypertension, anticoagulation, and concurrent cardiopulmonary bypass contribute to the severity of the presentation. Untreated, the mortality approaches 20% from pulmonary bleeding, but is higher overall owing to underlying illness.

Chest radiographic findings of pulmonary PSA vary over time. Initially, a focal area of consolidation consistent with pulmonary hemorrhage may be seen. Over time, resolution of the hemorrhage may reveal a new lung mass. Retrospective review of serial radiographs may identify a Swan-Ganz catheter in a peripheral location that correlates with the new mass.

Pulmonary CTA can show a focal enhancing lesion surrounded by pulmonary parenchymal hemorrhage and bronchial blood. However, when this diagnosis is highly likely, proceeding directly to pulmonary angiography may be warranted because this provides an opportunity for definitive treatment. Frequently these patients are quite ill with multiple medical problems, so the number of stops in the radiology department should be kept to a minimum. Pulmonary angiography should be performed in the usual fashion.

Symptomatic peripheral pulmonary artery aneurysms, both true and false, can be safely embolized in a manner similar to AVMs. The location of the aneurysm determines the feasibility of embolization, which increases as the aneurysm becomes more peripheral. Large central aneurysms are often too big for current

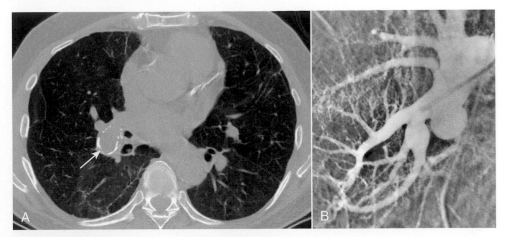

FIGURE 8-25. Pulmonary artery aneurysms in an adult with a history of tricuspid valvular bacterial endocarditis as a child. **A,** Axial computed tomography scan without contrast windowed to show a calcified right pulmonary artery aneurysm *(arrow).* **B,** Selective right pulmonary angiogram shows multiple aneurysms.

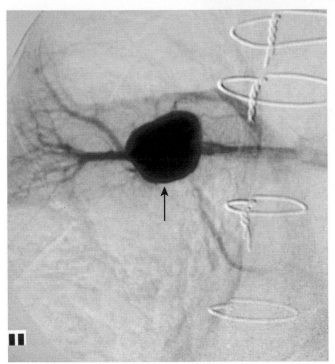

FIGURE 8-26. Pulmonary artery pseudoaneurysm due to a Swan-Ganz catheter placed in the operating room during coronary artery surgery. The patient developed intermittent massive hemoptysis in the postoperative period. Selective injection of the right upper lobe pulmonary artery shows a large pseudoaneurysm *(arrow),* which was successfully embolized with coils.

> ### Box 8-8. Conditions Leading to Bronchial Artery Hypertrophy
>
> Cystic fibrosis
> Chronic infection
> - Fungal
> - Tuberculosis
> - Pneumonia
> - Abscess
>
> Chronic granulomatous disease
> - Sarcoidosis
> - Wegener granulomatosis
>
> Bronchiectasis
> Congenital pulmonary stenosis/atresia with systemic pulmonary collaterals
> Acquired pulmonary artery stenosis/occlusion
> Tumor (rare)
> Systemic to pulmonary arterioarterial malformation

embolic materials or involve major proximal branches. Unlike embolization of AVMs, the risk of paradoxical embolization is low. However, fragile vasculitic aneurysms and PSAs are more prone to rupture during manipulation. Once the aneurysm is identified and localized, the pigtail catheter is exchanged for a guiding catheter. A selective catheter should then be used to deposit coils or plugs in the feeding artery. Because the pulmonary arteries are essentially end arteries, there is no concern for retrograde perfusion of the aneurysm. In some cases, coils can be gently packed into the aneurysm to promote thrombosis. Occlusion of the aneurysm is achieved in the majority of cases, with cessation of bleeding.

▬ BRONCHIAL ARTERY BLEEDING

Hypertrophy of the bronchial arteries usually occurs as a result of chronic inflammatory processes in the lung (Box 8-8). Bronchial

and parenchymal inflammatory processes derive their blood supply from the bronchial arteries rather than the pulmonary arteries (see Fig. 8-5). Chronic inflammation and hyperemia leads to enlargement of bronchial arteries and recruitment of collaterals from other systemic thoracic arteries (see Fig. 8-7 and Box 8-1). Pulmonary artery occlusion can also lead to bronchial and collateral artery enlargement due to systemic to pulmonary shunting (see Fig. 8-6).

Patients with enlarged bronchial arteries present with bleeding from the hypertrophied submucosal vessels. The triggering event for bleeding is frequently infection with mucosal inflammation and erosion. Patients typically can sense and localize the onset of bleeding. Endobronchial blood is very irritating to the airway, leading to coughing productive of large clots intermixed with sputum. Patients should lie with the source lung dependent during acute bleeding.

The definition of massive hemoptysis differs from that employed in most other types of arterial bleeding. Airway compromise and aspiration of blood are of greater risk to the patient than exsanguination. Hemoptysis of more than 300 mL of blood in 24 hours is therefore considered massive. Intervention should not be delayed until the patient has a measurable drop in hematocrit or hypotension.

Patients with suspected bronchial artery bleeding require immediate evaluation. A chest radiograph followed by emergency bronchoscopy should be obtained when patients have unexplained massive hemoptysis for the first time. Selective mainstem intubation or a bifurcated double-barrel endotracheal tube may be necessary to protect the non-bleeding lung. Correction of any underlying coagulopathy is essential. Exclusion of any alternative diagnoses is important before proceeding to angiography and embolization (Box 8-9).

CTA and MRA have no role in acutely bleeding patients, but can be very informative in stable situations. The presence of abnormal bronchial arteries and the nature of the underlying pulmonary pathology can be evaluated.

In the acute situation, angiography is performed for both diagnosis and therapy (by embolization) of bronchial artery bleeding. Airway protection is a major concern in actively bleeding patients because they must lie on their back during the procedure and be sedated. In addition to the usual risks of angiography and embolization, patients should be counseled on the risk (albeit low) of paralysis from inadvertent embolization of a spinal artery. Knowledge of the suspected side of bleeding (based on prior CT scan, bronchoscopy, the patient's history) is useful to direct the study. The angiographic technique is described earlier.

Hypertrophied bronchial arteries characteristically are tortuous with numerous branches to the lung and hilum, and contain rapid flow (see Fig. 8-5). When abnormal, these vessels are so large that they are readily visible from an aortogram (normal bronchial arteries are small and difficult to see). A parenchymal blush, as well as shunting to the pulmonary arteries and pulmonary veins through the parenchyma, may be seen, but extravasation is rare even in bleeding patients. Selective injection of the subclavian artery,

thyrocervical trunk, internal mammary artery, anterior chest wall arteries (e.g., long thoracic artery), intercostals arteries, and phrenic arteries may be necessary in patients with extensive pulmonary pathology, prior embolizations, or prior surgery. Bronchial, intercostal, and thyrocervical angiograms must be carefully inspected for branches to the anterior spinal artery. A normal diameter bronchial artery with absent parenchymal staining or shunting essentially excludes a systemic arterial etiology of hemoptysis unless the patient has a lung tumor (see Fig. 8-4). When an arterial source cannot be identified, pulmonary angiography should be considered in patients with cavitary lung lesions or a history of recent Swan-Ganz catheterization.

Embolization is the accepted therapy for patients with recurrent massive hemoptysis that is not responding to conservative measures. The risks of embolization unique to the bronchial arteries is the potential for spinal cord ischemic due to inadvertent embolization of an anterior spinal artery arising from a bronchial artery or other branch. This occurs in far less than 1% of patients. Pulmonary infarction, myocardial infarction (from aberrant communications to the coronary artery) stroke, and pericardial pain are extremely rare.

The goal of embolization of bronchial arteries (or hypertrophied collateral arteries) in patients with hemoptysis from benign disease is to decrease blood supply without infarcting tissue (Fig. 8-27). Owing to the chronic nature of the underlying pathology, embolization often controls the acute episode of bleeding but is rarely definitive. Particulate agents between 200 and 700 μm should be delivered through a selective catheter (frequently a microcatheter) that is securely placed in the artery. Glue and Onyx can also be used. When it is necessary to embolize a bronchial artery that gives rise to a spinal artery, the catheter should be advanced beyond the critical branch, and large particles (500-700 μm) should be used. The particles should be injected with fluoroscopic monitoring to avoid reflux into the aorta or critical side branches. The endpoint of embolization is stasis of flow in the target vessel. Alcohol, Ethiodol, and fine powders are contraindicated. Coils should not be used in the ostium of the artery because repeat embolization may be necessary. In certain vessels (e.g., internal mammary artery), placement of a coil or Gelfoam plug distal to the origin of the collateral branches to the bronchial arteries redirects the flow of embolic agent and prevents nontarget embolization of abdominal or chest wall soft tissues.

Technical and clinical success in embolization for hemoptysis depends on successful selective catheterization of the bronchial blood supply. The first embolization procedure usually has the best results, with greater than 90% technical and clinical success. Each subsequent procedure becomes more difficult and riskier as smaller and smaller collateral branches from other thoracic arteries are recruited. More intensive selective catheterization is required for repeat embolizations. The long-term success varies with the underlying etiology, but rebleeding is frequent in patients with

---

Box 8-9. Differential Diagnosis of Hemoptysis

PULMONARY
Bronchial artery (e.g., chronic inflammatory processes)
Pulmonary infarct
Pulmonary artery pseudoaneurysm
Pulmonary artery arteriovenous malformation
Malignancy
Mitral stenosis
Autoimmune (e.g., Goodpasture syndrome, Wegener granulomatosis)
Pneumonia
Aortopulmonary fistula

OROPHARYNGEAL
Inflammatory
Trauma (intubation)
Malignancy
Carotid blowout
Aspirated from nasal airway (e.g., epistaxis)

GASTROINTESTINAL
Aspirated from upper GI tract

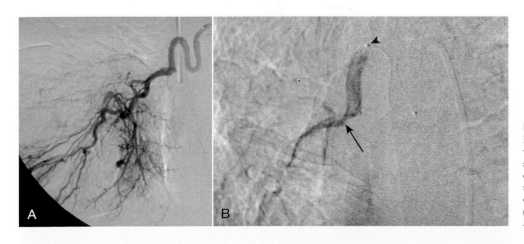

FIGURE 8-27. Embolization of a right lower lobe bronchial artery in a patient with cystic fibrosis. **A,** Digital subtraction angiogram before embolization shows an enlarged artery with dense parenchymal stain. **B,** Selective injection following embolization through a microcatheter *(arrowhead)* with Ivalon particles (300-500 μm) shows stasis of flow *(arrow).*

ongoing chronic inflammatory processes. Ultimately, pulmonary resection may be required, but it can have a high mortality owing to dense vascular pleural adhesions.

Patients with primary and metastatic cancer to the lung can present with bronchial bleeding. The bronchial arteries are often not hypertrophied in these patients, making embolization more challenging. Patients with intractable bleeding should be considered for embolization as a palliative measure. The transcatheter chemoembolization of unresectable lung cancer, through either pulmonary arteries, bronchial arteries, or both, is performed in some centers.

■■■ SUGGESTED READINGS

Abe T, Mori K, Shiigai M, et al. Systemic arterial supply to the normal basal segments of the left lower lobe of the lung—treatment by coil embolization—and a literature review. *Cardiovasc Intervent Radiol.* 2011;34:S117-S121.

Banovac F, Buckley DC, Kuo WT, et al. Reporting standards for endovascular treatment of pulmonary embolism. *J Vasc Interv Radiol.* 2010;21:44-53.

Blackmon SH, Rice DC, Correa AM, et al. Management of primary pulmonary artery sarcomas. *Ann Thorac Surg.* 2009;87:977-984.

Bounameaux H, Perrier A, Righini M. Diagnosis of venous thromboembolism: an update. *Vasc Med.* 2010;15:399-406.

Bussières JS. Iatrogenic pulmonary artery rupture. *Curr Opin Anaesthesiol.* 2007;20:48-52.

Castañer E, Gallardo X, Rimola J, et al. Congenital and acquired pulmonary artery anomalies in the adult: radiologic overview. *Radiographics.* 2006;26:349-371.

Chun JY, Morgan R, Belli AM. Radiological management of hemoptysis: a comprehensive review of diagnostic imaging and bronchial arterial embolization. *Cardiovasc Intervent Radiol.* 2010;33:240-250.

Daliri A, Probst NH, Jobst B, et al. Acta Radio. *Bronchial artery embolization in patients with hemoptysis including follow-up.* 2011;52:143-147.

Grosse C, Grosse A. CT findings in diseases associated with pulmonary hypertension: a current review. *Radiographics.* 2010;30:1753-1777.

Henzler T, Barraza Jr JM, Nance Jr JW, et al. CT imaging of acute pulmonary embolism. *J Cardiovasc Comput Tomogr.* 2011;5:3-11.

Jaff MR, McMurtry MS, Archer SL, et al. Management of massive and submassive pulmonary embolism, iliofemoral deep vein thrombosis, and chronic thromboembolic pulmonary hypertension: a scientific statement from the American Heart Association. *Circulation.* 2011;123:1788-1830.

Kadir S. Pulmonary angiography. In: Kadir S, ed. *Diagnostic Angiography.* Philadelphia: WB Saunders; 1986:584-616.

Iva SP. Bronchial artery embolization. *Tech Vasc Interv Radiol.* 2009;12:130-138.

Kearon C, Akl EA, Comerota AJ, et al. Antithrombotic therapy for VTE disease: Antithrombotic Therapy and Prevention of Thrombosis, 9th ed: American College of Chest Physicians Evidence-Based Clinical Practice Guidelines. *Chest.* 2012;141:e419S-494S.

Khattar RS, Fox DJ, Alty JE, Arora A. Pulmonary artery dissection: an emerging cardiovascular complication in surviving patients with chronic pulmonary hypertension. *Heart.* 2005;91:142-145.

Kuo WT, Gould MK, Louie JD, et al. Catheter-directed therapy for the treatment of massive pulmonary embolism: systematic review and meta-analysis of modern techniques. *J Vasc Interv Radiol.* 2009;20:1431-1440.

Lee KH, Sung KB, Yoon HK, et al. Transcatheter arterial embolization of pulmonary sequestration in neonates: long-term follow-up results. *J Vasc Interv Radiol.* 2003;14:363-367.

Ley S, Grünig E, Kiely DG, van Beek E, Wild J. Computed tomography and magnetic resonance imaging of pulmonary hypertension: Pulmonary vessels and right ventricle. *J Magn Reson Imaging.* 2010;32:1313-1324.

Nchimi A, Ghaye B, Noukoua CT, et al. Incidence and distribution of lower extremity deep venous thrombosis at indirect computed tomography venography in patients suspected of pulmonary embolism. *Thromb Haemost.* 2007;97:566-572.

Nguyen ET, Silva CI, Seely JM, et al. Pulmonary artery aneurysms and pseudoaneurysms in adults: findings at CT and radiography. *AJR Am J Roentgenol.* 2007;188:W126-W134.

Pelage JP, El Hajjam M, Lagrange C, et al. Pulmonary artery interventions: an overview. *Radiographics.* 2005;25:1653-1667.

Piazza G, Goldhaber SZ. Chronic thromboembolic pulmonary hypertension. *N Engl J Med.* 2011;364:351-360.

Ramsey J, Amari M, Kantrow SP. Pulmonary vasculitis: clinical presentation, differential diagnosis, and management. *Curr Rheumatol Rep.* 2010;12:420-428.

Sadigh G, Kelly AM, Cronin P. Challenges, controversies, and hot topics in pulmonary embolism imaging. *AJR Am J Roentgenol.* 2011;196:497-515.

Stein PD, Chenevert TL, Fowler SE, et al. PIOPED III Investigators. Gadolinium-enhanced magnetic resonance angiography for pulmonary embolism: a multicenter prospective study (PIOPED III). *Ann Intern Med.* 2010;152:434-443.

Stein PD, Fowler SE, Goodman LR, et al. PIOPED II Investigators. Multidetector computed tomography for acute pulmonary embolism. *N Engl J Med.* 2006;354:2317-2327.

The PIOPED Investigators. Value of the ventilation/perfusion scan in acute pulmonary embolism: results of the prospective investigation of pulmonary embolism diagnosis (PIOPED). *JAMA.* 1990;263:2753-2759.

Trerotola SO, Pyeritz RE. PAVM embolization: an update. *AJR Am J Roentgenol.* 2010;195:837-845.

CHAPTER 9

Thoracic Aorta

John A. Kaufman, MD, MS, FSIR, FCIRSE

Thoracic aortic diseases can be among the most challenging vascular problems to manage. The organs that are supplied directly by this segment of aorta (heart, brain, and spine) are intolerant of ischemia for more than a few minutes. Flow disturbances in the aorta impact the entire body. Surgical access requires a thoracotomy or sternotomy, and often cardiopulmonary bypass. The high morbidity of open repair of thoracic aortic pathology makes endovascular approaches appealing. Imaging and percutaneous intervention in the thoracic aorta is one of the most exciting areas of interventional radiology.

NORMAL ANATOMY

The thoracic aorta begins at the heart, at the level of the aortic valve. The thoracic aorta becomes the abdominal aorta at the diaphragm, just proximal to the celiac artery origin, usually at the T12 vertebral body. The thoracic aorta is divided into ascending, transverse, and descending portions (Fig. 9-1). The ascending aorta extends from the aortic valve to the origin of the first great vessel, usually the innominate (also known as brachiocephalic) artery. The transverse aorta is also termed the *aortic arch,* the segment that contains the origins of the great vessels. The descending thoracic aorta begins just distal to the left subclavian artery, ending at the diaphragm. The descending thoracic aorta is fixed adjacent to the spine, whereas the ascending aorta and arch have limited mobility.

The normal area of the aortic valve is 2.5-3.5 cm^2. There are usually three valve leaflets, named for the coronary artery that originates in the coronary sinuses (sinuses of Valsalva) above each leaflet; the right, left, and noncoronary. The coronary sinuses have a characteristic slight bulge in contour (see Fig. 9-1). Immediately above the coronary sinuses the ascending aorta is typically 2.5-3.5 cm in diameter. The transverse and descending thoracic aorta are frequently slightly narrower than the ascending aorta, with diameters rarely greater than 2.5 cm in normal individuals.

The major noncoronary branches of the thoracic aorta are (in order) the innominate artery, the left common carotid artery, and the left subclavian artery. The innominate artery bifurcates into the right common carotid and right subclavian arteries. Rarely (<1%) a small artery to the isthmus of the thyroid (the thyroid ima) may arise from the aortic arch. This vessel arises more commonly from the innominate artery (3%) or right common carotid artery (1%) (see Fig. 5-2).

The proximal descending thoracic aorta frequently has a slight bulge in contour along the inner anterior surface just distal to the left subclavian artery, termed a *ductus bump* (see Fig. 9-1). This is

the location of the fetal ductus arteriosus, the structure that connects the fetal pulmonary circulation to the aorta. Rarely, a small portion of the ductus remains patent in adults, resulting in an outpouching of the aorta at this point, termed a *ductus diverticulum"* (Fig. 9-2). This structure invariably has a broad mouth and totally smooth walls, important features to consider when evaluating patients for aortic trauma.

The descending thoracic aorta gives origin to a number of small, but clinically important arteries. These vessels supply the bronchi, esophagus, intercostal muscles, and the spinal cord. The bronchial arteries are discussed in Chapter 8 (see Figs. 8-4 and 8-5). The intercostal arteries arise from the posterolateral aspect of the thoracic aorta from the level of the T3 vertebral body to T12 (see Fig. 9-1). The arteries to the first through the third intercostal spaces usually arise from a pair of common trunks on each side of the aorta, termed the *supreme intercostals arteries.* From T4 to T12 each intercostal space has its own pair of arteries. These vessels have multiple anastomoses, including the internal mammary arteries anteriorly and the chest wall arteries laterally. Less constant are anastomoses to the anterior spinal and bronchial arteries.

The arterial supply to the thoracic portion of the spinal cord is derived from the upper and lower thoracic aorta. The anterior spinal artery at the T4-T5 level is variably supplied from intercostal and bronchial arteries. The anterior spinal artery at the level of the T6-T12 vertebral bodies, the artery of Adamkiewicz, originates from the intercostal arteries (usually the left) in 75% of individuals at these levels (Fig. 9-3). Spinal arteries have a characteristic appearance with a hairpin turn and a midline course.

There are many important variants of thoracic aortic arch anatomy, usually involving branching patterns of the great vessels and location of the descending thoracic aorta in relation to the spine. Familiarity with these variants is crucial to avoid diagnostic errors and therapeutic misadventures. A brief review of the embryology of the thoracic aorta makes understanding the variations easy. The thoracic aorta is derived from the embryonic primitive ventral and dorsal aortae that are connected by six paired branchial arches (Fig. 9-4). Between the sixth and eighth weeks of life, specific arches appear and regress, resulting in a single aorta with three major noncoronary branches. The first arch forms the maxillary and external carotid arteries. The second arch forms the stapedial arteries. The third arch forms the carotid arteries, while the fourth arch forms the aortic arch and the proximal subclavian arteries. The fifth arch is present in only 50% of fetuses and regresses completely. The sixth arch forms the pulmonary

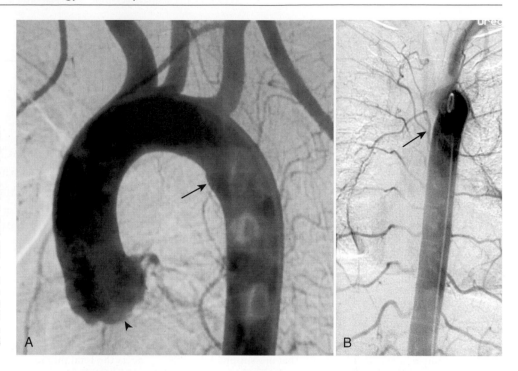

FIGURE 9-1. Normal thoracic aorta. **A,** Digital subtraction angiogram (DSA) of the aorta in the left anterior oblique (LAO) projection with the catheter positioned just above the aortic valve *(arrowhead)*. The ascending aorta, transverse arch, great-vessel origins, and proximal descending aorta are well visualized in this projection. The subtle bulge in the proximal descending thoracic aorta is a *ductus bump (arrow)*. Note the smooth contours. (The oval lucencies projected over the distal aorta are subtraction artifacts from the spine.) **B,** DSA aortogram in the anteroposterior (AP) projection with the catheter positioned just distal to the left subclavian artery. The paired intercostal arteries are well visualized, with the arteries to the upper ribs arising from common trunks *(arrow)*.

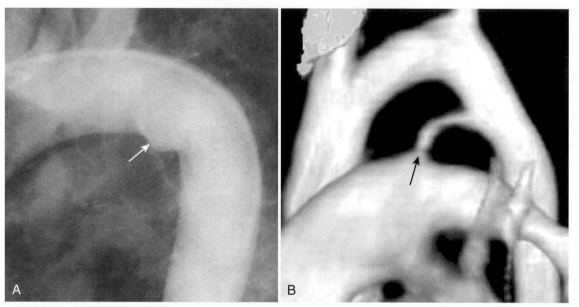

FIGURE 9-2. The ductus region of the thoracic aorta. **A,** In comparison to Figure 9-1A, a more defined, focal bulge is termed a *ductus diverticulum (arrow)*. Again note the smooth contours and lack of acute angles. **B,** Patent ductus arteriosus *(arrow)* seen on volume rendering of a computed tomography angiogram.

arteries. All of the anomalies of aortic branching can be traced to variations of branchial arch regression.

The most common variant (20%) of aortic arch anatomy is the left common carotid artery arising from the innominate artery ("bovine arch") (Table 9-1). Other frequent variants include direct origin of the left vertebral artery from the arch between the left common carotid and left subclavian arteries, and aberrant origin of the right subclavian distal to the left subclavian artery (Fig. 9-5). Aberrant right subclavian arteries lie posterior to the esophagus in 80% of patients, between the esophagus and trachea in 15%, and anterior to both in 5%. This vessel is more prone to aneurysm formation than normally located right subclavian arteries (see Fig. 6-22). Similarly, in a patient with a right-sided aortic arch, the left subclavian artery may arise aberrantly from the descending thoracic aorta.

The arch and descending thoracic aorta lie to the right of the spine in fewer than 1% of individuals (Fig. 9-6). This anomaly is the result of regression of left-sided rather than right-sided branchial arches. Most healthy adults with right-sided arches have variant great-vessel anatomy, commonly an aberrant left subclavian artery. When the branching pattern of the right sided arch is normal ("mirror image"), there is a 90% probability of a severe congenital cardiac defect.

Bilateral ("duplicated") aortic arches are a rare variant that result from failure of regression of branchial arches on both sides (Fig. 9-7). The arches may be equal or disproportionate in size, with variable great-vessel branching patterns. The arch segments arise from a single ascending aorta, pass lateral to both sides of the trachea and esophagus, and join posteriorly to form the descending thoracic aorta. Duplicated arches account for more

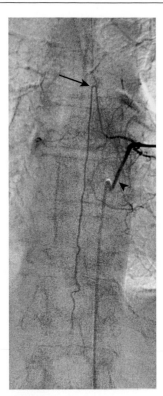

FIGURE 9-3. Artery of Adamkiewicz *(arrow)* seen on selective digital subtraction angiogram of the left T9 intercostal artery *(arrowhead)*. Note the classic hairpin turn in the spinal artery.

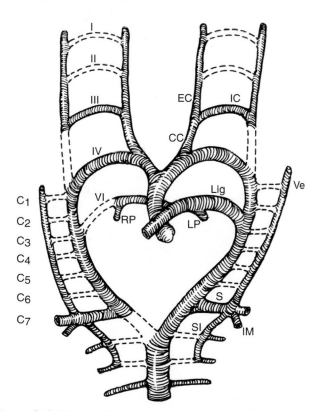

FIGURE 9-4. Diagram illustrating the development of the thoracic aorta, great vessels, and pulmonary arteries. I, II, III, IV, VI, Paired branchial arches between the ventral and dorsal aorta; C1-C7, cervical intersegmental arteries; CC, common carotid artery; EC, external carotid artery; IC, internal carotid artery; IM, internal mammary artery; Lig, ligamentum arteriosus; LP, left pulmonary artery; RP, right pulmonary artery; S, subclavian artery; SI, superior intercostal artery; Ve, vertebral artery. (From Kadir S. *Atlas of Normal and Variant Anatomy.* Philadelphia: WB Saunders, 1991, with permission.)

TABLE 9-1 Aortic Arch Variants

Variant	Incidence
Common origin innominate and left common carotid arteries	20%
Left vertebral arising from aorta *of which:*	5%
Between left common carotid and left subclavian artery	4%
Distal to left subclavian artery	<1%
Common origin carotid arteries	1%
Aberrant right subclavian artery (left arch)	1%
Right aortic arch *of which:*	<0.1%
Mirror image	0.06%
Aberrant left subclavian/other variation great vessel origin	0.03%
Duplicated arch	<0.1%
Cervical arch (right more common than left)	<0.1%
Coarctation	<0.1%

than 40% of all cases of thoracic vascular rings. Found most often in infancy or childhood, symptoms include recurrent pneumonia, stridor, apnea, choking, and dysphagia due to compression of the encircled trachea and esophagus. Other etiologies of vascular rings include right aortic arch with a left ligamentum arteriosum (25%), right aortic arch with anomalous innominate artery (17%), and pulmonary artery sling (5%).

Additional arch variants include a cervical arch, in which the aortic arch is derived from the third rather than the fourth branchial arch (Fig. 9-8). These arches are recognizable by their unusually high location in the chest, frequently in the apex of the hemithorax. Additionally, cervical arches tend to be somewhat ectatic and elongated, with associated anomalous great vessel origins.

▬ KEY COLLATERAL PATHWAYS

Obstructive lesions of the thoracic aorta are uncommon, but when present the collaterals are determined by the location of the lesion. In the unusual situation of coarctation of the aorta between the left common carotid and left subclavian artery origins, there is low or reversed flow in the left subclavian artery (see Coarctation below). The descending thoracic aorta also receives collateral supply from right subclavian artery branches through communication with mediastinal and intercostal arteries. The lower extremities receive blood via communication between the right internal mammary artery and the inferior epigastric artery in the anterior abdominal wall. The right subclavian artery and its branches can become quite enlarged in patients with longstanding distal arch coarctation.

The more common location for coarctation is the proximal descending thoracic aorta just beyond the left subclavian artery (Fig. 9-9). This results in hypertrophy of both subclavian arteries and their muscular branches. There is reversal of flow in intercostal arteries distal to the obstruction (usually beginning with the intercostal artery pair at T4), which are supplied from the internal mammary and other chest wall muscular arteries. In this situation, both internal mammary arteries supply the lower extremities via the epigastric arteries.

▬ IMAGING

Chest radiographs provide useful information about thoracic aortic anatomy and pathology. This is probably the only vascular bed

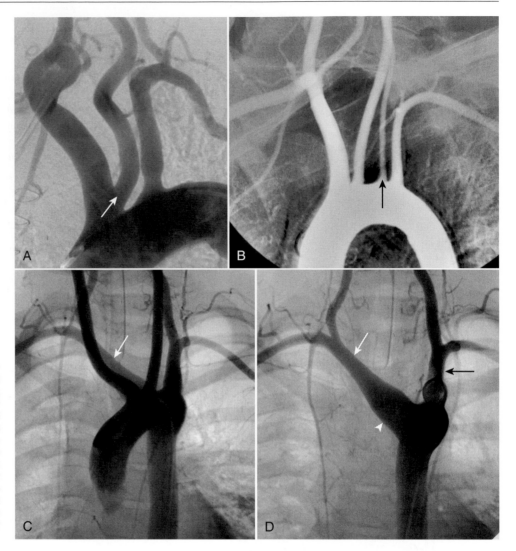

Figure 9-5. Variant anatomy of great-vessel origins. **A,** Bovine arch, with the left common carotid artery *(arrow)* arising from the brachiocephalic artery rather than the aortic arch. **B,** Origin of the left vertebral artery *(arrow)* directly from the aortic arch. **C,** Aberrant right subclavian artery *(arrow)* arising distal to the left subclavian artery. **D,** The same patient with the catheter positioned in the descending thoracic aorta. The right subclavian artery *(white arrow)* has a patulous origin *(arrowhead)* termed a *diverticulum of Kommerell*. The left subclavian artery *(black arrow)* is normal.

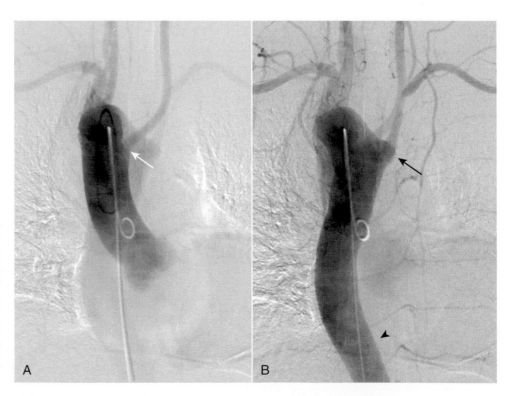

Figure 9-6. Digital subtraction angiogram in the anteroposterior projection of a patient with a right aortic arch and aberrant great vessel anatomy. **A,** Early image showing filling of the ascending thoracic aorta. The left common carotid artery (CCA) is the first branch *(white arrow)*, followed by the right CCA, right subclavian artery, and then the left subclavian artery. **B,** Later image showing the left subclavian artery origin *(black arrow)* as the last branch arising from the arch. The descending thoracic aorta *(arrowhead)* lies to the right of the spine.

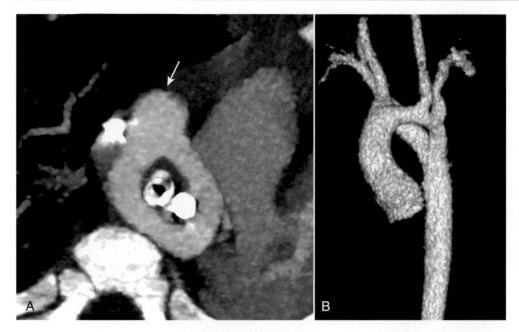

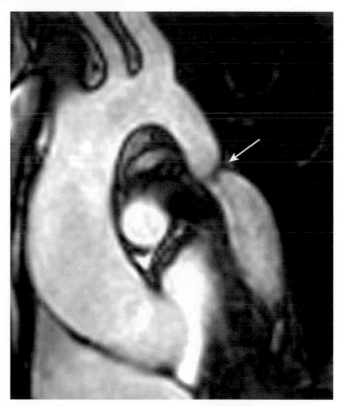

FIGURE 9-7. Duplicated arch in an infant demonstrated on contrast-enhanced computed tomography. **A,** Axial multiplanar reformat showing the ascending aorta *(arrow)* bifurcating into two arches that rejoin posteriorly. Endotracheal and nasogastric tubes show the trachea and esophagus surrounded by the vascular ring. **B,** Oblique three-dimensional volume rendering showing that each arch gives rise to a carotid and subclavian artery before coalescing into a single descending thoracic aorta.

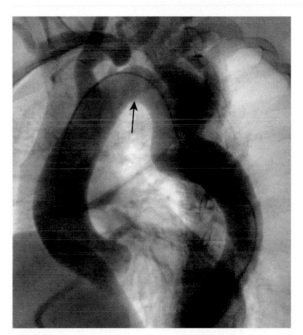

FIGURE 9-8. Cervical arch demonstrated on thoracic aortic angiogram in the left anterior oblique projection showing the elongated aorta *(arrow)* extending into the left lung apex.

FIGURE 9-9. Descending thoracic aortic coarctation. Oblique sagittal contrast-enhanced magnetic resonance angiogram shows the weblike coarctation *(arrow)* in the proximal descending thoracic aorta. See also Figure 9-32.

in which plain radiographs have an important role in imaging. Views should be obtained in both the anteroposterior (AP) and lateral projections, in full inspiration (Fig. 9-10). The location of the arch impression on the trachea is a clue to the relationship of the arch to the spine (the side of the impression indicates the side of the arch). The diameter of the aorta, presence of calcification, width of the mediastinum, deviation of mediastinal structures, and presence of pleural effusion should be evaluated. The bony structures should also be carefully inspected for evidence of prior surgery (e.g., sternal wires or rib resections), or enlarged collateral arteries (e.g., scalloping of the inferior margins of the lower ribs due to hypertrophied intercostals arteries in coarctation). As is always the case with imaging studies, comparison with old studies is crucial.

Computed tomography (CT)/CT angiography (CTA) is an excellent modality for evaluation of the thoracic aorta (Fig. 9-11). A high-quality CT scan is frequently sufficient for definitive diagnosis and planning of an intervention. Before injection of contrast, a noncontrast acquisition should almost always be obtained. This allows assessment for wall calcification, intramural hematoma, and other high-density lesions that may be obscured by the presence of contrast (see Intramural Hematoma later). The collimation for

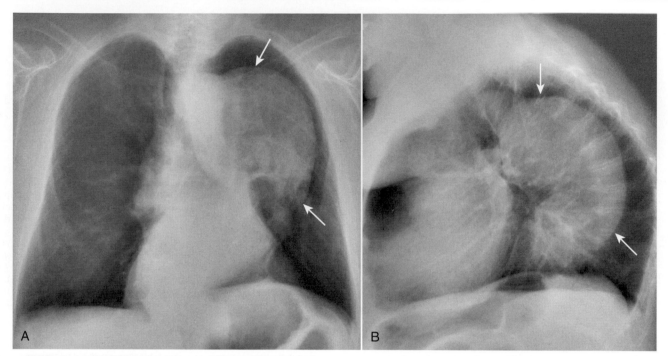

FIGURE 9-10. Chest radiograph in an older adult presenting with recurrent pneumonia. **A,** Anteroposterior view showing a large mass in the left chest *(arrows)* that displaces the trachea to the right and obscures the aortic arch. **B,** Lateral view of the same patient showing that the mass *(arrows)* is a large aneurysm of the descending thoracic aorta.

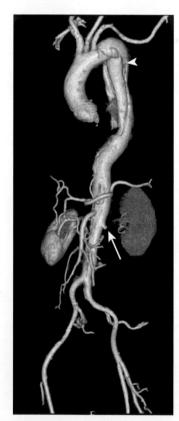

FIGURE 9-11. Oblique volume rendering of aortic computed tomography angiogram in patient with acute type B aortic dissection. The dissection plane can be seen in the proximal descending thoracic aorta *(arrowhead)*. There is acute thrombosis of the left renal artery *(arrowhead)* due to the dissection, with a markedly diminished left renal nephrogram compared to the right.

the noncontrast scan can be relatively thick in order to reduce time and radiation exposure. The contrast-enhanced scan should be performed with rapid injection of contrast (3-5 mL/sec for total volume of 80-120 mL), the arms raised over the patient's head, and with an appropriate scan delay. When using a peripheral intravenous access, injection from the right arm will decrease streak artifact from dense contrast in the left brachiocephalic vein. Collimation of less than 1 mm can be achieved with most scanners, which when combined with cardiac gating provides extremely detailed images (see Fig. 3-20). Careful inspection of other thoracic structures frequently yields important additional findings. Postprocessing is essential when evaluating tortuous or aneurysmal aortas.

Magnetic resonance (MR) of the thoracic aorta provides excellent anatomic (MR imaging, or MRI) and vascular (MR angiography, or MRA) images (Fig. 9-12; see also Fig. 9-9). Fast pulse sequences, cardiac gating, and breath-hold techniques optimize image quality. Anatomic images are acquired in orthogonal planes (axial, sagittal, and coronal), and in an oblique orientation through the arch. These images are essential for determining true aortic size, evaluating for pleural effusion, mediastinal hematoma, and other pathology. MRA is usually performed with a three-dimensional (3-D) fast-gradient echo acquisition and injection of gadolinium. The acquisition plane varies with the type of pathology and area of interest in the aorta, but generally a coronal slab is adequate. Slice thickness should be as thin as feasible in order to maximize resolution but without compromising anatomic coverage. As with CT, peripheral injection of contrast should be from the right upper extremity when possible. The absence of calcium on MR images is an advantage compared to CT, but artifact from metal remains a major limitation. In addition, certain patients, such as those with MRI-incompatible pacemakers, cannot undergo MR scans. Postprocessing is necessary to create angiographic views.

Ultrasound of the thoracic aorta can be performed with external (transthoracic) and internal (transesophageal) probes. Transthoracic ultrasound requires no patient preparation and, usually, no sedation. The ability to evaluate the distal arch and the descending thoracic aorta is limited owing to the distance from the anterior chest wall and surrounding lung. Insertion of transesophageal echocardiography (TEE) probes requires some patient preparation and sedation, but the ability to visualize the deeper aortic structures is greatly improved over transthoracic probes. Both studies are highly operator-dependent for acquisition of diagnostic images and require 30-45 minutes to complete.

Catheter angiography has a limited role in the diagnosis of thoracic aortic diseases (Table 9-2). The noninvasive modalities described have supplanted catheter angiography in most patients. Angiography is usually performed from a femoral approach, although the axillary artery can also be used. When using an axillary artery approach, the right should be chosen in patients with aortic dissection or when injections will be limited to the ascending aorta or arch. For catheter placement in the descending thoracic aorta only, the left axillary artery approach is preferable (see Fig. 2-38). Injection rates for contrast vary from 20 to 35 mL/sec for 2 seconds, so a reasonably sized pigtail catheter (5- to 7-French) is necessary. In young trauma patients with high

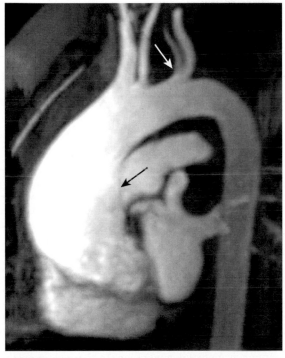

FIGURE 9-12. Oblique sagittal maximum intensity projection of a gadolinium-enhanced three-dimensional magnetic resonance angiogram showing a dilated ascending aorta *(black arrow)* in a patient with a bicuspid aortic valve. Note the left vertebral artery *(white arrow)* arising anomalously from the origin of the left subclavian artery. (Image courtesy of Barry Stein, MD, Hartford Hospital, Hartford, Conn.)

cardiac outputs, larger catheters and injection rates of 40-45 mL/sec for 2 seconds may be required. The first view that should be obtained when evaluating the thoracic aorta is the left anterior oblique projection with the catheter approximately 2 cm above the aortic valve (see Fig. 9-1). This view opens the aortic arch and places the great-vessel origins in profile. By carefully positioning the pigtail above the aortic valve, the risk of inadvertent injection into a coronary ostium or the left ventricle if the catheter jumps forward and unwinds can be minimized. Other views are obtained depending upon the anatomy and pathology. The field of view should encompass from the proximal great vessels to the diaphragm for initial injections. The catheter should be positioned at the level of the pathology whenever additional views are necessary.

Breath-holding is necessary for catheter aortography. Digital subtraction acquisitions (DSA) with rapid filming (minimum of 4-6 frames/sec) are desirable, especially in young, hyperdynamic patients. For patients with slow flow or suspected dissection, extended filming for as long as 30 seconds may be necessary. Full-strength contrast (at least 30% iodine) should be used unless patient factors require diluted contrast. In patients with large aneurysms and sluggish flow, slower filming with an elongated contrast injection (increased total volume over a longer period of time) improves opacification, but these are frequently the least satisfactory studies. Mask and pixel shifting are usually necessary even in cooperative patients who remain motionless during the injection, as cardiac motion introduces noticeable artifacts. The patient's arms should be raised over the head for biplane and true lateral filming unless contraindicated by clinical circumstances (e.g., trauma). Careful and frequent double flushing of the catheter is essential to avoid catheter-related embolic complications. Carbon dioxide gas is contraindicated as a contrast agent in the thoracic aorta.

ANEURYSMS

Aneurysms are less common in the thoracic than the abdominal aorta, but the range of etiologies is broader. The majority of thoracic aneurysms (80%) are degenerative in etiology (Box 9-1). Age, systemic atherosclerosis, hypertension, chronic obstructive pulmonary disease, a family history of aneurysms, and a personal history of aneurysms in other locations are frequent associations. Aneurysms in younger patients are typically nondegenerative in origin, such as vasculitis, inherited or acquired connective tissue abnormalities, and posttraumatic false aneurysms. Degenerative thoracic aortic aneurysms are often asymptomatic and discovered on chest imaging performed for other reasons (see Fig. 9-10). Large aneurysms may become clinically evident due to compression of adjacent structures, such as the central airways, pulmonary arteries, and superior vena cava (Box 9-2 and Fig. 9-13). Paralysis of a vocal cord can result from stretching of the recurrent laryngeal nerve by a large aneurysm. Rapid expansion of an aneurysm can cause pain in an otherwise stable patient, while

TABLE 9-2 Thoracic Aortography

Projection	Catheter Position*	Injection (mL/sec)†	Filming (frames/sec)	Application
LAO	Ascending	30-40	4-8	Trauma; aneurysm; dissection
RAO	Ascending	30-40	4-8	Trauma; aneurysm; dissection
LAO	Arch	20-30	4-8	Great-vessel origins
AP, lateral	Distal arch	20-30	4-8	Trauma; dissection; aneurysm; localization of bronchial arteries

*Pigtail catheter 5- to 7-Fr for injection in the ascending aorta; 5-French can be used when injection is limited to arch or descending aorta.
†For 2 seconds.
AP, Anteroposterior; LAO, left anterior oblique; RAO, right anterior oblique.

Box 9-1. Etiologies of Thoracic Aortic Aneurysms

Degenerative (associated with atherosclerosis)
Genetic
  • Marfan syndrome
  • Loeys-Dietz syndrome
  • Turner syndrome
  • Vascular Ehlers-Danlos
Bicuspid aortic valve
Chronic dissection
Arteritis
  • Giant-cell
  • Takayasu
  • Rheumatoid
  • Ankylosing spondylitis
Infection
Posttraumatic
Postcoarctation repair
Postcoronary bypass

Box 9-2. Complications of Thoracic Aortic Aneurysms

Rupture
Distal embolization
Compression of adjacent structures
  • Trachea
  • Esophagus
  • Pulmonary artery or vein
  • Superior vena cava
Stretching of recurrent laryngeal nerve
Fistula
  • Trachea or bronchus
  • Superior vena cava
  • Esophagus
Infection
Erosion of adjacent vertebrae

TABLE 9-3 Locations of Thoracic Aortic Aneurysms

Location	Percentage
Ascending aorta	40%
Aortic arch	15%
Descending thoracic aorta	35%
Thoracoabdominal aorta	10%

rupture presents with chest pain, hypotension, and cardiovascular collapse. The differential diagnosis in these patients includes acute myocardial infarction, pulmonary embolism, and other aortic emergencies such as dissection, intramural hematoma, or penetrating aortic ulcer.

Thoracic aortic aneurysms are described by their location: ascending aorta, arch, or descending aorta (Table 9-3). Aneurysm location has a major impact upon management, in that both the surgical and endovascular approach to repair is determined by the relationship of the aneurysm to the aortic valve, the great-vessel origins, and the abdominal visceral arteries. Aneurysms distal to the left subclavian artery may be treated with stent-grafts or surgically through a left thoracotomy with a clamp placed distal to the great-vessel origins. Ascending aortic or arch aneurysms are generally repaired through a median sternotomy with cardiopulmonary bypass, although branched endografts are becoming available.

Cross-sectional imaging of thoracic aortic aneurysms with CT or MR frequently provides satisfactory information for following progression of the aneurysm or planning intervention. When angiographic sequences are employed, both imaging modalities can allow precise delineation of extent of the aneurysm, status of the great vessels, and associated thoracic pathology. It is actually much easier to image thoracic aortic aneurysms with cross-sectional techniques than with conventional angiography. Careful postprocessing of images yields excellent diagnostic information. The large capacity of the aorta, slow flow, tortuosity of the anatomy, and cardiac motion conspire to make conventional angiography difficult.

Ascending Aortic Aneurysms

The etiology of ascending aortic aneurysms determines, in the majority of cases, the appearance on imaging studies. The age of the patient is also helpful in predicting the etiology, with collagen vascular and inflammatory diseases most often found in younger patients. The most common underlying pathology in older patients is medial degeneration. In these patients, the aortic valve is usually normal in diameter, with fusiform dilation of the aneurysm beginning distal to the sinotubular ridge (see Fig. 9-12). Severe aortic valvular stenosis may lead to post-stenotic dilatation of the ascending aorta. Most aneurysms 6 cm or more in diameter warrant consideration for surgical repair.

Dilation of the aortic valve and effacement of the sinotubular ridge is characteristic of Marfan syndrome, but may be seen with other connective disorders as well (see Fig. 1-37). Other features of Marfan syndrome include autosomal dominant inheritance (but spontaneous mutation accounts for 15%-30% of cases), asthenic body habitus, arachnodactyly, pectus deformities, subluxation of the lens, and increased risk of aortic rupture or dissection. Isolated ectasia of the aortic root can occur without other manifestations of Marfan syndrome. Less commonly, dilation of the aortic root and sinotubular ectasia can be seen in other heritable and some connective tissue diseases, such as osteogenesis imperfecta, Ehlers-Danlos syndrome, and rheumatoid arthritis.

Fusiform ascending aortic aneurysms are rare manifestations of Takayasu arteritis. Thickening of the aortic wall is characteristic. Syphilitic aortitis occurs in 10% of patients with untreated tertiary syphilis and was, at one time, the most common cause of thoracic

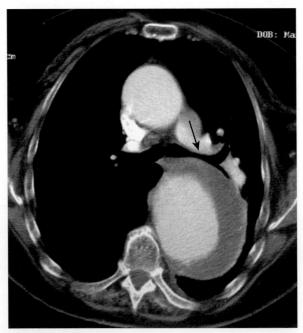

FIGURE 9-13. Axial computed tomography scan showing compression of the left main bronchus *(arrow)* by a large descending thoracic aortic aneurysm (same patient as in Fig. 9-10). Note the mural thrombus lining the aneurysm.

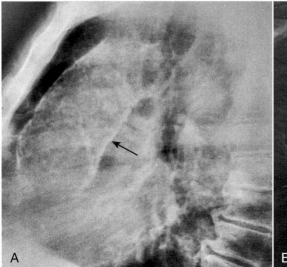
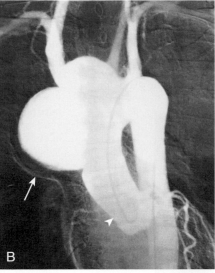

FIGURE 9-14. Syphilitic aortic aneurysms. **A,** Lateral chest radiograph shows dilatation and dense calcification of the ascending thoracic aorta *(arrow)*. **B,** Angiogram in the anteroposterior projection from another patient showing a lobulated aneurysm *(arrow)* of the ascending aorta and arch with preservation of the aortic valve and sinuses of Valsalva *(arrowhead)* and the descending thoracic aorta.

aortic aneurysm (Fig. 9-14). The characteristic features of syphilitic aneurysms are sparing of the sinotubular junction (although aortic regurgitation and aneurysms of the sinus of Valsalva can occur), saccular aneurysms in 75% with fine linear calcification, and shaggy "tree-bark" intima with superimposed atherosclerotic disease. The finding of extensive calcification of the ascending aorta on a chest radiograph strongly suggests syphilitic aortitis. Half of the aneurysms are located in the ascending aorta, one-third in the arch, one-fifth in the descending thoracic aorta, and rarely in the abdominal aorta.

Aneurysms of the sinus of Valsalva may be due to acute or chronic infection, vasculitis (e.g., Kawasaki), and following valvular surgery. Large focal saccular aneurysms of the ascending aorta at the implantation sites of coronary artery grafts or cannulation sites may represent pseudoaneurysms, often mycotic.

The treatment of ascending aortic aneurysms remains surgical replacement. The status of the aortic valve, coronary arteries, and great vessels influences the extent of the repair. In the future, endografts that can accommodate the ascending aorta, aortic valve, and coronary arteries may be feasible.

Aneurysms of the Transverse Arch

Fusiform aneurysms of the transverse aortic arch are almost always degenerative in nature, and contiguous with either an ascending or descending aortic aneurysm. Common features are intimal calcification with bulky plaque or mural thrombus, tortuosity and elongation of the arch, and deviation of mediastinal structures such as the trachea or esophagus. The most critical feature with respect to operative repair is the relationship of the aneurysm to the great-vessel origins.

Saccular aneurysms of the transverse arch are also most commonly degenerative in origin, but several additional etiologies should be considered. A focal aneurysm in an otherwise normal diameter but atherosclerotic aortic arch may be a contained rupture due to a penetrating ulcer. An "aortic blister" may result from deep excavation of an aortic plaque, with formation of a localized aneurysm without rupture. Mycotic aneurysms are usually associated with an irregular contour and perianeurysmal inflammatory changes. As noted, one third of syphilitic aneurysms occur in the arch and are most commonly saccular in appearance.

Aneurysms involving the transverse arch most often are managed with surgical repair and reimplantation of the great vessels. Hybrid debranching procedures using conventional thoracic endografts offer an alternative to traditional reconstructive arch surgery. In these procedures, surgical grafts are placed to the great

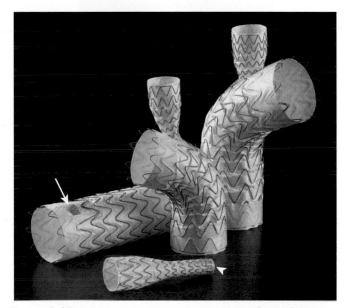

FIGURE 9-15. Branched thoracic endograft (GORE® TAG® Thoracic Branch Endoprosthesis) designed to allow perfusion of one major arch branch. The endograft has an opening *(arrow)* that can accommodate a side-branch graft *(arrowhead)*. (Image © W. L. Gore & Associates, Inc.)

vessels from the ascending aorta via median sternotomy, usually without cardiopulmonary bypass. This is followed by endograft placement across the arch from the ascending to the descending aorta, thus excluding the arch aneurysm. Although performed in only a few centers, the results of these procedures have been very good with low rates of stroke and paralysis. Thoracic endografts with one or more side branches are just becoming available and will one day obviate the hybrid debranching procedure except in unusual cases (Fig. 9-15).

Aneurysms of the Descending Thoracic Aorta

Most aneurysms of the descending thoracic aorta in patients older than 60 years are degenerative in origin. These may be localized or diffuse, but are usually fusiform in contour, have calcified intima, have some associated aortic tortuosity or redundancy, and often contain mural thrombus (Fig. 9-16, see also Fig 9-13). This tortuosity is often most notable at the diaphragmatic hiatus, where the descending thoracic aorta may actually make a 90-degree turn, run parallel to the diaphragm for a short distance, and then make another 90-degree turn to pass through the hiatus. Aortic diameters measured from axial images in areas of tortuosity are easily overestimated if the long diameter of an in-plane segment of vessel is measured. As a rule, always take the shorter diameter of noncircular segment of vessel as the true diameter.

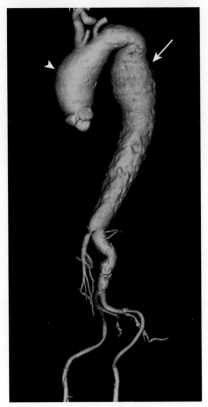

FIGURE 9-16. Ascending and descending thoracic aortic aneurysms in a 67-year-old woman shown on volume rendering of a computed tomography angiogram. The ascending aneurysm *(arrowhead)* measures 6 cm in maximum diameter and extends into the arch to the left subclavian artery. The proximal descending thoracic aorta is elongated and acutely angulated, and then becomes aneurysmal *(arrow)* measuring 6.4 cm in diameter at the widest point. The celiac artery is occluded.

As with ascending thoracic aortic aneurysms, aneurysms less than 6 cm in diameter are usually observed. Focal proximal aneurysms are simpler to repair with endovascular than surgical techniques. When the aortic dilatation extends below the diaphragm, the aneurysm is termed *thoracoabdominal* (Fig. 9-17). These are generally more complex to treat in that the abdominal visceral arteries are included in the aneurysm.

Fusiform descending thoracic aortic aneurysms may be found in patients with Takayasu arteritis, other vasculitides, and Marfan syndrome. These patients are generally young, without evidence of coexistent atherosclerotic disease.

Saccular aneurysms of the descending thoracic aorta are usually not simple atherosclerotic lesions. When localized to the proximal descending thoracic aorta, chronic aortic transection should be a strong consideration in a young patient, particularly if the aneurysm is heavily calcified with normal adjacent aorta (Fig. 9-18). Aneurysms that arise from the underside of the proximal descending aorta and burrow into the middle mediastinum toward the pulmonary artery may be aneurysms of the ductus remnant, termed a *ductus aneurysm*. Focal pseudoaneurysms in otherwise normal-caliber but atherosclerotic aortas may occur due to penetrating ulcers. An important differential in this situation is a mycotic aneurysm, which may have a similar appearance but is often multilobulated (Fig. 9-19; see also Fig. 1-35). Vasculitis (e.g., Behçet) may also result in focal saccular descending thoracic aortic aneurysms (see Fig. 1-18).

When imaging any thoracic aortic aneurysm, it is essential to know whether the patient has symptoms of pain, acute onset of hoarseness, hemoptysis, or dysphagia. These symptoms suggest an active process, such as rapid expansion or rupture. For example, a new left pleural effusion in a patient with a descending thoracic aortic aneurysm and acute onset of back pain suggests impending rupture. Stranding of the soft tissues in the mediastinum, or extravascular blood in the presence of a degenerative aneurysm, suggest rapid expansion or contained rupture, respectively. Mycotic aneurysms are by definition contained ruptures and may have a prominent inflammatory response in the surrounding soft tissues. In acute situations, CT is the preferred imaging modality for assessing the thoracic aorta.

The relationship of the aneurysm to the left subclavian artery and the abdominal visceral arteries greatly impacts the approach and complexity of treatment. Involvement of these major aortic branches in the aneurysm increases the difficulty and morbidity of intervention. In general, operative repair of descending thoracic aortic aneurysms has a mortality of 5%-10%. Paraplegia due

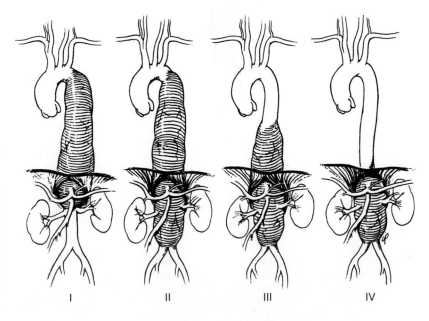

FIGURE 9-17. The Crawford classification of thoracoabdominal aneurysms. *I:* Descending thoracic aorta to suprarenal aorta. *II:* Proximal descending thoracic aorta to infrarenal aorta. *III:* Mid-descending thoracic aorta at or below the sixth intercostal artery to infrarenal aorta. *IV:* Supravisceral aorta at the twelfth intercostal space to the aortic bifurcation. (From Cambria RP. Management of thoracoabdominal aortic aneurysms. In: Gewertz BL, Schwartz LB, eds. *Surgery of the Aorta and Its Branches.* Philadelphia: WB Saunders, 2000, with permission.)

I   II   III   IV

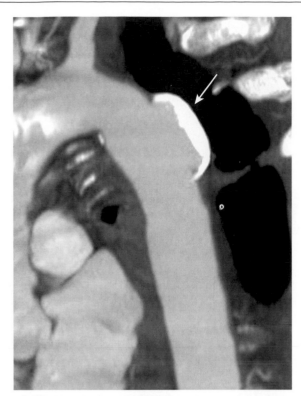

FIGURE 9-18. Pseudoaneurysm due to chronic untreated aortic transection in a 33-year-old man 12 years after a high-speed motor vehicle accident. A calcified proximal descending thoracic aneurysm was noted on a chest radiograph obtained to rule out pneumonia. Sagittal multiplanar reformatted computed tomography shows the eccentric, heavily calcified proximal descending thoracic aortic aneurysm *(arrow)*.

to spinal cord ischemia occurs in 5%-10% of patients, depending on such factors as the location of the aneurysm (distal increases risk), extent of repair (longer increases risk), number of patent intercostal arteries (more increases risk), presence of prior abdominal or thoracic aortic repair, and age of the patient. Other major morbidities include renal failure, stroke (about 3%), and respiratory failure.

Endovascular repair of descending thoracic aortic aneurysms is an attractive alternative to open surgical repair (Fig. 9-20). Although the paraplegia and stroke rates are only slightly lower than open repair, patients benefit greatly from the elimination of the thoracotomy and cross-clamping of the aorta. Patients with aneurysms that have 1.5-2 cm of normal aorta distal to the left subclavian or left common carotid artery and proximal to the celiac artery are potential candidates for conventional stent-grafts (Box 9-3). When the distance between the left subclavian artery and the aneurysm is shorter than 1.5 cm, the endograft can be placed across the left subclavian artery origin provided that the left vertebral artery is in continuity with the basilar artery. In elective cases, or when the left vertebral artery ends in the posterior inferior cerebral artery, left carotid to subclavian artery bypass is recommended before stent-graft coverage. In general, there is a 1% risk of stroke and 30% risk of symptomatic left arm ischemia with stent-graft overlay of the left subclavian artery.

A similar length of normal aorta is required for the distal end of the stent-graft. There is limited but positive experience with intentional endograft overlay of the celiac artery origin in patients with short distal landing zones. A patent superior mesenteric artery and pancreaticoduodenal arcade are essential. A larger accumulation of experience is needed to assess the safety of celiac artery occlusion during endograft procedures.

Endograft repair of thoracoabdominal aneurysms requires either a combined procedure with surgical debranching of the

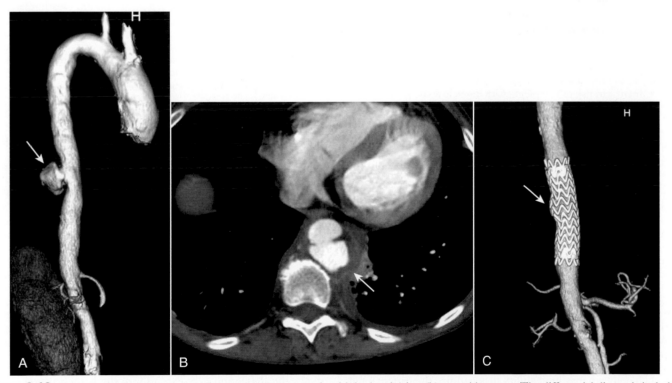

FIGURE 9-19. Focal descending thoracic pseudoaneurysm (symptomatic with back pain) in a 56-year-old woman. The differential diagnosis includes penetrating aortic ulcer and mycotic aneurysm. This patient had pneumonia 3 months earlier but all blood cultures were negative. **A,** Lateral view of volume rendering of a computed tomography angiogram (CTA) the thoracoabdominal aorta showing the focal aneurysm *(arrow)*, in essence a contained rupture of the distal descending thoracic aorta. **B,** Axial contrast-enhanced computed tomography showing the focal aneurysm and surrounding soft tissue reaction *(arrow)*. **C,** Oblique view of volume rendering of a CTA obtained after deployment of a stent graft showing exclusion of the pseudoaneurysm *(arrow)*. The patient remained on lifelong oral antibiotics.

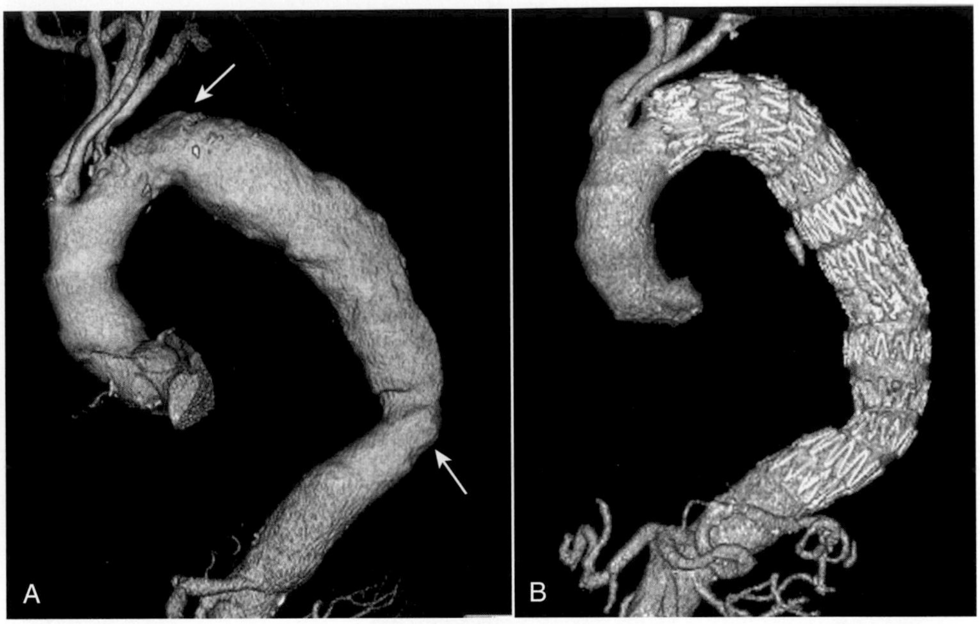

FIGURE 9-20. Descending thoracic aortic aneurysm treated with an endograft. **A,** Oblique volume rendering image from a computed tomography angiogram (CTA) showing the extent of the aneurysm *(arrows)*. The size of the aneurysm is greater than appears on the volume rendering in that the mural thrombus is not visualized. **B,** CTA of same patient after placement of an endograft. Note that the endograft extends proximal and distal to the aneurysm.

Box 9-3. Stent-Graft Repair of Thoracic Aortic Aneurysm

Proximal landing zone:
- 1.5-2 cm normal aorta distal to left subclavian artery or left common carotid

If left subclavian artery must be covered and cannot be sacrificed:
- Subclavian-carotid artery bypass

Distal landing zone:
- 1.5-2 cm normal aorta above celiac artery

Acceptable landing zone diameters:
- Varies with device

Severe angulation of proximal or distal aorta:
- Better results with longer landing zones

Prior abdominal aortic aneurysm repair:
- Increased risk of paraplegia with thoracic aortic stent-graft

Patency and caliber of pelvic arteries:
- Large delivery systems may require direct access to common iliac artery or abdominal aorta

Spinal cord protection:
- Consider lumbar drain before procedure

---

abdominal aorta followed by endograft placement, or branched endografts. Debranching procedures are major surgical interventions, because construction of bypasses (usually from the iliac arteries) to all of the visceral arteries is time consuming (see Fig. 3-18). The long-term patency of the bypass grafts is greater than 90%, but the 30-day mortality of the procedure (usually from cardiovascular and pulmonary causes) is about 15%. Branched endografts are less invasive for the patient but are time-consuming and require advanced interventional skill sets (see Fig. 10-17).

An important adjunct for thoracic aortic aneurysm repair, particularly when the distal aorta is treated, is a lumbar cerebrospinal fluid drain. This should be placed before undertaking the procedure (a bloody tap may limit ability to heparinize the patient), and usually remains in place for 24-48 hours. Spinal drainage (pressures less than 10 mm Hg) and maintenance of mean arterial pressure greater than 90 mm Hg dramatically decrease the risk of spinal cord ischemia. Patients in whom acute chord ischemia develops after an endograft should have urgent placement of a lumbar drain.

Delivery systems for thoracic stent-grafts tend to be large, so assessment of the iliac arteries and abdominal aorta is necessary when evaluating a patient for one of these procedures. Surgical placement of a temporary graft to the common iliac artery or distal aorta (termed a *conduit*) may be required to deliver the endograft in patients with small or diseased pelvic arteries. Antegrade insertion through the subclavian or carotid arteries, or the ascending aorta, is an unusual but feasible access option.

Approximately 85% of aneurysms undergo thrombosis after placement of a stent-graft, with type II endoleaks being the most common explanation of continued sac perfusion. Death related to the aneurysm is rare after successful endograft repair. Reintervention (embolization of an endoleak or placement of an additional endograft) is required in only 5%-7% up to 2 years after treatment. With the introduction of branched stent-grafts and the development of stent-grafts with aortic valves, this technology will become applicable to arch and ascending aortic aneurysms.

■ AORTIC DISSECTION

Aortic dissection occurs at a rate of approximately 3/100,000 persons per year, with men afflicted twice as often as women (Table 9-4). Dissection is essentially delamination of the arterial wall, with separation of the intima from the media. Usually, blood at systemic arterial pressure fills this new space (see Fig. 1-9). The lumen lined by intima is the "true" lumen, while blood in the media forms the "false" lumen. In most instances, extensive aortic dissection can occur only if the media is abnormal, such as in patients with longstanding atherosclerosis, Marfan syndrome, or other connective tissue disorders (Box 9-4). The presumed etiology is an acute defect in the intima that allows blood to enter the media. This defect may be a linear tear, or a penetrating ulcer in an aortic atherosclerotic plaque. Pressurized blood then dissects antegrade, retrograde, or in both directions (Fig. 9-21). As the intima is peeled away from the media, small tears ("fenestrations") occur at the origins of branch vessels. In these instances, the blood supply to the branch vessel may be entirely from the false lumen. Alternatively, the dissection may extend into the branch vessel, causing compromised flow or leading to thrombosis, termed *static obstruction*. The critical physiology of dissection is that the false lumen tends to remain at near systolic pressure throughout the cardiac cycle, owing to poor outflow. This results in progressive enlargement of the false lumen and compression of the true lumen during diastole (Fig. 9-22). When a critical branch vessel is supplied from a compressed true lumen, organ ischemia can result, termed *dynamic obstruction*.

Aortic dissection is classified according to the location of the entry tear and the extent of the false lumen (see Fig. 9-21). Classification systems for aortic dissection are based on the clinical outcomes. Dissection involving the ascending aorta is usually repaired surgically on an emergent basis owing to involvement of the aortic valve and coronary ostia, and the high risk of rupture into the pericardium or pleural cavity. Dissection isolated to the descending thoracic aorta is usually managed medically with aggressive blood pressure control unless critical organ ischemia is present. With time, the false lumen may thrombose if there is no outflow.

Patients with acute aortic dissection present with sudden onset of severe anterior or posterior chest pain, often described as "tearing." These same symptoms may be found in patients with ruptured thoracic aortic aneurysms, acute myocardial infarction, pulmonary embolism, and other thoracic emergencies. The pain may wax and wane. Patients are usually hypertensive on presentation; hypotensive patients have a worse prognosis. Associated symptomatic branch vessel occlusion, such as stroke, spinal cord ischemia, abdominal pain, or limb ischemia, occurs in up to 28% of patients and is also an indicator of worse prognosis. Rarely, organ or limb ischemia may be the only presenting symptom. The majority of patients with dissection are in their sixth through

TABLE 9-4 Aortic Dissection*

	Percentage
Origin in ascending thoracic aorta	60%
Origin in descending thoracic aorta	35%
Origin in abdominal aorta	5%
Mortality at 2 weeks:	
Origin in ascending thoracic aorta	33%
Origin in descending thoracic aorta	
Uncomplicated	10%
Symptomatic organ/limb ischemia	30%
Five-year survival from hospital discharge (management)	
Origin ascending thoracic aorta (surgery)	90%
Origin descending thoracic aorta (medical)	78%
Origin descending thoracic aorta (surgical)	83%
Origin descending thoracic aorta (endovascular)	76%

*The male to female ratio is 2:1.

Box 9-4. Conditions Associated with Aortic Dissection

Hypertension
Atherosclerosis
Inherited disorders
- Marfan syndrome
- Ehlers-Danlos syndrome
- Loeys-Dietz syndrome
- Osteogenesis imperfecta
- Turner syndrome
- Polycystic kidney disease
Autoimmune disorders
- Giant-cell arteritis
- Relapsing polychondritis
- Systemic lupus erythematosus
Pregnancy (etiology of 50% of dissections in women <40 years)
Congenital vascular anomalies
- Coarctation
- Bicuspid/unicuspid aortic valve
Iatrogenic causes
- Aortic catheterization
- Aortic surgery
- Intraaortic balloon pump
Cocaine/methamphetamine abuse

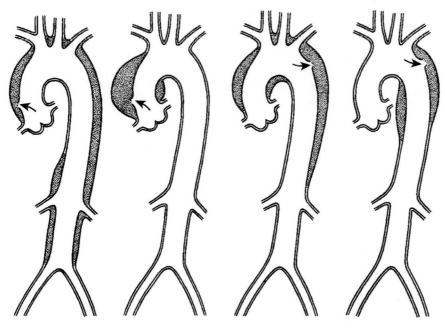

DeBakey:	Type I	Type II	Type III A	Type III B
Stanford		Type A		Type B

FIGURE 9-21. Classification of aortic dissection. Arrows indicate site of entry tear. (From Gertler JP, Tsukurov O. The spectrum of thoracoabdominal aortic disease. In: Gewertz BL, Schwartz LB, eds. *Surgery of the Aorta and Its Branches.* Philadelphia: WB Saunders, 2000, with permission.)

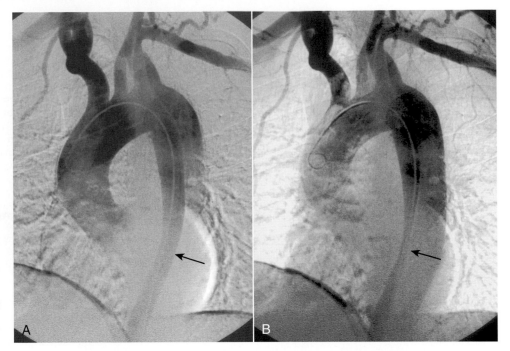

Figure 9-22. True and false lumen physiology of acute aortic dissection. **A,** Digital subtraction aortogram in the left anterior oblique projection of a patient with a dissection of the descending thoracic aorta extending into the left subclavian artery. The false lumen fills slowly owing to lack of a distal communication with the true lumen. During systole the true lumen *(arrow)* is partially distended. **B,** During diastole the false lumen depressurizes slower than the true lumen, leading to compression of the true lumen *(arrow)*.

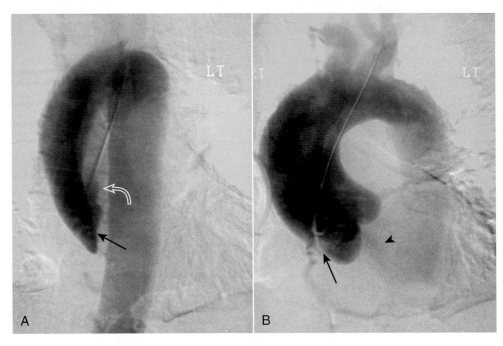

Figure 9-23. Catheter positioning in angiography of aortic dissection. **A,** Digital subtraction angiogram performed from the left axillary approach with injection into the false lumen. The catheter has inadvertently been inserted through an intimal tear *(curved arrow)* into the false lumen *(arrow)*. Note that the aortic valves, coronary arteries, and great vessels are not visualized. **B,** After repositioning the catheter in the true lumen, the dissection flap is visible *(arrow)* as are both the true and false lumens. There is slight aortic valve regurgitation *(arrowhead)*. This is the desired catheter position.

eighth decades, with underlying atherosclerosis and hypertension. Aortic dissection in a young individual is suspicious for an inherited abnormality of the arterial wall or a connective tissue disorder.

CT, without and with contrast, is an excellent modality for imaging of patients with acute aortic dissection (see Figs. 9-11 and 1-28). The value of the noncontrast scan is the conspicuity of acute intramural blood, which may be less obvious after administration of contrast. Other acute aortic pathologies, such as ruptured aneurysm, are easily distinguished from dissection on CT. A normal aortic CT in a patient with suspected dissection effectively excludes the diagnosis, provided that the quality of the study is satisfactory. In the region of the aortic root, artifacts due to motion, metal, and dense contrast in the superior vena cava can make interpretation difficult. Nevertheless, the overall sensitivity and specificity exceeds 95% for contrast-enhanced multidetector CT. MR with angiographic sequences has similar sensitivity and specificity, but can be difficult to obtain in an acute situation.

MRI is an excellent modality for long-term follow-up of dissections because of the ability to acquire images in multiple planes, avoid nephrotoxic contrast agents, and radiation (see Figs. 1-28 and 3-8). TEE is also an excellent imaging technique for dissection, but requires sedation and is not as readily available as CT. TEE has about 80% overall sensitivity and specificity, with better results for ascending aorta dissection.

Conventional angiography can be safely performed in patients with acute dissection, but is rarely necessary unless part of an intervention. The common femoral artery approach usually allows access to the true lumen, because dissections rarely extend distal to the external iliac arteries. However, if the true lumen cannot be entered from below, the right upper extremity frequently provides access to the true lumen in the ascending aorta. Opacification of both the true and false lumen, especially in the ascending aorta, is important to determine involvement of critical aortic branches and the aortic valve by the dissection (Fig. 9-23; see Fig. 9-22).

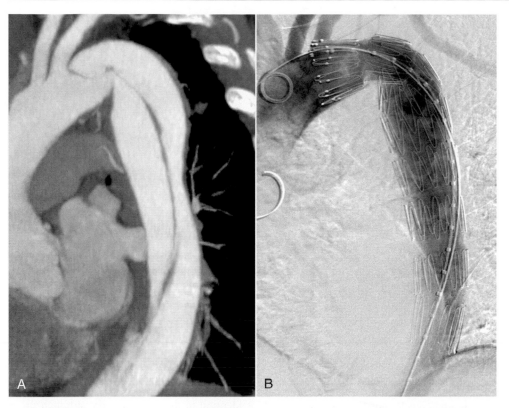

FIGURE 9-24. Stent-graft treatment of type B aortic dissection in a patient with visceral and renal malperfusion (same patient as in Fig. 9-11). The goal of therapy is to seal the entry tear, allowing depressurization and thrombosis of the false lumen with improved perfusion of the true lumen. **A,** Oblique reformat of CT angiogram of the proximal descending thoracic aorta shows that the dissection is distal to the left subclavian artery. **B,** Angiogram after placement of a stent-graft over the entry tear in the true lumen of the descending thoracic aorta. The true lumen has a normal diameter and the false lumen no longer fills.

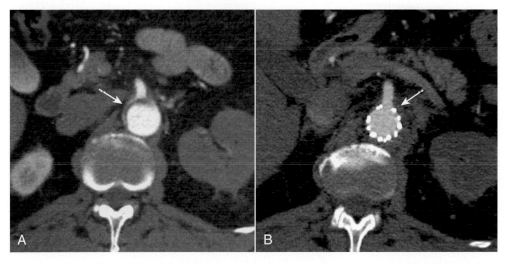

FIGURE 9-25. Treatment of compressed true lumen complicating a type B dissection with large bare metal stents in the true lumen. This is the same patient as in Figure 9-24, in whom a covered stent was placed proximally to cover the entry tear. **A,** Axial computed tomography (CT) scan before treatment showing marked compression of the true lumen *(arrow)* at the level of the superior mesenteric artery (SMA). **B,** CT scan 4 months after treatment with a stent-graft proximally and large bare stents *(arrow)* in the true lumen in the abdominal aorta. The size relationship of the true and false lumens has reversed, so that the true lumen now has a normal diameter. Note the widely patent SMA.

The traditional therapy for type A dissection is emergent surgical replacement of the ascending aorta, with or without valve replacement. This stabilizes the process in the ascending aorta, but distally the false lumen remains patent in 90%. The mortality of surgical repair is 26%. Approximately 15% of patients will have late aneurysmal change of the remaining dissected aorta. Type B dissections are usually managed medically (blood pressure control) in the acute phase unless pain is unremitting, there is branch vessel compromise, or rupture has occurred. In patients managed medically mortality is less than 10% and the dissection becomes chronic in 95% with subsequent aneurysmal change in 25%. In patients requiring surgery for complicated acute type B dissection the in-hospital mortality is almost 30%. In all patients surviving to discharge, the long-term risk of rupture of an aneurysmal chronic dissection is estimated to be approximately 10% per year but increases to 30% when the aortic diameter is more than 6 cm.

Several percutaneous options for management of acute dissection are available. Placement of a stent-graft over the entry tear has been shown to acutely depressurize the false lumen and restore normal flow dynamics in the true lumen (Fig. 9-24). Over time there is thrombosis of the false lumen adjacent to the stent-graft in almost all cases, although the false lumen often remains patent distally. When possible, the proximal end of the endograft should be placed in nondissected aorta. The endograft should be sized to the estimated diameter of the true lumen, not the overall diameter of the dissected aorta. Postdeployment balloon molding of the endograft should be minimized because new intimal tears can be created at the edges of the endograft. Initial results with this technique in patients with complicated type B dissection have been promising, with a 30-day mortality of about 5%, a paraplegia rate of 1%, and few major procedural complications such as stroke or retrograde dissection into the arch. Large bare stents to reinforce the true lumen and stabilize the intimal flap can be used in combination with a proximal endograft to enhance remodeling of the dissected aorta and preserve flow to the visceral branches (Fig. 9-25). Prospective studies to confirm improved long-term outcomes of endograft repair, especially compared to medical management in uncomplicated dissections, are needed.

Critical organ ischemia due to dynamic obstruction of a branch vessel may be relieved by covering the entry tear with an endograft. When this is unsuccessful, and in cases of static obstruction, placement of bare stents from the true lumen of the aorta into the true lumen of the branch vessel may restore flow. Percutaneous fenestration of the aortic flap (intentional creation of a large distal exit tear) can decompress the false lumen and relieve obstruction of the true lumen, but is no longer the first-line endovascular technique as mortality can be as high as 25% at 30 days. Fenestration is accomplished by crossing the intimal flap with an intravascular needle using fluoroscopy or intravascular ultrasound to guide the puncture. Large angioplasty balloons are then inflated across the flap to create an exit tear, which may then be supported with stents (see Fig. 10-32).

The role of aortic endografts versus surgery in the management of chronic dissection complicated by aneurysmal change is also promising but as of yet unproven. The false lumen reduces in diameter in approximately 80% of patients at 2.5 years, although late aneurysm rupture occurs in up to 3%.

INTRAMURAL HEMATOMA

An important variant of dissection is acute intramural hematoma (IMH), which is defined as blood in the medial layer with intact overlying intima (Fig. 9-26). This is found as an alternative diagnosis in about 5%-15% of patients with suspected aortic dissection. The etiology is suspected to be spontaneous hemorrhage into abnormal media in the absence of an intimal defect. Thrombus in the wall of the aorta can be seen in patients with dissection or penetrating aortic ulcer (see later), but the entity termed IMH refers specifically to the situation of intramural blood without identifiable communication with the lumen. The risk factors and symptom complex are identical to that of dissection. The most common location is in the proximal descending thoracic aorta, but mortality is highest when the ascending aorta is involved. Progression to dissection with development of an intimal tear and flow in a false lumen occurs in approximately 35%. This suggests that IMH may be the precursor for many dissections. A smaller percentage will develop subsequent aortic rupture. The closer to the aortic valve, the higher the in-hospital mortality rate (33% in the ascending thoracic aorta, and 13% in the descending).

Management of IMH is similar to that of dissection: surgery for IMH involving the ascending aorta and medical management for IMH when localized to the descending aorta. Expansion of the hematoma, continued pain, development of left bloody pleural effusion, or rupture requires more aggressive management of descending thoracic aortic IMH. Endograft placement is a good alternative to surgery in these patients, although why this works is less obvious than in dissection or aneurysms. Extensive coverage of the aorta from subclavian to celiac may be necessary because of the lack of a focality of the IMH. Minimal balloon molding is important when the endograft starts and ends on IMH to avoid creating an intimal tear at the end of the graft.

PENETRATING AORTIC ULCERS

Penetrating aortic ulcers (PAUs) are the result of unroofing of an atherosclerotic aortic intimal plaque, resulting in a focal partial or full thickness defect in the aortic wall. Approximately 6%-10% of patients with suspected acute aortic dissection are found to have PAU. The ulcer almost always occurs in the setting of preexisting aortic atherosclerosis, usually in the descending thoracic aorta, with one third of patients having more than one ulceration. The aortic diameter is often normal. A characteristic punched-out, undermined appearance is seen on imaging studies. Evidence of intramural blood, periaortic stranding, pleural effusion (30%), focal aneurysm formation, or periaortic hematoma should also be present (see Fig. 9-19). Irregular, even excavated-appearing aortic plaque is a prevalent finding in asymptomatic patients with severe atherosclerotic disease, so correlation with other imaging findings and clinical presentation is essential to avoid overcalling lesions. The symptom complex of PAU is identical to that of dissection, although up to 20% of patients present with focal aortic rupture. Medial fibrosis limits the extent of the intramural hematoma in some patients. The differential diagnosis of this lesion should always include mycotic aneurysm and trauma.

The initial management of PAU is medical (blood pressure and pain control) unless the lesion is in the ascending thoracic aorta. Ascending aortic ulcerations are managed like type A dissections with surgery. About 60% of patients with descending thoracic aortic ulcerations can be stabilized with medical management; however, continued pain, enlarging pleural effusion, expansion of the ulcer, or rupture warrants intervention. Some authors have suggested that a symptomatic ulceration that is 20 mm in diameter or greater, or 10 mm in depth, should be managed aggressively. Descending thoracic aortic PAU is often an ideal lesion for endograft repair. Covering the ulcer prevents progression, controls pain, and can be accomplished with a single short endograft.

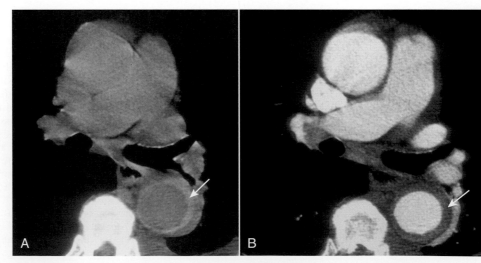

FIGURE 9-26. Intramural hematoma. **A,** Noncontrast axial computed tomography (CT) image shows high density *(arrow)* in the wall of the descending thoracic aorta representing an intramural hematoma. **B,** Contrast-enhanced axial CT image at the same level. No intimal flap is visible. Relative to the contrast-enhanced blood, the wall of the aorta now appears thickened by low density *(arrow)*. This underscores the importance of always obtaining an initial noncontrast scan before giving contrast when evaluating a patient for acute aortic pathology.

TRAUMA

Thoracic aortic injury may result from rapid deceleration, crush injuries, penetrating wounds, or instrumentation during surgical or angiographic procedures. In general, suspected aortic injury requires rapid evaluation, and, if found, active management.

The majority of thoracic aortic injuries are due to blunt trauma. When the outside of a rapidly moving person suddenly comes to a halt, the insides keep moving. Organs pull and twist against tether points, and impact against each other. In addition, compression of the thorax may also sharply increase intraaortic pressure and rigidity. Lastly, there may be shearing of the aorta between the head of the clavicle and the spine (the "osseus pinch"). The complex forces acting on the thoracic aorta are incompletely understood, but the result can be either partial or complete tear through the layers of the aortic wall. This is termed *traumatic transection*. These patients often have multiple injuries to the head, spine, and abdomen.

Patients with transection of the ascending aorta are rarely encountered in that these lesions are almost uniformly lethal in the field. The lack of surrounding connective tissue results in rapid exsanguination, or bleeding into the pericardial space and acute tamponade. Approximately 25% of patients with descending thoracic aorta transection survive when the adventitial or periadventitial mediastinal tissues can contain the bleeding in a pseudoaneurysm. This injury is located most often distal to the origin of the left subclavian artery (Table 9-5 and Fig. 9-27). The pseudoaneurysm is unstable, with risk of rupture when untreated that exceeds 90% within a month.

Aortic transection in a trauma patient can be reliably excluded if the chest radiograph is pristinely normal. However, in reality, supine chest radiographs in patients with massive trauma are rarely normal. Numerous chest radiograph findings have been evaluated that suggest aortic transection (Box 9-5). Diagnosis requires confirmatory imaging, most often with contrast-enhanced CT (see Fig. 9-27). Mediastinal blood should raise the suspicion of aortic injury, but may be due to bony trauma or disruption of venous structures. A normal-appearing aorta on a good-quality multidetector CT scan with satisfactory vascular enhancement reliably excludes aortic injury, with greater than 98% sensitivity and specificity. Irregularity of the aortic lumen or an obvious pseudoaneurysm seen on CT scan is consistent with transection. In many cases, postprocessing of the CT scan provides sufficient information to plan repair, such

TABLE 9-5 Aortic Injury Due to Blunt Trauma Seen at Imaging

Location	Incidence
Proximal descending thoracic aorta	90%
Great-vessel origin (innominate artery most common)	7%
Mid or distal descending thoracic aorta	2%
Ascending thoracic aorta	<1%

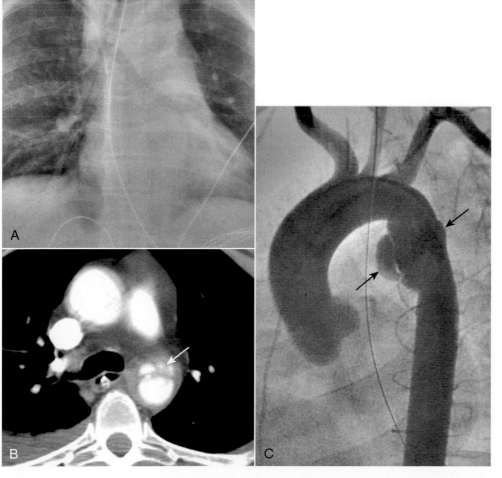

FIGURE 9-27. Transection of the proximal descending thoracic aorta. **A,** Chest radiograph of a patient after a high-speed motor vehicle accident. The arch is obscured, there is a left apical cap, the left mainstem bronchus is depressed, and the mediastinal tubes are displaced to the right. **B,** Axial computed tomography image of the same patient shows mediastinal hematoma and irregularity of the aortic lumen *(arrow)*. **C,** Digital subtraction aortogram in the left anterior oblique projection showing circumferential transection of the proximal descending thoracic with a large pseudoaneurysm *(arrows)*.

as identification of additional aortic injuries and arch anomalies. Conventional aortography should be obtained in any patient with an equivocal CT scan. In general, it is far wiser to perform an angiogram rather than try to be definitive on the basis of a marginal CT scan. Intravascular ultrasound can be used to identify subtle aortic wall injuries and small intimal flaps.

At aortography, a transection appears as an irregular collection of contrast beyond the normal aortic lumen (Fig. 9-28; see

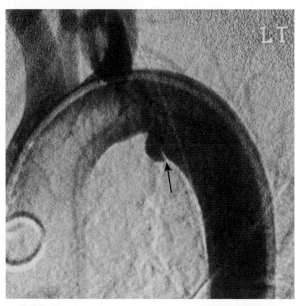

FIGURE 9-28. Focal aortic transection, surgically proven. This lesion can be differentiated from a ductus diverticulum (see Fig. 9-2) by the presence of sharp contour *(arrow)*.

Fig. 9-27). The tear may be partial (55%) or circumferential (45%), and more than one vascular injury may be present. Along the underside of the aorta just distal to the left subclavian artery there is frequently a slight bulge in the region of the ductus, the "ductus bump." These always have smooth walls, with a very gentle contour, and no acute angles or irregularity (see Fig. 9-1). Rarely, a small true saccular outpouching or even an aneurysm is found at this location, termed a *ductus diverticulum* (see Fig. 9-2). These are broad-mouthed, with smooth walls, and no sharp angles. Differentiation from a transection can be difficult when there is a large surrounding mediastinal hematoma from other injuries, but the presence of any sharp or irregular contour represents a transection until proven otherwise (see Fig. 9-28). Rarely, patients with undiagnosed aortic transection survive to present years later with focal calcified descending thoracic aortic aneurysm (see Fig. 9-18).

The initial management of the patient with a contained aortic transection is blood pressure and heart rate control with correction of other active life-threatening injuries. If necessary, patients with multiple injuries can be managed this way for several days or weeks until an intervention can be performed safely, although progression to rupture is seen in 5%-10% of cases. The traditional therapy of aortic transection is surgical placement of an aortic interposition tube graft. This surgery has a 2%-10% risk of spinal cord ischemia (decreased with spinal cord protection techniques such as a lumbar drain), and an overall mortality rate of approximately 12%. This surgery requires a left thoracotomy and usually partial or full cardiopulmonary bypass.

Stent-grafts are increasingly used to exclude traumatic aortic pseudoaneurysm (Fig 9-29). The procedure can be performed quickly, often percutaneously, in the patients with multiple injuries who would be at high risk for surgical repair. Challenges in this population include small-diameter aortas (compared to aneurysm and dissection patients), tight radius of the arch, and a paucity of devices designed for trauma. In the past, components from abdominal aortic endograft systems were widely used to overcome these limitations. Increasingly, small-diameter, flexible thoracic endografts are becoming available for use in aortic trauma.

In order to obtain an adequate proximal seal, the left subclavian artery must be covered in up to 30% of patients. Confirmation of a patent right vertebral artery and normal left vertebral artery is important to decrease the risk of posterior fossa stroke when the left subclavian artery is covered. Transposition of the left subclavian artery to the left common carotid artery (or carotid-subclavian bypass) should be performed in advance in patients at risk for this complication. Paraplegia is rare (3% or less) after endograft repair, and the mortality rate appears to be only about 9% (usually

FIGURE 9-29. Stent-graft repair of traumatic aortic transection. **A,** Angiogram prior to stent-graft placement shows a pseudoaneurysm *(arrow)* of the proximal descending thoracic aorta. Note sharp angulation between the arch and the descending thoracic aorta, and the variant branching anatomy with the vertebral artery arising from the arch rather than the left subclavian artery. **B,** Angiogram following stent-graft placement. The pigtail catheter was placed from the left arm approach to ensure that the endograft was deployed distal to the subclavian artery. The pseudoaneurysm is excluded. Note that the inferior lip of the proximal end of the stent graft is slightly elevated ("bird-beaked"), a common issue with stent-grafts in tight aortic arches.

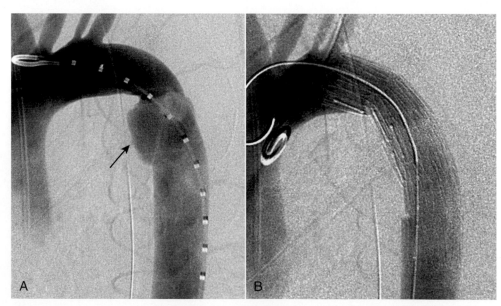

related to systemic complications of the original trauma). Catastrophic collapse of the graft has occurred when oversized devices are used in small aortas. The long-term follow-up of patients with endografts for traumatic aortic injury includes serial imaging with CT and chest radiographs. The extended outcomes of this approach are not known, particularly in individuals who will continue to grow if they survive. In adolescent and pediatric patients, surgical repair is still the preferred approach.

Penetrating aortic and great vessel injury is thought to be present in up to 5% of gunshot and 2% of knife wounds to the chest. Patients present with cardiac arrest, hypotension, hemothorax, hemomediastinum, or pseudoaneurysm. In the stable patient, CT angiography can provide a definitive diagnosis and important information about related injuries (Fig. 9-30). Endovascular repair with stent-grafts may be possible for injuries of the proximal great vessels or descending thoracic aorta. The majority of patients require immediate thoracotomy, but even so mortality rates remain above 80%.

VASCULITIS

Occlusive disease of the thoracic aorta due to atherosclerosis is virtually nonexistent. Whenever a patient presents with stenoses in the descending thoracic aorta that are not due to coarctation, dissection, or prior surgery, the most likely etiology is vasculitis (Table 9-6). Patients usually have additional signs of vasculitis, such as constitutional and joint symptoms, abnormal rheumatologic profiles, aortic wall thickening, and findings in other arteries consistent with vasculitis.

Long, smooth stenoses of varying severity are typical of arteritis. On cross-sectional imaging, a thickened aortic wall that enhances with contrast indicates an active process (Fig. 9-31; see Fig. 1-13). A thick, calcified wall with little or no enhancement after contrast administration suggests a "burned-out" or treated vasculitis. These findings can be made at both contrast-enhanced CT and MRI. The lack of signal from calcium makes MRI easier to read, but

calcification can be an important clue for a correct differential diagnosis and assessment of the activity of the disease. At angiography, these lesions have an appearance and location atypical for atherosclerotic disease, and may be associated with other unusual lesions such as great-vessel stenoses, aortic aneurysms, pulmonary artery aneurysms or stenoses, or abnormalities of the abdominal aorta. When performing conventional angiography as part of a vasculitis workup, images from the aortic valve to the femoral arteries should be acquired, with selective injection of any suspicious-appearing visceral or other branch vessel (see Figs. 1-14 through 1-16).

The therapy for thoracic aortic vasculitis is first medical with antiinflammatory agents, and only secondarily surgical with bypass procedures. Angioplasty and stent placement can successfully relieve ischemic symptoms, but a normal-appearing lumen is rarely achieved due to fibrotic nature of the lesions.

COARCTATION

Coarctation of the thoracic aorta is a congenital fibrous narrowing of the distal arch or, most often, the proximal descending thoracic aorta distal to the left subclavian artery (see Fig. 9-9). The narrowing can be variable in severity, but with hemodynamic significance manifests as upper extremity hypertension with decreased lower extremity pressures in young patients. Aortic dissection is a recognized complication. Hypertrophy of collateral arteries a hallmark of a severe stenosis. Untreated, this condition leads to left ventricular hypertrophy with subsequent dysfunction (Box 9-6). In older hypertensive adults, the descending thoracic aorta may become elongated and tortuous, simulating a congenital coarctation. The lack of a significant pressure gradient (<20 mm Hg) distinguishes this entity as a pseudocoarctation.

TABLE 9-6 Thoracic Aortic Vasculitis

Condition	Aortic Manifestation
Takayasu arteritis	Long segment stenoses, also involving proximal great vessels; rarely, focal aneurysms, dissection
Giant-cell arteritis	Aneurysm; dissection; rupture
Rheumatoid arthritis	Aortic insufficiency; ascending aortic aneurysm
Ankylosing spondylitis	Aortic insufficiency; sinotubular ectasia
Relapsing polychondritis	Aneurysm; dissection
Behçet disease	Focal aneurysms
Polymyalgia rheumatica	Aneurysm; dissection

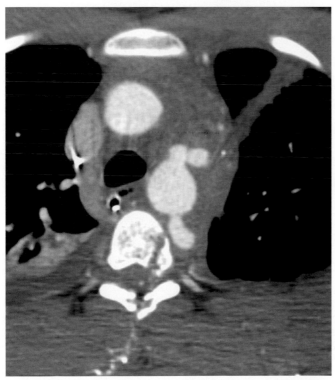

FIGURE 9-30. Gunshot wound to the descending thoracic aorta. Reformatted axial image showing the path of the bullet through the lung and vertebral body, and the pseudoaneurysms arising from the anterior and posterior aspect of the descending thoracic aorta. This was repaired percutaneously with an endograft.

Box 9-6. Thoracic Aortic Coarctation

6%-8% of all congenital cardiac disease
Bicuspid aortic valve in 40%
Other associated congenital cardiac anomalies
  • Patent ductus arteriosus
  • Ventricular septal defects
  • Mitral valve abnormalities
Life expectancy (untreated) is 35 years
Complications
  • Hypertension (upper body)
  • Left ventricular failure
  • Aortic dissection
  • Bacterial endocarditis
  • Mycotic aneurysm
  • Intracranial berry aneurysms
  • Intracranial hemorrhage

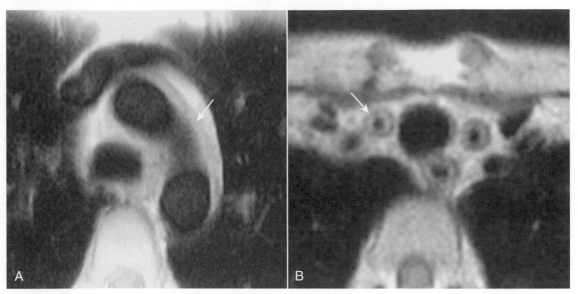

FIGURE 9-31. Takayasu arteritis. **A,** Axial T1-weighted magnetic resonance image (MRI) at the level of the aortic arch shows a thickened aortic wall *(arrow)* with intermediate signal intensity. **B,** Axial T1-weighted MRI through the proximal great vessels shows similar findings *(arrow on left,* common carotid artery). (Courtesy David Bluemke, MD, Johns Hopkins University Hospital, Baltimore, Md.)

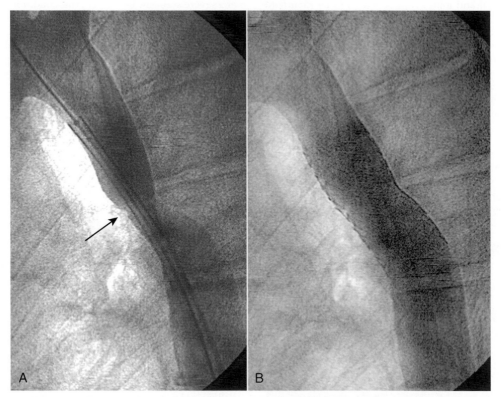

FIGURE 9-32. Treatment of symptomatic coarctation with a balloon-expandable stent. This is the same patient as in Figure 9-9. **A,** Oblique angiogram with the stent mounted on a balloon positioned across the coarctation *(arrow)*. **B,** Angiogram immediately after stent deployment showing greatly improved diameter of the aorta at the site of the coarctation.

Intervention for coarctation is based on the presence of a 20 mm Hg peak-to-peak pressure gradient or imaging evidence of significant collateralization. Surgical repair with either a patch or interposition graft has a very low mortality with a 10%-15% rate of late restenosis and 5%-8% aneurysm formation. The latter can be successfully managed with endograft placement. Angioplasty alone has a high rate of restenosis, whereas results for stent placement for both native and postsurgical recurrent coarctation approach those for surgical repair (Fig. 9-32). There is a small risk of aortic rupture with catheter-based techniques. An advantage

with balloon-expandable stents is the ability to be dilated as the patient grows. In general, surgery is still preferred for children younger than 5 years, whereas stent placement can be offered for older patients with focal native or recurrent coarctations.

THORACIC DUCT LEAK EMBOLIZATION

The thoracic duct originates at the cisterna chyli and is most often a single structure located anterior to the thoracic spine, usually on the right. The thoracic duct enters the left subclavian vein in the

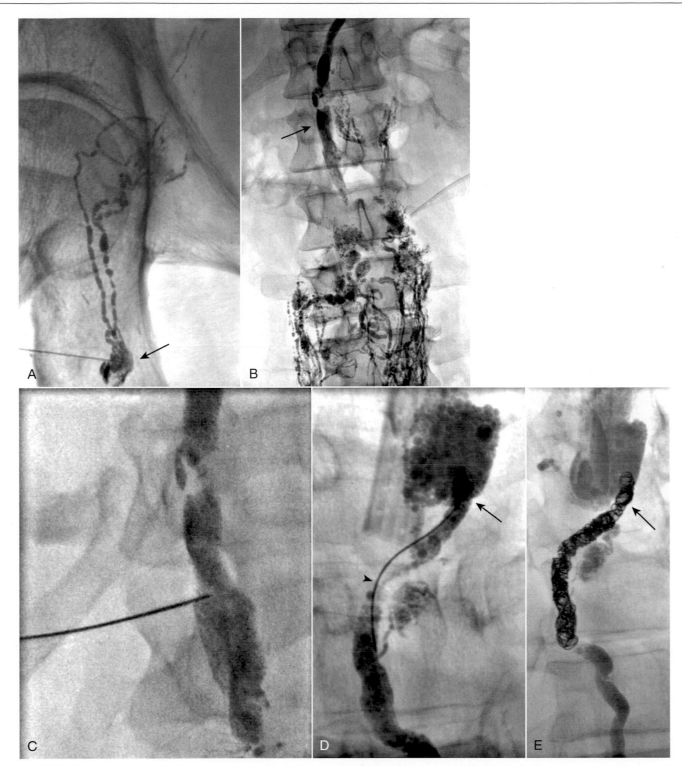

FIGURE 9-33. Thoracic duct embolization in a patient with a high-output lymph leak following esophagectomy. **A,** Direct intranodal injection of Lipiodol into an inguinal lymph node *(arrow).* Access was with ultrasound guidance. **B,** Spot radiograph of the upper abdomen showing coalescence of the opacified retroperitoneal lymphatics into the cisterna chyli *(arrow)* and the beginning of the thoracic duct. **C,** Puncture of the cisterna chyli with a 21-gauge needle introduced transabdominally. The intervening structures are ignored. **D,** Guidewire *(arrowhead)* in the thoracic duct. There is a large leak *(arrow)* adjacent to the Penrose drain. Note the droplets of oil contrast material. **E,** Multiple coils have been placed in the thoracic duct starting at the point of extravasation *(arrow).* This was followed by more coils and nBCA glue.

region of the sternoclavicular joint. This structure is the conduit for all of the lymph from the lower body—up to 4 L per day. Injury to this structure occurs most commonly during thoracic or neck surgeries (up to 3% of esophagectomies) but is also seen after thoracic trauma. Spontaneous chyle leaks are rare. The lymph accumulates in the chest, resulting in chylous pleural effusions. Chest

tube outputs of greater than 1 L per day are considered high output and have a 50% mortality with conservative treatment. The traditional management is to initiate parenteral hyperalimentation with fat-free nutrition for low-output leaks. If the low-output leak does not close spontaneously, then surgical ligation of the duct is performed. In patients with high-output leaks, early intervention

---

Box 9-7. **Thoracic Duct Embolization**

Patient should be fasting
Review abdominal computed tomography or magnetic
resonance imaging scan

DIRECT NODAL INJECTION
Localize groin lymph nodes with ultrasound
Local anesthetic
Access with 21-gauge or smaller needle under ultrasound
  • Between cortex and hilum of node
Hand injection of Lipiodol 1 mL per 5 minutes,
  total 3-6 mL
  • Reposition if extravasation or intravascular contrast seen
Chase with normal saline at same rate if cisterna not seen

TRADITIONAL LYMPHANGIOGRAM
Isosulfan blue, 0.5 mL first and third web spaces
  (bilateral)
  • Wait about 30-60 minutes until blue lymphatic
    channels visualized
0.5 % buffered Lidocaine without epinephrine dorsum
  of feet
Longitudinal incision over blue lymphatic channels
Isolate a lymphatic
  • Be sure this is not a small vein!
Cannulate with 27- or 30-gauge lymphangiography needle
  • Secure needle with suture around duct and Steri-Strips
    to skin
Lipiodol infusion, 6 mL/hr
  • Use standard power injector
  • Maximum 20 mL if no leak
    • Risk of oil pneumonitis with larger volumes
Serial spot films until cisterna chyli opacified

THORACIC DUCT EMBOLIZATION
Prophylactic intravenous antibiotics
Fluoroscopic localization for subcostal access keeping
  cisterna against the spine
Local anesthetic
20- to 21-gauge needle advanced under fluoroscopic
  guidance to cisterna
Puncture cisterna against spine
Insert 0.018-inch guidewire
Catheterize thoracic duct
Exchange for 3-French microcatheter; stiffer is better
Embolize with coils and n-BCA glue
Remove catheter
Remove lymphangiography needles and close foot incisions

---

is performed. The options include surgical ligation, Talc pleurode-sis, and more recently percutaneous thoracic duct embolization.

Percutaneous embolization of the thoracic duct, conceived and introduced by Cope, has an approximately 80% success rate in controlling chylous effusions due to thoracic duct injury. Access to the thoracic duct is through transabdominal catheterization of the cisterna chyli. The cisterna is punctured using local anesthetic and fluoroscopic guidance after opacification with iodized oil during a lymphangiogram (Fig. 9-33 and Box 9-7). No attempt is made to avoid any intervening abdominal viscera or vascular structures. Some operators attempt to disrupt the cisterna with multiple nee-dle passes if they are unable to catheterize the structure. When access to the thoracic duct is gained, a microcatheter is advanced

as close to the leak as possible. Embolization is performed with multiple coils and N-butyl cyanoacrylate (n-BCA) glue. As much duct as possible should be occluded, in that success relies on creat-ing a physical obstruction to the flow of chyle. Chest tube outputs may take several days to decrease satisfactorily. Failed emboliza-tions occur because of inability to perform the lymphangiogram, failure to access the cisterna (absent in about 2% of patients), and incomplete embolization of the thoracic duct.

SUGGESTED READINGS

Bondy CA. Aortic dissection in Turner syndrome. *Curr Opin Cardiol.* 2008;23: 519-526.
Booher AM, Eagle KA. Diagnosis and management issues in thoracic aortic aneurysm. *Am Heart J.* 2011;162:38-46.
Broberg C, Meadows AK. Advances in imaging: the impact on the care of the adult with congenital heart disease. *Prog Cardiovasc Dis.* 2011;53:293-304.
Chung JH, Ghoshhajra BB, Rojas CA, et al. CT angiography of the thoracic aorta. *Radiol Clin North Am.* 2010;48:249-264.
Cope C, Kaiser LR. Management of unremitting chylothorax by percutaneous embolization and blockage of retroperitoneal lymphatic vessels in 42 patients. *J Vasc Interv Radiol.* 2002;13:1139-1148.
Dake MD, Miller DC, Semba CP, et al. Transluminal placement of endovascular stent-grafts for the treatment of descending thoracic aortic aneurysms. *N Engl J Med.* 1994;331:1729-1734.
Dake MD, Kato N, Mitchell RS, et al. Endovascular stent-graft placement for the treatment of acute aortic dissection. *N Engl J Med.* 1999;340:1546-1552.
Eggebrecht H, Plicht B, Kahlert P, Erbel R. Intramural hematoma and penetrating ulcers: indications to endovascular treatment. *Eur J Vasc Endovasc Surg.* 2009;38:659-665.
Ehlert BA, Durham CA, Parker FM, et al. Impact of operative indication and surgical complexity on outcomes after thoracic endovascular aortic repair at National Surgical Quality Improvement Program Centers. *J Vasc Surg.* 2011;54:1629-1636.
Golledge J, Eagle KA. Acute aortic dissection. *Lancet.* 2008;372:55-66.
Hellinger JC, Daubert M, Lee EY, Epelman M. Congenital thoracic vascular anomalies: evaluation with state-of-the-art MR imaging and MDCT. *Radiol Clin North Am.* 2011;49:969-996.
Hoffer EK, Forauer AR, Silas AM, Gemery JM. Endovascular stent-graft or open surgical repair for blunt thoracic aortic trauma: systematic review. *J Vasc Interv Radiol.* 2008;19:1153-1164.
Holmes 4th JH, Bloch RD, Hall RA, et al. Natural history of traumatic rupture of the thoracic aorta managed nonoperatively: a longitudinal analysis. *Ann Thorac Surg.* 2002;73:1149-1154.
Itkin M, Kucharczuk JC, Kwak A, et al. Nonoperative thoracic duct embolization for traumatic thoracic duct leak: experience in 109 patients. *J Thorac Cardiovasc Surg.* 2010;139:584-589.
Khoynezhad A, Rao R, Trento A, Gewertz B. Management of acute type B aortic dissections and acute limb ischemia. *J Cardiovasc Surg.* 2011;52:507-517.
Khandelwal N, Kalra N, Garg MK, et al. Multidetector CT angiography in Takayasu arteritis. *Eur J Radiol.* 2011;77:369-374.
Kische S, Schneider H, Akin I, et al. Technique of interventional repair in adult aortic coarctation. *J Vasc Surg.* 2010;51:1550-1559.
McMahon MA, Squirrell CA. Multidetector CT of Aortic Dissection: A Pictorial Review. *Radiographics.* 2010;30:445-460.
Nadolski GJ, Itkin M. Feasibility of Ultrasound-guided intranodal lymphangiogram for thoracic duct embolization. *J Vasc Interv Radiol.* 2012;23:613-616.
Shiga T, Wajima Z, Apfel CC, et al. Diagnostic accuracy of transesophageal echocardiography, helical computed tomography, and magnetic resonance imaging for suspected thoracic aortic dissection: systematic review and meta-analysis. *Arch Intern Med.* 2006;166:1350-1356.
Slobodin G, Naschitz JE, Zuckerman E, et al. Aortic involvement in rheumatic diseases. *Clin Exp Rheumatol.* 2006;24:S41-S47.
Steenburg SD, Ravenel JG, Ikonomidis JS, et al. Acute traumatic aortic injury: imaging evaluation and management. *Radiology.* 2008;248:748-762.
Thrumurthy SG, Karthikesalingam A, Patterson BO, et al. A systematic review of mid-term outcomes of thoracic endovascular repair (TEVAR) of chronic type B aortic dissection. *Eur J Vasc Endovasc Surg.* 2011;42:632-647.
Williams DM, Lee DY, Hamilton BH, et al. The dissected aorta: percutaneous treatment of ischemic complications - principles and results. *J Vasc Interv Radiol.* 1997;8:605-625.
Williams DM, Lee DY, Hamilton BH, et al. The dissected aorta: III. Anatomy and radiologic diagnosis of branch-vessel com-promise. *Radiology.* 1997;203: 37-44.
Zabal C, Attie F, Rosas M, Buendia-Hernandez A, Garcia-Montes JA. The adult patient with native coarctation of the aorta: balloon angioplasty or primary stenting? *Heart.* 2003;89:77-83.

CHAPTER 10

Abdominal Aorta and Pelvic Arteries

John A. Kaufman, MD, MS, FSIR, FCIRSE

The abdominal aorta and pelvic arteries supply blood to all of the structures below the diaphragm. The pathologic processes that involve these vessels are varied and have major morbidity. This chapter covers aortic-iliac arterial diseases, including the male and female reproductive organs. The renal and mesenteric arteries are discussed in separate chapters.

NORMAL AND VARIANT ANATOMY

Abdominal Aorta

The abdominal aorta begins at the level of the diaphragmatic crura and terminates at the bifurcation into the common iliac arteries. This bifurcation is usually in the vicinity of the L4-L5 disk interspace. The major blood supply to the abdominal viscera is derived from the aorta (Fig. 10-1). The aorta is constant in location and presence, although there is extensive variability of the anatomy of the branch vessels. The average diameter of the abdominal aorta is 1.5-2 cm at the diaphragm and 1.5 cm below the renal arteries. The anterior branches of the abdominal aorta are the celiac, superior mesenteric (SMA), gonadal, phrenic, and inferior mesenteric arteries (IMA). The lateral branches are the renal and middle adrenal arteries (Table 10-1). The posterior branches are the lumbar arteries (one pair for each lumbar vertebra) and the middle sacral artery (arising at the aortic bifurcation). Clinically, the abdominal aorta is divided into supra (above) and infra (below) renal artery segments. The impetus for this division is the higher incidence of atherosclerotic and aneurysmal disease in the infrarenal abdominal aorta, and the increased complexity of interventions that involve the suprarenal portion.

The anatomy of the testicular and ovarian arteries is similar in the abdomen, but divergent in the pelvis. In 70% of individuals, the gonadal arteries arise from the anterior surface of the abdominal aorta just below the renal arteries (see Fig. 10-1). The most common variant location for gonadal artery origins is the renal arteries (20%), followed by the adrenal, lumbar, or even iliac arteries. The gonadal arteries pass to the pelvis along the anterior surface of the psoas muscles, adjacent to the gonadal veins and the ureters, and anterior to the iliac vessels.

In the male pelvis, the testicular arteries have a lateral course, entering the spermatic cord to continue into the scrotum. These arteries are the sole blood supply to the testes. In the female pelvis, the ovarian arteries have a more medial path, through the suspensory ligament of the ovary. The ovarian artery provides branches to the ovary and fallopian tubes. The artery then continues medially to the uterus, where it anastomoses with the uterine artery in the broad ligament.

The lumbar arteries are paired vessels that arise from the posterior wall of the abdominal aorta at the levels of the lumbar vertebrae. The origins of the paired lumbar arteries may be separate, or conjoint. These vessels anastomose with the intercostal and other chest wall arteries superiorly, the epigastric arteries anteriorly, and the internal iliac arteries inferiorly. These anastomoses can form the basis of collateral supply to the lower extremities in cases of distal aortic occlusive disease. The lumbar arteries supply the musculature of the back and abdominal wall, as well as the branches to the vertebral bodies and the contents of the spinal canal. This is of paramount concern whenever embolization of a lumbar artery for a nonneurologic indication is contemplated. In a small percentage of patients, the lower anterior spinal artery (artery of Adamkiewicz) will arise from an L1 or L2 lumbar artery.

The median sacral artery arises from the posterior wall of the aorta just proximal to the aortic bifurcation or as a common trunk with the L5 lumbar arteries (see Fig. 10-1). Occasionally, the median sacral artery will arise from a common iliac artery. This artery maintains a midline course in the pelvis, providing branches to the sacrum and coccyx. The median sacral artery is distinguished angiographically from the superior hemorrhoidal branch of the IMA by its posterior location and lack of a terminal bifurcation. The median sacral artery branches often anastomose with iliolumbar and rectal arteries.

Iliac Arteries and Their Branches

The aorta usually bifurcates between the L3-4 and L4-5 disk space into the right and left common iliac arteries (Fig. 10-2; see Fig. 10-1). In 2% of patients, the aorta divides over the L3 vertebral body, resulting in a steep bifurcation that is challenging to cross angiographically. The common iliac arteries are symmetric structures that usually have no major side-branches. In the adult, the average common iliac artery is 8-10 mm in diameter and 3-6 cm in length. The course of the artery is caudal, lateral, and slightly posterior into the pelvis. The right common iliac artery lies anterior and across the left common iliac vein. If seen, a small branch arising from a common iliac artery and taking a superior course into the abdomen will most likely be an accessory lower

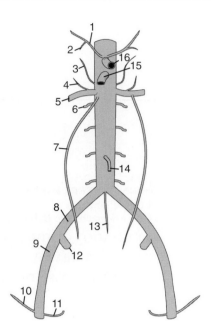

Figure 10-1. Drawing of the abdominal aorta and iliac arteries. *1*, Superior phrenic artery. *2*, Superior adrenal artery. *3*, Middle adrenal artery. *4*, Inferior adrenal artery. *5*, Renal artery. *6*, Lumbar artery. *7*, Gonadal artery. Note that in this drawing the left gonadal artery has variant origin from the left renal artery. *8*, Common iliac artery. *9*, External iliac artery. *10*, Deep iliac circumflex artery. *11*, Inferior epigastric artery. *12*, Internal iliac (hypogastric) artery. *13*, Median sacral artery. *14*, Inferior mesenteric artery. *15*, Superior mesenteric artery. *16*, Celiac artery.

Table 10-1 Major Branches of the Abdominal Aorta

Artery	Approximate Level of Origin
Celiac	T12-L1
Superior mesenteric	L1-L2
Renal	L2
Inferior mesenteric	L3-L4
Common iliac	L4-L5

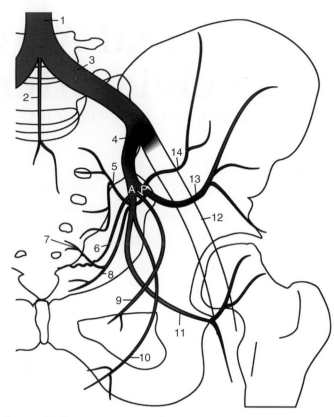

Figure 10-2. Drawing of conventional internal iliac artery anatomy (female). There is extensive variability of the anatomy of this vessel. *1*, Aorta. *2*, Median sacral artery. *3*, Common iliac artery. *4*, Internal iliac artery (A = anterior division; P = posterior division). *5*, Lateral sacral artery. *6*, Uterine artery. *7*, Middle rectal (hemorrhoidal) artery. *8*, Vesical artery. *9*, Obturator artery. *10*, Internal pudendal artery. *11*, Inferior gluteal artery. *12*, External iliac artery. *13*, Superior gluteal artery. *14*, Iliolumbar artery. (Courtesy R. T. Andrews, MD, Seattle, Wash.)

Box 10-1. Branches of the Internal Iliac Artery

ANTERIOR DIVISION ARTERIES
Inferior gluteal
Obturator
Internal pudendal
Uterine (females)
Prostatic (males)
Vesical

POSTERIOR DIVISION ARTERIES
Superior gluteal
Iliolumbar
Lateral sacral

pole renal artery. Occasionally, a median sacral artery may arise from a common iliac artery.

The common iliac arteries terminate when they bifurcate into the internal and external iliac arteries. The bifurcation is a point of fixation of the iliac arteries in the pelvis. The internal iliac (also known as the *hypogastric*) artery originates posterior and medial from the common iliac artery. This vessel is 1-4 cm in length, traveling in a posterior and inferior direction into the bony pelvis. The internal iliac artery then bifurcates into an anterior and posterior division (see Fig. 10-2). The divisional arteries then give rise to the major visceral and muscular arteries of the pelvis (Box 10-1). There is great variation in the branching patterns of the pelvic arteries. When these variants are encountered, identification of vessels should be based on what they supply rather than their point of origin.

The branches of the posterior division are the iliolumbar, superior gluteal, and lateral sacral arteries. The iliolumbar artery is usually the first branch, although it may arise from the proximal internal iliac or, rarely, the common iliac artery. The iliolumbar artery courses superiorly along the sacroiliac joint. There is usually an anastomosis between this artery and the lowest lumbar artery. The superior gluteal artery is the largest component of

the posterior division. This artery exits the bony pelvis through the greater sciatic foramen, superior to the piriformis muscle, to supply the muscles of the posterior pelvis. The lateral sacral arteries are named for their origins relative to the sacrum, rather than their course in the pelvis. These arteries are small in caliber and frequently multiple. They travel medially toward the sacrum, with anastomoses to the median sacral artery and the opposite lateral sacral vessels.

The anterior division of the hypogastric artery supplies the visceral and muscular contents of the pelvic cavity. The visceral branches are the internal pudendal, vesicle, middle rectal, and in females, the uterine and vaginal arteries (Fig. 10-3; see Fig. 10-2). Discrete superior and inferior vesicle arteries are usually

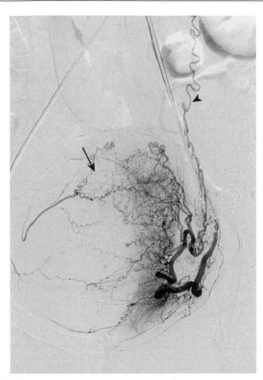

FIGURE 10-3. Selective injection of the left uterine artery in a patient with fibroids shows the hypervascular benign tumor *(arrow)* and reflux into the left ovarian artery *(arrowhead)*. (Courtesy Hal Folander, MD, St. Luke's Hospital & Health Network, Bethlehem, PA.)

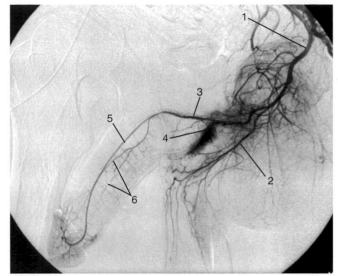

FIGURE 10-4. Normal internal pudendal arteriogram in a male. The arterial anatomy is usually symmetric. *1,* Internal pudendal artery. *2,* Perineal artery. *3,* Common penile artery. *4,* Normal bulbo-spongiosal blush. *5,* Dorsal penile artery. *6,* Deep penile artery (in this individual both arise from the left).

present. In females, the inferior vesicle artery becomes one of the vaginal arteries. The middle rectal artery, frequently a branch of the inferior vesicle artery, anastomoses with the IMA through the superior hemorrhoidal artery. The uterine artery courses medially in the broad ligament superior to the ureter. At the uterus the artery assumes a characteristic corkscrew configuration as it travels parallel to the uterine body. The uterus is a very vascular organ that stains or enhances intensely at angiography, particularly in premenopausal women. The uterine arteries anastomose with both the ovarian artery and the vaginal arteries. The internal pudendal artery supplies the external genitalia. Accessory pudendal branches may arise from other anterior division arteries or from external iliac artery branches. The internal pudendal artery exits the floor of the pelvis between the piriformis and coccygeus muscles, after which it travels anteriorly along the lateral border of the pelvis. The inferior rectal artery arises as a branch of the internal pudendal in this region. In males, the internal pudendal artery bifurcates into the perineal artery (to the scrotum) and a common penile artery (Fig. 10-4). The common penile artery bifurcates into deep penile (in the center of the corpus cavernosum) and dorsal penile (along the dorsal surface of the corpus cavernosum) arteries as it travels beneath the pubic symphysis. The prostatic artery arises as branch of the internal pudendal artery in about 50% of men, as a discrete branch of the anterior division in approximately 25%, and as branches of the obturator or inferior gluteal artery in the remainder. The prostatic artery often gives rise to branches to the bladder and seminal vesicles. At the prostate the artery usually bifurcates into posterior and anterior capsular arteries. In 25% of males, the anterior capsular artery anastomoses with distal branches of the internal pudendal artery. In females, the internal pudendal artery supplies the labia and the clitoris.

The obturator and inferior gluteal arteries are the primary musculoskeletal branches of the anterior division of the internal iliac artery (see Fig. 10-2). Both vessels frequently provide branches to the bladder. The obturator artery arises from the anterior division in 50% of individuals. This vessel exits the pelvis through the obturator canal, where it has a characteristic bifurcation. In approximately 15% of people, the artery may take its origin from the inferior gluteal or the internal pudendal arteries. The obturator artery arises from the superior gluteal artery (a branch of the posterior division) in 20% of individuals and from the common femoral or inferior epigastric arteries in 20%. The inferior gluteal artery is a branch of the anterior division in 75% of individuals and of the posterior division in 25%. The artery exits the pelvis between the piriformis and the coccygeus muscles in the lower portion of the sciatic notch. The inferior gluteal artery accompanies the sciatic and posterior femoral cutaneous nerves, terminating in branches to the buttocks and posterior thigh.

The external iliac arteries provide blood supply to the lower extremities. The typical diameter of the external iliac artery is 5-7 mm. The artery angles anteriorly and laterally from the common iliac artery bifurcation, passing under the inguinal ligament to form the common femoral artery. The angulation between the common and external iliac arteries can become severe in patients with redundant atherosclerotic arteries. The only branches of the external iliac artery are usually the circumflex iliac arteries (deep and superficial) arising laterally, and the inferior epigastric artery medially (see Fig. 10-1). These branches demarcate the transition from the external iliac to common femoral arteries. As noted above, the obturator artery is replaced to the external iliac artery in 20% of individuals, usually arising from a common trunk with the inferior epigastric artery.

▬ KEY COLLATERAL PATHWAYS

A large number of potential collateral arterial pathways are present in the abdomen and pelvis (Table 10-2). The pathway that becomes dominant in a particular patient depends upon the location and length of the obstruction, and whether one or both sides of the pelvis are affected (Fig. 10-5). Multiple collateral pathways frequently coexist in the same patient.

The collateral supply to the uterus in the presence of uterine artery occlusion is from the gonadal, vaginal, vesicle, and unnamed arteries in the broad ligament. In general, central pelvic structures may be supplied by branches from either side of the pelvis, the distal aorta, the IMA, the gonadal arteries, and even branches of the profunda femoral artery. Structures lateral to and including the iliac bones may be supplied by multiple branches of the internal

TABLE 10-2 Collateral Pathways in Aortoiliac Arterial Occlusion

Source	Example
Thoracic aorta	1. Superior to inferior epigastric to common femoral arteries
	2. Intercostal to lumbar arteries to aorta
Mesenteric arteries	Inferior mesenteric to hemorrhoidal to internal iliac to external iliac arteries (see Chapter 11)
Lumbar arteries	1. Lumbar to iliolumbar to internal iliac to external iliac arteries
	2. Lumbar to iliac-circumflex to common femoral arteries
Median sacral artery	Median sacral to lateral sacral to internal iliac to external iliac artery
Internal iliac artery	To opposite side of pelvis: internal iliac to lateral sacral and anterior division arteries cross midline to same arteries on contralateral side
	To common femoral artery on same side of pelvis when external iliac artery occluded:
	1. Internal iliac to posterior division branches to iliac circumflex to ipsilateral common femoral artery
	2. Internal iliac to both anterior and posterior divisions to profunda femoris branches to common femoral artery

iliac artery, lumbar arteries, or branches of the distal external iliac artery or the common femoral artery. Conversely, the ovaries can receive collateral supply from the uterine arteries.

IMAGING

Ultrasound of the abdominal aorta is an excellent modality for screening for abdominal aortic aneurysms (AAA). Reliable evaluation of aortic occlusive disease is more difficult with ultrasound. In large patients, the aorta is a deep structure, surrounded by air-filled bowel, making ultrasound imaging technically difficult. Tortuosity of the aorta and mural calcification can also limit ultrasound imaging. These same restrictions apply to ultrasound imaging of the common and especially the internal iliac arteries. With the addition of intravenous ultrasound (IVUS) contrast agents, this modality may become more useful in the evaluation of aortoiliac arterial occlusive disease.

Perhaps the single most useful cross-sectional imaging modality for the abdominal aorta is computed tomography angiography (CTA). Aortic vascular studies should begin with a noncontrast scan to assess calcification and detect fresh hemorrhage. Contrast-enhanced CT scans should be performed with a power injector (3-5 mL/sec contrast for a total volume of 70-90 mL) on a high-speed scanner using thin (0.5-2 mm) effective collimation. The scanning delay for contrast injection can be empiric or determined with a test bolus or automated triggering software. The field of view should be reduced to emphasize the central vascular structures. Images obtained in this manner can be postprocessed into elegant CT angiograms (see Fig. 3-21).

CTA has excellent sensitivity and specificity (each >99%) for detection of abdominal and iliac artery aneurysms. Aortic and iliac occlusive disease is readily evaluated with CTA. Heavily calcified iliac arteries, particularly tortuous and small external iliac arteries, can be difficult to evaluate for occlusive disease with confidence with CTA. Contrast is required for CTA, limiting utility in patients with chronic renal insufficiency.

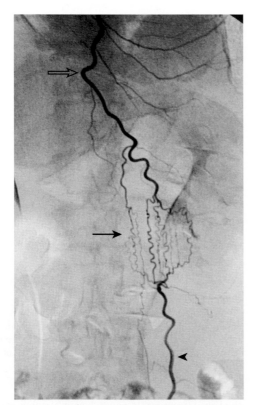

FIGURE 10-5. Internal mammary artery *(open arrow)* angiogram centered over the abdomen in a patient with aortoiliac occlusion showing collateralization *(arrow)* to the inferior epigastric artery *(arrowhead)*, providing blood supply to the left lower extremity. This is known as "nature's axillofemoral bypass."

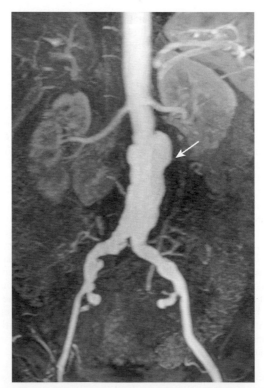

FIGURE 10-6. Coronal maximum-intensity projection (MIP) of gadolinium-enhanced three-dimensional magnetic resonance angiogram showing an infrarenal abdominal aortic aneurysm *(arrow)*.

TABLE 10-3 Abdominal Aortography

Parameter	Recommendations
Catheter	4- or 5-French pigtail or equivalent
Catheter position	T12-L1
Contrast	30% Iodine or greater
Injection rate	20-25 mL/sec for 2 seconds
Views	Anteroposterior and lateral
Filming rate	4-6 frames/sec
Additional views	10-15 degrees left anterior oblique with catheter at renal origins

TABLE 10-4 Pelvic Angiography

Parameter	Recommendations
Catheter	4- or 5-French pigtail or equivalent
Catheter position	2-3 cm proximal to aortic bifurcation
Contrast	30% Iodine or greater
Injection rate	7-15 mL/sec for 2-4 seconds
Views	Anteroposterior, 30-45 degrees oblique (bilateral)
Filming rate	2-6 frames/sec

TABLE 10-5 Abdominal Aortic Aneurysm

Factor	Reported values
Male: female	4:1
Prevalence	5%-9% males aged 65
Average rate of growth	0.2-0.4 cm/yr
Risk of rupture (male)	
<5.5 cm diameter	1%/yr
5.5-5.9 cm diameter	9.4%/yr
6-6.9 cm diameter	10.2%/yr
>7 cm diameter	32.5%/yr

Magnetic resonance imaging (MRI) of the abdominal aorta is relatively straightforward and accurate. With the exception of an inability to demonstrate calcium and artifact from metal, there are few limitations of this modality. The aortic wall can be evaluated from T1-weighted images in three orthogonal planes, but the best vascular imaging is obtained with gadolinium-enhanced three-dimensional (3-D) MR angiography (MRA) (Fig. 10-6). The volume of gadolinium ranges from 20 to 40 mL, injected at 2-3 mL/sec. The injection timing can be determined using automated triggering software or a test bolus of 2-3 mL. In patients with chronic renal insufficiency, the abdominal aorta and iliac arteries can be imaged with noncontrast MRA. The 3-D volume can then be postprocessed into angiographic images. Metal clips, orthopedic and spinal hardware, and certain stents can create artifacts that obscure vascular segments (see Fig. 3-15).

BOX 10-2. Causes of Aortoiliac Aneurysms

Degenerative
Chronic dissection
Inflammatory
Vasculitis
- Behçet disease
- Takayasu arteritis
Mycotic
Marfan syndrome
Ehlers-Danlos syndrome
Anastomotic pseudoaneurysm
Traumatic pseudoaneurysm

Conventional angiography of the abdominal aorta is usually performed with a 4- or 5-French pigtail or other flush catheter. The tip of the catheter is positioned at or just above the origin of the celiac artery (usually the T12-L1 interspace) (Table 10-3). If the renal artery origins are not well visualized, repositioning the catheter at the level of the renal arteries and filming with 10- to 15-degree left anterior oblique angulation will often display these vessels to best advantage (Fig. 10-7). In patients with contraindications to iodinated contrast, CO_2 or gadolinium can be used, although CO_2 may become trapped in large aneurysm sacs.

Non-selective pelvic angiography can be performed with the same catheter positioned 2-3 cm proximal to the aortic bifurcation to ensure that all of the side-holes are in the aorta (Table 10-4). The area included in the field of view should extend from the distal aorta to just below the common femoral artery bifurcation. Oblique views are crucial owing to the natural tortuosity of the pelvic arteries and to visualize the internal iliac artery origins. The posterior oblique projection usually displays the internal iliac artery origin to best advantage (Fig. 10-8; see also Fig. 2-52).

Angiography of the internal iliac artery or its branches requires a selective end-hole catheter. Usually both internal iliac arteries can be selected from a single femoral artery access. The contralateral internal iliac artery is selected in an antegrade fashion with a Cobra 2 or other angled catheter by crossing the aortic bifurcation, usually in conjunction with an angled steerable hydrophilic guidewire. The ipsilateral internal iliac artery can be selected from the same femoral artery access with a pull-down technique using a Waltman loop or a Simmons-shaped catheter, or sometimes by antegrade cannulation with an angled catheter (see Fig. 2-17). The posterior oblique projection is most useful to visualize the origin of the internal iliac artery (see Fig. 10-8). However, the anterior oblique view opens up the anterior and posterior division origins. In young patients, especially women, the internal iliac branches are prone to spasm, so gentle manipulation and generous utilization of intraarterial nitroglycerin (150- to 200-μg aliquots) may be necessary. Injection rates for these vessels vary, but are usually 3-5 mL/sec for 2-3 seconds.

ANEURYSMS

Etiologies of aortic and iliac artery aneurysms are listed in Box 10-2. Degenerative aneurysms are the most commonly encountered type in clinical practice, occurring in older patients with generalized atherosclerotic disease (Table 10-5; see also Fig. 3-17). Age, male gender, smoking, and family history heavily influence the risk of AAA. The size of the aneurysm determines timing of elective therapy, and the extent of involvement of the aorta, visceral arteries, and pelvic arteries determines the treatment approach. Aneurysms involving the descending thoracic as well as the abdominal aorta are more difficult to treat with endovascular techniques and require more extensive surgical exposure than aneurysms confined to the infrarenal aorta. In general, degenerative aortoiliac aneurysms are asymptomatic until they rupture, so that preemptive treatment is desirable.

The etiology of degenerative aortoiliac aneurysms is multifactorial and incompletely understood. The different potential mechanisms are detailed in Chapter 1, but include familial, enzymatic, and possibly infectious causes. Atherosclerotic changes including calcification of the intima are prominent features of these aneurysms. An AAA is defined as a fusiform or saccular enlargement of the aorta that is 1.5 times greater in diameter than a normal aorta, or more than 3 cm in diameter. Common and internal iliac arteries larger than 1.5-2 cm in diameter are considered aneurysms. Aneurysms are frequently lined with mural thrombus, although the volume and distribution are variable (see Fig. 3-17).

The most feared complication of AAA is rupture, which typically occurs without warning, often in a patient unaware of the presence of the aneurysm (see Fig. 1-10). The risk of rupture is proportional to aneurysm diameter, but is thought to be negligible when diameter is less than 5 cm. These patients undergo regular surveillance ("watchful waiting") with yearly aortic ultrasound. Elective repair of aneurysms is usually performed when the diameter exceeds 5.5 cm, although this number continues to

be debated. Women may be at higher risk for rupture at a smaller diameter than men. Other than rupture, other complications are rare but include distal embolization of mural thrombus, thrombosis, infection, and aortoenteric fistula.

Aortic aneurysms that occur in young patients, in unusual locations, or under unusual circumstances are usually not degenerative in etiology. Underlying connective tissue disorders, trauma, vasculitis, and infection are more common in these patients. Often these are actually pseudoaneurysms, which are at greater risk of rupture than similar sized degenerative aneurysms.

Degenerative aneurysms of the iliac arteries usually involve the common and/or the internal iliac arteries. Aneurysms of the external iliac artery are rare, possibly explained by the separate embryologic origin (iliofemoral) from the common and internal iliac arteries (sciatic). Isolated degenerative common iliac artery aneurysms account for 2% of abdominal aneurysms; most are found in association with AAA (Fig. 10-9). The male-to-female ratio for isolated iliac artery aneurysms is 7:1, and 50% are bilateral. In general, common iliac aneurysms warrant repair when

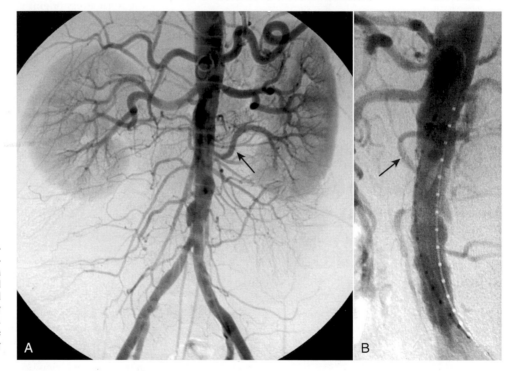

FIGURE 10-7. Digital subtraction aortography in a patient with diffuse aortic atherosclerosis. **A,** Anteroposterior angiogram obtained with a pigtail catheter placed just proximal to the level of the renal arteries. Incidentally, there is an accessory lower pole renal artery on the left *(arrow)*. **B,** Lateral view in the same patient. Note the course of the accessory renal artery *(arrow)*.

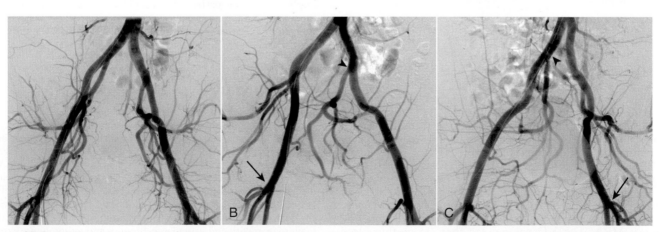

FIGURE 10-8. Digital subtraction angiogram anteroposterior and oblique views of the pelvis. **A,** Anteroposterior view. **B,** Right anterior oblique view portrays the left common iliac artery origin, the left common iliac bifurcation *(arrowhead)*, and the right common femoral artery bifurcation *(arrow)* to best advantage. **C,** Left anterior oblique view displays the right common iliac artery origin, the right common iliac artery bifurcation *(arrowhead)* and left common femoral artery bifurcation *(arrow)* to best advantage.

they reach a diameter of 3 cm. Isolated internal iliac artery aneurysms are even less common than isolated common iliac aneurysms (< 0.5%) (Fig.10-10).

Inflammatory aneurysms comprise 5% of all AAA. These are not infectious aneurysms. The characteristic appearance is an enhancing mantle of tissue circumferentially or partially surrounding the infrarenal aorta (Fig. 10-11). This distinguishes an inflammatory aneurysm from a localized rupture, in which the periaortic tissue will not enhance on contrast-enhanced CT or MRI scan. The etiology is unknown, occurring in slightly younger patients than bland degenerative AAA. The presenting symptoms may be abdominal pain and aortic tenderness, similar to a contained aortic rupture. The inflammatory mantle involves the duodenum in 90%, the inferior vena cava (IVC) and left renal vein in 50%, and ureters in 25%.

Aneurysm rupture can be either free, contained, or into an adjacent venous structure (Figs. 10-12 and 10-13; see also Fig. 1-10). Most free ruptures are associated with large retroperitoneal hematomas as well as intraperitoneal blood. Early or small ruptures may be subtle, with the only evidence being stranding in the periaortic fat. In comparison, chronic contained ruptures are usually focal saccular contour abnormalities associated with localized disruption of intimal calcification and little or no surrounding soft tissue reaction. Patients with rupture into an adjacent vein (left renal vein, IVC, or common iliac vein) may present with hematuria, flank pain, or high-output cardiac failure. When acute AAA rupture is suspected in a hemodynamically stable patient, CT scan is the imaging modality of choice. This should be performed first without contrast, followed by contrast. Common iliac and internal iliac artery aneurysms can also present with rupture.

Imaging of aortoiliac aneurysms has several objectives: detection of aneurysms, monitoring size, preintervention planning, and postintervention follow-up. Preprocedural planning requires evaluation of specific anatomic features of the aneurysm (Box 10-3).

Ultrasound is an excellent and inexpensive modality for detection and monitoring of AAA, with somewhat less success in the iliac arteries (especially internal iliac). However, ultrasound cannot provide sufficient information for planning intervention. Both CT with CTA and MRI with MRA can provide most of the information needed to plan interventions, as well as detection and monitoring of AAA. Postprocessing of good quality studies is necessary to obtain the pertinent information to determine suitability for and plan an endograft procedure. However, aneurysm size is best measured from raw or reformatted images, because volume and surface renderings may show only the opacified lumen (see Fig. 3-21). MRI is limited by an inability to show calcification, so a noncontrast CT scan is frequently also obtained when planning an endovascular repair using MR.

Conventional angiography is not necessary in most patients undergoing repair of AAA. Aneurysm size is not accurately depicted, because mural thrombus can reduce the diameter of the patent lumen so that the true vessel diameter is not appreciated. Conventional angiography can be useful in the evaluation of patients with complex AAA, such as juxtarenal or suprarenal aneurysms, unusual renal artery anatomy such as horseshoe kidney, suspected visceral artery occlusive disease, and iliac occlusive disease. A graduated measuring catheter should be used for these studies. IVUS can also be used to measure the internal diameters of vessels and distances.

Treatment of infrarenal AAA is by placement of a stent-graft or surgery. Surgical repair, though performed less and less often, is still the most durable treatment. Briefly, this involves a transabdominal or retroperitoneal incision, placement of a proximal clamp on the aorta (preferably infrarenal), placement of a distal clamp, incision of the aneurysm with evacuation of mural thrombus, suture ligation of patent lumbar arteries and the IMA, suturing of a synthetic graft that extends from the proximal clamp to either the distal aorta, common iliac or femoral arteries, and then closure of the incisions (Fig. 10-14). Surgical repair of suprarenal AAA is more difficult and morbid because a supraceliac clamp is required and the major visceral branches must be reimplanted. The mortality rate is 3%-6% for elective surgery and 25%-50% for emergent repair of a ruptured aneurysm. Acute severe complications include bowel ischemia (2%), limb ischemia (0.5%),

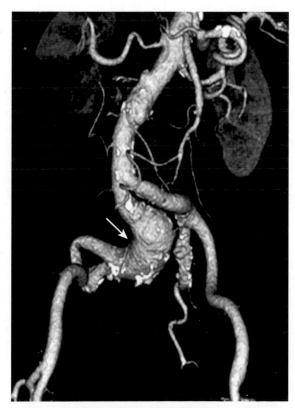

FIGURE 10-9. Right common iliac artery aneurysms. Volume rendering of a computed tomography angiogram showing a right common iliac artery aneurysm *(arrow)*. The aneurysm extends to the common iliac bifurcation. The abdominal aorta is normal in diameter.

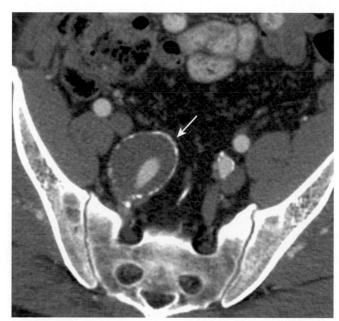

FIGURE 10-10. Axial contrast-enhanced computed tomography image showing an isolated right internal iliac artery aneurysm *(arrow)*. Note the intimal calcification and extensive mural thrombus.

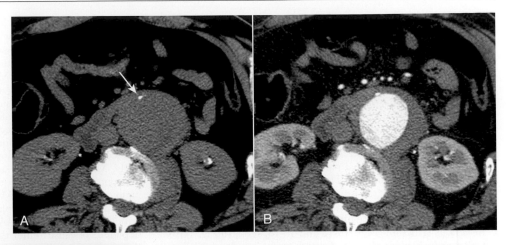

FIGURE 10-11. Inflammatory abdominal aortic aneurysm in a 53-year-old man. **A,** Axial computed tomography (CT) scan without contrast shows a thick rind external to the intimal calcium *(arrow)* around the aortic aneurysm. Note that the periaortic fat is free of stranding or other inflammatory signs. The density of the rind was 42 HU. **B,** Axial CT scan with contrast at the same level. Although difficult to tell without density measurements, the inflammatory rind enhances (now 64 HU). Hematoma related to abdominal aortic aneurysm rupture would not enhance.

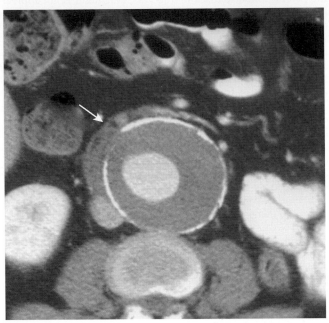

FIGURE 10-12. Subtle rupture (surgically proven) of the abdominal aorta in an older man with an episode of acute back pain. There is focal increased density of the periaortic soft tissues *(arrow)* adjacent to an interruption in the intimal calcification. Compare with Figure 1-10.

and cardiopulmonary disorders (15%). Repair of inflammatory aneurysms is more difficult owing to the periaortic rind.

Late complications of surgical repair are infrequent (Box 10-4). The two that are most dreaded are graft infection and aortoenteric fistula. Graft infection may present as sepsis, a draining wound, graft thrombosis, abscess formation, or an anastomotic aneurysm. Aortoenteric fistula usually occurs at the proximal anastomosis and presents as upper gastrointestinal bleeding (usually duodenal) of catastrophic proportions. By definition, graft material involved in aortoenteric fistulas is infected, but massive bleeding dominates the clinical scenario. Graft enteric fistulas can occur anywhere along the graft and present with chronic bleeding and infection (Box 10-5).

Endovascular repair of infrarenal AAA with stent-grafts is used in up to 75% of patients in some practices (Box 10-6). Aortic stent-grafts have three basic configurations (Fig. 10-15). Patients must meet anatomic criteria involving the proximal and distal attachment sites, angulation and tortuosity of the aorta and pelvis, and presence of calcification and occlusive disease in the access arteries. The specific requirements vary for each manufacturer. The bifurcated devices are usually modular in construction; that is, the endograft is assembled in the patient. The materials used in construction of endografts are biocompatible metals, such as nitinol, stainless steel, and Elgiloy, and proven vascular graft materials. Endografts function by depressurizing the aneurysm sac. Two critical differences between endovascular repair and surgery are the absence of sutured anastomoses to blood vessels, and the potential for continued patency of branch vessels arising from the sac such as lumbar arteries and the IMA. Most patients treated with current devices receive bifurcated endografts. Approximately 10%-15% of patients require a percutaneous intervention such as embolization of an internal iliac or accessory renal artery, or iliac angioplasty, in order to become anatomically suitable for a standard endograft (Box 10-7). Approximately 30% of patients who undergo internal iliac artery embolization develop transient buttock claudication. Recent innovations include an endograft with an external "endo-bag," which obliterates the aneurysm lumen, and a remote pressure sensor that can be deposited within the AAA during the procedure to allow subsequent pressure measurements during follow-up (Fig. 10-16).

Endografts that can accommodate branch arteries are becoming available and increase both the spectrum of patients that can be treated and the complexity of the procedures (Fig. 10-17). These devices use either small endograft appendages that are connected to the branch arteries with smaller endografts, or carefully positioned scallops or fenestrations in the main body that are positioned over the orifice of the branch. An endograft or bare stent is often placed through the fenestration into the branch artery. Alternatively, insertion of a small endograft into a branch vessel so that it runs cephalad between the main endograft and the aortic wall (the "snorkel" technique) has been used to allow placement of endografts over critical branch vessels origins (Fig. 10-18). These approaches further expand the treatment options for patients with aneurysms that involve the visceral artery segment of the abdominal aorta or the common iliac arteries.

The exact technique of endograft placement varies with each device, but certain commonalities exist. Most important is careful preprocedural planning, especially device selection, in that none is retrievable. For most manufacturers, the diameters of the device at the attachment sites should be at least 10%-15% greater than the artery (measured either adventitia-to-adventitia or intima-to-intima depending on the device). Excellent intraprocedural imaging is mandatory. Precise localization of critical branch vessels such as the renal and internal iliac arteries prevents inadvertent occlusion by graft overlay. In general, an aortogram is obtained centered on the renal arteries, followed by deployment of the proximal portion of the device (Fig. 10-19). Once this has been accomplished, the distal portion is deployed after localization of the internal iliac arteries. Most modular bifurcated devices require catheterization of at least one limb stump, usually from the opposite common femoral artery, to complete construction of the endograft.

The device delivery systems range in size from 12 to 21 French. Percutaneous insertion of endografts using the "pre-close"

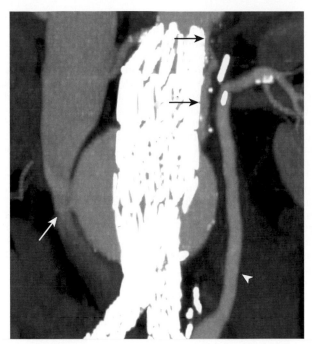

FIGURE 10-13. Aortocaval fistula. Coronal reformat of a computed tomography angiogram in a patient treated with a stent-graft for abdominal aortic aneurysm (AAA) rupture into the inferior vena cava. The aortocaval fistula *(white arrow)* is visible despite the presence of the stent-graft because of the proximal type I endoleak *(black arrows)* that allows continued perfusion of the AAA (for definition of endoleak, see Table 10-6 below). The patient had a left iliorenal bypass *(arrowhead)* before the stent-graft procedure to allow coverage of the left renal artery origin.

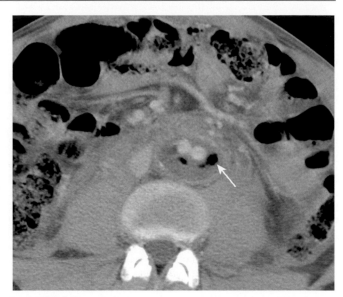

FIGURE 10-14. Axial computed tomography scan with contrast obtained 48 hours after surgery for aortic aneurysm. Perigraft gas *(arrow)* is present around the graft within the aneurysm sac, but is a normal finding up to 3 weeks after surgery. Compare with Figure 1-36. It is essential to know the date of surgery when interpreting postoperative scans.

Box 10-3. Preintervention Evaluation of Abdominal Aortic Aneurysms

Maximum diameter of aneurysm
Diameter and quality of normal infrarenal aorta
Quality and anatomy of renal and visceral arteries
Relationship of aneurysm to renal arteries:
  • Infrarenal: >1 cm length normal aorta below renal arteries
  • Juxtarenal: Aneurysm begins within 1 cm of renal arteries
  • Suprarenal: Aneurysm extends above renal arteries
Diameter and length of normal aorta distal to aneurysm (if present)
Relationship of aneurysm to aortic bifurcation
Distance from lowest renal artery to aortic bifurcation
Associated common and internal iliac artery aneurysms
Diameter and length of common iliac arteries
Diameter of external iliac artery
Presence of occlusive disease in iliac and common femoral arteries
  • Calcification, tortuosity, stenosis
Venous anatomy
  • Inferior vena cava, left renal vein
Renal anatomy
  • Horseshoe, pelvic kidney

Box 10-4. Complications of Surgical Aortic Aneurysm Repair

Bowel ischemia (usually acute, inferior mesenteric artery distribution)
Graft thrombosis
Aneurysm formation above or below graft
Anastomotic pseudoaneurysm (frequently at more than one anastomosis)
Aortoenteric fistula
Graft infection
Graft degeneration

Box 10-5. Aortoenteric Fistula

Clinical presentation includes massive hematemesis, lower gastrointestinal tract bleeding, sepsis, abdominal pain
Usually at anastomotic suture lines (<1% aortic repairs), but can occur with native aneurysm
Duodenum most common site, but can occur at any point where bowel and graft are in contact
On computed tomography, no definable fat plane between graft and bowel; ± perigraft gas
Angiography may be negative, small "nipple" at anastomosis, or aneurysm; extravasation rare
At upper endoscopy, graft may be visible in base of duodenal erosion

---

technique (see Chapter 2, Box 2-10) is becoming increasingly common, but surgical exposure of the common femoral artery is used whenever the artery is diseased, of questionable size, or a surgical graft is present. When femoral access is not feasible, direct access to the common iliac artery or placement of a conduit may be necessary. Endograft procedures can be performed under general anesthesia, regional block, or sedation with local anesthesia.

Placement of endografts is successful in more than 95% of attempts, as long as patients are carefully selected. The major complication rate is less than 5%, with most related to the vascular access. Patients usually are discharged home the first or second postprocedure day. Early mortality (<2%) has been shown to be lower with endograft repair of AAA when compared with surgery in prospective randomized trials. There have been three major randomized trials of endovascular versus open surgical repair: EVAR 1 (Endovascular Aneurysm Repair trial 1),

DREAM (Dutch Randomized Endovascular Aneurysm Management Trial), and OVER (Open Versus Endovascular Repair). After 2 years, there is equivalent survival and freedom from aneurysm rupture. In approximately 25% of patients with endografts, additional endovascular procedures are required within 8 years to maintain clinical success compared to 10% of patients undergoing surgery. This makes endograft repair more expensive overall.

Continued opacification of the aneurysm sac by contrast following endograft placement (termed *endoleak*) is found on CT scans in 30%-40% of patients acutely and 20%-40% during follow-up (Table 10-6 and Fig. 10-20; see Fig. 10-13). The etiology of the majority of early and late sac perfusion is type II, with types I and III being less common. Type IV perfusion is now uncommon and generally resolves spontaneously within 48 hours of endograft placement. Type V endoleaks ("endotension") are a diagnosis of exclusion, in that continued sac expansion is documented but no perfusion of the sac can be detected with any imaging modality.

Treatment of endoleaks is based on the risk of AAA rupture. Type I and III perfusion should be treated when discovered, because these have a strong correlation with AAA enlargement and potential rupture. These can often be treated with percutaneous methods, such as insertion of endograft extensions for type I leaks and insertion of endograft "patches" for type III perfusion.

However, careful assessment of the endograft is important, in that a failing device may fail again.

The management of type II endoleaks is more problematic. Currently, enlargement of the aneurysm in the presence of type II perfusion is considered an indication for intervention. Stable or shrinking aneurysms can be monitored, but it is often disconcerting to see continued perfusion in the aneurysm on CT or MRI scan. In the future, implantable pressure sensors will be placed in the aneurysm sac during the endograft procedure may have an important role in determining which patients with type II perfusion to treat (i.e., those with near systemic pressure in the aneurysm sac).

Type II endoleaks are analogous to arteriovenous malformations (AVMs), in which there are multiple feeding vessels to a single central nidus. With type II perfusion, the "nidus" is usually a channel or space within the intraaneurysmal thrombus that communicates with lumbar, median sacral, IMA, gonadal, or accessory renal arteries. As with treatment of an AVM, occlusion of the branch arteries is not sufficient, because additional arteries will be "recruited" over time. To effectively treat the type II perfusion, the central space must be obliterated. Access to this space can be retrograde through one of the branches (e.g., SMA to left branch of middle colic to IMA, or hypogastric to iliolumbar to lumbar artery) or by direct puncture of the aneurysm under fluoroscopic, CT, ultrasound, or IVUS guidance. Embolization may be with coils, Gelfoam soaked in thrombin, glue, or Onyx (Fig. 10-21). The long-term success of treatment of large type II endoleaks (i.e., multiple feeding arteries at multiple levels) has not been well described in the literature, but it is better than 50%.

Box 10-6. Indications and Contraindications for Endografts in Abdominal Aortic Aneurysm

INDICATIONS
AAA ≥5 cm diameter
Rapidly expanding (>5 mm/yr) smaller AAA
Contained-rupture AAA
Inflammatory AAA
High risk for complication with open repair

CONTRAINDICATIONS
No suitable proximal/distal attachment site
Severe, uncorrectable iliac occlusive disease
Mycotic aneurysm*
Marfan syndrome
Ehlers-Danlos syndrome
Indispensable IMA
Life-threatening contrast allergy
Poor compliance with follow-up

*Relative, may be used when surgical alternative is not feasible
AAA, Abdominal aortic aneurysm; IMA, inferior mesenteric artery.

Box 10-7. Adjunct Procedures Before or During Endovascular Repair of Aneurysms

Branch vessel embolization (internal iliac, accessory renal, or inferior mesenteric artery)
Angioplasty of iliac artery stenosis during device delivery
"Snorkel" to preserve branch artery perfusion
Placement of intraaneurysm remote pressure sensor
Stent reinforcement of endograft limb
Stent for access artery dissection
Stent-graft extension or surgical bypass for access artery rupture
Surgical placement of conduit graft to common iliac artery or aorta

---

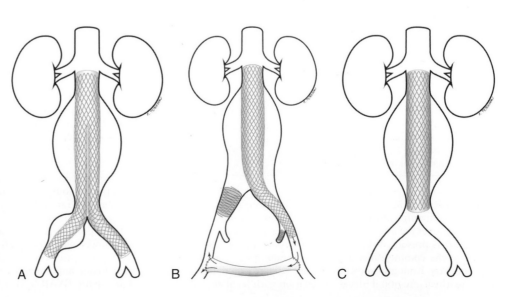

FIGURE 10-15. Endograft configurations. **A,** Bifurcated extending into either the common or external iliac arteries. This is the most common type of endograft. **B,** Aortounilateral iliac (AUNI) graft with surgical femoral-femoral bypass. This type is used when the patient's anatomy is not suited to a bifurcated graft. **C,** Tube graft. This is rarely used owing to the lack of adequate distal landing zones in the aorta below the aneurysm. (From Kaufman JA, Geller SC, Brewster DC, et al. Endovascular repair of abdominal aortic aneurysms: current status and future directions. *Am J Roentgenol.* 2000;175:289-302, with permission.)

The most important outcome of endografts is freedom from AAA rupture. Delayed rupture is reported in fewer than 0.1% of patients. The mortality rate is the same as for patients with rupture of unrepaired aneurysms. Most patients have stabilization or decrease in the volume of the aneurysm sac (see Fig. 4-25).

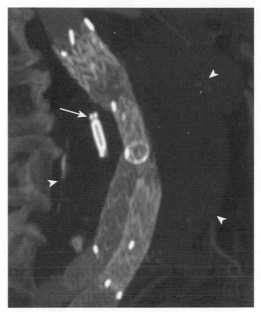

FIGURE 10-16. Remote pressure sensor *(arrow)* (CardioMEMS, Atlanta, Ga.) placed within the abdominal aortic aneurysm (AAA) sac *(arrowheads)* during endograft procedure to allow external determination of intrasac pressures. The device is a passive transmitter that emits a signal calibrated to the patient's AAA sac pressure when interrogated with a dedicated radiofrequency instrument.

However, continued sac growth is seen in at least 5% of patients. Long-term outcomes may be device specific. Shrinkage of the perianeurysmal fibrosis after endograft placement has been reported in patients with inflammatory aneurysms.

Plain films as well as CT scans (or some other reproducible imaging technique such as ultrasound) are essential parts of the follow-up of these patients. Patients must be studied at regular intervals for the remainder of their lives after endograft placement. As the AAA sac decreases in volume, the endograft may become distorted, with limb kinking, separation, and even disengagement from attachment sites. The incidence of complications is increasing as longer follow-up accumulates (Fig. 10-22). The future role of endografts for AAA remains to be determined as these late outcomes become known.

Isolated degenerative common iliac artery aneurysms can be managed with stent-grafts, often percutaneously. The same principles apply as for AAA endografts: adequate proximal and distal attachment sites, and the ability to deliver the device through the external iliac artery. Embolization of the proximal internal iliac artery is frequently required to avoid a type II endoleak unless a branched graft is available. Internal iliac artery aneurysms can be effectively managed by embolization of all outflow branches, followed by embolization of the proximal internal iliac artery or overlay by a stent-graft extending from the common to external iliac arteries.

OCCLUSIVE DISEASE

The most common cause of aortoiliac occlusive disease is atherosclerosis (Box 10-8). Isolated aortic lesions are unusual, occurring in 5% of patients with symptoms of chronic lower extremity arterial insufficiency. These manifest as calcified bulky intraaortic plaque ("coral reef" plaque) usually in the visceral artery segment, or focal infrarenal stenoses (Figs. 10-23 and 10-24). Combined aortic and iliac artery occlusive disease is the most common pattern, with associated infrainguinal occlusive disease in 65% (Fig. 10-25). When the occlusive disease

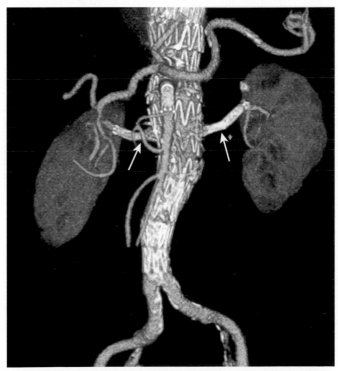

FIGURE 10-17. Branched endograft. Volume rendering of a computed tomography angiogram scan showing a branched aortic endograft (Zenith, Cook, Bloomington, Ill). There are extensions into both renal arteries *(arrows)*, the superior mesenteric artery, and celiac artery. (Courtesy Roy Greenberg, MD, Cleveland, Ohio.)

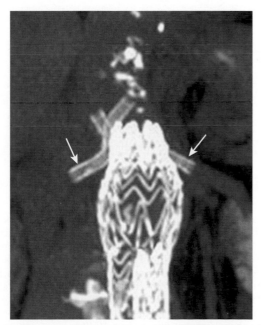

FIGURE 10-18. Conventional aortic endograft with bilateral renal artery "snorkels" *(arrows)*. The patient had a juxtarenal abdominal aortic aneurysm and in order to obtain a proximal seal the aortic stent-graft was deployed covering the renal artery origins. Covered stent-grafts were placed in both renal arteries adjacent to the aortic endograft as part of the procedure to allow continued renal artery perfusion. (Courtesy Constantino Pena, MD, Miami, Fla.)

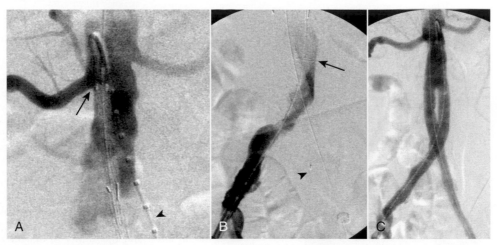

FIGURE 10-19. Basic elements of deployment of a modular bifurcated endograft, in this case a Gore Excluder (Flagstaff, Ariz.). **A,** Magnified digital subtraction angiogram (DSA) with craniocaudad angulation centered over the renal arteries. The top of the endograft *(arrow)* is positioned at the lowest renal artery before deployment. A graduated-marker pigtail catheter *(arrowhead)* has been inserted from the other femoral artery to guide the procedure. **B,** After deployment of the main body of the endograft from the left side, the contralateral limb gate *(arrow)* has been catheterized and a guidewire placed from the right. Contrast is injected from the right femoral sheath to determine the correct length for the contralateral limb. The distal end of the left iliac limb is indicated by the arrowhead. **C,** Final DSA aortogram showing exclusion of the aneurysm and excellent endograft position. The criss-cross of the limbs is a common configuration for this device that makes catheterization of the contralateral limb gate easier. The left internal iliac artery was chronically occluded before the procedure.

TABLE 10-6 Endoleak Classification

Type	Definition
I	Attachment: lack of seal between endograft and wall of artery A: Proximal B: Distal C: Leak around iliac occluder with aortounilateral graft
II	Branch-to-branch: retrograde flow in inferior mesenteric artery, lumbar, gonadal, or median sacral artery A: Simple—inflow without outflow from sac B: Complex—inflow and outflow vessels from sac
III	Device integrity: hole in graft material, separation of modular elements A: At modular connection B: Fabric disruption
IV	Porous graft material: "bleed-through" due to interstices in fabric of graft material
V	Endo-tension: No visible contrast or flow in aneurysm sac, but continued expansion
Early	Within 30 days of procedure
Late	After 30 days

is limited to the aortoiliac segment, the male-to-female ratio is 1:1. This ratio becomes 6:1 when there is also infrainguinal occlusive disease. With occlusion of the distal aorta, there is retrograde propagation of thrombus to the level of the next proximal patent aortic branch vessel. When this vessel is a lumbar or inferior mesenteric artery, the lumen of the aorta tapers to the origin of that vessel. Retrograde thrombosis to the level of the renal arteries results in an occlusion just at or immediately below the renal artery orifices (Fig. 10-26).

Patients with aortoiliac occlusive disease usually present with leg claudication or ischemia. Symptoms can be unilateral or bilateral depending on the level of obstruction and collateral pathways. Patients may complain of upper thigh claudication and proximal leg weakness with severe pelvic occlusive disease. Bilateral buttock claudication, impotence, and diminished femoral pulses in men is termed "Leriche syndrome," usually indicating severe disease of the distal aorta and common iliac arteries. This constellation of symptoms is present in up to one third of men with severe aortoiliac occlusive disease but is frequently not discussed. Aortic and iliac plaque can also be a source of distal atheroemboli ("blue-toe syndrome") (see Fig. 1-34). An iliac source should be suspected when there are recurrent episodes involving one foot; an aortic or more proximal source is suggested when both feet are involved.

Noninvasive studies of patients with isolated aortoiliac occlusive disease reveal diminished femoral pulses, decreased ankle-brachial indices, and reduced segmental pressures or pulse volume recordings (PVRs) in the thigh, with normalized distal waveforms (see Noninvasive Physiologic Evaluation in Chapter 15). However, PVRs cannot precisely localize the level of proximal disease, because common femoral artery occlusion produces the same distal waveform and pressure abnormalities as a more proximal lesion. Imaging of aortoiliac occlusive disease with ultrasound is less accurate than other modalities owing to iliac artery tortuously, the depth of the vessels in the pelvis, and calcification. Contrast-enhanced MRA detects aortoiliac disease with greater than 95% sensitivity and specificity (see Fig. 10-26). A coronal gadolinium-enhanced 3-D acquisition centered on the aortic bifurcation usually covers from the renal arteries to the femoral artery bifurcation. The presence of intravascular metal stents (particularly those made from stainless steel) can create artifact that obscures the vessel lumen so that MRA may not be useful in these patients (see Fig. 3-15). CTA has similar sensitivity and specificity, but also tends to overestimate the degree of stenosis. Unlike MRA, intravascular stents do not degrade CTA, but heavy calcification can obscure the lumen of a small-diameter vessel. Greater image postprocessing is required with CTA than MRA to eliminate bone and surrounding soft tissues. MRA and CTA can be used to both diagnose occlusive disease and plan for an intervention. In particular, patients with absent femoral pulses should be studied with MRA or CTA before undergoing arteriography from an axillary approach.

Conventional angiography should be obtained when intervention is required or when a diagnostic dilemma exists that cannot be resolved with noninvasive techniques. Angiography provides accurate morphologic as well as physiologic information. Care is required in interpretation of digital subtraction

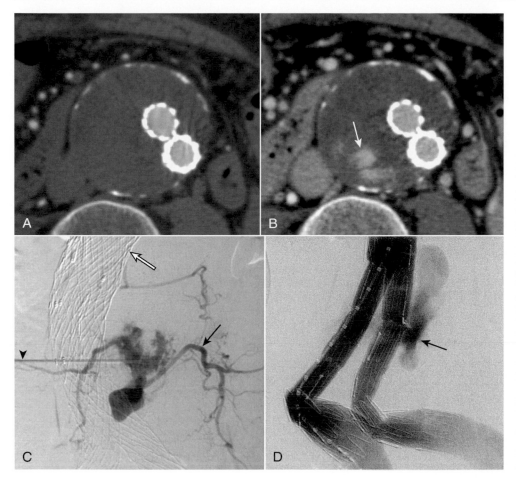

FIGURE 10-20. Sac perfusion after endograft placement ("endoleaks"). **A,** CT scan 12 months after endograft placement during the arterial phase. No contrast is seen in the sac (see next image). **B,** Image at the same level from the delayed phase (90 seconds after contrast injection) now shows contrast in the sac consistent with an endoleak *(arrow)*. This illustrates the importance of the delayed scan when evaluating endografts. **C,** Type II perfusion. Digital subtraction angiogram after direct sac puncture in the same patient as **A** and **B** showing filling of an intraaneurysmal space with communication with the lumbar arteries *(arrow)*. The access needle *(black arrowhead)* passes behind the graft *(open arrow)*. The pressure in the sac was near systemic. **D,** Type III perfusion in a different patient. Selective injection in the limb of a bifurcated modular endograft showing separation of the limb elements and reperfusion of the aneurysm sac *(arrow)*. The patient presented with aneurysm rupture. The leak was treated by placement of a short endograft across the gap.

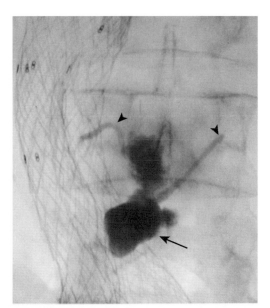

FIGURE 10-21. Digital image of the same patient as in Figure 10-20, **A-C,** following embolization of the sac with N-butyl cyanoacrylate. Glue has filled the space in the sac *(arrow)* and occluded the proximal lumbar arteries *(arrowheads)*.

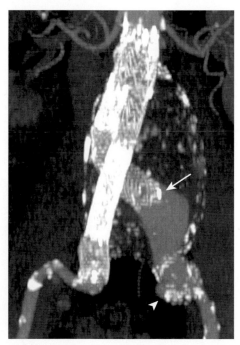

FIGURE 10-22. Late endograft complication. Coronal multiplanar reformation of a computed tomography angiogram obtained 4 years after stent-graft repair of an abdominal aortic aneurysm (AAA) shows the left limb *(arrow)* retracted into the AAA sac. The left common iliac artery *(arrowhead)* is short and aneurysmal, which contributed to the limb "pull-out". This is a type I endoleak (distal, or B), and the AAA had grown 1.3 cm in a year.

angiograms, because artifacts can be caused by motion, dense bone, and bowel gas (see Fig. 2-50). Bowel gas artifact in the abdomen can be minimized by intravenous injection of 1 mg glucagon before aortography. Oblique views are essential when evaluating the iliac arteries (see Figs. 2-52 and 10-8). Pressure measurements (preferably simultaneous with pharmacologic induction of distal hyperemia) obtained across lesions allows

---

Box 10-8. Etiologies of Aortoiliac Occlusive Disease

Atherosclerosis
Hypoplastic aorta syndrome
Vasculitis
Radiation arteritis
Dissection
Neurofibromatosis
Fibromuscular dysplasia

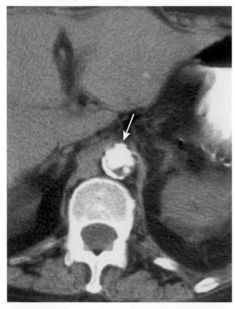

Figure 10-23. Bulky aortic plaque ("coral reef") in a patient with chronic postprandial abdominal pain. Axial noncontrast computed tomography scan at the level of the celiac artery origin showing heavily calcified intraluminal plaque *(arrow)*. The dense calcium in the aorta could have easily been overlooked if the noncontrast scan had not been obtained before contrast.

definitive determinations of severity and need for intervention (see Fig. 4-8). When necessary, IVUS can be used to further evaluate a lesion (see Fig. 2-54).

The indications for intervention in patients with aortoiliac occlusive disease are disabling claudication, threatened limb loss, or correction of a hemodynamicaly significant proximal lesion prior to a distal revascularization procedure. Patients with stable or mild claudication should undergo exercise therapy first. Supervised exercise is an effective intervention for increasing walking distance, as shown in the only randomized trial of best medical treatment compared to endovascular treatment of claudicants with iliac occlusive disease, the Claudication: Exercise Versus Endoluminal Revascularization (CLEVER) trial. All patients should be counseled for risk factor modification, smoking cessation if applicable, and evaluation for antiplatelet and statin therapy. Cilostazol, a phosphodiesterase III inhibitor, has been shown to increase walking distance and time to claudication by 50% but should not be used in patients with severe congestive heart failure.

Recommendations for the type of intervention based on lesion morphology and distribution are listed in Box 10-9. The surgical options include aortofemoral bypass, axillofemoral bypass, femoral-femoral bypass, and aortic endarterectomy (Figs. 10-27 and 10-28). An end-to-side proximal anastomosis is employed when residual flow in the native aorta is to be preserved. The femoral anastomoses are also usually end-to-side, with the graft material anterior to the native artery (see Fig. 2-33). The best long-term surgical results are for aortofemoral bypass or aortic endarterectomy (almost 90% primary 10-year patency), although the latter is rarely performed in most centers. Axillofemoral and femoral-femoral bypasses (both considered "extraanatomic" in that the grafts do not follow the natural course of the arteries that they replace) have lower patency rates owing to factors that include external compression and length of the graft. These are much less morbid surgeries that are therefore useful in debilitated or high-risk patients. Complications are similar to those listed in Boxes 10-4 and 10-5.

Angioplasty of aortic stenosis can be performed with a single low-profile low-pressure large-diameter balloon (10-16 mm) from one arterial access, or two smaller balloons (8- to 10-mm diameter) with "kissing" technique from bilateral access. Kissing technique is commonly used for aortic lesions that also involve the common iliac artery origins (see Fig. 4-16). The long-term results of angioplasty of focal aortic stenoses are excellent, but these are rare lesions. Stent placement is indicated for eccentric lesions, recanalization of complete occlusions, or lesions that are believed to be a source of atheroemboli. Stent-grafts may be used to exclude symptomatic ulcerated plaque, but otherwise currently have little role for aortic occlusive disease.

Figure 10-24. Focal aortic stenosis. **A,** Digital subtraction angiogram (DSA) of the distal abdominal aorta showing a focal atherosclerotic stenosis *(arrow)*. There was a 50-mm Hg gradient across the stenosis. **B,** Following angioplasty with a 12-mm diameter balloon there is persistent stenosis *(arrow)* with only slight reduction in the gradient. **C,** DSA after placement of a balloon-expandable stent *(arrow)*. The gradient was obliterated.

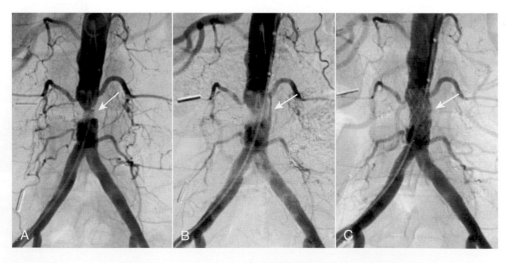

Isolated, concentric, and focal iliac stenoses that are at least 1 cm from the aorta or iliac artery bifurcation respond well to angioplasty alone, with a 4-year patency of almost 80% with initial procedural success. In general, stents should be required only in approximately 50% of cases when strict hemodynamic criteria are followed (Box 10-10). However, most lesions are not

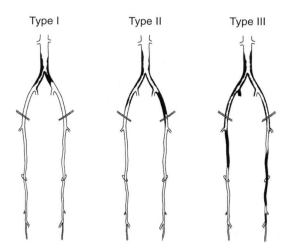

FIGURE 10-25. Patterns of aortoiliac occlusive disease. Type 1: Distal aorta and common iliac arteries. Type 2: Aorta and generalized pelvic arterial disease with intact distal runoff. Type 3: Multilevel disease including the aorta, pelvis, and distal runoff. This pattern carries the worst prognosis. (From Brewster DC. Direct reconstruction for aortoiliac occlusive disease. In: Rutherford RB, ed. *Vascular Surgery*, 5th ed. Philadelphia: WB Saunders, 2000, with permission.)

Box 10-9. Trans-Atlantic Intersociety Consensus II Recommendations for Iliac Interventions

Lesion type A—endovascular is treatment choice
- Unilateral or bilateral stenosis of CIA
- Unilateral or bilateral single stenosis (≤3 cm) of EIA

Lesion type B—endovascular preferred
- Short (≤3 cm) stenosis of infrarenal aorta
- Unilateral CIA occlusion
- Single or multiple stenosis totaling 3-10 cm involving the EIA not extending into the CFA
- Unilateral EIA occlusion not involving the origins of the IIA or CFA

Lesion type C—surgical treatment preferred
- Bilateral CIA occlusion
- Bilateral EIA stenosis 3-10 cm long not extending into the CFA
- Unilateral EIA stenosis extending into the CFA
- Unilateral EIA occlusion that involves the origins of the IIA and/or CFA
- Heavily calcified unilateral EIA occlusion with or without involvement of the origins of the IIA and/or CFA

Lesion type D—surgery is treatment of choice
- Infrarenal aortoiliac occlusion
- Diffuse disease involving the aorta and both iliac arteries requiring treatment
- Diffuse multiple stenoses involving the CIA, EIA, and CFA
- Unilateral occlusion of both CIA and EIA
- Bilateral EIA occlusions
- Iliac stenosis in patients with AAA requiring treatment and not amenable to endograft placement or other lesions requiring open aortic or iliac surgery.

AAA, Abdominal aortic aneurysm; CFA, common femoral artery; CIA, common iliac artery; EIA, external iliac artery; IIA, internal iliac artery.

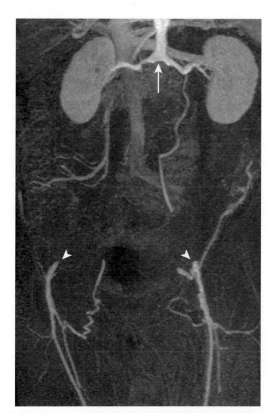

FIGURE 10-26. Chronic proximal aortic occlusion. Coronal maximal intensity projection of gadolinium-enhanced magnetic resonance angiogram showing occlusion of the abdominal aorta just below the renal arteries *(arrow)* and reconstitution of the distal runoff at the level of the common femoral arteries *(arrowheads)*.

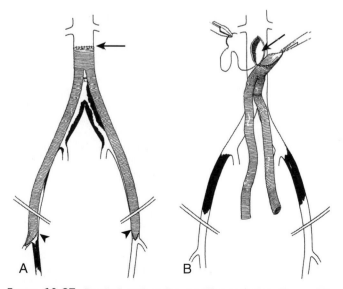

FIGURE 10-27. Surgical options for aortoiliac occlusive disease. The distal anastomosis is typically to the common femoral artery or lower when bypass is performed for occlusive disease. **A,** Aortobifemoral graft with end-to-end proximal *(arrow)* and end-to-side distal anastomoses *(arrowheads)*. **B,** Aortobifemoral graft with an end-to-side proximal anastomosis *(arrow)* that preserves flow to the distal lumbar and pelvic arteries. The femoral anastomoses are usually end-to-side. (From Brewster DC. Direct reconstruction for aortoiliac occlusive disease. In: Rutherford RB, ed. *Vascular Surgery*, 5th ed. Philadelphia: WB Saunders, 2000, with permission.)

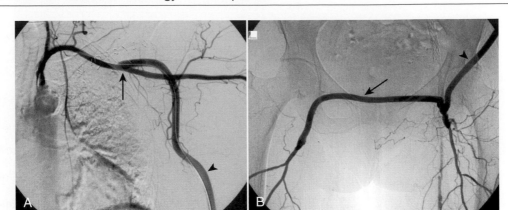

Figure 10-28. Axillobifemoral graft. **A,** Digital subtraction angiogram (DSA) of the proximal left upper extremity arteries showing the proximal anastomosis *(arrow)* of an axillobifemoral bypass *(arrowhead)*. **B,** DSA of the pelvis showing the axillofemoral bypass graft *(arrowhead)* with a cross femoral bypass *(arrow)* to the right profunda femoris artery.

Box 10-10. Indications for Stent Placement in the Aorta and Iliac Arteries

Failed angioplasty (residual pressure gradient >10 mm Hg at rest, 15 mm Hg with distal vasodilatation, or residual stenosis ≥ 30%)
Common iliac artery origin lesion
Recurrent stenosis
Anastomotic stenosis
Occlusive dissection flap
Recanalization of total occlusion
Ulcerated plaque
Planned distal revascularization procedure

---

ideal for angioplasty alone, and it is very hard to suppress the "oculostenting reflex," so most iliac lesions are treated primarily with stents. Typical balloon diameters for the common iliac artery are 8-10 mm. When a lesion involves the proximal common iliac artery or the origin, a second access from the opposite side is useful (see Fig. 4-17). This allows control injections for precise positioning of the stent, simultaneous pressure measurements, and inflation of an undersized balloon in the normal common iliac artery orifice during stent deployment to prevent distal embolization of plaque. Bilateral stent placement may be required to protect a relatively normal contralateral common iliac artery when treating origin disease. Treatment of disease involving both common iliac artery origins involves reconstruction of the aortic bifurcation with bilateral stents that extend equally into the distal abdominal aorta (Fig. 10-29; see Fig. 4-16).

Common iliac artery occlusions can be crossed from either a retrograde or antegrade approach. Generally, a retrograde approach is easier because the path from the access to the lesion is short and straight (Fig. 10-30). An angled catheter and a straight or angled hydrophilic guidewire can be used to probe the lesion for a "soft spot." Working over the bifurcation in an antegrade fashion requires a sturdy recurved catheter that allows probing of the occlusion (Fig. 10-31). Failure to cross the lesion occurs in about 5% of cases. Reentry devices can be used when a subintimal path has been created (see Fig. 4-6). Aggressive recanalization using the back end of a guidewire or even a long needle from a transjugular transhepatic portal access kit (see Fig. 14-18) can be used for stubborn lesions, although there is increased risk of vessel perforation. When fresh thrombus is present or suspected, a short course of thrombolysis reduces the risk of distal embolization during stent placement. Stent placement in occlusions have improved patency rates over angioplasty alone equal to that of stented stenoses (Table 10-7).

Internal iliac artery origin lesions can be treated through a sheath placed across the aortic bifurcation from the opposite groin. This provides an antegrade approach to the internal iliac artery, as well as proximal contrast injections during the procedure. Angioplasty or stent placement can be performed, but stents should be positioned carefully to avoid extension into the common iliac artery.

External iliac artery angioplasty and stent placement is technically similar to the treatment of common iliac artery lesions. The external iliac artery is more prone to rupture than the common iliac artery, so balloon sizing should be less aggressive (see Fig. 4-18). Extension of stents over the internal iliac artery origin usually does not jeopardize the patency of that vessel. However, placement of stents in the common femoral artery has generally been avoided owing to the relative ease of open endarterectomy of this vessel, and concerns about future percutaneous access and flexion across the hip joint.

Stent-grafts have an increasing role in iliac artery occlusive disease. These can be either balloon-expandable or self-expanding (see Fig. 4-24A and B). The indications include primary treatment of ulcerated plaque or recanalization of occlusion; angioplasty-induced iliac artery rupture; and treatment of in-stent restenosis of bare stents. Placement of kissing stent-grafts when performing bilateral common iliac artery origin revascularization may reduce restenosis in this location. Intimal hyperplasia at the ends of the stent-graft remains a problem.

Major complications of aortoiliac angioplasty and stent placement include distal dissection, embolization, thrombosis, and rupture. These occur in fewer than 5% of patients, but are more frequent when recanalizing occlusions. These complications can be minimized by attention to details, careful balloon selection, heparinization during the intervention, and remembering the dictum that "the enemy of good is better" (see Fig. 4-3).

DISSECTION

Isolated spontaneous dissection of the abdominal aorta and iliac arteries is extremely rare (Box 10-11). A dissection in this vascular territory is usually an extension of a spontaneous thoracic aortic dissection, or iatrogenic following a surgical or angiographic procedure (see Figs. 9-11 and 9-21). Rarely, abdominal or limb symptoms due to acute branch vessel occlusion are the first presentation of a dissection originating in the thoracic aorta. Patients may have vague abdominal or low back pain, or full-blown visceral or limb ischemia. Symptoms due to branch vessel involvement occur in almost one third of patients with aortic dissection (see Fig. 9-25). Ischemic symptoms are characteristically severe owing to the acuity of onset, but may wax and wane as the true lumen perfusion changes. Rupture of the false lumen of a dissected aorta in the abdomen is much less common than in the thorax.

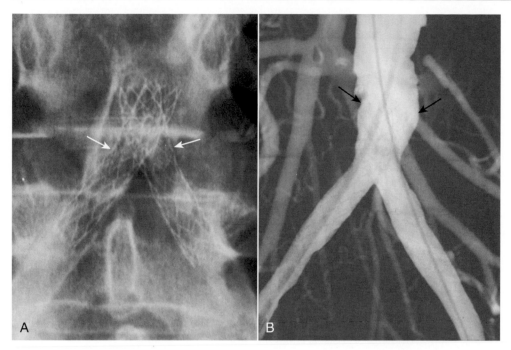

FIGURE 10-29. "Kissing" common iliac artery stents. **A,** Digital image showing crossing stents *(white arrows)* used to treat bilateral common iliac artery origin stenoses. **B,** Angiogram showing that the proximal ends of the stents *(black arrows)* extend into the distal aorta.

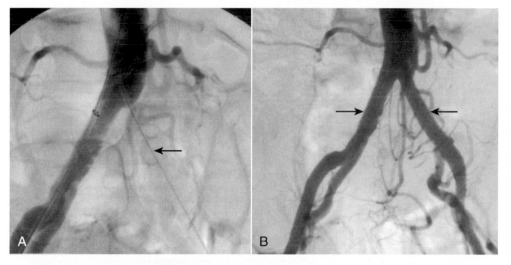

FIGURE 10-30. Occluded left common iliac artery recanalized in a retrograde fashion. **A,** Angiogram obtained after occlusion has been crossed *(arrow)* in a retrograde fashion from the left common femoral artery with hydrophilic guidewire and an angled catheter. The proximal occlusion is flush with the origin of the common iliac artery; compare with the occlusion in Fig. 10-31. **B,** Angiogram after bilateral common iliac artery stent placement *(arrows)*. The right stent was necessary because the left stent extended into the distal aorta.

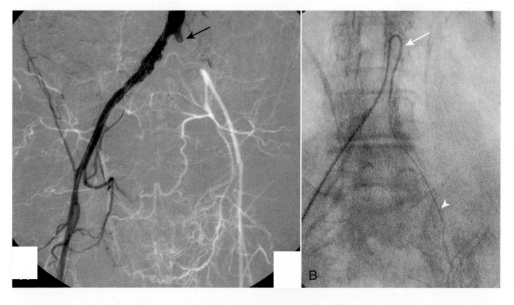

FIGURE 10-31. Crossing a common iliac artery occlusion using antegrade technique. **A,** Digital subtraction angiogram masked to demonstrate left common iliac occlusion *(arrow)* with late reconstitution of the left external iliac artery via retrograde flow in the internal iliac artery. **B,** The occlusion has been crossed by pulling a Simmons 1 catheter *(arrow)* into the "nipple" of the occlusion and advancing a hydrophilic guidewire *(arrowhead)* through the occlusion.

Table 10-7 Results of Focal Aortoiliac Angioplasty and Bare Stents (Generalized)

Iliac Artery Lesion	Procedure	Initial Success	4-Year Primary Patency
Stenosis	Angioplasty	90%	65%
Stenosis	Stent	95%	77%
Occlusion	Angioplasty	75%	54%
Occlusion	Stent	85%	61%

Box 10-11. Etiologies of Abdominal Aortic and Iliac Artery Dissection

Atherosclerosis (extension thoracic aorta)
Marfan syndrome (extension thoracic aorta)
Penetrating atherosclerotic ulcer
Trauma
Fibromuscular dysplasia (iliac arteries)
Athletes (iliac arteries)
Iatrogenic
- Angiography/intervention
- Fogarty balloon embolectomy
- Clamp injury

Box 10-12. Dissection of the Aorta and Iliac Arteries: Information Needed from Imaging

Proximal and distal extent of dissection
Aortic arch anatomy
Relationship of major branches to dissection lumens
Patency of major branches
Patency of false lumen
Overall size of aorta
Evidence of end-organ ischemia

Iatrogenic retrograde dissections created during angiographic procedures are frequently innocuous, because the false lumen tends to collapse rather than expand (see Fig. 2-32). However, occlusive antegrade dissection may occur following angioplasty or stent placement, particularly in the external iliac arteries.

Imaging of aortoiliac artery dissections should answer specific questions (Box 10-12). Ultrasound can detect dissection flaps in the abdominal aorta, but cannot adequately evaluate the status of the major branch arteries. Both MRA and CTA are excellent modalities for evaluation of dissection in this vascular bed. The 3-D data sets can be postprocessed on workstations to resolve complex anatomic issues.

Conventional angiography is usually indicated only in symptomatic patients before intervention. The diagnosis of aortic dissection is usually readily apparent on cross-sectional imaging studies. The stronger femoral pulse should be punctured (aortic dissections rarely extend beyond the common iliac arteries). Manipulation with a selective catheter may be required to find the true lumen. Midstream injection of contrast in the dissected abdominal aorta may not opacify both lumens unless fenestrations exist (Fig. 10-32). Sequential selective injection of both the true and false lumen, or repositioning of the catheter in the thoracic aorta proximal to the entry tear, is required in this situation. The lateral aortogram is particularly useful for evaluation of the visceral arteries.

The surgical management of symptomatic abdominal aortic dissection is resection of a small portion of the intimal flap, usually in the infrarenal aorta. A short aortic interposition graft may or may not be used as well. This creates a reentry point that decompresses the false lumen, allowing perfusion of the major branches that arise from the true lumen. Dissections isolated to the iliac arteries are treated surgically with bypass or placement of an interposition graft.

Occlusive symptoms of aortoiliac dissection can be effectively and quickly managed with percutaneous techniques. Compromise of blood flow may be due to compression of the aortic true lumen by the false lumen, extension of the dissection into the branch vessel, thrombosis, or any combination. These complications can be relieved by stent-graft placement over the entry tear in the thoracic aorta, followed in some instances by placement of large bare stents in the abdominal aortic true lumen and/or smaller stents in branch arteries (see Figs. 9-24 and 9-25). The initial step is always careful review of cross-sectional imaging to

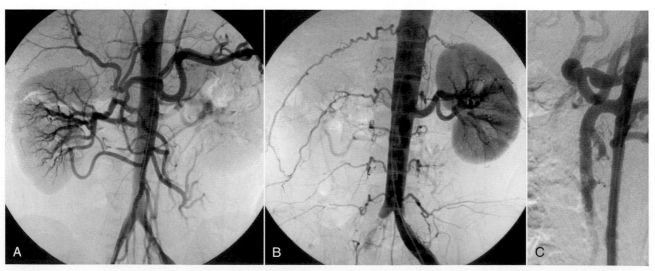

Figure 10-32. Abdominal extension of type B dissection. **A,** Digital subtraction angiogram (DSA) true lumen aortogram in the anterior projection shows filling of the visceral arteries and right kidney. The left kidney and lumbar arteries are not visualized. **B,** DSA false lumen aortogram in the same projection. The left kidney and lumbar arteries are visualized, but the visceral arteries and right kidney are not. **C,** DSA true lumen aortogram in the lateral projection showing filling of the visceral vessels.

identify the extent of the dissection and the anatomy of the target branch vessels.

Percutaneous aortic fenestration is another option when perfusion of the true lumen is compromised by a distended false lumen. Performed less often since the advent of stent-grafts, this remains in important technique. The essential components are identification of the true and false lumens, intravascular puncture through the dissection flap from one lumen to the other, and then balloon dilatation to enlarge the fenestration (Fig. 10-33). As with any dissection intervention, review of CT or MR studies before the procedure helps determine the orientation of the two lumens. Although it is often possible to identify each lumen with direct catheterization, sometimes only the true lumen can be accessed from a femoral approach. IVUS is a useful tool in these circumstances to localize the false lumen and guide the intervention. Re-entry devices designed for peripheral arterial interventions can be utlized to puncture across the dissection flap. Alternatively, a long needle (such as one used for transjugular intrahepatic portosystemic shunts) is inserted through a long protective sheath to the desired point of fenestration. A short thrust is usually sufficient to cross the flap. Entry into the false lumen is confirmed by injection of contrast, followed by insertion

of a guidewire. Puncture of the outer wall of the aorta is usually inconsequential, as long as the needle is simply withdrawn back into the aorta. The goal of the fenestration is to create a large communication between the two lumens, so large balloons with diameters equal to that of the aorta should be used. The final goal is normalization of pressures in both lumens, allowing reexpansion of the true lumen and improved perfusion of branch vessels.

▬ INFECTION

Native aortic infection presents with episodic fever, chills, and positive blood cultures. Mycotic pseudoaneurysm formation is associated with pain, distal embolization, and rupture. Patients may undergo an extensive evaluation for fever of unknown origin before arriving at the diagnosis of intravascular infection. Mycotic aneurysms of the native abdominal aorta can occur in any location. Organisms typically responsible for vascular infections are listed in Table 1-15. Almost one third of patients with mycotic aneurysms present with rupture.

Early in the infectious process of the native aorta, the imaging findings may be subtle or absent. Rarely, gas may be observed in the vessel wall or lumen (Fig. 10-34). Perivascular stranding

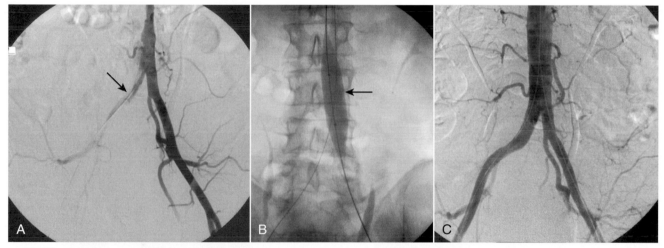

FIGURE 10-33. Percutaneous fenestration in a patient with a chronic type B dissection and right leg ischemia. **A,** Digital subtraction angiogram (DSA) over the pelvis with injection into the compressed true lumen of the distal abdominal aorta showing minimal flow in the right iliac arteries *(arrow)*. **B,** Using intravascular ultrasound guidance in the false lumen, a long sheathed needle was used to puncture the intimal flap from the true into the false lumen. A wire was advanced from the true to the false lumen and a 14-mm diameter balloon inflated across the fenestration *(arrow)* to enlarge the hole in the flap. **C,** DSA of the distal aorta after fenestration showing excellent filling of both sides of the pelvis. The patient had restoration of normal bilateral femoral pulses and relief of symptoms.

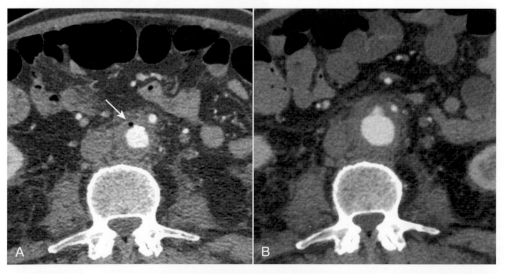

FIGURE 10-34. Axial computed tomography images of a patient with rapidly progressive aortic infection due to hematogenous seeding of clostridial perfringens from a colonic carcinoma. **A,** Image demonstrating intramural gas *(arrow)* and periaortic stranding. **B,** Three days later, image at the same level. The gas has resolved but the aorta is aneurysmal and the soft tissue stranding increased.

representing an inflammatory process precedes aneurysm formation. Ultimately, the arterial wall is digested and a pseudoaneurysm forms. Typically, mycotic aneurysms have a lobulated, wild-looking appearance, with extensive surrounding soft tissue reaction and hematoma (see Fig. 1-35). Adjacent major branch vessel origins are often consumed by the infectious aneurysm.

Infection of aortic graft material may occur from hematogenous seeding, direct extension from adjacent abscesses, and erosion into gastrointestinal or genitourinary (usually the ureter) structures. Graft infection also presents with fever, chills, and positive blood cultures. In addition, drainage from surgical incisions (especially in the groin), graft thrombosis, gastrointestinal bleeding, and anastomotic pseudoaneurysms may occur. Gastrointestinal bleeding results from graft erosion into bowel (chronic occult lower tract blood loss) or rupture of a proximal anastomotic pseudoaneurysm into the duodenum (massive acute upper gastrointestinal bleeding). When graft infection manifests as an anastomotic pseudoaneurysm, synchronous involvement of more than one anastomosis should be excluded. Rarely, vascular stents can become infected, resulting in a focal mycotic aneurysm as well as other characteristic symptoms of intravascular sepsis.

Infection of prosthetic graft material is suggested by perigraft fluid and/or air (see Fig. 1-36; compare with Fig. 10-14). Following aortic surgery, perigraft air should be reabsorbed within 2-3 weeks, and perigraft fluid within 2-3 months. Delayed appearance or persistence of perigraft fluid and air on CT or MRI are highly suggestive of infection. Soft-tissue stranding, lack of fat planes between graft material and bowel, graft thrombosis, and anastomotic pseudoaneurysms are also suggestive imaging findings. At conventional angiography the graft may appear completely normal, but intraluminal irregularities, focal anastomotic outpouchings, and (very, very rarely) opacification of bowel may be seen (Fig. 10-35).

The initial treatment of native aortoiliac vessel or graft infection is intravenous antibiotics. The longer the patient can be treated with antibiotics before intervention the better the survival, but all patients will ultimately need some kind of aortic repair. The traditional approach is surgical resection of the infected aorta, bypass (through a sterile bed if possible), and continuation of antibiotics (Fig. 10-36). Axillofemoral bypass with delayed aortic reconstruction, or direct vascular reconstruction with antibiotic-impregnated synthetic grafts, homograft, or autogenous femoral vein may be used. There is a small but growing experience with treatment of mycotic aortic aneurysms with stent-grafts. Lifelong antibiotics are often necessary in these patients.

EMBOLIC OCCLUSION

Acute aortoiliac arterial occlusion can be due to several diverse causes (Box 10-13). Embolic occlusion is sudden in onset in previously asymptomatic individuals, often resulting in profound ischemia. There is no associated chest or back pain to suggest a dissection. More than half of patients with symptomatic arterial emboli will have a cardiac arrhythmia at the time of presentation. More than 20% of emboli lodge at the aortic bifurcation, resulting in bilateral lower extremity ischemia. Smaller emboli may occlude

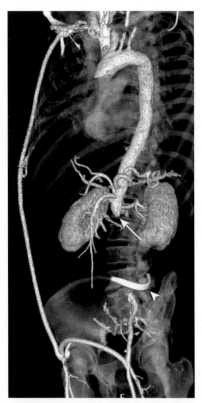

FIGURE 10-36. Volume rendering of CTA of the same patient as Fig. 10-34 obtained after resection of the infrarenal aorta *(arrow)* and placement of a right axillary-to-femoral and a right-to-left femoral-to-femoral bypass to perfuse the pelvis and legs. A surgical drain *(arrowhead)* can be seen in the retroperitoneum.

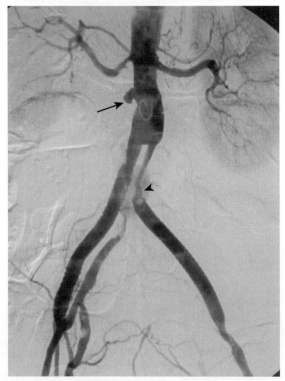

FIGURE 10-35. Aortoenteric fistula several years after aortobiiliac (onlay) graft for occlusive disease. The patient presented with fever, septicemia, and occult blood in his stool. Digital subtraction aortogram reveals a small proximal anastomotic pseudoaneurysm *(arrow)* and collapse of the left limb of the graft *(arrowhead)* with an intraluminal filling defect.

Box 10-13. Causes of Acute Aortic Occlusion

Embolus
Thrombosis of underlying stenosis
Dissection
Thrombosis of surgical graft
Hypercoagulable state
Trauma
Iatrogenic

one or both common iliac or common femoral arteries (see Table 1-13). Acute global ischemia of both limbs, with sudden return of one or more femoral pulses but persistent distal ischemia, may indicate fragmentation and distal embolization of a large aortic embolus. In contrast to embolic occlusion, thrombosis of a preexisting native arterial stenosis or a surgical graft is often preceded by a history of claudication and rarely results in critical ischemia owing to the presence of preexisting collaterals.

Patients with embolic occlusion of the aortoiliac arteries and profound ischemia have a surgical emergency (Fig. 10-37). Imaging should be expedient and accurate, in that rapid revascularization is essential to save limb and life. Many patients undergo emergent surgical embolectomy without antecedent imaging because the delay would compromise limb viability. When the limbs are viable, CT/CTA or MRA can exclude an alternative diagnosis such as dissection, demonstrate the level of occlusion, and detect other evidence of emboli such as renal infarcts. Conventional angiography demonstrates abrupt occlusion of the aorta or pelvic arteries by an intravascular filling defect, evidence of emboli and visceral arteries, and poor opacification of distal vessels with absence of developed collaterals. An axillary artery approach may be required when femoral pulses are absent, although the common femoral artery can be punctured with ultrasound.

There is little role for percutaneous techniques in patients with profound ischemia due to an embolus. When limbs are threatened but still viable, thrombolysis can be considered, although the risk of distal embolization during the procedure is high. In general, aortoiliac emboli are too large to be managed quickly and effectively with standard percutaneous techniques.

VASCULITIS

Aortoiliac occlusive disease is a well-recognized feature of Takayasu arteritis. Patients are atypical in age and risk factors for atherosclerotic disease (see Table 1-5). The process is diffuse, involving the visceral, renal, and common iliac arteries. Patients may present with hypertension, symptoms of mesenteric ischemia, or claudication.

Aortic wall thickening with a narrowed lumen is evident on CT or MRI, with wall enhancement by contrast. Aneurysms can also occur. The degree of wall calcification can be variable. At conventional angiography, long smooth stenosis of the aortoiliac arteries with extension into visceral and renal arteries is seen (Fig. 10-38).

Therapeutic options include surgical bypass, and, in some patients, angioplasty with stent placement. The lesions of Takayasu arteritis are fibrotic and extensive, so it is unlikely that a normal arterial caliber will be achieved with percutaneous methods, especially in the abdominal aorta. Information on long-term results of stent placement is scant, but promising.

Radiation vasculitis can involve the aorta and iliac arteries. The type and location of tumor treated, as well as contributory risk factors such as smoking, influence the severity. Diffuse aortic stenosis can occur in children following radiation for abdominal tumors. Isolated iliac artery disease can be seen after pelvic irradiation for genitourinary malignancy.

Behçet disease can present as multiple AAAs, and the thoracic aorta may also be involved (see Fig. 1-18). Patients have a characteristic constellation of clinical findings, including genital ulcers and uveitis.

MISCELLANEOUS

Hypoplastic aorta syndrome, also known as *abdominal aortic coarctation*, is believed to be a congenital disorder of unknown etiology and prevalence. Primarily found in young female patients, symptoms may not occur until middle age. Patients in this age group frequently have risk factors for atherosclerotic disease,

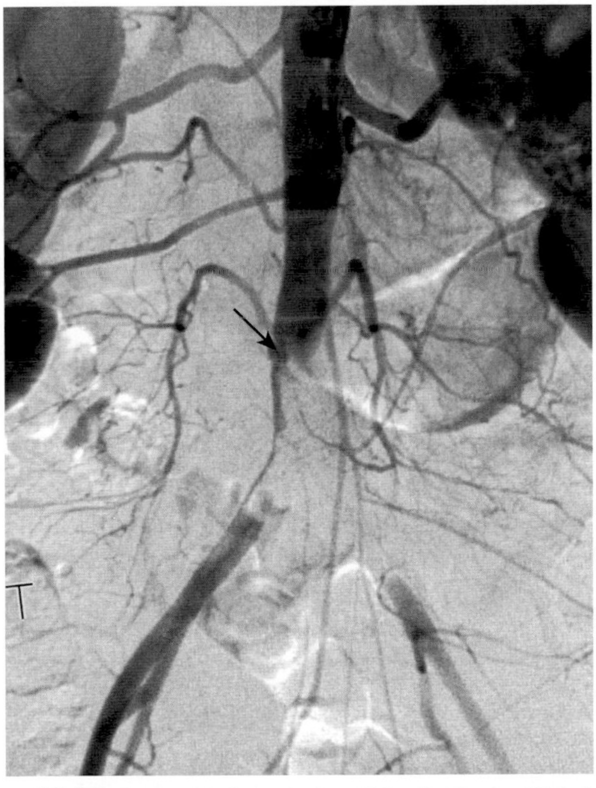

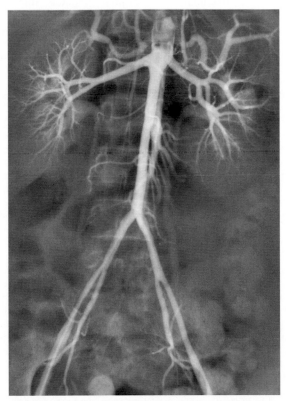

FIGURE 10-37. Acute embolic occlusion of the distal aorta. Digital subtraction aortogram showing embolic occlusion *(arrow)* of the distal abdominal aorta extending into both common iliac arteries. This was treated with surgical embolectomy. The source was cardiac.

FIGURE 10-38. Angiogram showing the findings of Takayasu arteritis of the abdominal aorta in a teenaged girl with aortic arch involvement. There is diffuse stenosis of infrarenal aorta and iliac arteries. This appearance is similar to that of hypoplastic aorta syndrome seen in middle-aged women in whom vasculitis workup is negative.

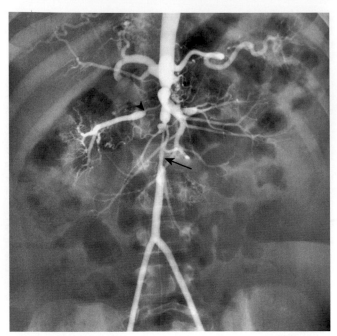

FIGURE 10-39. Abdominal aortic coarctation in a child with neurofibromatosis, hypertension, and diminished peripheral pulses. Aortogram showing renal artery stenosis *(arrowhead)* and diffuse narrowing of the infrarenal aorta *(arrow)*. The celiac and superior mesenteric artery origins were also severely stenotic.

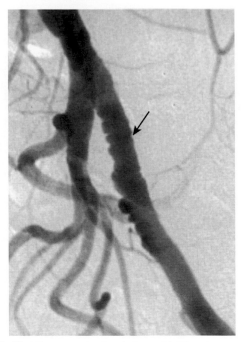

FIGURE 10-40. Fibromuscular dysplasia, medial fibroplasia type (asymptomatic) of the external iliac artery *(arrow)* in a middle-aged woman. The findings were bilateral.

such as smoking, diabetes, and hyperlipidemia. Atherosclerotic occlusive disease is frequently superimposed upon the already small aorta and iliac arteries in these patients. The angiographic appearance is striking, with a disproportionately small infrarenal abdominal aorta and iliac arteries. The differential diagnosis includes vasculitis (see Fig. 10-38), radiation injury, and neurofibromatosis. Visceral and renal artery involvement occurs when the lesion is centered in the mid portion of the abdominal aorta. Disease localized to the infrarenal aorta and common iliac arteries spares the visceral and renal arteries. Owing to the small caliber of the arteries and diffuse disease, surgical bypass is the preferred therapy.

Neurofibromatosis is associated with diffuse narrowing of the abdominal aorta, with concurrent visceral and renal artery stenoses. Pathologic study shows neurogenic cells are present in the media and adventitia. The appearance is similar to Takayasu arteritis and hypoplastic aorta syndrome, except patients are much younger at presentation and have other stigmata of neurofibromatosis (Fig. 10-39).

The iliac arteries are the third most common location for fibromuscular dysplasia (FMD) (Fig. 10-40). The typical patient is female, but older than those who present with renal artery FMD, probably because this is usually an incidental finding at angiography for other reasons. However, patients can present with occlusive symptoms or, less often, spontaneous dissection. Occlusive symptoms respond well to angioplasty, and dissection can be treated with stent placement.

Iliac artery endofibrosis is a rare condition manifesting as unilateral or bilateral external iliac artery stenoses in young athletes (Fig. 10-41). The etiology may be linked to repetitive motion of the legs while flexed at the hip, such as during competitive cycling. The lesions are fibrotic in nature and usually only produce a gradient only during extreme exercise. Only one side is affected in 85% of patients, with the remainder having bilateral lesions. The diagnosis is difficult to make, because the arteries may appear normal at imaging unless maximal provocative maneuvers are used. Management is by behavior modification, or surgical repair (endarterectomy with patch angioplasty),

or less often stent placement. Angioplasty alone is usually unsuccessful.

Ilioureteric fistula is a rare complication of chronic ureteral stents, which presents as intermittent massive hematuria. The typical patient has pelvic malignancy or other chronic indications for ureteral stents. The fistula usually occurs where the ureter crosses over the distal common or proximal external iliac artery. These patients can be managed with iliac endograft placement and long-term antibiotics.

■ TRAUMA

Most patients with out-of-hospital penetrating injuries to the abdominal aorta die immediately of exsanguination. Only 15% of patients are thought to survive long enough to undergo emergency surgery, for which the mortality rate is 61%. Bleeding is contained in these patients by adjacent retroperitoneal tissues. Associated bowel or visceral organ injuries are universal, and the IVC is also injured in 25%. In most cases, these patients require laparotomy for control of bleeding and repair of the multiple injuries.

Iatrogenic aortoiliac penetrating injury can occur during spinal surgery and laparoscopic procedures. These injuries may result in pseudoaneurysms or arteriovenous fistula (Figs. 10-42 and 10-43). Percutaneous treatment with an iliac artery endograft is an elegant solution to these problems.

Blunt injury to the aorta can result in an intimal tear with dissection or thrombosis, but injuries to major branch vessels (especially the renal arteries) are more common (Fig. 10-44). Most injuries to the infrarenal aorta are caused by seat belts during car accidents. Associated bowel and/or visceral organ injury are also universal in these patients as in those with penetrating injury.

Pelvic fracture can be associated with major bleeding from injured arteries, veins, or cancellous bone. Arterial bleeding related to pelvic fracture is well suited to management with interventional radiology techniques. Pelvic fractures can be grouped by the causative forces: (1) lateral compression, (2) anteroposterior compression, (3) vertical shear, and (4) combined mechanisms. A 3-cm diastasis of the symphysis pubis doubles the potential volume of the pelvis to 8 L. Most patients with

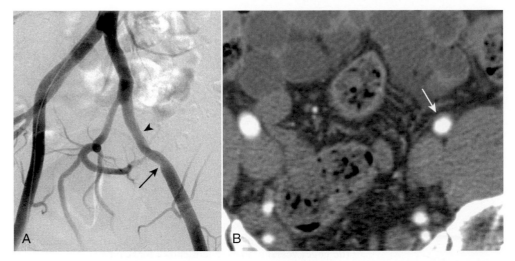

FIGURE 10-41. Iliac artery endofibrosis in a 37-year-old competitive cyclist with left leg cramping and weakness with extreme exertion. **A,** Digital subtraction angiogram of pelvis in the right anterior oblique projection depicts a small left external iliac artery *(arrowhead)* relative to the right, and a focal area of caliber change *(arrow)*. **B,** Axial computed tomography angiogram of the same patient showing that the left external iliac artery *(arrow)* is smaller than the right and has wall thickening.

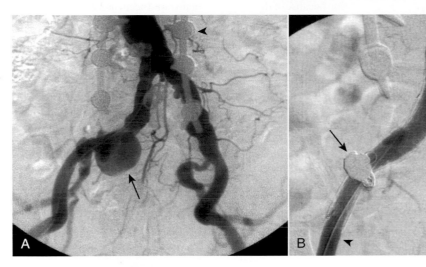

FIGURE 10-42. Posttraumatic common iliac artery pseudoaneurysm. **A,** New isolated saccular common iliac artery aneurysm *(arrow)* that appeared shortly after spinal surgery *(arrowhead)* consistent with an iatrogenic pseudoaneurysm. Computed tomography scan showed that the aneurysm arose from the back wall of the common iliac artery just proximal to the origin of the internal iliac artery. **B,** Successful exclusion of the aneurysm with a stent-graft *(arrowheads)*. The internal iliac origin was occluded with coils before stent-graft placement *(arrow)* to prevent retrograde filling of the pseudoaneurysm.

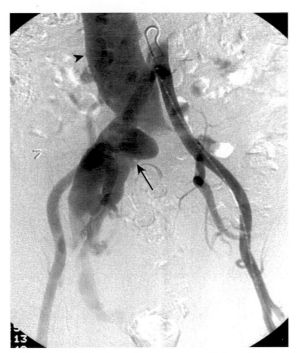

FIGURE 10-43. Digital subtraction angiogram of the pelvis showing a right common iliac artery to iliac vein fistula *(arrow)* in a patient in whom high-output cardiac failure developed following discectomy. Note the distended inferior vena cava *(arrowhead)* filled on aortic injection.

bleeding from pelvic fractures can be stabilized with pelvic fixation devices. Bleeding is controlled in this manner in 99% of patients with lateral compression injuries, which comprise 65% of all patients with pelvic fractures. Anteroposterior, vertical shear, and combined force injuries to the pelvis are less common but result in unstable injuries with bleeding unresponsive to pelvic fixation in 18%-22% of cases.

Arterial injury results from shearing of vessels against fixed ligamentous structures, avulsion of vessels attached to a displaced pelvic segment, or penetrating injury from a shard of bone (Box 10-14 and Fig. 10-45). A coagulopathic state induced by hypothermia or massive transfusion is a common complicating factor.

There is some debate about the optimal sequence of imaging and intervention in unstable patients with pelvic fractures. Peritoneal lavage, abdominal ultrasound, or abdominal and pelvic CT with contrast are performed early. If these studies are positive for intraperitoneal hemorrhage, the patient proceeds to surgery. Only abdominal injuries are repaired, even if a large expanding retroperitoneal hematoma is discovered. Surgery in the confined space of the pelvic retroperitoneum is extremely difficult, and decompressing the hematoma can lead to catastrophic blood loss. Pelvic fixation is performed externally in the emergency department or at the time of laparotomy. If the patient remains hemodynamically unstable, or has a transfusion requirement that exceeds 4-6 units of packed red blood cells in 24 hours, angiography is performed emergently.

In general, the threshold to proceed to angiography for embolization is decreasing. Stable patients with a hematoma and

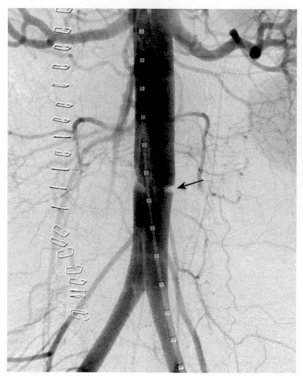

FIGURE 10-44. "Seat-belt injury" of the aorta in a young female involved in a high-speed motor vehicle accident. The patient also had bowel injuries (which had been repaired earlier that day) and lumbar spine fractures. Digital subtraction angiogram of the aorta shows a circumferential intimal flap *(arrow)* in the infrarenal abdominal aorta. This was treated percutaneously with an endograft, and the patient subsequently had fixation of the lumbar spine injury.

Box 10-14. Arteries Injured in Pelvic Fractures in Decreasing Order of Frequency

Superior gluteal
Internal pudendal
Obturator
Inferior gluteal
Lateral sacral
Iliolumbar
External iliac
Deep circumflex iliac
Inferior epigastric

---

extravasation documented on CT scan, or unstable patients with injuries isolated to the pelvis, can proceed directly to angiography. Earlier intervention is associated with improved outcomes because patients avoid the metabolic and hematologic derangements associated with massive blood loss.

Angiography in hemodynamically unstable patients with pelvic fractures should (1) rapidly evaluate potential sources of arterial bleeding and (2) proceed expeditiously to embolization. Review of plain films and CT scans of the pelvis helps direct the initial angiogram. A pelvic arteriogram with a pigtail catheter in the distal abdominal aorta positioned to fill the lower lumbar arteries should be performed to quickly determine the arterial anatomy and identify massive extravasation (see Fig. 1-29). Injuries that cause hemodynamic instability manifest angiographically as free extravasation, pseudoaneurysm, or large arteriovenous fistula. The absence of these findings on the flush pelvic injection does not exclude their presence. Selective bilateral internal and external iliac artery injections, with

oblique views if necessary, should be performed as a routine. Recognition of important pelvic arterial anatomic variants such as replacement of the obturator artery to the inferior epigastric artery origin (the "corona mortis", named because it can be the source of lethal bleeding if overlooked) is critical. Investigation of lumbar, circumflex iliac, profunda femoris, and gonadal arteries may be necessary. Extended filming may be needed to visualize pelvic arterial extravasation. The normal uterine blush in premenopausal women and the bulbospongiosal stain at the base of the penis in males can be confused with extravasation.

The primary goal of embolization in patients with pelvic fractures is to quickly decrease the pressure in the injured arteries to a level that will allow natural hemostasis. Complete devascularization of the pelvis or infarction of tissue is not desirable. Superselective catheterization should be used only in stable patients to avoid unnecessarily prolonging the procedure. The longer the patient bleeds, the sicker he or she becomes.

Gelfoam (Upjohn, Kalamazoo, Mich.) cut into pieces to match the target vessel is an excellent choice for branch vessel embolization because of the ability to obtain rapid occlusion and the potential for recanalization after several weeks. Typical pledget dimensions range from 1-mm cubes to 1- × 2- × 5-mm rectangles. In patients with multiple bleeding points, a slurry of Gelfoam cubes can be injected proximally in the hypogastric branches or trunk. Very small particles (Gelfoam powder, Ivalon, spheres) and alcohol should not be used. Embolization continues until extravasation is no longer visualized. Coils are useful when large vessels are transected, or in stable patients with pseudoaneurysms or arteriovenous fistulas when a precise embolization may be desired. Successful embolization is frequently clinically evident with sudden improvement in the patient's hemodynamic status. Careful completion angiography is important to exclude bleeding from a collateral source of blood supply (Fig. 10-46). Midline bleeding can be supplied from either internal iliac artery, and lateral bleeding may be supplied from lumbar, iliac circumflex, or profunda femoris artery branches as well as the internal iliac artery. If the patient remains hemodynamically unstable after a technically successful embolization, bleeding may be from either venous sources or another arterial source such as a liver or splenic laceration.

Most complications of percutaneous embolization of massive traumatic pelvic bleeding are acceptable compared to the alternative. Reflux of embolic material into the ipsilateral lower extremity can occur if the catheter is not well seated in the internal iliac artery. Emboli that lodge in the profunda femoris artery or other muscular branches are usually clinically silent. Occlusion of the superficial femoral or popliteal artery may result in a severely ischemic limb that requires urgent revascularization. Organ infarction (colon, bladder, uterus) is extremely rare.

■ UTERINE ARTERY EMBOLIZATION

Uterine Fibroids

The most common indication for selective uterine artery angiography is during embolization of symptomatic fibroids. This has become an extremely important procedure in many interventional practices. Fibroids are common benign leiomyomatous neoplasms of the uterus that occur in women in their reproductive years. Tumors may be single, multiple, small, or large (Table 10-8). Fibroids are vascular tumors that grow in size and increase in prevalence with age throughout a woman's reproductive life. Although almost half of women aged 40 years have fibroids (black women have triple the risk compared to white women), fewer than 20% are symptomatic. The uterus may become so enlarged by fibroids that it fills the pelvis and distends the abdomen. The natural history of uncomplicated fibroids is involution following menopause. Leiomyosarcoma of the uterus is rare during reproductive years (<0.5% of rapidly growing fibroids), but should be suspected when fibroid enlargement occurs in a postmenopausal woman.

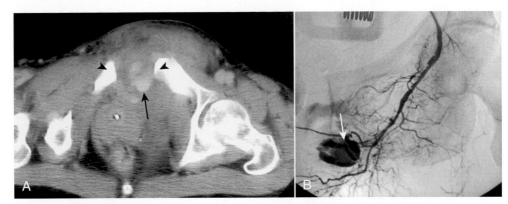

FIGURE **10-45**. "Open book" pelvic fracture in a middle-aged male motorcycle rider occurring when he collided with an ambulance. He was hemodynamically stable but required aggressive fluid resuscitation despite application of a compression belt. **A**, Axial computed tomography scan with contrast showing diastasis of the symphysis pubis *(arrowheads)* and extravasation *(arrow)* of contrast into a pelvic hematoma. **B**, Selective left internal pudendal digital subtraction angiogram showing extravasation *(arrow)*. This was embolized with Gelfoam pledgets. The right hypogastric artery was injected after embolization to confirm absence of cross-filling.

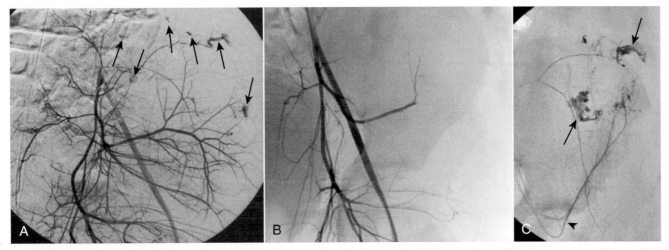

FIGURE **10-46**. Young child with left iliac wing fracture and hypotension despite massive fluid resuscitation following a motor vehicle accident. **A**, Digital subtraction angiogram of left internal iliac artery injection showing numerous points of extravasation *(arrows)*. **B**, Control angiogram following embolization with a spray of small Gelfoam cubes in the superior gluteal artery. There is cessation of bleeding. However, the patient remained hemodynamically unstable. **C**, Selective injection of the deep circumflex iliac artery *(arrowhead)* showing continued extravasation *(arrows)* from collateral supply to the area of trauma. This was successfully embolized with Gelfoam pledgets.

TABLE 10-8 Classification of Fibroids by Location

Location	Definition
Submucosal	Protruding into endometrial cavity
Intramural	Within the myometrium
Subserosal	Based in the myometrium, but covered by parietal peritoneum
Pedunculated	Attached to uterus by small stalk
Cervical	Located in uterine cervix

The indications for intervention are symptomatic fibroids that cause heavy, prolonged periods (menorrhagia), pelvic pain, dyspareunia, and pressure symptoms on adjacent structures (bladder, bowel, and ureters). Hormonal manipulation with oral contraceptives, antiprogestins, or progesterone-secreting intrauterine devices can control symptoms in up to three-fourths of women, but long-term compliance is poor due to frequent side effects. Pharmacologic induction of menopause with GnRH agonists results in amenorrhea and significant reduction in fibroid size, but this therapy cannot be continued indefinitely due to symptomatic hypoestrogenism and osteoporosis, and fibroids enlarge once medication is stopped.

Conventional surgical procedures include hysterectomy and myomectomy, using open, laparoscopic, or hysteroscopic techniques. Hysterectomy is the most definitive surgical option, with a major complication rate of approximately 7.5% (bleeding, urinary tract injury, pelvic floor disturbance, and infection). The recovery after hysterectomy varies with the surgical access (transabdominal, transvaginal, and laparoscopic), ranging from 4 to 6 weeks.

Myomectomy, the surgical removal of individual fibroids, can be accomplished via laparotomy, laparoscopy, or hysteroscopy (when the fibroids are largely intracavitary). The major complication rate is lower than for hysterectomy. Large and multiple fibroids can be difficult to treat, particularly if little normal myometrium is present. Conversion to hysterectomy occurs in only 1% of patients. The initial clinical success rate is approximately 80%. The recurrence rate of detectable fibroids is as high as 60% at 10 years, and up to 25% of women require repeat intervention.

Uterine artery embolization (UAE) is an alternative approach to management of fibroids. The basic principle is selective infarction of the fibroids with particulate embolic materials delivered directly into the uterine arteries. The indications are identical to those for surgery, that is, symptomatic fibroids that have not

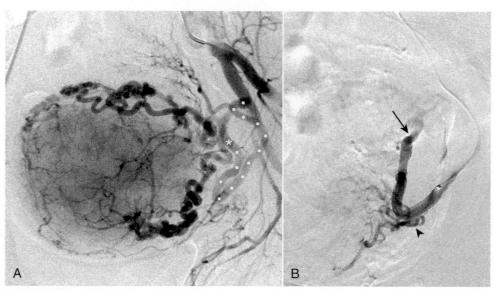

FIGURE 10-47. Fibroid embolization. **A,** Digital subtraction angiogram of the left internal iliac artery in the left anterior oblique projection shows the uterine artery *(white squares)* arising from the anterior division. There is a large hypervascular fibroid. Embolization was performed with a microcatheter positioned at the white asterisk, well within the ascending portion of the uterine artery. **B,** Left uterine angiogram following embolization. There is stasis in the ascending uterine artery *(arrow)*. The cervical and vaginal arterial supply *(arrowhead)* is preserved. Embolization of the right side was then performed.

responded to conservative therapy. The number of fibroids is not a limitation for UAE. Fibroids that are largely intracavitary may be expelled after embolization, but are not a contraindication. Although considered a complication of UAE, these patients can have the most dramatic positive response if the fibroid is expelled completely. Very large fibroids (>10-12 cm in diameter) are considered a contraindication by some interventionalists, but this point remains debated. Patients with suspected active pelvic or genitourinary infection, pregnancy, fibroids enlarging after menopause, vaginal bleeding after menopause, or suspected pelvic malignancy should not be embolized. There is no age cutoff for UAE, but young patients who desire pregnancy should be counseled that there can be a 2%-3% incidence of premature menopause following the procedure. In the author's experience, this has only occurred in perimenopausal patients with large fibroids. The estimated radiation exposure (Dose Area Product) with UAE varies with the patient's body mass index, fibroid volume, and embolization technique, but ranges from 1900 to 5600 cGY*cm².

Patients should be seen in consultation by the interventionalist before the procedure to review the history, explain the procedure, determine whether it is appropriate, and order any additional testing. The patient's fertility goals should be specifically discussed and documented, in that embolization of one or both ovarian arteries is necessary in up to 5% to devascularize the fibroids. Patients should have a pelvic examination, endometrial biopsy (if bleeding has occurred between periods—metrorrhagia), a PAP smear within 12 months, and either an ultrasound or MRI scan before the procedure. GnRH analogues should be stopped, if possible, for several weeks before the procedure. Currently, the procedure is not performed for nonfibroid causes of pelvic pain other than selected cases of adenomyosis. Embolization of massive fibroids before conventional surgery is also an accepted indication.

On the day of the procedure a serum pregnancy test should be obtained, and a Foley catheter placed to keep the bladder empty. Antibiotics (usually a broad-spectrum cephalosporin) and intravenous analgesics (narcotic and nonsteroidal) are administered before the embolization. Fluoroscopy should be set to the lowest pulse-mode possible; often a rate as low as 4 pulses per second is achievable with experience. Careful coning, limited use of magnification, and short angiographic runs at 1 frame per second contribute to minimizing ovarian exposure to radiation. An initial pelvic angiogram with a pigtail catheter positioned at the level of the renal arteries shows the pelvic circulation as well as the presence of enlarged gonadal arteries, one of the potential causes of clinical failure. Hypogastric angiography in the ipsilateral anterior oblique projection often allows identification of the uterine artery origin from the anterior division branch. The uterine arteries are usually hypertrophied, tortuous, and can be traced to the hypervascular masses in the uterus. Staining of the fibroid is common, but arteriovenous shunting is not and suggests a different pathology (e.g., arteriovenous malformation or tumor). The uterine arteries can be selected with an angled 4- or 5-French catheter (e.g., Cobra), but spasm can be a problem, so microcatheters are preferred by many interventionalists (see Fig. 10-3). The choice of embolic material is a matter of operator preference and of much discussion. Permanent particles in the 300- to 1200-μm diameter range (irregular or spheres) are common. The vascularity of the fibroids and the risk of nontarget embolization (especially reflux into ovarian artery collaterals) determines the choice of embolic size. The author has found that a stepwise approach using initially 700- to 900-μm acrylic spheres through a high-flow microcatheter positioned deep in the uterine artery beyond cervical and vaginal branches until there is very sluggish flow, followed by 900- to 1200-μm Ivalon spheres until there is stasis of flow, is an expeditious and effective embolization strategy (Fig. 10-47). Sometimes Gelfoam pledgets are used at the end of the procedure to occlude the uterine arteries, although some interventionalists perform the entire procedure with this material. Coil occlusion of the uterine artery is not necessary. Bilateral embolization is mandatory unless convincing evidence of unilateral blood supply to the fibroids is present. This is usually accomplished from a single arterial access by forming a Waltman loop or selecting the ipsilateral internal iliac artery with a recurved catheter, but bilateral femoral artery access is also used.

Pain control during the embolization is usually not difficult, because the procedure is often over before onset of significant cramping. Pretreatment with nonsteroidal antiinflammatory agents for several days before the procedure, superior hypogastric nerve block, and intraarterial lidocaine have all been described as means of reducing postprocedure pain (Fig. 10-48).

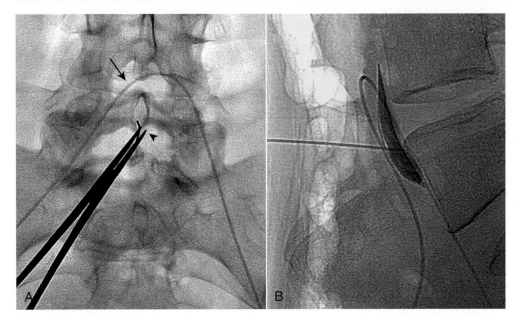

FIGURE **10-48**. Superior hypogastric nerve block performed at the time of uterine artery embolization. **A,** Digital spot film showing the position of the 21-gauge needle *(arrowhead)* on the anterior sacrum just below the aortic bifurcation. The needle is inserted under fluoroscopic guidance from an anterior approach regardless of the intervening structures. An intraarterial catheter *(arrow)* positioned over the aortic bifurcation is used for localization. **B,** Lateral digital spot film after injection of a small test dose of contrast to confirm appropriate needle position. Dilute local anesthetic is then injected to provide the nerve block. (Courtesy Prof. Christoph Binkert, MD, MBA, Winterthur, Switzerland.)

TABLE **10-9** Complications of Fibroid Embolization

Complication	Incidence
Permanent amenorrhea (age ≤ 45 yr)	0-3%
Permanent amenorrhea (age > 45 yr)	20-40%
Expulsion of fibroid	3%-15%
Sepsis	1%-3%
Emergent hysterectomy	<1%
Venous thromboembolism	<1%
Death	<1%

Data from Stokes LS, Wallace MJ, Godwin RB. Quality improvement guidelines for uterine artery embolization for symptomatic leiomyomas. *J Vasc Interv Radiol.* 2010;21:1153-1163.

Patients experience severe pelvic cramping for 12-24 hours following the procedure, followed by gradually decreasing cramping for 7 days. Sequential compression devices applied to the lower legs may reduce the risk of deep vein thrombosis. Most patients are managed overnight in the hospital for pain, but can be sent home the next day on oral medications. Patients should begin nonsteroidal antiinflammatory analgesics immediately after the procedure and continue afterward. Stool softeners are important because narcotics tend to cause constipation. Postembolization syndrome is common, manifested as fatigue, low-grade fevers, nausea, and anorexia. This gradually dissipates over the same time period, but can persist for many weeks. In general, the larger the fibroid volume embolized, the longer the recovery, but this is patient dependent. Severe complications are rare, but uterine infarction and death have been reported (Table 10-9). Fibroid tissue can be expelled for up to a year after the procedure. Rarely, dilatation and curettage is required if fibroid tissue becomes impacted in the endocervical canal. Endometritis manifests as a foul, purulent discharge, but is fortunately rare and can often be managed successfully with antibiotics. The interventionalist should follow up with the patient after the procedure, because postembolization syndrome can easily be confused with infection or other complication by other physicians.

Embolized fibroids shrink on average 50%-60% in volume, with satisfactory results in 85%-90% of patients (slightly more for bleeding and pain, slightly less for bulk symptoms). The reported range of success is wider (65%-90%) for patients treated primarily for adenomyosis. Approximately 25%-30% of patients will require an additional intervention to achieve sustained clinical success. Recurrent symptoms can be due to incomplete embolization, collateral supply from the gonadal or accessory uterine arteries, development of new fibroids, and coexistent pathology such as adenomyosis or endometriosis. Several large randomized prospective studies (UAE versus Surgery for Symptomatic Uterine Fibroids [REST], Embolization versus Hysterectomy [EMMY]) have demonstrated equivalence of UAE to surgical treatment in terms of initial clinical outcomes with faster recovery times, although reintervention directly related to fibroids is significantly higher over time with UAE.

High-intensity focused ultrasound (HIFU) can effectively ablate fibroid tissue in a noninvasive manner. This procedure is performed using MRI guidance to target the fibroids. A small area of tissue is destroyed during each activation, so that several hours may be required to treat a large fibroid volume. The procedure is essentially painless, with a very short recovery. Patients with numerous small fibroids may not be good candidates, nor are patients with scars in the ultrasound path or bowel overlying the fibroids (due to increased risk of heat injury). The overall initial clinical success (control or improvement of symptoms) is 95% with a recurrence rate of approximately 10% at 1 year. Complications occur in fewer than 15%, and include skin edema or burns, abdominal muscle injury, low back pain, and transient sciatica.

Other Gynecologic Indications

Pelvic embolization is sometimes required in women with uncontrollable vaginal bleeding due to postpartum uterine atony, obstetric or gynecologic surgery, unresectable gynecologic tumors, or rarely dysfunctional uterine bleeding. Postoperative arterial bleeding is visualized as extravasation or a pseudoaneurysm at angiography, whereas postpartum and tumor bleeding usually is not seen. In fact, tumors may even appear relatively avascular.

The principles of angiographic evaluation for these types of gynecologic bleeding are the same as for pelvic trauma. Patients with postpartum bleeding can be very unstable with massive blood loss. A pelvic angiogram followed by selective internal iliac injections should be obtained. Postpartum bleeding from uterine atony or placental abnormalities can be managed with Gelfoam or other particulate embolization until there is stasis of the uterine arteries. The uterine arteries may be constricted if the patients have undergone extensive resuscitation including oxytocin.

Ovarian failure is extremely rare in these patients, and the surgical option is emergent hysterectomy, so aggressive embolization is warranted. Localized postoperative bleeding can be embolized with coils following general embolization principles. Small permanent particles (e.g., 300-500 μm) can be used to devascularize tumors. Because the bleeding sites are almost always in the midpelvis with the potential for shared blood supply, careful evaluation of both internal iliac arteries is necessary at completion.

An unusual indication for UAE is ectopic cervical pregnancy. Implantation of the embryo in the endocervical canal occurs in 1 in 9000 of pregnancies overall and is the site of fewer than 1% of ectopic pregnancies. This is an extremely treacherous ectopic pregnancy, in that curettage can lead to intractable bleeding in the cervix controllable only with hysterectomy. Systemic methotrexate and fetal intracardiac potassium results in complete obliteration of the ectopic with normalization of serum β-hCG in 80% of patients. Patients who fail these measures should be considered for embolization. At angiography, the ectopic can appear as a focal hypervascular region in the cervix (Fig. 10-49). Bilateral uterine artery embolization prior to curettage of the pregnancy helps reduce bleeding and the incidence of emergent hysterectomy. Embolization with large particles or Gelfoam until stasis is adequate. Patients can reliably conceive following this procedure.

Abnormal placentation (accreta: placental villi attached on myometrium; increta: villi invading myometrium; percreta: villi reach or are through uterine serosa) occurs more commonly in patients with prior cesarean delivery and advanced maternal age, and requires emergency postpartum hysterectomy due to uncontrollable bleeding in up to 25% of patients. Placement of bilateral internal iliac artery balloon occlusion catheters before cesarean delivery allows intraoperative control of the hypogastric arteries (Fig. 10-50). The balloons are positioned from bilateral common femoral artery access into the contralateral internal iliac arteries and secured in place with sutures and tape. A syringe with the predetermined occlusive volume is left attached to each balloon lumen, so that they can be quickly inflated if needed without the need for fluoroscopy.

▬ EMBOLIZATION OF THE BLADDER

Unresectable bladder tumors or refractory severe cystitis may result in unrelenting substantial bleeding. Vesical artery embolization is occasionally indicated in these patients when all other measures have failed. There is limited published experience with this procedure, but success in 90% of patients is reported when the vesical arteries can be identified. Vesical arteries can arise as discrete branches of the anterior division of the hypogastric artery, as well as branches from the pudendal and uterine arteries. Abnormal hypervascularity or even a mass may be seen at angiography, but visualization of extravasation is unusual. Embolization with particles has a small risk of bladder infarction due to the rich blood supply of the organ.

▬ PENILE ANGIOGRAPHY

The indications for penile angiography are the evaluation of impotence and trauma. Approximately 50% of men older than age 40 years experience some degree of erectile dysfunction. There are numerous possible causes, including neurologic, endocrine, pharmacologic, psychologic, and vasculogenic. The least common cause is vasculogenic, which should be pursued only after other etiologies have been excluded. There are two potential vascular causes of impotence, venous leak (inability to trap blood in the corpus cavernosum) and arterial insufficiency. Vasculogenic impotence has a venous etiology in one third of cases, arterial in one third, and combined venous and arterial in the remainder. Patients with venous leak tend to respond well to pharmacologic therapies. Severe arterial insufficiency is more difficult to treat effectively, but in rare patients internal iliac or internal pudendal artery angioplasty or microvascular bypass to the penile arteries may be effective.

Duplex ultrasound of penile arterial flow in response to a pharmacologically induced erection can be used to screen for arterial insufficiency or venous leak. Dynamic cavernosometry and cavernosography can be used to diagnose a venous leak. When arterial insufficiency is suspected, angiography is indicated.

Before the angiogram, a Foley catheter is placed, and the patient is given an intracorporal injection of either prostaglandin E1 or papaverine to induce an erection. The penile arteries in the flaccid state are contracted and difficult to opacify at angiography.

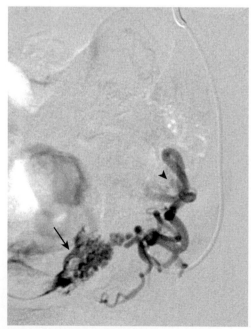

FIGURE 10-49. Cervical ectopic pregnancy. Selective left uterine artery digital subtraction angiogram showing abnormal vascularity of the cervix *(arrow)* in a patient with a cervical ectopic pregnancy who failed methotrexate therapy. The *arrowhead* denotes the ascending portion of the uterine artery along the body of the uterus. Embolization was performed bilaterally with small Gelfoam particles.

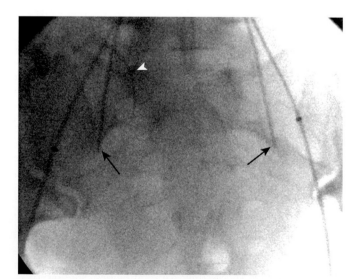

FIGURE 10-50. Bilateral internal iliac artery occlusion balloon catheters *(arrows)* in a patient about to undergo cesarean section for placenta increta. The catheters were placed though 6-French sheaths in each common femoral artery, positioned over the bifurcation into each internal iliac artery, and balloons left deflated. The fetal skull *(arrowhead)* is visible on the right. The poor quality of the image is due to the use of saved fluoroscopic images rather than digital spot films to minimize radiation to the fetus and mother.

Care should be taken to inject at 3 or 9 o'clock on the shaft to avoid injury to the dorsal penile artery. In general, a little less is better than a little more, because too rigid an erection will compromise arterial flow. Pelvic angiograms in the anteroposterior projection and both obliques are obtained with the catheter at the aortic bifurcation to exclude correctable inflow disease of the common and internal iliac arteries. Selective internal pudendal arteriography is performed with a 4-5-French Cobra-2 diagnostic catheter

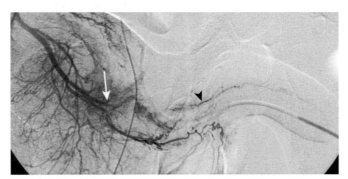

FIGURE 10-51. Vasculogenic (arterial) impotence following penile fracture. Selective right internal pudendal angiogram shows abrupt distal occlusion *(arrow)* with reconstitution of the deep cavernosal arteries via small collaterals *(arrowhead)*. Similar findings were present on the left.

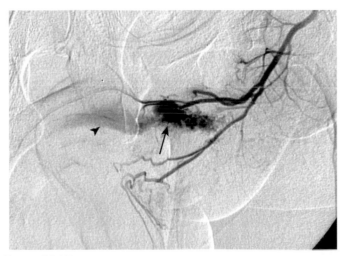

FIGURE 10-52. High-flow priapism following blunt perineal trauma in a skateboarder. Selective left internal pudendal angiogram showing extremely dense bulbar stain *(arrow)* with shunting into the corpora *(arrowhead)*. This was successfully embolized through a superselective microcatheter with autologous blood clot.

or a high-flow micro-catheter catheter (Fig. 10-51; see Fig. 10-4). Usually only one femoral access is required, and a Waltman loop is used to select the ipsilateral internal pudendal artery. Filming in the anterior oblique with the phallus oriented toward the opposite hip provides visualization of the entire internal pudendal artery including the penile supply. Injection of 200 µg of nitroglycerin into the internal pudendal artery immediately before angiography (4-5 mL/sec for 5 seconds) improves visualization. Bilateral angiograms should be obtained. Focal occlusion of the internal pudendal or common penile artery represents a correctable lesion.

Blunt and penetrating perineal trauma may result in an arteriovenous fistula of a cavernosal artery (Fig. 10-52; compare to Fig. 10-4). Clinically this presents as priapism, usually painful. When it is unresponsive to conventional measures, angiography and embolization may be warranted. Selective internal pudendal angiography is performed as described earlier. When a pseudoaneurysm or arteriovenous fistula is identified, embolization with a resorbable substance such as Gelfoam pledgets or autologous clot can be performed. Great care is needed not to confuse the normal bulbospongiosal stain with a vascular injury.

▬ PROSTATIC EMBOLIZATION FOR BENIGN HYPERPLASIA

Selective arterial embolization of the prostate for patients with symptomatic benign prostatic hyperplasia (BPH) is a new procedure. BPH is common in adult males, present in 50% of males by age 50 years. The prostate becomes enlarged (benign prostatic enlargement, BPE) and can cause urinary symptoms (lower urinary tract symptoms) as a result of bladder obstruction (bladder outlet obstruction, BOO) due to the enlarged prostate. Symptoms include difficulty initiating and maintaining micturition, frequent low-volume urination, urgency, and nocturia; collectively these are known as lower urinary tract symptoms (LUTS). Patients with BPH also have increased risk of infection and impotence. The conventional management initially is with medications, and subsequently transurethral resection, microwave, laser, and other ablative techniques when patients have impaired quality of life, large postvoid residuals (>25%), or bladder dysfunction. Selective embolization is a potential alternative treatment, although the experience is currently limited.

Patients undergo urologic evaluation to ensure that their symptoms are due to BOO related to BPE, bladder contractility is normal, there is no evidence of prostatic cancer or infection, and alternative therapies are not indicated. Because these patients often have atherosclerotic disease and variant prostatic arterial anatomy is common, preprocedural evaluation with CTA is helpful. The angiographic tools are similar to those used for uterine artery interventions. Selective internal iliac angiography with 5-French catheters is followed by prostatic angiography with microcatheters (Fig. 10-53). The enlarged prostate is hypervascular, although

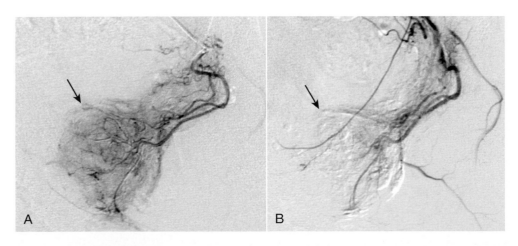

FIGURE 10-53. Embolization of the prostate for symptomatic benign prostatic hyperplasia. **A,** Selective prostatic artery digital subtraction angiogram (DSA) showing a hypervascular prostate gland *(arrow)*. **B,** DSA after embolization with 200 micron Ivalon particles showing staining of the prostate gland *(arrow)* with pruning of the intraprostatic artery branches. Contrast is seen refluxing into surrounding pelvic artery branches because the flow in the prostatic artery is very slow. (Courtesy Prof. Joao Pisco, MD, Lisbon, Portugal.)

portions of the bladder, rectum, and penis may be visualized due to collaterals or shared arterial supply. When selective embolization of the prostate can be assured, 100-300 μ particles are utilized until there is decreased vascularity rather than stasis.

Patients report rapid decrease in obstructive symptoms. There is usually little or no pain, and the risk of infection is low. Transient hematuria, transient rectal bleeding, and hematospermia have been reported in up to 10% of patients. Long-term results are pending, but early reports are encouraging for a durable response.

▓▓▓ Suggested Readings

Biffl WL, Smith WR, Moore EE, et al. Evolution of a multidisciplinary clinical pathway for the management of unstable patients with pelvic fractures. *Ann Surg.* 2001;233:843-850.

Bergqvist D. Pharmacological interventions to attenuate the expansion of abdominal aortic aneurysm (AAA)—a systematic review. *Eur J Vasc Endovasc Surg.* 2011;41:663-667.

Borge MA. Penile arteriography. *Tech Urol.* 1999;5:81-86.

Burke CT, Funaki BS, Ray Jr CE, et al. ACR Appropriateness Criteria® on treatment of uterine leiomyomas. *J Am Coll Radiol.* 2011;8:228-234.

Canaud L, Hireche K, Joyeux F, et al. Endovascular repair of aorto-iliac artery injuries after lumbar-spine surgery. *Eur J Vasc Endovasc Surg.* 2011;42:167-171.

Ciampalini S, Savoca G, Buttazzi L, et al. High-flow priapism: treatment and long-term follow-up. *Urology.* 2002;59:110-113.

Connolly JE, Wilson SE, Lawrence PL, Fujitani RM. Middle aortic syndrome: distal thoracic and abdominal coarctation, a disorder with multiple etiologies. *J Am Coll Surg.* 2002;194:774-781.

Coscas R, Kobeiter H, Desgranges P, Becquemin JP. Technical aspects, current indications, and results of chimney grafts for juxtarenal aortic aneurysms. *J Vasc Surg.* 2011;53:1520-1527.

Ehsan O, Darwish A, Edmundson C, et al. Non-traumatic lower limb vascular complications in endurance athletes. Review of literature. *Eur J Vasc Endovasc Surg.* 2004;28:1-8.

Delgal A, Cercueil JP, Koutlidis N, et al. Outcome of transcatheter arterial embolization for bladder and prostate hemorrhage. *J Urol.* 2010;183:1947-1953.

Donas KP, Schwindt A, Pitoulias GA, et al. Endovascular treatment of internal iliac artery obstructive disease. *J Vasc Surg.* 2009;49:1447-1451.

Ganguli S, Stecker MS, Pyne D, et al. Uterine artery embolization in the treatment of postpartum uterine hemorrhage. *J Vasc Interv Radiol.* 2011;22:169-176.

Gonsalves M, Belli A. The role of interventional radiology in obstetric hemorrhage. *Cardiovasc Intervent Radiol.* 2010;33:887-895.

Goodwin SC, Spies JB. Uterine fibroid embolization. *N Engl J Med.* 2009;361:690-697.

Gorny KR, Woodrum DA, Brown DL, et al. Magnetic resonance-guided focused ultrasound of uterine leiomyomas: review of a 12-month outcome of 130 clinical patients. *J Vasc Interv Radiol.* 2011;22:857-864.

Hirsch AT, Haskal ZJ, Hertzer NR, et al. ACC/AHA 2005 Practice Guidelines for the management of patients with peripheral arterial disease (lower extremity, renal, mesenteric, and abdominal aortic). *Circulation.* 2006;21(113):e463-e654.

Mwipatayi BP, Thomas S, Wong J, et al. A comparison of covered vs bare expandable stents for the treatment of aortoiliac occlusive disease. *J Vasc Surg.* 2011;54:1561-1570.

Moss JG, Cooper KG, Khaund A, et al. Randomised comparison of uterine artery embolisation (UAE) with surgical treatment in patients with symptomatic uterine fibroids (REST trial): 5-year results. *B J Obstet Gynecol.* 2011;118:936-944.

Murphy TP, Cutlip DE, Regensteiner JG, et al. Supervised exercise versus primary stenting for claudication resulting from aortoiliac peripheral artery disease: six-month outcomes from the claudication: exercise versus endoluminal revascularization (CLEVER) study. *Circulation.* 2012;125:130-139.

Nordon IM, Hinchliffe RJ, Loftus IM, et al. Pathophysiology and epidemiology of abdominal aortic aneurysms. *Nat Rev Cardiol.* 2011;8:92-102.

Norgren L, Hiatt WR, Dormandy JA, et al. Inter-Society Consensus for the Management of Peripheral Arterial Disease (TASC II). *J Vasc Surg.* 2007;45:S5-67.

Pisco JM, Pinheiro LC, Bilhim T, et al. Prostatic arterial embolization to treat benign prostatic hyperplasia. *J Vasc Interv Radiol.* 2011;22:11-19.

Popovic M, Puchner S, Berzaczy D, et al. Uterine artery embolization for the treatment of adenomyosis: a review. *J Vasc Interv Radiol.* 2011;22:901-909.

Ramirez JI, Velmahos GC, Best CR, et al. Male sexual function after bilateral internal iliac artery embolization for pelvic fracture. *J Trauma.* 2004;56:734-739.

Rasuli P, Jolly EE, Hammond I, et al. Superior hypogastric nerve block for pain control in outpatient uterine artery embolization. *J Vasc Interv Radiol.* 2004;15:1423-1429.

Slonim SM, Miller DC, Mitchell RS, et al. Percutaneous balloon fenestration and stenting for life-threatening ischemic complications in patients with acute aortic dissection. *J Thorac Cardiovasc Surg.* 1999;117:1118-1126.

Stokes LS, Wallace MJ, Godwin RB. Quality improvement guidelines for uterine artery embolization for symptomatic leiomyomas. *J Vasc Interv Radiol.* 2010;21:1153-1163.

Thevenet A, Latil JL, Albat B. Fibromuscular disease of the external iliac artery. *Ann Vasc Surg.* 1992;6:199-204.

Tyburski JG, Wilson RF, Dente C, et al. Factors affecting mortality rates in patients with abdominal vascular injuries. *J Trauma.* 2001;50:1020-1026.

Uberoi R, Tsetis D, Shrivastava V, et al. Standard of practice for the interventional management of isolated iliac artery aneurysms. *Cardiovasc Intervent Radiol.* 2011;34:3-13.

United Kingdom Small Aneurysm Trial Participants. Long-term outcomes of immediate repair compared with surveillance of small abdominal aortic aneurysms. *N Engl J Med.* 2002;346:1445-1452.

Vallejo N, Picardo NE, Bourke P, et al. The changing management of primary mycotic aortic aneurysms. *J Vasc Surg.* 2011;54:334-340.

van der Kooij SM, Hehenkamp WJ, Volkers NA, et al. Uterine artery embolization vs hysterectomy in the treatment of symptomatic uterine fibroids: 5-year outcome from the randomized EMMY trial. *Am J Obstet Gynecol.* 2010;203:105:e1-13.

Zakaria MA, Abdallah ME, Shavell VI, et al. Conservative management of cervical ectopic pregnancy: utility of uterine artery embolization. *Fertil Steril.* 2011;95:872-876.

CHAPTER 11

Visceral Arteries

John A. Kaufman, MD, MS, FSIR, FCIRSE

The arterial anatomy of the gastrointestinal tract is the most variable of all vascular beds. In addition, there is great diversity in the types of diseases that involve the gastrointestinal arteries and organs. Many visceral disorders, vascular and otherwise, can be treated effectively with endovascular techniques. As a result, visceral arterial diagnosis and intervention continues to be an important aspect of interventional radiologic practice.

■ NORMAL ANATOMY

Celiac Artery

The celiac artery arises from the anterior surface of the abdominal aorta at the level of the T12-L1 disk space (Fig. 11-1). In most individuals, the inferior phrenic arteries arise from the aorta in close proximity to the upper rim of the celiac artery orifice, but sometimes from the very proximal celiac artery. The celiac artery (also known as the celiac trunk) courses inferiorly under the posterior fibers of the diaphragmatic crura for a distance of 1.5-3 cm. There is frequently an indentation upon the superior aspect of the celiac artery caused by the fibers of the diaphragm (Fig. 11-2), which is made worse and can even occlude the lumen with expiration. Branches of the celiac artery supply the stomach, pancreas, liver, and spleen (Fig. 11-3).

The first branch of the celiac artery is usually the left gastric artery, arising superiorly distal to the diaphragmatic crura. Distal to the left gastric artery, the celiac artery bifurcates into the common hepatic and splenic arteries. A large branch to the pancreas, the dorsal pancreatic artery, may arise from the celiac, proximal hepatic, or splenic arteries. Conventional celiac artery anatomy is present in only 70% of individuals. A wide range of variants can occur (Table 11-1). An awareness of these variations and knowing where to look for celiac branches that may have anomalous origins are essential for visceral vascular imaging. Specific examples are provided in the following sections. As a rule, any of the celiac branches can arise independently from the aorta, or (with the exception of the left gastric artery) from the superior mesenteric artery (SMA). Rarely, the entire celiac artery can be replaced to the SMA. These variants are explained by the common embryology of the contents of the peritoneal cavity. For the same reason, celiac branches cannot arise anomalously from the renal arteries, because these organs are retroperitoneal in origin.

Liver (Arterial Supply)

The liver parenchymal anatomy is most often described using the Couinaud segments, based upon hepatic and portal venous anatomy (see Fig. 14-1). This chapter focuses on the arterial anatomy.

One third of the blood flow to the liver is arterial, but this supplies two thirds of the organ's oxygen. Conversely, the portal vein supplies two thirds of the blood volume, but only one third of the oxygen. The common hepatic artery arises from the celiac artery in more than 95% of individuals. The terminal branches of this artery are the gastroduodenal and proper hepatic arteries (see Fig. 11-3). In a little over half of patients, the proper hepatic artery gives rise to the entire arterial supply of the liver (Table 11-2). The proper hepatic artery continues for a short distance, and then divides into the left and right hepatic arteries. A separate branch to segments 4a and 4b, the middle hepatic artery, is often present. The left hepatic artery has a characteristic forked appearance that allows ready identification. The hepatic arteries are located anterior to the portal vein within the liver parenchyma.

The most common variants of hepatic arterial supply are replacement of part or all of the right hepatic artery from the SMA, or the left hepatic artery replaced to the left gastric artery (Fig. 11-4). These variants can occur in isolation or together. In general, 45% of patients have some variation in their hepatic arterial supply.

The cystic artery (to the gallbladder) is usually a branch of the right hepatic artery, although it may arise from the common hepatic, left hepatic, or even the superior mesenteric arteries (see Fig. 11-3).

Spleen

The spleen derives its blood supply from the celiac artery primarily via the splenic artery (see Figs. 2-21 and 11-3). This vessel courses posterior to the pancreas, and anterior and superior to the splenic vein. The splenic artery is much longer than the hepatic artery, and frequently several millimeters larger in diameter. The splenic artery gives rise to many small branches to the pancreas and stomach. The splenic artery divides into multiple branches, usually in the hilum of the spleen but sometimes in a more proximal location.

Stomach

The stomach is supplied by numerous arteries, all of which communicate with each other (see Fig. 11-3). The left gastric artery is usually the first branch of the celiac artery but can also arise directly from the aorta or rarely from the left hepatic artery. The left gastric artery supplies the gastroesophageal junction, fundus of the stomach, and a portion of the lesser curve. The lateral fundus is also supplied by short and posterior gastric arteries arising from the splenic artery and splenic hilum. These arteries anastomose with the left gastric artery.

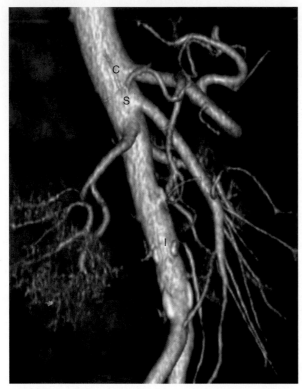

FIGURE 11-1. Oblique volume rendering of a computed tomography angiogram showing the origins of the celiac artery (C), superior mesenteric artery (S), and inferior mesenteric artery (I). There is moderate stenosis of the inferior mesenteric artery origin.

The body of the stomach is supplied by the gastroepiploic artery, which is located along the greater curvature of the stomach (see Fig. 11-3). The gastroepiploic artery has origins from the gastroduodenal artery (where it is called the right gastroepiploic artery) and the distal splenic artery (where it is called the left gastroepiploic artery). The lesser curvature of the body of the stomach is supplied by branches from the right gastric artery and branches of the left gastric artery (Fig. 11-5). The right gastric artery usually arises from the left or common hepatic arteries, and is a much smaller vessel than the left gastric artery.

The antrum and pylorus are supplied by the right gastroepiploic and right gastric arteries. In addition, the pancreaticoduodenal arteries (branches of the gastroduodenal artery) provide blood supply to this part of the stomach.

Pancreas

The pancreatic blood supply is derived from both the celiac artery and the SMA. The head of the pancreas is supplied by the pancreaticoduodenal arteries (see Figs. 11-3 and 11-6). These vessels are paired arteries anterior and posterior to the pancreatic head. They are further divided into superior and inferior vessels. The superior pancreaticoduodenal arteries arise from the gastroduodenal artery, while the inferior pancreaticoduodenal arteries arise from a common trunk off the proximal SMA.

The body of the pancreas is supplied by the dorsal pancreatic artery, usually a proximal branch of the splenic artery or the celiac artery, which contributes to the transverse pancreatic artery running the length of the gland (see Figs. 11-3 and 11-6). Less commonly, the dorsal pancreatic artery will arise from the common hepatic artery, the SMA, or the aorta. This is a small but important artery, in that it can contribute to the blood supply of the transverse colon via an accessory or a replaced middle colic artery in 1%-2% of patients (Fig. 11-7). The pancreaticoduodenal arteries also supply the body of the pancreas through the transverse pancreatic artery.

There are numerous small arteries that arise directly from the splenic artery to supply the body and tail of the pancreas. These are termed, aptly, *small pancreatic arteries*. The largest and most distal of these vessels is the pancreatica magna artery. All of these arteries communicate with the transverse pancreatic artery. The left gastroepiploic artery may provide small branches to the tail of the pancreas.

Superior Mesenteric Artery

There are usually four sources of arterial supply to the small bowel and colon: the gastroduodenal branches from the celiac artery, the SMA, the inferior mesenteric artery (IMA), and the anterior divisions of the internal iliac arteries. The SMA supplies the

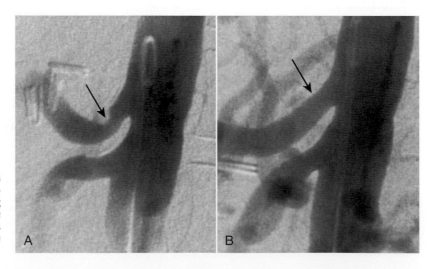

FIGURE 11-2. Crus impression upon the celiac artery. This is usually of no clinical significance. **A,** Lateral digital subtraction angiogram (DSA) of the aorta in expiration showing extrinsic compression on the superior aspect of the celiac artery *(arrow)* with post-stenotic dilatation. **B,** Repeat DSA in the same patient with inspiration showing absence of the stenosis *(arrow)*.

duodenum, small bowel, and the colon as far as the splenic flexure (Fig. 11-8). The IMA supplies the left colon, sigmoid colon, and proximal rectum (Fig. 11-9). The internal iliac arteries provide supply to the rectum and anus (see Fig. 10-2). The vasculature of the bowel is, in essence, one long multitiered arcade. The most peripheral continuous vessel in this arcade runs along the mesenteric border of the bowel. In the colon, this vessel is usually well developed and termed the *marginal artery of Drummond*. The equivalent vessel in the small bowel is less prominent and unnamed. The classic areas of overlap (watershed areas) of the bowel vascular supply are the splenic flexure of the colon (Griffith point) and the superior rectum.

The SMA arises from the anterior abdominal aorta 1-2 cm distal to the celiac artery (see Figs. 11-1 and 11-2). The SMA is typically 6-8 mm in diameter at its origin. The SMA passes behind the body of the pancreas and over the left renal vein, and runs through the mesentery slightly to the right and posterior to the superior mesenteric vein (SMV). The first major branch of the SMA is either the inferior pancreaticoduodenal artery trunk or the middle colic artery. These two vessels can also arise conjointly. The middle of the SMA supplies the small bowel from the third portion of the duodenum to the terminal ileum through multiple branches that usually arise from the left border of the vessel. These are termed *jejunal* or *ileal* branches based upon the portion of small bowel that they supply. The right side of the artery gives rise to the right colic artery, which supplies the ascending colon. The SMA terminates in the ileocolic artery, which supplies the terminal ileum and the cecum. A small appendiceal artery may arise from the ileocolic artery or directly from the distal SMA. The middle and right colic arteries bifurcate at the mesenteric border of the colon; the right into ascending and descending branches, and the middle into right and left branches. Of particular importance is the left branch of the middle colic, in that this artery anastomoses with the left colonic branches of the IMA.

In fewer than 1% of patients, the celiac artery and SMA share a common origin from the aorta. This is termed a *celiacomesenteric trunk*. The SMA frequently gives rise to an accessory or replaced right hepatic artery (20%), or less commonly a replaced proper or common hepatic artery (2%) (see Fig. 11-4). In fewer than 1% of patients, the splenic, transverse pancreatic, or dorsal pancreatic arteries may arise from the SMA. A persistent direct fetal communication between the celiac artery and the SMA, in conjunction with or distinct from the dorsal pancreatic artery, occurs in fewer than 1% of patients and is termed the *arc of Buhler* (see Figs. 11-6 and 11-8). A separate origin of some of the jejunal,

ileal, or colic branches from the anterior surface of the aorta between the SMA and IMA, known as a *middle mesenteric artery*, is extremely rare. If you find a case, please send it to me!

Inferior Mesenteric Artery

The IMA arises from the left side of the anterior distal abdominal aorta at the level of the L3 vertebral body, approximately 2-3 cm above the aortic bifurcation (see Fig. 11-1). This artery is much smaller than the SMA in diameter, usually no more than 3 mm. The artery has a sharply caudal course through the sigmoid mesentery (see Fig. 11-9). The first branch of the IMA is the left colic artery, from which a large branch ascends through the mesentery to meet the left branch of the middle colic artery at the splenic flexure. The blood supply of the sigmoid colon is provided by the IMA. The terminal branch of the IMA is the superior hemorrhoidal artery to the superior rectum. This is located in the center of the pelvis. On conventional angiography, the distal superior hemorrhoidal artery has a characteristic forked appearance, which distinguishes it from the straight median sacral artery. On a lateral view, the hemorrhoidal artery is in the middle of the pelvis, whereas the median sacral artery lies close to the anterior surface of the sacrum. The remainder of the rectum is supplied by the middle and inferior rectal arteries, terminal branches of the anterior division of the internal iliac arteries.

TABLE 11-1 Celiac Artery Anatomy

	Incidence
Left gastric, splenic, common hepatic arteries from celiac trunk	70%
Above plus dorsal pancreatic artery from celiac trunk	10%
Splenic, common hepatic arteries from celiac trunk; left gastric from aorta	2%
Splenic, left gastric arteries only from celiac trunk	3%
Common hepatic, left gastric arteries only from celiac trunk	<1%
Celiacomesenteric trunk (shared origin celiac and superior mesenteric arteries)	<1%
All branches individually from aorta	<1%
Splenic artery from aorta	<1%
Splenic artery from superior mesenteric artery	<1%

TABLE 11-2 Hepatic Arterial Anatomy

	Incidence
All branches from common hepatic artery	55%
Right hepatic artery from superior mesenteric artery (SMA)	12%
Accessory right hepatic artery from SMA	6%
Left hepatic from left gastric artery	11%
Accessory left hepatic from left gastric artery	11%
Right hepatic from SMA and left hepatic from left gastric artery	2%
Common hepatic artery from SMA	2%
Common hepatic artery from aorta	2%
Right hepatic artery from celiac	<1%

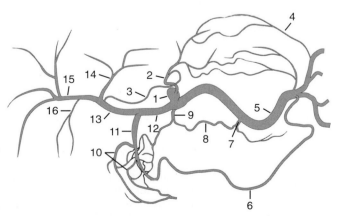

FIGURE 11-3. Anatomy of the celiac artery and its branches. *1,* Celiac trunk. *2,* Left gastric artery. *3,* Right gastric artery. *4,* Short gastric artery. *5,* Splenic artery. *6,* Gastroepiploic artery. *7,* Pancreaticomagna artery. *8,* Transverse pancreatic artery. *9,* Dorsal pancreatic artery. *10,* Superior pancreaticoduodenal arteries. *11,* Gastroduodenal artery. *12,* Common hepatic artery. *13,* Proper hepatic artery. *14,* Left hepatic artery. *15,* Right hepatic artery. *16,* Cystic artery.

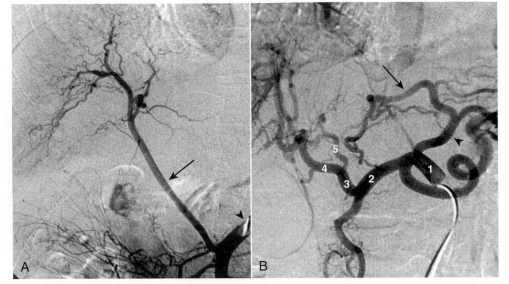

FIGURE 11-4. Hepatic arterial anatomic variants. **A,** Right hepatic artery replaced *(arrow)* to the superior mesenteric artery *(arrowhead)* in this patient with advanced cirrhosis. Note the characteristic corkscrew appearance of the intrahepatic arteries. **B,** Celiac angiogram showing the left hepatic artery *(arrow)* replaced to the left gastric artery *(arrowhead)*. The left hepatic artery has a characteristic forked appearance. *1,* Celiac artery; *2,* common hepatic artery; *3,* proper hepatic artery; *4,* right hepatic artery; *5,* middle hepatic artery (to segment 4).

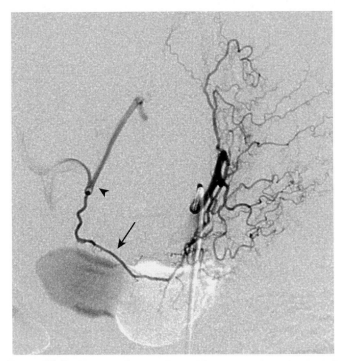

FIGURE 11-5. Right gastric artery *(arrow)* demonstrated on selective left gastric angiogram. The artery travels along the lesser curve of the stomach (note the gastric air bubble) to the origin of the left hepatic artery *(arrowhead)* in this patient.

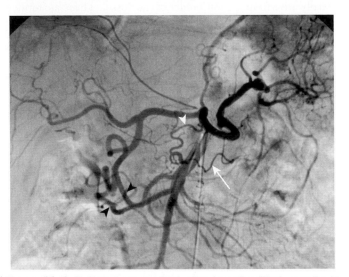

FIGURE 11-6. Enlarged pancreaticoduodenal arteries *(black arrowheads)* in a patient with occlusion of the celiac artery origin. The pancreaticoduodenal arteries are a collateral pathway between the superior mesenteric artery (SMA) and the celiac artery. The dorsal pancreatic artery *(white arrowhead)* communicates with both the proximal SMA and the transverse pancreatic artery *(white arrow)*.

KEY COLLATERAL PATHWAYS

Celiac Artery

The pancreaticoduodenal arteries from the SMA are the dominant collateral supply to the celiac artery (see Fig. 11-6). Primitive transpancreatic communications from the SMA through the dorsal pancreatic artery, such as the arc of Buhler, can exist in some individuals. These same circuits can provide collateral supply to the SMA from the celiac artery.

Spleen

The spleen receives collateral blood supply from the left gastric artery via the short gastric arteries, the right gastroepiploic to the left gastroepiploic arteries, arteries from the tail of the pancreas, and omental collaterals (arc of Barkow). Proximal splenic artery occlusion is usually well tolerated owing to the richness of this collateral bed.

Liver

Occlusion of the common hepatic artery results in reversal of flow in the gastroduodenal artery from the pancreaticoduodenal and gastroepiploic arteries. The left gastric artery can also provide collateral supply through the right gastric artery (see Fig. 11-5). The right gastric artery is an important collateral in the setting of proper hepatic artery occlusion. Over time, small unnamed collateral arteries may form in the porta hepatis. Within the liver parenchyma, the right and left hepatic arteries have a rich potential collateral network (Fig. 11-10). Occlusion of intrahepatic arterial branches is well tolerated for this reason.

The liver can recruit arterial supply from phrenic, intercostal, and internal mammary arteries. This is most often encountered in the setting of a vascular liver tumor.

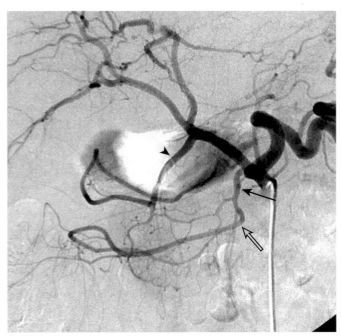

FIGURE 11-7. Right branch of the middle colic artery *(open arrow)* arising from the dorsal pancreatic artery *(solid arrow)*. The gastroduodenal artery *(arrowhead)* arises from the common hepatic artery as usual.

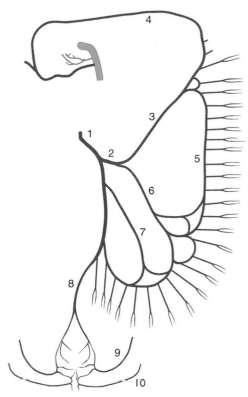

FIGURE 11-9. Drawing of the inferior mesenteric artery. *1*, Inferior mesenteric artery. *2*, Left colic artery. *3*, Ascending branch of left colic artery. *4*, Left branch of middle colic artery. *5*, Marginal artery. *6*, Descending branch of left colic artery. *7*, Sigmoid artery. *8*, Superior hemorrhoidal artery. *9*, Middle hemorrhoidal artery. *10*, Inferior hemorrhoidal artery.

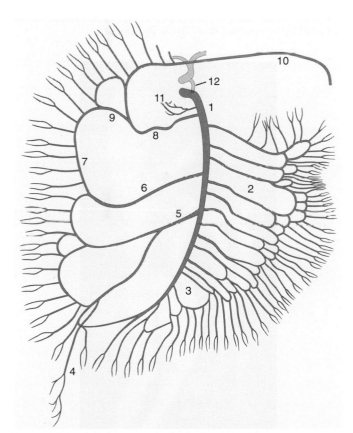

FIGURE 11-8. Drawing of conventional anatomy of the superior mesenteric artery. *1*, Superior mesenteric artery. *2*, Jejunal branches. *3*, Ileal branches. *4*, Appendicular artery. *5*, Ileocolic artery. *6*, Right colic artery. *7*, Marginal artery. *8*, Middle colic artery. *9*, Right branch of middle colic artery. *10*, Left branch of middle colic artery. *11*, Inferior pancreaticoduodenal arteries. *12*, Arc of Buhler.

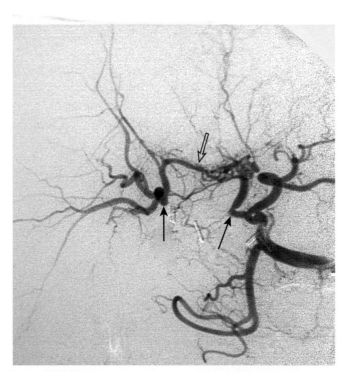

FIGURE 11-10. Digital subtraction angiogram of the hepatic artery showing intrahepatic collateralization *(open arrow)* around a right hepatic artery occlusion *(black arrows)*.

Superior Mesenteric Artery

The collateral pathways to the SMA from the celiac artery branches are described above (see Celiac, this section). The other major collateral pathway is from the IMA (Fig. 11-11). The ascending branch of the left colic artery communicates with the left branch of the middle colic artery at the splenic flexure through the arcade of Riolan. The marginal artery of Drummond also joins the left branch of the middle colic artery at the splenic flexure (see Fig. 11-9). Rarely, the dorsal pancreatic artery has a branch that continues to the transverse colon. Unnamed retroperitoneal collaterals from the aorta to the SMA can develop in some patients.

Inferior Mesenteric Artery

In the setting of IMA occlusion, the left branch of the middle colic artery is the major source of collateral blood supply. In addition, the anterior division of the internal iliac artery can supply the left colon through the hemorrhoidal arteries. This pathway is extremely important in patients with IMA occlusion undergoing right hemicolectomy, in which the anastomosis between the middle colic artery from the SMA and the left colic artery from the IMA is disrupted. In patients with intact collateral pathways and slowly progressive occlusive disease, a well-developed hypogastric collateral bed can supply the IMA, SMA, and ultimately celiac artery.

▬ IMAGING

The proximal celiac artery and SMA are amenable to interrogation by ultrasound (color-flow and duplex ultrasound) in most patients. The IMA is difficult to image in some patients owing to the small size of the artery. The velocities and directions of flow within the celiac artery and SMA are essential elements of the study. Flow in the celiac artery and its major branches has a low resistance pattern. Peak systolic velocities greater than 200 cm/sec in the celiac artery origin is indicative of at least 70% stenosis. The baseline waveform in the proximal SMA is high resistance. A postprandial state induces a high-flow, low-resistance waveform in the SMA. A peak systolic velocity at least 275 cm/sec and end-diastolic velocities of at least 45 cm/sec have both been shown to be predictive of SMA stenosis. In expert hands, ultrasound has an 89% sensitivity and 92% specificity for identification of stenoses greater than or equal to 70% of the SMA. Retrograde flow in the common hepatic artery is the best predictor of hemodynamically significant celiac artery stenosis. Ultrasound is less successful in the evaluation of distal branches of the SMA.

Magnetic resonance angiography (MRA) has excellent sensitivity and specificity for visceral artery ostial and proximal disease (Fig. 11-12). Three-dimensional (3-D) acquisitions in the coronal plane, centered on the aortic bifurcation, include the visceral arteries as well as the hypogastric artery origins. The ability to view vessel origins in multiple planes is useful when anatomy is complex or anatomic variants are present. Heavy calcification, metallic clips, and patient motion can cause artifacts. Small vessel disease is difficult to visualize with current technology.

Multidetector computed tomography angiography (CTA) of the visceral arteries, particularly with 64-channel equipment or better, can provide excellent depiction of even small visceral arterial branches. When performed for occlusive or inflammatory disease, the study should include a noncontrast scan. Heavily calcified plaque can be obscured by dense arterial opacification on contrast-enhanced sequences (see Fig. 10-23). Enhancement in the arterial wall is an important sign of vasculitis. Image postprocessing is essential to evaluate the visceral arteries (see Figs. 11-1 and 11-13). In addition to blood vessels, CTA provides valuable additional information about the perfusion of the visceral organs and bowel that can contribute to the diagnosis.

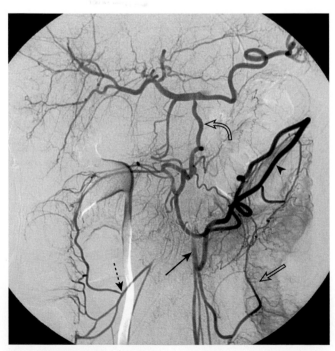

FIGURE 11-11. Filling of the celiac artery from the inferior mesenteric artery (IMA) *(black solid arrow)* via the dorsal pancreatic artery *(open curved arrow)* in a patient with superior mesenteric artery and celiac artery origin occlusions. IMA angiogram showing an intact marginal artery of Drummond *(open arrow)* and enlarged arc of Riolan *(arrowhead)* filling the middle colic artery and ultimately branches of the ileocolic artery *(dashed arrow)* via the marginal arcade of the right colic artery.

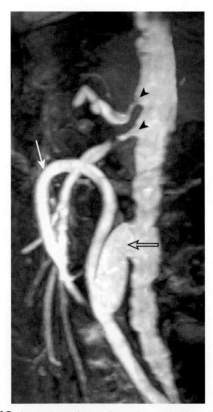

FIGURE 11-12. Lateral maximum intensity projection of gadolinium-enhanced three-dimensional magnetic resonance angiogram in a patient with a bypass graft *(solid white arrow)* to the superior mesenteric artery (SMA) arising from an onlay aortobifemoral graft *(open arrow)*. The patient had chronic mesenteric ischemia due to celiac artery and SMA stenoses *(arrowheads)* and an occluded inferior mesenteric artery.

Visceral angiography requires knowledge of a wide range of catheter shapes and guidewires. A quick fluoroscopic examination of the abdomen is useful in patients undergoing elective examinations with a history of recent oral or rectal contrast. Residual barium or Gastrografin in the colon may degrade the quality of the study. The best means of viewing the visceral artery origins is with a lateral aortogram. A pigtail catheter (4- to 5-French) should be placed with the tip at the T12-L1 vertebral interspace to visualize the celiac artery and SMA origins (see Figs. 10-7 and 11-2). A lower position (below the renal arteries) with a slight left posterior oblique angulation depicts the IMA origin. Selective catheters for the visceral arteries range from generic cobra shapes to complex curves designed for specific branch vessels. In general, vessels that arise with angles 45-100 degrees from the aorta can be engaged with simple curved selective catheters (Table 11-3; see Figs. 2-10 and 2-18 through 2-20). When the artery arises at an acute angle, such as the IMA, a recurved catheter is the best

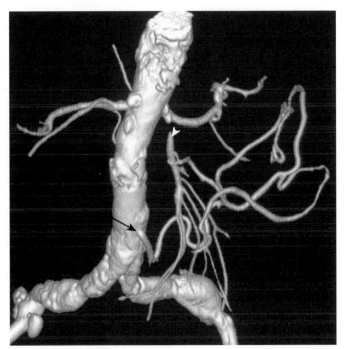

FIGURE 11-13. Volume rendering of computed tomography angiogram in a patient with celiac artery and superior mesenteric artery (SMA) origin occlusion showing collaterals from the inferior mesenteric artery *(black arrow)* to the SMA *(white arrowhead)*.

choice. Review of prior CTA and MRA data when available can guide catheter selection. Visceral vessels are easily traumatized by catheters and guidewires, so gentle technique is required at all times. Leading with the soft tip of a guidewire when pulling or pushing into a vessel reduces spasm and the risk of dissection (see Fig. 2-46). Coaxial microcatheters are almost always necessary for selection of small branch vessels for the reasons listed earlier (see Fig. 2-21). High-flow microcatheters that are designed for power injection of contrast at 2-3 mL/sec are very useful for super-selective visceral angiography.

The left gastric artery represents a specific challenge for selective catheterization when the vessel arises from its normal location—the upper surface of the celiac artery. A recurved pull-down catheter such as a Simmons 1 or a Sos can be pulled into the celiac artery so that the tip is advanced beyond the left gastric artery origin. Continued downward traction on the catheter forces the tip upward against the superior wall of the celiac artery. As the catheter is withdrawn further, the tip moves retrograde along the superior wall of the celiac artery until the orifice of the left gastric artery is engaged. The Rösch left gastric catheter is used in a similar fashion. Another technique is to form a Waltman loop in the splenic or hepatic artery with a braided 4- or 5-French Cobra-2 catheter (see Fig. 2-17). Once formed, the looped catheter is slowly pushed into the aorta until the tip engages the left gastric artery orifice. Occasionally, a left gastric artery that arises close to the origin of the celiac trunk can be selected directly with an angled catheter and a selective guidewire.

Celiac artery injections can be filmed in the anteroposterior projection (see Fig. 11-4B). Delayed filming is useful for visualization of the splenic and portal veins. The right anterior oblique projection is useful for selective common or proper hepatic artery injections to visualize the intrahepatic arteries. Complete coverage of the SMA may require overlapping fields of view to ensure visualization of the splenic flexure and small bowel in the pelvis. Complete coverage of the IMA also frequently requires two injections to include both the splenic flexure and the anal verge. A left posterior oblique projection will open the sigmoid colon flexure.

Several measures can be taken to improve the quality of visceral angiograms. Adequate injection rates and volumes are essential to fill this vast vascular bed. Glucagon (1 mg intravenously) before injection of contrast decreases bowel motion artifact on digital subtraction angiography studies, but is relatively short acting. Outside of the United States, hyoscine butylbromide (20 mg intravenously) provides durable bowel paralysis without the central nervous system side effects of scopolamine. This can be repeated if necessary to achieve cessation of peristalsis. Lastly, a series of masks obtained during a single respiratory cycle provides optimal subtraction when extended filming of injections is required, because most patients will have difficulty holding their breath.

TABLE 11-3 Injection Rates for Visceral Angiography

Artery	Typical Catheters	Injection (mL/sec/total volume)	Filming
Celiac	Cobra-2, Rösch celiac, Sos Omni	5-7/30-60	2-4/sec × 10 sec, then 1/sec
Splenic	Cobra-2, Simmons-2	5-6/30-50	Same
Hepatic	Cobra-2, Rösch hepatic, Simmons-2	4-5/15-30	Same
Left gastric	Simmons-1, Rösch left gastric, Cobra-2 (Waltman loop)	3-4/6-16	Same
Gastroduodenal	Cobra-2, Rösch celiac	3-4/6-16	Same
Superior mesenteric artery	Cobra-2, Rösch celiac, Sos Omni	5-7/30-60	Same; may require two injections with overlapping upper and lower fields to include all of bowel
Inferior mesenteric artery	Sos Omni, Rösch IMA Simmons-1	3-5/9-20	Same; for gastrointestinal bleed, use left posterior oblique projection and include anal verge on image

IMA, inferior mesenteric artery.

■ ACUTE MESENTERIC ISCHEMIA

Acute mesenteric ischemia is one of the most potentially devastating visceral arterial emergencies. A variety of causative mechanisms have been described (Box 11-1). More than 50% of cases are due to embolic occlusion of the SMA, one fifth are caused by thrombosis of a preexisting stenotic lesion, one fifth occur during a period of low flow or hypotension (nonocclusive mesenteric ischemia), and about 5% can be due to mesenteric venous thrombosis. Acute occlusion of the SMA is tolerated poorly, even in the presence of a widely patent celiac artery and IMA with intact collaterals. Time is the primary determinant of survival for these patients. In most series, the mortality rate exceeds 60% without early and aggressive intervention. Delay in diagnosis equals death.

The classic presentation of acute intestinal ischemia is sudden onset of generalized abdominal pain out of proportion to the physical findings. This scenario is particularly suggestive of acute mesenteric ischemia of embolic origin in patients with cardiac arrhythmias. The pain may also be subacute or stuttering in onset. Nausea, vomiting, and diarrhea are common subsequent symptoms. Despite the severe abdominal pain, bowel sounds remain present and peritoneal signs are absent until the ischemia is advanced. The development of peritonitis heralds sepsis, shock, and onset of multiorgan system failure. The white blood cell count may be elevated, but there are no laboratory tests specific for bowel infarction. Elevated serum lactate, amylase, and phosphate levels are found in many patients. Metabolic acidosis and a history of acute onset of abdominal pain should be considered highly suspicious for advanced acute mesenteric ischemia.

The patient's prior surgical history should be reviewed, with particular attention to the details of vascular reconstructions and bowel resections. The difficulty in imaging many patients with suspected acute mesenteric ischemia is that usually several other possible diagnoses are being considered at the same time. The plain film findings of early acute mesenteric ischemia are nonspecific. Gas in the bowel wall or portal vein indicates bowel infarction and is a late sign. Contrast-enhanced CT scan is an excellent initial imaging modality that allows evaluation of arterial and venous structures, as well as the bowel wall (Fig. 11-14). However, presence of oral contrast in the colon from the CT can degrade subsequent angiograms.

Conventional angiography remains an essential diagnostic modality in suspected acute mesenteric ischemia. A lateral aortogram should be obtained first to inspect the celiac artery and SMA origins (Fig. 11-15). The classic findings of an embolus are

contrast outlining a convex filling defect causing partial or complete luminal obstruction. An aortogram in the anteroposterior projection is valuable to assess the aorta and exclude associated renal artery emboli. Selective injection of the SMA to exclude peripheral pathology is mandatory if the origin is normal on the

---

Box 11-1. Etiologies of Acute Mesenteric Ischemia

Embolus (cardiac or aortic source)
Thrombosis existing atherosclerotic lesion
Dissection (aortic or localized to visceral artery)
Cholesterol embolization
Low-flow state (nonocclusive mesenteric ischemia)
Vasculitis
Iatrogenic (e.g., low placement of intraaortic balloon pump)
Mesenteric venous thrombosis

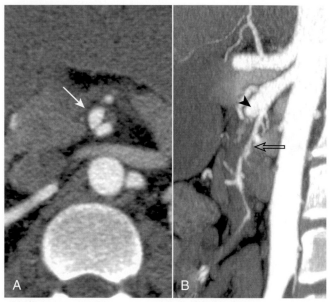

FIGURE 11-14. Acute spontaneous dissection of the superior mesenteric artery (SMA). **A,** Axial computed tomography image showing expansion of the SMA *(arrow)* with contrast on two sides of an intimal flap. **B,** Thick sagittal maximal intensity projection showing the origin of the dissection in the SMA *(arrowhead)* with thrombosis of the false lumen and a compressed but patent true lumen *(open arrow)*.

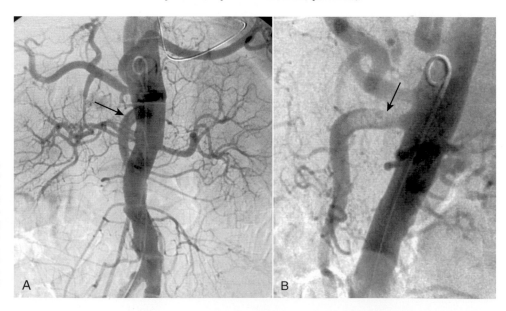

FIGURE 11-15. The lateral aortogram is the most useful view for visualizing the origins of the celiac artery and superior mesenteric artery (SMA). This patient had atrial fibrillation and acute simultaneous onset of abdominal pain and left leg ischemia. **A,** Digital subtraction aortogram (DSA) in the anteroposterior projection. The visceral artery origins are obscured *(arrow,* SMA.) **B,** Lateral DSA aortogram shows a filling defect in the origin of the SMA *(arrow)*.

aortogram (Fig. 11-16). Filming should continue through the portal venous phase to assess the patency of the SMV. Celiac artery and IMA injections may be performed if the SMA is normal, but rarely are these culprit vessels in acute mesenteric ischemia.

Large emboli may lodge at the SMA origin. As many as 85% of emboli will then progress distally in the SMA, usually stopping just beyond the origin of the first major branch. These emboli result in profound ischemia, because major potential collateral pathways (either from the celiac artery via the pancreaticoduodenal arteries or the IMA via the middle colic artery) are obstructed. Simultaneous embolization to other organs is common. When the clinical examination and radiographic findings suggest that bowel remains viable, catheter-based intervention may be considered. These include thrombolysis and suction embolectomy (see Fig. 11-16). In most patients, emergent surgical embolectomy or bypass with resection of any portions of nonviable bowel is necessary.

Thrombosis of a previously symptomatic or asymptomatic visceral artery stenosis may cause acute ischemia if collaterals are poorly formed or nonexistent. This tends to occur during episodes of hemodynamic stress or derangement, such as during acute myocardial infarction or severe dehydration. A heavily calcified aorta or SMA on CT is indicative of underlying atherosclerosis. Thrombolysis (catheter-directed) with subsequent angioplasty and stent can be attempted when full-thickness bowel ischemia has not occurred. Surgical bypass with resection of any portions of nonviable bowel remains the standard therapy in acutely ill patients.

Nonocclusive mesenteric ischemia is a syndrome of low flow in the SMA in the absence of a fixed lesion (Fig. 11-17). Most often associated with acutely ill patients on multiple vasopressor agents or digitalis, it can also be seen in the setting of cardiogenic shock and sepsis. Mortality is very high, usually from the precipitating conditions rather than the bowel ischemia. At angiography, vasoconstriction of the SMA and its branches, often with interposed areas of normal-caliber vessel, is characteristic. Injection of a vasodilator directly into the SMA, such as nitroglycerin, may break the spasm and can be used as a diagnostic test. Direct infusion of papaverine (0.5-1 mg/min) can be used to treat spasm until the patient's condition stabilizes. There is little role for surgical intervention in these patients.

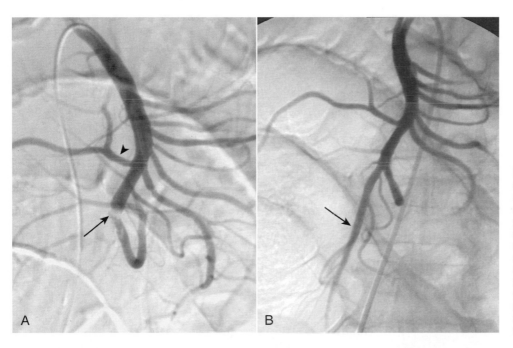

FIGURE 11-16. Aspiration thrombectomy of a distal superior mesenteric artery (SMA) embolus. **A,** Selective digital subtraction angiogram (DSA) of the SMA in a patient with several days of intermittent abdominal pain, a normal physical examination, and small bowel wall thickening on computed tomography scan. There is occlusion of the SMA by an embolus *(arrow)* distal to the right colic artery *(arrowhead)*. **B,** DSA obtained following percutaneous aspiration thrombectomy during the same procedure showing reperfusion of the distal SMA *(arrow)*.

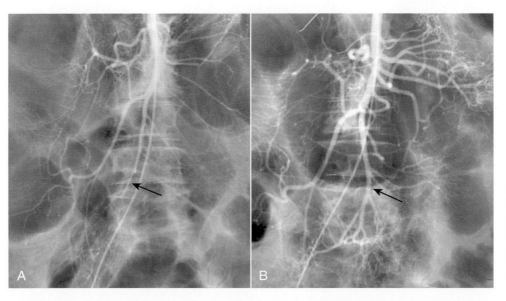

FIGURE 11-17. Nonocclusive mesenteric ischemia in a patient with abdominal pain following cardiac surgery. **A,** Selective SMA angiogram showing diffuse narrowing of all of the mesenteric vessels. For example, note the appearance of the ileocolic artery *(arrow)*. **B,** Angiogram repeated after infusion of papaverine showing marked improvement in the caliber of the arteries *(arrow)*.

▬ CHRONIC MESENTERIC ISCHEMIA

The symptoms of chronic mesenteric ischemia are completely different from those of acute ischemia. The onset is gradual, often months to years in duration. Postprandial pain is the defining symptom. Termed *intestinal angina*, the pain occurs 30-60 minutes following a meal, is poorly localized, resolves after 2-3 hours, and may be associated with nausea, vomiting, or diarrhea. Patients usually report weight loss and fear of eating (Box 11-2). Progression to acute ischemia can occur if patients are not treated.

The visceral arteries are well collateralized, so that chronic occlusion of the IMA or celiac artery in isolation are often well tolerated. Generally, the diagnosis of chronic mesenteric ischemia is only entertained if the SMA is abnormal, either alone or in combination with the celiac artery. A number of conditions can be associated with chronic mesenteric ischemia (Box 11-3). Ostial

---

Box 11-2. Risk Factors Associated with Chronic Mesenteric Ischemia

Age 50-70 years
Female-to-male ratio 3:2
Tobacco abuse
Generalized atherosclerosis
Hypertension
Chronic renal insufficiency
Diabetes
Past history of abdominal or vascular surgery

Box 11-3. Etiologies of Chronic Mesenteric Ischemia

Atherosclerosis
Dissection
Vasculitis
Median arcuate ligament syndrome
Fibromuscular dysplasia
Thoracoabdominal aneurysm
Iatrogenic
Abdominal aortic coarctation

---

atherosclerotic lesions may be aortic wall rather than visceral arterial plaque. Bulky, calcified intraluminal aortic plaque ("coral reef aorta") may cause physical obstruction of the visceral artery orifices (see Fig. 10-23). Although atherosclerosis is often limited to the proximal few centimeters of the vessels, symptomatic distal occlusive disease also occurs.

Median arcuate ligament syndrome is a somewhat controversial variant of chronic mesenteric ischemia that tends to occur in young, thin, female patients. The celiac artery is severely compressed by the median arcuate ligament, but the SMA and IMA are usually normal. The symptoms are typical of those of other forms of chronic mesenteric ischemia, with postprandial pain and even weight loss. Hemodynamically it is hard to explain the symptoms on the basis of ischemia when the SMA collateral pathways are intact.

The evaluation of patients with suspected chronic mesenteric ischemia should exclude other common causes of chronic abdominal pain (e.g., pancreatic, bowel, or biliary pathology). Arterial flow in the visceral arteries should be assessed first with duplex ultrasound. Careful interrogation of the visceral arteries is necessary to identify potentially confusing variant anatomy. Elevated fasting velocities, or less than 20% increase in the SMA peak systolic velocity after eating, are useful as diagnostic findings that can be used to follow up interventions. Both CTA and MRA provide exquisite anatomic information about the visceral artery origins (see Figs. 11-12 and 11-13). Conventional angiography remains essential for confirming the diagnosis and potential catheter-based therapy. In addition to the standard views, pressure gradients should be measured across any suspicious lesions.

The traditional therapy for chronic mesenteric ischemia is surgery. Transaortic endarterectomy, aorta-visceral artery bypass, and iliac-visceral are common operations for atherosclerotic lesions (see Fig. 11-12). These approaches are used more often for occlusions because, when possible, stenoses are treated with stents. Relief of symptoms improves as the number of vessels revascularized increases; surgical mortality is approximately 5%, and 5-year graft patency approaches 80%. Median arcuate ligament syndrome is treated with division of the overlying diaphragmatic crura and sympathectomy, as well as celiac artery reconstruction when necessary.

Percutaneous therapy of symptomatic atherosclerotic ostial and proximal visceral artery stenoses with stents is now usually considered the first treatment option. Angioplasty alone is rarely sufficient, because the plaque often involves the aortic wall (Fig. 11-18).

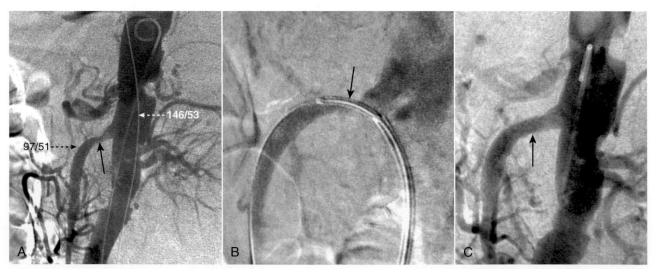

FIGURE 11-18. Superior mesenteric artery (SMA) stenosis treated with a stent in an older man with acute ischemic colitis in the splenic flexure during an episode of dehydration. The patient had a history of occasional postprandial abdominal pain after aortofemoral bypass graft for occlusive disease. **A,** Lateral digital subtraction angiogram (DSA) of the aorta showing a 60% proximal SMA stenosis *(arrow)* with a measured pressure gradient of 49 mm Hg systolic. The celiac is not well visualized on this image but was severely stenotic, and the IMA was occluded. **B,** DSA during positioning of a balloon-expandable stent *(arrow)* across the area of stenosis from a femoral approach. This was dilated to 7 mm. **C,** Lateral DSA of the aorta after stent placement. The gradient was 0 mm Hg, and the angiographic appearance was excellent *(arrow)*. The patient reported complete resolution of his postprandial pain.

Percutaneous techniques have also been successful in selected nonatherosclerotic etiologies such as Takayasu disease and isolated SMA dissection. The approach to the target artery is an important determinant of technical success. In many instances a femoral access with a curved guide catheter works well for selecting the artery and positioning devices. When the artery has a very steep downward angle from the aorta, a brachial artery access (usually left) facilitates selection and manipulation across the lesion. Long, precurved 5- to 7-French sheaths or guide catheters provide stability during the procedure and allow injection of contrast to monitor the intervention. A stiff working guidewire is essential, because devices must make an almost 180-degree turn into the artery in some cases. The tip of the guidewire should be observed at all times, because perforation of small arterial branches can occur. The choice of guidewire diameter is a matter of operator preference. Full heparinization is important to prevent catastrophic thrombotic complications. Balloon-expandable stents are used for ostial lesions. Self-expanding stents can be useful for lesions deeper in the SMA. Pressure gradients across visceral stenoses are often high, even after successful stent placement, and do not seem to reflect the clinical response. This may be due to the large and potentially low-resistance vascular bed supplied by the SMA and IMA. Approximately 80% of patients will have symptomatic relief with endovascular treatment; the more arteries that are abnormal before intervention, the higher the likelihood of clinical success with even one vessel revascularization. Restenosis by Duplex criteria occurs in two thirds, but only half of these (one third overall) develop recurrent symptoms over 3 years. The use of covered stents may decrease the incidence of symptomatic restenosis.

Stent placement in a stenotic IMA should be considered when this vessel is the dominant blood supply to the colon. The stenoses are usually very focal at the ostium, for which balloon-expandable stents should be used.

▬ GASTROINTESTINAL BLEEDING

Angiography for gastrointestinal bleeding was once a common study, often occurring at odd hours. Preventive pharmacologic therapy, endoscopic diagnosis and intervention, CT angiography, and improved medical interventions have decreased but not eliminated the need for angiography. This remains an important and often life-saving intervention. When a patient with gastrointestinal bleeding is referred, several key pieces of clinical information should be obtained (Box 11-4). This information determines the urgency, type, and sequence of diagnostic and therapeutic procedures. Be prepared to assume primary management responsibility for patients with gastrointestinal bleeding, especially in the middle of the night.

Acute Gastrointestinal Bleeding

Acute gastrointestinal bleeding resolves spontaneously in 85% of patients. The first goal of management is therefore to stabilize the patient with fluid resuscitation through large-bore venous lines,

placement of a nasogastric (NG) tube for upper gastrointestinal bleeding, airway protection if necessary, and a Foley bladder catheter. Correction of deranged clotting studies should be performed aggressively, and transfusion of blood products should be initiated. The patient's history should be carefully reviewed for clues, such as prior bleeding, known colonic pathology, previous gastrointestinal or vascular surgery, or liver disease. Vital signs should be followed closely, and when there is continued evidence of bleeding, further diagnostic and therapeutic measures are indicated.

The second key principle in the management of gastrointestinal bleeding (resuscitation of the patient is first) is localization. Without knowing where the bleeding is coming from, appropriate therapy is impossible. By convention, the ligament of Treitz divides the gut into upper and lower tracts. Bleeding is 5-8 times more common from the upper gastrointestinal tract, typically from ulcers and gastritis. Lower gastrointestinal bleeding is colonic in origin in 80% of patients, with one third from the right colon, one third from the transverse colon, and the remainder from the sigmoid colon and rectum. The most common etiology of colonic arterial bleeding in patients older than age 50 is diverticulosis, followed by angiodysplasia (see Vascular Malformations). In general, sources proximal to the ligament of Treitz manifest clinically as hematemesis, and those more distal as melena or hematochezia. This is not a hard rule, but when the NG tube aspirate is positive for blood, an upper gastrointestinal source is effectively ruled in (Boxes 11-5 and 11-6).

Patients with upper gastrointestinal bleeding should undergo endoscopy as their initial diagnostic evaluation. A source can be

---

Box 11-4. Key Clinical Information in Patients with Acute Gastrointestinal Bleeding

Which orifice is the blood coming from?
Hemodynamically stable or unstable?
What resuscitative measures have been undertaken?
Coagulopathy?
Has the patient undergone endoscopy?
Nasogastric tube in place?
Prior gastrointestinal or aortic surgery?
What is treatment plan following localization of bleeding?
Foley catheter in place?

Box 11-5. Etiologies of Acute Upper Gastrointestinal Bleeding

Peptic ulcer
Gastritis
Portal hypertension (varices)
Mallory-Weiss tear
Marginal ulcer
Iatrogenic (after biopsy, percutaneous gastrostomy)
Arteriovenous malformation/angiodysplasia
Dieulafoy lesion
Tumor
Pseudoaneurysm
Hemobilia
Hemosuccus entericus
Pseudo-gastrointestinal bleeding (swallowed blood from nasopharyngeal source)
Aortoenteric fistula

Box 11-6. Etiologies of Acute Lower Gastrointestinal Bleeding

Diverticulosis (most common etiology in older patients)
Hemorrhoids
Arteriovenous malformation/angiodysplasia
Postendoscopic polypectomy (can occur as late as 14 days)
Inflammatory bowel disease (most common etiology in young adults)
Ischemic bowel
Portal hypertension (colonic, rectal, stomal varices)
Tumor
Vasculitis
Radiation colitis
Infection (especially immunocompromised host)
Small bowel/colonic ulcers
Aortoenteric and graft-enteric fistula
Meckel diverticulum (children and young adults)

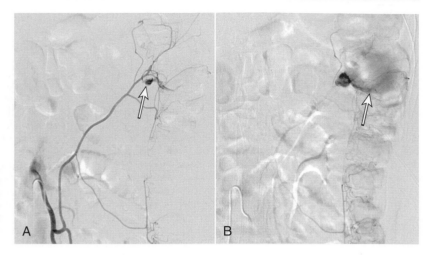

FIGURE 11-19. Angiographic demonstration of gastrointestinal bleeding. **A,** Selective inferior mesenteric artery angiogram showing extravasation of contrast *(arrow)* from a branch of the left colonic artery. **B,** Same patient, a few seconds later, showing persistent contrast that flows into lumen of the bowel *(arrow)*. This is consistent with a bleeding diverticulum.

identified more than 95% of the time, and in many cases treated with electrocautery, injection sclerotherapy, clip placement, or banding. Endoscopy in patients with lower gastrointestinal bleeding is more difficult, particularly when bleeding is brisk (overall 70% success rate in identifying a bleeding source). When a bleeding source is identified but cannot be controlled endoscopically, placement of clips around or on the lesion will facilitate localization at angiography. Contrast-enhanced CTA is increasingly being used as a noninvasive modality for diagnosis of lower gastrointestinal bleeding in stable patients. A triple phase study without oral contrast is required: noncontrast, arterial phase, and venous phase. Sensitivity and specificity are both greater than 95%. High attenuation material (fresh blood) or contrast extravasation into bowel are indicative of recent or active bleeding respectively. Although intravenous contrast is required for this study, a negative study obviates an angiogram, and a positive study allows a focused angiogram. Tagged red blood cell (technetium 99m) scans may also be used as a noninvasive study in stable patients. This study can detect bleeding at a rate of 0.1 mL/min, which is believed to be lower than the rate of bleeding (0.5-1 mL/min) visualized at angiography. However, localization of bleeding to a particular segment of bowel is possible in only about 50% of cases at nuclear medicine examinations.

In most centers, an angiographic intervention is performed following a positive CTA or bleeding scan. The likelihood of finding bleeding on an angiogram increases almost 10-fold when performed immediately after a positive bleeding scan compared to angiograms obtained without prior positive bleeding scan.

Angiography for acute gastrointestinal bleeding should begin with selective injection of the vessel supplying the most likely source of bleeding based on all available clinical, imaging or historical data. The suspected level of bleeding within the gastrointestinal tract determines which vessel to select: celiac artery for upper gastrointestinal sources, IMA for sigmoid and rectum, SMA for small bowel and right colon. With occlusion of the IMA, the SMA injection frequently suffices to evaluate the left colon and sigmoid. The anal verge must be included in the field of view on IMA injections. When bleeding is not identified on the first injection, selection of the next most likely artery is performed, and so on. A celiac injection should be included for lower gastrointestinal bleeding when SMA and IMA injections are negative because the middle colic artery is replaced to the dorsal pancreatic artery in 1%-2% of patients (see Fig. 11-7). A hypogastric artery injection may be necessary to exclude rectosigmoid bleeding when there is occlusion of the IMA.

Image acquisition should be rapid (3-6 frames/sec) during the arterial phase, and then slower for the venous phase. Visualization of the portal phase is mandatory, in that bleeding can be due to varices or mesenteric venous thrombosis. Intravenous glucagon decreases artifact from bowel gas on DSA examinations, an important source of artifacts. The use of CO_2 gas as a contrast agent has been reported to be extremely sensitive for depiction of gastrointestinal bleeding, but intraluminal gas artifact from bowel peristalsis is problematic. Flush aortography in patients with gastrointestinal bleeding is rarely indicated.

The angiographic diagnosis of gastrointestinal bleeding is based on visualization of extravasation of contrast into the bowel lumen. The contrast should appear during the arterial phase, persist through the venous phase, and change with time (Fig. 11-19). False-positive findings can be caused by preexisting barium in diverticula, bowel gas, densely enhancing veins, hyperemic bowel due to inflammation, or adrenal blushes. Digital images should be reviewed in both subtracted and unsubtracted modes to confirm the diagnosis. Extravasated contrast pooling in the rugae of the stomach or the haustra of the bowel may look like a vein (the "pseudo-vein sign"). This "pseudo-vein" persists beyond the venous phase of the injection (Fig. 11-20). False-negative studies can result from injection of inadequate volumes of contrast, failure to include all of the vascular bed in the imaging field, and failure to select the appropriate arteries. Foley catheter drainage of the bladder improves visualization of the distal sigmoid and rectum.

Therapy for gastrointestinal bleeding depends on the etiology and location. Management of variceal bleeding is discussed in Chapter 14. Cautery, clipping, or injection of upper gastrointestinal peptic ulcers, vascular malformations, and angiodysplasias are effective interventions in 85% of cases, with the highest success rates reported for gastric lesions. Surgical therapy is required in only 2%-5% of cases.

Catheter-based techniques for control of arterial gastrointestinal bleeding are highly effective, safe, and rapid. The two basic techniques used for arterial bleeding are embolization and, less often vasopressin infusion (Tables 11-4 through 11-6).

Embolization is commonly used for control of gastrointestinal bleeding because it is rapid and definitive. The basic objective of embolization in gastrointestinal bleeding is to decrease arterial pressure and flow sufficiently to allow hemostasis without creating tissue infarction. In general coils, pieces of Gelfoam, metamorphics (e.g., glue), or particles are used. The specific approach varies with the site of bleeding, the pathology, and the arterial anatomy. The rich collateral supply of the stomach allows embolization with relative impunity. Although identification of a bleeding source before embolization in the gastrointestinal tract is the rule, the left gastric artery is the exception and can be embolized empirically in patients with endoscopically proven fundal or gastroesophageal junction lesions (Fig. 11-21). Conversely, bowel bleeding should only be embolized after superselective catheterization confirms the precise site of

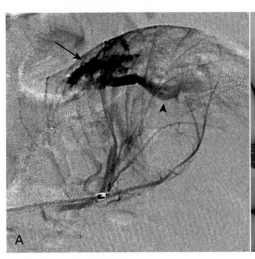 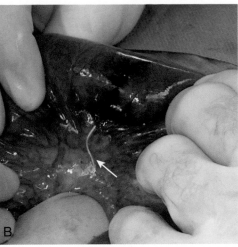

FIGURE 11-20. Dieulafoy lesion of the jejunum in a 3-year-old with massive lower gastrointestinal bleeding. **A,** Selective angiography through a microcatheter demonstrates extravasation of contrast *(arrow)* from an abnormal submucosal artery. The linear contrast in the bowel lumen is a "pseudo vein" *(arrowhead)*; contrast pooling within intraluminal thrombus or in between rugae. This did not wash away on later images. **B,** Intraoperative photograph showing staining with methylene blue of the segment of small bowel containing the bleeding. The microcatheter *(arrow)* is clearly seen through the transparent mesenteric peritoneum.

TABLE 11-4 Gastric/Duodenal Embolization for Gastrointestinal Bleeding

Indications	Ulcer, gastritis, pseudoaneurysm, Mallory-Weiss tear
Contraindication	Unidentified source of bleeding (except for empirical left gastric artery embolization), inability to select artery
Catheter location	
Fundal bleed/ gastroesophageal junction	Left gastric artery
Duodenal bleed	Gastroduodenal artery/inferior pancreaticoduodenal trunk
Preferred agents	Coils, Gelfoam pledgets, glue/Onyx, sometimes large particles for left gastric artery

TABLE 11-5 Colonic Embolization for Gastrointestinal Bleeding

Indication	Active lower gastrointestinal bleeding
Contraindications	Unidentified source of bleeding; ischemic bowel; inability to superselect bleeding artery
Catheter location	As close to bleeding site as possible
Preferred agents	Microcoils, Gelfoam pledgets, glue/Onyx

TABLE 11-6 Intraarterial Vasopressin Therapy

Indications	Colonic and small bowel bleeding not amenable to embolization
Contraindications	Active myocardial ischemia, limb ischemia, bowel ischemia, uncooperative patient
Catheter location	Proximal superior mesenteric artery or inferior mesenteric artery
Infusion	0.2-0.4 U/min
Protocol	Initiate at 0.2 U/min; repeat angiogram after 20-30 minutes to confirm cessation of bleeding; increase by 0.1 U/min every 20 minutes until bleeding is controlled or maximum dose (0.4 U/min) is given; infuse for 24 hours; taper to normal saline over 12-24 hours; pull catheter after 6-12 hours of no bleeding
Patient activity	Strict bedrest
Patient diet	Nil by mouth
Laboratory tests	Complete blood count and electrolytes every 12 hours
Troubleshooting	Is catheter still connected to pump? Is there a kink in the tubing? What is current dose? Has catheter become dislodged (check plain film or angiogram)

extravasation, because there is a small risk of bowel infarction (Fig. 11-22). In some cases a clip may have been placed on the mucosa adjacent to a bleeding lesion at endoscopy. This can be used to direct embolization when extravasation is not visualized. The duodenum represents a special situation, in that the blood supply is from both the celiac artery and SMA. Following embolization, injection of both arteries should be performed to confirm control of bleeding.

Embolic agents should be sized to occlude the target vessel. For empirical embolization of the left gastric artery, small Gelfoam cubes or large particles (up to 700-900 μm) are injected until stasis occurs (see Fig. 11-21). In most other instances a discrete feeding vessel can be identified, which can then be occluded with coils or Gelfoam. If the bleeding vessel cannot be reached with a catheter, embolization across origin of the

bleeding branch with coils is usually effective as long as no other collateral is present. Alternatively, embolization with a small volume of glue (NBCA) is very effective because flow directs the material to the site of bleeding (see Fig. 11-22). Bowel bleeding should always be embolized from the most selective position possible. If a superselective position with a coaxial microcatheter cannot be achieved or operative therapy is indicated, the catheter can be left in position and methylene blue injected at the time of resection to outline the segment of bowel responsible for the bleeding (see Fig. 11-20). Alternatively, a coil can be placed as close as possible to the bleeding site, which the surgeon can locate intraoperatively by palpation or transillumination of the mesentery.

Embolization is successful in more than 90% of cases, with few instances of bowel ischemia. In general, 80% of patients will not bleed again, but those with vascular lesions or ongoing inflammation are more likely to rebleed. Great care to avoid nontarget organ embolization is required. Patients undergoing bowel embolization should be monitored closely for evidence of acute bowel ischemia or delayed ischemic colonic strictures, but the combined incidence is less than 2%.

Vasopressin (pitressin) is a posterior pituitary hormone that causes both smooth muscle constriction and water retention. Infused into the proximal SMA or IMA, it can control acute diverticular bleeding, postpolypectomy, and mucosal bleeding in up to 90% of cases (Fig. 11-23). About half of these patients will not bleed again. Vasopressin infusion is a useful tool when the general vicinity of the bleeding is known, but selective catheterization is not possible. Infusion is from the proximal SMA or IMA so that the entire vascular bed is treated. Vasopressin should not be used for patients with bleeding due to pseudoaneurysms,

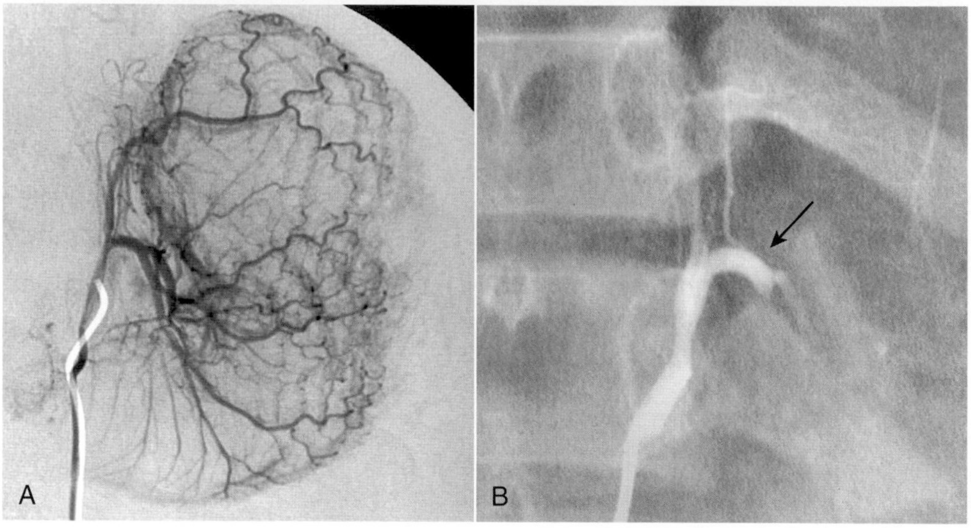

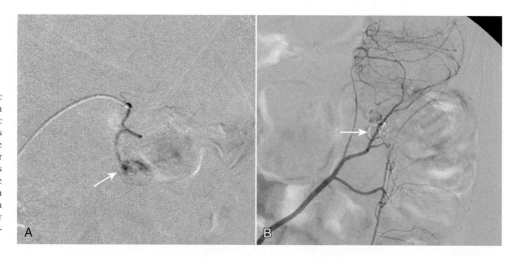

FIGURE 11-21. Empirical embolization of left gastric artery with Gelfoam pledgets in a patient with diffuse fundal abnormality on endoscopy. **A,** Left gastric artery digital subtraction angiogram showing hyperemic gastric fundus distended with thrombus but no extravasation. **B,** Injection in the left gastric artery following embolization with small Gelfoam pledgets showing truncation of the branches *(arrow)*.

FIGURE 11-22. Embolization of colonic bleeding. This is the same patient as in Figure 11-19. **A,** Superselective left colic angiogram through a microcatheter shows extravasation of contrast *(arrow)*. The catheter could not be advanced any closer to the site of bleeding so embolization was performed with n-butyl cyanoacrylate glue diluted 1:3 with iodized oil. **B,** Completion inferior mesenteric artery angiogram shows occlusion of the bleeding artery with glue *(arrow)*. The patient had no further bleeding and no complications.

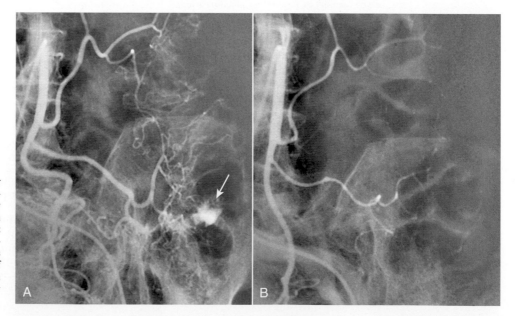

FIGURE 11-23. Management of lower gastrointestinal bleeding with vasopressin infusion. **A,** Inferior mesenteric artery (IMA) angiogram showing extravasation *(arrow)* from a diverticulum. **B,** Repeat IMA angiogram after infusion of vasopressin at 0.2 U/min for 30 minutes shows typical vasoconstriction and cessation of bleeding. The patient was maintained on vasopressin for 24 hours, then slowly weaned with no recurrence of bleeding.

ischemic bowel, or arteriovenous malformations. Patients experience initial abdominal cramping due to smooth muscle constriction in the bowel, often accompanied by evacuation of any blood in the bowel. This should not be mistaken for continued bleeding. Although very effective, vasopressin therapy requires monitoring in an intensive care unit. Rare complications include cardiac or digital ischemia from vasoconstriction, or hyponatremia from water retention. Vasopressin can also be used for bleeding from gastritis, although embolization of the left gastric artery is preferred by most angiographers. Duodenal bleeding responds poorly to vasopressin because of the dual blood supply (celiac artery and SMA).

Massive projectile upper gastrointestinal bleeding after aortic surgery (usually remote) should suggest an aortoenteric fistula. The usual location is at the proximal aortic anastomosis and the duodenum. Aortoenteric fistula can also occur after endograft repair of abdominal aortic aneurysm (AAA), from native aortic and common iliac aneurysms, and from necrosis of large periaortic tumors. Depending on the location of the fistula in the bowel or the volume of bleeding, bleeding may be from the lower gastrointestinal tract as well (Fig. 11-24). Stable patients should undergo upper endoscopy through the duodenum. Imaging with CT in the stable patient is often unrevealing, because loss of the fat plane between the duodenum and aortic grafts is seen in many patients postoperatively. Inflammatory changes, anastomotic pseudoaneurysms, fluid around the vascular prosthesis, or contrast extravasation all suggest the diagnosis. Treatment with aortic stent grafts can control bleeding, but most patients are currently managed with open repair. Long-term therapy with antibiotics is recommended because colonization by gastrointestinal bacterial flora of any prosthesis in this area is assumed.

Chronic Gastrointestinal Bleeding

There are numerous causes of chronic gastrointestinal bleeding (Box 11-7). Chronic gastrointestinal blood loss can be characterized as occult or overt. Occult bleeding tends to be due to colonic malignancies, polyps, and small arteriovenous malformations, as well as gastroduodenal peptic disease. Chronic overt bleeding can be due to diverticulosis, portal hypertension, and inflammatory diseases (Fig. 11-25). Graft-enteric erosions (not fistulas) should be considered in patients with prior aortoiliac surgery and chronic gastrointestinal bleeding of unknown etiology. Patients with chronic stomal bleeding and negative endoscopic examinations should be evaluated for occult portal hypertension and stomal varices (see Fig. 14-8).

Overall, failure to identify a bleeding source occurs in fewer than 5% of patients with chronic gastrointestinal bleeding. The majority of lesions in these patients are colonic in origin. The evaluation includes upper and lower endoscopy, capsule endoscopy, complete gastrointestinal radiography, CTA angiography,

and nuclear medicine bleeding scans (including a Meckel scan in young patients). The small bowel is the most difficult area to evaluate with these modalities.

A small percentage of patients will be referred for diagnostic angiography. Angiographic evaluation should be obtained only

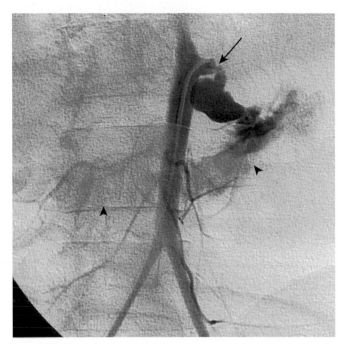

FIGURE 11-24. Selective digital subtraction angiogram of an aortoenteric fistula *(arrow)* showing opacification of the small bowel *(arrowheads)* in a patient with a necrotic retroperitoneal germ cell tumor and massive lower gastrointestinal bleeding. (Courtesy Robert Sheley, MD, and Oliver Ochs, MD, Good Samaritan Hospital, Portland, Ore.)

Box 11-7. Etiologies of Chronic Gastrointestinal Bleeding

Colonic carcinoma
Polyps
Arteriovenous malformation/angiodysplasia
Inflammatory bowel disease
Leiomyoma/leiomyosarcoma
Meckel diverticulum (young patients)
Graft-enteric erosion
Ulcer
Gastritis
Portal hypertension (varices)

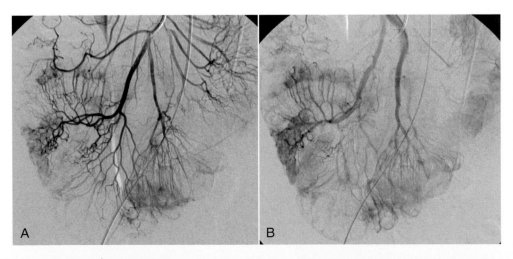

FIGURE 11-25. Crohn disease. Inflammatory bowel diseases are common causes of lower gastrointestinal bleeding in children and young adults. **A,** Superior mesenteric artery angiogram showing splaying of the mesenteric arcades and hyperemic ileum. **B,** Portal venous phase imaging in the same patient. There is no extravasation, but the small bowel remains densely staining, owing to inflammatory changes. Note the lack of bowel gas artifact in these images and in Figures 11-26 and 11-27 due to the use of bowel paralytic agent and multiple mask images. (Courtesy James Jackson, MD, London, United Kingdom.)

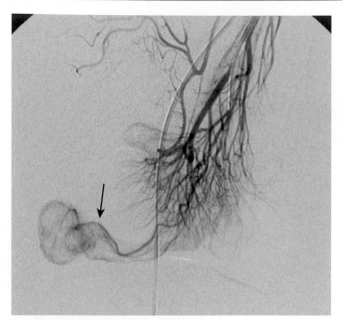

FIGURE 11-26. Demonstration of Meckel diverticulum on selective digital subtraction angiogram of the superior mesenteric artery. A characteristic vitelline artery is seen *(arrow)* extending beyond the border of the normal ileum. (Courtesy James Jackson, MD, London, United Kingdom.)

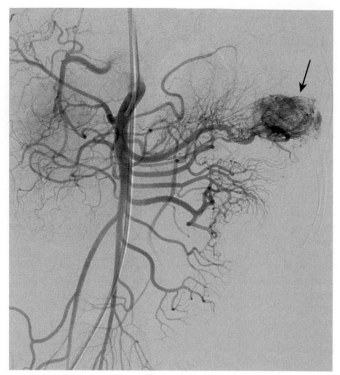

FIGURE 11-27. Angiographic appearance of small bowel gastrointestinal stromal tumors in a patient with chronic lower gastrointestinal bleeding. Selective superior mesenteric artery angiogram showing a densely staining mass in the left abdomen *(arrow)*. Incidentally, the patient has a replaced right hepatic artery. On the venous phase (not shown), the mass persists with dense staining and opacification of the draining vein. (Courtesy James Jackson, MD, London, United Kingdom.)

when all other studies are negative. Complete visceral angiography, with magnification views, should be performed. Careful bowel preparation, the use of smooth muscle paralytics, and magnification angiography are essential. Some operators advocate provocative angiography, with infusions of heparin or a thrombolytic agent into the SMA or IMA to try to trigger bleeding. This is not a common practice.

The lesions most often encountered are arteriovenous malformations and gastrointestinal stromal tumors (see later). Meckel diverticula have a characteristic arterial supply, the vitelline artery (Fig. 11-26). Treatment of most etiologies of chronic gastrointestinal bleeding is surgical.

■ NEOPLASM

Bowel

Neoplasms of the bowel are usually diagnosed by noninvasive imaging modalities or endoscopy. Rarely, the diagnosis is made at angiography during workup for gastrointestinal bleeding. The most common tumors found in this manner are either small bowel gastrointestinal stromal tumors (GIST) or leiomyomas/leiomyosarcomas (Fig. 11-27). These tumors constitute only about 2% of gastrointestinal tract malignancies, about 40% present with bleeding, and metastases are more common with lesions greater than 10 cm or with high mitotic rates. The most common location is the stomach (almost 50%), followed by the small bowel (30%), rectosigmoid (10%), duodenum (5%), and rarely the esophagus, mesentery, retroperitoneum, and omentum. The angiographic appearance is distinctive—a densely staining vascular mass that persists through the venous phase.

Primary colonic adenocarcinomas are usually avascular at angiography and difficult to detect unless large. An area of staining and irregularity of small arteries may be seen. Hypervascular metastases to the colon, such as melanoma, will appear as staining masses at angiography, and sometimes demonstrate arteriovenous shunting.

Carcinoid tumors of the bowel have a unique angiographic appearance, but are rarely diagnosed in this manner. These are rare (5/100,000) slow-growing tumors arising from enterochromaffin cells. Carcinoid tumors can occur in multiple locations, but the most common are the gastrointestinal tract (55%) and the lungs (about 33%). The prognosis is better with gastrointestinal tract carcinoids. In the gastrointestinal tract, 45% are located in the small bowel (usually the ileum), 20% in the rectum, 15% in the appendix, 10 % in the colon, and the remainder in the stomach and duodenum. Carcinoid and other well-differentiated neuroendocrine tumors release chromogranins, of which chromogranin A correlates well with tumor burden. Although the actual lesion is usually small, the associated dense fibrotic response results in retraction of the mesentery. At angiography, the contractile deformity of the mesenteric arterial and venous structures is characteristic (Fig. 11-28). Carcinoid tumors release serotonin and other vasoactive molecules, which are metabolized by the hepatocytes unless the source is from hepatic metastases or non-gastrointestinal carcinoid. The symptoms of flushing, hypertension, and diarrhea are indicative of release of serotonin by liver metastases. Somatostatin analogs (e.g., octreotide) are effective in controlling symptoms and appear to prolong survival in patients with metastatic disease. Up to two thirds of patients with carcinoid syndrome have right-sided cardiac disease (fibrosis) involving the tricuspid and pulmonary valves. This can result in right-sided heart failure and require operative valve replacement.

Pancreas

Pancreatic neoplasms are almost always diagnosed and staged by CT, ultrasound, or magnetic resonance imaging (MRI). Resectability is predicted from CT in almost all cases. The most common lesions are adenocarcinomas, although a variety of other primary and metastatic lesions can involve the pancreas. In

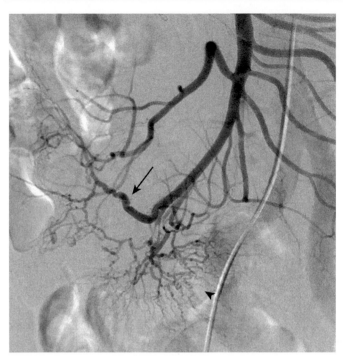

FIGURE 11-28. Selective superior mesenteric artery angiogram showing contraction of the mesentery *(arrowheads)* and arterial irregularity *(arrow)* due to a primary small bowel carcinoid.

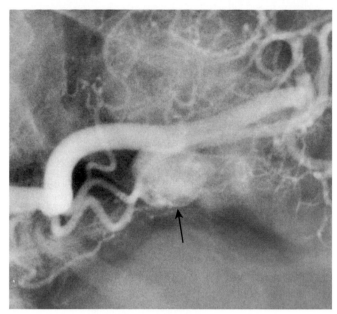

FIGURE 11-29. Typical hypervascular angiographic appearance of an islet cell tumor *(arrow)* in the body of the pancreas (in this case, insulinoma).

selected instances, angiography is used to define preoperative anatomy or to localize a small vascular lesion.

Resectability of adenocarcinoma of the head of the pancreas is determined partially by the degree of vascular involvement, particularly the portal vein, hepatic artery, and SMA. Venous encasement is manifested by narrowing of the portal vein confluence in the region of the mass (see Figs. 1-27C and **D**). Occlusion and venous thrombosis can occur. Arterial encasement of the hepatic, splenic, or superior mesenteric artery is almost always a late finding, indicating an unresectable lesion. Angiography is rarely indicated to determine resectability.

Pancreatic neuroendocrine tumors (NET) are a diverse group of lesions that, when functional, have a spectrum of symptoms related to the cell line of origin and degree of differentiation of cells. Almost one third of pancreatic NETs are functional. These lesions include carcinoid tumors (resulting in carcinoid syndrome when metastatic to the liver), insulinomas (hypoglycemia), glucagonomas (migratory rash, diabetes, diarrhea, deep venous thrombosis), somatostatinomas (diabetes, cholelithiasis, diarrhea with steatorrhea), gastrinomas (duodenal ulcers and diarrhea), and VIPomas (diarrhea, hypokalemia, and hypochlorhydria). Symptoms from carcinoid tumors, glucagonomas, and VIPomas respond to somatostatin analogs. Well-differentiated NETs are slow-growing, so that in nonfunctioning tumors symptoms may be determined by the presence of local invasion and metastases. For most NETs, patients are younger than those with pancreatic adenocarcinoma (median age 53 years), with a better prognosis (up to 6 years median survival for metastatic NET and carcinoid). The initial site of metastatic disease is usually the liver, followed by lung and bone.

Large islet cell tumors are readily diagnosed by CT, MRI, and ultrasound. Localization of small functioning lesions can be difficult. Thin-slice contrast-enhanced CT of the pancreas and endoscopic ultrasound have been used very successfully to identify small lesions, which appear as densely enhancing masses. Radiolabeled octreotide scans are useful to predict clinical response to somatostatin analogs and detect metastatic disease. Intraoperative ultrasound is also used to confirm the presence of a lesion before

Box 11-8. Localization of Pancreatic Gastrinomas, Insulinomas, and Nesidioblastosis with Stimulation

5-French catheter in right hepatic vein, multi-sidehole
Arteries to be selected
- Distal splenic
- Proximal splenic
- Dorsal pancreatic*
- Gastroduodenal
- Superior mesenteric artery
- Inferior pancreaticoduodenal*
- Proper hepatic (gastrinoma and insulinoma)

Angiogram in each position
Inject 1 mL 10% calcium gluconate (0.025 mEq/kg for nesidioblastosis) each location
Hepatic venous sampling
- 30 seconds before calcium injection
- 0, 30, 60, 90, 120, 190 seconds after

At least 5-minute intervals between calcium injections

*Optional depending on patient anatomy.

resection. Islet cell tumors are usually hypervascular masses, but angiography is rarely required to localize lesions (Fig. 11-29).

Occult functioning islet cell tumors (insulinoma and gastrinoma) can be localized by sampling of the hepatic veins following selective arterial injections of a secretagogue (Box 11-8 and Fig 11-30). A rise in the hepatic vein concentration of gastrin or insulin helps localize angiographically occult lesions. A proper hepatic angiogram and stimulation is performed to exclude the presence of hepatic metastases.

Pancreatic nesidioblastosis (pancreatic β-cell hypertrophy without a focal mass) is a rare complication of roux-en-Y gastric bypass for weight loss. The etiology is unknown, but patients present with symptomatic postprandial hypoglycemia rather than when fasting as in patients with insulinoma. Dietary modification, reversal of the bypass surgery, or partial or total pancreatectomy are potential treatments. Before pancreatectomy, nesidioblastosis can be localized by arterial injection of calcium gluconate, followed by hepatic venous sampling for insulin.

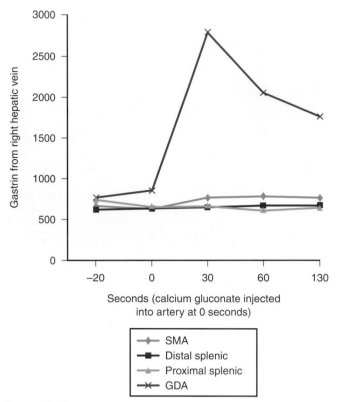

FIGURE 11-30. Graph of gastrin samples from the right hepatic vein following selective calcium gluconate arterial stimulation in a patient with Zollinger Ellison syndrome. A pancreatic mass could not be identified with cross-sectional imaging or angiography. The mass was localized to the gastroduodenal artery (GDA) injection, and at surgery a 0.5 cm gastrinoma was found in the wall of the duodenum. SMA, Superior mesenteric artery. Gastrin levels are in pg/mL.

Hepatic Neoplasms

Imaging

Routine diagnostic imaging of malignant and benign masses of the liver is performed with CT, MRI, positron emission tomography (PET) CT, and to a lesser extent ultrasound. Contrast-enhanced CT and MRI in at least three phases (noncontrast, arterial perfusion, portal venous phase) is preferred. The pattern of enhancement as well as the morphologic features of a lesion can suggest the identity of the mass. Extrahepatic metastases, the presence of portal hypertension, portal vein patency, and other findings that could alter therapy may be detected.

The role of conventional angiography in the diagnosis of hepatic masses is very limited, but interventionalists must be able to differentiate lesions because embolization has a major role in treatment (Table 11-7). Angiography is occasionally required to resolve a diagnostic dilemma. In addition to celiac, common or proper hepatic, and SMA injections through regular-sized catheters, selective and subselective injections of hepatic arterial branches through a high-flow microcatheter may be necessary to identify and characterize lesions. Patients who will undergo yttrium-90 radioembolization of liver tumors require careful investigation of the hepatic arterial blood supply, as well as identification of the cystic, right gastric, gastroduodenal, and replaced hepatic arteries.

The majority of liver tumors have hepatic arterial blood supply, but not all tumors are hypervascular. Vascular lesions may exhibit neovascularity, staining, shunting, and mass effect (Fig. 11-31). Arteriovenous shunting to the portal or hepatic veins, or the presence of tumor thrombus in the portal or hepatic veins, is highly suggestive of hepatoma (see Fig. 1-27**B**). Hypovascular lesions

TABLE 11-7 Angiographic Appearance of Malignant Liver Masses

Tumor	Vascularity	Angiographic Findings
Hepatoma	Vascular	Solitary or multifocal; neovascularity, parenchymal stain, arteriovenous shunting; hepatic and portal thrombus
Cholangiocarcinoma	Avascular	Venous and arterial encasement in porta hepatis
Metastatic adenocarcinoma (e.g., colon, pancreas, lung)	Avascular	Usually multiple; hypovascular area in parenchymal phase of angiogram; mass effect on adjacent blood vessels with large lesions; may have faint hypervascular rim with avascular center
Metastatic neuroendocrine tumors, ocular melanoma, renal cell carcinoma, sarcoma	Vascular	Multiple lesions; variable hypervascularity, parenchymal stain; arteriovenous shunting unusual; portal and hepatic venous thrombus rare

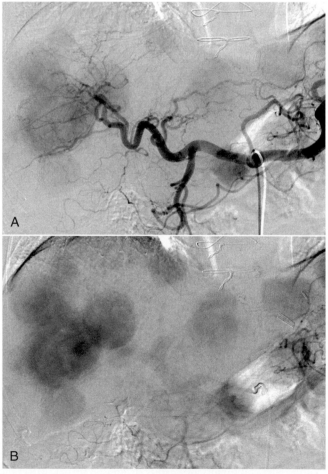

FIGURE 11-31. Angiographic appearance of hypervascular liver malignancy, in this case metastatic small bowel carcinoid tumor. **A,** Image from the arterial phase celiac artery angiogram of the same patient as in Figure 11-28 showing multiple hypervascular masses in the liver. **B,** Portal phase image showing persistent densely enhancing masses.

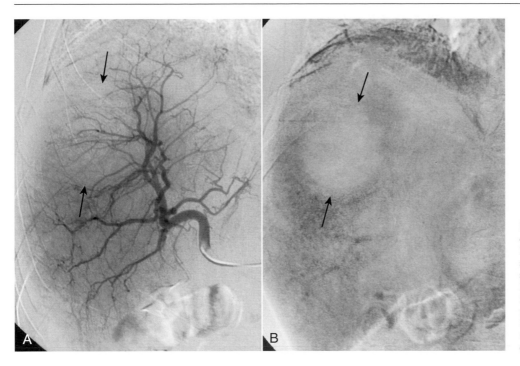

FIGURE 11-32. Angiographic appearance of a hypovascular malignant lesion in the liver. **A,** Metastatic colon carcinoma: selective right hepatic digital subtraction angiogram showing an area of hypovascularity *(arrows)* with splaying of surrounding vessels. **B,** Parenchymal phase from the same injection shows the hypovascular metastasis *(arrows)* with slight surrounding hyperemia believed to represent compressed normal liver tissue.

TABLE 11-8 Hepatoma

Average age	50-60 years
Male-to-female	3:1
Single lesion	50%
More than 5 lesions	10%-20%
One lesion > 5 cm	30%-50%
Portal vein thrombosis	30%
Distant metastases at time of diagnosis	10%

Box 11-9. Risk Factors for Hepatoma

Hepatitis B, chronic
Hepatitis C, chronic
Alcoholic cirrhosis
Nonalcoholic fatty liver disease
Hereditary hemochromatosis
α_1-antitrypsin deficiency
Autoimmune hepatitis
Porphyria
Wilson disease

TABLE 11-9 Eastern Cooperative Oncology Group Performance Scale

Performance Status	Definition
0	Fully active; no performance restrictions
1	Strenuous physical activity restricted; fully ambulatory and able to carry out light work
2	Capable of all self-care but unable to carry out any work activities. Up and about >50% of waking hours
3	Capable of only limited self-care; confined to bed or chair >50% of waking hours
4	Completely disabled; cannot carry out any self-care; totally confined to bed or chair

Adapted from Oken MM, Creech RH, Tormey DC, et al. Toxicity and response criteria of the Eastern Cooperative Oncology Group. *Am J Clin Oncol.* 1982;5: 649-655.

can cause mass effect on adjacent vascular structures, defects in the parenchymal phase of the angiogram, or vascular encasement (Fig. 11-32).

Hepatoma

Primary liver tumors (hepatoma) are the ninth most common cause of cancer death in the United States (Table 11-8). In many parts of the world, particularly Asian countries, hepatoma is the predominant hepatic malignancy. The major risk factor for hepatoma is chronic liver disease (Box 11-9). One subtype, fibrolamellar hepatoma, occurs in younger patients with no apparent risk factors. Tumors less than 20 mm in diameter have variable vascularity, but most larger than this are usually hypervascular in the

arterial phases of all contrast imaging modalities with "wash-out" during venous phase in cross-sectional imaging. When characteristic imaging findings are present, particularly on two different imaging modalities, then biopsy is not necessary for the diagnosis. Hepatoma is usually asymptomatic until very large, when it can cause pain, a palpable mass, or obstructive jaundice. Acute intraperitoneal rupture and hemorrhage occurs in 2%-3% of cases, usually in the setting of a subcapsular or exophytic lesion. Serum α-fetoprotein (AFP) is elevated in only 40% of patients with small hepatomas, so a normal level does not exclude hepatoma. Extremely high levels of serum AFP strongly suggests vascular invasion by tumor. There are several staging systems for overall performance status, hepatic reserve, disease burden, and prognosis (Tables 11-9 through 11-13). The MELD score, developed for patients undergoing transjugular intrahepatic portosystemic shunts (TIPS), is also used when describing patients with hepatoma (see Chapter 14).

The best treatment for hepatoma is liver transplantation, but fewer than 5% of patients qualify (single tumor no more than

TABLE 11-10 Child-Turcotte-Pugh Classification of Severity of Liver Disease in Cirrhosis

Variable	Points		
	1	2	3
Encephalopathy (grade)	0	I-II	III-IV
Ascites	None	Mild	Moderate
Bilirubin (mg/mL)*	<2	2-3	>3
Albumin (g/dL)	>3.5	2.8-3.5	<2.8
International normalized ratio	<1.7	1.7-2.3	>2.3

Score obtained by adding up the total points:
5-6 = Class A (well-preserved liver function, 95% 1-year survival).
7-9 = Class B (significant functional compromise, 80% 1-year survival).
10-15 = Class C (decompensated, 45% 1-year survival).
*Bilirubin points and values in patients with primary biliary cirrhosis: 1 = 1-4 mg/dL; 2 = 5-10 mg/dL; 3 = >10 mg/dL.

TABLE 11-11 Cancer of the Liver Program Score for Hepatoma

	Score		
	0	1	2
Child-Pugh stage	A	B	C
Tumor morphology	Uninodular and ≤ 50% total liver	Multinodular and ≤ 50% total liver	Massive, >50% total liver
α-Fetoprotein (ng/mL)	<400	≥400	
Portal vein thrombosis	No	Yes	

Early stage: 0 points, median survival 36 months.
Intermediate stage: 1 point, median survival 22 months; 2 points, median survival 9 months; 3 points, median survival 7 months.
Advanced stage: 4-6 points, median survival 3 months.
Adapted from Grieco A, Pompili M, Caminiti G, et al. Prognostic factors for survival in patients with early-intermediate hepatocellular carcinoma undergoing non-surgical therapy: comparison of Okuda, CLIP, and BCLC staging systems in a single Italian centre. *Gut.* 2005;54:411-418.

TABLE 11-12 Okuda Staging of Hepatoma

Criteria	Points	
	0	1
Tumor size	<50% of liver	>50% of liver
Ascites	No	Yes
Albumin (g/dL)	≥3	<3
Bilirubin (mg/dL)	<3	≥3

Okuda stage I: 0 points, 1-year survival 68%.
Okuda stage II: 1 or 2 points, 1-year survival 36%.
Okuda stage III: 3 or 4 points, 1-year survival 21%.
Adapted from Grieco A, Pompili M, Caminiti G, et al. Prognostic factors for survival in patients with early-intermediate hepatocellular carcinoma undergoing non-surgical therapy: comparison of Okuda, CLIP, and BCLC staging systems in a single Italian centre. *Gut.* 2005;54:411-418.

5 cm in diameter, or up to 3 tumors all less than 3 cm in diameter, no vascular invasion, no distant metastases). The recurrence rate after liver transplantation is 10%-15% over the lifetime of the patient. Resection of liver tumor (usually at least a segmentectomy, often more) is feasible in about 5% of patients with small, strategically located lesions without evidence of vascular invasion or distant metastases. After resection, the recurrence rate is 50% within 3 years, which is not surprising in that the entire liver is usually abnormal in these patients and at risk of developing hepatoma. Percutaneous ablation techniques are often used alone or in combination with other treatments; these are described in Chapter 25.

Transcatheter embolization with bland (TAE), chemotherapeutic (TACE), drug-eluting beads (DEBs), or Y-90 loaded microspheres are techniques for providing local control of liver tumors. There are few randomized prospective studies comparing the different embolization techniques, with local expertise and experience often determining which can be offered to a patient. In general, transcatheter therapies increase survival by approximately 50% compared to conservative management. This result further improved when combined with radiofrequency or other ablative technologies, especially when treating a focal lesion. Transcatheter therapies can be used to control disease while a patient is undergoing evaluation of transplant (the "bridge to transplant").

Sorafenib, a kinase inhibitor, was the first oral agent shown to improve survival in patients with diffuse hepatoma and preserved liver function. Survival increases by 2-3 months. Side effects including rash, gastrointestinal symptoms, and hand-foot-and-mouth disease occur in one third of patients.

Although the diagnostic role of angiography in hepatic malignancy is limited, the therapeutic potential is great. Most hepatomas derive the majority of their blood supply from the hepatic arteries. The dual nature of the hepatic blood supply allows arterial embolization to be performed safely. Furthermore, the direct delivery of antitumoral agents into the hepatic artery achieves a higher local tumor dose than could be administered peripherally.

Patients referred for transarterial therapy should be evaluated for liver function (including coagulation studies), patency of the portal vein, portal hypertension, the presence of biliary obstruction, or malignant ascites. There are no absolute guidelines for patient selection, but generally these include a Child-Pugh score of A or B, total bilirubin less than 2 mg/dL, absence of extrahepatic metastases, less than 50% replacement of the liver by tumor, good overall functional status, a lesion or lesions that are not amenable to surgical resection/transplant/percutaneous ablation, and a life expectancy of more than 6 months. Hepatic failure or the

presence of active liver infection is an absolute contraindication, because damage to some normal hepatic tissue is inevitable. Patients with indwelling biliary tubes, biliary obstruction, or biliary to enteric anastomoses are at increased risk for postembolization liver abscess and should receive 5-7 days of antibiotics before the procedure and 7-10 days of antibiotics afterward. Without antibiotics, the risk for infection is almost 25%. A drug with appropriate activity and bile excretion should be used. Occlusion of the portal vein by tumor or tumor thrombus is not a contraindication, but there is a risk of liver infarction with generalized lobar embolization. These patients can undergo selective embolization with an agent that will not be shunted into the vein, often demonstrating regression of the tumor thrombus. At the time of the procedure, all patients should receive antibiotics (Gram-negative coverage), steroids, and antiemetics.

Bland Embolization

Embolization with small (50-150 μ) permanent particles, such as polyvinyl alcohol without the addition of chemotherapeutic agents results in ischemia and infarction of tumor tissue. This can be an effective means of controlling hemorrhage from a ruptured hepatoma, but in most practices one of the following techniques is used for elective cases.

TABLE 11-13 Barcelona Clinic Liver Cancer Staging of Hepatoma

| BCLC Stage | PST* | Tumor Status | | Liver Function Status‡ |
		Tumor Stage	Okuda Stage†	
Stage A: early HCC	0			
A1	0	Single, <5 cm	I	No portal hypertension and normal bilirubin
A2	0	Single, <5 cm	I	Portal hypertension and normal bilirubin
A3	0	Single, <5 cm	I	Portal hypertension and abnormal bilirubin
A4	0	3 tumors <3 cm	I-II	Child-Pugh A-B
Stage B: intermediate HCC	0	Large multinodular	I-II	Child-Pugh A-B
Stage C: advanced HCC	1-2	Vascular invasion or extrahepatic spread	I-II	Child-Pugh A-B
Stage D: end-stage HCC	3-4	Any	III	Child-Pugh C

Stages A and B: All criteria should be fulfilled.
Stage C: At least one of the following: PST 1-2 or vascular invasion/extrahepatic spread.
Stage D: At least one of the following: PST 3-4, Okuda stage III, Child-Pugh C.
HCC, Hepatocellular carcinoma.
*PST, performance status: see Table 11-9
†Okuda stage, see Table 11-12.
‡Child-Pugh, see Table 11-10.
Adapted from Grieco A, Pompili M, Caminiti G, et al. Prognostic factors for survival in patients with early-intermediate hepatocellular carcinoma undergoing non-surgical therapy: comparison of Okuda, CLIP, and BCLC staging systems in a single Italian centre. *Gut.* 2005;54:411-418.

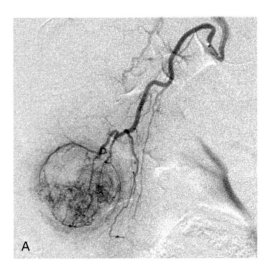
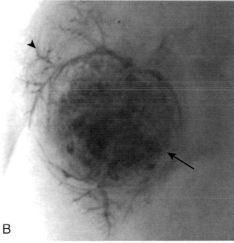

FIGURE 11-33. Chemoembolization of a right lobe hepatoma with iodized oil and doxorubicin. **A,** Selective angiogram through a microcatheter in the artery feeding the tumor. **B,** Digital spot image after embolization showing retained oil in the tumor *(arrow)* and shunting into the adjacent portal branches *(arrowhead),* an angiographic endpoint for the procedure.

Chemoembolization

Chemoembolization (TACE) is a widely available transarterial treatment for hepatoma. This usually involves injecting an emulsion of one or more chemotherapeutic drugs and iodized oil (see Chapter 4, Lipiodol) directly into the hepatic artery (Fig. 11-33). The mixture accumulates in and is retained by the hepatoma, which appears as a dense, persistent stain during the procedure and on subsequent x-ray imaging studies (see Fig. 4-47). The normal hepatocytes metabolize the lipiodol, so that liver tissue is preserved.

The drug is delivered as close to the tumor as possible (see Fig. 11-33). This often requires the use of a microcatheter, typically one that is high flow. Routine use of microcatheters reduces spasm during the procedure (which limits delivery of the drug) and dissection. With multifocal disease, or scattered small tumors, lobar embolization is used. One liver lobe at a time, rather than the whole liver, is embolized. Occasionally a single feeding artery is present to the tumor, in which case the entire dose can be delivered to a very limited area. In patients with abnormal liver function, selective embolization decreases the risk of subsequent liver failure.

There is tremendous variation between individuals, hospitals, and even countries in the details of how this procedure is performed. Catheter preferences, drugs used, drug ratios, amount of oil added, particulate or Gelfoam embolization during or after the delivery of the chemoembolic mixture, and procedural endpoints are greatly diverse. The optimal regimen has not been determined. At the Dotter Institute, hepatoma is treated with doxorubicin (50 mg) mixed in 7 mL of nonionic contrast and emulsified with 5-10 mL of iodized oil (more oil for more vascular or larger tumors), usually without particulate agents. A triple drug regimen of doxorubicin, mitomycin-C, and cisplatin is used in many centers.

Patients are usually admitted overnight for intravenous hydration, control of nausea, and pain medication. Some upper abdominal discomfort is normal, which should resolve in a few days. Severe abdominal pain or pain that persists longer than expected may indicate a complication such as chemical/ischemic cholecystitis, cholangitis, tumor rupture, or liver infarction. Patients are discharged with pain medication, antiemetics, and instructions to call if high temperature, dark urine, yellow eyes, or abdominal swelling occurs. Antibiotics are not routinely prescribed in our

TABLE 11-14 Complications of Chemoembolization

Specific Major Complication	Reported Rate (%)
Liver failure	2.3
Abscess with functional sphincter of Oddi	<1
Abscess with biliary-enteric anastomosis/ biliary stent/sphincterotomy	25
Postembolization syndrome requiring extended stay or readmission	4.6
Surgical cholecystitis	<1
Biloma requiring percutaneous drainage	<1
Pulmonary arterial oil embolus	<1
Gastrointestinal hemorrhage/ulceration	<1
Iatrogenic dissection preventing treatment	<1
Death within 30 days	1

Adapted from Brown DB, Cardella JF, Sacks D, et al. Quality improvement guidelines for transhepatic arterial chemoembolization, embolization, and chemotherapeutic infusion for hepatic malignancy. *J Vasc Interv Radiol*. 2006;17(2 Pt 1):225-232.

practice but are sometimes used in others. Liver function tests will be deranged for 7-10 days after the procedure (we do not usually check them unless we suspect that the patient is having a problem). Postembolization syndrome (low-grade fevers, fatigue, nausea) superimposed upon systemic effects of the chemotherapeutic agent are common but usually well tolerated by the informed patient. A scheduled visit in an outpatient office at 2 weeks allows assessment of recovery and planning for the next treatment.

Patients with multiple tumors or large lesions should undergo repeated embolizations. When lobar embolizations are performed, alternating lobes every 4-6 weeks (usually two treatments on the larger right lobe, one on the smaller left) allows adequate time for recovery of the normal hepatocytes. Lesions are followed by contrast-enhanced CT or MRI, with absence of enhancement and decreasing size being indicators of satisfactory embolization. Accumulated lipiodol in hepatoma is extremely dense on CT scan, and can been easily misinterpreted as a calcified lesion by someone unfamiliar with the patient's history (see Fig. 4-47B). Imaging is obtained as a matter of course after 3 embolizations, or whenever a treatment endpoint appears to have been reached. Patients who have stable disease can undergo surveillance imaging every 3 months for 2 years, followed by every 6 months until active disease is again detected.

Fulminant hepatic failure occurs in fewer than 1% of patients undergoing chemoembolization (Table 11-14). However, this complication can be lethal. Risk factors for liver failure include a total bilirubin higher than 2 mg/dL, tumor that replaces more than 50% of the liver, presence of a TIPS, and portal vein occlusion without vigorous cavernous transformation. Selective TACE can be performed in the presence of a TIPS when liver function is preserved, but the overall prognosis is worse than that for either TIPS or TACE alone. In the absence of biliary obstruction, biliary-enteric anastomoses, and indwelling biliary stents or catheters, the risk for infection is about 1%. Chemical or ischemic cholecystitis due to chemoembolization is rare (also less than 1%) and usually managed expectantly. Late biliary ductal dilatation without obstruction can be seen in some patients.

Long-term outcomes of TACE, as reported in the literature, encompass a wide range of disease burdens, patient comorbidities, and variations in technique. TACE does not cure hepatoma. Ultimately, patients develop and die of recurrent or new lesions, liver insufficiency, and sometimes extrahepatic disease.

Drug-Eluting Beads

Microspheres that can be loaded or coated with chemotherapeutic agents may provide more controlled delivery of drugs to the liver than conventional TACE (see Chapter 4). There are a number of different types of beads available, with different affinities and elution rates for the various chemotherapeutic agents. The precise dose of chemotherapy released by the beads remains difficult to predict. The general indications for DEBs are the same as for TACE, but are expanded to include patients with vigorously shunting tumors or invasion of the portal or hepatic veins. Selection of the DEB size and quantity depends on the vascularity of the tumor and the desired level of occlusion. In the PRECISION V trial, two vials loaded with a total of 150 mg of doxorubicin (75 mg each) were used. The bead size first vial delivered was 300-500 μ, and in the second 500-700 μ. Single vial treatments and lower doses of doxorubicin can be used for more focal, less vascular lesions. The DEBs are mixed with aqueous contrast, which allows controlled delivery similar to TACE although focal accumulation of contrast in the tumor, as with iodized oil, does not occur.

Delivery of DEBs follows the same principles as TACE. Lobar or selective treatment is preferred to whole liver embolization. Beads are delivered until the entire dose has been administered or flow becomes sluggish. Slow delivery of dilute concentrations of beads, and smaller sizes such as 100-300 micron diameter, are thought to improve penetration into the tumor and avoid premature termination of the procedure due to early stasis from clumping in larger vessels. The management of patients after embolization with DEBs is similar to that of TACE patients, with pain and nausea control, hydration, and antibiotics when biliary prostheses or enteric anastomoses are present. Major complication rates are similar to TACE. Follow-up CT shows hypovascular lesions without accumulation of contrast as with iodized oil (Fig. 11-34).

Experience with DEBs in hepatoma is very promising. The results of the PRECISION V trial comparing doxorubicin-loaded DEBs with doxorubicin TACE plus Gelfoam showed a trend toward improved tumor response rates with lower complication rates. The cost of DEBs is higher than inert spheres or lipiodol but far less than Y-90–loaded spheres.

Yttrium-90 Radioembolization

Embolization with radioactive embolic materials (usually Y-90–impregnated beads) is an alternative to TACE for primary and metastatic liver tumors (see Chapter 4). Operators in the United States must have U.S. Nuclear Regulatory Commission Authorized User status in order to deliver this agent. Most patients who can undergo TACE can also potentially undergo radioembolization. Portal and hepatic vein invasion are not considered a contraindication to radioembolization provided that the shunt fraction is acceptable (see below). Patient selection depends on anatomic, logistical, and cost factors. Because of the highly radioactive nature of the embolic material, the method of delivery is very different than for TACE. The embolic material must be ordered from an outside supplier for each patient and must be contained in specialized shielded containers during delivery. Radioactive spheres are not radiopaque and should not be mixed with contrast or lipiodol. This makes visualization of the progress of embolization procedure difficult. Usually, with glass spheres the entire dose is delivered without interruption because the embolic load is low. With resin spheres, intermittent injection of contrast is necessary because the embolic load is high and stasis or even reflux can occur before the entire dose is delivered. The spheres must be carefully flushed through the catheter before contrast can be injected. Repositioning of catheters during dose delivery is discouraged due to the risk of operator exposure from residual activity in the catheters and contamination of the field.

The most important anatomic information for determining candidacy for radioembolization is the arterial blood supply to the tumor and the degree of shunting through the tumor into the portal or systemic veins. Careful planning angiography is necessary

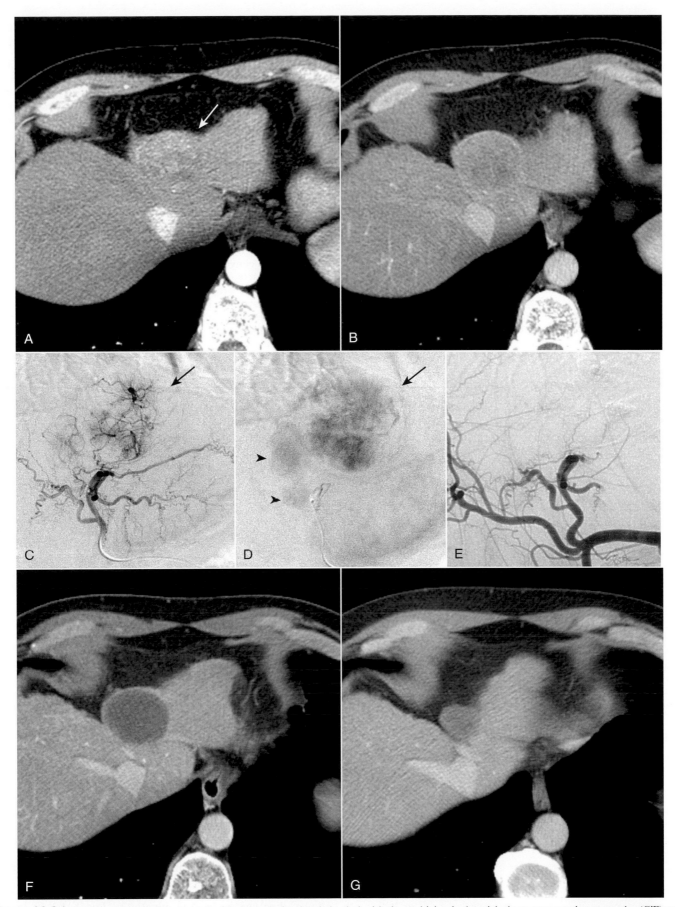

FIGURE 11-34. Segment 4 hepatoma treated with drug-eluting beads loaded with doxorubicin. **A,** Arterial phase computed tomography (CT) scan showing the enhancing exophytic lesion *(arrow)*. **B,** Portal phase image from the same study showing classic tumor washout and a hypervascular rim. **C,** Left hepatic angiogram showing hypervascularity and neovascularity of the hepatoma *(arrow)*. **D,** Later phase image from the same injection showing the persistent tumor staining *(arrow)*. Two satellite lesions are also seen *(arrowheads)*. **E,** Celiac angiogram following selective embolization of the left hepatic artery with drug-eluting beads. The tumor is no longer visible, and there is diminished perfusion of the left lobe relative to the right. **F,** Portal phase CT scan 1 month later shows lack of enhancement. **G,** Portal phase CT scan 3 years later shows contraction of the embolized tumor. There was no measured enhancement.

to understand the hepatic arterial anatomy. At the same time a test dose of Tc-99 macroaggregated albumin (MAA) is delivered into the hepatic artery at the likely site of Y-90 embolization. The Tc-99 MAA is theoretically the same size as the Y-90 spheres and simulates their distribution. Soon after injection of the Tc-99 MAA, the patient undergoes gamma camera scanning of the chest and abdomen to determine the shunt fraction to the lungs and/or portal system. A pulmonary shunt fraction that would result in a dose of greater than or equal to 30 Gy in a single treatment (50 Gy cumulative) or uncorrectable vascular anatomy that would allow nontarget organ exposure are usually contraindications to radioembolization because of the risk of radiation pneumonitis or gastrointestinal ulceration. The need for planning angiography and the nuclear medicine evaluation are unique to radioembolization.

During planning angiography, selective injections of the SMA, celiac artery, left gastric artery, right hepatic, and left hepatic artery are performed (see Figs. 11-4 and 11-5). The cystic, right gastric, gastroduodenal, and any anomalous branches to the stomach, intestine, or diaphragm should be identified. Depending on the type of sphere used and the intended site of delivery of the Y-90, coil embolization of these branches may be necessary. More aggressive embolization is recommended when using the resin spheres because the number of particles infused is very high and the risk of reflux greater. Glass spheres are loaded with a higher activity of Y-90, so that the total number of particles infused is much lower, resulting in less risk of nontarget organ embolization. Coil occlusion of the cystic artery is usually well tolerated because there are numerous small collaterals to the gallbladder through the liver parenchyma forming the gallbladder fossa.

The treatment schedule is similar to that for TACE, in that lobar or even segmental embolization is performed rather than whole-liver radioembolization. When using glass spheres the target dose for each lobe is 100-120 Gy based on CT-based liver volume calculations. Dosing with resin spheres is based on body surface area estimates. With vascular tumors, the actual dose may be much higher in the lesion than in the normal liver parenchyma. Patients can undergo multiple treatments of the same lobe as long as the maximum cumulative dose or lung shunt are not exceeded.

There are fewer systemic side effects of radioembolization than for TACE (Table 11-15). Patients are usually discharged to home the same day of the procedure. Use of arterial closure devices facilitates early discharge. Close contact with small children and pregnant women should be avoided for several days. Patients commonly report fatigue for a few weeks but little else in the way of postembolization syndrome. As of yet, there are no randomized prospective comparisons with conventional TACE. Limitations of Y-90 radioembolization include the overall expense of the spheres and nuclear medicine evaluation, and the need for preparatory coil embolization of gastrointestinal branches.

Colon Metastases

The most common hepatic malignancy in the United States is metastatic colon cancer. There are approximately 150,000 new

TABLE 11-15 Complications of Y-90 Radioembolization for Hepatoma

Radiation hepatitis	0%-4%
Cholecystitis	1%
Gastrointestinal ulceration	<5%
Postembolization syndrome requiring extended stay or readmission	<1%
Pain, fatigue, nausea	20%
Biliary (focal dilation, biloma)	10%

cases each year. Almost 10% of all cancer deaths in this country are due to metastatic adenocarcinoma of the colon. Hepatic metastatic disease eventually occurs in up to 75% of patients with colorectal cancer, with 20% present at the time of initial diagnosis. Unlike hepatoma patients, underlying liver disease is usually absent. Also unlike hepatoma, systemic chemotherapy is effective and is usually the initial treatment. Intraarterial infusion through implanted hepatic arterial catheters is an alternative to intravenous therapy. Hepatic resection is performed when disease is limited to one hepatic lobe and adequate hepatic reserve is present. In some patients, presurgical embolization of the portal vein in the liver segments to be resected is performed to induce hypertrophy of anticipated future liver remnant (see Chapter 14). Percutaneous ablation of hepatic metastases is described in Chapter 25.

Transarterial liver directed therapies are considered when patients fail conventional systemic therapy. These include TACE, DEBs, and Y-90 radioembolization. Angiographically, colon metastases are much less vascular than hepatoma and metastatic neuroendocrine tumors (compare Figs. 11-31 through 11-33). The indications, contraindications, and technical details of delivery of each embolic agent are similar to those described for hepatoma. Although chronic liver disease is usually absent at the time of initial diagnosis, multiple rounds of chemotherapy can limit hepatic reserve. Extrahepatic disease is not a contraindication to liver-directed therapy when the liver tumor burden dominates the clinical outcome. When performing TACE, a three-drug regimen is preferred (cisplatinum, 100 mg; mitomycin C, 30 mg; and doxorubicin, 30 mg). There is frequently less oil uptake in colon metastases than with hepatoma. Drug-eluting beads are usually loaded with 25 mg of irinotecan; the size most commonly used is 100-300 microns. The Y-90 dosing is the same as for hepatoma, as are the pretreatment diagnostic angiography and shunt calculation withTc-99 MAA. Protective embolization of visceral branches is required before Y-90 embolization. With all of these therapies the embolic endpoint of sluggish flow or stasis is arrived at sooner than in treatment for hepatoma.

The results of transarterial liver-directed therapy for metastatic colon cancer in patients who have failed two different lines of conventional chemotherapy are promising, with doubling of 2-year survival over patients who continue systemic therapies. The postprocedure complication rates are similar to when the procedure is performed for hepatoma. Randomized comparisons of TACE, DEBs, and Y-90 are lacking.

Neuroendocrine Metastases

Metastatic neuroendocrine tumors represent approximately 10% of all hepatic metastatic disease, and occur in more than 50% of patients with neuroendocrine tumors. Patients often eventually succumb to their liver disease. At angiography the lesions are usually hypervascular and can be quite bulky (see Fig. 11-31). A miliary pattern can also be seen. The relatively indolent nature of these tumors compared to hepatoma and other metastatic disease and the typical absence of chronic liver disease permits aggressive therapy. Surgical resection of isolated or limited hepatic metastases or debulking improves survival in selected patients. Liver transplantation has been described in highly selected patients. Systemic therapy with somatostatin analogs (octreotide or lanreotide) or sunitinib and everolimus (kinase inhibitors) increases survival in patients with disseminated disease.

Patients with progressive liver disease despite systemic therapy may benefit from liver directed therapies. Bland embolization, TACE, DEBs, and Y-90 radioembolization have all been employed to control hepatic metastases. For TACE, a three-drug regimen is preferred (cisplatinum [100 mg], mitomycin C [30mg], and doxorubicin [30mg]). Drug eluting beads are usually loaded with doxorubicin; the size most commonly used is 100-300 microns. The Y-90 dosing and treatment are the same as for hepatoma and colorectal carcinoma metastases. Protective embolization of selected visceral branches is also required prior to Y-90 embolization, but the hypervascular nature of neuroendocrine metastases decreases the risk of reflux of radioactive beads.

All patients with neuroendocrine tumors should receive 500 μg of octreotide either subcutaneously or intravenously at least 20 minutes before undergoing angiography or embolization. Patients with a history of carcinoid crisis can be managed with an octreotide drip started the night before the procedure and continued for 12-24 hours after embolization. The dosage is titrated to prevent carcinoid symptoms but patients must be on telemetry because bradycardia can occur. The dosing range is usually 100-200 μg/hr, but can be higher for severe symptoms.

Other Metastatic Tumors

Breast, ovarian, sarcomas, and other hepatic metastases can all be treated with liver-directed therapies when conventional treatments have failed. The specific therapeutic modality will vary by tumor, patient clinical status, and availability.

Primary ocular melanoma is a rare disease (5-6 cases/million), with a 50% 10-year survival. Death is usually due to metastatic disease to the liver, but also the lung and brain, often within a year of detection of metastatic disease if untreated. There are no effective systemic therapies for metastatic uveal melanoma. Liver-directed therapy for these patients appears to improve survival and includes TACE, immunoembolization, radioembolization, and isolated hepatic perfusion with melphalan.

Cholangiocarcinoma

The incidence of cholangiocarcinoma is approximately 10-20 million in the United States, with patients with primary sclerosing cholangitis at highest risk. The overall 5-year survival is about 5%. Surgical resection is feasible when the tumor is localized or, when intrahepatic, confined to one side of the liver. Liver transplantation has been reported in select patients. Transarterial liver-directed therapy with TACE (gemcitabine and cisplatin) and DEBs (doxorubicin), as well as Y-90 radioembolization have been used to treat patients with unresectable disease. These patients require antibiotic coverage before (5-7 days) and after (1-2 weeks) embolization because they often have indwelling biliary tubes and are at increased risk for liver abscess. Modest survival benefits are reported with liver-directed therapy of cholangiocarcinoma.

Benign Tumors

A wide range of benign lesions are found in the liver (Box 11-10). As with malignant liver lesions, CT, MRI, and ultrasound are usually diagnostic. Several lesions have characteristic angiographic appearances, but this modality is rarely necessary for diagnosis.

Hepatic cysts are present in at least 5% of individuals. Usually asymptomatic, they are avascular at angiography but may cause displacement of arterial and venous structures.

Hemangiomas are found in 7%-20% of the adult population, more often in women than men, with a predilection for the right lobe of the liver. Hemangiomas can vary in size and number, with those larger than 5 cm considered "giant." These lesions are comprised of large blood-filled spaces with little stromal tissue. Asymptomatic in the majority of patients, large hemangiomas can bleed spontaneously (reportedly up to 2%), cause mass effect, or lead to consumptive coagulopathy (Kasabach-Merritt syndrome). The angiographic appearance of hepatic hemangiomas is perhaps the most distinctive of all hepatic lesions: normal feeding arteries, with early pooling of contrast that increases and persists with time ("comes early and stays late") (Fig. 11-35). TACE (Lipiodol and 16-24 mg bleomycin) of symptomatic giant lesions is an alternative to surgical resection

Infantile hemangioendothelioma, though rare, is the most common benign hepatic tumor in infants. More frequent in females, patients present with hepatomegaly and high-output congestive heart failure in up to two-thirds of cases. The lesions are histologically benign; biopsy is not necessary unless the first appearance is after 1 year of age or atypical on imaging studies. Although lesions respond to steroids and alpha-interferon, embolization or surgical resection may be required. At angiography, recruitment of collateral arterial supply from phrenic, intercostal, abdominal wall, splenic, superior mesenteric, and renal arteries may be found (Fig. 11-36). Embolization with Gelfoam pledgets or

---

***Box 11-10.* Benign Liver Masses**

Simple cyst
Hemangioma
Adenoma (considered premalignant)
Focal nodular hyperplasia
Regenerating nodule
Abscess

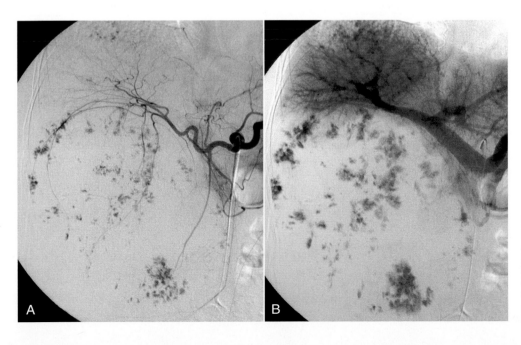

FIGURE 11-35. Giant hepatic cavernous hemangioma in a middle-aged woman. **A,** Celiac digital subtraction angiogram showing a large liver mass with absence of neovascularity but multiple areas of fluffy staining. **B,** Image from the portal phase showing progressive increase in enhancement ("comes early, stays late") pathognomonic of cavernous hemangiomas.

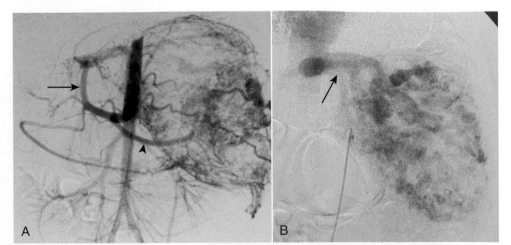

FIGURE 11-36. Infantile hepatic hemangioendothelioma causing high-output congestive heart failure in a week-old female. **A,** Digital subtraction angiogram aortogram showing a large shunting hypervascular mass supplied by the left hepatic artery *(arrow)*, splenic artery *(arrowhead)*, as well as numerous other collaterals. **B,** Later image from the same injection shows drainage through the left hepatic vein *(arrow)*.

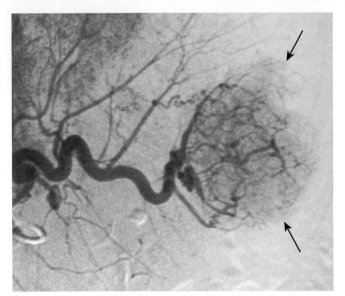

FIGURE 11-37. Hepatic digital subtraction angiogram of proven hepatic adenoma *(arrows)* in the left lobe of the liver in a woman taking birth control pills. There is neovascularity and parenchymal staining of a well circumscribed lesion.

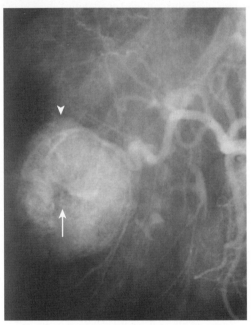

FIGURE 11-38. Hepatic angiogram of proven focal nodular hyperplasia *(arrowhead)* showing the characteristic central scar *(arrow)*.

cyanoacrylate glue is frequently curative. Small particles should be avoided owing to the risk of shunting through the mass.

Hepatic adenomas are well-circumscribed encapsulated masses comprised of hepatocytes. These lesions are found in women of childbearing age, and are associated with oral contraceptive use (3/1,000,000 women on contraceptives). Spontaneous rupture with intraperitoneal bleeding can occur, particularly during pregnancy. It has been estimated that up to 40% of patients experience symptomatic bleeding from hepatic adenomas (especially those with large lesions), with a 20% mortality if intraperitoneal rupture occurs. The risk of malignant transformation may be as high as 10%-15%. The angiographic findings are a sharply defined hypervascular mass with enlarged feeding vessels (Fig. 11-37). This angiographic appearance is not unique, and hepatoma should be considered in the differential diagnosis. The usual treatment is surgical resection because of the risk of rupture and malignancy, but bland embolization or TACE can be performed when this is not possible.

Focal nodular hyperplasia is usually a solitary mass of hepatocytes, Kupffer cells, bile ducts, and connective tissue. Found most often in young women, the lesions are usually asymptomatic, with little propensity for bleeding or rupture. A hypervascular mass with a central scar ("spoke-wheel") is a characteristic imaging finding on CT, MRI, and angiography (Fig. 11-38).

Hepatic abscesses can have a hypervascular rim of compressed and inflamed normal tissue surrounding a hypovascular center. Diagnosis by angiography is unusual.

Although not a focal mass lesion, peliosis hepatis is considered in this section because it is a rare benign condition with a distinctive angiographic appearance. Peliosis consists of cystic dilatations of the hepatic sinusoids that communicate with innumerable 1- to 3-mm diameter blood-filled spaces throughout the hepatic parenchyma. The cause is unknown, although associated with certain medications (steroids, oral contraceptive, tamoxifen) as well as acquired immunodeficiency syndrome. The clinical course is usually benign. Complications such as portal hypertension and rupture have been reported. A distinctive diffuse patchy appearance of the liver parenchyma at angiography is produced by the lacunar spaces in the liver (Fig. 11-39).

■ LIVER TRANSPLANTATION

Liver transplantation is a curative procedure for patients with end-stage liver disease and small hepatomas (a single tumor less than 5 cm in diameter, or no more than three tumors, none greater than 3 cm in diameter). Current 5-year survival exceeds 60%-80%

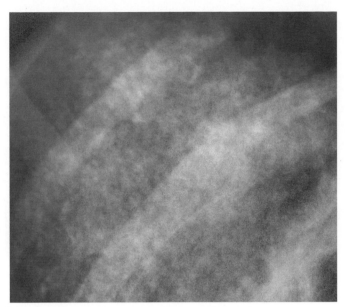

FIGURE 11-39. Angiogram showing peliosis hepatis in young woman taking birth control pills. There are innumerable small areas of hypervascularity throughout the right lobe of the liver.

Box 11-11. Vascular Complications of Liver Transplantation

Hepatic artery thrombosis
Hepatic artery stenosis
Hepatic artery pseudoaneurysm
Portal vein stenosis
Portal vein thrombosis
Intrahepatic inferior vena cava (IVC) stenosis
Suprahepatic IVC stenosis
IVC thrombosis
Hepatic vein stenosis
Hepatic vein thrombosis

---

overall (slightly less for patients transplanted for hepatocellular carcinoma), although the complication rates continue to be high.

The preoperative vascular imaging goals are largely directed at confirming vascular anatomy and patency of the hepatic arteries, the portal veins, and the inferior vena cava (IVC). In addition, a careful search for intrahepatic and extrahepatic malignancy is necessary. This workup rarely requires conventional angiography, in that ultrasound, CTA, and MRA can usually provide all required vascular information. Once restricted to evaluation of recipients, the same evaluation is applied to living related donors when available.

Imaging of the patient after liver transplantation requires knowledge of the vascular anastomoses created during the transplantation. Review of the surgical record or a conversation with the surgeon is the best way to get this information. For example, the donor celiac artery may be anastomosed directly to the recipient common hepatic artery or to the aorta. Portal vein anastomoses are usually end-to-end. A variety of systemic venous anastomoses may be used (see Fig. 14-39).

Vascular complications occur in 5%-15% of liver transplants (Box 11-11). The presentation may be liver failure, breakdown of biliary anastomoses, necrosis of the intrahepatic bile ducts, or nonspecific. Duplex ultrasound is the primary modality used to evaluate the vasculature of the transplanted liver. Absence of flow in the hepatic artery, a waveform with slow or absent systolic upslope, or focal high velocity suggests stenotic complications. Anastomotic arterial pseudoaneurysms occur in 1%-2% of

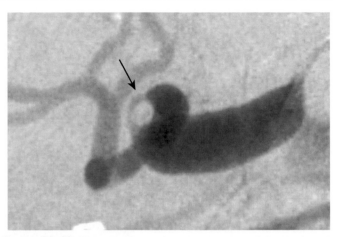

FIGURE 11-40. Stenosis of transplant hepatic artery. Selective hepatic artery digital subtraction angiogram in a transplant patient with new onset of hepatic dysfunction showing a severe stenosis *(arrow)* in a tortuous segment of artery. This had minimal improvement with angioplasty and was successfully treated with a stent.

patients. Angiography should be obtained to confirm and localize abnormalities detected by ultrasound. Transplant hepatic artery stenoses can be successfully treated with angioplasty and stent placement (Fig. 11-40). Thrombosis of a transplant artery can be treated with thrombolysis and either stent placement or surgical revision (Fig. 11-41). Early thrombosis suggests a technical issue such as an arterial kink.

In addition to arterial abnormalities, stenosis and thrombosis can occur in the portal vein, hepatic veins, and the IVC (see Figs. 14-32 and 14-35).

TRAUMA

Liver

Hepatic vascular trauma can result from penetrating or blunt injury. An important etiology is iatrogenic injury from biopsies or interventional radiologic procedures. A classification system has been devised to describe the overall degree of hepatic injury (Table 11-16). The overall mortality for lower grades of liver trauma is approximately 10%. High-grade injury carries a mortality that exceeds 50% owing to hepatic vascular trauma and injury to other organs. The imaging modality most often used to evaluate patients with abdominal trauma is CT. Conventional angiography is rarely obtained for diagnosis, but often for therapy.

Hepatic vascular trauma can present as intraperitoneal bleeding, subcapsular hematoma, arteriovenous (hepatic or portal) fistula, hemobilia, pseudoaneurysm, and thrombosis (Figs. 11-42 and 11-43). Patients with known liver injury and persistent bleeding should undergo angiography with the intent to perform embolization. A thorough diagnostic angiogram should be performed, including as a minimum celiac artery, proper hepatic artery, and SMA injections with rapid initial filming and slower filming through the portal phase. Identification of the origin of the bleeding site may require superselective injections in multiple projections. Focal injuries may manifest as extravasation or arteriovenous shunting. In the setting of large parenchymal hematomas or subcapsular hematomas, a diffuse pattern of punctate extravasation may be seen, which are referred to as the "starry night" (Fig. 11-44).

The intrahepatic arteries are not end arteries, but have potential collateral supply from other intrahepatic arteries. This is a critical concept when treating intrahepatic arterial bleeding, because occlusion proximal to the injury may result in persistent bleeding from distal reconstitution of the artery. Whenever possible, the artery on both sides of a focal abnormality should be occluded.

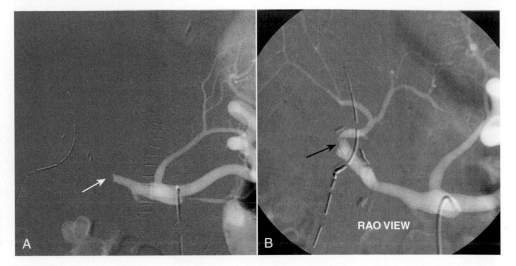

FIGURE 11-41. Acute thrombosis of a transplant hepatic artery. **A,** Celiac digital subtraction angiogram showing abrupt occlusion of the hepatic artery *(arrow)*. **B,** Following thrombolysis with 500,000 U of urokinase over 2 hours, the hepatic artery is now patent with a visible kink *(arrow)*. This required surgical revision.

TABLE 11-16 Liver Injury Scale of the American Association for the Surgery of Trauma

Grade	Injury Description
I	
Hematoma	Subcapsular; ≤10% surface area
Laceration	Capsular tear; ≤1 cm parenchymal depth
II	
Hematoma	Subcapsular; 10%-50% surface area Intraparenchymal; <10 cm diameter
Laceration	1-3 cm parenchymal depth; <10 cm length
III	
Hematoma	Subcapsular; >50% surface area or expanding Ruptured subcapsular or parenchymal hematoma Intraparenchymal hematoma; >10 cm or expanding
Laceration	>3 cm parenchymal depth
IV	
Laceration	Parenchymal disruption of 25%-75% of hepatic lobe or 1-3 Couinaud segments
V	
Laceration	Parenchymal disruption of > 75% of hepatic lobe or > 3 Couinaud segments
Vascular	Juxtahepatic venous injuries (i.e., inferior vena cava or central hepatic veins)
VI	
Vascular	Hepatic avulsion

Coils can be used for selective embolization, but particles may be necessary when injury is diffuse or selection is not possible owing to complex anatomy. Although the presence of a patent portal vein reduces the risk of liver infarction, these patients are often hypotensive and already suffering from hypoxic liver injury. Diffuse bleeding that requires embolization of large segments of the liver is often associated with subsequent liver dysfunction.

When evaluating a patient with suspected bleeding from a biliary drainage tube, it may be necessary to retract the tube briefly over a guidewire to unmask the injured vessel (Fig. 11-45). It is critical to leave the biliary guidewire in place during angiography, in that reinsertion of the tube is the best means of acutely controlling bleeding.

Spleen

The primary clinical manifestations of splenic injury are vascular (hemorrhage or infarction). Organ malfunction is not a clinical concern. Many splenic injuries can be managed conservatively with close observation, thus preserving the spleen and avoiding a laparotomy. This strategy is of particular importance in children, in whom maintaining the immunologic properties of splenic tissue is desirable. A grading system has been devised to describe the extent of splenic injury to help guide management (Table 11-17). Grade I and II lesions are usually managed conservatively, although delayed rupture can occur in up to one-third of patients. More severely injured spleens usually require intervention owing to hemodynamic instability of the patient or ongoing bleeding.

The conventional treatment of severe splenic injury is splenectomy. Embolization is an alternative in patients with a severely injured but viable spleen (Fig. 11-46). The optimal technique has not been determined, but both selective occlusion of sites of obvious vascular injury or proximal occlusion of the main splenic artery with coils have been described. Theoretically, selective embolization addresses the point of injury and preserves splenic tissue, but risks focal infarction. Embolization of the main splenic artery is thought to reduce bleeding by decreasing the arterial pressure in the splenic pulp, while avoiding splenic infarction due to preservation of collateral supply. Patients should receive routine antibiotics during embolization, but vaccinations for *Pneumococcus, Haemophilus influenzae,* or *Neisseria meningitides* are not necessary because splenic tissue is almost always preserved. The overall success rate in patients with grade 3 and 4 injuries is 80%-90% in avoiding splenectomy for rebleeding or infarction.

Bowel

Bowel injury occurs in fewer than 5% of cases of blunt trauma to the abdomen, but is found in 80% of patients with traumatic aortoiliac artery injuries. Vascular injury such as thrombosis, arteriovenous fistula, pedicle avulsion, or transection can occur. These injuries rarely require conventional angiography for evaluation or therapy.

▬ VISCERAL ARTERY ANEURYSMS

Aneurysms of the visceral arteries are rare in comparison to aortic and iliac, femoral, and popliteal artery aneurysms. The most commonly affected arteries are the splenic, hepatic, and celiac; multiple aneurysms have been found in one third of patients in some series (Table 11-18). The etiology of the aneurysm has a great influence on whether it will be a true or false aneurysm

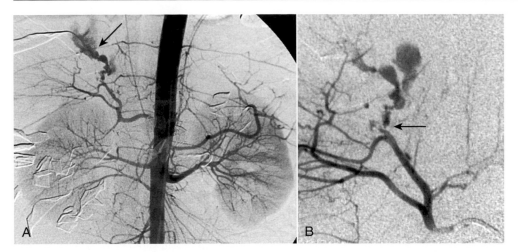

FIGURE 11-42. Arterial bleeding from traumatic laceration of the liver. **A,** Digital subtraction aortogram showing massive extravasation *(arrow)* in the right upper quadrant. The aortogram was obtained in this trauma patient because of the absence of any prior imaging. Note the generalized vasoconstriction of the visceral and renal arteries consistent with shock. **B,** Selective hepatic digital subtraction angiogram showing extravasation from a right hepatic arterial transection *(arrow)*. The objective of embolization in this setting is rapid control of bleeding to save the patient's life. This was successfully accomplished with coils and Gelfoam plugs.

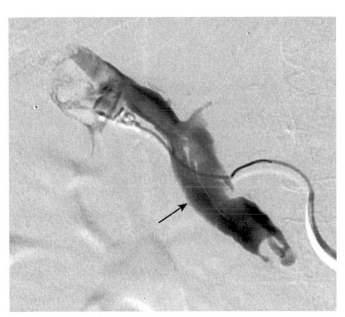

FIGURE 11-43. Patient with sudden onset of gastrointestinal bleeding and right upper quadrant pain several months after hepatic laceration due to blunt trauma. Superselective digital subtraction angiogram of a branch of the right hepatic artery through a microcatheter shows opacification of the common bile duct *(arrow)*.

(Box 11-12). Aneurysms related to degenerative processes, fibromuscular dysplasia (FMD), inherited disorders of the vascular wall, segmental arterial mediolysis, and vasculitis are true aneurysms unless they have ruptured. Aneurysms related to pancreatitis, infection, trauma, or surgery are always pseudoaneurysms. The majority of visceral aneurysms are asymptomatic until first presenting with rupture. The indications for intervention in asymptomatic true aneurysms must be individualized to the patient and the artery involved. There are no set rules for management of these lesions. Pseudoaneurysms almost always require intervention, because the risk of rupture is high. The mortality of ruptured visceral artery aneurysms can approach 80%.

Bleeding from arterial pseudoaneurysms occurs in approximately 5% of patients with pancreatitis. This diagnosis should be suspected when a pseudocyst contains high-density material consistent with thrombus on CT scan or increases suddenly in size in association with acute hypotension. Angiographic evaluation requires selective injections of all arteries that could potentially supply the pancreas and pseudocyst. The findings may be relatively subtle, such as an area of slight enlargement and irregularity in the artery. Endovascular management with embolization or stent-graft placement is preferred to surgery (Fig. 11-47).

Splenic artery aneurysms occur in approximately 0.8% of the population and 8%-10% of patients with portal hypertension. The incidence in women is four times higher than in men (Fig. 11-48). Women with a history of multiple pregnancies are at highest risk. Splenic artery aneurysms are also frequently found in patients with massive splenomegaly. Most splenic artery aneurysms are found incidentally, but patients may complain of epigastric, left upper quadrant abdominal, or back pain. The risk of rupture has not been quantified, but is highest in young patients (especially pregnant women) and older adults. Rupture of true aneurysms is most often into the lesser sac or adjacent venous structures. Splenic artery pseudoaneurysms due to pancreatitis can rupture into a pancreatic pseudocyst, adjacent bowel or stomach, or the peritoneal cavity.

Intervention is probably warranted in any pregnant patient with a splenic artery aneurysm, or any symptomatic aneurysm. There are no firmly defined size criteria for intervention in asymptomatic nonpregnant patients, but 2 cm in diameter has been recommended as the threshold for intervention, especially in young women. Endovascular treatment options include placement of a stent-graft in the splenic artery or embolization. A stent-graft preserves in-line flow to the spleen. Embolization is easier when the artery is tortuous. Packing of the aneurysm with coils, and/or placement of coils or plugs distal and proximal to the aneurysm effectively exclude it from arterial flow. With splenic artery embolization, the collateral blood supply to the spleen usually prevents global infarction, although microinfarcts are seen in 10%.

True aneurysms of the pancreaticoduodenal arteries are rare lesions associated with celiac artery or SMA occlusive disease and increased collateral flow in the peripancreatic arcade (Fig. 11-49). Rupture of these aneurysms can result in gastrointestinal bleeding, a large hematoma at the base of the mesentery, hypotension, and exsanguination. Selective embolization with placement of coils on both sides of the aneurysm can be life saving. There are usually more than enough additional collateral arteries to preserve adequate flow between the SMA and the celiac artery.

Mycotic aneurysms of mesenteric vessels are most often embolic in origin. Cardiac valvular sources are typical, although paradoxical septic emboli have been reported.

Patients who have undergone surgical resection of pancreatic head cancers (Whipple procedures) can develop a characteristic type of delayed postoperative bleeding from gastroduodenal or pancreatic artery pseudoaneurysms. Bleeding occurs in approximately 5%-8% of patients with a 15%-20% mortality. Early bleeding (within 24 hours) usually indicates a technical error. Delayed bleeding (after 24 hours but in our experience usually after the fifth postoperative day) often presents with a "sentinel" or "herald bleed" from a drain, the gastrointestinal tract, or both (Fig. 11-50). Patients with significant bleeding (e.g., hypotension, transfusion requirement) should undergo angiography at that time to look for a pseudoaneurysm, because subsequent bleeding occurs in most patients. When the origin is the GDA stump, stent-graft placement preserves hepatic arterial flow. When this is not feasible, coil embolization of the hepatic artery across the GDA stump is usually well tolerated if the portal vein is patent. Pancreaticoduodenal artery pseudoaneurysms can usually be coil embolized.

▬ FIBROMUSCULAR DYSPLASIA

The visceral arteries are the sixth most frequent site affected by FMD. Spontaneous dissection, focal aneurysm formation, and distal embolization can occur. The SMA, hepatic, and splenic arteries can be affected (Fig. 11-51). In asymptomatic patients, no treatment is required. Patients with complications of FMD may require interventions including stent or endograft placement, or surgical bypass.

▬ SEGMENTAL ARTERIAL MEDIOLYSIS

Segmental arterial mediolysis (SAM) is a rare disorder of unknown etiology occurring in middle-aged patients (Fig. 11-52).

Some authors consider it a precursor to or variant of FMD. The visceral arteries are most often involved, but cases of carotid and intracranial arterial disease have been reported. The lesion begins with vacuolization and lysis of the outer media. This weakens the artery wall and external elastic lamina, forms gaps, and allows separation of adventitia and media. Patients are symptomatic with pain (60%) and spontaneous hemorrhage (50%). Arterial dissection and multiple aneurysms are seen on imaging studies. There is no systemic treatment, although ruptured aneurysms can be embolized. Arteries may return to normal over time, but mortality is high (40%) particularly when there is progressive involvement, as is seen in more than one third of patients.

▬ DISSECTION

Dissection of the visceral arteries is often an extension of aortic dissection, but may be focal and spontaneous, iatrogenic, or traumatic in origin. Symptomatic visceral artery compromise from aortic dissection occurs in approximately 6% of patients, with a 25%-50% mortality at 30 days despite intervention. Up to 15% of acute deaths from aortic dissection are due directly or indirectly to mesenteric ischemia. MRA and CTA are highly sensitive and specific for diagnosis of aortic dissection and involvement of proximal visceral arteries (see Fig. 9-25). The celiac artery, SMA, and right renal artery are often supplied by the true lumen, whereas the left renal artery may arise from the

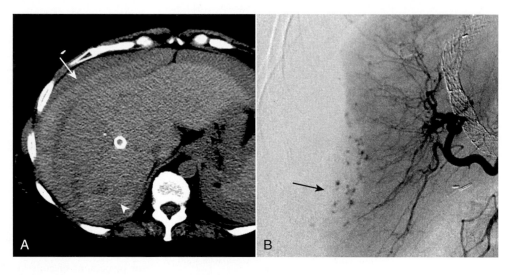

FIGURE 11-44. "Starry night" pattern of diffuse bleeding. **A,** Noncontrast computed tomography scan of the liver the night following transjugular intrahepatic portosystemic shunt procedure showing an acute parenchymal hematoma *(arrowhead)* and a large per-hepatic hematoma *(arrow).* **B,** Celiac angiogram showing multiple areas of punctate extravasation *(arrow)* in the region of the parenchymal hematoma. Embolization with multiple Gelfoam particles was successful in controlling bleeding. The patient had a protracted recovery due to hepatic dysfunction.

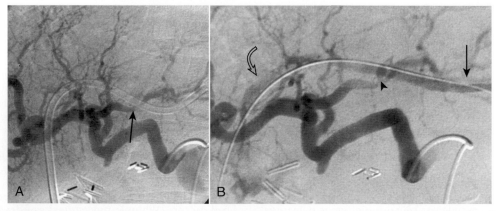

FIGURE 11-45. Patient with remote liver transplant and a chronic left-sided biliary drainage tube had brisk, pulsatile bleeding from the tract during a routine catheter change. **A,** Hepatic digital subtraction angiogram (DSA) with the tube in place showing slight narrowing of the left hepatic artery *(arrow)*, but no active extravasation. The gastroduodenal artery was ligated during the transplant surgery. **B,** Repeat DSA after removal of the tube over a guidewire showing a pseudoaneurysm *(arrowhead)*, with extravasation into the bile ducts *(curved arrow)* and the parenchymal track of the tube *(arrow)*. Coils were placed in the left hepatic artery on both sides of the pseudoaneurysm. The patient has since undergone numerous uneventful tube changes.

false lumen or have shared perfusion from both lumens (see Fig.10-32). Compression of the true lumen and/or extension of the dissection into the visceral artery results in visceral ischemia (Fig. 11-53). Stent-graft or surgical repair of the thoracic aortic entry tear often results in improved perfusion of the visceral vessels (see Fig. 9-24). Fenestration of the flap in the visceral segment, percutaneously or surgically, sometimes augmented with stent placement in the visceral artery is an alternative or additional approach (see Fig. 10-33).

Spontaneous localized dissection of a visceral artery is rare, occurring most commonly in middle-aged men. More than one artery may be involved, with the SMA in 60%, celiac artery in 35%, hepatic arteries in 10%, and splenic artery in 5% (see Fig. 11-14). Predisposing factors include FMD, connective tissue disorders, segmental arterial mediolysis, trauma, and hypertension. Patients present with acute onset of pain related to the

dissection and visceral ischemia. The usual initial management is anticoagulation, but this fails in 30%-50% of patients. Stent or endograft placement, or surgical bypass may be necessary to improve organ perfusion. Late complications include aneurysmal change of the false lumen, thrombosis, rupture, and distal embolization.

VASCULAR MALFORMATIONS

True vascular malformations of the liver, spleen, and pancreas are rare lesions, found in fewer than 1% of adults undergoing abdominal ultrasound. Most often these are asymptomatic lesions. Liver malformations may be arterioportal, arteriovenous, or portovenous. Ultrasound, CTA, and MRA are usually excellent modalities for diagnosis of liver arteriovenous malformations and distinguishing them from shunting vascular tumors. Localized lesions may be embolized when symptomatic, especially in neonates, but hepatic necrosis is a significant risk.

Liver arteriovenous malformations are found in up to 60% of patients with hereditary hemorrhagic telangiectasia (HHT), but are usually asymptomatic. Liver involvement is diffuse rather than focal. Patients can present with high-output cardiac failure, portal hypertension, or biliary disease (Fig. 11-54). Biliary strictures, dilation, and cysts are thought to be due to bile duct ischemia from arterial shunting. Attempted embolization or TIPS can lead to liver failure. Often liver transplantation is the best therapy for severely symptomatic patients.

A wide variety of vascular lesions can affect the stomach, small bowel, and colon (Box 11-13). The typical presentation is gastrointestinal bleeding, either chronic or acute. Angiodysplasia is a common lesion at endoscopy consisting of dilated, thin-walled, submucosal veins, venules, and capillaries. They are frequently multiple, can be located anywhere from the stomach to the rectum, and are not associated with a systemic or generalized syndrome or disorder. Several segments of bowel may be affected synchronously, with the most common colonic location in the cecum. These are usually lesions of mature adults (older than 60 years) without gender specificity. Angiodysplasia is usually treated endoscopically with cautery or injection. The classic angiographic appearance is vascular tuft or tangle with an early and dense draining vein (Fig. 11-55). Extravasation was classically reported in 10%, but is rarely seen in current practice. Embolization of angiodysplasia has been reported, but surgical resection of lesions not amenable to endoscopic therapy remains the mainstay of therapy.

Gastric antral vascular ectasia ("watermelon stomach") is a rare lesion usually found in older women with iron deficiency anemia. Extensive submucosal venous dilatation in the antrum results in

TABLE 11-17 Spleen Injury Scale of the American Association for the Surgery of Trauma

Grade	Injury Description
I	
Hematoma	Subcapsular; <10% surface area
Laceration	Capsular tear; <1 cm parenchymal depth
II	
Hematoma	Subcapsular; 10%-50% surface area Intraparenchymal; <5 cm diameter
Laceration	1-3 cm parenchymal depth not involving trabecular vessel
III	
Hematoma	Subcapsular; >50% surface area or expanding Ruptured subcapsular or parenchymal hematoma Intraparenchymal hematoma; >5 cm or expanding
Laceration	>3 cm parenchymal depth or involving trabecular vessels
IV	
Laceration	Laceration involving segmental or hilar vessels producing major devascularization (>25% of spleen)
V	
Laceration	Completely shattered spleen
Vascular	Hilar vascular injury which devascularizes the spleen

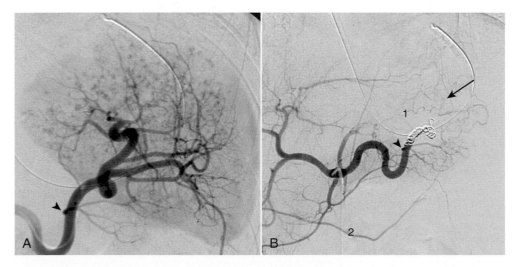

FIGURE 11-46. Splenic artery embolization for trauma in a patient with splenic injury following a motor vehicle accident. The objective of embolization in this stable patient is to decrease the overall splenic arterial flow but preserve viability of the organ. **A,** Selective splenic angiogram showing multiple areas of punctate staining in the region of the injury. Note the artery to the tail of the pancreas *(arrowhead)*. **B,** Celiac angiogram following coil embolization of the distal main splenic artery showing reconstitution of intrasplenic arteries *(arrow)* via *(1)* left gastric to short gastric arteries, *(2)* the right gastroepiploic to left gastroepiploic arteries, and the pancreatic arteries *(arrowhead)*.

characteristic parallel red stripes. Diagnosis and therapy does not require angiography.

The Dieulafoy lesion is an abnormally large artery (1- to 3-mm diameter) close to the mucosal surface of the bowel. Originally described in the stomach in older adult patients (male-to-female ratio 2:1), it is thought to account for 2%-5% of acute upper gastrointestinal bleeding. In modern series, up to one third of lesions are found in the colon, small bowel, and even the esophagus (see Fig. 11-20). Single lesions are typical.

TABLE 11-18 Artery of Origin of Visceral Artery Aneurysms

Splenic artery	60%
Hepatic artery	20%
Superior mesenteric artery	6%
Celiac artery	4%
Jejunal, iliac, colic arteries	4%
Pancreaticoduodenal arteries	2%
Gastroduodenal artery	2%
Inferior mesenteric artery	<1%

Box 11-12. Etiologies of Visceral Artery Aneurysms

Degenerative
Vasculitis
Pancreatitis
Trauma
Ehlers-Danlos syndrome
Fibromuscular dysplasia
Segmental arterial mediolysis
Mycotic
Behçet disease
Iatrogenic (surgery, percutaneous interventions)
Celiac artery or SMA stenosis/occlusion (pancreaticoduodenal artery aneurysms)
Splenomegaly (splenic artery aneurysms)

Dieulafoy lesions are usually diagnosed and treated at endoscopy, with mortality due to bleeding less than 5%. When endoscopic management fails, angiographic localization of bleeding and embolization is usually successful. Placement of metallic clips endoscopicaly on the mucosa around the artery can be helpful during angiographic localization.

Arteriovenous fistulas in the liver, spleen, pancreas, and bowel can occur after blunt or penetrating trauma, infection, or invasive procedures. In the liver, communication may be with the hepatic or portal vein, or the bile duct (see Fig. 11-43). Portal hypertension, variceal bleeding, and high-output cardiac failure may result from large fistulas. Endovascular treatment with embolization or small stent-grafts is frequently effective.

■ VASCULITIS

Polyarteritis nodosa is the most common vasculitis to affect the peripheral visceral arteries (Fig. 11-56). Stenoses and aneurysms may be found; the aneurysms are prone to rupture. Takayasu arteritis can cause stenosis of the visceral artery origins. SAM may mimic the angiographic appearance of vasculitis (see Fig. 11-52).

■ HYPERSPLENISM

The syndrome of platelet sequestration by an enlarged spleen is termed *hypersplenism*. Primary hypersplenism is rare. Secondary hypersplenism can be due to portal hypertension, neoplasm, Gaucher disease, or myeloproliferative disorders. More commonly symptomatic in children, hypersplenism also occurs in adults.

The conventional treatment of hypersplenism is correction of the underlying disorder or splenectomy. Although the latter is definitive, it is a major procedure that leaves the patient at risk for overwhelming sepsis from encapsulated bacteria. Partial embolization of the spleen (70%-80% of the total parenchyma) results in elevation of the platelet count and preservation of sufficient splenic pulp for maintenance of clinically relevant reticuloendothelial activity. Embolization should be from a distal position rather than proximal coil occlusion. Gelfoam pledgets soaked in antibiotics that provide coverage of both gram-positive and gram-negative organisms have been widely used. Patients require pain control for usually 48 hours owing to infarction of splenic tissue, and broad-spectrum antibiotic prophylaxis for 10-14 days following the procedure. Platelet counts

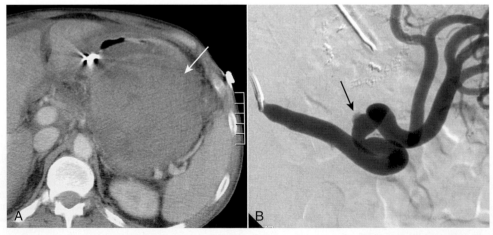

FIGURE 11-47. Splenic artery bleeding due to necrotizing pancreatitis. **A,** Computed tomography (CT) scan showing high-density thrombus *(arrow)* filling a known pseudocyst arising from the body of pancreas in a patient with acute abdominal pain and a drop in hematocrit level. **B,** Splenic artery digital subtraction angiogram showing the probable site of bleeding *(arrow)*. The arterial abnormality is subtle compared to the CT finding as the pseudocyst is filled with acute thrombus. This splenic artery was embolized by placing coils distal and proximal to the defect. The spleen remained well perfused by short gastric and gastroepiploic collaterals.

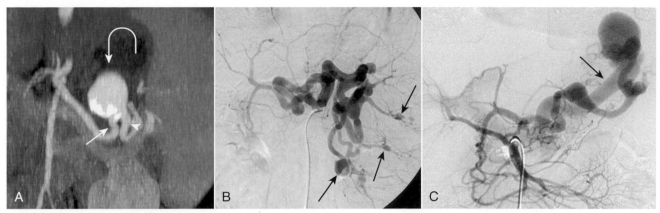

FIGURE 11-48. Splenic artery aneurysms. **A,** Thin coronal maximum intensity projection (MIP) of a computed tomography angiogram showing a partially calcified splenic artery aneurysm *(curved arrow)*. The inflow *(arrow)* and outflow *(arrowhead)* are clearly identified, providing important information for planning therapy (in this case coil embolization distal and proximal to the aneurysm). The stairstep appearance of the image is due to lack of sufficient overlap of the slices used for the MIP. **B,** Celiac digital subtraction angiogram in a patient with massive splenomegaly showing multiple small splenic artery aneurysms *(arrows)*. **C,** Angiogram in a patient with a multiple splenic artery aneurysms, one of which has ruptured into the splenic vein *(arrow)* causing portal hypertension. Note that the superior mesenteric artery has been injected and the splenic artery is filled via the pancreaticoduodenal arcade and the arc of Buhler due to a celiac origin stenosis. What is the variant of hepatic arterial anatomy?

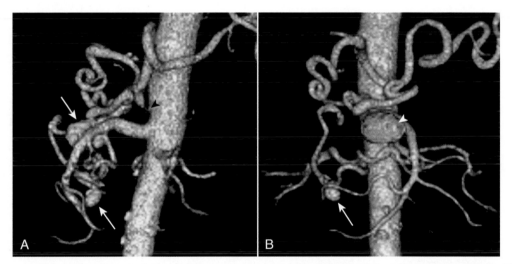

FIGURE 11-49. Aneurysms of the collateral arteries between the superior mesenteric artery (SMA) and the celiac artery in a patient with celiac artery stenosis. **A,** Lateral view of a volume rendering of an abdominal computed tomography angiogram showing the severe celiac artery stenosis *(arrowhead)* and two aneurysms *(arrows)* within the enlarged collateral arteries to the celiac artery. **B,** Frontal view of the same reconstruction. The lower aneurysm *(arrow)* is in the inferior pancreaticoduodenal arteries. The upper aneurysm *(arrowhead)* is larger, calcified, and arises in a massively enlarged arc of Buhler connecting the SMA through the dorsal pancreatic artery to the celiac artery.

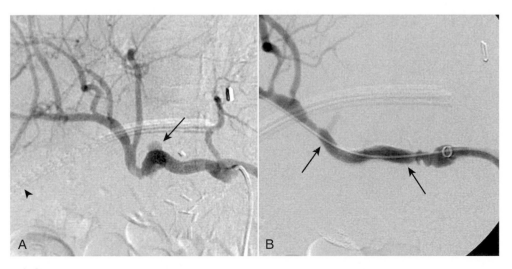

FIGURE 11-50. Gastroduodenal artery (GDA) stump blowout after Whipple procedure. The patient had intermittent massive bleeding from the Jackson-Pratt (J-P) drain. **A,** Celiac angiogram showing a pseudoaneurysm of the hepatic artery *(arrow)* at the expected location of the GDA origin. Note the proximity to the J-P drain *(arrowhead)*. **B,** Angiogram after placement of a 5-mm diameter stent-graft *(arrows)* across the GDA origin. The irregularity in the common hepatic artery is spasm due to the large sheath (8-French) and stiff guidewire used for this procedure.

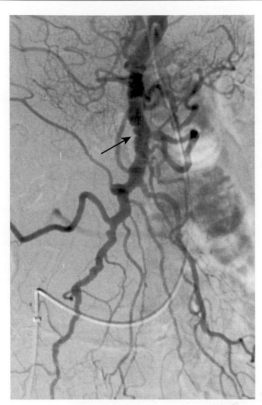

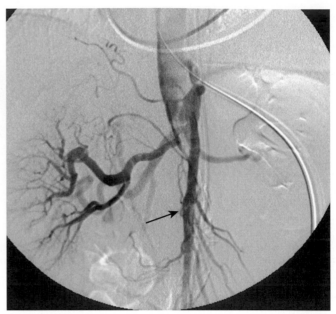

FIGURE 11-53. Visceral artery compromise due to thoracic aortic dissection extending into the abdomen. Digital subtraction angiogram in the true lumen, showing extreme compromise of the lumen and filling of the superior mesenteric artery *(arrow)*, right kidney, and faint opacification of the common hepatic artery. This is the "floating visceral arteries" sign. Compare with Figure 10-32.

FIGURE 11-51. Fibromuscular dysplasia of the superior mesenteric artery (SMA). Selective SMA digital subtraction angiogram showing irregular beaded contour *(arrow)* of medial fibroplasia.

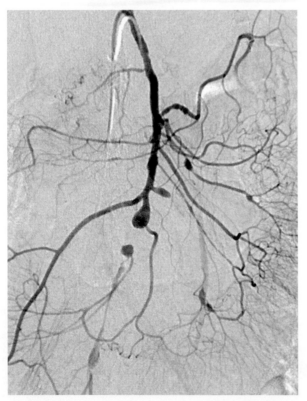

FIGURE 11-52. Segmental arterial mediolysis (SAM) in a 57-year-old woman who presented with a hematoma in the mesentery and multiple small SMA aneurysms seen on CT. Onset was sudden and rheumatologic workup was negative. Angiogram of the SMA shows multiple areas of focal dilatation and stenosis throughout the left colic and marginal arteries. The short occlusion is postoperative after emergency laparotomy with ligation of a bleeding artery.

should rise within 24 hours, peak within 2 weeks, and then stabilize after 2 months.

Improvement in platelet counts after embolization is proportional to the volume of residual splenic tissue. A final target of 70%-80% infarction (when the initial splenic volume is between 400 and 700 mL) or a residual volume of less than 170 mL achieved over two or more embolizations when the splenic volume is greater than 700 mL provides durable results with fewer complications. With larger spleens, the volume of infarcted tissue should be 390-540 mL per session. Complications are increased in patients with Child C cirrhosis and infarction of more than 540 mL of splenic tissue in a single session. These complications include splenic abscess, increased ascites or pleural effusions, and variceal bleeding.

Complete embolization (infarction) of the spleen is an alternative therapy for patients in whom splenectomy is required but is high risk, for example in a patient with a hostile abdomen and splenic vein occlusion and bleeding isolated gastric varices. Peripheral embolization and antibiotic coverage is necessary to prevent formation of a splenic abscess, which may occur in up to 40% of cases. In patients amenable to splenectomy, preoperative embolization with coils in the distal main splenic artery is beneficial to limit blood loss when the spleen is huge.

Patients who undergo total splenic embolization should be immunized against encapsulated bacteria (*Pneumococcus, H. influenzae* type b, and *Meningococcus*). When feasible, this should be performed 2-3 weeks before total embolization.

▬ SPLENIC STEAL SYNDROME

A rare complication of orthotopic liver transplantation, splenic steal occurs when a large spleen "sumps" blood from the liver allograft, leading to hepatic dysfunction. Coil embolization of the middle or distal splenic artery improves hepatic arterial perfusion with minimal risk of splenic infarction.

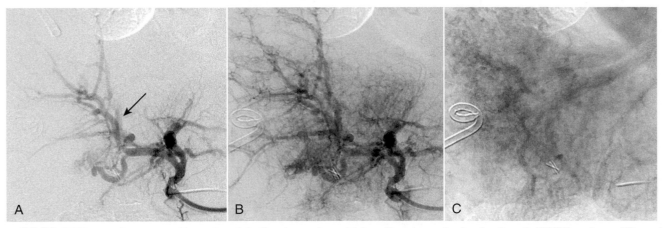

FIGURE 11-54. Diffuse arteriovenous malformation of the liver in a patient with hereditary hemorrhagic telangiectasia (HHT) syndrome. The patient first presented with multiple infected biliary cysts. During percutaneous drainage opacification of the hepatic artery was noted. A diagnosis of HHT was subsequently made. **A,** Early image from hepatic angiogram shows filling of portal vein branches *(arrow)*. **B,** A few seconds later the diffuse nature of the arteriovenous malformation is appreciated. **C,** Late image shows the hepatic veins. Note the pigtail drain in the right lobe biliary cyst. The patient eventually underwent liver transplantation.

Box 11-13. Vascular Lesions Contributing to Gastrointestinal Bleeding

Vascular ectasia
Angiodysplasia
Hereditary hemorrhagic telangiectasia (GI bleeding in 15%)
CREST syndrome
Gastric antral vascular ectasia ("watermelon stomach")
Hemangioma
- Isolated, sporadic (90%)
- Intestinal hemangiomatosis
- Blue rubber bleb syndrome (cutaneous and intestinal cavernous hemangiomas)

Klippel-Trenaunay-Weber syndrome
Arteriovenous malformations
Dieulafoy lesion

CREST, Calcinosis, Raynaud phenomenon, esophageal hypomotility, sclerodactyly, telangiectasia.

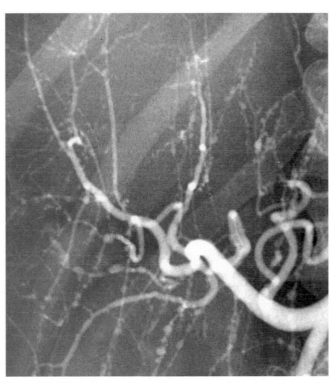

FIGURE 11-56. Celiac angiogram in a patient with polyarteritis nodosa showing innumerable small aneurysms.

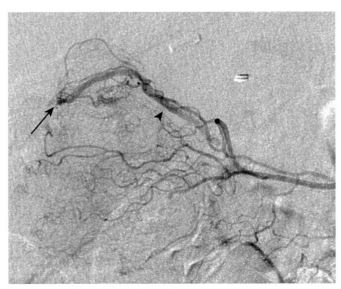

FIGURE 11-55. Selective middle colic angiogram showing right colonic angiodysplasia *(arrow)* with a small tuft of vessels and an early draining vein *(arrowhead)*.

SUGGESTED READINGS

Asensio JA, Forno W, Roldan G, et al. Visceral vascular injuries. *Surg Clin N Am.* 2002;82:1-20.

de Baere T, Deschamps F. Arterial therapies of colorectal cancer metastases to the liver. *Abdom Imaging.* 2011 Dec;36(6):661-670.

Bardou M, Benhaberou-Brun D, Le Ray I, Barkun AN. Diagnosis and management of nonvariceal upper gastrointestinal bleeding. *Nat Rev Gastroenterol Hepatol.* 2012;9:97-104.

Brown DB, Cardella JF, Sacks D, et al. Quality improvement guidelines for transhepatic arterial chemoembolization, embolization, and chemotherapeutic infusion for hepatic malignancy. *J Vasc Interv Radiol.* 2006;17(2 Pt 1):225-232.

Burrows PE, Dubois J, Kassarjian A. Pediatric hepatic vascular anomalies. *Pediatr Radiol.* 2001;31:533-545.

Covey AM, Brody LA, Maluccio MA, Getrajdman GI, Brown KT. Variant hepatic arterial anatomy revisited: digital subtraction angiography performed in 600 patients. *Radiology.* 2002;224:542-547.

Cui Y, Elahi D, Andersen DK. Advances in the etiology and management of hyperinsulinemic hypoglycemia after Roux-en-Y gastric bypass. *J Gastrointest Surg.* 2011;15:1879-1888.

Duffy AJ, Panait L, Eisenberg D, et al. Management of median arcuate ligament syndrome: a new paradigm. *Ann Vasc Surg.* 2009;23:778-784.

El-Serag HB. Hepatocellular carcinoma. *N Engl J Med.* 2011;365:1118-1127.

European Association for the Study of the Liver. European Organisation for Research and Treatment of Cancer. EASL-EORTC Clinical Practice Guidelines: Management of hepatocellular carcinoma. *J Hepatol.* 2012;56:908-943.

Filippone EJ, Foy A, Galanis T, et al. Segmental arterial mediolysis: report of 2 cases and review of the literature. *Am J Kidney Dis.* 2011;58:981-987.

Garcia-Tsao G, Korzenik JR, Young L, et al. Liver disease in patients with hereditary hemorrhagic telangiectasia. *N Engl J Med.* 2000;343:931-936.

Geffroy Y, Rodallec MH, Boulay-Coletta I, et al. Multidetector CT angiography in acute gastrointestinal bleeding: why, when, and how. *Radiographics.* 2011;31:E35-E46.

Gomes AS, Lois JF, McCoy RD. Angiographic treatment of gastrointestinal hemorrhage: comparison of vasopressin infusion and embolization. *Am J Roentgenol.* 1986;146:1031-1037.

Grieco A, Pompili M, Caminiti G, et al. Prognostic factors for survival in patients with early-intermediate hepatocellular carcinoma undergoing non-surgical therapy: comparison of Okuda, CLIP, and BCLC staging systems in a single Italian centre. *Gut.* 2005;54:411-418.

Hayashi H, Beppu T, Okabe K, et al. Therapeutic factors considered according to the preoperative splenic volume for a prolonged increase in platelet count after partial splenic embolization for liver cirrhosis. *J Gastroenterol.* 2010;45:554-559.

Health Resources and Services Administration (HRSA). MELD calculator. http://optn.transplant.hrsa.gov/resources/MeldPeldCalculator.asp?index=98.

Huo TI, Hsia CY, Huang YH, et al. Selecting a short-term prognostic model for hepatocellular carcinoma: comparison between the model for end-stage liver disease (MELD), MELD-sodium, and five cancer staging systems. *J Clin Gastroenterol.* 2009;43:773-781.

Jackson JE. Angiography and arterial stimulation venous sampling in the localization of pancreatic neuroendocrine tumours. *Best Pract Res Clin Endocrinol Metab.* 2005;19:229-239.

Kalva SP, Athanasoulis CA, Greenfield AJ, et al. Inferior pancreaticoduodenal artery aneurysms in association with celiac axis stenosis or occlusion. *Eur J Vasc Endovasc Surg.* 2007;33:670-675.

Kalva SP, Somarouthu B, Jaff MR, Wicky S. Segmental arterial mediolysis: clinical and imaging features at presentation and during follow-up. *J Vasc Interv Radiol.* 2011;22:1380-1387.

Kennedy A, Nag S, Salem R, et al. Recommendations for radioembolization of hepatic malignancies using yttrium-90 microsphere brachytherapy: a consensus panel report from the radioembolization brachytherapy oncology consortium. *Int J Radiat Oncol Biol Phys.* 2007;68:13-23.

Lammer J, Malagari K, Vogl T, et al. Prospective randomized study of doxorubicin-eluting-bead embolization in the treatment of hepatocellular carcinoma: results of the PRECISION V study. *Cardiovasc Intervent Radiol.* 2010;33:41-52.

Levine SM, Hellmann DB, Stone JH. Gastrointestinal involvement in polyarteritis nodosa (1986-2000): presentation and outcomes in 24 patients. *Am J Med.* 2002;112:386-391.

Lim EH, Jung SW, Lee SH, et al. Endovascular management for isolated spontaneous dissection of the superior mesenteric artery: report of two cases and literature review. *J Vasc Interv Radiol.* 2011;22:1206-1211.

Llovet JM, Bruix J. Systematic review of randomized trials for unresectable hepatocellular carcinoma: chemoembolization improves survival. *Hepatology.* 2003;37:429-442.

Madoff DC, Denys A, Wallace MJ, et al. Splenic arterial interventions: anatomy, indications, technical considerations, and potential complications. *Radiographics.* 2005;25:S191-S211.

Marti M, Artigas JM, Garzon G, et al. Acute lower intestinal bleeding: feasibility and diagnostic performance of CT angiography. *Radiology.* 2012;262:109-116.

Mitchell AW, Spencer J, Allison DJ, Jackson JE. Meckel's diverticulum: angiographic findings in 16 patients. *Am J Roentgenol.* 1998;170:1329-1333.

Moore EE, Cogbill TH, Jurkovich GJ, et al. Organ injury scaling: spleen and liver [1994 revision]. *J Trauma.* 1995;38:323.

Mozes MF, Spigos DG, Pollak R, et al. Partial splenic embolization, an alternative to splenectomy: results of a prospective, randomized study. *Surgery.* 1984;96:694-702.

Oken MM, Creech RH, Tormey DC, et al. Toxicity and response criteria of the Eastern Cooperative Oncology Group. *Am J Clin Oncol.* 1982;5:649-655.

Park WM, Gloviczki P, Cherry KJ, et al. Contemporary management of acute mesenteric ischemia: factors associated with survival. *J Vasc Surg.* 2002;35:445-452.

Pinter M, Hucke F, Graziadei I, et al. Advanced-stage hepatocellular carcinoma: transarterial chemoembolization versus sorafenib. *Radiology.* 2012;263:590-599.

Puppala S, Patel J, McPherson S, et al. Hemorrhagic complications after Whipple surgery: imaging and radiologic intervention. *AJR Am J Roentgenol.* 2011;196:192-197.

Riaz A, Lewandowski RJ, Kulik LM, et al. Complications following radioembolization with Yttrium-90 microspheres: a comprehensive literature review. *JVIR.* 2009;20:1121-1130.

Rösch J, Dotter CT, Brown MJ. Selective arterial embolization. A new method for control of acute gastrointestinal bleeding. *Radiology.* 1972;102:303-306.

Salem R, Lewandowski RJ, Gates VL, et al. Research reporting standards for radioembolization of hepatic malignancies. *J Vasc Interv Radiol.* 2011;22:265-278.

Schnüriger B, Inaba K, Konstantinidis A, et al. Outcomes of proximal versus distal splenic artery embolization after trauma: a systematic review and meta-analysis. *J Trauma.* 2011;70:252-260.

Shah RP, Brown KT, Sofocleous CT. Arterially directed therapies for hepatocellular carcinoma. *AJR Am J Roentgenol.* 2011;197:W590-W602.

Turba UC, Saad WE, Arslan B, et al. Chronic mesenteric ischaemia: 28-year experience of endovascular treatment. *Eur Radiol.* 2012;22:1372-1384.

Walker TG, Salazar GM, Waltman AC. Angiographic evaluation and management of acute gastrointestinal hemorrhage. *World J Gastroenterol.* 2012;18:1191-1201.

Waltman AC, Courey WR, Athanasoulis C, Baum S. Technique for left gastric artery catheterization. *Radiology.* 1973;109:732-734.

Wu JS, Saluja S, Garcia-Tsao G, et al. Liver involvement in Hereditary Hemorrhagic Telangiectasia: CT and clinical findings do not correlate in symptomatic patients. *AJR.* 2006;187:W399-W405.

Zeller T, Rastan A, Sixt S. Chronic atherosclerotic mesenteric ischemia (CMI). *Vasc Med.* 2010;15:333-338.

Zeng Q, Li Y, Chen Y, et al. Gigantic cavernous hemangioma of the liver treated by intra-arterial embolization with pingyangmycin-Lipiodol emulsion: a multi-center study. *Cardiovasc Interv Radiol.* 2004;27:481-485.

CHAPTER 12

Renal Arteries

John A. Kaufman, MD, MS, FSIR, FCIRSE

The kidneys receive almost 15% of the cardiac output, although they account for less than 5% of the total body mass. Obstructive arterial diseases of the kidney have both functional (e.g., decreased creatinine clearance) and hormonal (angiotensin-mediated hypertension) implications. There are few organs that have such a complex response to vascular disease and potentially rewarding results with intervention.

ANATOMY

Renal Arteries

The kidneys are paired organs that originate in the pelvis and ascend into the abdominal cavity in a retroperitoneal location. As each kidney travels cephalad it is supplied sequentially by a series of arteries from the aorta that regress spontaneously. Ultimately, each kidney is usually supplied by a single renal artery that originates from the aorta below the superior mesenteric artery (SMA) at roughly the L1-L2 disk space in about two thirds of individuals. The right renal artery orifice is located on the anterolateral wall of the aorta, frequently quite close to the SMA origin. The right renal artery courses posterior to the inferior vena cava (IVC), and assumes a position posterior to the right renal vein in the retroperitoneum (Fig. 12-1). The left renal artery originates in a more lateral location, and courses through the retroperitoneum posterior to the left renal vein. With an understanding of the typical locations of the renal artery orifices, the operator will avoid much frustration during selective angiography.

The renal artery is usually 4-6 cm long and 5-6 mm in diameter. Each renal artery gives rise to a small proximal branch to the adrenal gland (the inferior adrenal arteries) and the renal capsule (Fig. 12-2). In the region of the renal pelvis, the artery bifurcates into anterior and posterior divisions. The anterior division supplies the upper and lower poles and the anterior portion of the mid-kidney. The posterior division supplies primarily the posterior renal parenchyma, with supplemental supply to the upper and lower poles. The divisional arteries divide into segmental arteries (apical, upper, middle, lower, and posterior), which quickly give rise to the lobar and then interlobar arteries. At the corticomedullary junction, the interlobar arteries divide into the arcuate arteries. The terminal branches of the renal artery are the interlobular arteries, which ultimately supply the glomeruli.

Variations in number, location, and branching patterns of the renal arteries are present in more than 30% of people (Fig. 12-3). These vessels can enter the kidney through the hilum or travel directly to a renal pole (termed *polar artery*) (Table 12-1). Supernumerary renal arteries can arise from the abdominal aorta and iliac (usually common) arteries. Renal artery origins arising above the SMA origin are extremely rare. Congenital anomalies of renal position and configuration are often associated with aberrant locations of renal artery origins and supernumerary vessels. In particular, horseshoe kidney has a 100% incidence of multiple renal arteries. The fused lower poles of a horseshoe kidney, termed the *isthmus*, are trapped under the inferior mesenteric artery as the kidneys ascend out of the pelvis (Fig. 12-4). The isthmus can derive arterial blood supply from the distal aorta and iliac arteries.

The renal pelvis and proximal ureters are supplied by small branches of the segmental and distal main renal arteries. The middle portions of the ureters are supplied by the gonadal arteries (see Fig. 10-1). The distal ureters are supplied by terminal branches of the internal iliac arteries, most notably the cystic artery.

Adrenal Arteries

The adrenal glands are retroperitoneal organs that receive their blood supply from the renal arteries, directly from the aorta, from the inferior phrenic arteries, and rarely from the celiac artery or SMA. There are usually three adrenal arteries; the inferior, middle, and superior (see Fig. 10-1). In many instances these vessels are linked to capsular renal branches, and therefore are potential pathways for collateral blood supply to the kidney.

The inferior adrenal artery arises directly from the proximal renal arteries in two thirds of people. The middle adrenal arteries are small vessels that usually arise directly from the aorta. These arteries are slightly more common on the left than the right. The origins of the middle adrenal arteries may be replaced to the celiac artery or SMA in 2%-5% of patients. The superior adrenal arteries are constant branches of the inferior phrenic arteries. However, the origins of the inferior phrenic arteries are less predictable than their adrenal branches. These arteries arise from the aorta or the celiac artery in two thirds of patients, but may also originate from the renal arteries or the left gastric artery.

KEY COLLATERAL PATHWAYS

The renal arteries are end arteries. In contrast to the colonic and hepatic vasculature, the intrarenal collateral pathways are poorly developed. In the presence of slowly progressive proximal renal artery stenosis, renal capsular, ureteral, adrenal, and other retroperitoneal arteries may enlarge sufficiently to provide enough collateral blood supply to keep the kidney alive, but not functioning normally (Fig. 12-5). Acute proximal occlusion of a previously normal renal artery results in profound ischemia owing to the inadequate preexisting collateral supply.

▬ IMAGING

Renal Arteries

Ultrasound is an excellent modality for imaging renal parenchyma, and for detection of nephrolithiasis, and hydronephrosis.

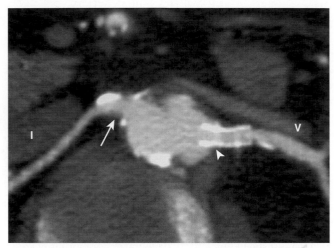

FIGURE 12-1. Thin curved maximum intensity projection of computed tomography angiogram viewed in the axial projection showing the renal arteries. The right renal artery origin *(arrow)* is located slightly anterior on the aorta, while the left *(arrowhead)* is lateral. This helps pick the best angiographic projection to visualize the renal artery origins. There is a patent stent in the left renal artery that protrudes slightly into the aortic lumen. I, Inferior vena cava; V, left renal vein.

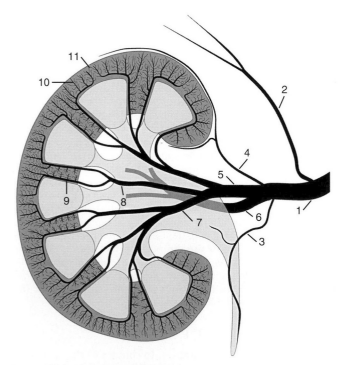

FIGURE 12-2. Drawing of typical renal artery anatomy. *1*, Main renal artery. *2*, Inferior adrenal artery. *3*, Ureteric artery. *4*, Capsular arteries. *5*, Anterior division. *6*, Posterior division. *7*, Segmental artery. *8*, Lobar artery. *9*, Interlobar artery. *10*, Arcuate artery. *11*, Interlobular artery.

The renal size should always be noted. A long axis kidney measurement of less than 8 cm in an adult in the setting of renal artery stenosis suggests a hemodynamically significant and longstanding stenosis. Color-flow duplex ultrasound is required to image the renal arteries. Main renal arteries are reliably depicted in 95% of patients, but the detection of small accessory renal arteries is less accurate. The normal renal artery is a low-resistance vessel, with antegrade flow present throughout the cardiac cycle and a peak systolic velocity less than 180 cm/sec (see Fig. 3-2). Evaluation of Doppler waveforms and velocities is required to identify stenoses in the main and segmental renal arteries (see Renal Artery Occlusive Disease and Fig. 3-3).

The resistive index (RI) has been variably successful in predicting functional outcomes of renal revascularization:

$$RI = (\text{peak systolic velocity} - \text{end diastolic velocity})/ \text{peak systolic velocity}$$

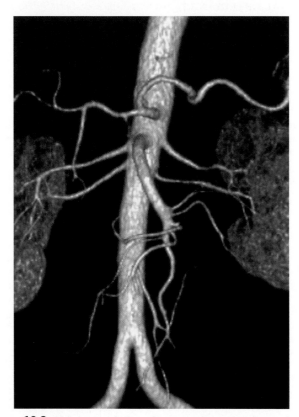

FIGURE 12-3. Volume rendering of computed tomography angiogram showing bilateral accessory renal arteries. Note the close proximity of the upper renal arteries to the superior mesenteric artery origin.

TABLE 12-1 Renal Artery Anatomy

Description	Incidence (%)
Single renal artery bilaterally	55
Proximal bifurcation main renal artery	17
Polar branch directly from aorta	12
Two hilar arteries directly from aorta	12
Three or more hilar arteries directly from aorta	2
Multiple renal arteries, one kidney	32
Multiple renal arteries, both kidneys	10

Measured from the arcuate or interlobar arteries, normal values should be less than 0.7; borderline increased resistance is 0.7-0.8; abnormal resistance is greater than or equal to 0.8. In children, RI of greater than 0.7 may be normal up to age 4 years. In adults, a high RI suggests chronic parenchymal disease that will not improve with revascularization. Blood pressure control response to intervention is not predicted by the RI.

Nuclear medicine studies can provide functional information and infer the presence of occlusive vascular lesions. Occasionally, nuclear medicine studies are obtained in patients with renal masses or nonocclusive vascular lesions to assess renal function.

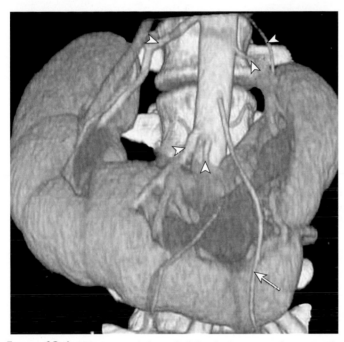

FIGURE 12-4. Volume rendering of abdominal computed tomography angiogram showing a horseshoe kidney with multiple renal arteries *(arrowheads).* Note the inferior mesenteric artery *(arrow)* draped over the isthmus of the kidney.

A number of imaging agents are available, including technetium-99m mercaptoacetyltriglycine (MAG3), and diethylenetriamine-pentaacetate (DTPA). An abnormal study with any of these agents after administration of an angiotensin-converting enzyme inhibitor such as captopril is highly suggestive of proximal renal artery stenosis.

Multidetector computed tomography angiogram (CTA) has a very high sensitivity and specificity for identification of renal arteries and detection of vascular pathology (see Fig. 12-3). A noncontrast scan should be obtained first to evaluate for nephrolithiasis, calcified renal artery lesions, and hyperdense renal masses such as hemorrhagic cysts. A thin-collimation breath-hold contrast-enhanced scan from the diaphragm to the common femoral arteries is required for a complete evaluation of the renal arteries. A good contrast bolus is essential. The celiac artery should be included for patients with suspected renovascular disease as hepatorenal or splenorenal bypasses are potential surgical options for treatment of proximal renal artery occlusive disease. The aorta is evaluated for concomitant occlusive or aneurysmal disease. The iliac arteries are included to detect accessory renal arteries and evaluate for occlusive disease that could impact treatment decisions. The renal parenchyma is inspected carefully for mass lesions. The presence of an adrenal mass in a hypertensive patient should raise the question of a pheochromocytoma or aldosteronoma (Conn disease). When evaluating a patient as a potential donor for renal transplantation, a delayed scan is obtained for venous and collecting system anatomy. Careful postprocessing of the three-dimensional (3-D) volumes improves sensitivity for small accessory vessels

Magnetic resonance imaging (MRI) of patients with renal vascular disease involves both anatomic and flow sequences. In the future, physiologic information will also be obtained during MRI of the kidney. With current techniques, anatomic sequences provide information about renal size and the presence of masses. Contrast-enhanced 3-D sequences provide excellent delineation of the renal vasculature (Fig. 12-6). However, patients with renal insufficiency are at increased risk for nephrogenic systemic sclerosis from the gadolinium (see Chapter 2). Several noncontrast MRA sequences have been developed particularly for patients with renal insufficiency (see Fig. 3-14). MRA is very sensitive and specific for ostial and proximal renal artery pathology (>90% sensitivity

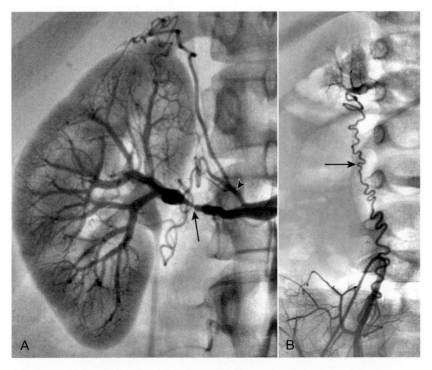

FIGURE 12-5. Renal artery collateral supply. **A,** Selective right renal angiogram of a young patient with hypertension due to fibromuscular dysplasia (probably intimal fibroplasia) *(arrow)* showing prominent capsular and peripelvic collaterals from the inferior adrenal artery *(arrowhead).* **B,** Selective injection of the right hypogastric artery showing retrograde flow in an enlarged ureteric artery *(arrow)* to the distal renal artery in a different child with renal artery stenosis. (Courtesy Frederick Keller, MD, Dotter Interventional Institute, Portland, Ore.)

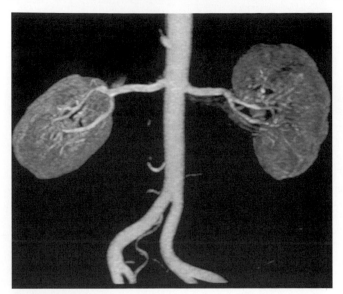

FIGURE 12-6. Coronal maximum intensity projection of a gadolinium-enhanced three-dimensional magnetic resonance angiogram of the abdomen showing normal renal arteries.

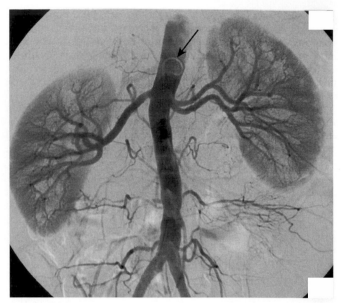

FIGURE 12-7. Digital subtraction angiogram of the abdominal aorta to evaluate the renal arteries. The catheter tip *(arrow)* is just proximal to the renal artery origins, and images are acquired with slight left anterior oblique angulation. With the catheter in this position there is minimal opacification of potentially confusing mesenteric arteries. The field of view includes the proximal iliac arteries. There are two left renal arteries arising adjacent to each other from the aorta.

and specificity for good quality studies). Subtle abnormalities in peripheral arteries, such as mild fibromuscular dysplasia (FMD), can be difficult to image with MRA.

Conventional angiography is usually performed following non-invasive imaging of some type with the specific goal of intervention. Previous studies should be reviewed before the procedure. Conventional angiographic evaluation of the renal arteries begins with an aortogram. The number and location of renal arteries, and the condition of the ostia and proximal renal arteries, can be determined from this study. To perform an aortogram for renal arteries, a pigtail or other catheter designed for high-volume aortic injection is positioned with its tip just at or slightly above the renal arteries (Fig. 12-7). The image intensifier should be positioned in a slight left anterior oblique projection to best visualize the renal artery origins. The most advantageous angle can be determined from review of prior cross-sectional imaging studies. Sufficient contrast injection (15-25 mL/sec for 2 seconds) and rapid filming (3-6 frames/sec) are necessary to obtain optimal images of the proximal renal arteries. The right renal artery can arise in a very anterior position, so that a steep left anterior oblique, or even a lateral view, may be necessary to visualize this ostium. Selective angiography is required to fully evaluate the branches of the renal artery and renal parenchymal masses. When multiple renal arteries are present, the renal parenchyma in the watershed areas between arteries typically has an irregular, indistinct contour on selective angiography (Fig. 12-8).

A wide variety of selective catheters can be used for renal angiography, but the basic choices are a curved selective catheter such as a Cobra-2, Rösch Celiac, or a recurved catheter such as a Sos selective. The curved catheter shape is chosen when the renal artery arises at close to a 90-degree angle from the aorta, whereas a recurved catheter can be used to pull down into a renal artery that arises at an acute angle (see Figs. 2-10 and 2-18 to 2-20). A radial or brachial approach is used to select a renal artery when there is a steep angle of origin, severe infrarenal aortic tortuosity, or aortoiliac occlusion. Injection rates of 5-6 mL/sec for 2-3 seconds provide excellent opacification of intrarenal branches. Rapid filming (3-6 frames/sec) is necessary. Oblique and craniocaudad oblique views are frequently required to optimally display the renal vasculature, but studies must be tailored to each patient. In general, an ipsilateral anterior oblique view presents the kidney enface. Administration of glucagon to reduce artifact from bowel motion on DSA may be helpful in some patients.

Adrenal Arteries

In most cases, the adrenal glands can be evaluated for mass lesions using ultrasound, CT, or MRI. The need to visualize the arterial supply of the adrenals is rare, but the only way is with conventional angiography. The adrenal arteries are too small and variable in location to be reliably evaluated with noninvasive techniques. For the same reasons, selective angiography of the adrenal gland is also difficult. Flush injections of the abdominal aorta, and selective renal and phrenic arterial injections, will aid in identification of the inferior and superior adrenal arteries. The middle adrenal artery, which arises directly from the aorta, can be selected with a recurved catheter. Hand injections of contrast should be used, because rupture of the artery and adrenal infarction can occur. The normal adrenal gland appears as a dense wedged-shaped suprarenal stain.

■ RENAL ARTERY OCCLUSIVE DISEASE

There are many causes of obstructive lesions of the renal artery, but the most common are atherosclerosis (90%) and FMD (Box 12-1). The clinical manifestations of renal artery occlusive disease are hypertension or renal failure, or both. Although it is convenient to separate these clinical presentations for the purposes of discussion, this is not always possible in clinical practice.

The majority (90%-98%) of patients with elevated blood pressure have primary or essential hypertension. No structural lesion can be identified in these patients. Hypertension caused by a renal artery stenosis is on of the causes of *secondary hypertension* and accounts for only 1%-5% of patients with hypertension. Many more patients have renal artery stenosis than have renovascular hypertension; most have some degree of primary hypertension as well. Nevertheless, carefully selected patients may benefit from treatment of the obstructing renal artery lesion. The basic mechanism of hypertension in renal artery stenosis is activation of the renin-angiotensin-aldosterone system (Box 12-2). However, there are likely many other dimensions to this problem. The clinical presentation of patients with symptomatic renal artery stenosis

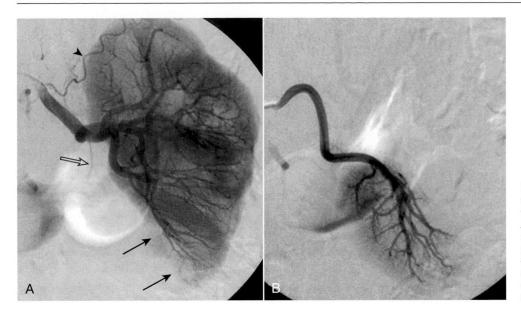

FIGURE 12-8. Selective renal artery digital subtraction angiogram in a patient with an accessory lower pole renal artery. **A,** Selective injection of the main left renal artery shows an indistinct lower pole margin *(arrows)*. Also seen are the capsular artery *(arrowhead)* and ureteric artery *(open arrow)*. **B,** Selective injection of the lower pole accessory renal artery shows the missing segment of the kidney.

Box 12-1. Causes of Renal Artery Stenosis

Atherosclerosis
Fibromuscular dysplasia
Dissection
Vasculitis
Neurofibromatosis
Developmental (abdominal aortic coarctation)
Compression of kidney by mass or hematoma
Iatrogenic

Box 12-2. Renin-Angiotensin-Aldosterone System

Renin (kidney) → Angiotensinogen (liver) → Angiotensin I
→ Angiotensin II (lung) → Increased aldosterone secretion
→ Hypertension

Box 12-3. Clinical Signs of Renovascular Hypertension

Sudden-onset severe hypertension
Sudden increased severity of hypertension
Onset of hypertension younger than 30 or older than
    55 years of age
Hypertension unresponsive to, or poorly controlled by,
    multiple drug therapy
Unexplained advanced renal failure
Renal failure in response to angiotensin-converting enzyme
    inhibitors or angiotensin II-receptor blocking agents
Episodes of recurrent severe unexplained pulmonary
    edema
Unexplained atrophic kidney or long axis size discrepancy
    > 1.5 cm

---

is variable, but in general features severe hypertension that is extremely difficult to control (Box 12-3).

Patients with atherosclerotic renal artery stenoses are usually in their sixth decade or older and are more likely to be male than female. Most patients with renal artery stenoses found at angiography are asymptomatic. Atherosclerotic stenoses are typically located within the first few centimeters of the origin of the renal artery. In most patients the stenosis is at or within 1 cm of the origin of the artery from the aorta (Fig. 12-9). These lesions are caused by aortic plaque encroaching upon the origin of the vessel and are termed *ostial stenoses*. Fewer than 10% of atherosclerotic lesions are truly confined to the renal artery proper (greater than 1 cm from the ostium). These are termed *proximal stenoses* (Fig. 12-10). In patients with severe atherosclerosis or longstanding hypertension, the smaller intrarenal branches may also be diseased (Fig. 12-11). Almost half of patients with atherosclerotic renal artery stenosis also have a stenotic lesion in the opposite renal artery.

Atherosclerotic renal artery disease is a progressive disorder, but predicting outcomes for individual patients is difficult. Approximately half of patients show progression of the degree of stenosis over 5 years, and as many as 12%-20% of stenoses greater than 75% will occlude within 1 year. However, many of these events will be clinically silent.

In contrast to atherosclerosis, hypertension due to renal artery FMD is found in young patients (usually in the third to fifth decade) and more commonly in females. Medial fibroplasia is the pathologic type present in 80% of patients with FMD, particularly in adults (Fig. 12-12; see also Fig. 1-11). The multiple small webs obstruct blood flow, resulting in hypertension. Other forms of FMD result in stenoses in young patients and can be difficult to distinguish from disease such as Takayasu arteritis and neurofibromatosis (see Fig. 4-7). Spontaneous intrarenal dissection is a rare complication of renal artery FMD that presents with acute flank pain, hematuria, and hypertension. Wedge-shaped renal infarcts are seen on CT or MRI, but angiography is often necessary to exclude emboli or vasculitis (Fig. 12-13).

FMD of the medial fibroplasia type is usually located in the distal main renal artery and extends into the first order branches in 25% of patients. About half of patients have bilateral disease, but when the disease is unilateral the right renal artery is involved in more than two thirds. The true rate of progression of FMD is unknown, but about one third of patients have progressive disease. Renal artery aneurysms are found in up to 9% of patients with FMD.

Other vascular causes of renovascular hypertension are less prevalent. Aortic dissection involving the renal artery, vasculitis, neurofibromatosis, and compression of the renal parenchyma by a large subcapsular hematoma can all result in hypertension (see Figs. 10-32 and 10-39). The regional variations in etiologies of renovascular hypertension are striking; in Asia, Takayasu disease is responsible for two thirds of the cases of secondary hypertension, especially in children, whereas FMD is most common in North America and Europe.

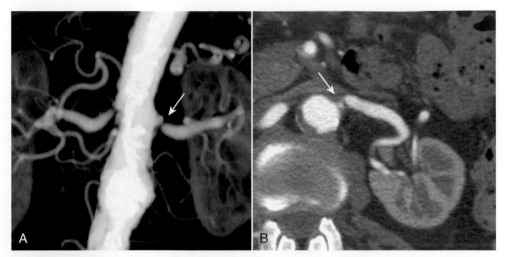

FIGURE **12-9**. Ostial atherosclerotic stenoses of both renal arteries. **A,** Computed tomography (CT) angiogram showing severe bilateral ostial renal artery stenoses. On the left *(arrow),* the stenosis appears to be slightly distal to the renal artery ostium. **B,** Axial image from the same CT at the level of the left renal artery origin showing that the stenosis is caused by aortic wall plaque *(arrow).*

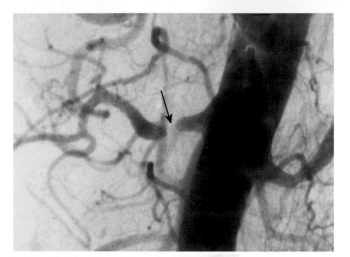

FIGURE **12-10**. Atherosclerotic renal artery stenosis. Aortic injection (digital subtraction angiogram) showing true proximal (>1 cm from the origin) renal artery stenosis *(arrow).* The tiny residual lumen is not seen on this nonselective injection.

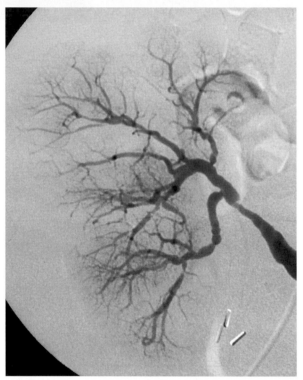

FIGURE **12-11**. Selective right renal digital subtraction angiogram of a transplant kidney showing focal severe stenosis of the main renal artery as well as diffuse disease of the small intrarenal branches and patchy parenchymal enhancement. The kidney had functioned well for 22 years after transplantation.

Renal artery occlusive disease that results in renal insufficiency (ischemic nephropathy) is almost always the result of atherosclerotic plaque. Renal artery obstruction is thought to be the underlying etiology of 8%-10% of patients requiring long-term hemodialysis. Bilateral renal artery stenosis is more likely to result in renal failure than a unilateral lesion, as long as the contralateral kidney is normal. Renal failure due to FMD is unusual, although uncontrolled hypertension can result in nephrosclerosis and renal insufficiency.

The choice of techniques used for diagnosis of renovascular disease is influenced by the clinical history. Children with severe hypertension should undergo careful evaluation for essential hypertension, pheochromocytoma, vasculitis, coarctation, chronic renal parenchymal injury, and other more common causes of elevated blood pressure. Angiography may be necessary to evaluate for subtle abnormalities such as stenotic accessory and intrarenal arteries not detectable with noninvasive imaging. Young adults with normal renal function and suspected renal artery hypertension based on clinical presentation should undergo angiography, because subtle or peripheral FMD can be missed by noninvasive imaging modalities. Furthermore, treatment with balloon angioplasty can be performed at the same time. Adults with suspected renal vascular hypertension should first have at least one noninvasive test before angiography. When carefully performed, color-flow duplex ultrasound can detect renal artery stenosis (>60% reduction in luminal diameter) with roughly 95% sensitivity and specificity. Multiple criteria exist for interpretation of duplex data, with no clear superiority of one over the other (Table 12-2). An RI less than 0.8 is predictive of a positive outcome with renal revascularization when performed for renal insufficiency, but it has little impact on hypertensive response.

Both MRA and CTA have excellent sensitivity and specificity for detection of ostial and proximal renal artery stenosis (>90% in each category). Reduction in luminal diameter greater than 75%, post-stenotic dilatation, and decrease in renal mass are indicative of hemodynamically significant disease. These techniques allow evaluation of the artery in multiple planes, a distinct advantage over conventional angiography (see Fig. 12-9). The

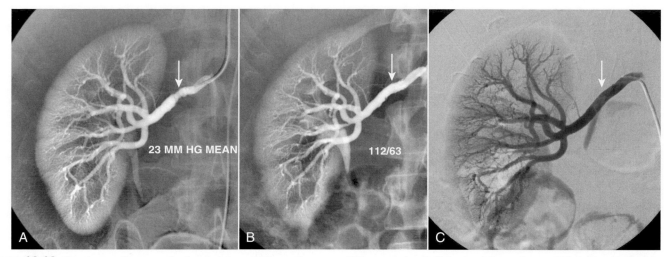

FIGURE 12-12. Renal artery fibromuscular dysplasia in a middle-aged woman with hypertension. **A,** Selective right renal artery digital subtraction angiogram showing irregular beaded appearance *(arrow)* of medial fibroplasia in the proximal right renal artery. There was a 23-mm Hg gradient across this lesion. **B,** Angiogram after angioplasty with a 6-mm diameter balloon. The artery has a normal diameter with typical postangioplasty irregularity of the intima *(arrow).* **C,** Selective angiogram obtained 4 years later shows a normal-appearing right renal artery *(arrow).*

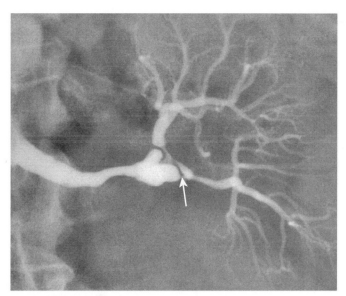

FIGURE 12-13. Selective renal angiogram of a middle-aged man with acute onset of left flank pain showing spontaneous intrarenal dissection *(arrow)* typical of fibromuscular dysplasia. The aorta was normal.

TABLE 12-2 Duplex Criteria (Main Renal Artery) for Renal Artery Stenosis

Stenosis	Renal Artery PSV (cm/s)	Renal Artery PSV/Aortic PSV
0%	<180	<3.5
<60%	≥180	<3.5
≥60%	≥180	≥3.5
100%	0	NA

PSV, Peak systolic velocity; NA, not applicable owing to renal artery PSV of 0 cm/sec.

reliable evaluation of small accessory renal arteries and intrarenal branches is not possible yet with these techniques. In patients with normal renal function, captopril scintigraphy has similar sensitivity and specificity but does not provide sufficient anatomic information for planning a procedure.

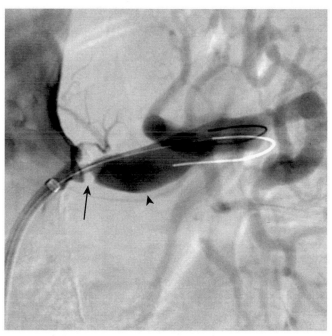

FIGURE 12-14. Angiographic signs of hemodynamically significant renal artery stenosis include luminal narrowing *(arrow)* and post-stenotic dilation *(arrowhead).* This is the same patient as in Figure 12-9.

The angiographic diagnosis of renal artery stenosis is suggested by the degree of luminal narrowing (50%-75%), post-stenotic dilatation, slow flow distal to the lesion, presence of collateral circulation, and decreased renal mass (Fig. 12-14). Delayed filming may be necessary to visualize a reconstituted artery distal to a proximal occlusion (Fig. 12-15). The location of the lesion (ostial or proximal) should be carefully determined, as should the extent of the disease. One of the greatest advantages of angiography is the ability to measure pressure gradients across stenoses. A mean systolic pressure gradient greater than 10 mm Hg or peak systolic gradient greater than 20 mm Hg between the aorta and the renal artery distal to the lesion is suggestive of a hemodynamically significant stenosis. Generally the larger the gradient, the more confident one can be that treating the stenosis will benefit the patient. However, a catheter through a moderate lesion in a small artery may further decrease the cross-sectional area of the lumen

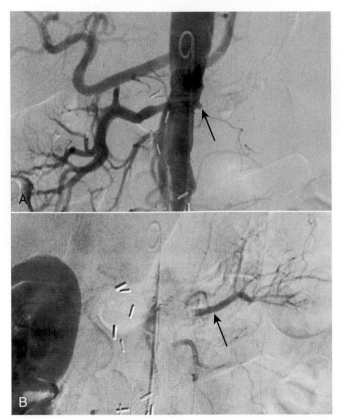

FIGURE 12-15. Delayed opacification of renal artery distal to an occluded stent. **A,** Digital subtraction angiogram of the aorta shows the stump of the occluded left renal artery *(arrow)*. **B,** Late image from the same injection shows the distal renal artery reconstituted *(arrow)* through small retroperitoneal branches.

---

and induce a pressure gradient. Low-profile pressure-sensing guidewires may be useful in this situation. Borderline gradients require careful assessment before treatment, including close correlation with the patient's clinical presentation.

Sampling of the renin directly from the renal veins is occasionally helpful to establish the diagnosis of renal vascular hypertension and identify which kidney is responsible. A curved selective catheter (e.g., Cobra-2) or a straight catheter with a tip deflecting wire can be used. A single side hole should be punched near the tip of the catheter. Blood samples are obtained from each renal vein, and from the IVC above and below the renal veins. On the left, the catheter tip should be lateral to the orifice of the left gonadal vein. Samples need not be simultaneous, but they should be collected within a short period of time. Renin levels from one kidney that are at least 1.5 times that of the contralateral kidney are indicative of renovascular hypertension. A rise in renin between the infrarenal and suprarenal IVC is further evidence of renovascular hypertension. When multiple renal veins are present, samples should be obtained from each vein.

The indications for intervention in renal artery stenosis differ slightly for hypertension and ischemic nephropathy (Box 12-4). All symptomatic lesions that cannot be managed medically require intervention in patients with reasonable life expectancies. Asymptomatic lesions are generally not treated unless the kidney is solitary.

There are numerous surgical options for revascularization of the renal arteries (Box 12-5). Ostial and proximal atherosclerotic renal artery lesions are easier to deal with than distal main or segmental artery lesions. The overall mortality for surgical intervention is approximately 4%, with hypertension cured in 18%, improved in 71%, and unchanged or worse in 11%. In patients with renal failure, improvement can be expected in 50% of patients, no change is seen in 39%, and in 11%, the condition deteriorates.

Box 12-4. Indications for Intervention in Renal Artery Stenosis

Severe hypertension* with:
    Unilateral or bilateral renal artery stenosis
    Mean pressure gradient >10 mm Hg or peak systolic
      gradient > 20 mm Hg
    Atherosclerosis, fibromuscular dysplasia, Takayasu disease,
      dissection
Renal failure with:
    No other explanation for severe azotemia
    Bilateral stenosis†
    Mean pressure gradient >10 mm Hg or peak systolic
      gradient > 20 mm Hg
    Atherosclerosis, dissection

*See Box 12-3 for signs of hypertension likely due to renal artery disease.
†Unilateral renal artery stenosis is unlikely to cause renal failure when the contralateral kidney is normal.

Box 12-5. Surgical Approaches for Renal Artery Stenosis

Aortorenal bypass
Hepatorenal bypass (right kidney)
Splenorenal bypass (left kidney)
Aortorenal endarterectomy
Ileorenal bypass
Autotransplantation to pelvis
Nephrectomy

Angioplasty and stent placement are the techniques used most often in treatment of obstructive lesions of the renal artery. Atherosclerotic lesions are almost always managed with a stent, whereas FMD almost always responds to angioplasty alone. These procedures should be approached in a careful, planned manner, as they can be among the most difficult arterial interventions. Patients scheduled for renal artery intervention for hypertension should stop or decrease long-acting antihypertensive medications before the procedure if possible. Successful angioplasty or stent placement may lead to profound hypotension when drug effects persist after acute renal revascularization. Patients should be instructed to drink fluids until 2 hours before the procedure, at which time intravenous fluids should be initiated at a brisk pace. Some interventionalists administer a calcium-channel blocking agent before the procedure to prevent vasospasm. Patients with preexisting renal failure can be treated beforehand with a renal protective strategy (see Table 2-7). An aortogram should be obtained in all cases; CO_2 gas can be used in patients with azotemia. Once the decision to intervene is made, syringes containing heparin (1000 U/mL) and nitroglycerin (100 µg/mL) are placed on the angiography table. A long curved 6- or 7-French sheath, or a 7- or 8-French curved guiding catheter, is inserted. The curve of the sheath or guide catheter is selected to match the angle of the renal artery as it arises from the aorta (see Fig. 2-18). Manipulation in the aorta should be minimized to decrease the risk of cholesterol embolization. Heparin (5000-10,000 units) is administered before selecting the renal artery. For ostial lesions, the image intensifier is angled to display the renal artery ostium in profile. A selective 5-French catheter appropriate for the configuration of the renal artery is used to find the renal artery origin. A gentle puff of contrast confirms catheter position. Ostial lesions are gently probed with an atraumatic but steerable guidewire. Extremely tight ostial lesions can sometimes only be crossed with microwires. When using a pull-down catheter, leading with 1-2 cm of a Bentson guidewire minimizes the risk of subintimal dissection.

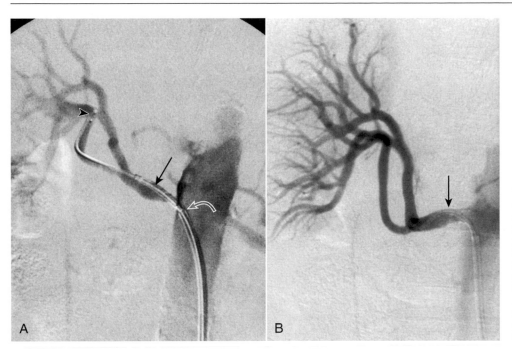

FIGURE 12-16. Guidewire straightening of a renal artery during stent placement. **A,** Control digital subtraction angiogram (DSA) obtained through the sheath *(curved arrow)* while positioning a balloon-mounted stent *(arrow)* across the ostial renal artery stenosis. A Rosen guidewire is in the posterior division *(arrowhead)*. **B,** DSA after stent deployment and removal of the guidewire. Note the change in angle of the main renal artery *(arrow)* relative to the aorta compared to the previous image.

Once the selective guidewire has crossed the lesion, the catheter is advanced until it, too, has crossed the lesion. The guidewire is removed, blood is aspirated, and a small amount of contrast is injected, followed by 100-200 μg of nitroglycerin. When there is complete stasis of the intrarenal branches due to obturation of the lesion by the catheter, additional heparin can be delivered directly into the renal artery. A working wire is then carefully inserted. A moderately stiff 0.035-inch guidewire with a short straight floppy tip, or 0.014-0.018-inch stiff guidewires with short soft platinum tips are preferred by the author. J-tipped guidewires are more likely to induce spasm or cause dissection of intrarenal branches. A stiff guidewire can change the angle of the renal artery, facilitating the procedure (Fig. 12-16). Careful control of guidewires at all times is critical, because straight-tipped guidewires can perforate the kidney.

Embolic protective devices can be used in patients with suitable anatomy and lesions (see Fig. 4-19). A dedicated renal artery protection device is not currently available. The evidence supporting the benefit of renal protection is evolving at this point, but enthusiasm is great.

The guiding catheter or sheath should be brought as close as possible to the renal artery ostium to provide added stability to the system. In addition, contrast can be injected through the sheath or guiding catheter to monitor the progress of the procedure (see Figs. 12-14 and 12-16). Ostial lesions almost always require stent placement, because the stenosis is caused by aortic rather than renal artery plaque. Predilatation with an undersized balloon facilitates positioning of stents when the lesion is very tight or irregular. Stents mounted on 0.018-inch or smaller systems have a low crossing profile and can often be advanced "bare-back" through the lesion. Sometimes the sheath or guiding catheter must be advanced through the lesion to facilitate positioning of the stent.

The ideal stent design for renal artery ostia has not been determined, but most often a balloon-expandable stent is used. Whether bare or covered stents provide superior results is unknown. Typical diameters for renal artery ostia are 5-7 mm. Stent lengths are usually 1.2-2 cm. The stent should be deployed so that it protrudes into the aorta a few millimeters to ensure adequate displacement of the aortic plaque (Fig. 12-17; see also Figs. 12-1 and 3-19). "Flaring" the aortic end of the stent with a slightly larger balloon is cosmetically appealing but of unproven benefit.

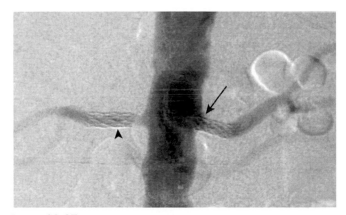

FIGURE 12-17. Proper and improper stent positioning. Digital subtraction angiography after bilateral renal artery stent placement shows excellent position on the left with slight protrusion into the aortic lumen *(arrow)*. The stent on the right ends within the renal artery *(arrowhead)*. To completely cover the lesion, this stent should also extend to the aortic lumen.

Proximal renal artery atherosclerotic lesions (i.e., those that are located more than 1 cm from the aortic lumen) respond well to angioplasty alone, but in practice are now routinely stented. All of the same precautions described for intervention in ostial lesions should be exercised. A large branch in the vicinity of the stenosis can be protected by placing a 0.018-inch guidewire through the sheath or guiding catheter alongside the working wire and into the branch during the angioplasty. When the lesion occurs at a bifurcation of the renal artery, kissing balloons or stents may be necessary (Fig. 12-18).

Drug-eluting stents can be used when treating smaller (≤3.5 mm) renal arteries such as accessory or segmental arteries. Data supporting this practice have yet to be developed, but bare stents in renal arteries less than 5 mm in diameter have poor long-term patency.

Renal artery FMD of the medial fibroplasia type responds well to simple angioplasty with excellent long-term results (see Fig. 12-12). Best results occur in patients younger than 50 years of age with duration of hypertension less than 8 years and no evidence of

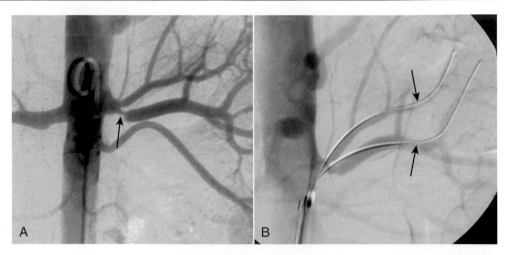

Figure 12-18. Early bifurcation of the left main renal artery with a proximal stenosis of the lower branch in a young patient with hypertension. **A,** Digital subtraction aortogram before angioplasty showing the proximal renal artery stenosis *(arrow)* that begins at the bifurcation of the renal artery. **B,** Aortic injection after angioplasty of the stenosis using the kissing technique (a small protective balloon in the upper artery and a 5-mm diameter balloon in the lower artery) showing the placement of the guidewires *(arrows).*

Table 12-3 Complications of Renal Artery Angioplasty and Stents

Complication	Incidence (%)
Death (30 days)	0.5
Renal artery rupture	<1
Renal artery thrombosis	<1
Cholesterol embolization (systemic)	1
Branch artery occlusion	3
Flow-limiting dissection	5
Renal failure	5
Puncture site*	5
Stent infection	Anecdotal

*Hematoma, pseudoaneurysm.

peripheral arterial disease. The technical success rate is approximately 90%, with one third to one half of patients experiencing a cure (i.e., normalization of blood pressure), about one third experience improved blood pressure control with medications, and up to 15%-20% experience no change. Restenosis occurs in up to 20% and should undergo repeat angioplasty. Stents are rarely necessary in treatment of the medial fibroplasia form of FMD. There is less experience with other forms of FMD, but these lesions tend to be more fibrotic and elastic.

Involvement of intrarenal branches commonly occurs with FMD, increasing the complexity of the procedure. However, because FMD tends to be found in young patients with normal iliac arteries and aortas, some of the technical aspects of the procedure can be less demanding than with atherosclerotic renal artery stenosis. FMD of segmental and smaller renal artery branches requires small-diameter balloons and 0.18-inch or smaller guidewires.

Renal angioplasty and stent placement is a challenging procedure owing to the types and locations of lesions, the size of the vessels, and the angles between the aorta and the renal arteries. In addition, renal arteries are deep in the body, move with respiration, are poorly collateralized, and supply an organ that does not tolerate acute ischemia well. In general, complications occur more frequently with stent placement (15% of patients) than with angioplasty alone (5%-10% of patients) (Table 12-3). The lowest complication rates occur with angioplasty for FMD, and the highest occur with stent placement in patients with diffuse aortic and renal

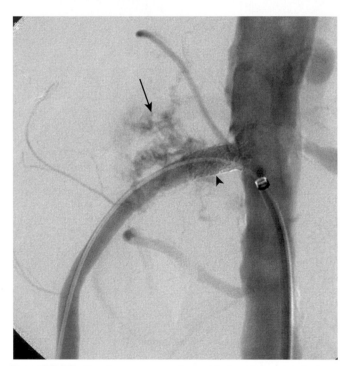

Figure 12-19. Renal artery rupture *(arrow)* during placement of a 6-mm diameter stent *(arrowhead)* in a hypertensive older woman. This is a very rare complication, probably due to oversizing of the stent for this particular patient. After stent deployment the patient was hemodynamically stable and pain free; the rupture was only discovered on the completion angiogram. Note that the guidewire had been left in place until the final angiogram was obtained, allowing for quick placement of a covered stent.

artery atherosclerosis. The most severe complication, renal artery rupture, is minimized when balloon sizes are carefully selected. Prompt recognition with reinflation of a balloon across the rupture is life-saving (Fig. 12-19). Once stabilized, either stent-graft placement or surgery can be considered. Complications may occur at any point during renal artery revascularization from balloons, stents, and even guidewires (Fig. 12-20). For this reason, meticulous attention to detail and technique is required throughout the procedure. Bilateral lesions, particularly in azotemic patients, can be treated several days apart to minimize contrast load.

Renal artery interventions for atherosclerotic disease causing hypertension and/or azotemia have different goals. In hypertension, improvement is proportional to the baseline systolic pressure. A performance goal of 10-15 mm Hg reduction for pretreatment systolic pressures of 155-180 mm Hg, or a target of 165 mm Hg

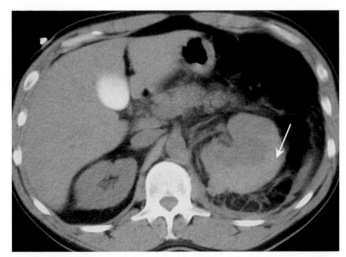

FIGURE 12-20. Renal capsular hematoma *(arrow)* presumably due to guidewire perforation of the kidney during angioplasty (same patient as in Fig. 12-18). The patient developed flank pain several hours after the angioplasty.

for pretreatment systolic pressures greater than 180 mm Hg have been suggested for renal artery stents. Reduction in the number of medications required to maintain blood pressure control is also an indicator of clinical success. For patients treated for advanced renal failure due to atherosclerotic renal artery stenosis, stabilization of improvement of renal function is considered a success. In this population, a low RI may predict a good clinical result with intervention.

There have been several large prospective trials of renal artery interventions in atherosclerotic disease. The Dutch Renal Artery Stenosis Intervention Cooperative (DRASTIC) study compared angioplasty to medical therapy for hypertension. The study has been criticized for a high crossover rate (medical therapy to angioplasty), but showed more sustained blood pressure control and fewer renal artery occlusions at 12 months in the angioplasty patients. The Stent Placement in Patients with Atherosclerotic Renal Artery Stenosis and Impaired Renal Function (STAR) trial randomized patients with creatinine clearances less than 80 mL/min/m² and well-controlled blood pressure to medical therapy or medical therapy plus stents. Stent placement did not lead to improved outcomes, but the study was underpowered; one third of the patients had stenosis less than or equal to 70%, and more than half had unilateral disease. The Angioplasty and Stenting for Renal Artery Lesions (ASTRAL) trial was much larger (806 vs. 140 patients), and randomized patients to medical therapy or medical therapy plus catheter-based intervention. The primary outcome was renal function, whereas blood pressure control was a secondary endpoint. The study failed to show improved renal preservation or blood pressure control with renal artery stents, and there was increased morbidity in the intervention group due to procedural complications. However, this study also has limitations in that 41% of patients had stenosis less than or equal to 70%, patients whom referring clinicians wanted treated with stents were not enrolled, and procedural success rates were low (82%). The Cardiovascular Outcomes in Renal Atherosclerotic Lesions (CORAL) trial has completed enrollment of 1080 patients randomized to best medical therapy or stenting plus best medical therapy. Results are pending.

The results of these and other studies underscore the importance of careful patient selection for renal artery interventions for hypertension or renal function. In patients with hypertension, renal artery stent placement for atherosclerotic lesions has a high technical success rate, but the hypertension is rarely cured (Table 12-4). Approximately two thirds of properly selected patients should experience improved blood pressures with or

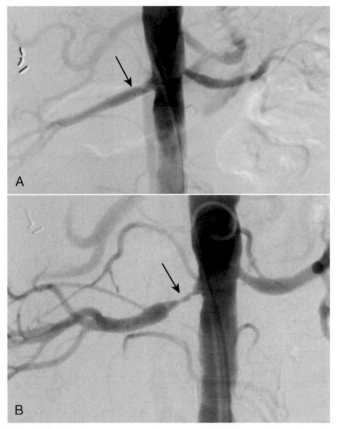

FIGURE 12-21. Recurrent stenosis of a renal artery stent due to intimal hyperplasia in a patient with hypertension. **A,** Digital subtraction angiogram (DSA) after right renal artery stent placement *(arrow)* shows an excellent result. The patient had an excellent clinical response. **B,** DSA 6 months later, when the patient returned for evaluation of worsening hypertension, shows diffuse intimal hyperplasia causing stenosis within the stent *(arrow)*. This was treated by placement of a second stent inside the first.

without fewer medications. About one third will not respond, and in up to 5%, the condition will worsen. The restenosis rate of stents is about 15% at 12 months.

Angioplasty and stent placement for renal insufficiency have similar technical success rates as procedures performed for hypertension, but lower overall success rates. In patients with atherosclerotic lesions, normalization of serum creatinine is the exception, with stabilization of renal function seen in approximately half of patients, mild improvement in about 20%, and continued deterioration in the remainder. The best clinical outcomes are in patients with rapidly deteriorating renal function, bilateral proximal stenoses, serum creatinine less than 3.0 mg/dL, normal sized kidneys, and few comorbid diseases. The reasons for the less impressive results in treatment of azotemia compared to hypertension are multifactorial and may include procedural cholesterol embolization, preexisting irreversible renal parenchymal disease, and the influence of comorbid medical conditions. Distal protection devices may have a role in renal artery interventions in these patients.

Intimal hyperplasia resulting in restenosis remains a major limitation of all renal artery interventions (percutaneous as well as surgical) (Fig. 12-21). Some degree of hyperplasia occurs after every intervention; therefore, the larger the initial postprocedural lumen, the better the long-term patency. When placing stents, the long-term results are best when the final diameter of the artery is 6 mm or more. Covered stents, drug-eluting stents, and brachytherapy, are all being investigated to improve the outcomes of renal artery revascularization.

TABLE 12-4 Results of Renal Artery Revascularization for Hypertension

Lesion	Technical Success (%)	Primary Clinical Success (%)*
Atherosclerosis (angioplasty)	85	60
Atherosclerosis (stent)	95	70
Fibromuscular dysplasia[†] (angioplasty)	90	85
Takayasu arteritis	85	85[‡]

*Hypertension improved at 12 months.
[†]Primarily medial fibroplasia type.
[‡]Limited number of patients.

RENAL DENERVATION FOR HYPERTENSION

The renal sympathetic system consists of efferent fibers that stimulate sodium reabsorption, renin release, and renal vascular smooth muscle contraction. The afferent fibers help sense renal injury (e.g., ischemia) and signal the hypothalamus, which then communicates to the kidney through the efferent fibers. Both sets of fibers form a network around the renal arteries within the adventitia.

Approximately 5%-7% of patients with hypertension have resistant hypertension; that is, failure to achieve a blood pressure less than 140/90 mm Hg in nondiabetic patients and 130/80 mm Hg in diabetic patients despite optimal three-drug therapy. When anatomic etiologies and other causes of severe hypertension such as primary aldosteronism have been excluded, sympathectomy may be considered.

Surgical sympathectomy for control of severe hypertension was performed between 1930 and the 1960s. Developed in an era before effective oral antihypertensive agents, it controlled blood pressure in 50% of patients. The procedure was associated with major morbidity (e.g., severe orthostatic hypotension and incontinence) and an operative mortality of 5%, leading to rapid abandonment once medications became available. Technologies that allow less invasive approaches to renal denervation have been developed, and there is renewed interest in this strategy for the treatment of resistant hypertension.

The new techniques for renal denervation disrupt the sympathetic plexus around the renal artery using imaging to guide the application of an ablative energy. For example, radiofrequency (RF) energy can be applied to the sympathetic plexus from the renal artery lumen using a dedicated RF catheter (Fig. 12-22). A curved guiding catheter at the renal ostium allows a steerable probe to be inserted into the renal artery. The tip is deflected against the intima for the treatments. With this device, the artery is treated in four to six locations between the renal artery bifurcation and the ostium in a spiral pattern to ensure circumferential interruption of the sympathetic nerve plexus. The patient is anticoagulated during the procedure, and requires analgesia because each RF activation is painful. Using current probes, the minimal length of normal renal artery is 2 cm, and ideally the patient has a single renal artery at least 4 mm in diameter. Patients with prior renal artery interventions or a single kidney have not been included in the studies published to date. Complication rates are low and include renal artery dissection and thrombosis. Other devices, such as a balloon-based RF delivery catheter or a high energy focused US approach, may expand the anatomic criteria for treatment.

The results of the two studies (Symplicity HTN1 and HTN2, using the Symplicity catheter, Medtronic, Mountain View, Calif.) have demonstrated that 84% of patients treated had a decrease in systolic blood pressure of at least 10 mm Hg. A target systolic blood pressure less than 140 mm Hg was achieved in 39% of treated patients compared to 6% of controls. Remarkably, these benefits appear to be sustained and to continue to improve over

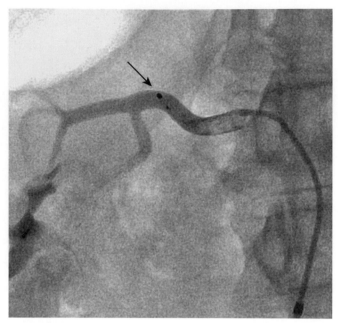

FIGURE 12-22. Renal denervation with a radiofrequency probe in a patient with refractory hypertension and normal renal arteries. The steerable probe is deflected against the wall of the renal artery prior to the ablation. A total of four to six treatments in different locations create a circumferential disruption of the adventitial sympathetic fibers (Courtesy Krishna Rocha-Singh, MD, Springfield, Ill.)

Box 12-6. Etiologies of Acute Renal Artery Occlusion

Embolus (cardiogenic)
Trauma
Aortic dissection
Spontaneous renal artery dissection
Iatrogenic
Hypercoagulable state
Thrombosis of existing stenosis
Thrombosis of renal artery aneurysm

---

time. In 10% of patients there was no response, and all patients continued to require medications. The long-term blood pressure control and the potential for late complications such as renal artery stenosis are not known.

ACUTE RENAL ISCHEMIA

The normal kidney with normal vasculature has no collateral blood supply of clinical relevance. Acute occlusion of a normal main renal artery results in an ischemic kidney that must be revascularized within 30 minutes in order to preserve substantial function ("warm ischemic time"). After that, recovery of renal function is time dependent, dropping rapidly for every additional minute of occlusion, such that after 90-120 minutes little function can be salvaged. The most common etiology of acute occlusion in older patients is an embolus from a cardiac source, whereas trauma is usually the cause in young patients (Box 12-6). Patients may complain of back pain, nausea, hematuria, and vomiting.

Thrombosis of a chronic hemodynamically significant renal artery stenosis rarely results in immediate loss of the kidney. In most cases, adequate collateral supply for renal preservation develops before the occlusive event. Renal artery occlusion in these patients is frequently clinically silent, but may manifest as sudden worsening of hypertension.

The short warm ischemia time for kidneys precludes successful revascularization unless the patient happens to be undergoing

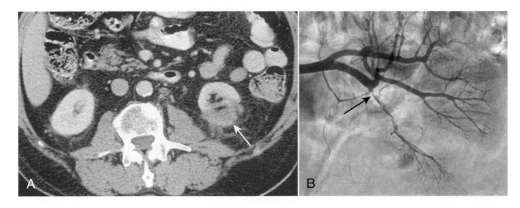

FIGURE 12-23. Focal renal infarction due to a small cardiac embolus. **A,** Axial computed tomography image with contrast showing a focal area of inhomogeneous enhancement *(arrow)* with associated perinephric stranding in an older patient who had acute onset of left flank pain several days earlier. **B,** Selective left renal artery digital subtraction angiogram showing a partially recanalized peripheral embolus *(arrow)*.

Box 12-7. **Etiologies of Renal Artery Aneurysms**

Fibromuscular dysplasia
Degenerative
Idiopathic
- Vasculitis
- Polyarteritis nodosa (small arteries)
- Behçet disease (large arteries)
Neoplasm (angiomyolipoma)
Trauma
Mycotic
Ehlers-Danlos syndrome
Iatrogenic (i.e., after biopsy, angioplasty)

---

surgery or angiography at the moment of occlusion. Nuclear medicine scans can be used to determine kidney perfusion in cases of suspected renal artery occlusion, but do not provide anatomic information. CT or MRI with contrast allows inspection of the aorta and main renal artery, renal parenchyma, and adjacent soft tissue structures. Focal areas of abnormal perfusion may be seen in patients with peripheral arterial emboli or main renal artery occlusion with patent accessory renal arteries (Fig. 12-23). CTA or MRA sequences may reveal aortic or renal artery dissection, evidence of multiple acute occlusions suggestive of emboli, or other structural abnormalities such as a renal artery aneurysm. At angiography, delayed filming well into the venous phase for both aortic injections and selective renal artery injections is necessary to detect distal reconstitution of the renal artery by collaterals (see Fig. 12-15). In cases of suspected embolic occlusion, both kidneys must be evaluated with selective injections, because bilateral renal artery emboli are found in almost a third of patients.

The management of acute renal artery occlusion depends on the etiology and timing. Occlusion due to dissection during angioplasty can be managed with stents if the true lumen can be entered distal to the dissection. Similarly, thrombosis during an intervention should be pursued aggressively with thrombolysis, mechanical displacement, or aspiration thrombectomy. Surgical revascularization may be necessary to avoid loss of the kidney.

▬ RENAL ARTERY ANEURYSMS

Renal artery aneurysms are rare lesions, found in approximately 0.1% of patients undergoing angiography (Box 12-7). Nonspecific "degenerative" and FMD-related aneurysms are typically located at extraparenchymal locations and bifurcations of first and second order renal artery branches in 90% of patients (Fig. 12-24). Aneurysms due to vasculitis (e.g., polyarteritis nodosa) or hematogenously disseminated infection occur in the peripheral intraparenchymal renal artery branches (see Fig. 1-15).

Degenerative aneurysms are symptomatic in fewer than 10% of patients, and fewer than 5% rupture (Fig. 12-25). The risk of

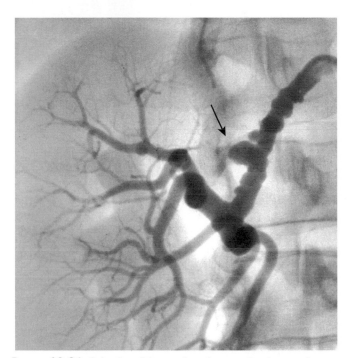

FIGURE 12-24. Selective right renal angiogram showing renal artery aneurysm *(arrow)* due to fibromuscular dysplasia (medial fibroplasia).

rupture is increased in pregnant patients and when the diameter of the aneurysm is 2 cm or greater. Although not substantiated, calcification of the aneurysm wall is believed to be somewhat protective. Rupture is associated with 10% mortality in nonpregnant patients and 55% in pregnant patients. Other complications of renal artery aneurysms include spontaneous dissection, renal infarction due to emboli, hypertension due to compression of the renal artery, flank pain, and spontaneous arteriovenous fistula.

Large renal artery aneurysms may be detected by any of the cross-sectional imaging modalities. CT and MRI allow assessment of the size of the aneurysm, presence of mural thrombus, and renal infarcts. Calcification of the aneurysm wall is believed to be a secondary rather than primary process. The other visceral arteries should be carefully inspected, because multiple aneurysms are present in some cases. Small and intraparenchymal renal artery aneurysms require angiography for definitive diagnosis. Angiography may also reveal characteristic findings of FMD.

The indications for treatment of these rare and usually asymptomatic lesions must be individualized for each patient (Box 12-8). The traditional approach to extraparenchymal aneurysms is surgical reconstruction, sometimes requiring removal of the kidney, repair of the aneurysm, and then autotransplantation. Endovascular techniques are advantageous because they are associated with less morbidity than a major reconstructive surgery is. Aneurysms

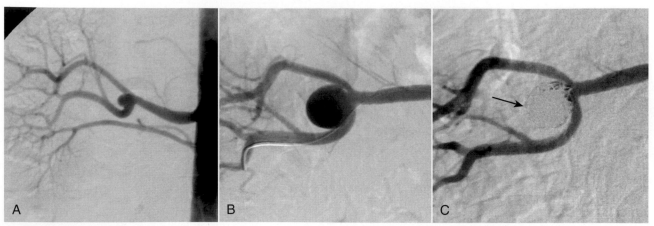

Figure 12-25. Degenerative renal artery aneurysm. **A,** Aortogram showing a small aneurysm at the bifurcation of the main right renal artery. There is an accessory lower pole artery as well. **B,** Selective right renal angiogram 9 years later showing a dramatic increase in size of the aneurysm. **C,** Selective right renal angiogram after placing a stent from the main renal artery into the larger of the two divisional arteries and packing of the aneurysm with coils *(arrow)*.

Box 12-8. **Indications for Intervention in Renal Artery Aneurysms**

Rupture
Size ≥ 2 cm
Renovascular hypertension
Expansion
Distal embolization
Symptomatic dissection
Flank pain
Woman of childbearing age/pregnancy

---

with narrow necks can be treated with the same techniques used for intracranial aneurysms, using detachable coils and sometimes bridging stents across the mouth of the aneurysm (see Fig. 12-25). When there is suitable length of normal artery on both sides of the aneurysm, a small stent-graft can be used. Aneurysms at branch points are more challenging, in that preservation of all of the branches may not be possible. Sacrifice of a small branch may be acceptable to achieve a successful percutaneous treatment. Ruptured intraparenchymal aneurysms can be coil-embolized to avoid nephrectomy. Intact intraparenchymal aneurysms due to a systemic disease are managed with control of the underlying disease process or nephrectomy.

NEOPLASM

A broad range of benign and malignant neoplasms can occur in the kidney (Tables 12-5 and 12-6). The role of vascular imaging for diagnosis of renal masses is limited, because cross-sectional imaging with ultrasound, CT, and MRI can detect and characterize most lesions. A detailed discussion of the diagnostic features of renal masses is beyond the scope of this chapter. However, certain characteristic features are important to remember. Venous invasion by any renal mass is highly indicative of malignancy, particularly renal cell carcinoma (RCC), although intravenous extension of angiomyolipoma (AML) has been reported. Venous invasion can be mimicked by inflow of unopacified blood from hepatic veins on CT; delayed images may be helpful to resolve this issue. Invasion of adjacent structures by a mass represents presumptive evidence of malignancy until proven otherwise.

Angiography is usually performed for intervention. An aortogram followed by selective injection of the renal arteries is required for complete staging of the arterial supply. Renal tumors can parasitize arterial supply from the renal capsule, renal collecting system, retroperitoneum, bowel, spleen, pancreas, and liver.

TABLE 12-5 Benign Renal Neoplasms

Lesion	Angiographic Appearance
Angiomyolipoma	Neovascularity, bizarre aneurysms, no shunting
Oncocytoma	Hypervascular mass, spoke-wheel appearance of arteries, central scar, no shunting
Metanephric adenoma	Hypovascular, may have calcifications

TABLE 12-6 Malignant Renal Neoplasms

Lesion	Angiographic Appearance
Renal cell carcinoma	Variable, but most often prominent neovascularity*, mass effect, hypervascularity, shunting, ± venous invasion
Transitional cell carcinoma	Neovascularity, mild hypervascularity, encasement, shunting unusual
Wilms tumor	Hypovascular or avascular mass, mild neovascularity, displacement, encasement
Lymphoma	Avascular mass, displacement of intrarenal branches
Metastatic carcinoma	Hypervascular (melanoma, sarcoma) or avascular (lung, breast, bowel)

*Avascular in 6%.

Selective injection of the arterial supply of these structures may be necessary. Occasionally, injection of 6-10 μg of epinephrine in the renal artery prior to contrast injection is used to constrict normal vessels so that the abnormal tumor vessels will be more evident. Occasionally IVC cavography and selective renal venography are performed to exclude the presence of venous invasion.

When the origin of a retroperitoneal tumor is uncertain from cross-sectional imaging, diagnostic angiography may be useful. Selective injection of renal and other visceral arteries can help identify the dominant arterial blood supply, and thus the organ of origin (see Fig. 1-26).

Angiomyolipoma

Angiomyolipomas (AML) are benign hamartomatous lesions that contain fat, smooth muscle, and blood vessels (Fig. 12-26). Patients

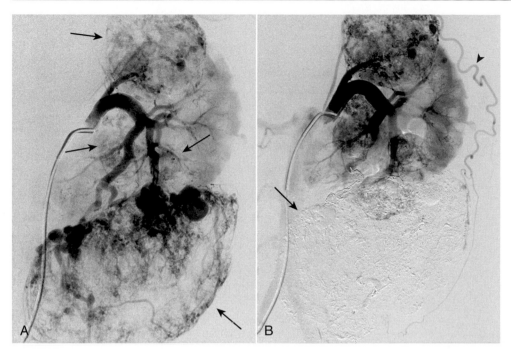

FIGURE 12-26. Multiple renal angiomyolipomas (AML) in a patient with tuberous sclerosis syndrome and prior spontaneous hemorrhage. His renal function was normal. **A,** Selective left renal angiogram showing multiple hypervascular masses within the kidney *(arrows)*. Note the enlarged main renal artery. The hypervascularity with aneurysms is typical for AML. The right kidney was similarly involved. **B,** The same patient after embolization of the giant lower pole AML with dehydrated alcohol mixed with lipiodol *(arrow)*, followed by a few coils in the largest feeding arteries. Visualization of the other AMLs and the renal parenchyma is improved after the giant lesion has been embolized. The enlarged capsular artery *(arrowhead)* was embolized after this image was obtained.

may be asymptomatic, or present with chronic pain, renal dysfunction (due to mass effect on normal tissue), and acute hemorrhage. When single, these are most often sporadic lesions; when bilateral, there is an 80%-90% correlation with tuberous sclerosis. Sporadic AML tends to occur in older patients (mean age 52 years), are single in 87% of patients, average 5.4 cm, and have a 14% rate of acute hemorrhage. Lesions associated with tuberous sclerosis occur earlier (mean age 30 years), are multiple in 97%, are often larger (mean 8.9 cm), and up to 45% of patients experience a spontaneous hemorrhage. This lesion is one of the 11 major diagnostic features of tuberous sclerosis complex, an autosomal dominant disorder. Genetic counseling and screening of relatives should be discussed with patients with multiple AML. Malignancy within an AML is rare (<1%), but is found in lesions that have predominantly epithelioid components. There is a higher incidence of epithelioid components in AML associated with tuberous sclerosis.

The angiographic appearance of AML is distinctive, with wild-appearing hypervascularity and intralesional aneurysms. Arteriovenous shunting is uncommon, as is venous invasion. The presence of aneurysms and lack of shunting and venous invasion helps distinguish these from RCC. Usually the diagnosis is already certain from CT or MRI.

When small (<3 cm), these lesions are usually asymptomatic. Acute spontaneous hemorrhage is a well-recognized complication of larger lesions and is usually a major clinical event with pain and hypotension. Embolization is an effective treatment for AML that has ruptured, and for large AML (>4 cm) to prevent rupture. When treating a patient whose AML has ruptured, particles and coils may be needed to control extravasation. Patients embolized prophylactically are usually treated with alcohol (in a ratio of 7 parts dehydrated alcohol to 3 parts lipiodol) or small particles (see Fig 12-26). With selective catheterization and controlled delivery of the embolic material, renal function is usually preserved, repeat embolization is required in 12% due to AML expansion or continued enhancement on imaging, and the long-term rate of bleeding is decreased to about 6%.

Oncocytoma

Oncocytomas are uncommon lesions found more often in middle-aged men (2:1 male-to-female). In most series these comprise about 5% of all renal masses and have an association with

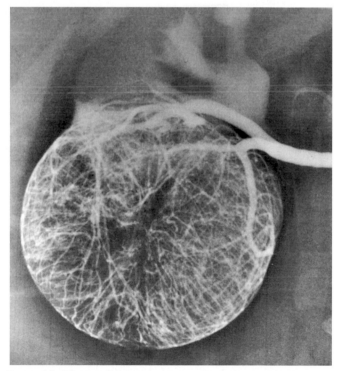

FIGURE 12-27. Renal oncocytoma in a patient with dual renal arteries. The mass is supplied entirely by the lower renal artery. Note the typical "spoke-wheel" pattern of neovascularity and the sharply defined borders of the mass. (Courtesy Frederick Keller, MD, Dotter Interventional Institute, Portland, Ore.)

Birt-Hogg-Dubé syndrome (benign skin tumors, oncocytomas, and spontaneous pneumothorax). The lesions have sharply defined borders, are vascular, and approximately one third have a central scar. About 10% are bilateral, and synchronous RCC has been reported in up to one third of lesions. Similar lesions are found in endocrine and exocrine organs such as the thyroid and pancreas (Fig. 12-27). The lesions are rarely metastatic; definitive diagnosis requires excision.

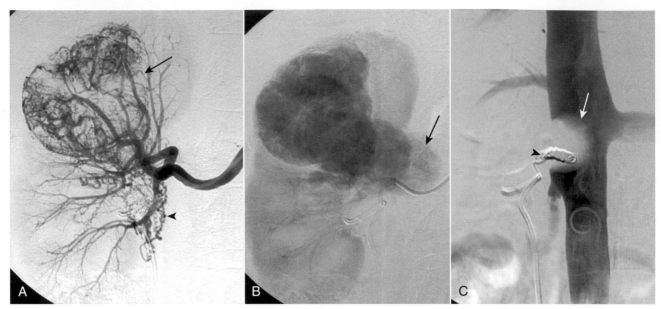

FIGURE 12-28. Renal cell carcinoma. **A,** Selective right renal artery digital subtraction angiogram showing a hypervascular mass *(arrow)* with wild neovascularity in the upper pole of the kidney. There is hypertrophy of the peripelvic arteries *(arrowhead)*, which provide collateral supply to the tumor. A ureteral stent is in place. **B,** Later image from the same angiogram showing extension of tumor thrombus into the right renal vein *(arrow)*. The kidney was embolized first with Gelfoam pledgets and then coils in the distal main renal artery. **C,** Inferior vena cavogram of the same patient showing tumor thrombus *(arrow)* growing out of the right renal vein orifice. Note the coils in the distal main renal artery *(arrowhead)*. The patient underwent nephrectomy the next day.

TABLE 12-7 TNM Staging of Renal Cell Carcinoma

Definition	TNM
Tumor < 7 cm confined by renal capsule	T1
4 cm or less	T1a
>4 cm but ≤7 cm	T1b
Tumor ≥ 7 cm confined by renal capsule	T2
>7 cm but ≤ 10 cm	T2a
>10 cm	T2b
Tumor extends beyond capsule or into ipsilateral adrenal gland but still within Gerota fascia	T3
Extends into renal vein or renal sinus fat	T3a
Extends into renal vein and IVC below diaphragm	T3b
Extends into renal vein and IVC above diaphragm	T3c
Lymph node involvement	
No regional lymph nodes	N0
Metastasis to regional lymph nodes	N1
Metastases	
None	M0
Distant	M1

T, Tumor stage; N, lymph node stage; M, metastases stage.

Metanephric Adenoma

Metanephric adenomas are rare lesions, found more commonly in women than men (2.6:1) and usually in middle age, although lesions can also occur in children. The lesions are most often single, less than 2 cm, symptomatic with pain or hematuria in about one third of cases, and associated with polycythemia vera. Diagnosis is almost always by CT or MRI, and management is with a renal tissue-sparing resection.

TABLE 12-8 Anatomic Staging of Renal Cell Carcinoma

Stage	T	N	M
I	1	0	0
II	2	0	0
III	1 or 2	1	0
	3	0 or 1	0
IV	4	0 or 1	0
	Any	0 or 1	1

T, Tumor stage; N, lymph node stage; M, metastases stage. See Table 12-7 for definition of TNM stages.

Renal Cell Carcinoma

RCC is increasing in frequency (about 65,000 new cases are diagnosed in the United States each year), but the average size at diagnosis is getting smaller and survival is improving. The majority of cases are now discovered incidentally during imaging for other reasons. In adults, RCCs comprise over 80% of all malignant renal masses, with transitional cell carcinoma of the renal pelvis (8%-10%), nephroblastoma (Wilms tumor, 5%-6%), and miscellaneous sarcomas (2%-3%) accounting for the remainder. RCCs are more common in males than females, may be multiple when associated with von Hippel-Lindau disease, and are typically found in patients 40 years or older. More than 90% of RCCs are epithelial in origin, of which 75% are clear cell, 15% papillary, and 5% chromophobe carcinoma. A grading system has been developed to describe RCCs (Fig. 12-28; Tables 12-7 and 12-8). At presentation, about 60% are localized, 20% have regional lymph node involvement, and 20% have distant metastases. Survival with localized disease is 70% at 5 years and is very dependent upon the histologic features of the tumor. Tumor invasion of the renal vein or IVC in the absence of metastasis has a 5-year survival rate of approximately 50% in patients undergoing radical nephrectomy with complete removal of IVC thrombus.

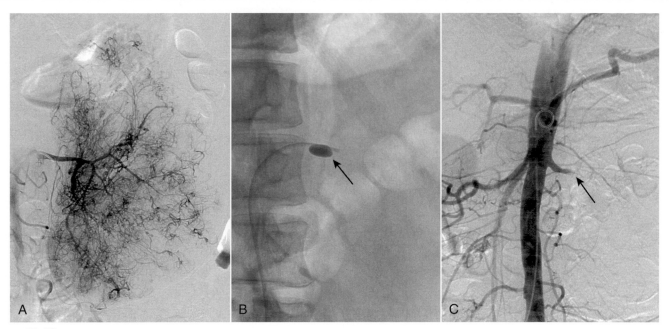

Figure 12-29. Alcohol ablation of the left kidney in a patient with a large renal cell carcinoma. **A,** Selective left renal angiogram shows hypervascularity and neovascularity replacing the entire left kidney. **B,** An occlusion balloon *(arrow)* has been inflated in the renal artery distal to the inferior adrenal artery. A total of 9 mL of dehydrated alcohol was infused. **C,** Aortogram after embolization showing the absence of flow in the left renal artery *(arrow)*.

The treatment options for small RCC include percutaneous ablation (see Chapter 25) and laparoscopic partial nephrectomy. Catheter-based interventions are reserved for large lesions before resection or as palliative treatment. The typical indication for angiographic intervention in RCC is preoperative embolization of the tumor (see Fig. 12-28). Large renal cell cancers and those with venous invasion can be difficult to resect owing to the extremely vascular nature of the mass. In these cases, embolization of the entire kidney before resection can reduce blood loss significantly. The timing for embolization varies from one center to another, but is generally performed within 24 hours of the surgery. Embolization 4-6 weeks in advance was once advocated because of theoretical induction of an autoimmune response, but that protocol is now rarely practiced. The goal of embolization is devascularization of the tumor and usually the kidney. For this reason, peripheral embolization is preferred. Dehydrated alcohol, small particles or spheres, Gelfoam powder, or Gelfoam pledgets can be used. The choice of particle size should be based on the presence of arteriovenous shunts. Smaller particles result in a longer procedure but a more peripheral embolization. Alcohol ablation using a balloon occlusion catheter for control in the main renal artery is favored by many interventionalists (Fig. 12-29). The volume of absolute alcohol required depends on the size and vascularity of the mass (see Chapter 4, Box 4-21). At the termination of the embolization, a few coils may be placed deep in the main renal artery. Coils placed in the proximal renal artery can be displaced into the aorta during surgical manipulation of the kidney. If coils are placed, the surgeon should be alerted to their presence.

Wilms Tumor

Wilms tumor is primarily a childhood lesion (8/1,000,000 children younger than 15 years of age), although there is a second peak incidence in the sixth decade. In children, the 5-year survival is 90% with lower stage tumors; in adults, 5-year survival is approximately 80%. Treatment includes resection, chemotherapy, and radiation therapy.

Box 12-9. Vascular Imaging Goals for Renal Donors

Number of renal arteries
Length of main renal arteries (preferred > 2 cm)
Quality of renal artery (presence of atherosclerosis or other
   pathology)
Renal vein anatomy
Quality of aorta

Metastatic Disease

Metastases to the kidney are seen in about 1% of all nonrenal cancers. The most common primary is lung carcinoma, with breast, gastrointestinal, and melanoma being the next most likely tumors of origin. Usually tumor involvement is bilateral and multiple, such that synchronous RCC is not a concern. Rarely metastases are single and isolated to the kidney, in which case clinical and imaging differentiation from primary RCC is difficult. In these cases, percutaneous ablation or surgical resection should be considered because survival is improved with treatment in the absence of other metastatic disease.

RENAL TRANSPLANTATION

Evaluation of the renal vasculature is an essential component of the workup of living donors and is frequently required when a transplanted kidney malfunctions or fails. The objectives of vascular imaging are different in each group. Vascular interventions are usually only necessary following transplantation.

The imaging of living renal donors is focused on detection of exclusionary vascular and parenchymal abnormalities or anomalies (Box 12-9). The left kidney is preferred by most surgeons because of the longer renal vein. In the past, when only open nephrectomy was performed, interest in the arterial anatomy was far greater than the renal veins. However, with laparoscopic donor nephrectomy, information about renal vein anatomy is of great importance. Most centers rely heavily on CT/CTA or MR/MRA, as these modalities

TABLE 12-9 Vascular Complications of Renal Transplantation

Complication	Incidence (%)
Renal artery stenosis	5-10
Renal artery thrombosis	1-2
Renal vein thrombosis	1-2
Postbiopsy pseudoaneurysm	1-2
Postbiopsy arteriovenous fistula	1-2
Anastomotic pseudoaneurysm	<1

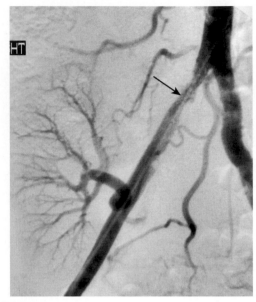

FIGURE 12-30. Common iliac artery (CIA) stenosis proximal to a renal transplant in a patient with new onset hypertension. Digital subtraction angiogram of the pelvis shows focal right CIA stenosis *(arrow)*, which produced a 46-mm Hg gradient. The transplant renal artery was normal in other views. The gradient was eliminated after stent placement in the common iliac artery and the patient's hypertension resolved.

provide information about renal parenchyma and the collection system in addition to the vascular structures (see Figs 12-3 and 12-4). Angiography is rarely necessary. When required (usually to exclude subtle renal artery pathology) flush aortography and selective angiography should performed.

Transplanted kidneys are usually placed in the recipient's iliac fossa. The renal vein is anastomosed to the iliac vein in an end-to-side fashion. Short saphenous or gonadal vein grafts may be necessary when the donor renal vein is inadequate. A variety of arterial anastomoses may be used, depending on the anatomy of the donor arteries and the recipient. Renal arteries of kidneys from living donors are usually anastomosed to recipient internal iliac artery in an end-to-end fashion, or end-to-side to the external iliac artery. Renal arteries from cadaveric donor kidneys may be anastomosed in similar fashions, or may include a portion of the donor aorta (termed a *Carrel patch*). This patch simplifies management of kidneys with multiple renal arteries, because the patch can be anastomosed directly to the external iliac artery rather than deal with each small artery separately. When performing imaging or interventions on renal transplants, it is critically important to know the details of the surgery.

The indications for vascular imaging of the transplanted kidney include deterioration of renal function and hypertension. The goal of imaging in these patients is to find a correctable vascular cause of symptoms. In many cases there is already some degree of renal dysfunction, and patients are on nephrotoxic immunosuppressive drugs such as cyclosporine. For these reasons, the initial examination in most patients is ultrasound with duplex color-flow. In addition to vascular information, the collecting system and perinephric tissues can be examined as well. Alternatively, MRA has proven very useful in detection of arterial and venous abnormalities. This modality allows evaluation of the arterial inflow from the aorta to the renal artery, and the venous outflow from the kidney to the IVC. Angiography can be performed following pretreatment with a renal protective strategy, or alternative contrast agent (CO_2). Knowledge of the surgical anatomy helps determine the angiographic approach (contralateral femoral access is preferred when the anastomosis is to the internal iliac artery). Complex oblique views may be necessary to visualize the transplant artery.

Vascular complications occur in up to 15% of patients with renal transplants (Table 12-9). Acute renal artery thrombosis usually occurs within the first month of transplantation and is associated with loss of the kidney in more than 90% of patients, owing to the lack of collateral supply to the transplanted kidney. Causes of thrombosis include technical factors related to the surgery, rejection, and postoperative hemodynamic instability. Late thrombosis is usually due to rejection or renal artery stenosis. Emergent surgical thrombectomy is usually required for renal salvage, although percutaneous mechanical techniques such as suction thrombectomy or thrombolysis may be indicated in selected cases.

Hemodynamically significant stenoses can also occur at any point in the arterial inflow to the kidney, including the common iliac artery (Fig. 12-30). Transplant renal artery stenosis usually occurs at the surgical anastomosis. Focal weblike stenoses immediately

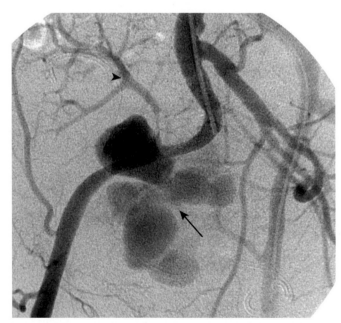

FIGURE 12-31. Mycotic pseudoaneurysm *(arrow)* of the arterial anastomosis of a transplanted kidney *(arrowhead)*. The wild, multilobulated appearance is characteristic of mycotic pseudoaneurysms.

adjacent to the anastomosis are believed to be hyperplastic lesions related to the intraoperative placement of clamps. Extensive intrarenal arterial stenoses are seen in chronic rejection, poorly controlled hypertension, diabetes, and atherosclerotic disease (see Fig. 12-11). Angioplasty with or without stent placement of transplant renal arteries has a technical success rate of approximately 90%, with a 1-year clinical success rate of approximately 75% for hypertension and 85% for renal function. More important, allograft survival is 85% at 10 years after intervention. When the stenosis is in a proximal inflow vessel, the long-term results are even better.

The presence of an anastomotic pseudoaneurysm should raise suspicion of infection (Fig. 12-31). Pseudoaneurysms in the renal

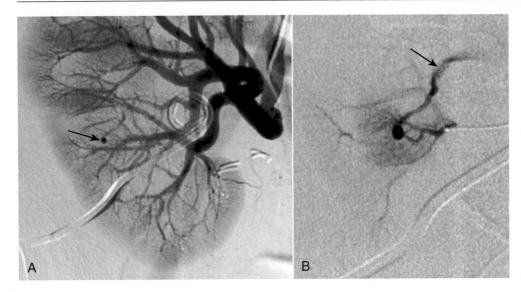

FIGURE **12-32**. Iatrogenic renal artery injury in a transplant kidney. The patient presented with anuria and acute clot obstruction of the renal pelvis and ureter one day after a percutaneous renal biopsy. The bleeding persisted after percutaneous placement of a nephrostomy tube. **A,** Transplant renal artery digital subtraction angiogram (DSA) showing a small pseudoaneurysm *(arrow)* in the region of the biopsy. **B,** Superselective DSA before embolization showing that there is also an arteriovenous fistula *(arrow* on vein).

parenchyma are usually related to percutaneous biopsy. Patients may present with a retroperitoneal hematoma, hematuria, renal dysfunction, or a pulsatile mass. Embolization is the preferred treatment, allowing maximal sparing of the renal parenchyma (Fig. 12-32). This is important, because most of these patients undergo biopsy because of suspected rejection as manifested by deterioration of renal function. The use of superselective coaxial micro catheters permits precise deployment of microcoils or glue near the origin of the pseudoaneurysm.

Arteriovenous fistulas in transplant kidneys are typically the result of percutaneous biopsies. These lesions may occur alone or in conjunction with a pseudoaneurysm. These may not present clinically until quite large, with a hypertrophied feeding branch that "steals" from the rest of the kidney. The treatment is embolization, with the goal being to preserve as much renal parenchyma as possible.

Venous thrombosis occurs early within the posttransplant period. Patients present with renal dysfunction, pain, hematuria, and proteinuria. Loss of the transplanted kidney is common. Late renal vein stenoses are rarely diagnosed, but may respond to angioplasty or stent placement.

▬ TRAUMA

The renal artery is injured in approximately 7% of penetrating abdominal wounds and in 15% of patients with major blunt abdominal trauma. The incidence of iatrogenic renal vascular trauma is not known, although it is thought to occur in as many as 2% of percutaneous nephrostomy procedures. In cases of blunt trauma, almost 80% of injuries consist of renal contusions or small corticomedullary lacerations with an intact renal capsule. The renal capsule is disrupted in 17% of lacerations, of which 7% communicate with the collecting system. Renal pedicle disruption and/or fragmentation of the kidney occur in only 3% of cases. A classification scheme for blunt trauma to the kidney has been developed to facilitate management decisions (Table 12-10). Patients with grade I though IV injuries are usually managed conservatively if there is no evidence of ongoing bleeding, but nephrectomy is ultimately required in 9% of grade III, 22% of grade IV, and 83% of grade V injuries. Patients with intermediate grade injuries may benefit from angiographic interventions to control hemorrhage or address nonocclusive arterial dissections.

By virtue of the mechanism of injury or required force, patients with community acquired renal trauma often have sustained multiple other injuries. CT scanning is the preferred imaging modality for these patients in most trauma centers to allow a generalized survey. The grade of the renal injury can be established quickly based

TABLE 12-10 Renal Injury Scale

Grade	Definition	Description
I	Contusion	Hematuria without visible injury
	Hematoma	Subcapsular, stable, no parenchymal injury
II	Hematoma	Stable perirenal hematoma
	Laceration	<1.0-cm depth renal cortex, no urinary extravasation
III	Laceration	>1.0-cm depth renal cortex, urinary extravasation
IV	Hematoma	Laceration involves cortex, medulla, and collecting system
	Vascular	Main renal artery and/or vein injury, contained hemorrhage
V	Laceration	Shattered kidney
	Vascular	Avulsion of renal hilum with devascularized kidney

Advance one grade for bilateral injuries up to grade III.

on the CT findings. A nonenhancing renal artery and kidney indicates thrombosis of the main renal artery due to dissection or transection (Fig. 12-33). Active extravasation and pseudoaneurysms may be seen in patients with fractured kidneys or penetrating trauma. Angiography is obtained when the diagnosis of a correctable vascular injury is uncertain, ongoing retroperitoneal bleeding that is amenable to embolization is suspected, or in patients with persistent hematuria (Fig. 12-34). Flush aortography is essential to determine the basic renal vascular anatomy and detect associated aortic, lumbar artery, and mesenteric artery injuries. Selective renal angiography is then performed to study the kidney.

When evaluating a patient for suspected arterial injury related to percutaneous nephrostomy placement, temporary removal of the tube over a guidewire may be the only way to visualize the injury (Fig. 12-35). If the angiogram is performed with the tube in place, the lesion can be tamponaded and difficult to visualize. The tube is readvanced into position as soon as filming stops to control the bleeding. After embolization, the tube is again backed out over a guidewire for the final control angiogram to confirm adequate treatment.

The full range of vascular injuries may be seen in patients with renal trauma. Selective embolization of extravasation, pseudoaneurysms, and arteriovenous fistulas is efficacious and spares more renal parenchyma than would be possible with open repair. Permanent agents that can be precisely deposited, such as coils or glue, are used in most cases. The use of microcatheters allows superselective embolization. However, in cases of massive extravasation and a hemodynamically unstable patient, rapid control of hemorrhage is more important than maximizing preservation of renal tissue. Embolization is successful in controlling bleeding in more than 95% of patients.

In some circumstances main renal artery dissections and obstructive intimal flaps can be treated with stents or stent-grafts. The overall success in preserving a functional kidney appears to be 50%, with early intervention for partially occlusive lesions having the best results. The likelihood of preservation of meaningful renal function with percutaneous recanalization of a thrombosed main renal artery is very low.

ARTERIOVENOUS MALFORMATIONS AND FISTULAS

Congenital renal arteriovenous malformation (AVM) is rare in the general population, with an incidence of approximately 4 per 10,000 individuals. Arteriovenous fistulas (AVFs) are almost always acquired, although the patient may not recall a specific

incident. More than 70% of AVFs are directly related to trauma or iatrogenic misadventures.

The majority of AVMs and AVFs are asymptomatic, and remain so throughout the life of the patient. Many post-traumatic AVFs close spontaneously. Symptomatic patients present with hematuria (72%), hypertension (more common with AVFs due to the "steal" phenomenon), and flank pain. Less common symptoms include high-output cardiac failure and spontaneous retroperitoneal hemorrhage.

Large lesions may be visible on CT or MR studies, but in general these examinations are most useful to exclude more common causes of hematuria. Angiography is required for the definitive diagnosis of renal AVMs and AVFs. Following flush aortography, selective angiography should be performed. When extremely high-flow lesions are present, balloon occlusion angiography may be necessary to adequately visualize the lesion.

Percutaneous embolization with coils, glue, or alcohol is the preferred treatment for most symptomatic lesions (Fig. 12-36). Surgery for very large AVFs may be necessary when appropriate embolic agents are not available.

RENAL ABLATION

Transarterial ablation of a kidney as an alternative to nephrectomy can be accomplished with selective embolization provided that the renal artery is patent. Indications include intractable renal bleeding due to unresectable tumors, nephrotic syndrome with unmanageable proteinuria, end-stage polycystic kidneys causing mass effect or pain, and severe hypertension related to a nonfiltering kidney. Global embolization of the kidney with small particles or alcohol is usually effective. In patients with polycystic kidney disease, the decrease in overall renal size is approximately 50% at 6 months. Placement of a few coils in the main renal artery without distal embolization may result in delayed reperfusion of the offending organ.

PHEOCHROMOCYTOMA

Pheochromocytoma is a rare (0.8 per 100,000) functional adrenal tumor that can cause severe and unpredictable hypertension. Up to one fourth of patients have a hereditary syndrome (e.g., multiple endocrine neoplasia types 2 A and B, neurofibromatosis type 1, and von Hippel-Lindau syndrome). These tumors are typically 2 cm or greater in size; 5%-10% are multiple. CT, MRI, or ^{131}I-meta-iodobenzylguanidine (MIBG) nuclear medicine scan are used for diagnosis. Angiography is rarely required. Extra-adrenal,

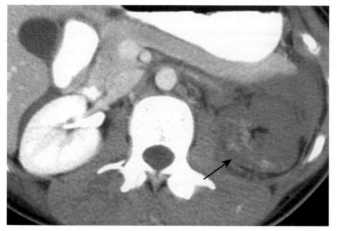

FIGURE 12-33. Traumatic left renal artery thrombosis after a motor vehicle accident (car + alcohol + tree). Axial computed tomography image with contrast showing lack of perfusion of the left kidney *(arrow)* and a perinephric hematoma.

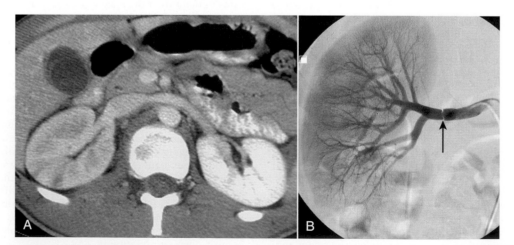

FIGURE 12-34. Focal renal artery injury due to blunt trauma in an 11-year-old male with no other injuries. **A,** Contrast-enhanced CT showing decreased enhancement of the right kidney relative to the left. **B,** Selective right renal digital subtraction angiogram (an aortogram was obtained first) showing a focal circumferential injury *(arrow)* in the distal main renal artery. There is slight dilation of the renal artery just proximal to the defect, suggesting disruption of the intima and media with a pseudoaneurysm. This was confirmed at surgery; in older or sicker patients, stent-graft repair is a good option.

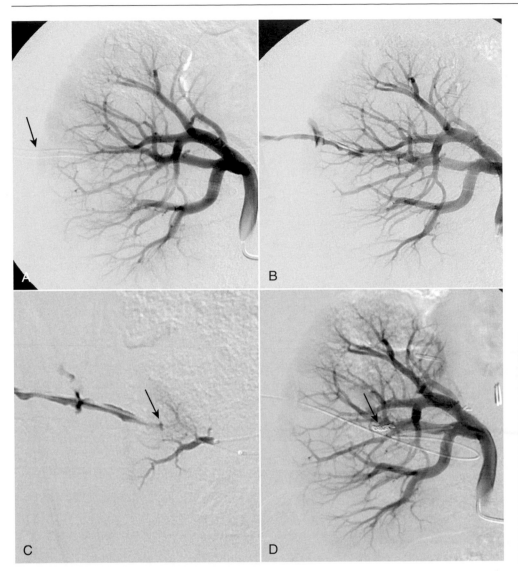

FIGURE 12-35. Renal artery injury due to nephrostomy placement in a transplant kidney. The patient had persistent hematuria with clots after nephrostomy for ureteral stricture. **A,** Selective angiogram with the nephrostomy tube in place *(arrow)* does not show an abnormality. **B,** Repeat angiogram after removal of the nephrostomy over a guidewire showing extravasation of contrast with drainage along the tube tract. **C,** Angiogram through a microcatheter shows the point of extravasation *(arrow)* from an interlobular artery. The microcatheter could not be advanced into the bleeding artery, so embolization with coils was performed of the feeding interlobar artery. **D,** Completion renal angiogram with the guidewire in place confirms absence of extravasation. *Arrow* = coils.

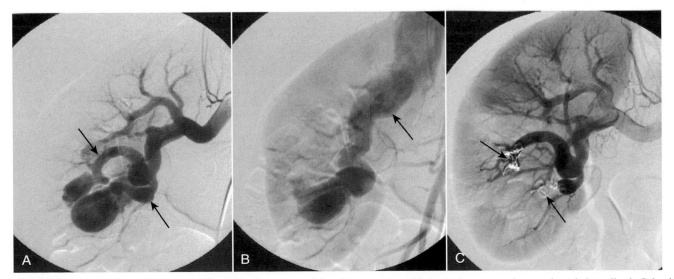

FIGURE 12-36. Right renal arteriovenous malformation in a teenaged female presenting with intermittent gross hematuria and clot colic. **A,** Selective right renal digital subtraction angiogram (DSA) showing dilated lower pole segmental renal arteries *(arrows)* with shunting to large veins through multiple small communications. **B,** A later image after the same injection showing dense opacification of the right renal vein *(arrow)*. **C,** DSA following coil embolization *(arrows)* of the two large feeding arteries showing absent filling of the malformation.

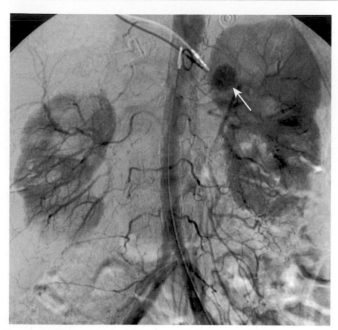

FIGURE 12-37. Pheochromocytoma appearance on angiogram. Late-phase digital subtraction aortogram showing a densely enhancing and staining left adrenal mass *(arrow)*.

metastatic, and bilateral pheochromocytomas are each found with an approximate incidence of 10%. Adrenal pheochromocytomas secrete epinephrine and norepinephrine. Primary pheochromocytomas located outside the adrenal gland, termed *paragangliomas*, are more likely to be malignant and secrete only norepinephrine. Common extraadrenal locations are the renal hilum, the vicinity of the origin of the inferior mesenteric artery (organ of Zuckerkandl), the bladder wall, and the posterior mediastinum.

Hypertensive crisis can be precipitated by contrast during angiography. Pretreatment with oral phenoxybenzamine (10 mg twice daily initially and increased to 20-40 mg twice daily until blood pressure is controlled) and careful procedural monitoring by an anesthesiologist is recommended whenever a patient with suspected pheochromocytoma receives iodinated contrast. Acute hypertensive crisis can be controlled with intravenous nitroprusside or 5 mg of phentolamine. Pheochromocytomas have a characteristic intense, prolonged parenchymal blush on arteriography (Fig. 12-37). The treatment is surgical resection of the tumor.

▬ SUGGESTED READINGS

Azizi M, Steichen O, Frank M, et al. Catheter-based radiofrequency renal-nerve ablation in patients with resistant hypertension. *Eur J Vasc Endovasc Surg.* 2012;43:293-299.

Baez JC, Jagannathan JP, Krajewski K, et al. Pheochromocytoma and paraganglioma: imaging characteristics. *Cancer Imaging.* 2012;12:153-162.

Bakal CW, Cynamon J, Lakritz PS, Sprayregen S. Value of preoperative renal artery embolization in reducing blood transfusion requirements during nephrectomy for renal cell carcinoma. *J Vasc Interv Radiol.* 1993;4:727-731.

Bastide C, Rambeaud JJ, Bach AM, Russo P. Metanephric adenoma of the kidney: clinical and radiological study of nine cases. *BJU Int.* 2009;103:1544-1548.

Bax L, Woittiez AJ, Kouwenberg HJ, et al. Stent placement in patients with atherosclerotic renal artery stenosis and impaired renal function: a randomized trial. *Ann Intern Med.* 2009;150:840-848.

Bishay VL, Crino PB, Wein AJ, et al. Embolization of giant renal angiomyolipomas: technique and results. *J Vasc Interv Radiol.* 2010;21:67-72.

Chimpiri AR, Natarajan B. Renal vascular lesions: diagnosis and endovascular management. *Semin Intervent Radiol.* 2009;26:253-261.

Cocheteux B, Mounier-Vehier C, Gaxotte V, et al. Rare variations in renal anatomy and blood supply: CT appearances and embryological background. A pictorial essay. *Eur Radiol.* 2001;11:779-786.

Cornelis F, Couzi L, Le Bras Y, et al. Embolization of polycystic kidneys as an alternative to nephrectomy before renal transplantation: a pilot study. *Am J Transplant.* 2010;10:2363-2369.

Crutchley TA, Pearce JD, Craven TE, et al. Clinical utility of the resistive index in atherosclerotic renovascular disease. *J Vasc Surg.* 2009;49:148-155.

Esler MD, Krum H, Sobotka PA, et al. Renal sympathetic denervation in patients with treatment-resistant hypertension (The Symplicity HTN-2 Trial): a randomised controlled trial. *Lancet.* 2010;376:1903-1909.

Hill GS. Hypertensive nephrosclerosis. *Curr Opin Nephrol Hypertens.* 2008;17:266-270.

Golwyn DH, Routh WD, Chen MY, Lorentz WB, Dyer RB. Percutaneous transcatheter renal ablation with absolute ethanol for uncontrolled hypertension or nephrotic syndrome: results in 11 patients with end-stage renal disease. *J Vasc Interv Radiol.* 1997;8:527-533.

Karagiannis A, Mikhailidis DP, Athyros VG, Harsoulis F. Pheochromocytoma: an update on genetics and management. *Endocr Relat Cancer.* 2007;14:935-956.

Krum H, Schlaich M, Whitbourn R, et al. Catheter-based renal sympathetic denervation for resistant hypertension: a multicentre safety and proof-of-principle cohort study. *Lancet.* 2009;373:1275-1281.

Kumbhani DJ, Bavry AA, Harvey JE, et al. Clinical outcomes after percutaneous revascularization versus medical management in patients with significant renal artery stenosis: A meta-analysis of randomized controlled trials. *Am Heart J.* 2011;161:622-630.

Lao D, Parasher PS, Cho KC, Yeghiazarians Y. Atherosclerotic renal artery stenosis-diagnosis and treatment. *Mayo Clin Proc.* 2011;86:649-657.

Leiner T, Michaely H. Advances in contrast-enhanced MR angiography of the renal arteries. *Magn Reson Imaging Clin N Am.* 2008;16:561-572.

Lopera JE, Suri R, Kroma G, et al. Traumatic occlusion and dissection of the main renal artery: endovascular treatment. *J Vasc Interv Radiol.* 2011;22:1570-1574.

Margey R, Hynes BG, Moran D, et al. Atherosclerotic renal artery stenosis and renal artery stenting: an evolving therapeutic option. *Expert Rev Cardiovasc Ther.* 2011;9:1347-1360.

Marini M, Fernandez-Rivera C, Cao I, et al. Treatment of transplant renal artery stenosis by percutaneous transluminal angioplasty and/or stenting: study in 63 patients in a single institution. *Transplant Proc.* 2011;43:2205-2207.

Master VA, McAninch JW. Operative management of renal injuries: parenchymal and vascular. *Urol Clin North Am.* 2006;33:21-31.

Murphy TP, Cooper CJ, Dworkin LD, et al. The Cardiovascular Outcomes with Renal Atherosclerotic Lesions (CORAL) study: rationale and methods. *Vasc Interv Radiol.* 2005;16:1295-1300.

Nelson CP, Sanda MG. Contemporary diagnosis and management of renal angiomyolipoma. *J Urol.* 2002;168:1315-1325.

Olin JW, Froehlich J, Gu X, et al. The United States Registry for Fibromuscular Dysplasia: results in the first 447 patients. *Circulation.* 2012;125:3182-3190.

Reinhard H, Aliani S, Ruebe C, et al. Wilms' tumor in adults: results of the Society of Pediatric Oncology (SIOP) 93-01/Society for Pediatric Oncology and Hematology (GPOH) Study. *J Clin Oncol.* 2004;22:4500-4506.

Rocha-Singh KJ, Novack V, Pencina M, et al. Objective performance goals of safety and blood pressure efficacy for clinical trials of renal artery bare metal stents in hypertensive patients with atherosclerotic renal artery stenosis. *Catheter Cardiovasc Interv.* 2011;78:779-789.

Sharfuddin A. Imaging evaluation of kidney transplant recipients. *Semin Nephrol.* 2011;31:259-271.

Simmons MN, Schreiber MJ, Gill IS. Surgical renal ischemia: a contemporary overview. *J Urol.* 2008;180:19-30.

Singh AK, Sahani DV. Imaging of the renal donor and transplant recipient. *Radiol Clin North Am.* 2008;46:79-93.

Slovut DP, Olin JW. Fibromuscular dysplasia. *N Engl J Med.* 2004;350:1862-1871.

Textor S. Issue in renovascular disease and ischemic nephropathy: beyond ASTRAL. *Curr Opin Nephrol Hypertens.* 2011;11:139-145.

Tublin ME, Bude RO, Platt JF. Review. The resistive index in renal Doppler sonography: where do we stand? *AJR Am J Roentgenol.* 2003;180:885-892.

Tullus K. Renovascular hypertension - is it fibromuscular dysplasia or Takayasu arteritis? *Pediatr Nephrol.* 2013;28:191-196.

Wheatley K, Ives N, Gray R, et al. Revascularization versus medical therapy for renal-artery stenosis. *N Engl J Med.* 2009;361:1953-1962.

van Jaarsveld BC, Krijnen P, Pieterman H, et al. The effect of balloon angioplasty on hypertension in atherosclerotic renal-artery stenosis. Dutch Renal Artery Stenosis Intervention Cooperative Study Group. *N Engl J Med.* 2000;342:1007-1014.

Verschuyl EJ, Kaatee R, Beek FJ, et al. Renal artery origins: best angiographic projection angles. *Radiology.* 1997;205:115-120.

Willoteaux S, Faivre-Pierret M, Moranne O, et al. Fibromuscular dysplasia of the main renal arteries: comparison of contrast-enhanced MR angiography with digital subtraction angiography. *Radiology.* 2006;241:922-929.

CHAPTER 13

Inferior Vena Cava and Tributaries

John A. Kaufman, MD, MS, FSIR, FCIRSE

The inferior vena cava (IVC) and its tributaries are frequent sites of vascular pathology. Diseases of organs that drain into the IVC may first become clinically apparent when the cava becomes involved. IVC imaging and intervention are prominent components of current interventional radiology practice.

NORMAL ANATOMY

The IVC is formed by the confluence of the common iliac veins at the level of the L5 vertebral body (Fig. 13-1). In the abdomen, the IVC is usually located to the right of the midline and the aorta, anterior to the lumbar and lower thoracic spine. The IVC is a posterior structure for much of its course. The retrohepatic IVC resides in a groove or tunnel in the bare area of the liver encompassed posteriorly by suspensory ligaments of the liver and the diaphragm. The IVC exits the abdomen through a diaphragmatic hiatus, with a slight anterior course before draining through the inferoposterior wall of the right atrium. Frequently there is a membranous lip at the junction of the IVC with the right atrium, termed the *eustachian valve* (Fig. 13-2). The supradiaphragmatic portion of the IVC is frequently intrapericardial.

The IVC typically has an oval shape in cross-section, but is easily deformed by adjacent abdominal or retroperitoneal masses. The average diameter of the infrarenal IVC is approximately 23 mm, although the intrarenal segment is usually slightly larger. The IVC is a valveless elastic structure that responds to increased venous volume or pressure by dilatation, and responds to decreased volume or increased intraabdominal pressure by collapsing. The dynamic nature of the IVC should be considered when interpreting imaging studies or contemplating interventions.

The IVC is a single, right-sided structure in approximately 97% of individuals (Table 13-1). The embryology of the IVC is complex in that the antecedent structures are paired and segmented. Anomalies of the IVC can be explained by aberrations of regression of these segments. The three pairs of fetal veins that become the IVC are the posterior cardinal, the subcardinal, and the supracardinal (see Fig. 13-1). The posterior cardinal veins normally involute completely, although persistence on the right results in a retrocaval right ureter. The subcardinal veins form the intrahepatic IVC, and contribute to the renal veins and suprarenal segment of the IVC. Regression of the right subcardinal vein results in azygos or hemiazygos continuation of the IVC

(Fig. 13-3). The infrarenal IVC and the azygos veins are derived from the supracardinal veins. Duplication of the infrarenal IVC results from failure of regression of the left supracardinal vein, while a left-sided IVC results from regression of the right supracardinal vein (Fig. 13-4). When there is caval duplication, each iliac vein is usually isolated and drains through its own IVC, although communication at the normal level of the iliac vein confluence may also occur. The left side of a duplicated IVC drains into the left renal vein, which then usually crosses the aorta in the normal location to join the right IVC, forming a normal single suprarenal IVC. When there is only a single left-sided IVC, both iliac veins drain into the IVC, which usually crosses the aorta at the level of the left renal vein to form a normally located suprarenal IVC (see Fig. 13-4). Thus, unless there is an associated anomaly of the subcardinal veins, duplicated or left-sided IVCs usually revert to a normal location above the level of the renal veins.

The major tributaries of the IVC are the hepatic, renal, gonadal, and common iliac veins (see Fig. 13-1). Smaller tributaries include the lumbar, right adrenal, and phrenic veins. The common and external iliac veins are discussed in Chapter 16, and the hepatic veins in Chapter 14.

The most common pattern of renal vein anatomy is a single vein from each kidney, with the left renal vein passing anteriorly between the aorta and the superior mesenteric artery (SMA) to join the IVC opposite the right renal vein at the level of the L2 vertebral body. The orifice of the normal left renal vein is anterior, while that of the right is posterior. The right renal vein is shorter than the left, with average lengths of 3 cm and 7 cm, respectively (Fig. 13-5). Renal veins rarely have valves, but commonly connect to other retroperitoneal veins such as the lumbar, azygos, and gonadal veins. In patients with portal hypertension these connections may enlarge to allow drainage of portal blood from the splenic and short gastric veins into the left renal vein.

Variations in renal vein anatomy are present in almost 40% of individuals (see Table 13-1) due to the complex embryologic relationships of the kidneys and the veins. In the fetus, the subcardinal and supracardinal veins form a web of veins that surround the aorta. As the kidneys rise out of the pelvis between the sixth and ninth weeks of gestation, their blood supply is constantly changing. Persistence of any of the venous elements may result in an anomaly, of which multiple right renal veins are the most common (28%) (Fig. 13-6). The next most common anomaly is a circumaortic left renal vein (5%-7%), in which the

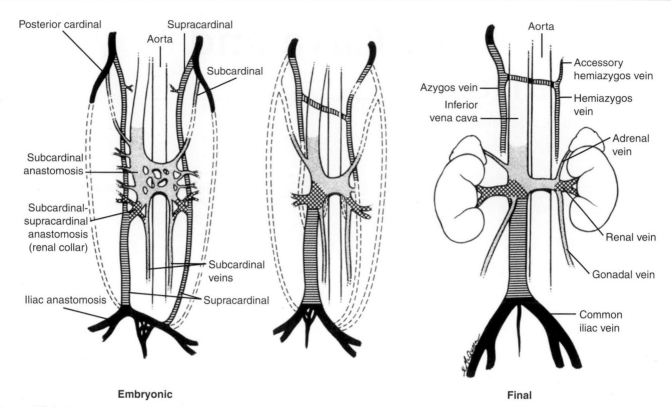

Embryonic   **Final**

FIGURE 13-1. Development and normal anatomy of the inferior vena cava (IVC). (From Lundell L, Kadir S. Inferior vena cava and spinal veins. In: Kadir S, ed. *Normal and Variant Angiographic Anatomy*. Philadelphia: Saunders, 1991, with permission.)

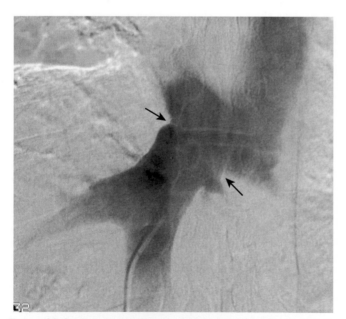

FIGURE 13-2. Digital subtraction venogram of the suprahepatic inferior vena cava showing the eustachian valve *(arrows)*.

TABLE 13-1 Anatomic Variants of the Inferior Vena Cava and Renal Veins

Variant	Incidence (%)
Duplicated IVC	1.0
Left-sided IVC	0.5
Absent IVC	0.1
Azygos/hemiazygos continuation of the IVC	0.5
Circumaortic left renal vein	7
Retroaortic left renal vein	3
Multiple right renal veins	28

IVC, Inferior vena cava.

the vessels. This fact is crucial when considering gonadal vein interventions. The right gonadal vein drains into the anterior surface of the IVC just below, or at the level of, the right renal vein in most individuals (see Fig. 13-1). In fewer than 10% the right gonadal vein empties directly into the right renal vein. In the majority (>99%) of individuals the left gonadal vein empties into the left renal vein just before the renal vein crosses the aorta. Rarely, the left gonadal vein empties directly into the IVC. Usually, there is a valve present just at or below the orifice of the gonadal veins.

Four to five pairs of lumbar veins drain the vertebral column and the surrounding musculature. These veins empty into the posterolateral aspect of the IVC at the levels of the L4-L1 vertebral bodies. The lumbar veins anastomose with the ascending lumbar veins, paired structures that lie deep to the psoas muscles, parallel to the IVC (Fig. 13-7). The ascending lumbar veins originate from the superior aspect of the common iliac veins. In

left renal vein has both a preaortic and a retroaortic component. The latter may enter the IVC close to the level of the normal preaortic vein, or as low as the confluence of the iliac veins. In 3% of individuals a single left renal vein passes behind (retroaortic) the aorta to reach the IVC.

The gonadal veins ascend from the pelvis anterior to the psoas muscle as companions of the gonadal arteries and the ureters. There are multiple small anastomoses between the gonadal veins and other retroperitoneal veins along the entire length of

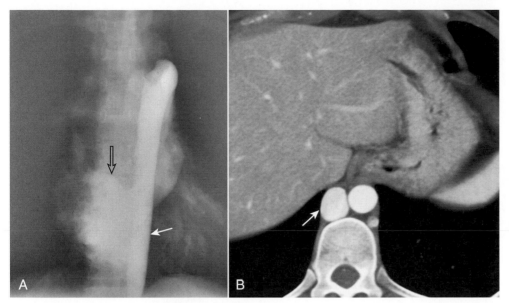

FIGURE 13-3. Hemiazygos and azygos continuation of the inferior vena cava (IVC). **A**, Venogram performed by injection in the IVC shows absence of the suprahepatic IVC and drainage via the hemiazygos vein *(solid arrow)* into a left-sided superior vena cava. Contrast is present in the right atrium *(open arrow)*. **B**, Axial computed tomography scan from another patient showing a dilated azygos vein *(arrow)* adjacent to the descending thoracic aorta and absence of the intrahepatic IVC.

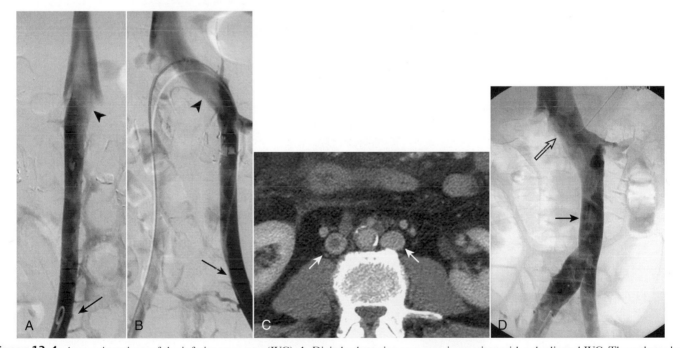

FIGURE 13-4. Anatomic variants of the inferior vena cava (IVC). **A**, Digital subtraction cavogram in a patient with a duplicated IVC. The catheter has been inserted from the right femoral vein. There is absent inflow from the left iliac vein *(arrow)*, the IVC appears smaller than usual, and there is prominent inflow from the left renal vein *(arrowhead)*. **B**, The same patient after catheterization of the left IVC *(arrow)*, which empties into the left renal vein *(arrowhead)*. **C**, Axial computed tomography scan from a different patient showing typical appearance of a duplicated IVC *(arrows)*. There is thrombus in the right-sided IVC. **D**, Left-sided IVC *(black arrow)* that crosses to the right at the level of the left renal vein *(open arrow)*.

the thorax, the ascending lumbar veins become the azygos vein on the right and the hemiazygos vein on the left. The ascending lumbar veins interconnect with other retroperitoneal veins, such as the intercostal and renal veins.

The pelvic structures drain through veins named in a manner analogous to the arterial supply. The superior gluteal, inferior gluteal, and obturator veins coalesce into the internal iliac veins, which drain into the common iliac vein. The visceral structures of the pelvis drain by the middle and inferior rectal (also known as hemorrhoidal), vesical, uterine, vaginal, and prostatic veins. These veins are all interconnected with each other, so that precise labeling of structures is not always possible. In addition, the middle hemorrhoidal vein anastomoses with the portal venous system through the superior hemorrhoidal vein.

The testicle drains initially into the pampiniform plexus, a complex of venous sinuses contained in the scrotum. The anterior pampiniform plexus drains into the internal spermatic vein, the middle plexus drains around the ductus deferens, and the posterior plexus drains along the posterior edge of the spermatic cord into branches of the internal pudendal veins. The three components of the pampiniform plexus anastomose and allow collateral drainage.

The internal spermatic (gonadal) vein traverses the retroperitoneum as described earlier and enters the renal vein on the left and the IVC on the right. The internal spermatic vein is a single vessel in only about 50% of individuals. Valves are usually present in these veins (see Fig. 13-1). Rarely, the internal spermatic vein may communicate with the portal veins.

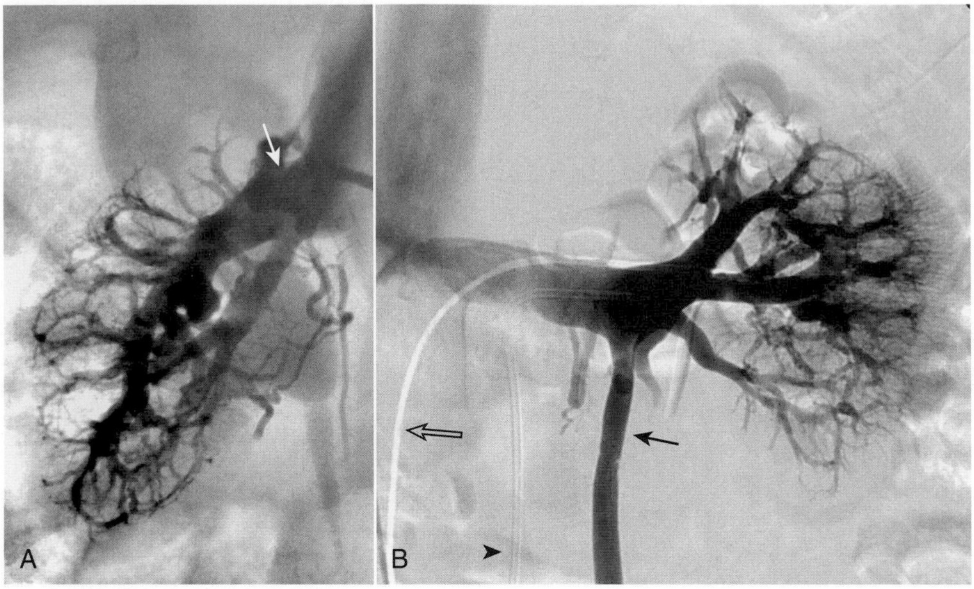

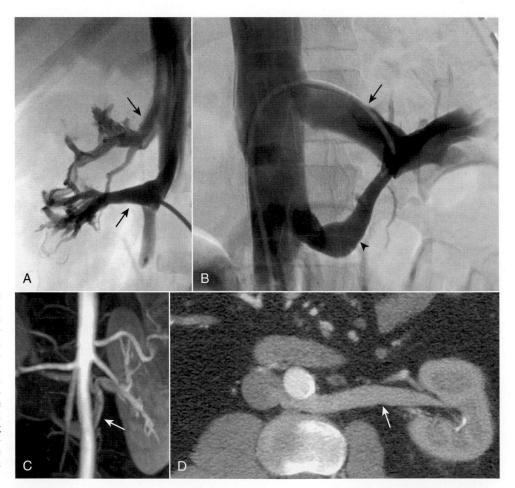

FIGURE 13-5. Normal conventional renal venograms. **A,** The right renal vein *(arrow)* is short with a caudal angulation. **B,** The left renal vein is long, crossing anterior to the aorta and posterior to the superior mesenteric artery to join the inferior vena cava. Note reflux of contrast into the left gonadal vein *(arrow)*. There is a catheter in the renal artery *(arrowhead)*, through which 10 μmg of epinephrine was injected to temporarily decrease arterial flow just before injection through the venous catheter *(open arrow)*.

FIGURE 13-6. Anatomic variants of the renal veins. **A,** Conventional venogram showing multiple right renal veins *(arrows)*. **B,** Digital subtraction study showing a circumaortic left renal vein with preaortic superior *(arrow)* and retroaortic inferior *(arrowhead)* components. **C,** Coronal maximum intensity projection of a contrast-enhanced magnetic resonance angiogram showing a retroaortic left renal vein *(arrow)* that courses caudad and posterior to the aorta before joining the inferior vena cava. **D,** Oblique reformatted computed tomography image showing the anatomic relationships of a retroaortic left renal vein *(arrow)*.

The uterus has a prominent venous plexus that drains through the broad ligaments to the uterine veins. The uterine veins primarily drain into the internal iliac veins, but also through the gonadal veins and through the perineum along the vagina to the labial veins. In pregnancy, the uterine plexus dilates enormously and is often associated with prominent gonadal and labial veins. The ovarian (gonadal) veins drain into the IVC at the level of the renal veins. Valves are present in 85% of left and 95% of right ovarian veins. In a manner analogous to the internal spermatic veins, the ovarian veins may be single or multiple, and have multiple communications with other retroperitoneal veins (Fig. 13-8).

In most individuals, the adrenal glands are each drained by a single vein. Both adrenal veins communicate with renal capsular and retroperitoneal veins. Multiple adrenal veins are the exception, but do occur. The right adrenal vein empties directly into the IVC 2-5 cm above the right renal vein, usually between T11

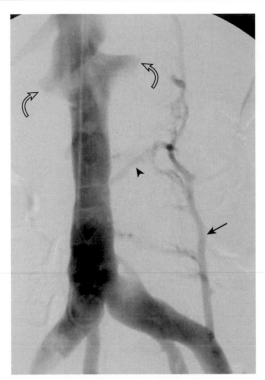

FIGURE 13-7. Digital subtraction cavogram performed from a jugular vein approach. The left ascending lumbar vein *(arrow)* communicates with a lumbar vein *(arrowhead)*. There is reflux into the orifices of both renal veins *(curved arrows)*.

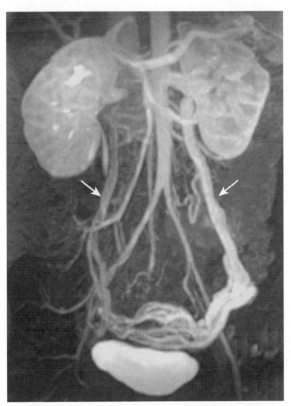

FIGURE 13-8. Maximum intensity projection of a gadolinium-enhanced three-dimensional magnetic resonance angiogram of a woman showing dilated ovarian veins *(arrows)*. The direction of flow is retrograde in the left ovarian vein, across the pelvis through the uterine plexus, and antegrade in the right ovarian vein. This patient presented with chronic pelvic pain (see Pelvic Congestion Syndrome). (Courtesy Barry Stein, MD, Hartford, Conn.)

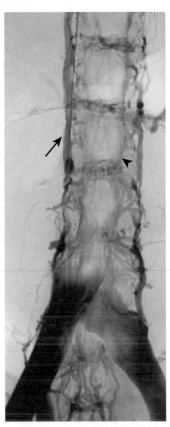

FIGURE 13-9. Digital subtraction cavogram of a patient with extrinsic compression of the inferior vena cava. There is filling of the para vertebral *(arrow)* and intravertebral *(arrowhead)* veins.

and L1 (see Fig. 13-1). The orifice of the vein is located on the right posterolateral wall of the IVC in three fourths of patients and on the left in about one fourth. The vein usually courses inferiorly toward the gland but may run superiorly in about 15% of patients. Rarely (approximately 8%) a small accessory hepatic vein drains into the right adrenal vein, or vice versa. The left adrenal vein drains into the superior aspect of the left renal vein 3-5 cm from the IVC. The left inferior phrenic vein forms a common trunk with the left adrenal vein before it joins the renal vein. The location of the left adrenal vein is extremely constant, but in unusual cases the vein may drain directly into the IVC. In 2% of patients, two left adrenal veins may be found.

■ KEY COLLATERAL PATHWAYS

The collateral drainage of the IVC varies with the level of the occlusion. Infrarenal obstruction results in drainage of the lower extremities via ascending lumbar, paraspinal, gonadal, inferior epigastric, and abdominal wall veins (Fig. 13-9). Retrograde or obstructed flow in the internal iliac veins results in drainage through gonadal, ureteric, and the inferior mesenteric veins (the latter through anastomoses between the hemorrhoidal veins). Occlusion of the IVC between the renal and hepatic veins can be drained by all of the collateral routes described for infrarenal obstruction. In addition, the azygos and hemiazygos veins assume an important role, particularly for drainage of the renal veins. Obstruction at the level of the suprahepatic IVC (above the hepatic vein orifices) results in collateral flow through all of the routes described, except the inferior mesenteric vein.

Renal vein obstruction on the right is drained via lumbar veins and the azygos vein. The ureteric vein may also hypertrophy in these patients. Renal vein obstruction on the left is drained by the lumbar veins, hemiazygos vein, and the left gonadal vein.

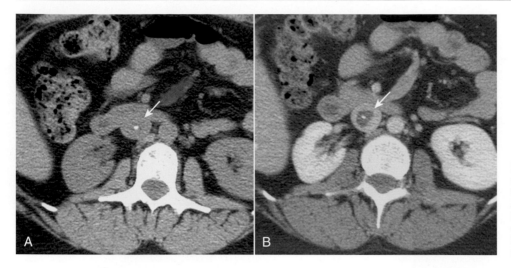

FIGURE 13-10. Computed tomography scan showing partially calcified subacute thrombus in the inferior vena cava (IVC). **A,** Noncontrast scan showing calcification in the IVC *(arrow)* at the level of the duodenum. **B,** Delayed contrast-enhanced image from the same patient showing the full extent of the thrombus *(arrow).*

The rich network of intercommunicating veins in the pelvis allows collateral drainage of occluded gonadal veins through transpelvic, ascending lumbar, and internal iliac veins. Obstruction of the adrenal veins results in drainage through small retroperitoneal collaterals such as renal capsular veins.

IMAGING

Evaluation of the IVC with ultrasound is inexpensive and widely available. The intrahepatic portion of the IVC can be consistently visualized. Duplex ultrasound can provide information about direction of flow. However, the depth of the vessel within the abdomen, bowel gas, and obesity make imaging of the infrarenal IVC with ultrasound more difficult. Renal vein anatomy can be difficult to evaluate for similar reasons.

Imaging of the IVC with multidetector computed tomography (CT) is simple and highly accurate for most forms of pathology. For dedicated CT of the IVC, a triple-phase study consisting of a noncontrast scan, an arterial-phase acquisition, and a delayed acquisition (1-2 minutes) during the venous enhancement phase should be used. Contrast can be injected through an upper extremity vein. The collimation can be thicker than that used for arterial studies, because the venous structures are larger in diameter. The noncontrast scan is useful for detection of high-attenuation abnormalities such as high-density acute thrombus or calcified chronic occlusions (Fig. 13-10). The late phase scan is necessary because mixing of opacified blood from the renal veins during the arterial phase can result in pseudo filling defects. Variant IVC and renal vein anatomy is depicted with sensitivity and specificity that exceeds 95%, particularly when studies are viewed on postprocessing workstations that allow reconstruction in multiple planes (see Fig. 13-6).

Magnetic resonance imaging (MRI) of the IVC and renal veins with venographic sequences (MRV) has similar accuracy, sensitivity, and specificity as contrast-enhanced CT. Anatomic sequences in at least two planes (axial and coronal) should be obtained, followed by flow sequences. Thick-sliced (5 mm) two-dimensional time-of-flight (2-D TOF) sequences acquired in the axial plane with superior saturation provide excellent images, although slow or retrograde flow in obstructed segments will suffer from signal loss. Gadolinium-enhanced breath-hold 3-D acquisitions of the IVC in the coronal plane are not susceptible to signal loss. These sequences are similar to those used for evaluation of the abdominal aorta. Imaging of the venous system is accomplished by repeating the same sequence after the arterial phase (Fig. 13-11).

Cavography should be performed with a pigtail catheter positioned just at or slightly below the confluence of the common iliac veins (see Figs. 13-4 and 13-7). When an abnormality is suspected higher in the IVC, the catheter can be repositioned at

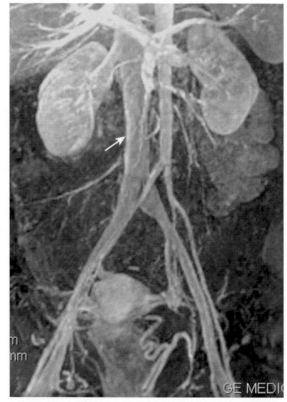

FIGURE 13-11. Maximum intensity projection of venous phase of gadolinium-enhanced three-dimensional magnetic resonance angiogram showing enhancement of the venous structures *(arrow,* IVC). (Courtesy Barry Stein, MD, Hartford, Conn.)

that level after the initial injection. Power injection of contrast (20-25 mL/sec for 2 seconds) and rapid filming (3-4 frames/sec) are necessary to adequately opacify the IVC. When the right femoral approach is used for catheter placement, reflux of contrast into the proximal left common iliac vein is indicative of a conventional single IVC. Injection in the left common iliac vein is advocated by some interventionalists to exclude a duplicated IVC. An unexpectedly small infrarenal IVC at cavography from either side also suggests the presence of a duplicated IVC (see Fig. 13-4). Brisk unopacified inflow of renal vein blood produces a changing flame-shaped filling defect in the IVC contrast that points toward the heart. This should not be confused with a renal vein thrombus; repeat injection with the pigtail in the intrarenal IVC will usually resolve this question. In patients with elevated

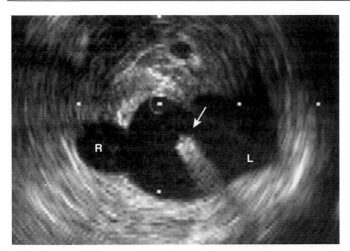

FIGURE 13-12. Intravenous ultrasound-guided inferior vena cava filter placement. The right (R) and left (L) renal vein origins are well visualized. The apex of the filter *(arrow)* was placed at this level.

right heart pressures, contrast may reflux into hepatic and renal veins. Whenever the identity or location of a tributary vein is in doubt, selective injection with a visceral catheter should be performed. The projection most commonly used for cavography is anteroposterior, but the lateral view is useful when evaluating for obstruction or intraluminal masses. In patients with renal insufficiency or contrast allergies, either CO_2 or gadolinium can be used as appropriate. Alternatively, intravascular ultrasound (IVUS) with a low-frequency probe can be used to image the IVC and guide interventions (Fig. 13-12). The major imaging IVUS landmarks of the IVC are the confluence of the iliac veins, the renal and hepatic veins, and the cavoatrial junction.

The renal veins have very high flow rates, which makes selective renal venography challenging. When the primary goals are localization of the renal veins or sampling, selective catheter shapes such as Cobra-2 or Simmons (1 for the right renal vein, 2 for the left) can be used. For diagnostic venography, catheters with multiple side holes should be used so that large volumes of contrast can be injected without traumatizing the vein. A multi-side hole straight or pigtail catheter directed into the renal veins with a deflecting guidewire is a useful combination for renal venography. When extensive filling of the intrarenal veins is required, injection of 10 μmg of epinephrine into the renal artery temporarily reduces venous outflow (see Fig. 13-5). Typical renal venography injection rates are 10-15 mL/sec for 2 seconds, with rapid filming (3-4 frames/sec).

Selective gonadal venography is simplified by the consistent location of the left gonadal vein orifice in the left renal vein. A left renal venogram often localizes the orifice of the left gonadal vein (see Fig 13-5B). Injection during the Valsalva maneuver or tilting the venography table in reverse Trendelenburg may be necessary to unmask reflux into the gonadal vein. A competent valve at the gonadal vein orifice can make selective placement of a catheter difficult. The right gonadal vein orifice is more difficult to localize as it originates from the IVC. When a femoral venous access is used, a Cobra-2 catheter can be used to select the left gonadal vein, and a recurved catheter such as a Simmons-1 can be used for the right (Fig. 13-13). From a jugular approach, a Headhunter-1 or similar angled catheter can be used to select each vein. Many angiographers prefer a jugular venous access for gonadal venography, particularly when an intervention is anticipated. A steerable angled hydrophilic guidewire is helpful to advance the catheter into the gonadal vein. Hand injection of 5-15 mL of contrast is usually sufficient to opacify a normal gonadal vein. Higher volumes may be necessary in dilated veins. Shielding of the gonads is not possible in female patients but should be considered in males.

Adrenal venography is usually only required to confirm catheter location during adrenal vein sampling (Fig. 13-14). Review of abdominal CT scans before the procedure can help localize the right renal vein. A single side hole is added near the tip of the catheter to facilitate aspiration of blood. The left adrenal vein is easily catheterized with a 5-French Simmons-2 or similar long recurved catheter. The tip of the catheter is placed in the left renal vein beyond the ostium of the left phrenic vein. The catheter is then slowly retracted so that the tip pushes against the superior wall of the renal vein. As the catheter is withdrawn, the tip will engage the phrenic vein, and allow selection of the adrenal vein. On occasion, a microcatheter is used to subselect the adrenal vein. On the right, a steeply angled 5-French catheter is used to find the right adrenal vein above the right renal vein. Small hepatic branches can be easily confused with the adrenal gland. A few milliliters of contrast should be slowly and gently injected to avoid rupture of the delicate adrenal veins. Patients may report a mild ache or sensation of fullness in the back with adrenal vein injections. This characteristic sensation can be used to help determine when the correct vein has been selected. Adrenal venography has many appearances; a well-defined wedge-shaped structure with arborizing veins, a delta pattern of veins, a triangular pattern of veins, spiculated veins in the shape of the gland, or even a nonspecific-appearing vein in the expected location of the adrenal vein. On the right, collateral drainage into a hepatic vein suggests that the selected vein is an accessory hepatic rather than adrenal vein.

▬ INFERIOR VENA CAVA OBSTRUCTION

The usual location (>90%) of IVC occlusion is in the infrarenal segment. Obstruction can be caused by intrinsic or extrinsic pathology (Box 13-1). The most common etiology of intrinsic obstruction is thrombosis, typically extension of iliac vein thrombus (Box 13-2). Isolated thrombotic occlusion of the IVC is unusual in the absence of a translumbar IVC line, an IVC filter, trauma, or surgery. Delayed thrombosis can occur following liver transplantation due to stenosis of the caval anastomoses.

Extrinsic compression of the IVC can be caused by tumor, adenopathy, aortic aneurysm, pericaval fibrosis, surgical ligation, and hepatic enlargement (see Fig. 13-9). In pregnant patients, positional obstruction of the IVC can be caused by the enlarged uterus. This is usually relieved when the patient is in the left lateral decubitus position.

The symptoms of IVC obstruction vary with the rapidity of the occlusion, the status of collateral veins, and the flow within the venous system. Gradual occlusion of the IVC may be asymptomatic if the collateral veins are intact and enlarged. Acute occlusion usually results in sudden onset of bilateral lower extremity edema. The swelling subsides, sometimes completely, as collateral veins become recruited and enlarge. In some patients, sudden interruption of venous return from the lower extremities may result in hypotension. This rare complication is most likely to occur in a patient with an IVC filter that becomes acutely occluded by a large embolus. In patients with disrupted or thrombosed collateral veins, even gradual occlusion may cause symptoms. Exercise, or creation of a lower extremity arteriovenous fistula, may unmask a previously asymptomatic obstruction by virtue of the increased venous flow.

On physical examination, the finding of bilateral lower extremity edema and dilated abdominal wall veins should suggest occlusion of the IVC. Patients with longstanding IVC occlusion can develop typical venous stasis changes of the lower extremities, such as brawny discoloration of the skin, woody edema, and ulcers.

Obstruction of the IVC can be suggested on duplex ultrasound examination when there is stasis of flow, loss of the normal respiratory variation, or thrombosis of the iliofemoral veins bilaterally (Fig. 13-15). A blunted or absent Doppler response to Valsalva is suggestive of central occlusion when the finding is bilateral. Direct interrogation of the IVC may be possible, but it cannot be reliably performed in the infrarenal segment in all patients.

Cross-sectional imaging with CT and MR allows diagnosis of IVC obstruction as well as evaluation of the adjacent soft tissues for possible causes. Expansion of the IVC implies an intrinsic occlusion, whereas compression is almost always associated with an obvious extrinsic mass lesion. High-attenuation material in the IVC on a noncontrast CT can be seen with acute thrombus. Enhancement of the wall of the IVC with a low-attenuation lumen after administration of contrast is diagnostic of an intrinsic occlusion (typically bland thrombus) (Fig. 13-16). Contrast may be visualized around an intraluminal filling defect at the proximal

and distal extent of an occlusion, or with incomplete obstruction. Intraluminal tumor may enhance with contrast (see Tumors). The extent of an occlusion may be overestimated if stagnant blood caudad to an obstruction does not enhance with contrast. Delayed scans help avoid this pitfall.

Diagnostic cavography provides less information about the etiology of an occlusion than ultrasound, CT, or MRI, but may be necessary to localize the pathology as intrinsic or extrinsic and determine the extent. Intraluminal occlusions have a characteristic appearance with contrast on both sides of a filling defect (Fig. 13-17). Extrinsic compression causes broadening or effacement of the lumen (see Fig. 13-9). Rarely, IVUS is required to make a conclusive diagnosis. Stenosis of the IVC can be evaluated with

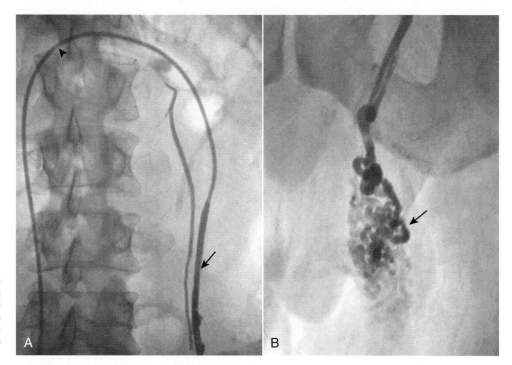

FIGURE 13-13. Selective left gonadal venogram in a patient with a varicocele. **A,** The left gonadal vein *(arrow)* has been selected with a catheter *(arrowhead)* from the right femoral approach **B,** Digital image showing a distended pampiniform plexus *(arrow)*.

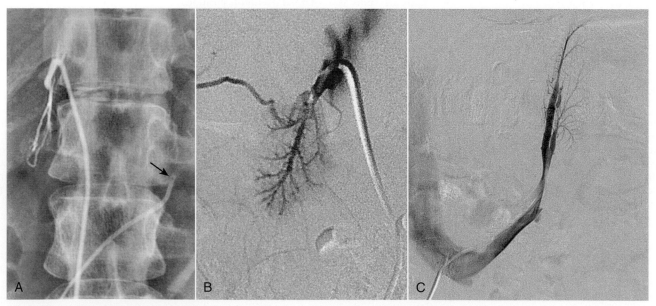

FIGURE 13-14. Adrenal venography. **A,** Unsubtracted digital image showing catheterization of both renal veins with injection of contrast on the right. Each catheter has a single side hole *(arrow)* near the tip to facilitate sampling. **B,** Digital subtraction image showing a normal right adrenal gland. **C,** Digital subtraction image showing a normal left adrenal gland.

measurement of a pressure gradient across the lesion. In the supine patient, the normal gradient should be less than 3 mm Hg. When performing cavography in a patient with obstruction, contrast should be injected as close to the lesion as possible to avoid overestimating the extent of occlusion. Contrast injected in a remote location such as a femoral vein preferentially opacifies the collateral veins rather than the obstructed IVC. Patients should not be instructed to perform Valsalva during injection of contrast, because the IVC lumen may be artifactually obliterated by the transient increase in intraabdominal pressure.

Acute thrombosis of the IVC is often linked to iliofemoral thrombosis, occlusion of an IVC filter, or a hypercoagulable condition. Therapy for IVC thrombosis is usually the same as that for lower extremity deep venous thrombosis. Anticoagulation, elevation of the extremities, and compression stockings are the traditional medical treatments. Surgical thrombectomy is rarely indicated. Catheter-directed thrombolysis or catheter thrombectomy with pharmacomechanical or mechanical techniques can provide rapid relief of symptoms. (This technique is discussed in Chapter 16.) One of the goals of thrombolysis or thrombectomy is the unmasking of underlying IVC pathology that may have precipitated the thrombosis (Fig. 13-18). There is a small risk (1%) of major pulmonary embolism (PE) during interventions for caval thrombus. Optional or temporary IVC filters may have a role in selected patients as a preventive measure.

Symptomatic stenoses of the IVC or other occlusive lesion can be stented to prevent recurrent thrombosis. A variety of stents have been used for this purpose, including both balloon-expandable and self-expanding. Stents with diameters in the range of 12-30 mm are required. The long-term results of IVC stents for benign stenoses in the absence of a hypercoagulable state have been excellent when large-diameter stents can be placed. The reported patency is 80% at 5 years.

Chronic occlusions of the IVC can be successfully recanalized using standard techniques. Evaluation with CT before the procedure is helpful to plan the procedure. The longer the occlusion, the more difficult it will be to recanalize successfully. Complete absence of a visible IVC remnant on CT is discouraging, but does not exclude successful recanalization. Simultaneous jugular and femoral vein access is often necessary to provide a visual target during recanalization and assist in delivering devices across the lesion. Stent placement is almost always necessary. Large-diameter self-expanding stents are preferred in this location. Longstanding occlusions may not initially dilate beyond 10 or 12 mm diameter due to atresia of the IVC remnant. These sometimes respond to gentle angioplasty and dilate further at a later date. Stents can be used in the presence of a chronically occluded IVC filter. In this situation, the stents are placed through the filter, pushing the filter elements to the side. Surgical approaches with embolectomy, bypass, and hybrid techniques that include stent placement have a 5-year primary patency of 40%-50%. Large studies with long-term results of

Box 13-1. Etiologies of Inferior Vena Cava Obstruction

INTRINSIC
Thrombosis
Stenosis
Tumor
• Primary
• Invasion from adjacent organ/retroperitoneum
Iatrogenic

EXTRINSIC
Enlarged liver
• Hypertrophy
• Tumor
• Regenerating nodules
Compression by retroperitoneal mass
• Adenopathy
• Tumor
• Aortic aneurysm
Pregnant uterus
Retroperitoneal fibrosis
Surgical ligation, clip
Abdominal compartment syndrome

Box 13-2. Risk Factors for Thrombosis of the Inferior Vena Cava

Hypercoagulable state
Instrumentation
Central venous access catheter (transfemoral or direct inferior vena cava [IVC])
Partial IVC interruption (filter or clip)
Surgery
Extrinsic compression
Tumor (primary IVC or invasion)
Chemotherapy

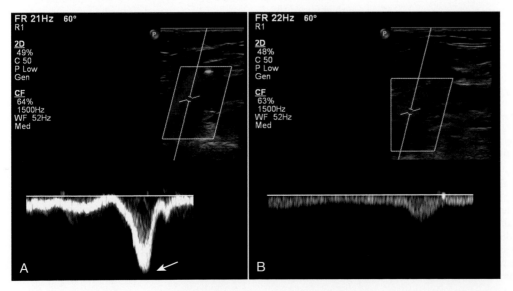

FIGURE 13-15. Duplex ultrasound showing indirect evidence of inferior vena cava occlusion. **A,** Image from the common femoral vein (CFV) of a normal patient showing phasic variation of flow with normal response to augmentation *(arrow).* **B,** Image from the CFV of a patient with central venous occlusion. There is loss of respiratory and cardiac variation of flow at the common femoral vein, with blunted response to augmentation. These findings were bilateral. The level of obstruction could be in the iliac veins as well as the inferior vena cava.

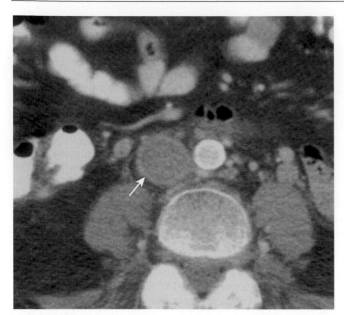

FIGURE **13-16**. Axial computed tomography scan showing a distended, thrombus-filled inferior vena cava *(arrow)* with enhancement of the vessel wall.

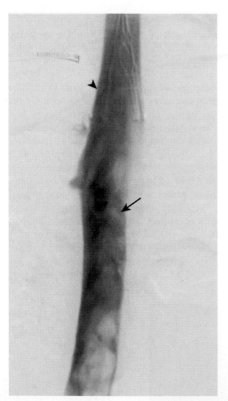

FIGURE **13-17**. Digital subtraction cavogram showing thrombus extending to the level of the renal veins *(arrow)*. The thrombus is visualized as an intraluminal filling defect outlined by contrast. A vena cava filter *(arrowhead)* was placed in the suprarenal inferior vena cava.

endovascular approaches are not available, but should have similar if not slightly better patency.

Treatment of symptomatic extrinsic compression of the IVC (massive lower extremity and scrotal/labial edema, abdominal wall edema, and ascites) should be directed, when possible, to the mass or lesion causing the compression. Resection of tumors, shrinkage of nodal masses with chemotherapy or radiation, or patience (especially in the case of compression of the IVC by a

pregnant uterus) may resolve symptoms. Diuretics, correction of hypoalbuminemia, compression stockings, and anticoagulation or antiplatelet therapy should be instituted when possible. When conservative measures fail or are not feasible, stent placement is an excellent option for patients with malignant or other terminal illnesses who seek improvement in the quality of their remaining life (Fig. 13-19). Large self-expanding stents should be used, sized to the normal diameter IVC. The stent should not protrude into the right atrium if possible, because this may induce arrhythmias and the motion may fracture the stents. Approximately two thirds of patients experience significant symptomatic relief. The average life expectancy of these patients when the compression is due to malignancy is well less than 6 months.

▬ VENA CAVA FILTERS

Vena cava filters prevent thrombotic pulmonary emboli (PE) by trapping the thrombus in the vena cava. Filters do not prevent the formation of thrombus, enhance anticoagulation, or treat PE that has already occurred. The conventional treatment for deep venous thrombosis (DVT) and PE is anticoagulation. Filters should be used when patients with venous thromboembolism (VTE) cannot be anticoagulated or when patients at high risk for development of DVT cannot be screened, monitored, or receive prophylaxis. Filters placed in patients who are at risk for but do not yet have VTE are considered prophylactic, a controversial but very common indication. There is no role for filters in stable patients with VTE who can be treated with anticoagulation (Box 13-3). Patients who receive filters should resume conventional treatment appropriate for their degree of VTE as soon as practical.

There are a large number of vena cava filters available (Figs. 13-20 and 13-21 and Table 13-2). Several are designed to be removable or convertible to a nonfiltration state as well. Most filters probably function equally well, so the criteria for selection of one device over another should be based on availability, access routes, and vena cava anatomy. Devices with smaller diameter delivery systems ("low-profile") have the greatest flexibility in terms of the number of potential access sites. Filters can be placed from the femoral, jugular, or upper arm veins. Most filters have an upper limit for the IVC diameter of 28-30 mm.

Permanent filters are thought to increase the risk for recurrent DVT. Furthermore, because the thresholds for placing these devices are lowered, patients are living longer after placement. This has stimulated interest in nonpermanent IVC filters. There are no randomized clinical trials to guide decisions about different filters. In general, a nonpermanent filter should be considered for any patient with either transient risk for PE and/or contraindication to anticoagulation and a life expectancy of more than 6 months.

Removable filters can be classified as either temporary (must be removed) or optional (can be left in place as a permanent filter). Most temporary filters are attached to a catheter or wire that facilitates removal but occupies a venous access site for 2-6 weeks. There is a 4%-5% risk of access site infection and a 10%-15% conversion rate to a permanent filter when these devices are used during lower extremity deep venous thrombolysis.

Filters that have been in place for a period of time are covered by a layer of fibrotic tissue and neointima wherever the filter touches the wall of the IVC. In addition, elements of the filter such as feet or arms can migrate through the wall of the IVC. The elements of the filter outside the IVC are usually covered by connective tissue that is contiguous with the IVC adventitia. Filter retrieval is accomplished by peeling the filter away from the wall of the IVC, sliding the filter out of the covering tissue, or a combination of both using a snare or other retrieval device. The duration of time that can pass before any one filter becomes so firmly attached to the IVC that it cannot be retrieved is not known with certainty because every patient is different and every filter placement unique. The more contact between the IVC and the filter,

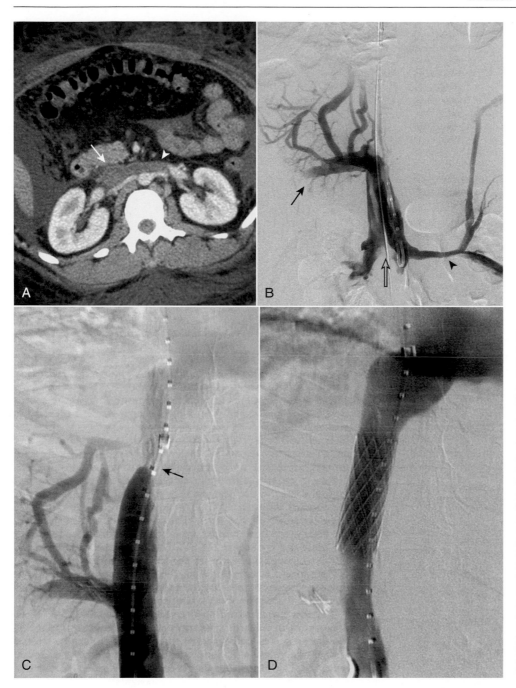

FIGURE 13-18. Acute inferior vena cava (IVC) thrombosis following cholecystectomy in young female with a previously undiagnosed hypercoagulable syndrome. **A,** Axial computed tomography image showing high-density thrombus in the IVC *(arrow)* extending into the left renal vein *(arrowhead).* The thrombus extended from the intrahepatic IVC retrograde to both femoral veins. Notice the extensive subcutaneous edema and ascites. **B,** Cavogram obtained from a jugular vein approach shows thrombus in the IVC *(open arrow).* There is retrograde flow into an accessory right hepatic vein *(solid arrow)* with collateral drainage through the liver to other hepatic veins due to occlusion of the intrahepatic IVC. Some contrast refluxes into the partially thrombosed left renal vein *(arrowhead).* **C,** After pharmacomechanical and infusion thrombolysis, the IVC thrombus has cleared revealing a tight stenosis *(arrow)* of the intrahepatic IVC above the accessory right hepatic vein. **D,** The stenosis did not respond to angioplasty, so an extra-large balloon-expandable stent was placed. (Courtesy Palmaz XL, Cordis, Warren, N.J.)

the less likely that it can be retrieved after a long duration if the dominant mechanism is to peel the filter rather than extract it.

Filter Placement

After determining the indication for the vena cava filter, review of existing cross-sectional imaging may reveal an important anatomic variant. A cavogram is performed to assess caval patency, anatomy, and dimensions (see Imaging for technical details). A key anatomic variant is a duplicated IVC, which occurs in fewer than 1% of the population (see Fig. 13-4). When the pigtail catheter is placed from the right common femoral or a jugular vein, reflux of contrast into the left common iliac vein helps exclude this anomaly. When a duplicated IVC is present, each common iliac vein usually drains only into the IVC on the same side. Multiple renal veins may also be present. When in doubt regarding IVC anatomy, selective catheterization should be used to investigate further.

The level of the lowest renal vein should be identified. The filter delivery sheath is then inserted over a guidewire into the IVC and the filter deployed. The ideal location for filter placement is a matter of much debate and opinion, but little fact. Cone-shaped filters can be placed with the apex just above or as close to the lower lip of the renal vein as possible (Fig. 13-22). The rationale for placement in this location is that the high flow from the renal veins will prevent thrombus formation or propagation above the filter. When a well-developed circumaortic left renal vein is present, this could be a potential circuit around the filter and placement below or across the lower, retroaortic component of the left renal vein is recommended. The specific steps for deployment vary with different filters and are explained in the package inserts. After deployment of the filter, a repeat cavogram through the delivery sheath, or at the minimum a digital spot film, is obtained to document the final position of the device.

When there is insufficient space below the renal veins owing to a short IVC or the presence of thrombus, the filter can be placed

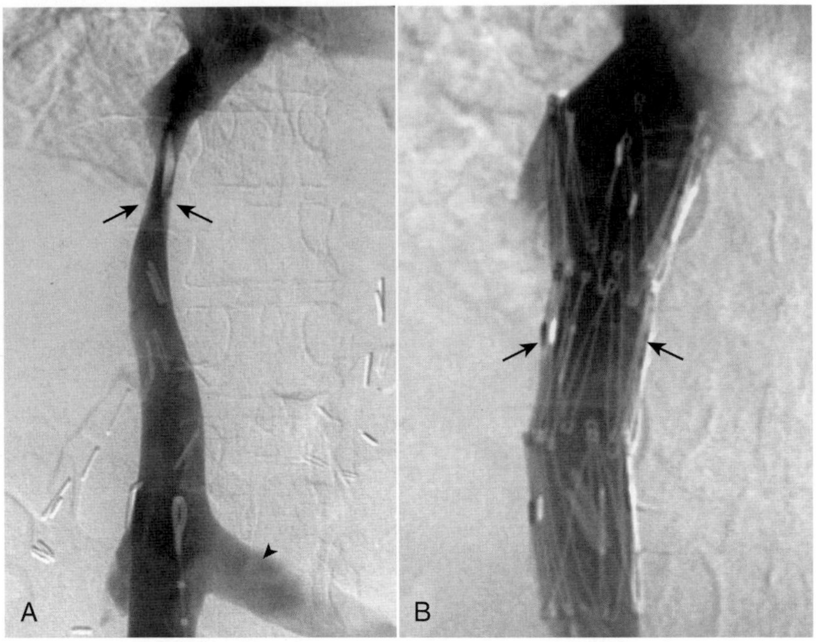

FIGURE 13-19. Intrahepatic inferior vena cava (IVC) stenosis due to metastatic carcinoid tumor to the liver. The patient had tense bilateral lower extremity edema. **A,** Digital cavogram showing compression of the intrahepatic IVC *(arrows)* and reflux into the left renal vein *(arrowhead)*. There was a 22-mm Hg gradient across the stenosis. **B,** Digital cavogram after placement of a 20-mm diameter Z-stent (courtesy Cook Group, Bloomington, Ind.) in the intrahepatic IVC *(arrows)*. The gradient was reduced to 2 mm Hg and the patient's edema resolved over the next few days.

Box 13-3. Indications for Vena Cava Filters

CLASSIC INDICATIONS (PROVEN VTE)
Contraindication to AC
Complication of AC
Inability to achieve/maintain therapeutic AC

EXTENDED INDICATIONS (PROVEN VTE)
Recurrent VTE (acute or chronic) despite adequate AC
Iliocaval DVT
Large, free-floating proximal DVT
Difficulty establishing therapeutic AC
Massive PE treated with thrombolysis/thrombectomy
Chronic PE treated with thromboendarterectomy
Thrombolysis for iliocaval DVT
VTE with limited cardiopulmonary reserve
Recurrent PE with filter in place
Poor compliance with AC medications
High risk of complication of AC (e.g., ataxia, frequent falls)

PROPHYLACTIC INDICATIONS (NO VTE*)
Trauma patient with high risk of VTE
Surgical procedure in patient at high risk of VTE
Medical condition with high risk of VTE

---

*Primary prophylaxis not feasible, e.g., as a result of high bleeding risk, inability to monitor the patient for VTE.
AC, Anticoagulation; DVT, deep vein thrombosis; PE, pulmonary embolism; VTE, venous thromboembolism.

---

in the segment of IVC between the renal and hepatic veins (known as a *suprarenal* placement) (see Fig. 13-17). The Bird's Nest filter (Cook, Bloomington, Ind.) should be avoided in a suprarenal location because the wire mesh, which frequently prolapses during deployment, can extend up into the heart, causing arrythmias. In the presence of a duplicated IVC, a filter should be placed in each IVC, or a single filter in a suprarenal location. When a mega cava is discovered (diameter > 28-30 mm), the Vena Tech LP (B. Braun, Bethlehem, Pa.) can be used off-label in the United States up to 35 mm. Only the Bird's Nest filter can be used on label up to 40 mm. Filters can be placed in septic

patients without fear of device infection, although this is listed as a contraindication by most manufacturers.

In pregnant patients in their first trimester, the entire procedure can be performed from a jugular approach if necessary to minimize radiation exposure. The classic teaching is to place the filter in the suprarenal location in pregnant women or women of childbearing age (to avoid compression of the filter by a gravid uterus), but there is no objective evidence to support this practice.

Rarely, patients with upper extremity venous thrombosis will require a filter in the superior vena cava (SVC). The majority of the patients requiring SVC filters reported in the literature have been extremely ill with short life expectancies. In this situation, the filter should be oriented appropriately with the apex toward the heart and the feet in the SVC just below the junction of the left brachiocephalic vein with the SVC (see Fig. 7-14). Because of the pericardial reflection along the SVC, a conical filter without secondary upper arms should be used to decrease the risk for perforation and acute pericardial tamponade.

The complications of IVC filters are listed in Table 13-3. When a patient with a filter experiences a documented recurrent PE, the first step is to determine whether the patient can be treated with anticoagulation. Patients who can be anticoagulated require no further evaluation, but should be treated with a full course of therapy. Patients who cannot be anticoagulated require evaluation for the origin of the PE. The discovery of new lower extremity DVT, trapped thrombus in the filter, or thrombus extending above the filter suggests filter failure. In these situations a second device should be placed, usually in the suprarenal IVC.

Other sources of emboli should be considered when PE recurs in a patient with an IVC filter without lower extremity DVT. Potential origins of emboli include internal iliac, gonadal, renal, and upper extremity vein thrombosis. Management of emboli from the renal and gonadal veins may require a suprarenal filter.

Symptomatic complete occlusion of the filter can be treated with anticoagulation or thrombolysis if the patient no longer has contraindications to these therapies. Otherwise, conservative measures such as elevation of the extremities and compression stockings are used. On very rare occasions IVC thrombosis after filter placement in the setting of extensive DVT (unilateral or bilateral) results in arterial ischemia (phlegmasia cerulea dolens) (see Fig. 16-12). A difficult problem to treat in patients who cannot be anticoagulated or undergo thrombolysis, this usually occurs soon after initial filter placement in a hypercoagulable patient.

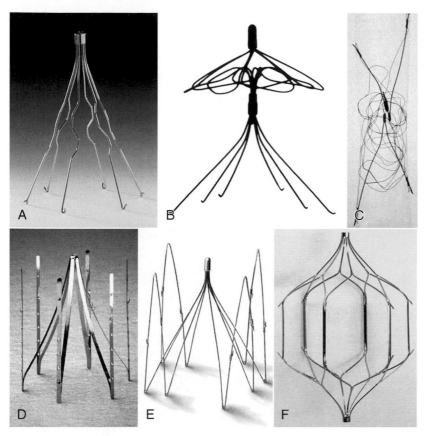

FIGURE 13-20. Examples of permanent inferior vena cava (IVC) filters. **A**, The 12-French stainless steel Greenfield (Boston Scientific). **B**, Simon Nitinol (C. R. Bard). **C**, Bird's Nest (Cook Medical). **D**, Vena Tech (B. Braun Medical). **E**, Vena Tech LP (B. Braun Medical). **F**, TrapEase (Cordis Corporation, 2003).

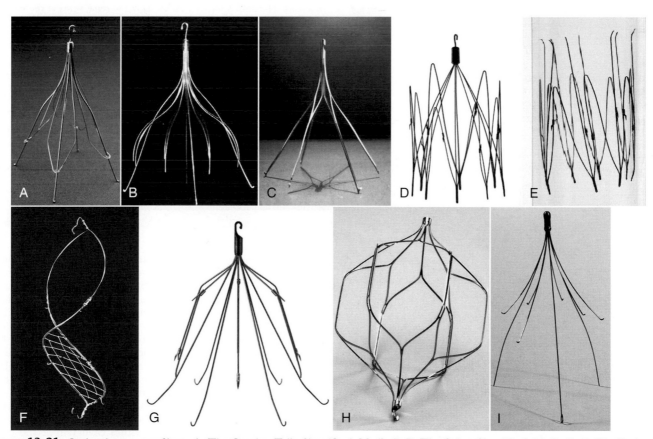

FIGURE 13-21. Optional vena cava filters. **A**, The Gunther Tulip filter (Cook Medical). **B**, The Celect filter (Cook Medical). **C**, The Option Filter (Argon Medical). **D**, The B. Braun Convertible filter in closed position (B. Braun Medical). **E**, The B. Braun Convertible filter with the cap removed (constrained within a plastic tube). **F**, The Crux filter; note that the filter is deployed with the filter element toward the patient's feet (Crux BioMedical). **G**, The Meridian filter (C.R. Bard, Inc. Used with permission. The trademark Bard and Meridian are the property of C.R. Bard, Inc.). **H**, The OptEase filter; note that the filter is deployed with the hook toward the patient's feet (Cordis Corporation, 2012). **I**, The ALN filter. (ALN Implants). Filters **A, B, C, F, G,** and **I** are retrieved from a jugular approach. Filter **H** is retrieved from the femoral approach. Filter **F** is retrievable from either approach. Filter **D** is converted from a jugular approach by retrieving the apical cap.

TABLE **13-2** Vena Cava Filters

Filter*	Introducer ID	Access	Maximum IVC Diameter (mm)	Metal
Permanent				
Simon Nitinol (CR Bard)	7	IJV, SV, AV, CFV	28	Nitinol
Greenfield (Boston Scientific)	12	IJV, CFV	28	Stainless steel
Vena Tech LGM (B. Braun)	10	IJV, CFV	28	Phynox
Vena Tech LP (B. Braun)	7	IJV, AV, CFV	28 (35 OUS)	Phynox
Bird's Nest (Cook Medical)	12	IJV, CFV	40	Stainless steel
TrapEase (Cordis)	6	IJV, AV, CFV	30	Nitinol
Optional				
ALN (ALN Implants)	7	IJV, BV, CFV	28 (32 OUS)	Stainless steel
Option (Argon Medical)	5	IJV, CFV	28 (32 OUS)	Nitinol
Meridian (CR Bard)	8	IJV, CFV	28	Nitinol
Vena Tech Convertible (B. Braun)	10	IJV, CFV	28	Phynox
Gunther (Cook Medical)	8.5	IJV, CFV	30	Conichrome
Celect (Cook Medical)	7 8.5	IJV CFV	30	Conichrome
OptEase (Cordis)	6	IJV, AV, CFV	30	Nitinol
Crux (Crux Biomedical)	9	IJV, CFV	28	Nitinol and ePTFE

*All filters are magnetic resonance imaging compatible to 3 T; Cook Medical recommends a 6-week interval between placement and scanning with the Bird's Nest. AV, Antecubital vein; BV, basilic vein; CFV, common femoral vein; ID, internal diameter in French; IJV, internal jugular vein; OUS, outside the United States; SV, subclavian vein.

Surgical venous thrombectomy and even amputation may be necessary, but the mortality rate is generally high.

Filter Retrieval or Conversion

Optional filters should not be removed or converted until the patient is no longer at risk for PE. Physicians placing these devices should determine at the time of insertion whether the patient is a candidate for future removal or conversion, and actively participate in patient follow-up. This should not be left to the patient or their primary physician.

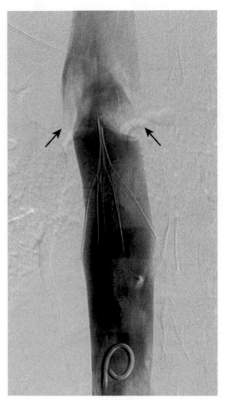

FIGURE **13-22**. Infrarenal position of a cone-shaped filter (Option, Argon Medical). The arrows indicate inflow from the renal veins at the level of the apex of the filter.

TABLE **13-3** Complications of Inferior Vena Cava Filters

Outcome	Incidence (%)
Recurrent pulmonary embolism	5
Symptomatic complete inferior vena cava occlusion	5
Symptomatic insertion site thrombosis	2
Major filter migration (to heart, lungs, iliac veins)	<1
Filter fracture with clinical consequences	<1
Symptomatic perforation of adjacent structures	<1

Filter removal or conversion in the patient with VTE should not occur until the patient is back on full anticoagulation for at least 2 weeks. Patients who are subtherapeutic should delay the procedure until therapeutic for this period of time. The patient with a prophylactic indication should be either tolerating pharmacologic prophylaxis or have passed the period of risk. Patients who had the filter placed for prophylaxis, without known VTE (e.g., trauma), should have a documented negative lower extremity venous duplex ultrasound before the filter is removed. Filter removal can be safely performed in fully anticoagulated patients; anticoagulation should not be interrupted for the procedure.

Before removal or conversion, patients should have imaging of the filter to evaluate for trapped emboli. This can be with CT scan before the procedure or with a cavogram at the time of removal (Fig. 13-23). A small amount of adherent thrombus to filter elements is not usually a concern, but any fresh-looking thrombus should raise the questions of adequacy of anticoagulation in patients with VTE or the need for anticoagulation in patients who had the filter placed prophylactically. The procedure can be stopped at this point, patient workup or treatment

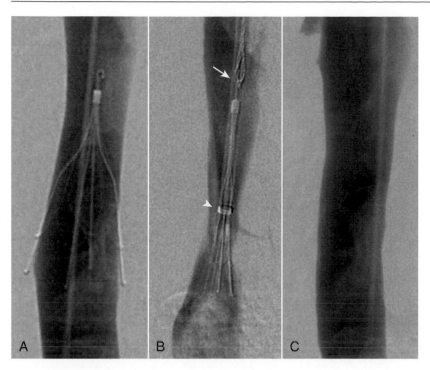

FIGURE 13-23. The process of filter retrieval. **A**, Initial cavogram confirming patency of the filter and IVC (Gunther Tulip, Cook Medical). Note that the feet appear outside of the contrast column, but are in reality covered by neointima. **B**, The filter has been snared *(arrow)* and the sheath *(arrowhead)* advanced part way down the device. Contrast injection shows the temporary collapse of the inferior vena cava (IVC) before the filter detaches from the wall. To remove the filter, traction is applied to the snare as the sheath is advanced over the feet. **C**, Completion cavogram after filter removal showing a normal IVC.

(extraction), or both (see Fig. 13-23). A considerable amount of force may be necessary when filters are well incorporated, and the patient may feel pain.

There are several techniques for dealing with filters that are difficult to engage or remove. During a difficult procedure, it is important to be sure that the patient is anticoagulated. Conebeam CT is very helpful to understand the relationship of the filter to the IVC wall. A stiff guidewire ("buddywire") through the sheath and filter alongside the snare can help align the sheath, snare, and filter. When the hook is against the IVC wall but there is still space between the filter apex and the wall, a snare can be constructed around the filter (see Fig. 4-53). A second catheter from the opposite approach to deflect the filter away from the wall may be useful; an angioplasty balloon between the filter apex and the IVC wall can also reposition the apex. Very adherent filter apices can be freed using rigid bronchoscopy forceps (with great care), and adherent filters can be extracted using a sheath rimmed with a laser, usually used for pacemaker lead extraction (Fig. 13-25).

When removal is difficult, it is always acceptable to stop the procedure and leave the filter permanently unless the filter itself is causing a problem and removal is the only treatment. Caval laceration, thrombosis, filter fracture, and filter embolization are rare but reported complications of difficult retrievals. Following retrieval, patients should be treated for their underlying extent of VTE.

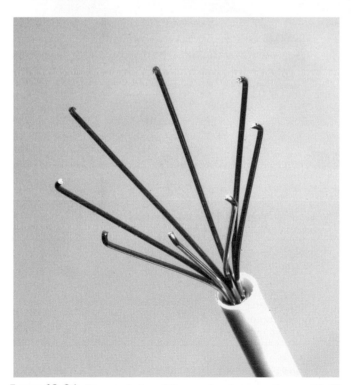

FIGURE 13-24. Forceps designed for grasping the apex of removable filters. (Courtesy ALN Implants, Bormes les Mimosa, France.)

for several weeks may be undertaken, and then removal can be attempted again.

Filter removal is from the jugular approach, the femoral approach, or both depending on the filter design. An initial cavogram is performed to assess for trapped thrombus and the orientation of the filter. A long sheath large enough to accommodate the filter and the grasping device are inserted. The usual removal tool is a snare or dedicated forceps (Fig. 13-24; see Fig. 4-51). Once the filter is securely engaged, it is removed by either sliding the sheath over the filter (peeling), pulling the filter into the sheath

▬ TUMORS

Primary tumors of the IVC are rare, with fewer than 1 per 34,000 seen at autopsy. These are almost always leiomyosarcomas. The most common location is the segment of IVC between the renal and hepatic veins (42%), followed by the infrarenal IVC (34%) and the intrahepatic IVC (24%). The tumors are mostly intraluminal, but extraluminal extension into the adjacent retroperitoneum is present in many cases (Fig. 13-26). Women are affected more often than men.

Tumors may invade the IVC directly through the wall, or by growing through a side branch (Boxes 13-4 and 13-5, and see Figs. 1-26 and 12-28). The most common etiology of intravascular tumor is renal cell carcinoma. Up to 20% of patients with renal cell

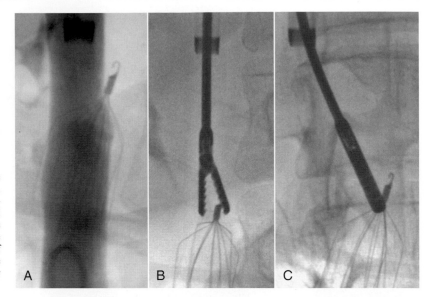

FIGURE **13-25**. Rigid bronchoscopy forceps used to free the apex of a filter. **A,** Cavogram showing a G2 filter (CR. Bard, N.J.), tilted with the apex outside the column of contrast indicating an overlying layer of fibrotic material and neointima. **B,** Oblique image of rigid bronchoscopy forceps in open position on the filter apex. The forceps were inserted through a large jugular vein sheath. **C,** Image of forceps during careful nibbling at the material overlying the filter apex. After freeing the apex, the filter was successfully removed with a snare and sheath.

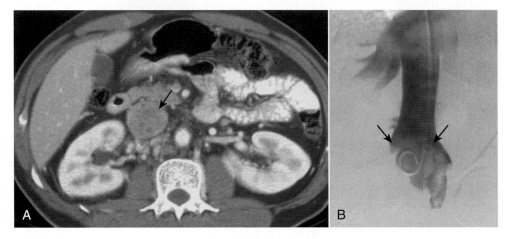

FIGURE **13-26**. Primary leiomyosarcoma of the inferior vena cava (IVC). **A,** Axial computed tomography image showing a heterogeneously enhancing mass expanding the IVC *(arrow)*. The kidneys and renal veins were normal. **B,** Digital subtraction image obtained during transvascular biopsy of the mass, showing an intraluminal filling defect *(arrows)* expanding the IVC.

Box 13-4. **Tumors That Encase the Inferior Vena Cava**

Liposarcoma
Retroperitoneal leiomyosarcoma
Malignant fibrous histiocytoma
Cholangiocarcinoma
Hepatocellular carcinoma
Hepatic metastatic lesions
Pancreatic carcinoma
Duodenal carcinoma

Box 13-5. **Tumors That Invade the Inferior Vena Cava**

Renal cell carcinoma
Hepatocellular carcinoma
Pheochromocytoma
Adrenal carcinoma
Uterine sarcoma
Germ cell tumor
Prostate carcinoma

---

carcinoma have tumor in the renal vein, and 4%-15% have extension into the IVC. In half of these, the tumor is located in the intrarenal IVC, and in 40%, in the intrahepatic IVC. Tumor extension into the right atrium occurs in as many as 10% of these patients.

The clinical presentation of patients with IVC involvement by tumor varies with the degree and acuity of the obstruction, the type of tumor, and the extent of intracaval tumor or associated thrombus. Primary IVC tumors are generally advanced before they become symptomatic with metastatic disease, iliofemoral thrombosis, renal vein obstruction, and hepatic vein obstruction. Secondary involvement of the IVC by malignancy is usually detected during workup of the primary lesion. Pulmonary embolism, cardiac arrhythmias, and Budd-Chiari syndrome can occur with intracaval tumor.

Imaging of patients with IVC involvement by malignancy is focused on determining the origin and stage of the malignancy,

localization of the level of IVC obstruction, and determination of the extent of intracaval tumor. CT and MRI are the preferred modalities for IVC imaging in these patients, in that both the pericaval and intraluminal structures can be imaged. Expansion of the IVC with enhancing intraluminal tissue is consistent with tumor rather than thrombus. Leiomyosarcoma of the IVC with retroperitoneal extension may be indistinguishable from a primary retroperitoneal lesion with caval invasion.

Cavography is reserved for patients with inconclusive findings on cross-sectional imaging. Occasionally, intravascular biopsy is performed to confirm the nature of the intraluminal process (Fig. 13-27).

Therapy of primary IVC leiomyosarcoma is radical resection and replacement of the IVC with synthetic graft material when

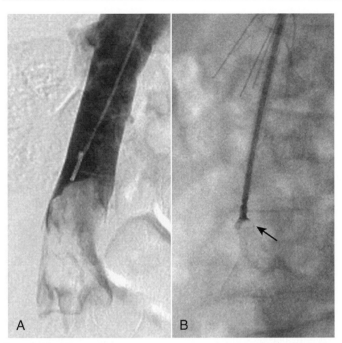

FIGURE 13-27. Biopsy of an intravascular mass. **A,** Cavogram showing a large intraluminal filling defect in the infrarenal vena cava. **B,** Clamshell biopsy *(arrow)* through a long sheath positioned just above the mass. A removable inferior vena cava filter was placed first because the initial diagnosis was iliocaval thrombosis. The biopsy revealed prostatic carcinoma, and the filter was subsequently removed.

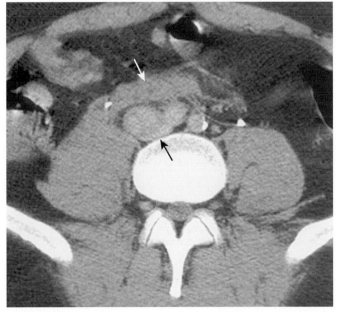

FIGURE 13-28. Traumatic laceration of the inferior vena cava (IVC) due to blunt trauma, surgically repaired. Axial computed tomography image showing an enlarged, irregular IVC *(black arrow)* and retroperitoneal hematoma *(white arrow).*

necessary. Operative mortality is as high as 13%, with a 5-year survival of only 28% and a high rate of local recurrence.

TRAUMA

The IVC and abdominal veins can be injured by penetrating or blunt trauma, surgery, or interventional procedures (Fig. 13-28). Though a low-pressure system, blood flow in the IVC and renal veins is substantial, with the potential for major blood loss. The

---

Box 13-6. Causes of Renal Vein Thrombosis

Hypercoagulable state
Membranous glomerulonephritis
Dehydration
Thrombosis of the inferior vena cava
Stenosis (transplant renal vein)
Extrinsic compression
Retroperitoneal tumor
Adenopathy
Retroperitoneal fibrosis
Nephrotic syndrome
Tumor thrombus
  • Renal cell carcinoma
  • Adrenal carcinoma

IVC is injured in 2% of abdominal gunshot wounds. More than 50% of patients with caval injuries die before arriving at the hospital; of those who survive to receive medical care, up to 50% also die. Multiple organ injuries are common in these patients, and 10% have associated major arterial injuries. The diagnosis is evident on CT scan, although rarely cavography may be required. Management is expectant when possible, because surgical repair or ligation of the traumatized IVC is extremely difficult owing to the difficult exposure and diaphanous nature of the vessel wall. Most bleeding from the IVC is tamponaded by surrounding structures when the retroperitoneum is intact. Owing to the 50% mortality rate from intraoperative exsanguination, surgery is reserved for patients with evidence of continued bleeding. Stent-graft treatment of this injury has been reported in a few patients, usually using components from abdominal aortic systems such as large aortic cuffs. This is a promising approach for an extremely challenging injury. Renal vein injuries are usually managed with ligation, which is tolerated well.

RENAL VEIN THROMBOSIS

There are many etiologies of renal vein thrombosis (Box 13-6). The rapidity of obstruction and degree of collateralization determine the symptoms (see Fig. 13-18). Acute thrombosis that extends into the renal hilum, obstructing collateral drainage pathways, results in renal dysfunction, back pain, and hematuria with congestion and edema of the kidney. These symptoms are similar to those caused by acute renal ischemia of arterial etiology. Extensive thrombosis can result in permanent ischemic damage to the kidney. Renal vein thrombus may be a source of pulmonary emboli. For this reason, identification of inflow of unopacified blood from the renal veins, indicating patent vessels, is critical when performing cavography before IVC filter placement.

Ultrasound, CT, and MRI are all useful imaging modalities in these patients, although CT has the disadvantage of requiring iodinated contrast. Variant renal vein anatomy may be difficult to detect by ultrasound in obese patients. An enlarged renal vein that lacks Doppler signal on duplex imaging or enhancement with contrast on CT or flow on MRV is conclusive for thrombosis. An obvious intraluminal mass that enhances with contrast is tumor, most likely from the kidney. Whenever renal vein thrombus is detected, the kidney should be carefully inspected for tumor. Imaging of suspected renal vein thrombosis with CTA or MRA should also include an assessment of the renal arterial supply. Small renal veins with diminished or absent flow may be seen in patients with longstanding renal failure.

Renal venography is rarely required for diagnosis of this disorder (see Imaging for technical details). When performed, venographic studies should begin with a cavogram, followed by selective injection of the renal veins. An intraluminal filling defect indicates acute thrombus. Webs, synechia, stenosis, and enlarged collateral veins connote chronic occlusion.

The conventional therapy of bland renal vein thrombosis in patients with stable renal function is anticoagulation. When anticoagulation is contraindicated, a suprarenal IVC filter should be placed. In patients with acute renal dysfunction due to renal vein thrombosis (especially those with renal transplants), thrombolysis with mechanical and pharmacologic techniques should be considered. Theoretically, combined renal vein and artery infusion of the thrombolytic agent maximizes delivery of the agent to the thrombus.

RENAL VEIN VARICES/NUTCRACKER SYNDROME

Renal vein varices are unusual lesions with a number of different etiologies (Box 13-7). Patients present with vague flank pain and hematuria. Varices are more common on the left than the right. Extrinsic compression of the left renal vein between the superior mesenteric artery and the aorta with the symptom complex described earlier is termed *nutcracker syndrome*. Although there is much disagreement about this condition, it is most often diagnosed in thin young women, particularly when there has been recent substantial decrease in weight.

Distended renal veins may be noted on ultrasound, CT, or MR studies. A careful search for an underlying cause is important. Venography reveals enlarged, tortuous hilar veins that drain into retroperitoneal veins (Fig. 13-29). The presence of high flow should suggest an arteriovenous malformation or arteriovenous fistula (see Fig. 12-36). A stenosis may be visualized at the orifice of the renal vein. A pressure gradient of at least 2 mm Hg between the renal vein and the IVC is suggestive of renal venous hypertension due to outflow obstruction.

Treatment of renal vein varices varies with the etiology. There is controversy about renal vein stent placement for nutcracker syndrome causing primarily flank pain because it is a diagnosis of

elimination; if the stent placement does not resolve the pain, the diagnosis is eliminated but the stent is permanent. When stents are placed, large self-expanding stents should be used, generally at least 6 cm long to minimize the risk of stent migration. Varices caused by high flow from an arteriovenous fistula or malformation often can be successfully managed with selective arterial embolization. Venous malformations are more difficult to treat, because they can be extensive with numerous points of communication with retroperitoneal veins.

PELVIC CONGESTION SYNDROME

Chronic pelvic pain is a perplexing and disturbingly frequent problem. An estimated 10 million women are affected, but an explanation can be found in fewer than half. The evaluation of these patients requires a thorough gynecologic workup, including laparoscopy in most cases. A wide variety of gynecologic conditions can be responsible for chronic pelvic pain, including endometriosis, chronic infection, adhesions, fibroids, adenomyosis, and pelvic varicosities. Nongynecologic pathology can cause chronic pelvic pain as well. Dilated ovarian and periuterine veins are the etiology of the pain in up to 30%, termed pelvic congestion syndrome. However, dilated ovarian and pelvic veins can be visualized with ultrasound, CT, and MRI in up to 50% of normal multiparous women; correlation with symptoms is therefore essential to make a diagnosis. The symptoms of pelvic congestion syndrome include pelvic pain, dyspareunia, menstrual abnormalities, vulvar varices, and lower extremity varicose veins. Symptoms are worse when standing, toward the end of the day, with sexual arousal, and during menstruation. Dilated pelvic veins in the absence of symptoms is not considered pelvic congestion syndrome.

Reflux of blood in ovarian veins is the dominant underlying etiology of pelvic varicosities in most patients. Almost half of the patients also have reflux in the internal iliac veins, and a subset have isolated internal iliac vein reflux. Rarely, pelvic arteriovenous malformations or fistulas may be encountered. Valves are present at the orifices of the ovarian veins in 85% of women, but are incompetent in about 40% on the left and 35% on the right. Unimpeded reflux of blood into the pelvis results in distention and engorgement of the periuterine veins. Predisposing conditions include prior pregnancy, but also include nutcracker syndrome, tubal ligation, and presence of an intrauterine device. Pelvic congestion syndrome is most often but not exclusively a condition of women of childbearing age.

Patients with suspected pelvic congestion syndrome should undergo a full gynecologic evaluation for other causes of chronic pelvic pain. This may include diagnostic laparoscopy and attempts at medical management. When other etiologies have been excluded, venous intervention may be warranted.

Box 13-7. Etiologies of Renal Vein Varices

Congenital venous malformation
Renal vein thrombosis
Obstruction of outflow ("nutcracker syndrome")
Spontaneous splenorenal shunt
Arteriovenous malformation
Arteriovenous fistula
- Intrarenal
- Aorta to left renal vein
Vascular renal tumor

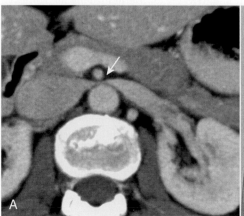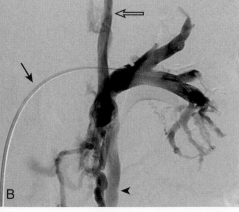

Figure 13-29. "Nutcracker syndrome" in a 25-year-old woman with chronic left flank pain and intermittent hematuria with a normal urologic workup. **A,** Computed tomography scan with contrast showing compression of the left renal vein *(arrow)* between the aorta and superior mesenteric artery. **B,** Selective left renal venogram showing varices *(solid arrow,* catheter from inferior vena cava [IVC]). The kidney drains entirely via retroperitoneal collateral veins including paralumbar, the left ovarian *(arrowhead),* and the hemiazygous *(open arrow)* veins. The pressure gradient between the IVC and the renal hilum was 7 mm Hg.

Preprocedural imaging is obtained with CT or MRI (see Fig. 13-8). These studies are usually performed with the patient supine, which may underestimate the degree of venous distention. The normal diameter of the gonadal veins is 5 mm or smaller. When abnormal, the diameter can easily exceed 10 mm. Enlarged parauterine veins and vulvar varices are often present. There is no good noninvasive test for assessing internal iliac vein reflux.

Ovarian and internal iliac venography remains the definitive diagnostic imaging modality for pelvic congestion syndrome (see Imaging for technical details). Ideally the patient should be studied on a tilting table in reverse Trendelenburg position. Flush cavography is not necessary before selection of the ovarian veins. Because the left ovarian vein is more commonly affected than the right, and because it is easier to catheterize, this vein should be addressed first. A left renal venogram should be obtained to demonstrate reflux into the ovarian vein as well as any associated renal vein pathology. Injection into an abnormal ovarian vein reveals retrograde flow into the pelvis and filling of the uterine plexus of veins, with drainage through the hypogastric veins or through a contralateral normal ovarian vein (Fig. 13-30). Similarly, injections into the internal iliac veins may identify reflux in to the pelvic veins.

There is no effective medical management of pelvic congestion syndrome. Surgical management includes ligation of the ovarian veins via a laparoscope and hysterectomy. These procedures are reportedly effective in controlling symptoms in almost 75% of cases. However, because most patients with pelvic congestion syndrome are relatively young, embolotherapy represents an attractive alternative (Box 13-8).

Embolization with a combination of a sclerosant in the parauterine venous plexus and coils or plugs in the ovarian and internal iliac veins achieves the best results. Access from either the femoral or jugular vein can be used, although the approach to the ovarian veins is antegrade with the latter. Recurved catheters and long curved guide catheters or sheaths are necessary when access is from the femoral vein (see Fig. 13-13). Ovarian and internal iliac venograms are obtained before embolization to confirm the anatomy and identify potential sources of collateralization and variant anatomy. When the valve at the orifice of an ovarian vein is competent, or there is absence of reflux in the internal iliac vein, embolization should not be performed. A 4- or 5-French catheter is preferred to facilitate delivery of embolics, but microcatheters can be advanced as deep into the pelvis as possible. A sclerosant (for example, 3% sodium tetradecyl sulfate diluted to a concentration of 2% with contrast) can be injected into the pelvic veins. This injection is monitored with a roadmap technique or fluoroscopy to minimize reflux into normal veins. Coils or plugs are then placed starting in the distal ovarian vein and along the length of the vein to just below the orifice. The ovarian veins often have duplicated segments, and these can be selectively catheterized and embolized along the way. Interruption of the ovarian veins at multiple levels prevents collateralization around the coils and recurrent symptoms (Fig. 13-31). This also decreases the chance of recanalization through the coiled segment. Spasm of the vein is common due to catheter manipulation, but can be reduced by injection of 150- or 200-µmg aliquots of nitroglycerin.

Treatment of this disorder is often staged, starting with ovarian vein embolization. If this does not resolve symptoms, embolization of refluxing internal iliac veins using a similar technique is warranted. This is required in up to 50% of patients according to some reports, but it has been required less often in the author's experience. The complexity and variability of the internal iliac vein anatomy makes this a challenging procedure. Oversizing of coils is important to avoid nontarget embolization to the pulmonary arteries.

Embolization reduces or eliminates symptoms at 5 years in up to 70% of cases, but careful patient selection is critical. Women may experience increased pelvic pressure or pain for days or

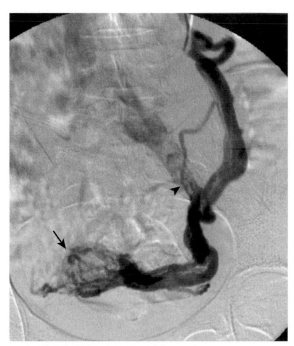

FIGURE 13-30. Digital subtraction left ovarian venogram in a patient with pelvic pain, showing filling of the uterine plexus *(arrow)* and drainage via the internal iliac vein *(arrowhead)*.

Box 13-8. Indications for Ovarian Vein Embolization

Pelvic varicosities with:
- Chronic pelvic pain and otherwise negative work-up
- Dyspareunia and otherwise negative work-up
- Severe labial and perineal varicosities

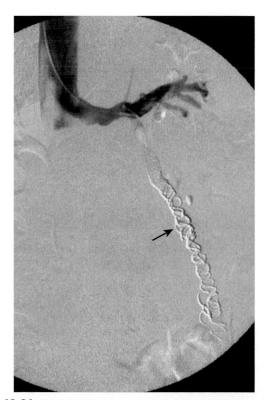

FIGURE 13-31. Digital subtraction venogram after embolization of the left ovarian vein for chronic pelvic pain. The coils extended to the renal vein.

weeks following embolization. This is probably related to venous thrombosis in the pelvis and almost always resolves with time. More serious complications are rare, but include thrombosis of the parent vein (renal or iliac) and pulmonary embolism.

■ VARICOCELE EMBOLIZATION

Dilatation of the pampiniform plexus, termed a *varicocele*, results from reflux of blood through incompetent gonadal vein valves in males. These are common lesions, found in 5%-17% of males, with a left-to-right ratio of 10:1. When present, varicoceles are bilateral in about 10%, and isolated to the right side in only 1%-7%. Varicoceles are associated with pain, infertility, and testicular hypoplasia. The etiology of varicoceles is unclear, but this abnormality is rare in prepubertal males. Sudden onset of any varicocele or an isolated right varicocele should prompt imaging of the retroperitoneum to exclude an abdominal or renal mass. Varicoceles may cause infertility (25% of males with varicoceles have abnormal semen), pain, testicular atrophy, or scrotal enlargement. Varicoceles are more common than infertility in males, but in some studies, sperm counts have been shown to increase after treatment of varicoceles.

The diagnosis of varicocele, unlike pelvic vein varicosities, is usually clinical. Patients present with a palpable scrotal abnormality that increases in size with Valsalva and diminishes in the supine position. A grading system is used to describe the physical examination (Table 13-4). Bilateral varicoceles can be due to transscrotal drainage, usually left to right. This can be excluded on physical exam by applying pressure over the left pampiniform plexus in a supine patient. When the patient stands, return of the right varicocele indicates reflux in the right gonadal vein. Ultrasound is the preferred imaging modality when a subclinical varicocele is suspected (e.g., in an infertile male with a normal physical examination). The finding of a dilated pampiniform complex is diagnostic, with 2 mm being the upper limit of normal diameter pampiniform veins. Reflux may be noted with Valsalva maneuver using Doppler or color-flow imaging. MRI is also used for imaging of the scrotal contents. Venography is only performed as part of an embolization procedure (see Fig. 13-13).

There is no effective medical treatment for varicoceles (Box 13-9). The goal of intervention is interruption of the reflux pathway (the internal spermatic vein). Surgical or laparoscopic ligation of the internal spermatic vein can be performed at multiple levels: high retroperitoneal (Palomo), low retroperitoneal (Ivanissevich), and microsurgical subinguinal. The recurrence rate is approximately 10%-20% following surgical ligation, usually due to collateral flow around the ligature, a missed additional internal spermatic vein, or a loose ligature.

TABLE 13-4 Varicocele Grades

Grade	Size
1	Small, palpable only with Valsalva
2	Moderate, nonvisible, but palpable when patient stands
3	Large, visible

Box 13-9. Indications for Internal Spermatic Vein Embolization

Varicocele with:
- Pain
- Testicular hypoplasia
- Infertility

Prevention of reflux into the anterior pampiniform plexus by percutaneous occlusion of the internal spermatic vein has many similarities to embolization of the ovarian vein to prevent reflux into the periuterine veins. The initial technical features are identical in terms of access, selection of the veins, and venography. Microcatheters may be required for the catheterization of the gonadal vein in the pelvis. A variety of agents can be used to occlude the vein, including coils, plugs, glue, and even boiling contrast material. Injection of sclerosant is very effective when performed through selective catheterization of the pampiniform plexus. Approximately 2-6 mL of 3% sodium tetradecyl sulfate is injected into the spermatic vein at the level of the ischiopubic bones while the patient performs a Valsalva maneuver and with compression over the pampiniform plexus below the injection site to prevent reflux into the scrotum. The patient should be in reverse Trendelenburg position on a tilt table, with an elastic scrotal compression applied for 1 minute after injection. The patient should then be repositioned into Trendelenburg position when compression is released. When coils are used, they should be placed first at the level of the inguinal canal, which usually corresponds to the superior pubic ramus. Multiple coils are then deposited along the entire length of the vein. When present, multiple internal spermatic veins should be individually embolized. In patients with bilateral varicoceles, only the largest (usually the left) should be treated. The patency of the middle and posterior pampiniform plexuses allow occlusion of the anterior plexus outflow without compromising testicular function. After the procedure, the patient should be instructed to avoid heavy physical activity for 7 days and follow a high-fiber diet with good hydration to avoid constipation.

The results of embolization of internal spermatic veins are similar to surgery, with a technical success rate that exceeds 90%, and a recurrence rate that approaches 10%. Pampiniform swelling occurs in about 10% and thrombosis in approximately 2%. Hydroceles are extremely rare. Failures of embolization occur due to missed additional veins, collateralization from perirenal and retroperitoneal veins, and recanalization of occluded segments.

■ ADRENAL VENOUS SAMPLING

Adrenal lesions rarely require catheter-based imaging for diagnosis. The majority of adrenal masses can be detected and evaluated with CT, MRI, or nuclear medicine studies. Masses of questionable etiology may be amenable to percutaneous CT-guided biopsy. The primary catheter-based procedure performed in patients with suspected functional adrenal pathology is venous sampling. These patients have confirmed endocrine disorders but require localization to an adrenal gland in order to guide surgery. Venous sampling should never be performed in order to make the diagnosis of an endocrine disease.

Primary Hyperaldosteronism

Aldosterone is a hormone secreted by the adrenal cortex that induces renal sodium retention and excretion of potassium. This is a normal response to renal artery stenosis, congestive heart failure, pregnancy, and cirrhosis, and is termed *secondary aldosteronism*. Primary aldosteronism (Conn syndrome) is hypersecretion of aldosterone by either an adrenal adenoma (two thirds of cases) or bilateral idiopathic adrenal hyperplasia (one third of cases) (Box 13-10). Adenomas are bilateral in 2% of cases, and in fewer than 1% of cases an adrenal carcinoma is the source of the aldosterone.

A serum potassium level less than 3.5 mEq/L in a patient with diastolic hypertension suggests Conn syndrome. Additional laboratory investigation includes plasma renin and aldosterone levels in the morning and randomly during the day, and urine sodium and potassium. Low renin levels and/or a high aldosterone-to-renin level (>30) suggests primary aldosteronism. An aldosterone suppression test may be performed with either a high sodium diet for 3 days or saline infusion over 4 hours. Imaging of the adrenal glands is performed with CT or MRI. When a unilateral adrenal mass is found in the setting of a very high aldosterone-to-renin ratio (>50), surgery may be considered without adrenal vein sampling. In most other instances of suspected primary hyperaldosteronism, adrenal vein sampling is performed to localize the hypersecreting nodule.

Evaluation of prior imaging is helpful to localize the right adrenal vein and its insertion upon the IVC. In addition, left renal vein and IVC variants can be identified that will impact sampling approach. The procedure is usually performed in the morning, with the patient fasting. The patient should be systemically heparinized after obtaining access in both common femoral veins. Catheters are then positioned in both adrenal veins (see Fig. 13-14) (see Imaging for technical details). Gentle contrast injections are the rule, in that the adrenal veins are weak and prone to rupture. Cone-beam CT is helpful to confirm catheter position, particularly on the right. Samples can be obtained sequentially or simultaneously from both adrenal veins and a peripheral (usually femoral) vein. Sampling protocols vary by institution, as does the use of adrenocorticotropic hormone (ACTH). Adenomas are sensitive to ACTH, whereas the normal adrenal gland in the setting of primary hyperaldosteronism is not. When used it can be given as a bolus, with or without subsequent infusion (0.25-mg bolus followed by infusion of 0.15-0.20 mg/hr). Sampling may be obtained before or after ACTH administration; serial or single samples can be obtained. The author's institution administers the IV bolus of ACTH, with sampling sequentially of the right, left, and then infraadrenal IVC starting 15 minutes after the ACTH administration. Although there is not a uniform standard, the technique should be consistent from procedure to procedure to minimize potential errors. A clear understanding of the volume of blood needed for the samples, the types of tubes, and the handling requirements is important to perform the study correctly. Strict attention to labeling of the tubes is necessary so that right/left confusion does not occur with the results.

Samples are submitted for both aldosterone and cortisol, because it is assumed that the production of the latter is the same for both glands. The cortisol test confirms that an adrenal vein has been sampled, allows correction for dilution of right adrenal vein samples, and can help distinguish between an adenoma and idiopathic adrenal hyperplasia. The ratio of adrenal catheter to peripheral sheath cortisol should be greater than 1. In patients with adenomas, the ratio of aldosterone/cortisol from the affected gland is high before and after ACTH administration, whereas the opposite gland is similar to the femoral vein samples at baseline and has a blunted response to stimulation. In patients with bilateral hyperplasia, there is no lateralization of ratios before or after ACTH administration. Some centers define lateralization as at least a threefold to fourfold difference in ratios from side to side. A less than twofold difference suggests bilateral adrenal hyperplasia. Sampling provides diagnostic information in more than 95% of cases.

Treatment for a unilateral adrenal adenoma is surgical resection. Bilateral hyperplasia is usually managed medically, because

bilateral adrenalectomy would result in adrenal insufficiency (Addison disease). Transcatheter ablative techniques have been described but are not widely utilized.

Other Disorders

Adrenal vein sampling is occasionally required in patients with Cushing syndrome, a distinctive clinical complex due to hypercortisolism (Box 13-11). The most common etiology is iatrogenic as a result of administration of glucocorticoids or adrenocorticotropic hormone. Endogenous Cushing syndrome has both central nervous system and peripheral etiologies (Table 13-5). The diagnosis is based on biochemical abnormalities. Urinary excretion of free cortisol is elevated, and plasma cortisol levels do not drop in response to a single dose of dexamethasone in patients with endogenous Cushing syndrome.

Localization of the cause of Cushing syndrome is of paramount importance in directing therapy. Patients with pituitary or ectopic sources of ACTH will have elevated serum levels of that hormone. Patients with elevated glucocorticoids and independently functioning adrenal masses (adenomas in 90%, adrenocortical carcinoma in 10%, and rarely bilateral or unilateral macronodular hyperplasia) have low serum ACTH levels because the pituitary negative feedback mechanisms are intact. The contralateral adrenal gland is frequently atrophic.

Imaging of the adrenal glands in patients with Cushing syndrome includes either a CT scan or MRI for detection of a mass. Selective catheterization of the adrenal veins for venous sampling for cortisol levels is occasionally required to confirm localization to the adrenal gland. Samples are obtained from both adrenal veins, the IVC above the adrenal veins, and below the renal veins. Stimulation is not required. The treatment of Cushing syndrome due to unilateral adrenal abnormality is surgical resection. Catheter ablation of the adrenal gland by forceful retrograde venous injection of contrast has been described in a few patients but appears to have limited durability.

Adrenal venous sampling for metanephrines and normetanephrines may be necessary in the evaluation of a patient with clinical findings of pheochromocytoma and ambiguous adrenal masses. These patients require preprocedural blood pressure control, and sampling is performed without a stimulating agent. Catecholamine levels are increased 4-5 times on the side of the tumor, with reversal of the ratio of metanephrines to normetanephrines.

Box 13-11. Symptoms of Cushing Syndrome

Hypertension	Peripheral edema
Muscle weakness	Glucose intolerance
Osteoporosis	Vascular fragility
Cutaneous striae	Hirsutism
Truncal obesity	Moon facies
Buffalo hump	Amenorrhea

TABLE 13-5 Etiology of Endogenous Cushing Syndrome

Etiology	Mechanism	Incidence (%)
ACTH-secreting anterior pituitary tumor	Adrenal hyperstimulation	65
Adrenal adenoma or carcinoma	Independent secretion	20
Ectopic ACTH secretion by tumor	Adrenal hyperstimulation	15

ACTH, Adrenocorticotropic hormone.

Box 13-10. Symptoms of Primary Aldosteronism (Conn Syndrome)

Diastolic hypertension
Hypokalemia
Hypernatremia
Hyperchlorhydria
Alkalosis

▬ Suggested Readings

Ahmed K, Sampath R, Khan MS. Current trends in the diagnosis and management of renal nutcracker syndrome: a review. *Eur J Vasc Endovasc Surg.* 2006;31: 410-416.

Angel LF, Tapson V, Galgon RE, et al. Systematic review of the use of retrievable inferior vena cava filters. *J Vasc Interv Radiol.* 2011;22:1522-1530.

Asciutto G, Asciutto KC, Mumme A, Geier B. Pelvic venous incompetence: reflux patterns and treatment results. *Eur J Vasc Endovasc Surg.* 2009;38:381-386.

Asghar M, Ahmed K, Shah SS, et al. Renal vein thrombosis. *Eur J Vasc Endovasc Surg.* 2007;34:217-223.

Barber B, Horton A, Patel U. Anatomy of the origin of the gonadal veins on CT. *J Vasc Interv Radiol.* 2012;23:211-215.

Bittles MA, Hoffer EK. Gonadal vein embolization: treatment of varicocele and pelvic congestion syndrome. *Semin Intervent Radiol.* 2008;25:261-270.

Broholm R, Jørgensen M, Just S, et al. Acute iliofemoral venous thrombosis in patients with atresia of the inferior vena cava can be treated successfully with catheter-directed thrombolysis. *J Vasc Interv Radiol.* 2011;22:801-805.

Brountzos EN, Binkert CA, Panagiotou IE, et al. Clinical outcome after intrahepatic venous stent placement for malignant inferior vena cava syndrome. *Cardiovasc Intervent Radiol.* 2004;27:129-136.

Buckman RF, Pathak AS, Badellino MM, Bradley KM. Injuries of the inferior vena cava. *Surg Clin North Am.* 2001 Dec;81(6):1431-1447.

Därr R, Eisenhofer G, Kotzerke J, et al. Is there still a place for adrenal venous sampling in the diagnostic localization of pheochromocytoma? *Endocrine.* 2011;40:75-79.

Daunt N. Adrenal vein sampling: how to make it quick, easy, and successful. *Radiographics.* 2005;25(S1):S143-58.

Decousus H, Leizorovicz A, Parent F, et al. A clinical trial of vena caval filters in the prevention of pulmonary embolism in patients with proximal deep-vein thrombosis. *N Engl J Med.* 1998;338:409-415.

Dewald CL, Jensen CC, Park YH, et al. Vena cavography with CO_2 versus with iodinated contrast material for inferior vena cava filter placement: a prospective evaluation. *Radiology.* 2000;216:752-757.

Fiore M, Colombo C, Locati P, et al. Surgical technique, morbidity, and outcome of primary retroperitoneal sarcoma involving inferior vena cava. *Ann Surg Oncol.* 2012;19:511-518.

Ganeshalingam S, Rajeswaran G, Jones RL, et al. Leiomyosarcomas of the inferior vena cava: diagnostic features on cross-sectional imaging. *Clin Radiol.* 2011;66:50-56.

Garg N, Gloviczki P, Karimi KM, et al. Factors affecting outcome of open and hybrid reconstructions for nonmalignant obstruction of iliofemoral veins and inferior vena cava. *J Vasc Surg.* 2011;53:383-393.

Hartung O, Loundou AD, Barthelemy P, et al. Endovascular management of chronic disabling ilio-caval obstructive lesions: long-term results. *Eur J Vasc Endovasc Surg.* 2009;38:118-124.

Iaccarino V, Venetucci P. Interventional radiology of male varicocele: current status. *Cardiovasc Intervent Radiol.* 2012;35:1263-1280.

Imberti D, Ageno W, Manfredini R, et al. Interventional treatment of venous thromboembolism: a review. *Thromb Res.* 2012;129:418-425.

Kahn SL, Angle JF. Adrenal vein sampling. *Tech Vasc Interv Radiol.* 2010;13:110-125.

Kalva SP, Chlapoutaki C, Wicky S, et al. Suprarenal inferior vena cava filters: a 20-year single-center experience. *J Vasc Interv Radiol.* 2008;19:1041-1047.

Kara T, Younes M, Erol B, Karcaaltincaba M. Evaluation of testicular vein anatomy with multidetector computed tomography. *Surg Radiol Anat.* 2012;34:341-345.

Kaufman JA, Waltman AC, Rivitz SM, Geller SG. Anatomical observations on the renal veins and inferior vena cava at magnetic resonance angiography. *Cardiovasc Interv Radiol.* 1995;18:153-157.

Kidane B, Madani AM, Vogt K, et al. The use of prophylactic inferior vena cava filters in trauma patients: a systematic review. *Injury.* 2012;43:542-547.

Kies DD, Kim HS. Pelvic congestion syndrome: a review of current diagnostic and minimally invasive treatment modalities. *Phlebology.* 2012;27(Suppl 1):52-57.

Kim HS, Malhotra AD, Rowe PC, et al. Embolotherapy for pelvic congestion syndrome: long-term results. *J Vasc Interv Radiol.* 2006;17:289-297.

Malaki M, Willis AP, Jones RG. Congenital anomalies of the inferior vena cava. *Clin Radiol.* 2012;67:165-171.

Menard MT. Nutcracker syndrome: when should it be treated and how? *Perspect Vasc Surg Endovasc Ther.* 2009;21:117-124.

Neglén P, Oglesbee M, Olivier J, Raju S. Stenting of chronically obstructed inferior vena cava filters. *J Vasc Surg.* 2011;54:153-161.

PREPIC Study Group. Eight-year follow-up of patients with permanent vena cava filters in the prevention of pulmonary embolism: the PREPIC (Prevention du Risque d'Embolie Pulmonaire par Interruption Cave) randomized study. *Circulation.* 2005;112:416-422.

Ratnam LA, Marsh P, Holdstock JM, et al. Pelvic vein embolisation in the management of varicose veins. *Cardiovasc Intervent Radiol.* 2008;31:1159-1164.

Razavi MK, Hansch EC, Kee ST, et al. Chronically occluded inferior venae cavae: endovascular treatment. *Radiology.* 2000;214:133-138.

Rossi GP. New concepts in adrenal vein sampling for aldosterone in the diagnosis of primary aldosteronism. *Curr Hypertens Rep.* 2007;9(2):90-97.

Rossi GP, Barisa M, Allolio B, et al. The Adrenal Vein Sampling International Study (AVIS) for identifying the major subtypes of primary aldosteronism. *J Clin Endocrinol Metab.* 2012;97:1606-1614.

Türkvatan A, Ozdemir M, Cumhur T, Olçer T. Multidetector CT angiography of renal vasculature: normal anatomy and variants. *Eur Radiol.* 2009;19:236-244.

Wang X, Zhang Y, Li C, Zhang H. Long-term result of endovascular treatment for patients with nutcracker syndrome. *J Vasc Surg.* 2012;56:142-148.

Yang DM, Kim HC, Nam DH, et al. Time-resolved MR angiography for detecting and grading ovarian venous reflux: comparison with conventional venography. *Br J Radiol.* 2012;85:e117-e122.

Zhang CQ, Fu LN, Xu L, et al. Long-term effect of stent placement in 115 patients with Budd-Chiari syndrome. *World J Gastroenterol.* 2003;9:2587-2591.

CHAPTER 14

Portal and Hepatic Veins

John A. Kaufman, MD, MS, FSIR, FCIRSE, and Peter J. Bromley, MD, FRCPC

Portal and hepatic venous interventions are increasing due to the growing population of patients with chronic liver disease and the application of more aggressive surgical approaches to hepatic malignancy. Catheter-based techniques are important for the diagnosis and management of these conditions.

ANATOMY

Hepatic Segmentation

The distributions of the right and left hepatic arteries and portal vein branches are not reflected by surface landmarks such as the ligamentum teres and falciform ligament. The most widely accepted schema is by Couinaud with a modification by Bismuth (Fig. 14-1). The liver is divided into right and left halves by a plane that passes through the inferior vena cava (IVC) and the gallbladder fossa along the path of the middle hepatic vein. Each liver half is then further divided into four portions for a total of eight hepatic segments. The left-sided segments are numbered from 1 to 4 beginning with the caudate lobe. The right-sided segments are 5-8. Bismuth's modification divides segment 4 into 4a (superiorly) and 4b (inferiorly).

Venous Anatomy

The portal and hepatic veins are distinct but interrelated systems responsible for the venous drainage of all of the abdominal viscera except the kidneys and adrenal glands. The linkage of the two systems occurs in the liver. Blood collected by the tributaries of the portal vein passes through the hepatic sinusoids. After traversing the sinusoids, blood is collected in the hepatic veins and flows to the right atrium. The portal vein supplies two thirds of the blood flow into the liver but carries only one third of the liver's oxygen supply. The hepatic artery provides the bulk of the liver's oxygen.

The portal vein is formed beneath the neck of the pancreas by the confluence of the splenic and the superior mesenteric veins and travels in the free edge of the gastrohepatic ligament (Fig. 14-2). The normal portal vein is about 8 cm in length and 10-12 mm in diameter. At the liver hilum (porta hepatis) the portal vein bifurcates into right and left branches that further ramify as they penetrate through the liver (Fig. 14-3). The portal vein bifurcation is extrahepatic in 40%-48% of individuals but is generally surrounded by dense fibrous connective tissue in the porta hepatis. A trifurcation of the main portal vein, resulting in absence of a right portal trunk, is encountered in about 11% of cases. Occasionally the left portal vein provides a branch to a portion of the right lobe of the liver (4%), usually the anterior segments (5 and 8). The left portal vein is critical to the fetal circulation, receiving blood from the placenta via the left umbilical vein and delivering it across the liver to the IVC via the ductus venosus. The ductus venosus eventually atrophies and becomes the ligamentum venosum while the umbilical vein becomes part of the ligamentum teres. Persistence of the ductus venosus is very rare (Fig. 14-4). Valves are present in the portal vein in utero but rarely persist into adult life.

Blood in the portal system is collected from the gastrointestinal tract, pancreas, and the spleen by a network of major tributaries (see Fig. 14-2). The superior mesenteric vein (SMV) collects blood from the small bowel and the right colon (cecum to the mid transverse colon). Pancreaticoduodenal veins drain both into the SMV and directly into the main portal vein. The inferior mesenteric vein (IMV) collects blood from the left colon (mid transverse colon to rectum). The IMV drains into the splenic vein in roughly two thirds of individuals and in the remaining one third enters the SMV at or just below the confluence. The splenic vein drains the spleen as well as portions of the stomach (short gastric veins) and pancreas. By convention, the terms *proximal* and *distal* in the venous system are based on the normal direction of flow, with blood traveling from a proximal (peripheral) to a distal (central) location. The proximal splenic vein is therefore that portion closest to the spleen, whereas the distal portion is closest to the portal confluence.

The left gastric vein, or coronary vein, is a major draining vein of the stomach and lower esophagus. The coronary vein drains into the main portal vein in about two thirds of individuals, and into the splenic vein in the remaining one third.

The common bile duct and common hepatic artery lie with the portal vein in the gastrohepatic ligament. The portal vein, hepatic artery, and bile ducts continue together into the liver parenchyma in a grouping referred to as "portal triads." There is actually a fourth element, the lymphatic ducts. The terminal branches of the portal vein join with the terminal branches of the hepatic artery to perfuse the hepatic sinusoids. Blood percolates through the sinusoids, where it is separated from the hepatocytes by a thin endothelial layer, and drains to the centrilobular hepatic veins. This forms the basic functional unit of the liver. The centrilobular veins join together, forming sublobular veins that unite

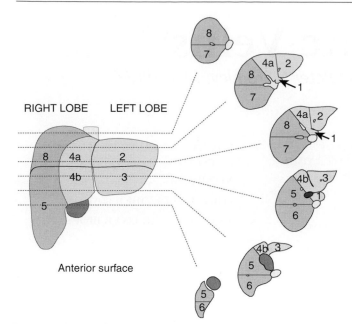

RIGHT LOBE   LEFT LOBE

Anterior surface

FIGURE 14-1. Drawing of hepatic segmentation. The right and left lobes are separated by a plane that passes through the inferior vena cava and the gallbladder fossa along the path of the middle hepatic vein. Segments 2 and 3 are separated from segment 4 by the ligamentum teres. The right-sided segments are numbered 5-8. The plane of the right hepatic vein separates the right posterior segments (6 and 7) from the right anterior segments (8 and 5). The superior segments (7 and 8 on the right and 4a and 2 on the left) are separated from the inferior segments (5 and 6 on the right and 4b and 3 on the left) by the planes of the right and left portal branches.

eventually to form the hepatic veins. The largest of the hepatic veins exit the posterosuperior surface of the liver and join the hepatic segment of the IVC just before it leaves the abdomen, usually about 2 cm below the right atrium. These are the right, middle, and left hepatic veins and are referred to by anatomists as the *upper group*. The left and middle hepatic veins are oriented anterior and anterolateral (respectively) while the right hepatic vein typically has a lateral or posterolateral orientation (Fig. 14-5). The middle and left hepatic veins form a common trunk before joining the IVC in 65%-85% of individuals. A second, lower group of hepatic veins arising from the caudate and right lobes are also present and vary in number. Large-caliber veins from the lower right lobe (inferior right hepatic veins) are seen in approximately 15% of individuals. These large veins are usually solitary but can be duplicated.

The quantity of blood flow in the portal vein is totally dependent on the perfusion of the spleen, pancreas, and gastrointestinal tract. After a meal, portal vein flow increases dramatically (postprandial portal hyperemia) as a consequence of increased perfusion of these organs. The direction of normal portal blood flow is toward the liver (hepatopetal).

▆ KEY COLLATERAL PATHWAYS

Two series of important collateral networks are recognized in the portal circulation. Portal-to-portal collaterals become apparent when focal occlusions develop within the portal circulation. Blood bypasses the occlusion but remains within the portal circulation. Three commonly encountered venous occlusions are in the splenic, portal, and superior mesenteric veins. When the splenic vein occludes, retrograde flow through the short gastric veins to the left gastric vein can occur (Fig. 14-6). Occlusion of

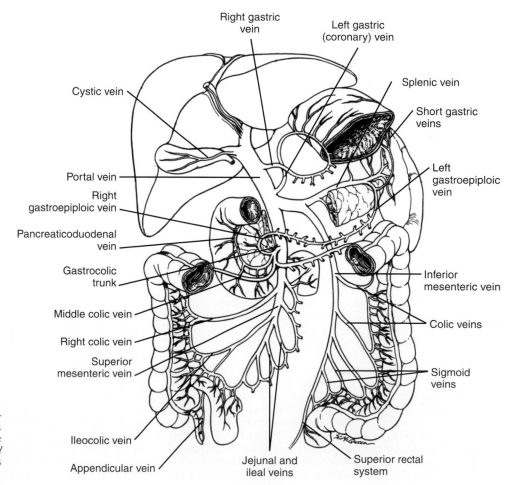

FIGURE 14-2. Drawing of portal and mesenteric veins. (From Lundell C, Kadir S. The portal venous system and hepatic veins. In Kadir S, ed. *Atlas of Normal and Angiographic Anatomy.* Philadelphia: WB Saunders, 1991, with permission.)

the central SMV can result in collateral drainage through mesenteric, paraduodenal, and marginal veins. The collateral pathways for splenic vein and SMV occlusion are frequently submucosal and are therefore prone to bleeding into the gastrointestinal tract. Occlusion of the portal vein results in enlargement of the pericholedochal and epicholedochal veins in the gastrohepatic ligament, termed *cavernous transformation* (Fig. 14-7). A small, residual, or recanalized main portal vein may exist within this network but can be difficult to identify.

Portal-to-systemic collaterals develop in the setting of portal hypertension and represent pathways for blood to escape the portal circulation and return to the systemic circulation (Fig. 14-8). Termed *varices*, the majority of these pathways represent enlargement of preexisting small communications between the portal and systemic veins. Unusual portal-to-systemic collaterals can form following abdominal surgery. Both portal-to-portal and portal-to-systemic collaterals may be present in the same patient.

Obstruction of the main hepatic veins frequently results in intrahepatic collateralization to other hepatic veins. If at least one hepatic vein remains patent, obstruction of main hepatic veins is usually well tolerated. Collateral drainage through capsular and diaphragmatic veins may also occur.

▄▄▄ IMAGING

Transabdominal ultrasound (US) with Doppler interrogation is an excellent noninvasive means for evaluating the patency of the portal vein, hepatic veins, and hepatic artery. Color-flow Doppler and power Doppler provide quick means for locating the vessels and confirming patency, with color-flow Doppler also providing directional information. Spectral Doppler should also be performed and the waveforms evaluated. Each vessel has a typical waveform (Fig. 14-9). The portal vein is a high flow, low pressure, low-resistance conduit characterized by a gentle phasic waveform with respiratory variation. The splenic and superior mesenteric veins have similar waveforms. Flow in the portal system increases dramatically after meals. The hepatic veins are characterized by a variable waveform influenced by right atrial contractions. The hepatic artery has a low-resistance arterial waveform. A structural evaluation of the liver should also be performed, noting the overall size and echotexture of the liver, parenchymal masses (cystic

or solid), and biliary dilatation. Ascites should be noted and the volume qualitatively estimated (minimal, moderate, large). Ultrasound can be technically demanding depending on the patient's body habitus, ability to cooperate, and severity of underlying liver disease.

Computed tomography angiography (CTA) is an excellent modality for imaging the hepatic and portal veins. Furthermore, detection of mass lesions is highly sensitive. The three-dimensional (3-D) relationships of the vascular structures (notably the portal vein and hepatic veins) can be easily appreciated from the axial CT images and postprocessed data (Fig. 14-10). Dedicated vascular CTA of the liver requires a minimum of two acquisition phases: hepatic arterial and portal venous. The first scan through the liver is obtained during the arterial phase of enhancement. Approximately 30-60 seconds after the initiation of the bolus, the scan should be repeated to obtain the portal venous phase. Addition of preliminary noncontrast and delayed postcontrast images optimizes evaluation of the hepatic parenchyma for any mass lesion (triple or quadruple phase examination). The arterial phase should be performed with thin effective collimation and overlapping slices to ensure longitudinal resolution appropriate for the size of the hepatic artery. Wider collimation can be used for the portal venous phase and to cover the remainder of the abdominal contents if necessary.

Magnetic resonance imaging (MRI) and MR venography (MRV) are also excellent tools for evaluating the portal venous system and hepatic veins, as well as the liver parenchyma. Dedicated anatomic sequences should be obtained in multiple planes for overall anatomic evaluation. The relatively slow and nonpulsatile flow in the portal venous system is well suited for MRV with time-of-flight (TOF) and phase-contrast (PC) techniques. However, the complex geometry of the vessels limits the utility of these sequences. Gadolinium-enhanced 3-D gradient echo volume

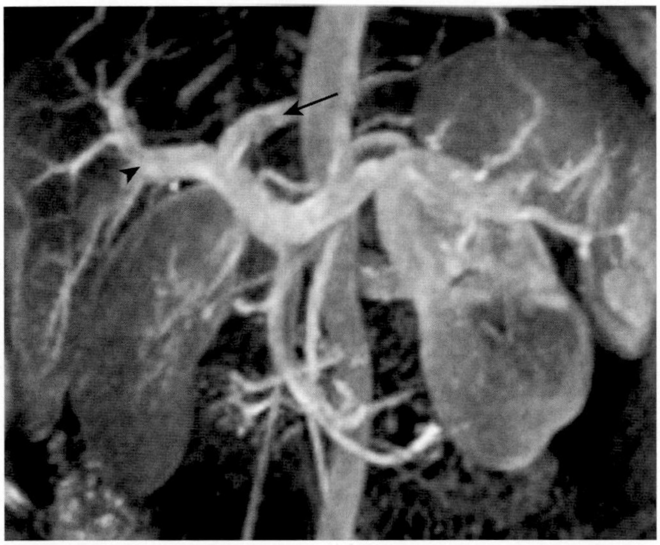

FIGURE 14-3. Gadolinium-enhanced three-dimensional magnetic resonance angiogram (maximum intensity projection) of the abdomen showing a normal portal venous system. The main portal vein bifurcation into the right *(arrowhead)* and left *(arrow)* portal veins is well visualized. (Courtesy Barry Stein, MD, Hartford, Conn.)

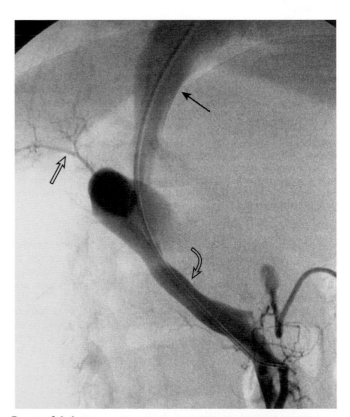

FIGURE 14-4. Patent ductus venosus. Digital subtraction angiogram showing that the portal vein *(curved arrow)* communicates directly with the inferior vena cava (IVC) *(straight arrow)* through the ductus venosus. The intrahepatic portal veins are diminutive *(open arrow)*.

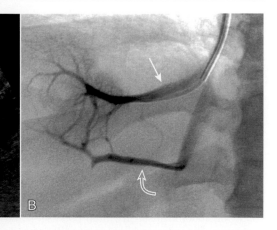

FIGURE **14-5**. Hepatic vein anatomy. **A,** Ultrasound showing the relationships of the hepatic vein orifices *(arrowhead,* right hepatic vein; *straight arrow,* middle hepatic vein; *curved arrow,* left hepatic vein.) **B,** Inferior right hepatic vein. Injection of a somewhat small right hepatic vein *(straight arrow)* opacifies a second, lower right hepatic vein *(curved arrow)* that drains directly into the IVC.

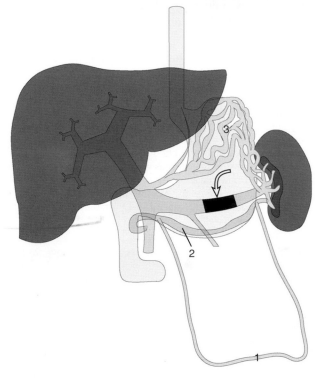

FIGURE **14-6**. Drawing of collateral pathways to the portal vein in the setting of isolated splenic vein obstruction *(curved arrow)* in a patient with normal portal pressures. *1,* Omental vein to gastroepiploic vein to superior mesenteric vein (SMV). *2,* Gastroepiploic veins to SMV. *3,* Short gastric veins to coronary vein.

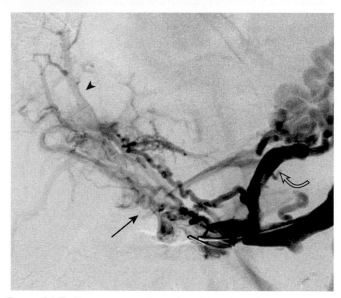

FIGURE **14-7**. Cavernous transformation of the portal vein demonstrated during injection of the splenic vein via transsplenic access. The extrahepatic portal vein is occluded, resulting in dilated paracholedochal and epicholedochal veins *(arrow)* that reconstitute the intrahepatic portal branches *(arrowhead).* The guidewire in the splenic vein is curled at the level of the portal vein occlusion. Note the retrograde filling of the coronary vein *(curved arrow)* and gastric varices.

acquisitions, in both arterial and portal venous phases, provide dramatic angiographic images of these structures unaffected by signal loss due to complex or in-plane flow (see Fig. 14-3). Image postprocessing is an essential tool when interpreting hepatic and portal venous MRV.

Hepatic venography can be performed from either the femoral vein or internal jugular vein approaches. Femoral venous access is convenient if no other procedure is to be performed. A Cobra-type curved catheter can be used; however, a recurved catheter such as a Simmons-1 is very effective for engaging the hepatic veins from the femoral approach. Access from the jugular vein is mechanically more advantageous, providing a direct line for the catheter into the hepatic vein. A multipurpose angled-tip catheter is generally effective in selecting the hepatic veins. The junction of the diaphragm with the right cardiac border represents a convenient fluoroscopic landmark for the hepatic vein orifices. The main trunk of the right hepatic vein is characteristically oriented in a lateral or slightly posterolateral direction while the middle and left hepatic veins are more anterior in orientation (see Fig. 14-5). A test injection of contrast should be performed by hand to ensure that the catheter tip is not wedged in a small hepatic vein branch. Some angiographers advocate the addition of a side hole near the tip of the catheter to prevent an inadvertent wedged injection. A formal venogram can then be obtained by injecting contrast at a rate of 5-6 mL/sec for a total of 15-18 mL during suspended respiration (Fig. 14-11).

Balloon occlusion hepatic venography can be used to image the small hepatic veins as well as the portal vein (Table 14-1). An 8- to 11-mm diameter occlusion balloon is gently inflated with 2-3 mL of dilute contrast (or room air for rapid deflation) until the hepatic vein wall is circumferentially engaged (see Fig. 2-26). Standard iodinated contrast material or carbon dioxide (CO_2) gas can then be injected through the catheter by hand. In a normal liver, the portal vein is usually not visualized because contrast drains into other hepatic vein branches. With cirrhosis, opacification of the portal vein and even retrograde flow may be seen. Because of its extremely low viscosity, CO_2 gas easily traverses the hepatic sinusoids, providing superior opacification of the portal vein. When sinusoidal hypertension (discussed later) is

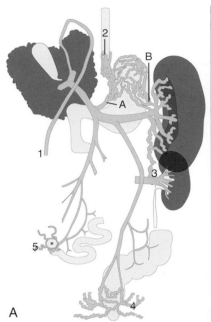

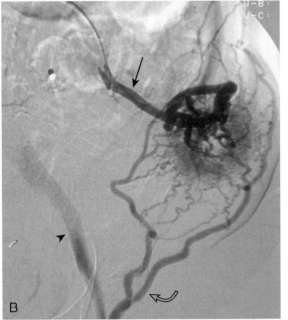

FIGURE 14-8. Portal-to-systemic collateral pathways. **A,** Drawing of portal-to-systemic collateral pathways. *1,* Recanalized umbilical vein (drains to anterior abdominal wall). *2,* Esophageal varices (drain to mediastinal veins), supplied by retrograde flow in left gastric vein (A) and retrograde flow in short gastric veins (B). *3,* Splenorenal varices that drain through the retroperitoneum from the splenic vein to the left renal vein. *4,* Inferior mesenteric to hemorrhoidal vein varices. *5,* Portal-to-systemic collaterals at sites of prior abdominal or pelvic surgery (in this case an ileostomy). **B,** Stomal varices in a patient with portal hypertension and an ileostomy. Digital subtraction angiogram of injection in a mesenteric vein *(straight arrow)* shows dilated peristomal veins that drain to the abdominal wall veins *(curved arrow)* through innumerable small communications. The *arrowhead* points to the external iliac vein.

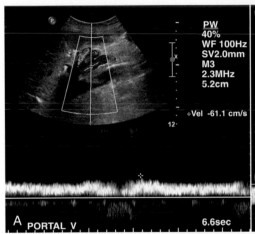

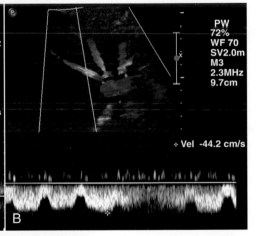

FIGURE 14-9. Normal Doppler waveforms of portal and hepatic veins. **A,** Normal left portal vein with monophasic hepatopetal flow. **B,** Normal left hepatic vein with triphasic hepatofugal flow.

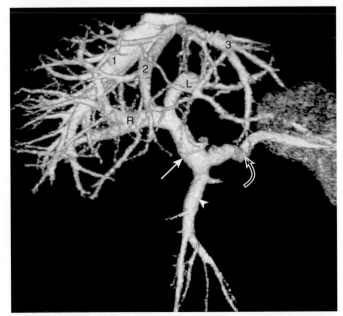

FIGURE 14-10. Volume rendering of portal and hepatic veins of the venous phase of a computed tomography angiogram. (*Arrowhead,* superior mesenteric vein; *arrow,* main portal vein; *curved arrow,* splenic vein.) R, right portal vein. L, left portal vein. *1,* right hepatic vein. *2,* middle hepatic vein. *3,* left hepatic vein.

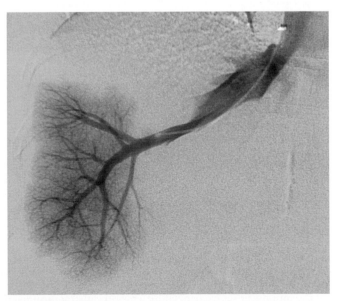

FIGURE 14-11. Normal free hepatic venogram showing typical ramification of the hepatic veins and a homogeneous liver parenchyma.

TABLE **14-1** Portal Venography

Technique	Catheter	Injection and Rate	Notes
Wedged hepatic	Balloon occlusion	20 mL iodinated contrast, 30-40 mL CO_2 gas	Hand injection
Transhepatic	Pigtail	12-15 mL for 36-45 mL	Transabdominal or transjugular access
Arterioportography	Visceral in SMA, celiac, or splenic artery	6-10 mL for 60-80 mL	Intraarterial Priscoline and/or nitroglycerin* (SMA only)
Splenoportography	18- to 21-gauge needle in splenic pulp	10-20 mL	Hand injection

*Priscoline = 25-50 mg injected through the superior mesenteric artery catheter immediately before contrast injection. Nitroglycerin = 200–300 µg before contrast injection. SMA, Superior mesenteric artery. Injection parameters for iodinated contrast if not otherwise specified.

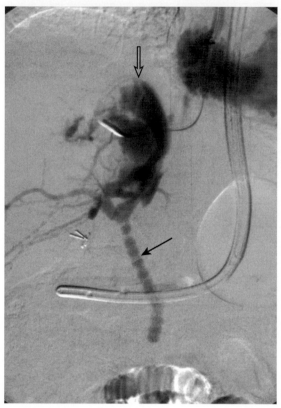

FIGURE **14-12**. Liver laceration *(open arrow)* and visualization of the common bile duct *(arrow)* caused by wedged hepatic venogram with CO_2 gas.

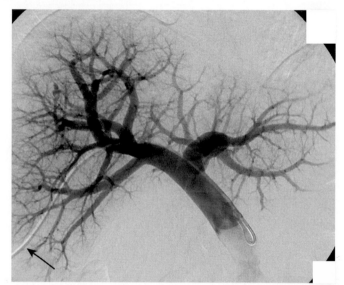

FIGURE **14-13**. Digital subtraction angiogram portogram using a 5-French catheter *(arrow)* inserted transhepatically from the right midaxillary line. The patient had normal coagulation studies and no ascites. The transhepatic tract was embolized with Gelfoam pledgets at the termination of the procedure.

present, the contrast enters the portal vein and a portal venogram can be obtained. Aggressive injection of either iodinated contrast or CO_2 gas can result in hepatic fracture, a potentially lethal complication (Fig. 14-12).

Direct opacification of the portal system can be accomplished with a transhepatic approach analogous to that employed during a transhepatic cholangiogram (Fig. 14-13). Local anesthetic is infiltrated into the skin and a narrow-gauge needle (typically 21-gauge) is advanced into the liver under fluoroscopic control. Transpleural puncture should be avoided, and the needle should pass over, not under, the rib. As the needle is slowly withdrawn, contrast is carefully injected with continuous fluoroscopic monitoring. The portal branches must be differentiated from hepatic arterial branches, because both flow in the same direction; arterial flow is faster with less arborization. Once a suitable portal vein radicle is opacified, a 0.018-inch guidewire can be introduced and the needle exchanged for a coaxial introducer set with a 4- or 5-French outer catheter. A 0.035-inch guidewire can then be inserted into the portal system and the introducer set exchanged for a pigtail catheter positioned deep in the splenic vein or SMV. The same transhepatic tract can be used to insert larger instruments if interventions are to be

performed. Depending on the size of the catheters used and the patient's coagulation status, it may be appropriate to embolize the tract with Gelfoam pledgets or coils at the end of the procedure to reduce the risk of intraperitoneal bleeding.

Transvenous portal access is obtained by using a special directional cannula introduced into a hepatic vein from the jugular vein (see Transjugular Intrahepatic Portosystemic Shunt). When performed correctly this method avoids puncture of the liver capsule and thus reduces the risk of bleeding complications. The portal system can also be opacified by inserting a needle percutaneously into the splenic pulp and injecting either iodinated contrast or CO_2. This method, known as splenoportography, is rarely used for diagnostic imaging but can be a useful alternative approach for splenic vein interventions. Lastly, percutaneous retrograde catheterization of a recanalized umbilical vein allows access to the left portal vein (Fig. 14-14).

Indirect opacification of the portal venous system can be achieved by arterioportography. Injection of the SMA and/or IMA results in opacification of the mesenteric tributary veins and portal vein as the contrast drains from the splanchnic capillary bed. The rate and density of opacification of these veins can be significantly improved by injecting a vasodilator such as nitroglycerin (NTG; 200-300 µg) through the arterial catheter immediately before the contrast injection. Dilution of the NTG to 50-100 µg/mL provides a sufficient volume. The NTG is injected through the selective SMA or IMA catheter, followed by 5-10 mL of saline flush. The angiogram should be performed immediately (5-8 mL/sec in the SMA and 2-4 mL/sec in the IMA

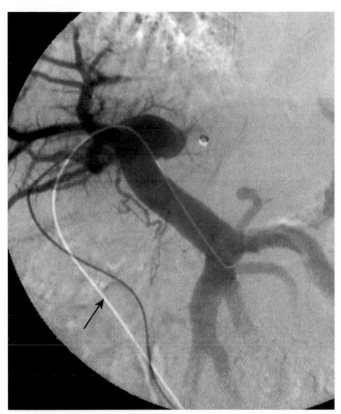

FIGURE 14-14. Digital subtraction angiogram portogram performed by retrograde catheterization of a recanalized umbilical vein *(arrow)*. Subtraction artifact due to respiration results in a double image of the catheter.

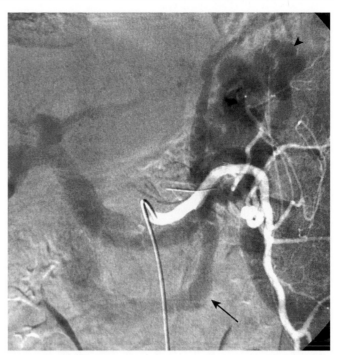

FIGURE 14-15. Visualization of the portal venous system from arterial injections. Late digital subtraction angiogram image from a splenic artery injection in a patient with portal hypertension masked to show the splenic artery in white and veins in black. The splenic vein is visualized just below the splenic artery with filling of the portal vein. In addition, there is filling of large gastric varices *(arrowhead)* with drainage into the left renal vein *(black straight arrow)* and inferior vena cava.

for 6-10 seconds), with rapid filming (at least 4 frames/sec) for a few seconds followed by 1 frame/sec during the venous phase. Breathholding is essential to minimize motion artifacts, and glucagon (1 mg intravenously) may be used to decrease peristalsis.

Injection of the celiac artery also opacifies the portal vein with blood draining from the spleen, stomach, and pancreas. Selective catheterization of the splenic artery results in greater portal venous opacification (Fig. 14-15). For selective splenic artery injections, volumes between 20 and 60 mL may be needed depending on the size of the spleen. Vasodilators are not of assistance in this vascular bed. This technique is less effective in the presence of congestive splenomegaly, which requires very large volumes of contrast and has significantly increased transit time through the spleen.

▀ PORTAL HYPERTENSION

Portal hypertension can be defined as an absolute portal venous pressure of greater than 10 mm Hg. More commonly, the pressure gradient between the portal and systemic veins is used to guide therapy; normal gradient is less than 5 mm Hg. Elevated pressures can exist in the entire portal venous system, or focally in isolated segments. Portal hypertension is just one manifestation of chronic liver disease (Box 14-1).

In industrialized countries, portal hypertension is most commonly encountered in patients with cirrhosis (schistosomiasis is the most common etiology globally). The usual diseases in industrialized nations leading to cirrhosis and portal hypertension are alcoholic liver disease, chronic viral hepatitis (hepatitis B and C viruses), and steatohepatitis (Box 14-2). The incidence of cirrhosis in the United States is 3.6/1000 adults. End-stage liver disease was the 12th leading cause of death in the United States in 2009. In at least 50% of these patients alcohol is the most significant cause of liver failure. Patients in whom a cause cannot be identified are said to have "cryptogenic cirrhosis."

Box 14-1. Physical Findings in Advanced Liver Disease

Ascites
Splenomegaly
Caput medusae
Spider nevi
Palmar erythema
Jaundice
Gynecomastia
Testicular atrophy

Box 14-2. Causes of Cirrhosis

HEPATOCELLULAR
Alcohol
Viral hepatitis (B, C)
Wilson disease
Hemochromatosis
α_1-antitrypsin deficiency
Glycogen storage disease type IV
Steatohepatitis
Drugs/toxins

CHOLESTATIC
Extrahepatic biliary atresia
Primary biliary cirrhosis
Primary sclerosing cholangitis
Choledochal cyst
Cystic fibrosis

VENOUS OUTFLOW OBSTRUCTION
Veno-occlusive disease
Budd-Chiari syndrome
Congestive heart failure
Constrictive pericarditis

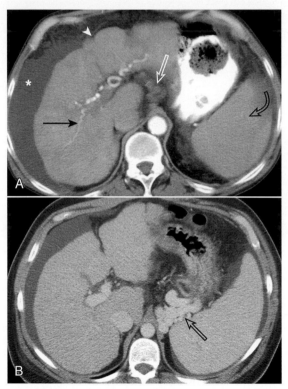

FIGURE 14-16. Imaging findings of portal hypertension on computed tomography. **A,** Axial computed tomography (CT) scan during the arterial phase of a patient with alcoholic cirrhosis, demonstrating many of the associated findings in portal hypertension: ascites (*), nodular contour of contracted liver *(arrowhead)*, tortuous "corkscrew" arteries due to contraction of the liver parenchyma *(straight closed arrow)*, gastroesophageal varices *(straight open arrow)*, and enlarged spleen *(open curved arrow)*. **B,** Axial CT scan during the venous phase in a different patient, showing opacification of gastroesophageal varices *(open arrow)*.

The many causes of portal hypertension are organized into three categories based on the level of obstruction: posthepatic, intrahepatic, and prehepatic (Box 14-3). Pathologists further divide the intrahepatic causes as presinusoidal, sinusoidal, and postsinusoidal on the basis of histologic findings. The level of obstruction in alcoholic cirrhosis is primarily sinusoidal. In schistosomiasis, a common cause of portal hypertension in parts of Africa and South America, the obstruction is presinusoidal.

The pathophysiology of portal hypertension in cirrhosis is a combination of increased resistance to blood flow through the liver and an increased volume of blood flow through the splanchnic circulation. As resistance and flow both increase, the direction of blood flow in the portal vein begins to reverse (hepatofugal flow—blood literally fleeing the liver). The portal blood returns to the systemic circulation through extrahepatic collaterals termed *varices*. These decompressive pathways are rarely sufficient to normalize the portal pressure.

Patients with portal hypertension and cirrhosis are described using the Child-Pugh and Model for End-Stage Liver Disease (MELD) scores (see Table 11-10). The MELD score was developed originally to predict risk for the transjugular intrahepatic portosystemic shunt (TIPS) procedure (see below).

Ascites is the most common complication of cirrhosis (Box 14-4 and Fig. 14-16). The pathogenesis of ascites is complex and multifactorial, involving multiple hormonal pathways responsible for sodium and free water regulation. Nonetheless, sinusoidal hypertension is thought to be a critical factor. The development of ascites in cirrhotic patients marks a very significant prognostic point in the progression of liver disease. About half of patients with cirrhosis develop ascites within 10 years; the 2-year survival after ascites develops is approximately 50%; and in patients with refractory ascites, 50% will be dead in 6 months. Refractory ascites is defined as fluid overload that is unresponsive to a sodium-restricted diet

and high-dose diuretic treatment and requires frequent large volume paracentesis. Patients who cannot tolerate medical therapy are also considered to have refractory ascites.

Portosystemic shunting results in enlarged thin-walled veins termed *varices* (see Fig. 14-8). Variceal blood flow is from the high-pressure portal system to the low-pressure systemic veins. Gastroesophageal varices are the source of gastrointestinal bleeding in 60%-90% of patients with cirrhosis and portal hypertension. Other causes of bleeding include peptic ulcer, hemorrhagic gastritis, and Mallory-Weiss syndrome. Splenorenal varices can contribute to gastrointestinal bleeding if there are communications with the gastric mucosa via short gastric veins. Up to 50% of patients with cirrhosis develop esophageal varices, and almost one third have gastric varices. Once present, the yearly rate of variceal bleeding is 5%-15%, with a mortality rate of 20% at 6 weeks. In general, a portosystemic gradient of 12 mm Hg or greater is associated with in increased risk of variceal bleeding. Approximately 70% of patients will rebleed without treatment, but aggressive

TABLE **14-2** Hepatic Encephalopathy

Grade	Definition
I	Mild confusion, shortened attention span, sleep disorders, mild asterixis, tremor
II	Lethargic or drowsy, variably oriented, personality changes, asterixis
III	Somnolent but arousable, confused, hyperreflexia, positive Babinski sign
IV	Comatose, decerebrate neurologic examination

endoscopic and pharmacologic management decreases the rate of rebleeding to about 20%. One third of all deaths in patients with cirrhosis and portal hypertension are the result of bleeding from gastroesophageal varices.

Hepatic encephalopathy is a neuropsychiatric condition that results from a combination of liver failure and portal-to-systemic shunting. Symptoms range from personality changes and sleep disturbance to coma (Table 14-2). Chemical substances produced in the intestine (likely by bacterial action) that are normally metabolized by a healthy liver are presumed to be responsible. Because portal-to-systemic shunting contributes to encephalopathy, this condition can be worsened by surgical or radiologic shunts performed to reduce portal pressure. Survival without liver transplantation for recurrent encephalopathy can be as low as 40% at 1 year.

Congestive splenomegaly results from chronic venous congestion secondary to portal hypertension, producing splenic enlargement and varying degrees of hypersplenism (thrombocytopenia being the most common manifestation). In a similar fashion, portal hypertensive gastropathy and portal hypertensive colopathy result from chronic venous congestion secondary to portal hypertension. These can lead to acute bleeding but more commonly cause chronic, low-grade blood loss associated with an iron-deficiency anemia.

Hepatorenal syndrome refers to renal failure in patients with advanced hepatic failure and portal hypertension, characterized by a very low glomerular filtration rate in the absence of other causes of renal impairment. The syndrome has been estimated to occur in 10% of hospitalized patients with cirrhosis and ascites. The kidney is histologically normal but subject to abnormal vasoconstriction. The pathophysiology of the syndrome appears to be closely tied to the same abnormal regulation of sodium, free water, and arterial blood volume that contributes to ascites formation.

Hepatic hydrothorax is the accumulation of a significant volume of pleural fluid (usually > 500 mL) in a patient with cirrhosis who has no cardiac or pulmonary disease that would otherwise account for the effusion. Other causes for effusion, including malignancy, should be ruled out before the diagnosis is established. Hepatic hydrothorax is usually right-sided and is thought to occur by the migration of fluid from the abdomen, across defects in the diaphragm. Ascites may or may not be present. In the latter situation, lymphatic fluid weeping from the bare area of the liver may be the source of the effusion. This condition is estimated to occur in 4%-10% of patients with cirrhosis.

Hepatopulmonary syndrome is characterized by the triad of liver disease, hypoxemia due to right-to-left shunting, and intrapulmonary vascular dilations. Patients characteristically become short of breath and/or desaturate when changing from a supine to upright position. Mortality is increased significantly with the development of hepatopulmonary syndrome. The treatment options are limited, with oxygen therapy a mainstay.

The imaging of patients with portal hypertension relies primarily on cross-sectional imaging with CT, MRI, and ultrasound

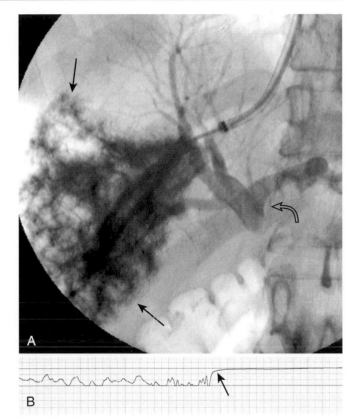

FIGURE **14-17**. Demonstration of portal hypertension with hepatic venogram and pressure measurements. **A,** Balloon-occlusion wedged hepatic venogram using iodinated contrast in a patient with cirrhosis and portal hypertension. The hepatic parenchyma *(straight arrows)* has a patchy ("moth-eaten") appearance (compare with Fig. 14-11). In addition, there is opacification of the portal vein *(curved arrow)*. **B,** Hepatic vein pressure tracing during free and wedged measurements using a balloon occlusion catheter. The free tracing (balloon deflated) has a low-pressure multiphasic waveform representative of the systemic venous system. With inflation of the occlusion balloon *(arrow)*, the pressure rises and becomes monophasic, reflecting the portal venous pressure.

(see Fig. 14-16). A small, nodular liver with associated varices and ascites is characteristic. The lateral segment of the left lobe of the liver may be hypertrophied in advanced cases. The diameter of the portal vein may be increased (>12 mm) in portal hypertension. On duplex color-flow ultrasound examination, demonstration of hepatofugal flow in the portal vein, umbilical vein, or the coronary vein is diagnostic. The hepatic veins may have diminished, monophasic flow. The portal vein should be carefully inspected for thrombus.

The angiographic demonstration of portal hypertension is usually incidental to other procedures such as chemoembolization of a liver tumor. Contraction of the liver, enlargement of the left lobe, and tortuous "corkscrew" appearance of the intrahepatic arteries are typical arterial findings (see Fig. 11-4**A**). Visualization of varices, retrograde flow in the IMV, increased size of the portal vein, and hepatofugal flow on venous phase images are all evidence of portal hypertension (see Fig. 14-15). Conventional hepatic venograms may reveal small hepatic veins with decreased flow in advanced cases. Wedged hepatic venograms demonstrate a patchy parenchymal stain and opacification of the portal vein with hepatofugal flow (Fig. 14-17).

Determination of the portal pressure is useful in the diagnosis and treatment of portal hypertension. In some cases, this may be the primary reason for hepatic venography. In most instances, direct measurement of portal venous pressures is not practical. The most convenient method is to obtain hepatic sinusoidal

TABLE 14-3 Hepatic Vein Pressure Measurements (Relative)

Level of Obstruction	FHVP	WHVP	HVPG
Prehepatic	Normal	Normal	Normal
Presinusoidal	Normal	Normal/slight increase	Normal/slight increase
Sinusoidal	Normal	Increased	Increased
Postsinusoidal	Normal	Increased	Increased
Posthepatic	Increased	Increased	Normal

FHVP, Free hepatic vein pressure; HVPG, hepatic vein pressure gradient; WHVP, wedged hepatic vein pressure.

pressure measurements using an occlusion-balloon catheter technique in combination with hepatic venography. This is analogous to evaluation of left heart pressures with pulmonary-artery wedge pressure measurements using a Swan-Ganz catheter. An occlusion balloon catheter is positioned in a hepatic vein but not inflated. A triphasic waveform should be observed on the transducer monitor and the mean pressure recorded (the free hepatic venous pressure, FHVP) (see Fig. 14-17). The occlusion balloon is then inflated using a small (3 mL) syringe. Once the balloon is wedged, the hepatic venous waveform flattens and becomes monophasic. The wedged hepatic venous pressure (WHVP) is then measured. The intrahepatic portal pressure is expressed as the hepatic vein pressure gradient (HVPG) or "corrected sinusoidal pressure":

$$HVPG = WHVP - FHVP$$

The normal HVPG is less than or equal to 5 mm Hg. An HVPG greater than 5 mm Hg is indicative of portal hypertension. An HVPG of 12 mm Hg or greater is associated with the development of variceal hemorrhage (Table 14-3). The pressure between the hepatic vein and the right atrium should also be measured to confirm the absence of a significant gradient.

More invasive means can be used to obtain the absolute portal pressure by percutaneous transhepatic or transjugular access of the portal vein. Direct percutaneous puncture of the spleen yields the splenic pulp pressure, which is indicative of the portal pressure. This latter method is rarely used.

The initial management of patients with portal hypertension is with medical therapy (Table 14-4). The treatment goals for stable patients is to eliminate factors contributing to cirrhosis and to reduce portal pressure by 20%, or less than 12 mm Hg. Aggressive medical intervention has decreased the incidence of ascites, bleeding, and encephalopathy in the past decade. Oral β-blockers are used to decrease portal pressure. Dietary restriction and diuretic therapy can successfully control ascites in 90% of cases. Patients with acute worsening of hepatic encephalopathy should be evaluated for occult gastrointestinal bleeding and bacterial peritonitis. Lactulose and Rifaximin are the mainstays of therapy. Acute esophageal variceal bleeding can be controlled in 90% of patients with combined endoscopic and medical therapy.

Surgical creation of portal-to-systemic venous shunts is rarely performed, but effectively lowers portal pressure and addresses many of the complications of portal hypertension (Table 14-5). A total shunt, in which the entire portal flow is diverted into the systemic veins through a large (15-25 mm diameter) communication have greater than 90% patency and minimal rebleeding. However, these shunts are associated with a 30%-50% incidence of encephalopathy and often lead to an acceleration of underlying liver disease. Partial shunts use smaller anastomoses (8-15 mm diameter) to reduce the portal-caval gradient to 12 mm Hg while preserving hepatopetal flow. Lower incidences of both encephalopathy and liver failure have been reported with these procedures, with

TABLE 14-4 Medical Therapy of Portal Hypertension

Complication	Medical Therapy
Hepatic encephalopathy	Dietary protein restriction Oral lactulose therapy Rifaximin
Ascites	Dietary sodium restriction Diuretic therapy Large-volume paracentesis

Variceal hemorrhage	Primary prevention:
	  Nonselective β-blockers
	Acute hemorrhage:
	  Volume resuscitation and management in an intensive care unit setting
	  Endoscopic sclerotherapy or variceal band ligation to control hemorrhage
	  Vasoactive drugs (e.g., terlipressin, somatostatin, octreotide, β-blockers, nitrates)
	Secondary prevention:
	  Endoscopic sclerotherapy or variceal band ligation to obliterate gastroesophageal varices
	  Nonselective β-blockade

Hepatic hydrothorax	Dietary sodium restriction Diuretic therapy Large-volume paracentesis Thoracentesis

TABLE 14-5 Surgical Portal-to-Systemic Shunts

Type	Description
Total	Large diameter (15-25 mm) portocaval (end-to-side or side-to-side portal vein to IVC), mesocaval (side-to-side superior mesenteric vein to IVC), central splenorenal*
Partial	Small diameter (8-15 mm) side-to-side portocaval or mesocaval
Selective	Distal splenorenal†

*Spleen is removed and splenic vein is anastomosed end-to-side to left renal vein, diverting portal flow.
†Spleen is retained and splenic vein is anastomosed end-to-side to left renal vein so that only splenic venous flow is diverted from portal circulation.
IVC, Inferior vena cava.

excellent control of bleeding. Selective shunts decompress only a portion of the portal system while preserving hepatopetal flow. The best known is the distal splenorenal shunt combined with ligation of the coronary and right gastroepiploic vein. Although usually effective in decompressing gastroesophageal varices and successful in maintaining forward flow to the liver, the sustained sinusoidal hypertension with this shunt does not improve ascites.

The ultimate surgical therapy for portal hypertension from chronic liver disease is liver transplantation. However, end-stage liver disease, not portal hypertension, is the indication for transplantation.

TRANSJUGULAR INTRAHEPATIC PORTOSYSTEMIC SHUNT

The TIPS procedure decompresses the portal venous system by the percutaneous creation of a low-resistance tract through the liver between the portal and hepatic venous systems. Conceived by Josef Rösch in 1969, TIPS did not become an important clinical technique until the introduction of metallic stents in the late 1980s.

The TIPS procedure is of documented benefit and indicated in patients with variceal bleeding and ascites who have failed

Box 14-5. Indications for TIPS

ESTABLISHED

Acute hemorrhage from varices not responsive to medical therapy

Recurrent variceal hemorrhage not responsive to medical therapy (Child's B and C)

Refractory ascites

Refractory hepatic hydrothorax

Budd-Chiari syndrome

PROMISING

Portal hypertensive gastropathy

Hepatorenal syndrome

TIPS for first variceal hemorrhage

Early TIPS for ascites

TIPS, Transjugular intrahepatic portosystemic shunt.

Box 14-6. Contraindications to TIPS

ABSOLUTE

Severe hepatic failure

Biliary or systemic sepsis

Isolated gastric varices with splenic vein occlusion

Severe left- or right-sided heart failure

Pulmonary hypertension

RELATIVE

Cavernous transformation of the portal vein

Severe hepatic encephalopathy

Biliary dilatation

International normalized ratio > 5

Platelet count < 20,000/cm^3

TIPS, Transjugular intrahepatic portosystemic shunt.

Box 14-7. TIPS for Acute Bleeding: Questions to Ask

Has patient undergone endoscopy to confirm source of bleeding?

Where are the varices located?

Has endoscopic therapy been tried?

Is patient hemodynamically stable?

Is medical therapy optimized, including correction of coagulopathies?

Is the portal vein known to be patent (and by what imaging test)?

Is airway protection necessary to prevent aspiration of blood during the procedure?

Is patient a candidate for liver transplant?

TIPS, Transjugular intrahepatic portosystemic shunt.

TABLE 14-6 TIPS Mortality Risk and MELD Score

MELD	Comment
0-12	Low risk
13-17	Some risk
18-25	High risk
>25	Compassionate application only

TIPS, Transjugular intrahepatic portosystemic shunt.

When tense ascites is present, a large-volume paracentesis immediately before the procedure allows the liver to assume a normal position in the peritoneal cavity. The TIPS procedure can be performed with conscious sedation, although general anesthesia is preferred by some interventionalists and most patients. In critically ill patients with acute bleeding, intubation is warranted for airway protection. Intravenous antibiotics (usually a third generation cephalosporin) are infused before the procedure. In elective cases, appropriate blood products should be transfused to keep the platelet count greater than 20,000/cm^3 and the international normalized ratio (INR) less than 2.

Creation of a TIPS results in characteristic hemodynamic changes. The shunt causes hepatic parenchymal portal perfusion to decrease and hepatic arterial flow to increase. Central venous pressures and cardiac index increase after TIPS, whereas systemic vascular resistance decreases.

Prediction of risk is difficult in patients with TIPS because the population of patients with portal hypertension is heterogenous. Patients treated for bleeding have better survival than those treated for ascites. In general, the higher the Child score, the worse the outcome. The MELD scoring system is often used to predict survival. Online MELD calculators are readily available, requiring the patient's total bilirubin, serum creatinine, and INR values. There is a higher risk of early mortality in patients with a MELD score of 18 or greater (Table 14-6). In general patients with compromised hepatic arterial blood supply (e.g., hepatic artery occlusion or multiple prior episodes of chemoembolization), or hepatic dysfunction manifested by a bilirubin level greater than 3 mg/dL are at risk of hepatic decompensation after TIPS. Patients with preexisting diastolic ventricular dysfunction benefit less from TIPS performed for ascites.

The TIPS procedure requires a dedicated portal vein access kit. In the kits are a long sheath that reaches from the jugular to the hepatic vein and an external directional indicator on the needle or needle guide to orient the puncture. Some kits contain an open needle; others contain a trocar sheath needle (Fig. 14-18). In addition, a dedicated covered stent may be used to create the shunt (Fig. 14-19). The core steps of the procedure are summarized in Box 14-8 and illustrated in Figure 14-20.

The traditional venous access for introduction of the TIPS set (with the intent to work through the right hepatic vein) is the right internal jugular vein, although either internal or external jugular vein can be used. A left-sided jugular access facilitates catheterization of the right hepatic vein and is preferred by the author, but awake patients may experience chest discomfort owing to the rigid devices in the mediastinum. Great care is necessary when advancing sheaths, metal cannulas, and needles through the heart. These maneuvers should be monitored fluoroscopically, even though they are performed over a guidewire, because lethal cardiac perforation can occur.

The hepatic vein is usually selected with an angled catheter and a 3-J or angled hydrophilic guidewire. The catheter should be rotated lateral and slightly posterior to locate the right hepatic vein. Contrast injection is important to confirm the identity of the vein, especially in patients with small livers or massive ascites that displace the liver and distort venous anatomy. Inadvertent selection of an accessory hepatic vein or the right renal vein will

medical management (Boxes 14-5 through 14-7). Stent-grafts have vastly improved durability and primary patency rates, such that surgical portocaval shunts are uncommon in many centers.

Patent portal and hepatic veins should be documented before TIPS is attempted. An ultrasound examination of the liver with Doppler interrogation of these veins is commonly used. Contrast-enhanced CT or MRI of the liver is preferred because the relationships of the hepatic and portal veins are clearly depicted, and these studies are more sensitive for coincident hepatoma or other liver masses. The bile ducts should be evaluated, because biliary obstruction is a relative contraindication to the procedure.

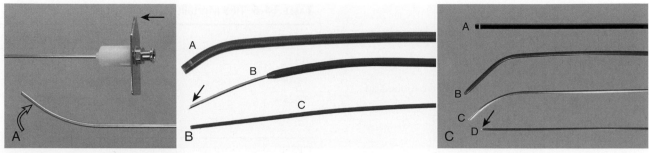

FIGURE 14-18. Components of transjugular intrahepatic portosystemic shunt kits. **A,** Directional marker *(straight arrow)* indicates the direction of the tip of the needle or cannula *(curved arrow)*. **B,** The Haskal kit: (A) 10-French angled introducer sheath; (B) assembled 9-French angled needle guide catheter with the curved 16-gauge access needle *(arrow)*—portal vein puncture is achieved with this needle; (C) straight 5-French Teflon catheter. **C,** The Rösch-Uchida kit: (A) Straight 10-French introducer sheath; (B) 10-French angled guide for cannula; (C) 14-gauge stiffening cannula that is inserted within B; (D) assembled 5-French catheter and 0.038-inch trocar stylet *(arrow)*—portal vein puncture is achieved with this assembly advanced coaxially through the 10-French catheter and stiffening cannula. The trocar stylet is then removed, leaving the 5-French catheter in the portal vein. (Both kits courtesy Cook Group, Bloomington, Ind.)

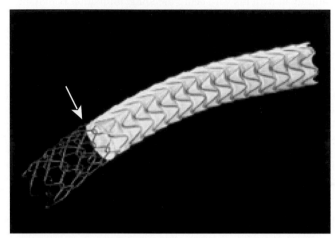

FIGURE 14-19. The most commonly used stent-graft for transjugular intrahepatic portosystemic shunt is the GORE® VIATORR® TIPS Endoprosthesis. The bare stent portion of the device is intended to reside in the portal vein. A radiopaque band *(arrow)* identifies the junction between the uncovered and covered portion. The graft material is ePTFE. (Image © 2013 W. L. Gore & Associates, Inc.)

Box 14-8. Basic Steps of the TIPS Procedure

Jugular vein access
Catheterization of hepatic vein (usually right)
Wedged hepatic venogram (usually with CO_2 gas)
Puncture from hepatic vein to intrahepatic portal vein (usually right portal branch)
Portal venogram to confirm patency (especially splenic vein)
Measure pressure gradient (means) between portal vein and right atrium
Dilatation of parenchymal tract (8 mm diameter, 3-4 cm long balloon)
Deployment of stent-graft (usually 10-mm diameter self-expanding)
Measure gradient:
    Bleeding: <12 mm Hg
    Ascites: 50% reduction
Further dilatation of shunt or extension if necessary to reduce gradient
Embolization of varices (in patients with active variceal bleeding)
Completion portal venogram

TIPS, Transjugular intrahepatic portosystemic shunt.

result in procedural failure and possible severe complication. The choice of hepatic vein is dictated by anatomic considerations. In most patients the right hepatic vein is large, easily catheterized, and has a downward slope that accommodates the curved metallic elements of the TIPS kit. However, the middle hepatic vein is also large and can be easily confused with the right hepatic vein when viewed in the anteroposterior projection. The left hepatic vein is often smaller with an anterior course and almost perpendicular axis relative to the IVC.

The next step is a wedged hepatic venogram to confirm the patency of the portal vein and provide a visual target for needle passes (see Figs. 2-26 and 14-17). This is most safely performed with a balloon occlusion catheter in the hepatic vein. In addition, the opacified hepatic parenchyma allows confirmation of the identity of the hepatic vein and localization of the border of the liver. This step is omitted with the Hawkins kit, with which injection of CO_2 into the liver parenchyma through the access needle is used to opacify the portal vein.

The ideal location in the hepatic vein from which to start the puncture depends on patient anatomy. The target on the portal side is the right or left portal vein just peripheral to the bifurcation of the main portal vein (see Fig. 14-20). Based on the wedged hepatic venogram and prior review of cross-sectional imaging, an entry point in the hepatic vein is selected, taking into consideration the target vein and the thickness of liver parenchyma. Peripheral starting points risk entry into peripheral portal branches or extracapsular puncture of the liver. Working through small portal branches can present technical challenges with respect to delivery of devices around sharp angles. Conversely, starting too central in the hepatic vein may result in puncture of the extrahepatic main portal vein, which can result in intraperitoneal hemorrhage (Fig. 14-21). In most cases, initiating punctures within 2-4 cm of the hepatic vein orifice result in successful TIPS creation. The needle is rotated either anteriorly or posteriorly depending on which hepatic vein is being used. The directional indicator on the hub of the needle or cannula provides useful directional information (Table 14-7; see also Fig. 14-18).

Locating the portal vein during the puncture is often the most difficult step of the procedure. An alternative to wedged hepatic venography is intravascular ultrasound (IVUS), particularly with a probe that images in a sagittal plane. When inserted from a femoral approach, this can provide real-time ultrasound guidance of this critical step (Fig. 14-22).

The actual technique of puncture with the Ross and trocar needles differs slightly. The curved 16-gauge modified Ross needle is rotated and thrust into the liver at the same time. Trocar-based systems, such as the Rösch-Uchida kit (Cook Group, Bloomington, Ind.), have a curved 14-gauge blunt metal cannula that is rotated to engage the wall of the hepatic vein, through which the 0.038-inch flexible trocar and 5-French catheter assembly are

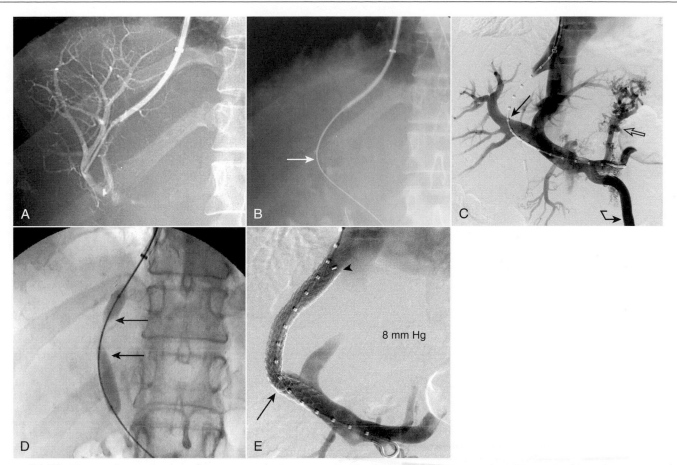

FIGURE 14-20. The transjugular intrahepatic portosystemic shunt procedure (in this case for refractory ascites). The wedged hepatic venogram with CO_2 is not shown (for an example, see Fig. 2-26). **A,** Puncture of right portal vein branch from right hepatic vein. Identity of the portal vein is confirmed with contrast injection. **B,** Guidewire *(arrow)* advanced into the portal system. **C,** Portogram with simultaneous injection of contrast through the sheath in the inferior vena cava (IVC). The catheter enters the right portal vein *(arrow)*. Note the retrograde flow in the inferior mesenteric vein (IMV) *(curved arrow)* and left gastric varices *(open arrow)*. The right renal vein orifice is well visualized. The pressure gradient was then measured between the portal vein and IVC (17 mm Hg). **D,** Balloon dilatation of the intrahepatic tract. The waist on the angioplasty balloon *(arrows)* identifies the length of the tract through the liver parenchyma between the right hepatic and portal veins. **E,** Portal venogram after placement of a self-expanding stent-graft (Viatorr, W. L. Gore & Associates, Inc.) across the tract, dilated to 8 mm. The varices no longer fill, the IMV is no longer seen, and there is some flow into the left portal vein. The *arrow* indicates the marker between the bare distal rings of the stent in the portal vein and the graft-covered portion of the stent in the liver parenchyma and hepatic vein. The stent protrudes slightly into the IVC *(arrowhead)*.

thrust into the liver parenchyma. With all kits, the needle should be advanced approximately 1 cm beyond the expected or known location of the portal vein unless using IVUS guidance. Periportal fibrosis, when present, results in a palpable "pop" when the portal vein is entered. However, overaggressive thrusts without consideration for the location of the portal vein target may result in puncture of the liver capsule and hemoperitoneum. The curve of the Ross needle and Rösch-Uchida cannula can be modified as needed, but the devices become difficult to advance through the sheath when the angles are too acute. The Ross needle is advantageous in hard livers, whereas the flexible Rösch-Uchida needle is easier to use when it is necessary to puncture at an acute angle. With the trocar system, the inner trocar is removed after the thrust, leaving the 5-French outer catheter in place.

The rotation of the needle or cannula should be maintained during all subsequent maneuvers. The natural tendency of the device is to orient itself to the hepatic vein, which moves the tip away from the portal vein. In addition, the operator should allow the puncture system to move slightly with inspiration and expiration, like a horseback rider in a saddle. When the device is held in a fixed position, the tip may migrate out of the portal vein as the liver moves up and down with each breath. Using a 10-mL syringe, the operator aspirates while slowly pulling the Ross needle or 5-French catheter back. When blood is freely aspirated,

contrast is gently injected under fluoroscopic guidance. One of three structures will be visualized: the portal vein, the hepatic vein, or the hepatic artery. Hepatic arterial flow is hepatopetal and brisk, whereas portal flow is slower and can be either hepatopetal or hepatofugal. Hepatic veins flow towards the heart. If the portal vein is not opacified, another syringe can be attached and the process of withdrawal with aspiration continued until the hepatic vein is reached. The puncture is repeated, varying the degree of rotation or starting location in the hepatic vein until the portal vein is found. Puncture of the hepatic artery within the hepatic parenchyma is usually inconsequential. Similarly, puncture of the biliary tree is typically without sequelae.

Once portal vein puncture is confirmed, a guidewire is advanced into the main portal vein. A 0.038-inch Bentson or angled hydrophilic guidewire may be used. The former guidewire tends to prolapse down the main portal vein, whereas the latter allows directional control. When the guidewire remains in an intrahepatic portal vein, a 5-French hydrophilic Cobra-2, Rösch inferior mesenteric, or Binkert catheter can be used to direct the guidewire into the main portal vein. Once the wire is deep in the portal system, the tapered black outer guide for needle or cannula can then be advanced over the wire into the portal vein. In an awake patient, this usually hurts more than the puncture, but provides maximum security when exchanging for a pigtail catheter.

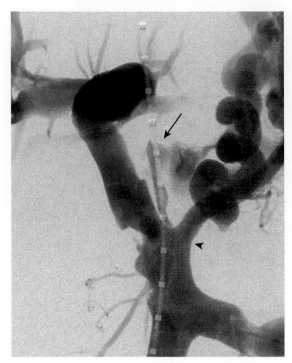

FIGURE 14-21. Extrahepatic puncture of the portal vein with extravasation of contrast *(arrow)*. The puncture was in the main portal vein just above the coronary vein *(arrowhead)*. The extravasation resolved with placement of the TIPS stent-graft.

TABLE 14-7 Needle Rotation During TIPS Puncture

Hepatic Vein	Portal Vein Target	Rotation of Needle
Right	Right	Anterior
Middle	Right	Posterolateral
Middle	Left	Posteromedial
Left	Left	Posteromedial

TIPS, Transjugular intrahepatic portosystemic shunt.

Pressure measurements are then obtained so that the opening gradient can be documented, followed by a portogram (preferably with the catheter in the splenic vein to confirm its patency).

Dilatation of the transhepatic tract is the next step. This is the most uncomfortable part of the procedure so it is helpful to alert the anesthesiologist or administer additional analgesics to the awake patient before inflating the balloon. A stiff 0.035-inch Amplatz wire should be used for this and all other maneuvers. A noncompliant balloon, 6-8 mm in diameter and 4-6 cm in length is positioned across the transhepatic tract and the sheath is withdrawn. The balloon is inflated with dilute contrast under fluoroscopic visualization. The initial waist produced by the hepatic parenchyma will give way, typically revealing two focal indentations on the balloon. These identify the length and location of the transhepatic tract, in that they represent the more resilient fibrous tissue surrounding the portal and hepatic veins. A digital spot film can be obtained and used as a reference for stent-graft selection.

Self-expanding stent-grafts have replaced bare stents as the preferred device for the TIPS tract. The only commercially available device in the United States is the Viatorr (W. L. Gore and Associates, Flagstaff, Ariz.). This is a nitinol-based ePTFE stent-graft that is 8-12 mm in diameter, variable in length, with 2 cm of bare stent at the portal end of the device (see Fig. 14-19). A radiopaque ring demarcates the junction between the covered and uncovered portions of the endograft. Mounted on the delivery catheter, the covered portion of the device is constrained by an ePTFE shroud, whereas the bare metal portion is constrained by a loading tube. The covered portion of the stent-graft should extend from entry site in the portal vein to the IVC. This reduces late stenosis at the hepatic vein end of the endograft. The 2 cm of bare metal are meant to be in the portal vein. A measuring portogram with simultaneous injection through the sheath in the hepatic vein is used to select the endograft length. The general rule of thumb is to measure portal vein to IVC distance and then add 1 cm to the desired covered length.

The endograft is deployed through a 10-French sheath that has been advanced well into the portal vein. The endograft is pushed to the end of the sheath, and then the sheath is withdrawn into the hepatic vein. This allows the bare metal portal end to expand while the covered portion remains contained in the shroud. The delivery catheter is then retracted until the bare metal stent rings are pulled tight against, but not into, the parenchymal tract. The endograft is deployed by pulling a string that releases the shroud.

Once deployed, the gradient should be checked to determine whether further expansion of the endograft is necessary. The target gradient is less than 12 mm Hg when the indication is bleeding varices, or 50% of the initial gradient for ascites. The stent-graft cannot be made larger in diameter than the manufactured maximum. Appropriate-sized balloons are used to fully expand the endograft as necessary. A venogram is performed with a pigtail catheter to document positioning, and the final pressure gradient across the shunt is determined. Additional stents or stent-grafts should be placed if the tract has not been adequately covered. If the gradient is still not adequate, consideration should be given to creating a second (double-barrel) TIPS.

When the TIPS is performed to control acute bleeding, embolization of gastroesophageal varices should be performed. Coil embolization of the main trunk of the varix will suffice, but a more distal embolization will be obtained by first injecting gelatin sponge pieces soaked in a sclerosant such as 3% sodium tetradecyl sulfate (STS), STS/iodized oil foam, or dehydrated alcohol into the varices (Fig. 14-23). Sometimes flow is so brisk that several coils should be placed first to slow flow, followed by injection of the sclerosing agent. However, should portal hypertension recur, new varices will form and old ones can recanalize.

The TIPS stent-graft expands over time to its maximum diameter because of the properties of the nitinol metal components. As a result, the gradient may continue to drop after the procedure. When TIPS is performed for ascites, the drop in gradient can be controlled by placing a short bare stent in the parenchymal tract before deployment of the stent-graft, which externally constrains the stent-graft at a predetermined diameter and allows incremental increases using angioplasty balloons (Fig. 14-24).

In some cases, access to the portal vein by transhepatic puncture can be difficult. Percutaneous insertion of a wire or catheter into the portal system has been used to provide a target. This can be introduced from a transhepatic intercostal approach or via a recanalized umbilical vein when present (see Fig. 14-14). Metallic coils can be placed percutaneously next to the right portal vein under CT guidance just prior to TIPS. CT has also been used to place guidewires through the liver, crossing the right portal vein and entering the IVC. The wire is snared from a jugular access and the shunt completed from that approach. Transabdominal and intravascular ultrasound can be used to guide portal vein puncture. Minilaparotomy with exposure of a mesenteric vein permits retrograde formation of the TIPS tract with puncture from the portal to the hepatic vein, rather than vice versa.

The complication rate from TIPS in experienced hands is less than 5% with a mortality rate of less than 2% (Table 14-8). The most serious and potentially lethal procedural complications of TIPS are nearly all related to the extracapsular puncture (see Fig. 14-21). Massive intraperitoneal bleeding from the liver can occur in patients with ascites or severe coagulopathy. Extrahepatic

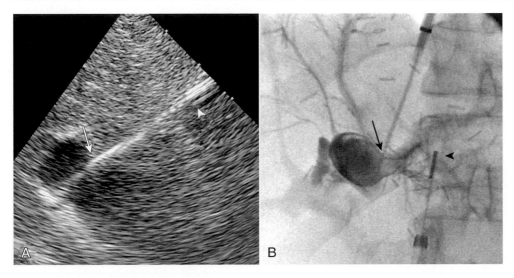

FIGURE 14-22. Intravascular ultrasound-guided transjugular intrahepatic portosystemic shunt (TIPS) using the 8-French AcuNav linear probe. (Courtesy Siemens, Munich, Germany.) **A,** Intravenous ultrasound image (IVUS) showing the TIPS needle entering the portal vein *(arrow)*. The TIPS cannula can be seen in hepatic vein *(arrowhead)*. **B,** Image from a TIPS procedure using IVUS guidance in a patient with prior right hepatectomy. The TIPS needle is in the portal vein *(arrow)*. The IVUS transducer *(arrowhead)* can be seen in the inferior vena cava.

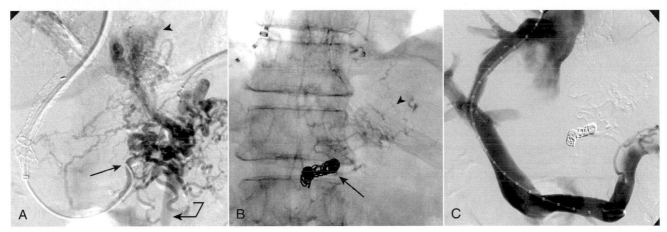

FIGURE 14-23. Embolization of left gastric vein and esophageal varices during a transjugular intrahepatic portosystemic shunt (TIPS) procedure. **A,** Selective left gastric venogram *(arrow)* after placement of the TIPS shows extensive gastric varices and filling of distal esophageal varices *(arrowhead)*. The vein heading off the bottom of the image *(bent arrow)* is a retroperitoneal collateral to the left renal vein. **B,** Single image after injection of 6 mL of 3% sodium tetradecyl sulfate foamed with 2 mL of room air and 1 mL of Lipiodol. (Courtesy Guerbet, Bloomington, Ind.) The sclerosant can be seen in the varices *(arrowhead)*. Coils were placed in the left gastric vein *(arrow)* after injection of the sclerosant. **C,** Completion portal venogram showing absence of filling of the varices.

puncture of the portal vein followed by angioplasty of the vein wall can also result in massive bleeding. Puncture of a hepatic artery branch is usually inconsequential, but bleeding or hepatic artery thrombosis can occur. Combined arterial and bile duct injury during needle passes can lead to a fistula and significant hemobilia and/or biliary obstruction. Careless manipulation of instruments in the right atrium can induce cardiac arrhythmias or perforate the atrium, causing cardiac tamponade.

Major acute postprocedural complications of TIPS creation include cardiac decompensation (from a combination of increased venous return through the shunt and elevation of right heart filling pressures), acceleration of liver failure, and precipitation or worsening of hepatic encephalopathy. A transient (weeks to months) hemolytic anemia has been described in approximately 10% of patients with bare stents, possibly due to fracture of red blood cells in the stent. This seems much less common with covered stents. Radiation-induced dermatitis has been described following very protracted cases. Endograft infection is rare, but can occur at any time after TIPS.

The technical success rate for TIPS for variceal bleeding averages about 97% (range 89%-100%). Causes of procedural failure include inability to access a hepatic or portal vein, hard liver parenchyma that prevents puncture with the needle, and occluded portal veins.

Shunt occlusion in the first 30 days is unusual. Technical problems, such as a residual stenosis in the stent-graft at the portal vein end, or hypercoagulability may be the cause. Percutaneous thrombectomy (as simple as sweeping the TIPS with an occlusion balloon) or thrombolysis with TIPS revision should be considered.

Initial clinical success varies with the indication; for recurrent variceal bleeding it is approximately 98% (range 97%-100%), whereas for intractable ascites approximately 60%-70% of patients respond. Numerous randomized prospective trials have confirmed that TIPS is superior to endoscopic therapies in the prevention of rebleeding. Variceal bleeding rates average 20% after TIPS (range 9%-41%) versus 49% for combined medical and endoscopic therapy (range 23%-61%). In the setting of refractory ascites, TIPS results in control of ascites in 79% of patients at 6 months compared to 24% of patients undergoing large-volume paracentesis. There is improved survival of patients with refractory ascites with TIPS compared to medical therapy, but also increased encephalopathy. Ultimately, all patients undergoing TIPS are likely to die of progressive liver failure or hepatoma unless transplanted.

There has been recent interest in applying TIPS earlier in the course of the patient's disease. The Early TIPS trial, a 31-patient randomized prospective single-center study of TIPS following the first variceal bleed versus conventional medical and endoscopic management, found a significant survival benefit at

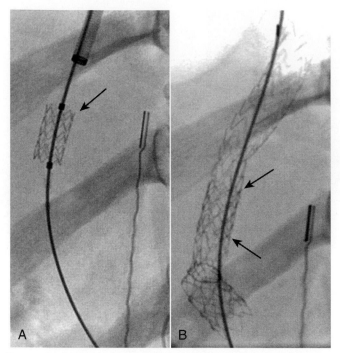

FIGURE 14-24. External restricting balloon-expandable stent used to control expansion of the 10-mm diameter self-expanding stent-graft in a patient at increased risk of encephalopathy after transjugular intrahepatic portosystemic shunt for ascites. Intravenous ultrasound guidance was used for this procedure. **A,** The balloon-expandable stent *(arrow)* has been deployed in the hepatic parenchymal tract. The diameter is 7 mm. **B,** The stent-graft has been deployed through the balloon-expandable stent *(arrows)*. The stent-graft was dilated to 8 mm to obtain the desired final gradient, and the external stent will ensure that it remains at that diameter unless enlarged with an angioplasty balloon.

TABLE 14-8 Complications of TIPS Procedure

Complication	Incidence (%)
Early	
Procedural mortality	<1
Intraperitoneal bleeding:	
Punctured liver capsule	5
Extrahepatic portal vein puncture	2
Hemobilia	2
Portal vein thrombosis	2
Stent migration/malplacement	2
Infection	2
Renal failure (contrast-induced)	5
Accelerated hepatic failure	1-5
Hemolysis	10
Worsened hepatic encephalopathy	20-30
Late	
Ascites, persistent requiring medical management	10-30
Recurrent variceal bleeding (bare stent)	15-25 (1 year)
Shunt stenosis (bare stent)	50 (1 year)

TIPS, Transjugular intrahepatic portosystemic shunt.
Adapted from Haskal ZJ, Martin L, Cardella JF, et al. Quality improvement guidelines for transjugular intrahepatic portosystemic shunts. SCVIR Standards of Practice Committee. *J Vasc Interv Radiol.* 2001;12:131-136

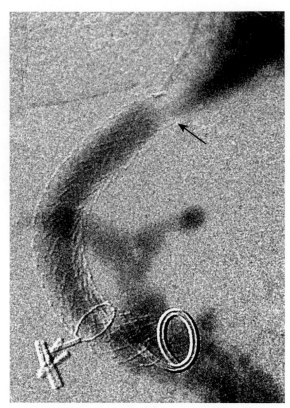

FIGURE 14-25. Symptomatic transjugular intrahepatic portosystemic shunt (TIPS) dysfunction with recurrent refractory ascites 24 months after the original procedure. CO_2 portal venogram shows stenosis in the hepatic vein at the end of the stent-graft *(arrow)*. Pressures were measured throughout the portal vein and TIPS, with a 21 mm Hg gradient localized to the hepatic vein end of the stent. This may have been avoided had the stent-graft extended in to the IVC. CO_2 was used as a contrast agent because the patient had renal insufficiency.

6 weeks and 1 year with TIPS, with a 50% reduction in recurrent bleeding. The broad applicability of these results is uncertain, in that the majority of the patients consumed alcohol up to the time of treatment and the overall prevalence of chronic viral hepatitis was low (16%).

Late TIPS dysfunction can be defined as stenosis or occlusion of the shunt, resulting in elevation of the portal-systemic pressure gradient and recurrent symptoms (Fig. 14-25). With bare metal stents, the reported 1-year primary patency of TIPS ranged from 25% to 66%. One-year primary unassisted patency is dramatically improved with stent-grafts, approaching 80%-90%, due to the reduction in late in-tract stenosis because of the ePFTE covering. When stenoses occur with stent-grafts, they are almost always in the hepatic vein when the endograft ends a little short (thus the recommendation that the endograft should extend slightly into the IVC). The hepatic vein stenosis can be treated with angioplasty and/or extension with placement of an additional stent.

Worsening of encephalopathy after TIPS occurs in 30%-50% of patients, with patients treated for ascites being at greatest risk. Encephalopathy seems to be less problematic with covered stents. Other risk factors include preexisting encephalopathy, increased age, hypoalbuminemia, and cirrhosis of nonalcoholic etiology. Fewer than 10% of patients have mental status changes refractory to medical treatments. Options in these patients include diminishing the shunt diameter by placing a "shunt-reducing" stent within the tract, shunt occlusion, or liver transplantation (Fig. 14-26). The same options apply to the occasional patient in whom rapidly deteriorating liver function develops after TIPS creation.

To detect shunt malfunction, duplex ultrasound and CT can be used for surveillance. Because air is trapped within the graft

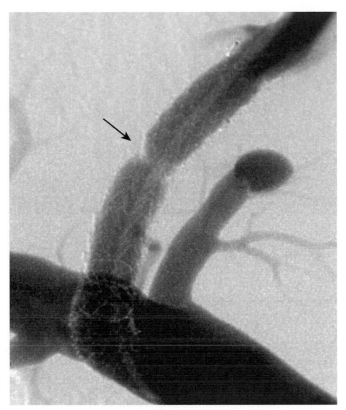

FIGURE 14-26. Reducing stent placed in a transjugular intrahepatic portosystemic shunt for hepatic encephalopathy. A Viatorr endograft (W. L. Gore & Associates, Inc.) was deployed on the sterile back table, constrained to 6 mm with a suture using an angioplasty balloon as a mandrill, reloaded into the sheath, and then deployed within the existing stent-graft. The waist in the new endograft *(arrow)* increased the gradient from 4 mm Hg to 14 mm Hg.

TABLE 14-9 Ultrasound Parameters for Follow-Up of TIPS

Doppler Parameter	Velocity (cm/sec)
Peak shunt velocity	< 90 or > 190
Change in peak shunt velocity	Decrease > 40 or increase > 60
Main portal vein velocity	<30

TIPS, Transjugular intrahepatic portosystemic shunt.

material in fresh Viatorr stent-grafts, ultrasound is useless for 1-2 weeks. Traditionally, follow-up examinations at 6 weeks, 3 months, and 6 months are then followed by examinations biannually (Table 14-9). The velocities within TIPS stent-grafts are somewhat higher than previously described for bare metal stents (Fig. 14-27). Alternatively, patients with Viatorr endografts can be managed expectantly with observation for either recurrent varices (with endoscopy) or ascites (physical exam).

When TIPS malfunction is suspected, venography with pressure measurements is the best way to resolve the question (and treat the patient at the same time). This should be performed whenever a screening ultrasound suggests a stenosis or in the setting of recurrent varices, bleeding, or ascites (see Fig. 14-25).

▬ DIRECT INFERIOR VENA CAVA TO PORTAL SHUNT

Direct puncture from the IVC through the caudate lobe to the main portal vein (DIPS; direct IVC-to-portal shunt) is an alternative approach to TIPS (Fig. 14-28). An IVUS probe placed from a femoral approach is used to guide the puncture. A modified Rösch-Uchida cannula with an exaggerated curve to provide stability in the IVC is inserted from a jugular access and used to guide the needle through the IVC just below the hepatic veins into the main portal vein under direct visualization with IVUS. The target is the portal vein just proximal to the bifurcation into the right and left branches. A standard trocar technique with a long 21-gauge hollow stylet needle that will accept a 0.018-inch guidewire is used. Most of the remaining steps of the procedure are the same as for conventional TIPS. A stent-graft is essential in that extrahepatic puncture of the portal vein is common with

this technique. This approach is very useful for patients with difficult hepatic or portal vein anatomy, hepatic parenchymal lesions that would obstruct a standard approach, or very small livers in whom extracapsular puncture is a concern. Patient selection can be made from contrast-enhanced CT before the procedure. Surgeons performing orthotopic liver transplants with "piggy-back" hepatic vein anastomoses (see Transjugular Liver Biopsy) should be alerted not to expect to find the stent-graft in the hepatic vein at the time of removal of the recipient's liver.

▬ BALLOON RETROGRADE TRANSRENAL OBLITERATION OF GASTRIC VARICES

Gastric varices are difficult to manage endoscopically. When these are the primary portosystemic collaterals, an alternative to TIPS is balloon occlusion retrograde transrenal vein obliteration of these varices (BRTO). Large gastric varices often drain into the systemic circulation through retroperitoneal collaterals to the left renal vein, usually in conjunction with the adrenal vein (see Figs. 14-15 and 14-23A). Catheterization of these collaterals from the left renal vein with an occlusion balloon and temporary obstruction of outflow allows retrograde injection of a sufficient volume of sclerosing agent to fill the gastric varices.

The anatomy of the gastrorenal collaterals can be complex, requiring coil embolization of small branches that drain into IVC, diaphragm, or the portal system. Careful review of the portal phase of a CTA is of great help in determining the anatomy and the size of the occlusion balloon needed.

Before the procedure, a Foley catheter should be placed because the sclerosant agents can cause hemolysis. Patients should also be vigorously hydrated with intravenous fluids. The left adrenal vein is selected using standard technique (see Fig. 13-14). The vein is usually enlarged because of the portosystemic shunting. A long sheath (30 cm is usually just right) large enough to accept the appropriate occlusion balloon is advanced in the vein. An occlusion balloon is then negotiated beyond the adrenal vein inflow and inflated (Fig. 14-29). Large occlusion balloons may be necessary, up to 20 mm or more. Contrast is injected through the occlusion balloon with sufficient volume to fill the gastric varices almost to the splenic and/or coronary vein.

The sclerosing agent can be injected through the balloon catheter or ideally a high-flow microcatheter advanced as deep within the varices as possible. Ethanolamine oleate mixed with contrast is used for BRTO in Asia, but this can cause clinically troublesome hemolysis. In our practice we have used a foam of 3% STS, iodized oil, and room air (10:1:1), injecting up to 40 mL. Higher concentrations of iodized oil can lead to balloon rupture as the oil dissolves some occlusion balloon membranes. Polidocanol (3%) foamed with iodinated contrast and air in a 1:2:1 ratio can also be used. Because of potential toxicity with the large volumes that would be required, dehydrated alcohol should not be used. The sclerosing agent is injected under fluoroscopic control until the gastric varices are completely filled or reflux is seen into a nontarget vein. The balloon remains inflated for at least 4 hours (some operators leave the balloon in overnight) to maximize exposure of the varices to the sclerosant. The remaining sclerosant is aspirated through the microcatheter and balloon catheter, and then

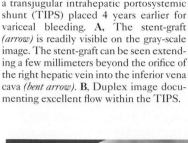

FIGURE **14-27**. Ultrasound follow-up of a transjugular intrahepatic portosystemic shunt (TIPS) placed 4 years earlier for variceal bleeding. **A,** The stent-graft *(arrow)* is readily visible on the gray-scale image. The stent-graft can be seen extending a few millimeters beyond the orifice of the right hepatic vein into the inferior vena cava *(bent arrow)*. **B,** Duplex image documenting excellent flow within the TIPS.

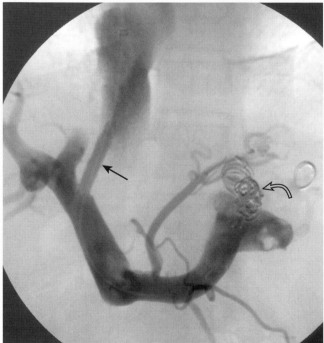

FIGURE **14-28**. Completion digital subtraction angiogram portogram following direct inferior vena cava–to–portal shunt (DIPS) with a stent-graft *(straight arrow)*. Large retroperitoneal varices arising from the splenic vein were occluded with coils *(curved arrow)*. (Courtesy Bryan Petersen, MD, Portland, Ore.)

contrast is gently injected. Thrombosis of the varices should be observed. No further treatment is needed and the balloon is deflated and removed.

Patients will experience upper abdominal discomfort related to the thrombosed gastric varices. This usually resolves over 2-3 weeks, but a vague discomfort may last for months. Upper endoscopy shortly after BRTO may not be able to distinguish between patent or thrombosed varices, but over time the varices should recede. CT is an excellent modality for following these patients noninvasively. Acute major complications occur in fewer than 5% and include thrombosis of the portal vein, pulmonary embolism from dislodged clot, and renal failure from extensive hemolysis. In experienced centers the success rate for controlling gastric variceal bleeding is more than 95% at 5 years. Predictably, other varices (usually esophageal) develop or progress in two thirds of patients since the underlying portal hypertension remains uncorrected. These can be managed medically and endoscopically, such that recurrent bleeding occurs in 10% of patients at 5 years.

The encephalopathy rate is low with BRTO, and liver function is usually not impacted.

▃ PARTIAL SPLENIC EMBOLIZATION

Splenomegaly with concomitant thrombocytopenia is common in portal hypertension. Partial splenic artery embolization to improve platelet counts can be performed as described in Chapter 11. The indications are primarily thrombocytopenia, although encephalopathy and liver function have been reported to improve post–partial splenic embolization, and risk of variceal bleeding decreases when combined with endoscopic ligation. Splenic embolization can also be used to treat patients with post–liver transplant splenic steal (see also Chapter 11).

▃ HEPATIC VEIN OBSTRUCTION/ BUDD-CHIARI SYNDROME

In the 19th century, Budd and Chiari separately described thrombotic occlusion of the major hepatic veins, defining a clinical syndrome that now bears their names. Since then, obstruction at a variety of levels has been included under the heading of Budd-Chiari syndrome (Box 14-9). Considered as a group, these disorders all have in common global obstruction of hepatic venous drainage. The incidence is between 0.2 and 0.8/1,000,000 per year. The syndrome has a variable presentation, ranging from minimal symptoms to fulminant liver failure. There are no specific laboratory findings. Symptoms usually do not develop if at least one hepatic vein can drain to the right atrium without impediment. Hepatic venous outflow obstruction leads to hepatic congestion and sinusoidal hypertension. Clinical findings can include abdominal pain, hepatomegaly, and ascites (Box 14-10). Hepatocellular injury can progress rapidly to necrosis, or more slowly, leading to cirrhosis. Patients with acute thrombotic occlusions are usually hypercoagulable (>80% have at least one risk factor, and 50% have two or more), either from an underlying coagulation disorder, pregnancy, oral contraceptive use, or a malignancy (Box 14-11).

The characteristic cross-sectional imaging findings of Budd-Chiari syndrome include massive ascites, hepatomegaly, splenomegaly, slitlike or obliterated hepatic veins, intrahepatic hepatic vein to hepatic vein collaterals, and hepatic venous or IVC webs. Patients with chronic Budd-Chiari syndrome may have hypertrophy of the caudate and atrophy of the right lobes of the liver, and gastroesophageal varices. On ultrasound, hepatic venous flow may be absent or dampened, with loss of transmitted atrial waves. Patchy, fan-shaped enhancement of the liver parenchyma ("nutmeg liver") with sparing of the caudate lobe is typical on contrast-enhanced CT or MRI (Fig. 14-30).

Venography for Budd-Chiari syndrome should include both cavography and selective hepatic venography. A pigtail catheter should be positioned below the infrahepatic IVC with injection

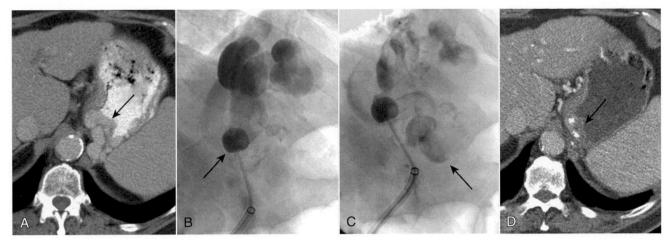

FIGURE 14-29. Balloon retrograde transrenal obliteration (BRTO) of gastric varices. **A,** Portal phase computed tomography (CT) image showing large gastric varices *(arrow).* **B,** Digital image obtained after inflation of an occlusion balloon *(arrow)* in the inferior phrenic vein proximal to the left adrenal vein and retrograde injection of sclerosant opacified with contrast through a microcatheter several centimeters above the balloon. **C,** Digital image obtained about 30 minutes later shows penetration of the sclerosant deep into the left gastric varices almost to the splenic vein. Thrombus is forming in the veins *(arrow).* The balloon was deflated after 4 hours. **D,** CT image obtained several months later shows collapse of the gastric varices with retained contrast material *(arrow).*

Box 14-9. Budd-Chiari Syndrome: Levels of Hepatic Vein Obstruction

Hepatic venules
Main hepatic veins
Hepatic vein orifices
Suprahepatic inferior vena cava

Box 14-10. Symptoms of Acute Budd-Chiari Syndrome

COMMON
Massive ascites
Hepatomegaly
Splenomegaly
Abdominal pain
Jaundice
Vomiting

LESS COMMON
Variceal bleeding
Lower extremity edema

Box 14-11. Risk Factors for Budd-Chiari Syndrome

Hypercoagulable syndromes
Oral contraceptives
Polycythemia
Connective tissue diseases
Paroxysmal nocturnal hemoglobinuria
Myelofibrosis
Pregnancy
Chemotherapy
Therapeutic irradiation
Liver transplantation (suprahepatic IVC)

---

of 20-25 mL of contrast for a total volume of 40-50 mL. The intrahepatic IVC is frequently narrowed due to compression by the swollen liver parenchyma. Hepatic venous inflow may be absent when the level of obstruction is at the hepatic veins (Fig. 14-31). Obstructing webs may be identified in the suprahepatic IVC

(Fig. 14-32). The classic venographic appearance of the hepatic veins in Budd-Chiari syndrome due to small vessel thrombosis is a spiderweb-like network of small, unnamed collateral and recanalized veins draining directly into the IVC (see Fig. 14-30). Stenoses and webs in the hepatic veins may also be found.

The standard management for patients with acute Budd-Chiari syndrome is anticoagulation and identification of prothrombotic risk factors. When a focal IVC or major hepatic venous stenosis can be identified, treatment with angioplasty or stents should be performed (see Figs. 14-31 and 14-32). Pressure gradients should be measured across hepatic veins or IVC webs (normal ≤ 2 mm Hg) to determine whether intervention is necessary. Acute thrombotic occlusions of the main hepatic veins and IVC can be treated with percutaneous mechanical thrombectomy or catheter-directed thrombolysis. Anticoagulation and correction of underlying stenotic lesions are important to ensure long-term success.

TIPS is indicated when there is diffuse venous obliteration and uncontrollable ascites or progressive cirrhosis despite anticoagulation. Occlusion of the hepatic veins makes the procedure more complex in that it can be hard to find a starting point for the puncture. The wedged hepatic venogram, if it can be performed, usually does not show the portal vein because the level of obstruction is postsinusoidal. IVUS guidance can be very helpful in these patients. In comparison to patients with alcoholic or viral cirrhosis, the liver in Budd-Chiari syndrome is often enlarged, which requires longer needle passes and often multiple stent-grafts. Careful review of CT scans before the procedure, IVUS guidance, arterial portography, or even a small platinum-tipped guidewire in the hepatic artery can help localize the portal vein during the procedure. Mesocaval shunt or liver transplantation may ultimately be necessary.

The long-term survival of patients with Budd-Chiari managed aggressively is excellent, with more than 90% alive at 5 years. These patients are at increased risk of developing hepatocellular carcinoma.

PREHEPATIC PORTAL VENOUS THROMBOSIS/OCCLUSION

Thrombotic occlusions within the extrahepatic portal system occur in patients with advanced cirrhosis or with normal livers and prothrombotic risk factors. The clinical presentation and management are different for these two groups, with cirrhotic patients usually more symptomatic from their liver disease, and patients without cirrhosis symptomatic from the acute venous occlusion. Thrombosis

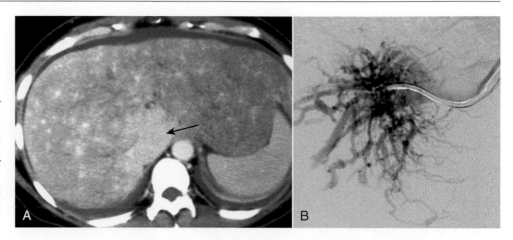

FIGURE 14-30. Classic appearance of Budd-Chiari syndrome due to thrombosis of the hepatic veins and venules. **A,** Contrast-enhanced computed tomography scan showing patchy enhancement of the liver parenchyma with the exception of a hypertrophied caudate lobe *(arrow).* **B,** Digital left hepatic venogram showing the classic "spiderweb" pattern. The recanalized and collateral branches of the hepatic vein have a deranged appearance.

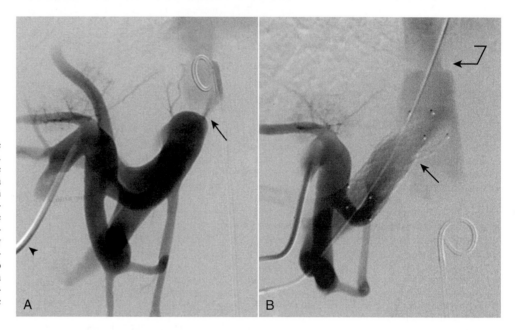

FIGURE 14-31. Budd-Chiari syndrome due to hepatic vein stenosis and IVC web. **A,** Focal severe stenosis at the orifice *(arrow)* of the middle hepatic vein with a 15-mm Hg gradient. The hepatic vein could only be accessed from a transhepatic approach *(arrowhead).* This was the only visible hepatic vein on cross-sectional imaging. **B,** Following angioplasty and stent placement *(arrow)* from a jugular approach, the gradient was reduced to 2 mm Hg. The web in the inferior vena cava *(bent arrow)* was treated with angioplasty alone. The patient had dramatic improvement of liver function.

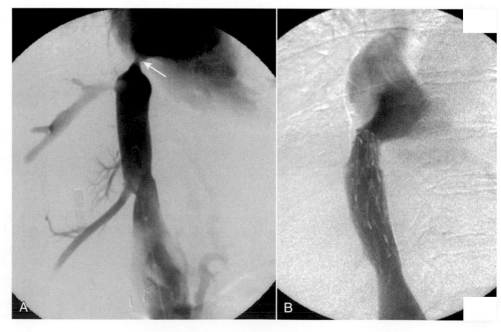

FIGURE 14-32. Budd-Chiari syndrome due to suprahepatic inferior vena cava (IVC) stenosis in a patient with a liver transplant. **A,** Digital subtraction angiogram (DSA) cavogram shows severe anastomotic stenosis *(arrow)* in the suprahepatic IVC and reflux into hepatic veins. The gradient was 12 mm Hg across the stenosis. **B,** DSA cavogram after angioplasty and stent placement using 20-mm diameter Z-stents. (Courtesy Cook Group, Bloomington, Ind.) As is often the case, angioplasty alone was not able to reduce the gradient, but after stent placement the gradient was eliminated. Note that the hepatic vein reflux has disappeared.

can occur in the portal, splenic, and mesenteric veins—or any combination of the three. The more veins involved, the more symptomatic the patient. Isolated portal vein or splenic vein thrombosis can be clinically silent until bleeding develops from varices.

Portal Vein Thrombosis

Portal vein thrombosis occurs in patients with uncompensated cirrhosis, malignancy, and hypercoagulable disorders. Cirrhotic patients should be carefully evaluated for hepatic malignancy. Portal vein thrombosis following liver transplant may be due to an underlying anastomotic stenosis. Patients with cirrhosis are frequently asymptomatic, with the diagnosis made on imaging

for other reasons, whereas patients without cirrhosis are usually symptomatic.

Isolated acute portal vein thrombosis in noncirrhotic patients presents with acute onset of upper abdominal pain with nonacute abdominal physical examination, fever, ascites, and abnormal liver enzymes. Evaluation with ultrasound or CT is definitive, and should include determination of the extent of the thrombosis, the presence of ascites, and a search for a responsible malignancy.

Anticoagulation is the standard therapy for benign acute portal vein thrombus in noncirrhotic patients. Approximately 40% of patients will resolve their portal vein thrombus. Severely symptomatic patients (ascites, abdominal pain, hepatic dysfunction) with acute thrombosis of the portal vein may benefit from endovascular recanalization of the portal vein using catheter-directed thrombolysis, mechanical thrombectomy, and/or stent placement. This can be performed from transhepatic and transjugular approaches, the latter combined with TIPS creation to provide outflow (Fig. 14-33).

Chronic portal vein thrombosis typically leads to an extensive system of dilated collateral channels in the gastrohepatic ligament and porta hepatis. This has been termed "cavernous transformation of the portal vein" and represents dilated paracholedochal and epicholedochal veins in the gastrohepatic ligament (see Fig. 14-7). These can become large enough to cause symptomatic extrahepatic biliary obstruction (portal biliopathy) in 4% of patients. When cirrhosis is present, the formation of portal-to-systemic collaterals, notably gastroesophageal varices, can subsequently bleed. Chronic portal vein thrombosis with cavernous transformation does not respond to thrombolysis. Recanalization from either a transhepatic, transjugular, or transsplenic approach can be performed (Fig. 14-34). Once the portal vein has been stented, a TIPS should be created to maintain patency.

Splenic Vein Thrombosis

Isolated thrombosis of the splenic vein occurs due to the same risk factors as portal vein thrombosis, although pancreatitis and pancreatic neoplasm are important additional etiologies. The initial management should be anticoagulation, which results in recanalization of the vein in approximately 80% of patients. Percutaneous catheter-based treatment is not common for acute splenic vein occlusion because the spleen has well-established collateral drainage.

With chronic occlusion, the short gastric veins become the major venous drainage of the spleen (see Fig. 14-6). Subsequently, acute upper gastrointestinal tract bleeding can occur

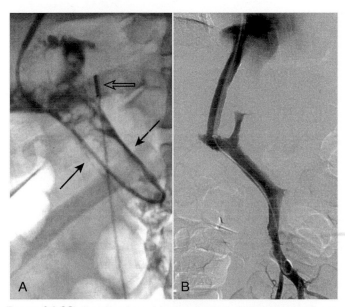

FIGURE 14-33. Portal and mesenteric vein thrombosis treated with transjugular intrahepatic portosystemic shunt (TIPS) and thrombolysis in a 41-year-old man with a hypercoagulable syndrome. **A,** Image during the TIPS after access to the portal vein using intravenous ultrasound guidance *(open arrow)* showing extensive thrombosis *(arrows)*. **B,** Final portal venogram after placement of the TIPS, pharmacomechanical thrombolysis, and thrombolytic infusion into the superior mesenteric vein and splenic vein for 2 days shows restored patency.

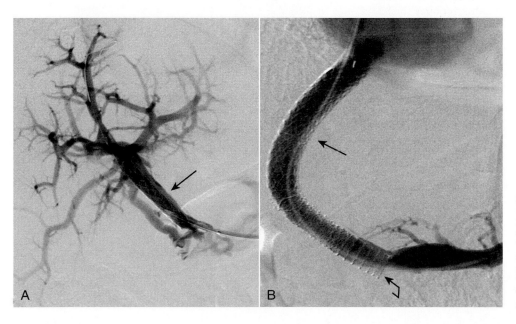

FIGURE 14-34. Recanalization of chronic portal vein occlusion (same patient as in Fig. 14-7). **A,** Portal venogram after placement of a stent in the portal vein *(arrow)* from a transsplenic approach. **B,** Portal venogram after completion of the transjugular intrahepatic portosystemic shunt *(arrow)*. The incomplete opacification of the bare stent in the portal vein is due to unopacified inflow from the superior mesenteric vein *(bent arrow)*.

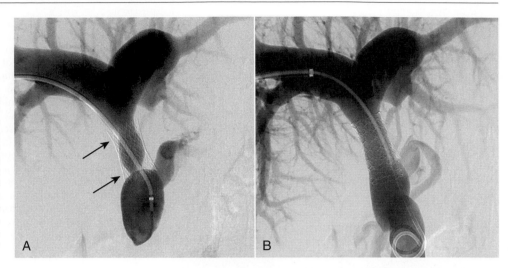

FIGURE 14-35. Portal vein anastomotic stenosis after liver transplant treated 7 years ago with a stent. The patient now has elevated velocities across the stent seen by duplex ultrasound. **A,** Transhepatic portogram showing tandem stenoses *(arrows)* within the stent. The pressure gradient was 14 mm Hg between the superior mesenteric vein and the intrahepatic portal vein. **B,** Portogram after placement of a second stent within the first. The gradient was reduced to 3 mm Hg, and the velocities normalized on follow-up duplex ultrasound.

from the resulting gastric varices. This is of particular importance because the clinical scenario may mimic variceal hemorrhage in cirrhotic patients. However, splenic vein thrombosis rarely results in esophageal varices unless cirrhosis is also present. Patients bleeding from isolated gastric varices must be evaluated for splenic vein occlusion before TIPS creation is contemplated, because TIPS does not provide benefit to these patients. Creation of a TIPS with the intent to recanalize the splenic vein should be considered, especially in patients with concomitant cirrhosis. Surgical splenectomy, splenic artery embolization, and BRTO are also potential treatments options.

Mesenteric Venous Thrombosis

SMV thrombosis is the most feared manifestation of extrahepatic portal vein thrombosis. This can lead to severe congestion in the affected segments of bowel, resulting in mesenteric ischemia. The mortality rate can be as high as 50%. In stable patients without peritoneal signs, anticoagulation is the first line of therapy with almost three fourths of patients achieving at least partial clearing of the thrombus. When patients have ongoing pain, bowel wall thickening, or other signs suggestive of progressive venous congestion, catheter-directed thrombolysis using direct transhepatic access successfully restores patency. In severe cases, the addition of indirect infusions through the SMA may promote clearing of thrombus in peripheral mesenteric veins. Intestinal infarction, as suggested by the development of peritonitis, requires surgical intervention. Chronic occlusion of the SMV may result in formation of mesenteric varices and intestinal bleeding. Short segment stenoses and occlusions may be amenable to stent placement, usually from a transjugular approach. Extensive occlusions (involving the main SMV and peripheral branches) may only be treatable with bowel resection or transplant.

POSTTRANSPLANT PORTAL VEIN STENOSIS

Portal vein complications occur in approximately 2% of patients undergoing liver transplantation. The donor portal vein is usually anastomosed to the recipient vein in an end-to-end fashion. Acute complications include portal vein thrombosis, kinks, and anastomotic strictures. Acute occlusion is frequently catastrophic with respect to viability of the transplant and requires urgent surgical revision. Intimal hyperplasia related to the anastomosis can result in late portal vein stenosis, which presents as presinusoidal extrahepatic portal hypertension. Ultrasound, CT/CTA, and MRI/MRV are excellent modalities for visualizing the portal vein anastomoses. In general, a 50% reduction in diameter of the anastomosis or an increase in flow velocity of greater than 3.5:1 compared to the portal vein proximal to the anastomosis is of concern.

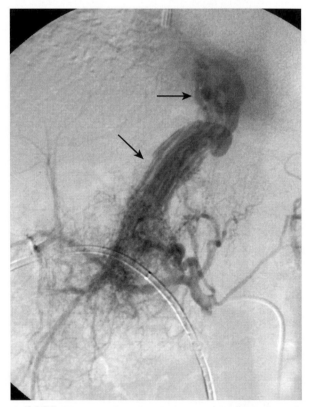

FIGURE 14-36. Hepatoma invading the hepatic vein. Early image from a selective hepatic artery digital subtraction angiogram shows a hypervascular mass invading the middle hepatic vein and extending into the inferior vena cava *(arrows)* with associated arteriovenous shunting. Note the typical "threads and streaks" in the tumor representing tumor neovascularity.

Direct transhepatic access to the portal vein allows measurement of gradients across the area of stenosis and treatment with stent placement (Fig. 14-35). Embolization of the parenchymal tract in the liver with Gelfoam and/or coils at the time of sheath removal prevents bleeding complications

NEOPLASM

Primary neoplasms of the portal and hepatic veins are extremely rare. Conversely, these veins are frequently involved by gastrointestinal tract malignancy.

Hepatoma has a characteristic propensity to invade the portal and hepatic veins and propagate within the lumen (Fig. 14-36).

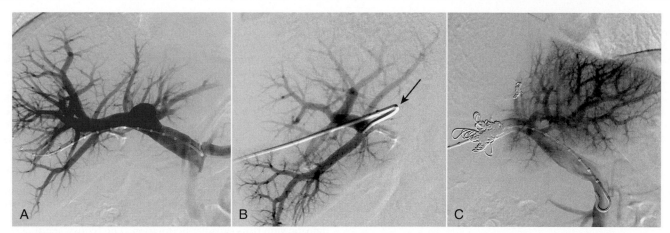

FIGURE 14-37. Transhepatic portal vein embolization prior to right hepatectomy for metastatic colon cancer. **A,** Portal venogram from the right transhepatic approach. **B,** Intraprocedural portal venogram showing how a recurved catheter *(arrow)* is used to select the ipsilateral portal vein branches. **C,** Late image from the completion portal venogram shows absence of perfusion of the right lobe. Embolization was performed with 100-micron particles followed by coils, all through the recurved catheter. The liver tract was then embolized with gelatin sponge and 3 mm coils.

Care should be taken to exclude the presence of hepatoma in cirrhotic patients presenting with portal vein thrombosis. Enhancement of intravascular "thrombus" on CT or MRI is diagnostic of tumor. Hepatic arteriography or percutaneous image-guided biopsy may be needed to make the distinction between bland thrombus and tumor thrombus in problem cases. Arterioportal shunting due to tumor can result in variceal bleeding (see Fig. 1-27B). Embolization of the tumor with permanent particles, rather than TIPS, is the initial treatment.

Carcinoid tumor is a member of the neuroendocrine group of tumors and occurs most frequently in the right lower quadrant, either in the appendix or the terminal ileum. A localized fibrotic reaction in the adjacent mesentery often occurs with carcinoid tumors and can obstruct the mesenteric veins (see Fig. 11-28).

Pancreatic adenocarcinoma characteristically obstructs the portal system by compression or malignant invasion of adjacent portions of the SMV, splenic vein, or portal vein (see Fig. 1-27C). Cholangiocarcinoma (Klatskin tumor) encases the portal vein producing stenoses in the intrahepatic portions of the portal vein. Neoplastic enlargement of lymph nodes in the gastrohepatic ligament and porta hepatis can also lead to obstruction of the main portal vein.

PORTAL VEIN EMBOLIZATION

Transhepatic embolization of portal vein segments to induce hypertrophy of the future liver remnant (FLR) before partial liver resections for localized primary or metastatic tumor improves surgical outcomes. Occlusion of peripheral intrahepatic portal vein branches triggers hepatocyte regeneration in nonembolized liver segments. This is due to multiple hepatotropic substances that increase in portal flow after embolization. Healthy liver regenerates faster than cirrhotic liver (12-21 cm³ per day at 2 weeks compared to 9 cm³ per day). The morbidity and mortality (related to hepatic insufficiency) after partial hepatectomy are decreased in patients who have undergone portal vein embolization before resection.

Portal vein embolization is most often necessary before resection of more than 3 Couinaud segments—usually a right hepatectomy. The estimated minimal residual volume of liver required to tolerate extended partial hepatectomy depends on the health of the liver, with greater volumes necessary in patients with underlying parenchymal disease (40%) or prior chemotherapy (30%) compared to those with a normal liver (20%). The preoperative estimation of the FLR is therefore a critical step in determining eligibility for portal vein embolization. There are two basic approaches to calculation of liver volumes, both of which require measurements of the liver from CT. When there are a few liver tumors, the tumor volume can be subtracted from the overall volumes and the FLR calculated:

$$FLR = (\text{total liver volume} - \text{total tumor volume})$$
$$- (\text{resected volume} - \text{tumor resected volume})/$$
$$(\text{total liver volume} - \text{tumor volume})$$

Alternatively, the total estimated liver volume (TELV) is first calculated based upon body surface area (TELV = [1267.28 × body surface area] – 794.41). The FLR is then measured from CT, and the FLR/TELV ratio calculated. This method, which is often referred to as the *standardized estimate*, accommodates for the different liver volumes required by different sized patients.

Severe portal hypertension, uncontrollable intrahepatic portal to hepatic vein shunts, occlusion of the portal vein by tumor, and occlusion of the portal vein in the FLR are contraindications to the procedure. When performed for hepatocellular carcinoma, some authors advocate chemoembolization of the tumor 2 weeks before portal vein embolization to maximize hypertrophy of the FLR.

The procedure is performed after careful review of CT and MRI for venous anatomy and tumor location. Antibiotic prophylaxis is recommended. Transhepatic percutaneous access through one of the segments that will ultimately be removed reduces the risk of damage to the portion of liver that will be preserved. Ultrasound guidance allows access of a peripheral portal vein segment, followed by placement of a 5-French sheath with a radiopaque marker band. A portal venogram and pressures are obtained (Fig. 14-37). The portal vein segments are then selectively catheterized. Recurved catheters are useful to select portal vein branches that are on the same side as the access. The entire portion of liver to be removed should be embolized, because hypertrophy of segments of the liver intended for resection has no clinical benefit and may decrease the amount of hypertrophy in the planned liver remnant. The lateral branches of segment 4 should be embolized when the planned resection will include this portion of the liver. Microcatheters may be necessary for precise selection. Many embolic agents have been used, including small particles, glue, gelatin sponges, alcohol, and coils. The goal is peripheral occlusion, so when particles are used, the size should be 100-200 μ, followed by coils in the larger segmental arteries. The capacity of the portal venous bed is enormous, so large quantities of particles may be needed. At the end of the procedure, coils are placed in the portal branch, through which access was obtained (if ipsilateral to the embolization), and coils or gelatin sponges are used to occlude the parenchymal tract.

Pain is uncommon after the procedure, but many patients have postembolization syndrome, including malaise and low-grade fever. The overall complication rate is about 2%-9%, including portal vein thrombosis, hemoperitoneum, subcapsular hematoma, pseudoaneurysm, and hemobilia. Many of the complications are related to the transhepatic access, prompting some interventionalists to prefer the ipsilateral transhepatic puncture.

The average volume increase achieved with extensive right lobe embolization depends on the presence or absence of preexisting liver disease and whether or not segment 4 embolization is included. In general, the FLR hypertrophy occurs over 3-4 weeks and peaks by 6 weeks. Using the standardized estimate, the increase in FLR volume ranges from 28% to 46% at 4 weeks' postembolization. The addition of embolization of segment 4 increases the hypertrophy of segments 2 and 3, but the overall FLR is smaller.

◼ TRANSJUGULAR LIVER BIOPSY

Transjugular liver biopsy is usually performed in patients with suspected diffuse parenchymal disease, such as cirrhosis, and when coagulopathy or ascites prevents safe performance of a percutaneous liver biopsy (Box 14-12). This procedure may also be performed in absence of coagulopathy or ascites when wedged hepatic vein pressures are needed in addition to a biopsy for initial workup of cirrhosis. A platelet count less than 50,000 or an INR above 1.5 are considered contraindications to percutaneous liver biopsy. The amount of ascites sufficient to exclude the percutaneous route is less well defined, but any volume of ascites that displaces the liver from the abdominal wall is of concern. The rationale for the transjugular technique is simple; jugular venous access can be safely obtained in the presence of coagulopathy, particularly with ultrasound guidance, and the biopsy needle never transgresses the liver capsule, thus eliminating the risk of intraperitoneal bleeding. Biopsy of discrete liver masses is difficult with this technique, unless they are large and immediately adjacent to a hepatic vein.

Box 14-12. Indications for Transjugular Liver Biopsy

Suspected hepatocellular disease with at least one of the following:
- Coagulopathy
- Ascites
- Wedged portal pressure also required

Transjugular liver biopsy uses a system very similar to the Rösch-Uchida TIPS set but smaller in caliber. The biopsy needle is a modified version of the same core biopsy devices routinely used for percutaneous organ biopsy (see Fig. 4-55A). Jugular and right hepatic vein access is obtained as for TIPS. A hepatic venogram is performed to confirm the identity and patency of the vein. The assembled rigid guiding cannula system and introducer sheath is inserted over a guidewire into the right hepatic vein. The cannula can be modified with gentle curves when there is angulation of the hepatic vein at the orifice. Alternatively, access from the left internal jugular vein often allows easy and secure cannulation of the right hepatic vein (Fig. 14-38). Biopsy from the middle or left hepatic vein can also be performed, with the needle rotated as described in Table 14-7. The optimal location from which to perform the biopsy from the hepatic vein is within 3-4 cm of the IVC. Biopsy from more peripheral locations in the hepatic vein risks capsular perforation. The biopsy needle is then introduced through the guiding cannula. The tip of the cannula is rotated such that the needle will be directed in an anterior and caudal direction. The biopsy needle is then advanced a few millimeters into the hepatic parenchyma and the spring-loaded mechanism is fired, deploying the cutting needle and obtaining the biopsy. The biopsy needle is then removed and the sample inspected. An assistant should carefully hold the guiding cannula in the hepatic vein while the sample is retrieved from the biopsy device because respiratory motion tends to displace the system from the hepatic vein. Additional samples can be obtained as required. After the procedure, frequent vital signs should be obtained for 4 hours.

Patients with whole liver transplants can present anatomic challenges for transjugular liver biopsy due to altered relationships of the hepatic veins to the IVC. There are three basic techniques for attaching orthotopic livers to the recipient systemic veins (Fig. 14-39). The most difficult anastomoses are the piggy back transplants, in which a window is created between the donor and recipient IVCs as they lie side-to-side. The donor hepatic veins may be very difficult or impossible to cannulate with the biopsy device from the jugular approach. In these patients, transcaval biopsy from either the jugular or femoral approach can be used.

Transjugular liver biopsy with a cutting needle is successful in obtaining hepatic tissue in at least 98% of cases and, in contrast to older transvenous techniques, yields samples of high diagnostic quality. Previous methods using a coring needle and suction, or grasping forceps, often produced crushed and/or fragmented specimens.

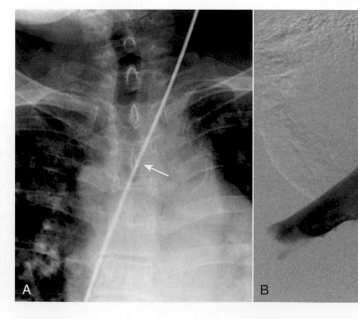

FIGURE 14-38. Transjugular liver biopsy from the left internal jugular vein in a patient with an orthotopic liver transplant. The right hepatic vein could not be securely engaged from a right jugular vein access. **A,** Spot image of the chest showing the course of the metal cannula *(arrow)* across the mediastinum. This was advanced into position over a stiff guidewire to prevent injury to the SVC or heart. **B,** Contrast injection through the biopsy cannula confirming the location in the hepatic vein.

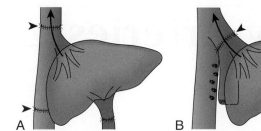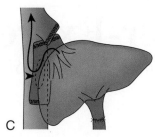

FIGURE 14-39. Whole-liver transplant hepatic venous anatomy that can impact transjugular liver biopsy. The *curved arrows* indicate hepatic venous flow. **A,** End-to-end inferior vena cava (IVC) anastomoses *(arrowheads)* preserve normal anatomic relationships. **B,** The donor IVC at the hepatic veins is anastomosed to the origins of the recipient hepatic veins *(arrowhead)*. Although overall anatomic relationships are similar to the pretransplant state, the donor IVC now forms a blind pouch. **C,** The "piggy-back" anastomosis. The recipient hepatic vein origins have been ligated, and the donor IVC anastomosed side-to-side *(arrowhead)* to the recipient IVC. This can be the most difficult anatomy when performing transjugular liver biopsy.

Capsular perforation is rare with this technique (2%-6%), but bleeding complications can be fatal. Inadvertent renal biopsy can occur either by hepatic capsular perforation or unrecognized catheterization of the right renal vein. Hemobilia with biliary obstruction is another rare potential complication that may indicate intrahepatic vascular injury. Patients who develop persistent abdominal pain following transjugular liver biopsy should be evaluated with an abdominal CT followed by angiography as necessary. A pseudoaneurysm, arteriovenous fistula, or extravasation may be evident and can be embolized selectively with coils.

▬ SUGGESTED READINGS

Akahoshi T, Hashizume M, Tomikawa M, et al. Long-term results of balloon-occluded retrograde transvenous obliteration for gastric variceal bleeding and risky gastric varices: a 10-year experience. *J Gastroenterol Hepatol.* 2008;23:1702-1709.

Albillos A, Bañares R, González M, et al. Value of the hepatic venous pressure gradient to monitor drug therapy for portal hypertension: a meta-analysis. *Am J Gastroenterol.* 2007;102:1116-1126.

Beckett D, Olliff S. Interventional radiology in the management of Budd-Chiari syndrome. *Cardiovasc Intervent Radiol.* 2008;31:839-847.

Bhogal HK, Sanyal AJ. Using transjugular intrahepatic portosystemic shunts for complications of cirrhosis. *Clin Gastroenterol Hepatol.* 2011;9:936-946.

Bittencourt PL, Couto CA, Ribeiro DD. Portal vein thrombosis and Budd-Chiari syndrome. *Hematol Oncol Clin North Am.* 2011;25:1049-1066.

Boyer TD, Haskal ZJ, American Association for the Study of Liver Diseases. The role of transjugular intrahepatic portosystemic shunt in the management of portal hypertension. *Hepatology.* 2005;41:386-400.

Boyer TD, Haskal ZJ, American Association for the Study of Liver Diseases. The role of transjugular intrahepatic portosystemic shunt (TIPS) in the management of portal hypertension: update 2009. *Hepatology.* 2010;51:306.

Carr CE, Tuite CM, Soulen MC, et al. Role of ultrasound surveillance of transjugular intrahepatic portosystemic shunts in the covered stent era. *J Vasc Interv Radiol.* 2006;17:1297-1305.

Clark TW. Stepwise placement of a transjugular intrahepatic portosystemic shunt endograft. *Tech Vasc Interv Radiol.* 2008;11:208-211.

de Baere T, Denys A, Madoff DC. Preoperative portal vein embolization: indications and technical considerations. *Tech Vasc Interv Radiol.* 2007;10:67-78.

Fanelli F, Bezzi M, Bruni A, et al. Multidetector-row computed tomography in the evaluation of transjugular intrahepatic portosystemic shunt performed with expanded-polytetrafluoroethylene-covered stent-graft. *Cardiovasc Intervent Radiol.* 2011;34:100-105.

Farsad K, Fuss C, Kolbeck KJ, et al. Transjugular intrahepatic portosystemic shunt creation using intravascular ultrasound guidance. *J Vasc Interv Radiol.* 2012;23:1594-1602.

Gaba RC, Khiatani VL, Knuttinen MG, et al. Comprehensive review of TIPS technical complications and how to avoid them. *AJR Am J Roentgenol.* 2011;196:675-685.

García-Pagán JC, Caca K, Bureau C, et al. Early use of TIPS in patients with cirrhosis and variceal bleeding. *N Engl J Med.* 2010;362:2370-2379.

Garcia-Tsao G, Bosch J. Management of varices and variceal hemorrhage in cirrhosis. *N Engl J Med.* 2010;362:823-832.

Giusca S, Jinga M, Jurcut C, et al. Portopulmonary hypertension: from diagnosis to treatment. *Eur J Intern Med.* 2011;22:441-447.

Glatard AS, Hillaire S, d'Assignies G, et al. Obliterative Portal Venopathy: Findings at CT Imaging. *Radiology.* 2012;263:741-750.

Haskal ZJ, Martin L, Cardella JF, et al. Quality improvement guidelines for transjugular intrahepatic portosystemic shunts. SCVIR Standards of Practice Committee. *J Vasc Interv Radiol.* 2001;12:131-136.

Hong R, Dhanani RS, Louie JD, Sze DY. Intravascular ultrasound-guided mesocaval shunt creation in patients with portal or mesenteric venous occlusion. *J Vasc Interv Radiol.* 2012;23:136-141.

Huang TL, Cheng YF, Chen TY, et al. Doppler ultrasound evaluation of postoperative portal vein stenosis in adult living donor liver transplantation. *Transplant Proc.* 2010;42:879-881.

Khan S, Tudur Smith C, Williamson P, Sutton R. Portosystemic shunts versus endoscopic therapy for variceal rebleeding in patients with cirrhosis. *Cochrane Database Syst Rev.* 2006:CD000553.

Kim HS, Patra A, Khan J, et al. Transhepatic catheter-directed thrombectomy and thrombolysis of acute superior mesenteric venous thrombosis. *J Vasc Interv Radiol.* 2005;16:1685-1691.

Kiyosue H, Mori H, Matsumoto S, et al. Transcatheter obliteration of gastric varices. Part 1. Anatomic classification. *Radiographics.* 2003;23:911-920.

Kiyosue H, Mori H, Matsumoto S, et al. Transcatheter obliteration of gastric varices: Part 2. Strategy and techniques based on hemodynamic features. *Radiographics.* 2003;23:921-937.

Koconis KG, Singh H, Soares G. Partial splenic embolization in the treatment of patients with portal hypertension: a review of the English language literature. *J Vasc Interv Radiol.* 2007;18:463-481.

Merkel C, Montagnese S. Hepatic venous pressure gradient measurement in clinical hepatology. *Dig Liver Dis.* 2011;43:762-767.

Olliff SP. Transjugular intrahepatic portosystemic shunt in the management of Budd-Chiari syndrome. *Eur J Gastroenterol Hepatol.* 2006;18:1151-1154.

Opio CK, Garcia-Tsao G. Managing varices: drugs, bands, and shunts. *Gastroenterol Clin North Am.* 2011;40:561-579.

Park H, Yoon JY, Park KH, et al. Hepatocellular carcinoma in Budd-Chiari syndrome: a single center experience with long-term follow-up in South Korea. *World J Gastroenterol.* 2012;18:1946-1952.

Petersen BD, Clark TW. Direct intrahepatic portocaval shunt. *Tech Vasc Interv Radiol.* 2008;11:230-234.

Plessier A, Rautou PE, Valla DC. Management of hepatic vascular diseases. *J Hepatol.* 2012;56(Suppl 1):S25-S38.

Saab S, Nieto JM, Lewis SK, Runyon BA. TIPS versus paracentesis for cirrhotic patients with refractory ascites. *Cochrane Database Syst Rev.* 2006:CD004889.

Saugel B, Phillip V, Gaa J, et al. Advanced hemodynamic monitoring before and after transjugular intrahepatic portosystemic shunt: implications for selection of patients–a prospective study. *Radiology.* 2012;262:343-352.

Tesdal IK, Filser T, Weiss C, et al. Transjugular intrahepatic portosystemic shunts: adjunctive embolotherapy of gastroesophageal collateral vessels in the prevention of variceal rebleeding. *Radiology.* 2005;236:360-367.

Testino G, Ferro C. Hepatorenal syndrome: a review. *Hepatogastroenterology.* 2010;57:1279-1284.

Thakrar PD, Madoff DC. Preoperative portal vein embolization: an approach to improve the safety of major hepatic resection. *Semin Roentgenol.* 2011;46:142-153.

Uflacker R, Reichert P, D'Albuquerque LC, et al. Liver anatomy applied to the placement of transjugular intrahepatic portosystemic shunts. *Radiology.* 1994;191:705-712.

Uflacker R. Applications of percutaneous mechanical thrombectomy in transjugular intrahepatic portosystemic shunt and portal vein thrombosis. *Tech Vasc Interv Radiol.* 2003;6:59-69.

Walser EM, Soloway R, Raza SA, Gill A. Transjugular portosystemic shunt in chronic portal vein occlusion: importance of segmental portal hypertension in cavernous transformation of the portal vein. *J Vasc Interv Radiol.* 2006;17:373-378.

Walser EM, Runyan BR, Heckman MG, et al. Extrahepatic portal biliopathy: proposed etiology on the basis of anatomic and clinical features. *Radiology.* 2011;258:146-153.

Woodrum DA, Bjarnason H, Andrews JC. Portal vein venoplasty and stent placement in the nontransplant population. *J Vasc Interv Radiol.* 2009;20:593-599.

Zimmerman MA, Cameron AM, Ghobrial RM. Budd-Chiari syndrome. *Clin Liver Dis.* 2006;10:259-273.

CHAPTER 15

Lower-Extremity Arteries

John A. Kaufman, MD, MS, FSIR, FCIRSE

The lower-extremity arteries are a common site for vascular diseases. The legs have a relatively large muscle mass and a prominent role in basic daily activities. Lesions in this vascular bed produce troublesome symptoms at an early stage. Advanced disease frequently results in limb loss, although often the underlying systemic disease has the greatest impact on mortality. Interventions in the lower extremities are increasing in frequency as techniques and devices improve.

ANATOMY

The blood supply to the lower extremities can be roughly divided into runoff vessels (inline flow to the foot) and musculoskeletal branches that terminate in the structures of the limb. In most instances, the status of the runoff vessels is the primary clinical concern. However, in the presence of occlusion of the runoff vessels, the musculoskeletal branches become the principal source of collateral blood supply.

The common femoral artery (CFA) is the continuation of the external iliac artery. This vessel is usually 6-9 mm in diameter and 5-7 cm in length, with frequent and variable small, unnamed muscular branches. The CFA extends from the inguinal ligament to the origins of the superficial femoral artery (SFA) and profunda femoris artery (PFA) just distal to the inferior margin of the femoral head (Fig. 15-1). In 10% of individuals, the artery bifurcates while it is still anterior to the femoral head (termed *high bifurcation*) (Fig. 15-2). The CFA is contained within the femoral sheath, a continuation of the abdominal wall fascia. The sheath is funnel shaped, with the broad base opening toward the abdomen. In addition to containing the artery, the sheath also contains the femoral vein (medial to the artery) and the femoral canal (the most medial structure). The femoral canal contains lymphatic channels and often a lymph node. The femoral nerve lies lateral to the femoral sheath, within the femoral triangle formed by the sartorius muscle laterally, the adductor longus muscle medially, the inguinal ligament superiorly, and the iliacus, psoas major, pectineus, and adductor longus muscles posteriorly.

The origin of the PFA has a lateral and posterior orientation relative to the SFA (see Fig. 10-8). The PFA provides proximal branches to the hip (the lateral and medial femoral circumflex arteries) before descending deep in the thigh adjacent to the medial edge of the femur. There are multiple branches from the PFA to the muscles of the thigh before it terminates above the adductor canal. These muscular branches anastomose with muscular branches of the SFA and popliteal arteries. Variations in the branching pattern and origin of the PFA are present in 40% of individuals. The most common variants are independent origins of the medial (20%) or lateral (15%) circumflex femoral arteries from the CFA.

The SFA is remarkable for the almost complete lack of variability (rather boring for anatomists but appreciated by interventionalists) (Table 15-1). The origin of the SFA from the CFA is anterior and medial to the PFA. The SFA runs beneath the sartorius muscle in the thigh, anterior to the femoral vein (Fig. 15-3). The artery passes through the adductor canal in the distal thigh, where it becomes the popliteal artery. The SFA is usually 5-7 mm in diameter, with many muscular branches along its length. The last large medial branch is named the *descending* or *supreme genicular artery*. The muscular branches of the SFA become important collateral pathways in the setting of occlusive disease.

One of the few variants of SFA anatomy is a persistent sciatic artery (0.025%). This vessel is a normal fetal branch of the internal iliac artery that continues into the lower-extremity posterior to the femoral head to supply the runoff vessels (Fig. 15-4). This artery usually regresses as the external iliac artery becomes the arterial supply of the lower limb. When persistent, the sciatic artery may terminate in the posterior thigh, in which case the runoff is through the SFA, or continue to the popliteal artery with a discontinuous or absent SFA. Persistent sciatic arteries are bilateral in 25% of patients. The posterior course of the artery renders it subject to repetitive trauma, resulting in occlusive disease or aneurysm formation.

The popliteal artery is the continuation of the SFA from the adductor canal to the origins of the tibial vessels below the knee (see Fig. 15-1). In clinical practice the joint line of the knee divides the artery into above-knee and below-knee segments. Although these are not official anatomic terms, the popliteal artery should always be described in this manner because the type of intervention and subsequent outcome are influenced by the level of disease.

The average diameter of the popliteal artery is 4-5 mm. The blood supply of the knee joint is provided by the superior and inferior (medial and lateral), and middle genicular arteries. These arteries are recognizable by their horizontal course around the knee. The posterior calf muscles are supplied by the vertically oriented sural arteries arising from the posterior aspect of the popliteal artery. The most common anatomic variation of the popliteal artery is a high origin of one or more of the tibial arteries. Usually, the popliteal artery bifurcates into the anterior tibial

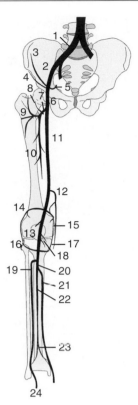

FIGURE 15-1. Drawing of lower-extremity arteries. *1*, Common iliac artery. *2*, External iliac artery. *3*, Deep iliac circumflex artery. *4*, Superficial circumflex iliac artery. *5*, Inferior epigastric artery. *6*, Common femoral artery. *7*, Profunda femoris artery (PFA). *8*, Medial femoral circumflex artery. *9*, Lateral femoral circumflex artery. *10*, Descending branch of PFA. *11*, Superficial femoral artery. *12*, Descending genicular artery. *13*, Popliteal artery. *14*, Lateral superior genicular artery. *15*, Medial superior genicular artery. *16*, Lateral inferior genicular artery. *17*, Medial inferior genicular artery. *18*, Sural arteries. *19*, Anterior tibial artery. *20*, Tibioperoneal trunk. *21*, Posterior tibial artery. *22*, Peroneal artery. *23*, Perforating branches to anterior and posterior tibial arteries. *24*, Dorsalis pedal artery.

TABLE 15-1 Anatomic Variants of the Lower-Extremity Arteries

Variant	Incidence (%)
Two or more PFA branches from CFA	2
Persistent sciatic artery	0.025
Duplication of SFA	<0.001
High origin of a tibial artery	5
Peroneal origin from the anterior tibial artery	1
True popliteal artery trifurcation (no tibioperoneal trunk)	2
Hypoplastic posterior tibial artery	3.8
Hypoplastic anterior tibial artery	1.6
Hypoplastic anterior and posterior tibial arteries	0.2

CFA, common femoral artery; PFA, profunda femoris artery; SFA, superficial femoral artery.

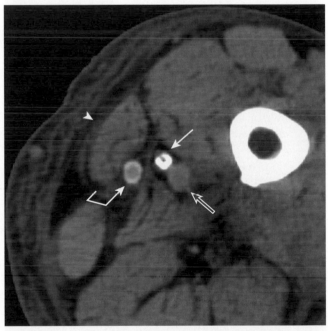

FIGURE 15-3. Axial computed tomography image of the thigh during the venous phase. The calcified and occluded superficial femoral artery *(white arrow)* lies beneath the sartorius muscle *(arrowhead)*, slightly anterior and medial to the femoral vein *(open arrow)*. The bent arrow indicates an ePTFE surgical bypass graft.

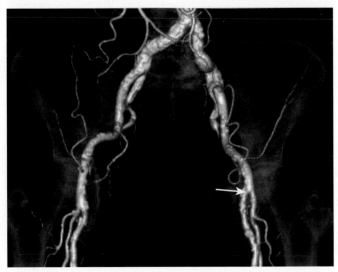

FIGURE 15-2. Computed tomography angiogram of the pelvis showing high bifurcation of the left common femoral artery *(arrow)* anterior to the femoral head. Compare to the common femoral artery bifurcation on the right relative to the femoral head.

artery and the tibioperoneal trunk at the distal edge of the popliteus muscle. In 5% of individuals, one of the tibial runoff vessels has an origin from the popliteal artery above this level (Fig. 15-5).

The runoff vessels in the calf consist of the anterior tibial, posterior tibial, and peroneal arteries. The anterior tibial artery arises from the popliteal artery just distal to the popliteus muscle. This artery passes anteriorly through the interosseous membrane and then descends to the foot medial to the fibula in the anterior fascial compartment of the calf (Fig. 15-6). In fewer than 1% of individuals, the peroneal artery originates from the anterior tibial artery. In most instances, the tibioperoneal trunk is a short artery of variable length that descends several centimeters beyond the anterior tibial artery origin before bifurcating into the posterior tibial and peroneal arteries. The posterior tibial artery courses deep to the soleus muscle to the medial

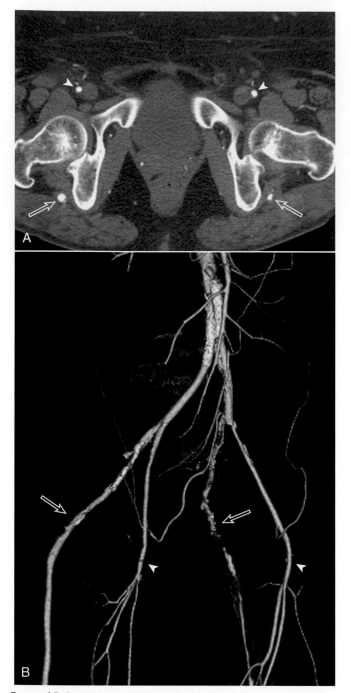

Figure 15-4. Bilateral persistent sciatic arteries. **A,** Axial image from a computed tomography angiogram showing small common femoral arteries *(arrowheads)* and bilateral persistent sciatic arteries posteriorly *(open arrows)*. **B,** Volume rendering of the same patient showing the persistent sciatic arteries *(open arrows)* originating from the internal iliac arteries *(arrowheads, common femoral arteries).* This patient has occlusive disease in the left persistent sciatic artery that was symptomatic with claudication.

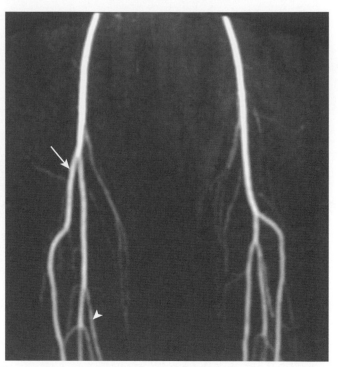

Figure 15-5. Coronal maximum intensity projection of a three-dimensional gadolinium-enhanced magnetic resonance angiogram at the level of the knees, showing high origin of the right anterior tibial artery *(arrow)* and low origin of the right posterior tibial artery *(arrowhead).* Compare with the normal left tibial artery origins.

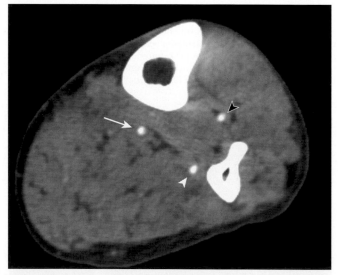

Figure 15-6. Axial computed tomography image during the arterial phase at the level of the calf. (*Black arrowhead,* anterior tibial artery; *white arrowhead,* peroneal artery; *white arrow,* posterior tibial artery.)

malleolus. The peroneal artery descends to the ankle posterior and medial to the fibula (see Fig. 15-6). At the ankle, the peroneal artery terminates in a characteristic fork created by the anterior and posterior perforating branches (see Fig. 15-1). The posterior tibial and peroneal arteries are contained within the deep posterior fascial compartment of the calf.

The anterior and posterior tibial arteries continue into the foot in 95% of individuals, while the peroneal artery terminates above the ankle in an equal percentage. In roughly 5% of individuals, one of the runoff vessels is absent. When either the anterior or

posterior tibial artery is congenitally absent in the calf, the peroneal artery may continue into the foot in its stead.

There is much variability of the arterial supply to the foot, similar to the hand. Rather than memorize minutiae, it is best to be familiar with the classic anatomy described and use it as a basis when interpreting imaging studies. The anterior and posterior tibial arteries provide the bulk of the arterial supply to the foot (Fig. 15-7). The anterior tibial artery continues into the foot below the level of the ankle joint as the dorsalis pedis artery. The medial and lateral tarsal arteries are large branches that arise from the proximal dorsalis pedis artery. At the level of the proximal

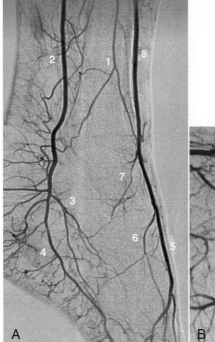

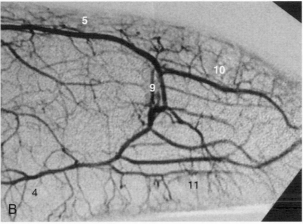

FIGURE 15-7. Pedal artery anatomy. **A,** Lateral digital subtraction angiogram (DSA) of the ankle and forefoot. *1,* Distal peroneal artery with anterior and posterior communicating branches. *2,* Posterior tibial artery. *3,* Medial plantar artery. *4,* Lateral plantar artery. *5,* Dorsalis pedis artery. *6,* Lateral tarsal artery. *7,* Medial tarsal artery. *8,* Anterior tibial artery. **B,** DSA of the forefoot. *4,* Lateral plantar artery. *5,* Dorsalis pedal artery. *9,* Arcuate artery. *10,* Dorsal metatarsal artery. *11,* Plantar metatarsal artery.

metatarsals, the dorsalis pedis bifurcates into a deep plantar branch and the arcuate artery. The arcuate artery curves toward the lateral edge of the foot along the dorsal aspect of the metatarsal bone bases, supplying the dorsal metatarsal arteries to the distal foot before anastomosing with distal branches of the plantar arteries. The posterior tibial artery passes posterior and inferior to the medial malleolus, and then bifurcates into the medial and lateral plantar arteries. The lateral plantar artery is usually the larger of the two, with a course diagonally across the plantar aspect of the foot. The lateral plantar artery forms a second, deep plantar arch that supplies the plantar metatarsal arteries. This arch anastomoses with the deep plantar branch of the dorsalis pedis artery between the first and second metatarsals. The medial plantar artery travels inferior to the first metatarsal bone to supply the great toe.

The blood supply of the foot can be considered in terms of three-dimensional anatomic units called *angiosomes*. These include skin as well as the underlying structures (Table 15-2). An understanding of angiosomes can help direct revascularization procedures when there is tissue loss in the foot.

KEY COLLATERAL PATHWAYS

The PFA is critically important in the collateral supply of lower-extremity arteries (Fig. 15-8). Occlusion of the CFA results in collateralization from the abdomen, pelvis, and the contralateral extremity to the PFA, which in turn reconstitutes the SFA (Box 15-1 and Fig. 15-9). These are the same collateral pathways that reconstitute the PFA when it is severely stenotic or occluded at its origin.

Proximal occlusion of the SFA results in hypertrophy of PFA branches, which in turn reconstitute the SFA via muscular branches in the thigh (Fig. 15-10). This can be an extremely effective collateral pathway, so much so that patients may have palpable distal pulses. When the distal SFA is occluded, the descending trunk of the PFA provides collateral flow to the popliteal artery through the lateral genicular arteries. Occlusion of the above-knee popliteal artery can be collateralized from both the distal SFA (via the descending genicular artery) and the PFA. In the presence of a below-knee popliteal artery occlusion, the sural and genicular arteries can reconstitute the tibial arteries.

TABLE 15-2 Angiosomes of the Foot

Artery	Arterial branches	Angiosome
PT	Medial calcaneal	Heel
	Medial plantar	Instep
	Lateral plantar	Lateral foot and forefoot
Peroneal	Anterior perforating	Lateral anterior upper ankle
	Lateral Calcaneal	Plantar heel
AT	Multiple branches	Anterior ankle
	Dorsalis pedis	Dorsum of the foot

AT, Anterior tibial artery; PT, posterior tibial artery.

Occlusion of the tibioperoneal trunk and the proximal tibial arteries results in collateral supply from the sural and genicular arteries. Each of the tibial arteries has the potential to provide collateral supply to the others. The peroneal artery is the most common source of collateral supply, in that it is frequently spared in occlusive disease and occupies a central location in the calf. At the ankle the peroneal artery has a constant bifurcation that can collateralize to the distal anterior or posterior tibial arteries (see Fig. 15-7).

Occlusion of either the dorsalis pedis or posterior tibial artery distal to the medial malleolus is well tolerated if the plantar arches are intact. Occlusion of both the proximal dorsalis pedis and the inframalleolar posterior tibial artery is collateralized by tarsal and metatarsal arteries.

NONINVASIVE PHYSIOLOGIC EVALUATION

Evaluation of lower-extremity arterial occlusive disease requires determination of physiologic impact as well as imaging. The severity of an obstructive lesion does not always correlate with the severity of the symptoms. Knowledge of the patient's past surgical history is important for accurate interpretation of physical examination and any test. Noninvasive physiologic testing provides an objective measure of disease that can be used to follow patients and document outcomes of interventions (Box 15-2).

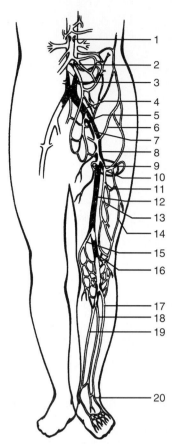

FIGURE 15-8. Diagram of collateral pathways to the lower-extremity arteries. Shaded areas are levels of obstruction. *1*, Superior mesenteric artery. *2*, Inferior mesenteric artery. *3*, Lumbar artery. *4*, Common iliac artery. *5*, Internal iliac artery. *6*, Deep iliac circumflex artery. *7*, External iliac artery. *8*, Common femoral artery. *9*, Medial femoral circumflex artery. *10*, Lateral femoral circumflex artery. *11*, Profunda femoris artery. *12*, Superficial femoral artery. *13*, Second perforator. *14*, Descending branch of lateral femoral circumflex artery. *15*, Descending genicular artery. *16*, Popliteal artery. *17*, Anterior tibial artery. *18*, Peroneal artery. *19*, Posterior tibial artery. *20*, Dorsalis pedis artery. (Modified with permission from Kempczinski RF. The chronically ischemic leg: an overview. In Rutherford RB, ed. *Vascular Surgery*, 5th ed. Philadelphia: WB Saunders, 2000.)

Box 15-1. Collateral Pathways in Common Femoral Artery Occlusion

Lumbar artery → circumflex iliac artery → PFA → SFA
Common iliac artery → internal iliac artery → PFA → SFA
Contralateral PFA → transpubic collaterals → PFA → SFA

PFA, Profunda femoris artery; SFA, superficial femoral artery.

The most basic physiologic assessment is the physical examination. Important information can be obtained from the patient history and by examining the limbs in question. The lower extremities should be evaluated for skin integrity, capillary refill, temperature, and palpable pulses. In diabetic patients, it is important to inspect between the toes for early skin breakdown and infection. The femoral, popliteal, dorsalis pedis, and posterior tibial arterial pulses should be checked in both legs, regardless of the laterality of symptoms. In addition, the carotid and radial pulses should be assessed.

The ratio of the systolic blood pressures of the ankle to the upper arm (the ankle-brachial index, ABI) is a basic measure of the status of the peripheral arteries. An appropriately sized blood

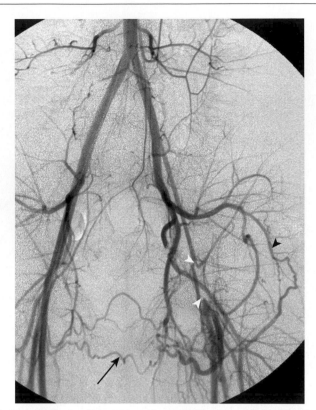

FIGURE 15-9. Collateralization around chronic left common femoral artery occlusion *(white arrowheads)* in an adolescent due to cardiac catheterization as an infant. The only symptom was leg-length discrepancy. There are well-developed collaterals from ipsilateral hypogastric branches *(black arrowhead)* and contra lateral external pudendal arteries *(black arrow)*.

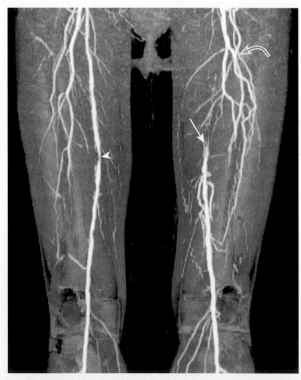

FIGURE 15-10. Collateralization of a superficial femoral artery (SFA) occlusion by enlarged profunda femoris artery (PFA). Coronal maximum intensity projection of a computed tomography angiogram showing an enlarged left PFA *(curved arrow)* that reconstitutes an occluded SFA in the midthigh *(straight arrow)*. Note the focal SFA stenosis *(arrowhead)* on the right.

Box 15-2. **Noninvasive Tests of Lower-Extremity Arterial Supply**

Physical examination
Ankle-brachial index (ABI)
Segmental limb pressures
Doppler waveforms
Plethysmography (volume or photo)

TABLE 15-3 Resting Ankle-Brachial Indices

ABI	Severity of Disease	Typical Symptoms
≥0.95	None	None
0.75-0.95	Mild, single segment	None, claudication
0.5-0.75	Moderate	Claudication
0.3-0.5	Moderate severe, usually multilevel	Severe claudication
<0.3	Critical, multilevel or acute occlusion	Rest pain, tissue loss

ABI, Ankle-brachial index (ratio of ankle systolic blood pressure and brachial systolic blood pressure).

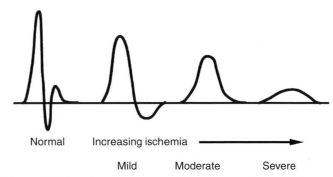

Normal   Increasing ischemia ⟶

Mild   Moderate   Severe

FIGURE 15-11. Schematic of changes in lower-extremity arterial Doppler waveforms with different levels of ischemia. Note that the normal pattern is triphasic (high peripheral resistance). (Adapted from Rholl K, Sterling K, Jones CS. Noninvasive vascular diagnosis in peripheral vascular disease. In Kaufman JA, Hartnell GA, Trerotola SO, eds. *Noninvasive Vascular Imaging With Ultrasound, Computed Tomography, and Magnetic Resonance.* Fairfax, Va: Society of Cardiovascular and Interventional Radiology, 1997, with permission.)

pressure cuff and a Doppler ultrasound probe are used to determine the systolic blood pressure at the ankle (dorsalis pedis or posterior tibial artery) and the brachial artery. The blood pressure in both arms should be obtained, and the highest used to calculate the ratio. Ratios are often slightly greater than 1 in normal individuals. In patients with occlusive disease, the ABI correlates roughly with the extent of disease and degree of ischemia (Table 15-3). This is a simple test that can be performed at the bedside or the procedure table before and after an intervention.

The ABI can be falsely elevated in patients with diabetes with noncompressible vessels due to calcific medial sclerosis. The digital arteries are not as severely affected by this process. In these patients, toe pressures are an important indicator of the severity of occlusive disease. The normal systolic blood pressure in the toe is greater than 50 mm Hg, with a toe-brachial index of at least 0.6. Toe pressures less than 30 mm Hg are incompatible with healing of ulcers or surgical incisions.

One of the major limitations of the ABI is that it does not provide any information about the level of the obstruction. A useful and simple modification is to obtain blood pressures at three or four different levels in the leg ("segmental limb pressures"). A Doppler probe is positioned over a pedal artery as cuffs over the thigh, calf, and ankle are inflated and deflated. The pressure at which signal reappears in the foot is noted as each cuff is deflated. Appropriately sized cuffs are used for each segment of the leg. The variability in limb circumference of the leg results in slightly higher pressure measurements with the thigh cuffs, especially in obese patients. In addition, diabetic patients may have falsely normal pressure measurements for reasons noted earlier. A drop in pressure of more than 20-30 mm Hg at any level suggests hemodynamically significant occlusive disease in that vascular segment. In addition, a difference in pressures from side to side of more than 20 mm Hg indicates occlusive disease at that level or proximal in the affected limb.

Segmental limb pressures are frequently combined with Doppler waveform analysis at each level (Fig. 15-11). This greatly enhances the utility of the study by providing an assessment of flow in addition to pressure. Changes in the shape and amplitude of the waveform reflect increasing severity of disease (Fig. 15-12). Precise identification of the insonated vessel is essential for accurate testing.

Additional noninvasive examinations for peripheral vascular disease are volume and photoplethysmography. These techniques measure the global perfusion of the extremity by

recording the minute changes in the volume of the extremity that occur throughout the cardiac cycle. The terms *volume plethysmographic recordings* (VPRs) or *pulse volume recordings* (PVRs) are essentially interchangeable. A series of blood pressure cuffs are applied to the extremity, and sequentially inflated to 60-65 mm Hg. The pressure in the cuff changes slightly as the volume of blood changes with systole and diastole. These changes are displayed as a waveform (Fig. 15-13). Abnormalities in the waveform indicate occlusive disease in the vascular segment proximal to the cuff. For example, an abnormal tracing at the thigh is not caused by SFA disease, but disease in the aorta, common iliac artery, or CFA. Medial sclerosis does not affect plethysmography, but patient motion does degrade the study.

The plethysmographic waveform can be analyzed for both contour and amplitude. The contour of the waveform is determined by the status of the arterial blood supply. As the degree of stenosis becomes more severe, the dicrotic notch is lost and the overall slope is flattened. The amplitude of the waveform reflects the underlying muscle mass. Fat and bone are relatively avascular, and contribute little to the change in volume during the cardiac cycle. This accounts for why the amplitude increases slightly at the calf in normal individuals owing to the lower amount of adipose tissue. Photoplethysmography can be used in the evaluation of vasospastic disorders by testing before and after temperature stimuli.

Patients with claudication and normal or near-normal pulse examinations and physiologic tests should undergo exercise testing. Occlusive lesions that are well compensated at rest may be unmasked by hyperemia created in the distal muscular bed during exercise. Testing is performed before and after walking on a treadmill at a grade of 10-12 degrees for 5 minutes at 1.5-2 miles per hour. The time to onset and features of the symptoms are recorded. Normally, the ABI remains unchanged or even increases with exercise, and the amplitude of the volume recording increases with preservation of the contour. An abnormal response indicates hemodynamically significant occlusive disease.

▬ IMAGING

A wide variety of imaging modalities can be applied to the lower-extremity arteries. Availability of a technique at a particular institution depends upon the presence of appropriate equipment and expertise. Regardless of the imaging modality, it is essential to know the patient's symptoms, past surgical history, and results of noninvasive testing before performing and interpreting a study.

Color-flow Doppler ultrasound can be used to image the lower-extremity arteries and surgical bypass grafts. A variety of criteria have been promoted to categorize occlusive lesions (Table 15-4).

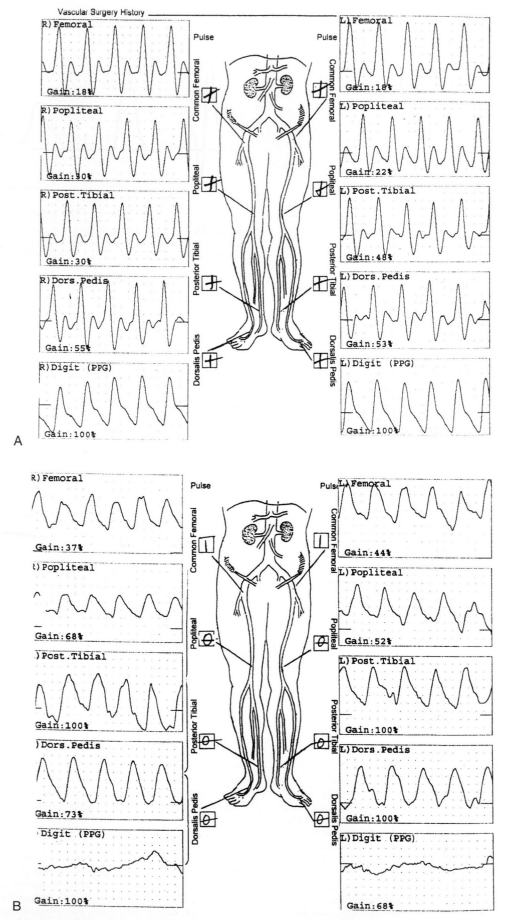

FIGURE 15-12. Normal and abnormal lower-extremity Doppler waveforms. **A,** Normal examination showing excellent waveforms and pressures at all levels. The pedal waveforms typically lose the triphasic pattern. **B,** Examination in a patient with severe ischemia. The arm/thigh blood pressures ratios were 0.53 on the right and 0.43 on the left, indicating bilateral inflow disease. The arm/calf pressure indices dropped to 0.35 on the right and 0.28 on the left, indicative of bilateral superficial femoral artery disease as well. The ankle-brachial index (ABI) was 0.28 on the right and 0.24 on the left. The waveforms are barely biphasic proximally and are essentially flat in the toes. These findings are consistent with severe bilateral multilevel disease.

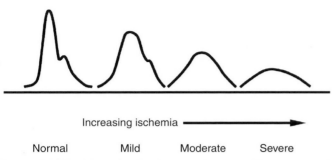

Increasing ischemia ⟶

Normal   Mild   Moderate   Severe

FIGURE **15-13**. Schematic of volume plethysmographic waveforms in relationship to degree of inflow disease. As disease progresses, the waveform becomes blunted and diminished in amplitude. (Adapted from Rholl K, Sterling K, Jones CS. Noninvasive vascular diagnosis in peripheral vascular disease. In Kaufman JA, Hartnell GA, Trerotola SO, eds. *Noninvasive Vascular Imaging With Ultrasound, Computed Tomography, and Magnetic Resonance.* Fairfax, Va: Society of Cardiovascular and Interventional Radiology, 1997, with permission.)

TABLE **15-4** Duplex Criteria for Native Lower-Extremity Arterial Stenosis

Stenosis	PSV (Sample Value)	Poststenotic Turbulence
None	Normal (100 cm/sec)	None
<50%	<2 × normal (<200 cm/sec)	Minimal
50%-75%	2-4 × normal (>200 cm/sec)	Moderate
76%-99%	>4 × normal (≥400 cm/sec)	Severe
100%	No flow	Not applicable

PSV, Peak systolic velocity.

Careful inspection of each abnormal vascular segment with gray-scale, color, and Doppler ultrasound is necessary to precisely localize abnormalities. Bypass grafts are particularly well suited to ultrasound imaging when they are superficial in location.

Magnetic resonance angiography (MRA) can detect luminal stenoses greater than 50% in the lower-extremity arteries with sensitivity and specificity that exceed 95%. The first technique to produce reliable imaging was two-dimensional time-of-flight (2-D TOF) MRA. This appeared to have the ideal quality of imaging blood flow rather than contrast enhancement, so that timing issues were nonexistent. However, overestimation of stenoses, saturation of inplane flow, and the long time span (1.5-2 hours) needed for a complete examination were among several serious limitations of 2-D TOF MRA. Gadolinium-enhanced three-dimensional (3-D) acquisitions have replaced 2-D TOF MRA in most instances. Stepping table technology permits true gadolinium-enhanced MRA runoffs. Bolus chase or multiple injections of gadolinium (usually no more than 30-40 mL in total) provide excellent images from the renal arteries to the ankle (see Fig. 3-12). Time-resolved techniques allow dynamic imaging of the blood flow in the extremity (see Fig. 3-13). Dedicated foot sequences are useful in the foot due to small vessel size (Fig. 15-14). An entire runoff from the renal arteries to the foot can now be acquired in a few minutes. In patients with renal insufficiency at high risk for nephrogenic systemic fibrosis from gadolinium, noncontrast MRA techniques are used.

Computed tomography angiography (CTA) of the lower-extremity arteries is widely available due to multirow detector technology. As the number of rows increases, the imaging of lower-extremity arteries improves. Depending upon the number of detector channels, reconstructed images of 0.5-2 mm thickness can be obtained from the renal arteries to the calf in less than 20 seconds (see Fig. 15-10). Contrast is injected at 3-5 mL/sec for a total volume of approximately 100-150 mL, although the volume

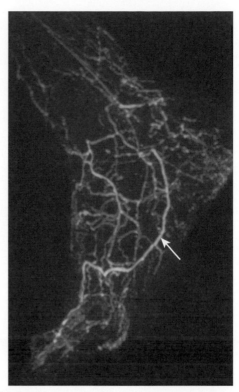

FIGURE **15-14**. Dedicated three-dimensional gadolinium-enhanced magnetic resonance angiogram of the foot in a patient with severe tibial artery disease demonstrates a patent lateral plantar artery *(arrow)*.

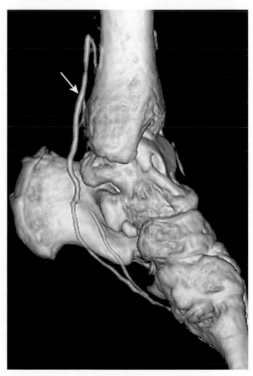

FIGURE **15-15**. Volume rendering of a CTA at the level of the foot showing a reconstituted distal posterior tibial *(arrow)* and plantar arteries.

needed decreases as the number of detector rows increases. Opacification is generally excellent from the renal to the tibial arteries. Venous enhancement and heavy calcification of small vessels are limitations in the calf and foot, but can sometimes be overcome by focused examinations (Fig. 15-15). Streak artifact from joint

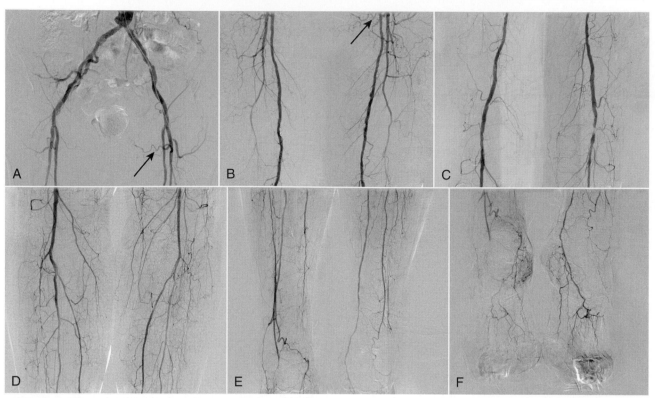

FIGURE 15-16. Bilateral lower-extremity runoff using bolus-chase digital subtraction angiogram technique. Each level was carefully programmed to have several centimeters of overlap with the previous level. The levels were changed during the acquisition by the angiographer who monitored arterial opacification on a live image during the injection. Contrast was diluted to two-thirds strength and injected at a rate of 10 mL/sec for a total duration of 10 seconds. **A,** Station 1, pelvis. A pigtail catheter has been positioned in the distal abdominal aorta. There are stents in both common iliac arteries and occlusion of the left internal iliac artery. The *arrow* is on a distinctive branch of the left profunda femoris artery (PFA). **B,** Station 2, thighs. The distinctive branch of the left PFA *(arrow)* is seen at the top of the image, confirming adequate overlap with the previous station. The superficial femoral arteries are diseased but patent. **C,** Station 3, knees. There is focal severe stenosis of the above-knee popliteal artery on the left. **D,** Station 4, proximal calves. Both anterior tibial arteries are occluded proximally. **E,** Station 5, distal calves. On the right, the anterior tibial artery reconstitutes distally but the dorsalis pedis artery is occluded. The right posterior tibial artery is occluded distally, and the plantar artery is reconstituted from the peroneal artery. On the left, the peroneal and posterior tibial arteries are diseased but continuous. **F,** Station 6, feet. On the right, the medial and lateral plantar arteries are filled from a posterior terminal branch of the peroneal artery. The dorsalis pedis artery is not visualized. On the left, the posterior tibial artery is continuous with the plantar arteries, but the dorsalis pedis artery is not visualized.

replacements can make interpretation of the adjacent arteries impossible. Postprocessing is necessary to remove bone and soft tissues.

The role of conventional angiography in the diagnosis of lower-extremity arterial disease has changed substantially with the improvement in noninvasive imaging techniques. Angiography was once obtained uniformly in all patients before surgery or intervention. Currently angiography is a secondary diagnostic imaging modality (used to resolve conflicting noninvasive test results or when CTA or MRA are not adequate), but the primary imaging modality during interventions.

Angiographic evaluation of the lower extremities includes, as a minimum, the aortic bifurcation to the ankle. In most patients, an abdominal aortogram with a pigtail or other high-flow nonselective catheter is performed before imaging the lower extremities, particularly when renovascular or visceral artery occlusive disease is suspected (see Fig. 10-7). The catheter should be positioned with the side holes in the visceral segment when the celiac artery and SMA are to be included. Pelvic arteriography is performed with the same catheter just proximal to the aortic bifurcation. Anteroposterior and bilateral oblique views should be obtained whenever iliac artery pathology is suspected (see Fig. 10-8). Typical pelvic angiographic injection parameters are 8-10 mL/sec of contrast injected for 2-3 seconds, with imaging at 2-4/sec. Pressure gradients should be obtained across any suspicious stenosis (see Fig. 4-8).

Positioning of the legs is an important consideration during runoff angiograms. The legs should be held as close together and as stationary as possible without tight straps or tape that could compress vessels and create artifactual occlusions. The latter is most likely to occur at the ankles and feet. Even though optimum positioning of the feet varies among departments, it is not critical because dedicated foot imaging can and should always be added when indicated.

Bilateral lower-extremity runoffs are obtained with the catheter at the aortic bifurcation using two basic strategies. The simplest is stationary imaging of overlapping areas of the legs. Small (10-20 mL) contrast injections are performed with filming at 1-2 frame/sec until all vessels are fully opacified at the level being imaged. Rapidly filling normal arteries and slowly filling reconstituted arteries are both easily imaged. The overall volume of contrast necessary is dependent upon the severity of disease; as the length and number of occlusions increase, more contrast is needed to opacify reconstituted distal vessels. This technique allows runoff imaging even with very basic C-arms and tables.

The second, more common approach is to image sequential overlapping levels of the pelvis and legs during a long continuous contrast injection using motorized tables, C-arms, or both. Although less overall contrast is typically used compared to stationary runs, the likelihood of underfilling of vessel segments is greater. A test injection of a small amount of contrast (10-20 mL) at the aortic bifurcation with imaging at the knees allows assessment of the symmetry of flow. The imaging stations, technique, and patient positioning are then set. Scout images of the legs are obtained followed immediately by contrast injection and digital subtraction imaging (Fig. 15-16). Manually activated changes in

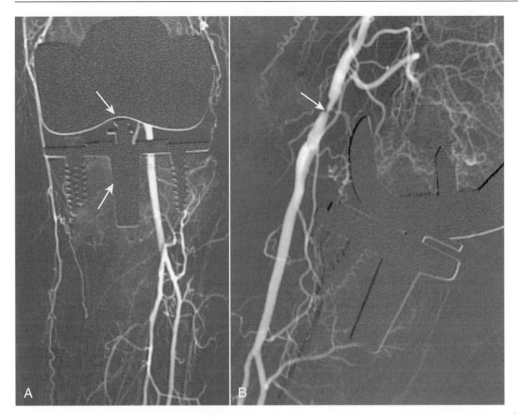

FIGURE 15-17. Importance of careful limb positioning and multiple views during angiography. Popliteal artery stenosis obscured by total knee prosthesis. **A,** Digital subtraction angiogram in the antero-posterior projection showing the above-knee popliteal artery obscured by the knee prosthesis *(arrows).* **B,** Lateral view of the same patient showing a focal stenosis *(arrow)* in the above-knee popliteal artery that was treated successfully with angioplasty.

table position ("bolus chase") are based on real-time assessment of vascular opacification. Single-phase injections use a constant rate of contrast injection, whereas dual phase injections use one rate in the pelvis followed by a lower rate during imaging of the extremities to increase the overall duration of the injection. A typical single-phase injection would be full-strength or diluted low osmolar contrast injected at 6-10 mL/sec for 10-12 seconds. A dual-phase injection might use 10 mL/sec when imaging the pelvis followed by 6 mL/sec during filming of the legs.

When there is a big disparity in the time that it takes contrast to reach both knees, reactive hyperemia effectively decreases the transit time on the slower side by half. This simple maneuver is performed by inflating a blood pressure cuff to a suprasystolic pressure at the ankle for 2-3 minutes. The cuff is then released and removed just before contrast injection.

Selective single-limb angiography provides excellent filling of vessels with less dilution of contrast. The inflow vessels should first be examined with pelvic (or aortic and pelvic) arteriography. Subsequently, when the access is from the ipsilateral CFA, a 5-French straight multiple side-hole or a tightly recurved end-hole catheter can be withdrawn into the external iliac artery. When the access is from the contralateral CFA, an end-hole catheter such as an Sos or Cobra-2 can be positioned over the aortic bifurcation in the common or external iliac artery. Contrast injection rates of 4 mL/sec provide excellent opacification using bolus chase or standing runs (see Fig. 15-7).

The origins of the SFA and PFA are usually best viewed from an ipsilateral anterior oblique projection (see Fig. 10-8). These views should be obtained when the vessel origins are not clearly seen in anteroposterior projections. Additional oblique and even lateral views of specific abnormalities are not usually obtained, but can be important to accurately grade stenoses, particularly in the tibial arteries where overlying bone can obscure vessels or create subtraction artifacts (Fig. 15-17).

Whenever there is pathology present in the foot, dedicated views are necessary. A single lateral view that includes the malleolus to the toes is usually sufficient, although an anteroposterior

projection may be necessary for specific indications (see Fig. 15-7). Positioning the catheter tip in the external iliac artery or SFA maximizes the delivery of contrast to the foot. The foot should be carefully taped in position (with special attention to delicate skin and pressure points). Extreme plantar flexion of the foot should be avoided to prevent artifactual occlusion of the dorsalis pedis artery (Fig. 15-18). In the presence of extensive proximal occlusive disease, it is important to use reactive hyperemia, prolonged image acquisition, and injection of full-strength low-osmolar contrast at 5 mL/sec for 4-6 seconds.

▬ CHRONIC OCCLUSIVE DISEASE

There are many causes of peripheral arterial occlusions (Box 15-3). This section focuses on atherosclerotic disease, which is the most common chronic pathology encountered in lower-extremity arterial circulation.

The prevalence of atherosclerotic peripheral arterial disease increases with age, from 3% in individuals aged 40-59 years to 20% in adults older than 70 years. Until age 65 years, men are affected more often than women. Fewer than half of people with atherosclerotic peripheral arterial disease are symptomatic, most commonly with atypical leg pain. Classic pain with ambulation (claudication) occurs in 10%-35%. Only 1%-2% have rest pain, tissue loss, or gangrene (critical limb ischemia; CLI) at presentation. Smoking, diabetes, hyperlipidemia, homocystinemia, advanced age, ethnicity, and hypertension are important risk factors.

Peripheral arterial disease is a marker of systemic atherosclerosis and increased risk of death from stroke and myocardial infarction. The estimated rate of nonfatal cardiovascular events in patients with confirmed peripheral arterial disease is 2%-4% per year. Approximately 65% of patients with lower-extremity arterial disease have abnormal cardiac stress tests, and 25% have carotid artery stenoses greater than 70%. The underlying cause of death in 60% of patients with peripheral vascular disease is a cardiac event. A diagnosis of peripheral vascular disease confers a mortality rate that is almost triple that of age-matched controls (Table 15-5).

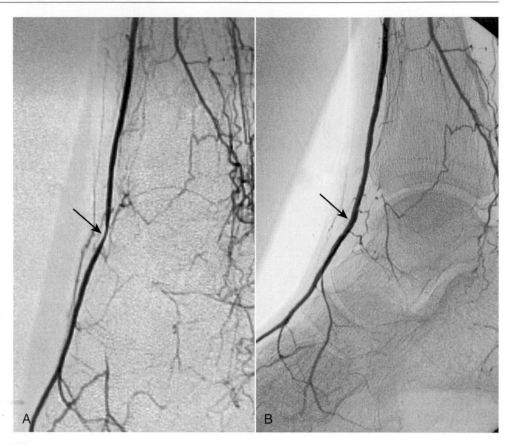

Figure 15-18. Artifactual stenosis of dorsalis pedis artery due to positioning of the foot ("ballerina sign"). **A,** Lateral digital subtraction angiogram of the foot in plantar flexion ("en pointe" like a ballerina) showing focal stenosis *(arrow)* of the dorsalis pedis artery. **B,** The angiogram was repeated with the foot in neutral position. The dorsalis pedis stenosis is now gone *(arrow)*. This same artifact can also be caused by tight straps or tape on a limb.

Box 15-3. Etiologies of Chronic Peripheral Vascular Occlusions

Atherosclerosis
Thromboangiitis obliterans (Buerger's disease)
Popliteal entrapment syndrome
Adventitial cystic disease
Radiation
Vasculitis
Ergotism
Trauma
Chronic embolism

Table 15-5 Survival in Patients with Peripheral Vascular Disease

Parameter	(%)
5-year survival, all patients	70
10-year survival, all patients	50
15-year survival, all patients	30
5-year survival, claudication managed conservatively	87
5-year survival, claudication requiring surgery	80
5-year survival, limb-threatening ischemia treated with surgery	48
5-year survival, reoperation for limb-threatening ischemia	12

The symptoms of chronic peripheral arterial occlusive disease are related to the level of the occlusion and the presence of comorbid conditions such as diabetes. Symptoms are typically manifested in the limb segment distal to the occlusive process. The classic chronic complaint is claudication, which is consistently described by patients as onset of muscular tightening or cramping with exertion. This should resolve within minutes with rest. Patients may often report atypical symptoms such as nonspecific leg weakness and numbness with exercise that also resolves with rest. As chronic ischemia progresses, skin changes such as scaling, hair loss, and atrophy occur.

Critical limb ischemia is manifested as rest pain, ulceration, and tissue necrosis. Rest pain in CLI is aggravated by elevation of the limb and relieved when the limb is dependent. The foot may be noticeably red when dependent, and pale when elevated. Ulceration is painful and usually occurs in the foot and toes following minor trauma. Spontaneous posterolateral lower leg ulceration can be seen with small vessel arterial disease. Severe ischemic changes can develop in diabetic patients in the presence of palpable pedal pulses, owing to extensive microvascular pathology. To facilitate communication about patients with peripheral vascular disease, the classification devised by Rutherford and associates should be used (Table 15-6).

Not all ulcers represent CLI. Patients with severe diabetic neuropathy can develop ulceration over pressure points such as the metatarsal head. These are usually painless and associated with callous formation. Venous ulcers are distinguished from lesions due to arterial insufficiency by their typical medial location around the medial ankles in the lower leg, rich vascularity, and associated manifestations of chronic venous stasis (see Fig. 16-19).

The distribution of lower-extremity atherosclerosis is symmetric in almost 80% of patients, although the severity of the lesions may not match (Box 15-4). Involvement of adjacent segments is common, with combined iliac artery and SFA disease in 46%, and femoropopliteal and tibial disease in 38%. The iliac arteries are diseased in 46% of patients with SFA and popliteal stenoses. There are several well-recognized patterns of distribution of disease, including normal inflow with severe infrapopliteal artery disease in patients with diabetes and renal failure; isolated distal aortic and bifurcation disease in middle-aged females; and iliofemoral disease in smokers (Fig. 15-19).

TABLE 15-6 Rutherford Categories of Chronic Limb Ischemia

Grade	Category	Clinical Description	Objective Criteria*
0	0	Asymptomatic	Normal treadmill or reactive hyperemia test
	1	Mild claudication	Completes treadmill test; ankle pressure after exercise > 50 mm Hg but at least 20 mm Hg lower than brachial pressure
I	2	Moderate claudication	Between categories 1 and 3
	3	Severe claudication	Cannot complete treadmill test; ankle pressure < 50 mm Hg after exercise
III	4	Ischemic rest pain	Resting ankle pressure < 60 mm Hg; flat or severely dampened ankle or metatarsal pulse volume recording; toe pressure < 40 mm Hg
III	5	Minor tissue loss; nonhealing ulcer, focal gangrene with diffuse pedal ischemia	Resting ankle pressure < 40 mm Hg; flat or barely pulsatile ankle or metatarsal pulse volume recording; toe pressure < 30 mm Hg
	6	Major tissue loss extending above transmetatarsal level; functional foot unsalvageable	Same as category 5

*Treadmill test is 5 minutes at 2 mph on a 12-degree incline.

> **Box 15-4. Typical Locations for Atherosclerotic Stenosis in the Lower Extremities**
>
> Superficial femoral artery in Hunter canal
> Common iliac artery
> Popliteal artery at joint line
> Tibioperoneal trunk
> Origins of tibial arteries

Most patients (70%-80%) have stable symptoms over 5 years, whereas 10%-20% note an increase in severity, and 5%-10% progress to CLI. Limb loss is one of the most clearly defined measures of outcome in peripheral vascular disease. Only 12% of symptomatic patients require amputation within 10 years of diagnosis, or roughly 1% of claudicants per year. Diabetes and continued smoking result in higher rates of amputation.

Patients presenting with CLI (about 1%-3% of newly diagnosed patients per year) have a worse prognosis than claudicants. Up to 25% require amputation at the time of presentation, more than half undergo revascularization, and the remainder can be managed medically. Within a year, 25% of these patients will have died, the same percentage will have undergone below- or above-knee amputations, and similar proportions will be symptom free or still in a state of CLI.

Management is conservative for most patients with claudication. Lifestyle modification (cessation of smoking being the most important), exercise programs, lipid management, and control of comorbid diseases such as diabetes are frequently successful in stabilization or slight improvement of symptoms in patients able to comply. A 6-month trial of conservative therapy is usually indicated before considering more aggressive treatment. Supervised exercise programs reliably reduce reported claudication symptoms and increase walking time. Few medications, however, have been shown to conclusively improve claudication symptoms. One that is effective is cilostazol, a phosphodiesterase inhibitor that can increase walking distance by up to 50% in some patients. The typical dose is 100 mg by mouth twice daily. Cilostazol is contraindicated in patients with congestive heart failure. Aspirin and other antiplatelet drugs reduce overall risk of cardiovascular events, but have little impact on claudication symptoms.

Patients with progressive symptoms or who are severely limited by their claudication may be considered for revascularization procedures. Patients with critical ischemia (rest pain, tissue loss, and gangrene) often require aggressive intervention to preserve the limb. As a general rule, healing of an ischemic foot ulcer will not occur in the absence of a pulse in at least one pedal artery.

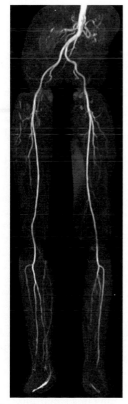

FIGURE 15-19. Gadolinium-enhanced three-dimensional magnetic resonance angiogram runoff in a patient with diabetes and foot pain with nonpalpable pedal pulses. The arteries are widely patent to the level of the distal tibial arteries where occlusions are seen of all three tibial arteries at various levels in the calves. (Courtesy Constantino Pena, MD, Miami, Fla.)

The workup of a patient with peripheral arterial disease begins with a history and physical examination. The nature and onset of the symptoms, comorbid conditions, and clinical evidence of cardiac or cerebrovascular disease should be determined. The physical examination is of paramount importance and includes a comprehensive pulse examination, careful inspection of the limb for evidence of ischemic disease, and detection of clues indicative of nonarterial causes of the presenting symptoms.

Physiologic testing is relatively inexpensive and has a major role in the diagnosis and follow-up of patients with symptomatic peripheral vascular disease. Patients with true claudication can be separated from patients with limb pain due to spinal stenosis and osteoarthritis. Progression of disease and effectiveness of interventions can be documented objectively. Exercise testing should be obtained in any patient with suspected claudication whose study results are normal or near-normal while at rest.

The decision to pursue imaging in a patient with peripheral vascular disease is dependent upon the management plan. Owing to the expense and potentially invasive nature of the imaging studies, these examinations should not be obtained unless a patient requires revascularization. The history, physical examination, and results of physiologic testing are sufficient to diagnose peripheral vascular disease in almost all patients.

Noninvasive imaging with ultrasound, MRA, and CTA has reported sensitivities and specificities for occlusive lesions exceeding 95% for all three modalities. MRA and CTA are particularly useful in imaging the lower-extremity runoff in patients with infrarenal aortic occlusions, in that both the arterial inflow and outflow can be visualized (see Fig. 10-26). Ultrasound does not reliably image aortic and iliac inflow, but can quantify flow through abnormal areas. The degree of a focal arterial stenosis is often overestimated on MRA and CTA, and metal in vascular clips or joint prostheses can create signal loss on MRA. Streak artifacts from joint prostheses seen on CTA can obscure adjacent blood vessels. In patients with mild renal insufficiency, allergy to iodinated contrast, and severe multilevel disease, MRA and ultrasound are excellent imaging choices.

Conventional angiography remains crucially important in the management of patients with symptomatic chronic peripheral vascular disease. Angiography is indicated when a percutaneous intervention is highly probable based on examination or noninvasive testing, or when discrepant results are obtained. Surgical bypass can be performed on the basis of high-quality ultrasound, MRA, or CTA.

Percutaneous access for angiography in patients with severe occlusive disease or prior surgery can be challenging. Posterior plaque in the CFA is common and can impede insertion of a guidewire. Patients with prior surgery or angiograms may have scarring of the soft tissues that prevents advancement of a catheter. In this situation, overdilation of the tract by 1 French size over a stout guidewire (e.g., Amplatz) is necessary before placement of the catheter. The presence of an aortobifemoral bypass graft can also complicate the initial access (see Fig. 2-33). When femoral access cannot be obtained, axillary, radial, or translumbar puncture may be required. Patients having undergone prior distal surgical bypass procedures may require additional views in opposing obliquities for a complete study. Surgical anastomoses frequently have a flared appearance ("the hood" of the graft) related to the manner in which the graft is attached to the native vessel (Fig. 15-20). Distal bypasses may arise from the CFA, PFA, SFA, or even the popliteal artery. The proximal anastomosis is usually on the anterior wall of the vessel when the origin is the CFA, PFA, or SFA; filming in a steep anterior oblique projection may be necessary for adequate visualization. Distal anastomoses vary in orientation depending upon the target vessel. The course of the bypass graft may be similar to the native artery or may be extraanatomic (see Fig. 15-3). Careful attention to coning and positioning during the angiogram is necessary to avoid inadvertently excluding a portion of the graft. When there is a severe stenosis in the mid or distal portion of the graft, contrast injected proximal to the graft may not opacify the stagnant column of blood in the graft. This "pseudo occlusion" should be suspected when a definite meniscus is not seen at the origin of the graft or when a pulse is known to be present in the nonvisualized bypass. Selective injection into the graft is necessary to determine the status of the graft in these cases.

The most common surgical interventions in patients with chronic occlusive disease are various bypass procedures. A number of surgical conduits have been investigated, but autogenous vein and polytetrafluoroethylene (PTFE) have proven the most successful, with single segment great saphenous veins having the best results. In general, synthetic grafts are used only when autogenous vein is not available. Veins may be harvested from either leg (great and small saphenous vein), or constructed from available lengths of arm veins (cephalic, basilic, brachial veins). An in situ great saphenous vein graft is created by fashioning proximal and distal arteriovenous anastomoses without removing the vein from the leg. Intraluminal cutting devices are used to destroy the intervening vein valves, and all side branches are carefully obstructed by direct ligation/clipping or endovascular coil embolization. The size of the vein at the anastomosis site approximates that of the artery. Reversed saphenous vein grafts are first harvested from the leg, followed by ligation of branches. The vein is then tunneled through the soft tissues in reverse orientation, so that the smaller (formerly most peripheral) end is at the CFA, and the larger (formerly most central) end is at the distal anastomosis. Local endarterectomy procedures alone or in combination with distal bypass are sometimes used, especially for lesions of the CFA and PFA origin.

Perioperative mortality for peripheral vascular bypass is 2%-5%, largely due to cardiac events. Early graft thrombosis (within 30 days) due to technical errors, such as kinking or a retained valve, or a hypercoagulable state occurs in 2%-7%. Intimal hyperplasia is the cause of most graft failures between 3 months and 2 years. In synthetic grafts this occurs at the anastomoses or at sites of clamp placement on native vessels. In addition to these locations, intimal hyperplasia can occur anywhere within a vein graft, but usually occurs at the sites of valves, branch vessels, or vein-to-vein anastomoses. Graft failure after 2 years is usually the result of progression of disease in the inflow or outflow vessels. However, vein bypass grafts can remain patent despite occlusion of

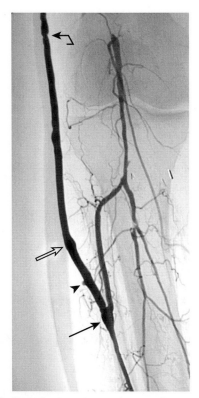

FIGURE 15-20. Digital subtraction angiogram of reversed great saphenous vein graft from the common femoral artery to the right anterior tibial artery. The course of the graft is posterior and lateral to the knee joint in an extraanatomic location to facilitate anastomosis to the anterior tibial artery. Proximally there is an area of stenosis *(bent arrow)* in the graft (which later underwent angioplasty); *open arrow* indicates the location of a venous valve; *arrowhead* identifies the stump of a ligated venous branch; *arrow* is pointing to the flared distal anastomosis of the vein end-to-side to the anterior tibial artery.

the native inflow. Graft infection and anastomotic pseudoaneurysms are additional complications. The overall results of surgical bypass grafts are listed in Table 15-7. Long-term rates of limb salvage and patient survival are best when the indication for surgery is severe claudication rather than critical ischemia.

Graft surveillance with ultrasound is important to prevent thrombosis and extend the life of the bypass. A decrease in the ABI of 0.15-0.2, or identification of a new hemodynamically significant stenosis at any point in the graft, should prompt further imaging. Focal stenoses are usually treated first with percutaneous angioplasty (see Fig. 15-20 and Fig. 15-21). These are fibrotic lesions and may require a cutting or scoring balloon. Long-segment lesions are best managed with graft revision or insertion of a jump graft around the stenotic area. Thrombolysis of an acutely thrombosed graft may unmask an underlying stenosis, although no lesion is found in up to one third of cases. When the graft crosses the knee joint and no stenosis is found after thrombolysis, flexion and stress views should be obtained to exclude kinking or external compression (Fig. 15-22).

TABLE 15-7 Results of Lower-Extremity Surgical Bypass

Procedure	5-Year Primary Patency (%)
Femoral to Popliteal Artery Bypass	
Synthetic above-knee	60
Synthetic below-knee	35
Saphenous vein above-knee	75
Saphenous vein below-knee	75
Femoral to Tibial Artery Bypass	
Synthetic	14
Saphenous vein	75
Femoral to Pedal Artery Bypass	
Saphenous vein	45

Percutaneous Superficial Femoral Artery and Popliteal Interventions

Percutaneous intervention for occlusive disease of the infrainguinal arteries has a long history; the first percutaneous angioplasty ever was performed in the leg (see Fig. 4-1). A wide variety of technologies have since been applied to this vascular bed, including angioplasty, stents, drug-eluting stents, stent-grafts, mechanical atherectomy, drills, freezing or drug-eluting balloons, and lasers. Devices for treatment of occlusive disease in this vascular segment are a focus of intense commercial activity.

Catheter-based interventions for SFA and popliteal artery occlusive disease have undergone numerous clinical trials, but until recently few were prospective and even fewer randomized. One challenge has been the rapid evolution in technology and clinical practice, such that multiyear trials may not produce results relevant to current practice. Nevertheless, these are the preferred interventions (over surgical bypass) in many situations (Box 15-5). Stenoses and occlusions of almost any length can be treated, but the initial technical success and long-term results are proportional to lesion length and multiplicity, with shorter and fewer being better.

Long occlusions can be treated either through the native lumen, or with subintimal angioplasty (see Fig. 4-5). Drug-eluting stents hold promise for use in long-segment recanalization of the SFA and popliteal artery, and for below-knee interventions. When fresh-appearing thrombus is present in an occlusion, a short trial of catheter-directed thrombolysis may convert it to a stenosis and decrease the risk of distal embolization (see Fig. 4-28).

The most direct approach to infrainguinal interventions is from an antegrade puncture in the ipsilateral CFA, which provides the greatest mechanical advantage and permits use of standard length delivery systems. Antegrade puncture is frequently not possible, however, because of a large abdominal pannus. From the contralateral approach, a 30- to 45-cm flexible sheath placed over the aortic bifurcation provides a stable platform for most interventions. Longer guidewires are often necessary with this access, especially when working in the distal SFA. Typical balloon diameters for the SFA are 5-7 mm, and for the popliteal artery 4-6 mm, on 5-French

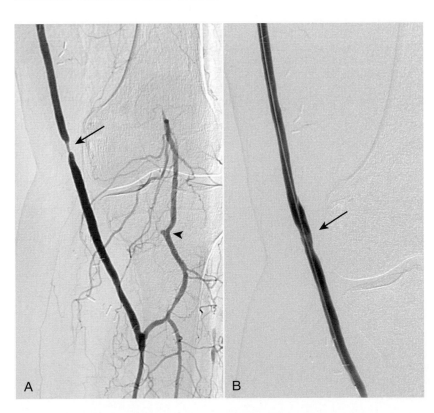

A   B

FIGURE 15-21. Angioplasty of a vein graft stenosis. **A,** Digital subtraction angiogram (DSA) showing focal stenosis *(arrow)* of a reversed saphenous vein bypass from the common femoral artery to the anterior tibial artery. The deviation in the popliteal artery *(arrowhead)* with an associated bulge is the site of the distal anastomosis of an old occluded graft to the popliteal artery. **B,** DSA after angioplasty of the stenosis showing an excellent result *(arrow)* that remained widely patent for several years.

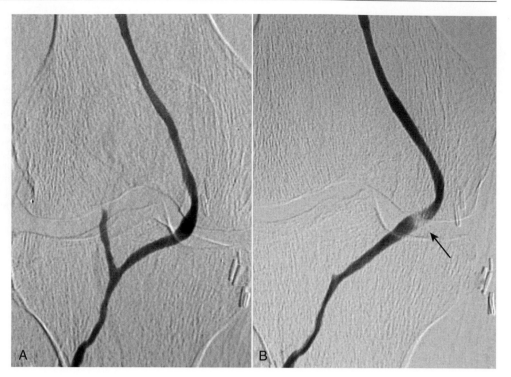

FIGURE 15-22. Graft entrapment in the popliteal fossa. **A,** Digital subtraction angiogram (DSA) in neutral position of a left femoral to below-knee popliteal artery saphenous vein bypass graft after successful thrombolysis of a graft thrombosis. Other views of the graft showed no evidence of stenosis. **B,** DSA with slight flexion of the knee shows compression of the graft *(arrow)* at the level of the knee joint consistent with graft entrapment. This was released surgically, and the graft has remained patent since.

Box 15-5. **Trans-Atlantic Inter-Society Consensus (TASC) II Recommendations for Femoropopliteal Interventions (2007)***

Lesion type A: Endovascular is treatment of choice
- Single stenosis ≤ 10 cm (unilateral/ bilateral)
- Single occlusion ≤ 5 cm length

Lesion type B: Endovascular frequently used but insufficient scientific evidence
- Multiple lesions, each ≤ 5 cm in length (stenoses or occlusions)
- Single stenosis or occlusion ≤ 15 cm in length, not involving the distal popliteal artery
- Heavily calcified occlusion ≤ 5 cm in length
- Single popliteal stenosis
- Single or multiple lesions in the absence of continuous tibial vessels to improve inflow for distal bypass

Lesion type C: Surgical treatment used more often but insufficient scientific evidence
- Recurrent stenoses or occlusions that need treatment after two prior endovascular interventions
- Multiple stenoses or occlusions totaling > 15 cm, ± heavy calcification

Lesion type D: Surgery is treatment of choice
- Chronic total occlusion of CFA or SFA (>20 cm), involving the popliteal artery.
- Chronic total occlusion of the popliteal artery proximal trifurcation vessels

---

CFA, Common femoral artery; POP, popliteal artery; SFA, superficial femoral artery.

*These recommendations are likely to change as stent-grafts, drug-eluting stents, drug-eluting balloons, and pharmacologic adjuncts become scientifically evaluated.

---

or smaller catheters. Balloon lengths of 20 cm or more are available for treatment of long-segment disease. Rapid-exchange balloon catheters are an advantage when working in the distal SFA or popliteal artery. Cutting and scoring balloons and debulking devices are useful for recalcitrant stenoses (see Figs. 4-15, 4-26, and 4-27).

Most operators judge the results of angioplasty visually, with rapid flow and decreased filling of collaterals, and by improvement of distal pulses if present. An irregular lumen with visible fissures in the plaque are common after adequate angioplasty and should not be interpreted as dissections requiring additional treatment when flow is brisk and distal perfusion improved (see Figs. 4-9 and 4-10). Intravascular ultrasound, transcutaneous ultrasound, and pressure measurements using special guidewires can provide more objective assessment of technical results.

When the results of angioplasty are unsatisfactory or when extensive disease is present, self-expanding bare metal stents or stent-grafts improve the lumen (Fig. 15-23). In many practices, stent placement is the norm. Balloon-expandable stents should not be used in the SFA or popliteal artery, because they can be crushed by external forces. The choice between bare metal stent and stent-graft is also often subjective. Stent-grafts usually require larger diameter delivery systems and exclude potential collateral branches, whereas bare metal stents are subject to restenosis over their entire length. (Fig. 15-24 and see Fig. 4-24) When placing either of these devices it is believed important to limit balloon inflations beyond the ends of the stent or stent-graft to decrease the occurrence of intimal hyperplasia in these locations. Intravascular brachytherapy and drug-eluting stents may decrease intimal hyperplasia.

The environment of the SFA is demanding, in that different forces act on different locations. The portion of the artery at the adductor canal is subject to compression, flexion, and rotation during normal bending and straightening of the knee. Stent fracture is a well-recognized event in this location, presumably related to these forces. The risk of fracture is linked to stent design and the number of stents placed (areas of overlap create rigid zones).

Crossing long-segment occlusions can be a particular challenge with SFA interventions, particularly with heavily calcified lesions. A number of tools have been developed to improve success rates. These can be used to get through or around occlusions (see Figs. 4-4 and 4-6). When a subintimal approach is used intentionally (or unintentionally), some of these devices can be used to facilitate reentry into the true lumen below the lesion.

Careful monitoring of guidewire tip position during SFA interventions reduces the risk of spasm in distal vessels. Intraprocedural heparin (3000-5000 U), nitroglycerin, and antiplatelet drugs

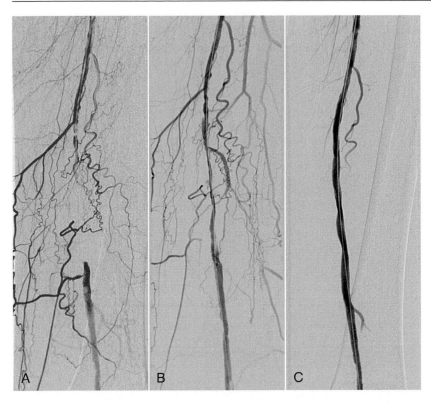

FIGURE 15-23. Recanalization of a distal superficial femoral artery (SFA) occlusion with a stent. **A,** Digital subtraction angiogram (DSA) before the intervention showing the well-collateralized occlusion of the distal SFA with reconstitution at the adductor canal. **B,** DSA after successfully crossing the lesion and angioplasty showing an unsatisfactory result with a narrow, irregular arterial lumen and continued filling of collaterals. **C,** DSA following self-expanding bare metal stent placement and repeat angioplasty. There is now excellent flow through the stented region without visualization of collaterals.

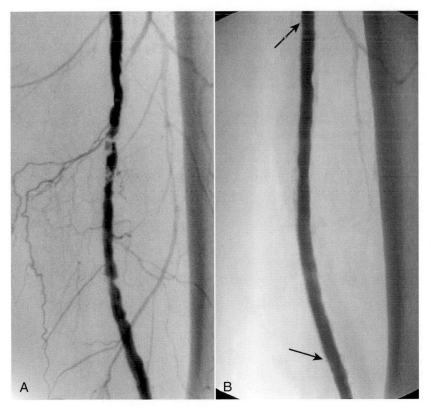

FIGURE 15-24. Long-segment superficial femoral artery (SFA) stenoses treated with ePTFE-covered stent graft. **A,** Digital subtraction angiogram (DSA) showing multiple stenoses in the distal SFA. Note the small muscular branches arising from the SFA. **B,** DSA following angioplasty and placement of a stent-graft (W. L. Gore & Associates, Inc.). The multiple small branches seen in the previous image are no longer present *(arrows).*

should be used. Larger doses of heparin should be used for longer segments of disease and longer interventions. Anticoagulation may be continued overnight when long-segment disease is treated or runoff is poor. As a minimum, patients should be discharged on aspirin 80-360 mg/day for life unless contraindicated. In addition, an oral platelet inhibitor such a clopidogrel 75 mg/day for 3 months may be beneficial.

The most common complications of SFA and popliteal interventions are intraprocedural thrombosis, occlusive dissection, and distal embolization. The overall rate of complications is less than 5% in most centers, but increases with the extent of preexisting disease, complexity of the procedure, and duration. The use of distal protection devices (see Fig. 4-19) should be considered when feasible in patients at risk for distal embolization, such as long segment interventions, irregular plaque with mobile components, or symptoms of distal embolization before the procedure. Intraprocedural thrombosis or embolization can be managed with thrombolysis, mechanical thrombectomy, or suction thrombectomy (see Fig. 4-33). Flow-limiting dissections are effectively treated with stent placement. Anticoagulation, gentle catheter and guidewire manipulation, and careful attention to guidewire and device positions minimize injury to the SFA or distal vessels.

The technical success rate for percutaneous SFA and popliteal interventions is greater than 95% for stenoses and 85%-90% for occlusions. The lower rate in occlusions is due to occasional failures to cross the lesion. Pressure gradients as a definition of technical success are usually not used in SFA and popliteal artery angioplasty. The degree of residual stenosis (<30%), qualitative assessment of flow, return of palpable distal pulses, or an ABI measured on the procedure table is used to determine the procedural endpoints.

The outcomes of SFA and popliteal artery interventions continue to be an area of intense investigation and redefinition. The easiest outcome to measure is freedom from amputation, but this may not be adequate for patients treated for severe claudication rather than critical ischemia. The Society of Vascular Surgery has recommended a composite endpoint for CLI of above-ankle amputation of the index limb or major reintervention (new bypass graft, jump/interposition graft revision, or thrombectomy/thrombolysis). This endpoint is termed a *major adverse limb event* (MALE). In patients treated for claudication, duration of symptomatic improvement and freedom from reintervention are important endpoints.

The BASIL (Bypass versus Angioplasty in Severe Ischemia of the Leg), a seminal multicenter trial comparing angioplasty to vein or synthetic conduit bypass demonstrated no difference in survival or amputation rates at 2 years (despite a 20% procedural failure rate for angioplasty). The vessels treated included the SFA and more distal arteries. However, after 2 years, patients randomized to bypass who had venous conduits had superior results with fewer reinterventions. The application of these results to current practice should be tempered, in that few interventionalists restrict SFA interventions to angioplasty alone.

Certain observations are consistent: interventions on short stenoses have the best outcome, with results deteriorating as lesions become longer and include occlusions; surgical bypass with good-quality single-segment saphenous vein has the best long term primary and secondary patency but is associated with longer recovery and more morbidity than percutaneous interventions; bare metal stents and stent-grafts improve long-term patency but restenosis remains a major issue (Table 15-8 and Fig. 15-25). Drug-eluting stents and drug-coated balloons show promise in reducing the incidence of restenosis by as much as 50%. The long-term data on these devices has yet to be developed. In summary, percutaneous intervention has become the preferred treatment option for many patients with femoropopliteal artery disease, but much work is needed to understand outcomes in different populations.

TABLE 15-8 Results of Superficial Femoral and Popliteal Artery Angioplasty and Stents

Procedure	Indication	Primary Patency at 3 Years (%)
Angioplasty (stenosis)	Claudication	62
Angioplasty (stenosis)	Limb salvage	43
Angioplasty (occlusion)	All	48
Bare stent, SFA	All	65
Stent-graft, SFA	All*	70

*Results for Viabahn (W. L. Gore) in long segment stenoses or occlusions.

Tibial Artery Angioplasty and Stents

Tibial artery interventions are considered separately from the SFA and popliteal arteries because both the clinical and technical challenges are different. The indications are usually limb salvage in the setting of CLI with impending or ongoing tissue loss, or preservation of runoff distal to a bypass graft. Tibial artery occlusive disease is rarely isolated, but frequently occurs in conjunction with SFA and popliteal artery disease. Almost three fourths of patients undergoing tibial artery angioplasty are diabetic.

The optimal approach to tibial artery intervention is antegrade from the ipsilateral CFA. When this is not possible, use of a long, flexible sheath or guiding catheter placed over the aortic bifurcation is necessary to provide stability and allow contrast injections. Positioning the sheath or guide catheter in the SFA improves delivery of contrast to the target area. When working in tibial arteries over the bifurcation, long guidewires and balloon catheters are required. Angioplasty in pedal arteries is possible with these extra-long shaft balloons. Rapid-exchange balloon catheters are especially useful in this environment (see Fig. 4-14). Combined retrograde access through the dorsalis pedis or posterior tibial artery and antegrade access from a femoral approach are useful advanced techniques, especially for subintimal recanalization of long-segment distal occlusions.

Typical balloon diameters for tibial arteries are 2-4 mm. These small vessel balloons often require 0.018-inch or smaller guidewires. Lesions at the origins of the tibial arteries can undergo angioplasty safely using "kissing balloons" in both arteries or a safety wire in one and the balloon in the other (Fig. 15-26). Long balloons (≥20 cm) are specifically designed for angioplasty of diffusely diseased tibial arteries (Fig. 15-27). Angioplasty through the pedal arch is feasible with these specialized balloons.

Stents are increasingly used in this vascular bed (Fig. 15-28). Drug-eluting stents may have an important role in these small-diameter arteries. Long-segment recanalization with subintimal techniques, atherectomy, or laser atherectomy improves procedural

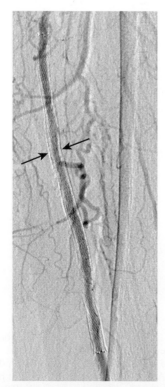

FIGURE 15-25. Intimal hyperplasia within a bare metal stent *(arrows)* in the superficial femoral artery. This is the same patient as in Figure 15-23, imaged 1 year later.

success but long-term outcomes are not known. Focal recalcitrant lesions can undergo angioplasty with cutting or scoring balloons

Intraprocedural thrombosis is of greater concern with tibial artery intervention than SFA or popliteal artery. Patients should be aggressively anticoagulated with heparin (ACT > 250) during the procedure. Addition of intravenous antiplatelet drugs, similar to the approach used in coronary interventions, is advocated by some interventionalists. Liberal use of intraarterial nitroglycerin is important to prevent spasm in these small vessels.

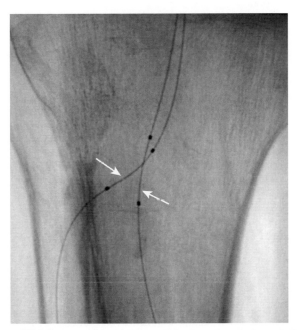

FIGURE 15-26. Spot film showing positioning of angioplasty balloons *(arrows)* for kissing balloon angioplasty of anterior tibial and tibioperoneal artery origin stenoses.

Intervention in these small, diseased arteries is more prone to complications than in other peripheral arteries. Vessel rupture is usually of little consequence although compartment syndrome can occur. Occlusive flaps, thrombosis, and distal embolization are seen on 5%-10% of patients.

The published literature on tibial artery intervention is scant in comparison to more proximal lesions. The technical success approaches 95%, particularly for focal disease in native vessels that have inline runoff to the foot (Table 15-9). Occlusions, stenoses of bypass graft anastomoses, and lesions in vessels with poor runoff have a lower technical success rate. Limb salvage is a more accurate measure of outcome than lesion patency, in that most tibial interventions are performed for this indication.

ACUTE LIMB ISCHEMIA

Acute limb ischemia is the sudden onset (less than 2 weeks) of a symptomatic limb due to arterial occlusion. The estimated incidence is 1.5 cases per 10,000 persons per year. Approximately 45% of patients will present with a viable limb, 45% with a threatened limb, and 10% with a nonviable limb. The acute, profoundly ischemic limb is a surgical emergency. Cell death begins after 4 hours of total ischemia and is irreversible after 6 hours. The clinical presentation can be summarized as the "six Ps" (Box 15-6). These symptoms reflect the greater sensitivity of nerves and muscle to ischemia than skin and subcutaneous tissues. The mortality of patients with acute limb ischemia within 1 year is almost 20% despite aggressive intervention; amputation is undertaken in 15% of those who survive.

There are numerous causes of acute limb ischemia (Box 15-7). A major diagnostic goal is the distinction between primarily embolic versus thrombotic occlusion (Table 15-10). Embolic occlusions tend to result in profound ischemia owing to the absence of developed collateral circulation (see Fig. 1-33). Thrombosis of a preexisting stenosis is generally better tolerated because the collateral circulation is already established.

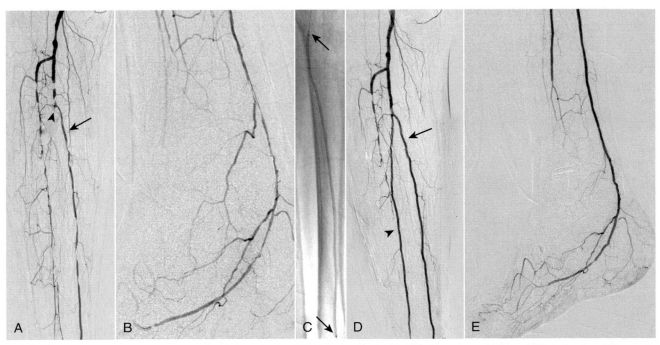

FIGURE 15-27. Tibial artery reconstruction in a patient with critical limb ischemia. **A,** Digital subtraction angiogram (DSA) showing diffuse occlusive disease of the tibial arteries. (*Arrow,* posterior tibial artery; *arrowhead,* occluded peroneal artery.) **B,** DSA of the foot showing the diseased distal posterior tibial artery supplying the plantar artery. **C,** Spot image of a 2 mm × 20 cm angioplasty balloon *(arrows)* in the posterior tibial artery. Angioplasty was also performed of the tibioperoneal trunk, the peroneal artery after recanalization with a guidewire, and the distal posterior tibial artery and lateral plantar artery. **D,** Completion DSA showing patent posterior tibial *(arrow)* and peroneal arteries *(arrowhead)* as well as the tibioperoneal trunk. **E,** Completion DSA of the foot.

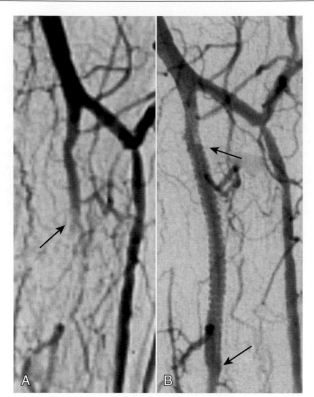

FIGURE 15-28. Stent placement in the peroneal artery. **A,** Digital subtraction angiogram obtained before intervention showing short occlusion of the peroneal artery *(arrow)*. Not shown are the distal occlusion of the anterior tibial artery and the occluded posterior tibial artery. **B,** During angioplasty of the peroneal artery an occlusive intimal flap occurred that was treated with a 2.75-mm diameter coronary stent *(arrows)*. The anterior distal anterior tibial artery was successfully recanalized with balloon angioplasty alone.

TABLE 15-9 Results of Tibial Artery Interventions

Parameter	Result (%)
Technical success	95
Primary patency angioplasty 1 year	40
Primary patency bare stent 1 year	50
Primary patency drug-eluting stent 1 year	85

Box 15-6. Six "P"s of Acute Limb Ischemia

Pulseless
Pain
Pallor
Paresthesia
Paralysis
Poikilothermia (cool limb)

A classification system has been devised for describing the degree of acute limb ischemia (Table 15-11). This classification is different from the one for patients with chronic ischemia, in that the clinical presentation and outcomes are different. For example, tissue loss and gangrene are late findings of ischemia, but paralysis and sensory loss indicate acute hypoxia of nerves and muscle.

Patients presenting with acute limb ischemia should be heparinized immediately to prevent propagation of thrombus

Box 15-7. Etiologies of Acute Limb Ischemia

Embolic
Trauma
Thrombosis of atherosclerotic stenosis
Thrombosis of surgical bypass graft
Thrombosis of degenerative popliteal aneurysm
Popliteal artery entrapment or cyst with thrombosis
Iatrogenic
Dissection
Vasospasm
Venous thrombosis (phlegmasia cerulea dolens)
Low-output cardiac state

TABLE 15-10 Differentiating Features of Acute Arterial Occlusion

	Embolic	Thrombotic
Identifiable source of emboli	Frequent	Rare
Preexisting claudication	Rare	Frequent
Physical examination	Normal proximal and contralateral pulses	Evidence of peripheral vascular disease in ipsilateral and contralateral limb
Degree of ischemia	Frequently profound	Frequently threatened but viable
Imaging findings	Normal vessels with abrupt occlusion (sometimes multiple), frequently at major bifurcation of vessel, no collaterals, meniscus sign	Diffuse atherosclerotic disease, well developed collaterals, usually midvessel occlusion

and provide a mild vasodilatory effect. The history of onset of symptoms frequently suggests the etiology of the occlusion. Examination of all of the peripheral pulses is important to gauge the presence of peripheral vascular disease or multiple emboli. The electrocardiogram may provide an important clue regarding the etiology of the occlusion (looking specifically for atrial arrhythmias or prior myocardial infarction).

The decision to obtain an imaging test is based upon the clinical status of the limb and the probable etiology of the occlusion. Patients with critically ischemic but viable limbs due to a presumed embolus or graft thrombosis should proceed directly to surgical exploration; the delay required to obtain imaging may jeopardize the ability to salvage the extremity. Intraoperative angiography can be performed in patients with profound ischemia when visualization of distal runoff is necessary. Patients with threatened but viable limbs and extensive underlying vascular disease or a complex vascular surgical history benefit from preoperative imaging. Patients with nonviable limbs are managed with amputation of the affected extremity.

Imaging with MRA and CTA can provide diagnostic information in cooperative patients. These modalities are not considered first in many patients because current therapeutic endovascular procedures are not routinely feasible with CT or MR guidance. Conventional diagnostic angiographic studies have the potential for becoming therapeutic interventions, such as thrombolysis or pharmacomechanical thrombectomy.

TABLE **15-11** Clinical Categories of Acute Limb Ischemia

Category	Definition	Prognosis	Physical Examination		Doppler Signals	
			Sensory Loss	Muscle Weakness	Arterial	Venous
I	Viable	Not immediately threatened	None	None	+	+
II	Threatened					
	a. Marginally	Salvageable with prompt treatment	Minimal (toes)	None	Occasional +, frequently −	+
	b. Immediately	Salvageable with immediate treatment	More than toes, rest pain	Mild to moderate	Rare +, usually −	+
III	Irreversible	Major permanent tissue loss	Anesthetic	Paralysis	−	−

The angiographic evaluation of a patient with acute ischemia should be tailored to the clinical situation. Standard catheters, guidewires, and injection rates can be used. Percutaneous access should be planned to support a possible intervention. In patients with suspected embolic disease, an aortogram may reveal silent emboli to renal or visceral branches, or pathology such as an aneurysm or large ulcerated plaque. As a minimum, imaging should span from the aortic bifurcation to below the level of the occlusion. Oblique views of the pelvis may demonstrate emboli in the hypogastric arteries, thus confirming the nature of the more distal occlusion. A dedicated, but reasonable effort should be made to image the reconstituted vessels distal to the occlusion to facilitate planning of interventions. However, in patients with poor collaterals this may be difficult or impossible.

Revascularization of the viable acutely ischemic limb is almost always indicated. Thrombectomy with Fogarty balloon catheters through limited CFA or popliteal artery incisions is an effective method to relieve acute obstruction, especially embolic obstruction. This can be accomplished with the patient under local anesthesia. Balloon catheters can also be passed in a retrograde manner into the pelvic inflow arteries. When embolectomy is unsuccessful in restoring sufficient flow for limb viability, bypass surgery can be performed. Fasciotomy may be necessary in patients in whom compartment syndrome (especially anterior calf) develops following surgery. Surgical interventions result in limb salvage in 75%-90% of patients and a 30-day mortality of 10%-15%. However, embolectomy is frequently incomplete, particularly in the tibial and pedal arteries, and may result in intimal injury.

Percutaneous interventions in patients with acutely ischemic but viable limbs (categories I, IIA, and IIB) are indicated when urgent surgery is not necessary and embolic occlusion is unlikely. The objectives of treatment are to rapidly restore flow and identify underlying lesions that subsequently can be corrected percutaneously or with surgery. Pharmacologic thrombolysis, mechanical thrombolysis, and aspiration thrombectomy are useful techniques in both embolic and thrombotic occlusions (see Fig. 4-28). Occlusions less than 14 days old are amenable to pharmacologic and mechanical thrombolysis. Mechanical thrombectomy devices are very useful for rapid restoration of flow. Subsequent pharmacologic thrombolysis may be used to clean up residual thrombus for optimal results. Aspiration thrombectomy should be considered for acute (<48 hours) occlusions, especially those occurring as complication of a revascularization procedure (see Fig. 4-33).

Thrombolysis or mechanical thrombectomy successfully restores antegrade flow in more than 95% of patients as long as the occlusion can be crossed with an infusion catheter or thrombectomy device. Causes of procedural failure include severe coexistent inflow or outflow disease, organized thrombus, or large atheromatous emboli. The results measured in terms of limb salvage range from 75% to 92% depending on the extent

TABLE **15-12** Sources of Atheroemboli

Source	Percentage of All Atheroemboli
Aortic or iliac stenosis	47
Aortic or iliac aneurysms	20
Upper extremity stenosis and aneurysm	14
Lower-extremity stenosis	12
Degenerating synthetic graft	7

of underlying disease and patient comorbid conditions. With thrombolysis, the majority of severe complications are hemorrhagic, occurring in 6%-9% of patients and more commonly with long infusions, in hypertensive patients, in patients older than age 80 years, and in patients with thrombocytopenia. Mechanical thrombectomy, pharmacomechanical thrombectomy, ultrasound-assisted thrombolysis, and aspiration thrombectomy can shorten overall procedure times and thus should reduce complication rates (see Figs. 4-31, 4-32, and 4-34). There are no recent randomized prospective trials of endovascular versus surgical treatment for acute limb ischemia. Based on older studies of catheter thrombolysis compared with surgery, long-term limb preservation with thrombolysis with or without surgery is identical to surgical therapy alone, but mortality may be lower owing to fewer cardiovascular complications.

◼ BLUE TOE SYNDROME

Spontaneous rupture of atheromatous plaque can result in distal embolization of cholesterol crystals, atheromatous debris, thrombus, and platelet aggregates (Table 15-12). The estimated incidence is 0.03% in hospitalized patients. Macroemboli are believed to occur in approximately 40% of patients and may present as acute limb ischemia (see previous section). In 60% of patients, the emboli are small or microscopic, measuring 200 μm or less in diameter. Lower-extremity microembolization presents with sudden onset of painful, localized red-purple discolorations of one or more toes ("blue toe syndrome") (Fig. 15-29). The region of discoloration may contain interlaced areas of discoloration and normal skin, known as *livedo reticularis*. Patients with microembolization frequently have intact pedal pulses, although combined microembolization and macroembolization occurs in 16% of patients overall. Embolization may be spontaneous or follow endovascular procedures or surgical manipulation. Extensive friable aortic plaque is a known (but unquantified) risk factor.

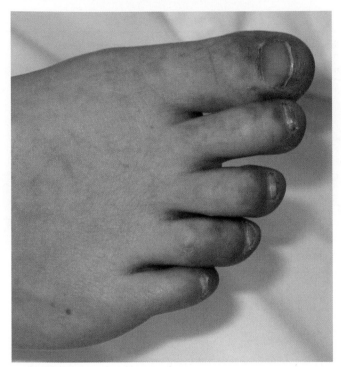

FIGURE 15-29. Blue toe syndrome from an embolizing plaque in the ipsilateral common iliac artery. Note the dusky distal toes and the surrounding erythematous areas. Angiography showed patent pedal arteries consistent with microemboli. The iliac lesion was treated with a covered stent.

The distribution of emboli may suggest the location of the source. Unilateral extremity symptoms usually indicate an inline source (common iliac artery or distal), especially when recurrent. Bilateral limb involvement is suggestive of an aortic or more proximal source. When renal failure occurs synchronously with the lower-extremity symptoms, a thoracic aortic source with concurrent cholesterol embolization of the kidneys should be suspected.

Imaging of patients with atheroembolism is directed at identification of a source. When the thoracic aorta is suspected, transesophageal echocardiography, CTA, and MRA are sensitive noninvasive modalities. Diffuse or localized plaque, ulcerations, or aneurysms are suspicious lesions in this setting, but it is often difficult to be conclusive. When an abdominal aortic source is suspected, CTA and MRA can be used in search of similar pathology. However, a "smoking gun" lesion may never be identified with certainty.

Angiography is obtained when noninvasive studies are inconclusive or when a pulse deficit is present. When the patient has unilateral embolization, the catheter should be inserted from the contralateral CFA. An irregular or severe stenosis, ulcerated plaque, or aneurysm may be found (Fig. 15-30). Intraluminal filling defects are not seen in patients with microembolism, because the occlusions are in vessels below the limits of resolution of the angiogram. Thus a normal angiogram does not rule out atheroembolism.

Patients who do not receive definitive treatment have recurrent embolization in up to 90% of cases within 5 years. Traditionally, surgical excision or bypass of the suspected source lesion has been the standard therapy. Surgical treatment of aortic lesions is associated with a 4% overall 30-day mortality and a 10% incidence of intraoperative embolization. Surgery for peripheral arterial sources carries a much lower risk. Percutaneous exclusion of aortic lesions with stent-grafts and treatment of iliofemoral artery lesions with angioplasty, bare stents, or stent grafts have been used with success. Interestingly, these procedures have not

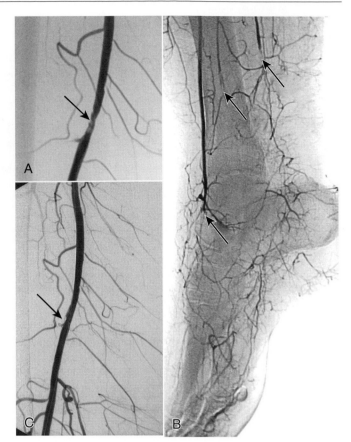

FIGURE 15-30. Tibial artery macroembolization due to an ulcerated superficial femoral artery (SFA) stenosis. **A,** Magnified view of SFA digital subtraction angiogram (DSA) showing a focal stenosis with an irregular surface *(arrow)*. **B,** DSA of the ankle and foot showing embolic occlusions of all three tibial arteries *(arrows)*. **C,** DSA of the SFA lesion following angioplasty shows marked improvement in the appearance of the lumen *(arrow)*. Repeat distal angiography showed no new emboli related to the angioplasty. The patient was maintained on anticoagulation and antiplatelet therapy.

Box 15-8. Etiologies of Peripheral Artery Aneurysms

Degenerative
Iatrogenic
- Catheterization
- Surgical anastomosis
- Intervention

Trauma
Infection
Behçet disease
Ehlers-Danlos syndrome

---

generally been associated with an acute periprocedural atheroembolism. The long-term outcomes of percutaneous interventions for atheroembolism are not known.

ANEURYSMS

Aneurysms of the lower-extremity arteries are less common than those of the abdominal aorta. There are numerous etiologies of peripheral aneurysms, but degenerative (true aneurysms) and iatrogenic (pseudoaneurysms) are the most common (Box 15-8). Degenerative popliteal artery aneurysms are slightly more common than CFA aneurysms and occur in patients with demographics typical of degenerative aneurysms. Aneurysms in otherwise

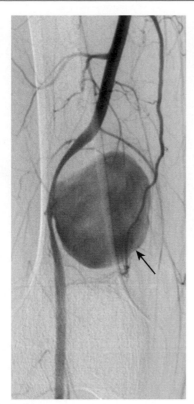

FIGURE 15-31. One of many peripheral pseudoaneurysms *(arrow)*, in this case in the above-knee popliteal artery, that occurred over a period of 3 years in a middle-aged man with Ehlers-Danlos type IV. The patient died of a ruptured iliac artery several years later.

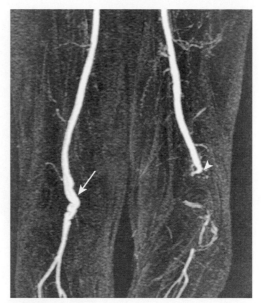

FIGURE 15-32. Coronal maximum intensity projection of gadolinium-enhanced three-dimensional magnetic resonance angiogram of a patient with acute onset of left calf claudication. There is abrupt proximal occlusion of the left popliteal artery *(arrowhead)* with distal reconstitution. On the right there is a patent right popliteal artery aneurysm *(arrow)*. An ultrasound confirmed a thrombosed popliteal artery aneurysm on the left that was bypassed surgically.

normal young patients or the SFA, PFA, and tibial arteries are rare and should prompt evaluation for an unusual etiology such as Ehlers-Danlos syndrome (Fig. 15-31).

Popliteal Artery Aneurysm

Popliteal artery aneurysms (artery diameter > 2 cm) are bilateral in 50%, with a male-to-female ratio of about 15:1 and association with concomitant CFA aneurysms in approximately 40%. About 40% of patients with unilateral popliteal aneurysms have concurrent abdominal aortic aneurysms (AAAs), whereas three fourths of patients with bilateral popliteal artery aneurysms have AAA. However, only 14% of patients with AAA have popliteal aneurysms. The etiology is degenerative in more than 90% of cases. Mural thrombus is common. On physical examination the popliteal artery pulse feels generous. Distal pulses may be diminished or reduced. The entire popliteal artery may be aneurysmal, but focal aneurysms most often involve the vessel above the joint line.

The most feared complications of popliteal artery aneurysms are acute limb ischemia (25%) due to thrombosis and distal embolization of mural thrombus. About 25% present with claudication and only 3% with rupture. Compression of the adjacent vein can cause deep vein thrombosis. Just over 40% of patients are asymptomatic.

Imaging of patients with suspected popliteal artery aneurysms should include the abdominal aorta and both popliteal arteries. The calcified wall of the aneurysm may be visible on plain radiographs. Ultrasound is an excellent initial diagnostic modality for patients with suspected popliteal artery aneurysms. The presence of mural thrombus in a large popliteal artery is diagnostic of an aneurysm even when the diameter is less than 2 cm. A proportionally large popliteal artery in the setting of diffuse arteriomegaly does not constitute an aneurysm. The entire length of the popliteal artery and the contralateral popliteal artery should be

studied. MRA (gadolinium-enhanced) and CTA can detect the aneurysm as well as image the tibial runoff (Fig. 15-32). Angiography is useful for accurate delineation of the runoff before intervention, but can fail to detect aneurysms that are noncalcified and lined with mural thrombus.

Popliteal artery aneurysms require treatment before development of symptoms. Almost half of patients with asymptomatic aneurysms develop distal ischemia within 5 years. Surgical excision and bypass was the traditional treatment for all symptomatic aneurysms and asymptomatic aneurysms that exceed 2 cm in diameter. Stent-grafts are increasingly being used to exclude popliteal artery aneurysms. Adequate segments of normal artery are necessary proximal and distal to the aneurysm. The stent-graft must cross the knee joint, so a flexible, compressible device is necessary (Fig. 15-33). Endograft repair of popliteal aneurysms has a primary assisted patency at 3 years of 87%, with 11% of patients experiencing graft thrombosis and a less than 4% rate of limb loss. Dual antiplatelet therapy has been recommended after endograft placement.

Thrombolysis of an acutely thrombosed popliteal artery aneurysm can be beneficial for recovery of distal runoff provided that degree of ischemia does not require immediate intervention. Coaxial systems are useful in this setting, in that a microinfusion catheter can be positioned in one of the tibial runoff arteries while the larger 5-French infusion catheter remains in the popliteal artery. However, it is not necessary to eliminate all of the thrombus in the aneurysm. These patients may be at higher risk for distal embolization during thrombolysis when there is a large amount of thrombus in the aneurysm.

Common Femoral Artery Aneurysm

True aneurysms of the CFA are usually degenerative in origin, whereas most pseudoaneurysms are related to angiographic procedures or surgical anastomoses. The clinical course of degenerative aneurysms is not well understood, but thrombosis in up to 15%, distal embolization in up to 10%, and rupture in 1%-5% have been reported. Patients can present with groin pain, a pulsatile mass, or compression of adjacent nerves or veins. Degenerative

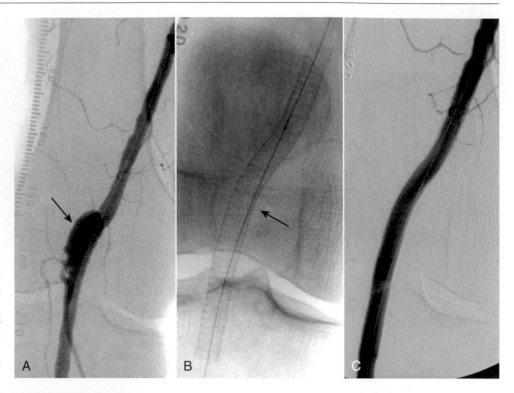

Figure 15-33. Endograft repair of a popliteal artery aneurysm. **A,** Digital subtraction angiogram (DSA) showing the popliteal artery aneurysm *(arrow)* with normal diameter artery above and below. **B,** Digital spot image after deployment of the stent-graft *(arrow)* and gentle balloon angioplasty at both ends. **C,** DSA confirming exclusion of the aneurysm by the endograft.

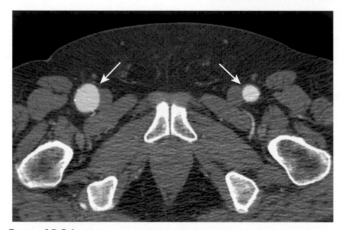

Figure 15-34. Contrast-enhanced computed tomography scan showing bilateral degenerative common femoral artery aneurysms *(arrows)* in a patient with an abdominal aortic aneurysm. The aneurysm is 2.7 cm in diameter on the right and 1.5 cm on the left.

aneurysms are found most often in older men and are bilateral in more than 70% of cases. The normal CFA averages about 9 mm in diameter in adult men. A diameter of 2 cm is therefore considered an aneurysm, and a diameter of 2.5 cm is considered an indication for intervention (Fig. 15-34). The imaging modality that is used most often to evaluate the CFA for aneurysms is ultrasound. In postoperative patients, an important distinction is the difference between the generous hood of a graft and an aneurysm; a diameter greater than 2 cm and the presence of mural thrombus are helpful clues that an aneurysm is present. When a degenerative or anastomotic aneurysm is found, MRA or CTA should be obtained to evaluate the aortic and pelvic vessels for additional aneurysms. Angiography may be required for complex lesions or when distal embolization is suspected. When possible, it is best to avoid percutaneous arterial access through a CFA aneurysm or pseudoaneurysm because compression can be difficult.

Postcatheterization false aneurysms occur in up to 5% of patients undergoing cardiac catheterization when arterial closure

devices are not used. The incidence is less than 1% in most interventional radiology practices. Patients present with groin or retroperitoneal hematomas, groin pain, a pulsatile mass, and a new bruit within 24-48 hours of the procedure (see Fig. 3-7). Patients with large groin hematomas may harbor pseudoaneurysms despite the lack of a palpable pulsatile mass. The artery of origin may be the CFA, SFA, PFA, or a small branch. Groin pseudoaneurysms (especially small) thrombose spontaneously in more than 90% of patients, but rupture can occur in up to 3%. Treatment with ultrasound-guided compression or ultrasound-guided thrombin injection can effectively obliterate up to 90% of puncture-related pseudoaneurysms (Fig. 15-35; see also Chapter 4). Patients with Ehlers-Danlos syndrome and Behçet disease are at particularly high risk for development of puncture-site pseudoaneurysms.

Anastomotic pseudoaneurysms occur in 3% of all femoral surgical anastomoses. The rate of complication (rupture, distal embolization, and thrombosis) is low when the diameter of the anastomotic aneurysm is less than 2 cm. Graft degeneration and infection are potential etiologies in this setting, so discovery of one anastomotic pseudoaneurysm should prompt evaluation of all anastomoses of the graft.

Persistent Sciatic Artery Aneurysm

The embryology of persistent sciatic arteries is described earlier under Anatomy (see Fig. 15-4). Aneurysmal degeneration complicates 50% of persistent sciatic arteries. These aneurysms occur distal to the sciatic notch, probably as a result of repetitive trauma to the superficially located anomalous vessel (Fig. 15-36). Patients present with thrombosis, distal embolization or a mass lesion in the buttock, but rupture is rare. The rate of limb loss is almost 18% in symptomatic patients.

The diagnosis of asymptomatic persistent sciatic artery is usually made during preintervention imaging in patients with claudication. On MRA and CTA, the SFA is hypoplastic or absent, while the internal iliac artery is enlarged and continues into the posterior thigh through the greater sciatic foramen to the popliteal artery. Aneurysms can be large, calcified, and filled with thrombus, and have been confused with soft tissue neoplasms. At angiography, a large posterior branch of the internal iliac artery

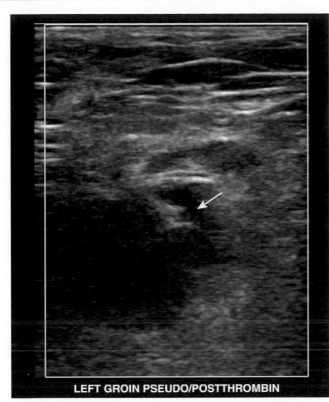

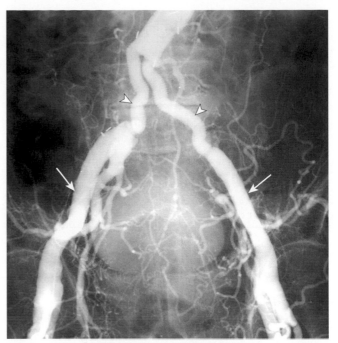

FIGURE 15-37. Pelvic angiogram of an older man with arteriomegaly. The patient was 5 feet 6 inches tall and had previously undergone aorto–bi-iliac graft placement *(arrowheads)* for abdominal aortic aneurysm. The diameter of the limbs of the surgical graft is 12 mm. The external iliac *(arrows)* and common femoral arteries dwarf the large surgical graft. The patient also had diffusely large superficial femoral arteries and bilateral popliteal artery aneurysms.

FIGURE 15-35. Color Doppler image of the same pseudoaneurysm as shown in Figure 3-7B 3 minutes after injection of 500 U of thrombin through a 21-gauge needle *(arrow)* introduced directly into the pseudoaneurysm using sterile technique, local anesthetic, and ultrasound guidance. There is no flow in the aneurysm. The concentration of thrombin was 1000 U/mL, and injection is performed slowly to prevent reflux into the normal artery. Injection should not be performed if there is an arteriovenous fistula associated with the pseudoaneurysm.

is seen continuing into the thigh, often with a small external iliac artery and CFA.

The treatment of persistent sciatic artery aneurysms has classically been surgical excision or exclusion with restoration of inline runoff to the popliteal artery. Stent-graft treatment in selected patients is feasible.

ARTERIOMEGALY

Arteriomegaly is a distinct condition of unknown etiology in which there is diffuse ectasia of the aorta, iliac, and femoropopliteal arteries (Fig. 15-37). As many as one third of patients also have focal, discrete aneurysms superimposed on generalized ectasia, especially of the femoral and popliteal arteries. Most common in men, this condition has been reported in up to 5% of patients undergoing imaging for aortic aneurysms.

TRAUMA

The extremities are the site of injury in one third of all civilian patients with vascular trauma. The predominant mechanisms are penetrating and blunt trauma. Penetrating trauma is more common in urban locations, whereas blunt injury is more prevalent in rural settings. The rate of limb loss with major injuries is less than 15%, but dysfunction due to associated bone and nerve injury occurs in about one fourth of the remaining patients.

Penetrating Trauma

Penetrating trauma from projectiles, stabbing devices, or bone fragments can cause a spectrum of vascular injuries (see Table 1-12). In the civilian population bullets are responsible for 64%, knives for 24%, and shotgun pellets for 12% of penetrating injuries.

The initial evaluation and management of a patient with penetrating extremity trauma should focus initially on diagnosis and

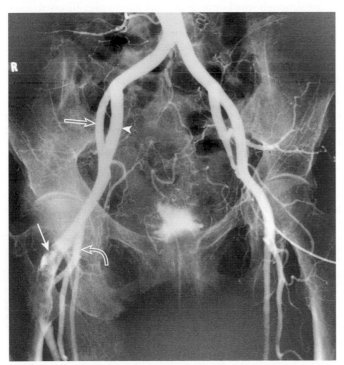

FIGURE 15-36. Angiogram of a persistent sciatic artery with aneurysmal degeneration. On the right the internal iliac artery *(arrowhead)* is larger than the external iliac artery *(open arrow)*. There is an aneurysm of the persistent sciatic artery partially filled with thrombus *(arrow)* in the upper posterior thigh. The right common femoral artery *(curved arrow)* is smaller than normal.

Box 15-9. Signs of Vascular Injury

HARD
Active arterial hemorrhage
Thrill or bruit
Expanding hematoma
Extremity ischemia
Pulse deficit

SOFT
Adjacent fracture
Adjacent nerve injury
Stable hematoma
Delayed or decreased capillary refill
History of hypotension or bleeding
Extensive soft tissue injury

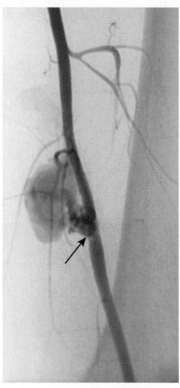

FIGURE 15-38. Digital subtraction angiogram of the extremity in a patient with a gunshot wound to the medial thigh and an expanding hematoma. Distal pulses were intact. There is a pseudoaneurysm *(arrow)* of the superficial femoral artery at the adductor canal.

treatment of lethal truncal or head injuries. Once these issues have been addressed, the mechanism of injury to the extremity should be ascertained if possible. The wound should be examined for bleeding, expanding hematoma, or other "hard" signs of vascular injury (Box 15-9 and Fig. 15-38). A complete pulse examination with determination of an ABI is crucial. Patients with a normal ABI (>1) and a normal physical examination have a 9% incidence of vascular injury. Almost all of these injuries are minor (e.g., small nonobstructing intimal flaps) or confined to branch vessels. The incidence of injury increases to 20% when patients have soft signs of injury or an ABI less than 1 (assuming baseline normal arteries). Patients with a pulse deficit, neurologic deficit, or shotgun injury have a 40% incidence of vascular injury (Fig. 15-39).

Angiography was at one time performed emergently on every patient presenting with a penetrating injury in the vicinity (within 1 cm of the expected course) of a major runoff vessel. The overall positive rate for clinically important vascular injuries was

less than 10%. Imaging of patients with penetrating extremity trauma is now reserved for those with clinical findings suggestive of injury (unless the mechanism of injury was a shotgun blast). All other asymptomatic patients with normal pulses do not require imaging regardless of the proximity of the injury to a major runoff vessel. These patients are observed for 12-24 hours and then released if the examination remains normal. Conversely, patients with a profoundly ischemic limb or active hemorrhage from the wound should proceed directly to surgery. Stable patients with viable limbs but a diminished ABI or clinical signs of vascular injury are suitable candidates for imaging.

The use of ultrasound has been investigated extensively as a diagnostic tool in this patient population. The sensitivity and specificity for major vascular injury are reported to each exceed 95% when a skilled sonographer performs and interprets the study. When patients are undergoing CT for evaluation of head or truncal injury, continuation of the scan through the area of interest may identify an injury. Dedicated lower-extremity CTA in trauma patients has more than 95% sensitivity and specificity for detecting clinically important arterial injury. Angiography is a useful examination in selected patients in whom catheter-based therapy such as stent-graft placement or embolization may be feasible.

Before angiography for extremity trauma, the entry and exit wounds should be identified to ensure that the entire region at risk is included in the imaging field. Inflow studies are only necessary when pulses proximal to the wound are abnormal. Penetrating injury in the upper thigh may involve branches of the profunda femoris or inferior gluteal arteries. At least two views through the area of suspected injury are necessary to exclude subtle intimal injuries. When a pulse deficit is present, the distal runoff should be imaged.

The treatment of penetrating injuries varies with the type and extent of the injury. Small intimal flaps and arteriovenous fistulas frequently heal spontaneously. Injuries to branch vessels can be effectively managed with coil embolization. Open repair is the standard treatment for major injuries to the SFA or popliteal artery, although small stent-grafts may have a role. Injury to a single tibial artery can be managed with coil occlusion or ligation if appropriate but open reconstruction is recommended when more than one artery is traumatically occluded.

Knee Dislocation

Knee dislocations receive special consideration in terms of the risk of vascular injury. The massive force required to create this injury, coupled with the fixed position of the popliteal artery in relation to the knee joint, results in arterial injury in 30%-40% of dislocations. Posterior dislocations have a higher risk for vascular injury than anterior dislocations (Fig. 15-40). Popliteal artery occlusion is tolerated poorly in normal individuals owing to the sparse collateral supply to the lower leg. Patients presenting with a critically ischemic limb after a knee dislocation have a 20% rate of amputation despite aggressive revascularization.

The physical examination should focus on the integrity of the distal pulses and the presence of hard signs of vascular injury. Only 2% of patients with entirely normal vascular examinations before and after reduction of the knee will have a vascular injury. The ABI should be greater than 0.9 in the absence of known peripheral arterial disease. However, a low threshold for imaging should be maintained when the physical examination is not absolutely satisfactory. Patients with an ischemic limb should proceed directly to surgery.

Most patients with knee dislocation with a suspected vascular injury by history or examination can be imaged with CTA or color-flow duplex ultrasound. The advantage of CTA is that the bony structures can be imaged as well to visualize fractures not seen on plain x-ray studies. Angiography is used when vascular injury is suspected but CTA or ultrasound is normal or equivocal.

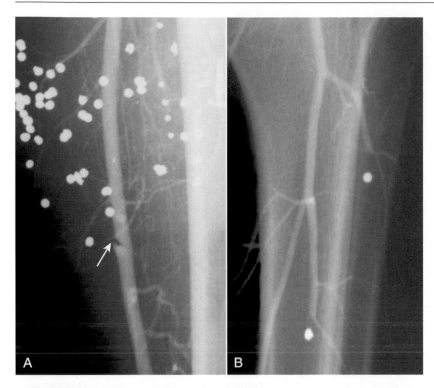

FIGURE 15-39. Patient with absent dorsalis pedis pulse following shotgun injuries to the thigh. **A,** Magnified view of superficial femoral artery (SFA) angiogram showing an intimal flap *(arrow)* in the proximal SFA. There are numerous lead pellets in the surrounding soft tissues. **B,** Magnified view of the proximal tibial arteries showing intraluminal pellets occluding the anterior tibial and peroneal arteries. The lead pellets entered the SFA through the proximal injury and became emboli.

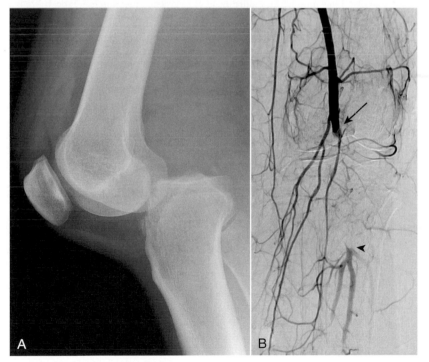

FIGURE 15-40. Arterial thrombosis associated with knee dislocation. **A,** Radiograph showing posterior dislocation of the knee. Following reduction, the distal pulses were not palpable and the foot was cool and pale. **B,** Digital subtraction angiogram showing thrombosis of the popliteal artery between the muscular branches proximally *(arrow)* and the origin of the anterior tibial artery *(arrowhead)*. At surgery the intima was disrupted in this region; the segment of popliteal artery was excised and a short vein graft was placed.

Multiple views, including a true lateral or steep oblique, should be obtained. Typical findings include intimal tears, spasm, and thrombosis. Minor intimal lesions may be managed conservatively with antiplatelet medications, whereas major injuries are treated surgically.

▬ VASCULITIS

The most prevalent large-vessel inflammatory-type disease of the lower extremities is thromboangiitis obliterans (Buerger disease). The incidence is thought to be 12.6/100,000 in the United States. The lower extremities are affected by thromboangiitis obliterans more often than the upper extremities. More than 60% of patients present with intermittent claudication, and 46% have ischemic ulcers. Thromboangiitis obliterans should be suspected in any patient presenting with symptoms of peripheral vascular disease before age 45 years. There is a strong association with tobacco abuse and male gender. Heavy cannabis use is associated with a similar pattern of peripheral arterial disease. The pathology of thromboangiitis obliterans is discussed in Chapter 1; in summary, the acute phase is characterized by inflammatory intraluminal thrombus, and the chronic phase is characterized by fibrosis with preservation of the internal elastic lamina.

Patients with thromboangiitis obliterans frequently have severe symptoms of peripheral vascular disease; critical limb ischemia is the presenting state in 80% of cases. Noninvasive testing usually indicates obstruction at the infrapopliteal level. There are no characteristic findings at MRA or CTA that distinguish thromboangiitis obliterans from conventional atherosclerosis other than the distribution of the disease. The conventional angiographic findings are striking (Box 15-10; see also Fig. 1-17). Cessation of smoking is crucial to arrest progression of disease, and intense wound care is required to heal ulcers. Recent reports of angioplasty of the tibial and pedal arteries with the goal of establishing inline flow to the foot through one artery suggest a role for endovascular therapy. Surgical bypass is more often performed with bypass to a target pedal vessel. However, amputation is common, especially when the patient continues to smoke, which reduces the already poor primary patency of surgical bypass at 1 year from 41% to 20%.

Other large vessel vasculitides are rare in the lower extremities, but include Behçet disease, acquired immunodeficiency syndrome–related vasculitis, and systemic lupus erythematosus.

■ POPLITEAL ARTERY ENTRAPMENT

Two forms of popliteal artery entrapment have been described: functional and anatomic. The normal anatomic relationships of the popliteal artery as it exits the popliteal fossa are to pass between the heads of the gastrocnemius muscles and posterior to the popliteus muscle (Fig. 15-41). Patients with functional entrapment syndrome have normal anatomy but hypertrophy of the plantaris, medial gastrocnemius, and soleus muscles. With plantar flexion, the former two muscles compress the artery against the lateral femoral condyle, and the latter muscle compresses the artery against the lateral soleal band. The arteries remain normal in these patients despite repetitive compression. In patients with anatomic entrapment, the popliteal artery has a different relationship to these muscles, which results in compression of the artery with exercise (Table 15-13). This leads first to adventitial thickening and fibrosis, followed by aneurysm formation, thrombosis, and distal embolization.

Anatomic and functional popliteal artery entrapments are mimicked by chronic recurrent exertional compartment syndrome, a more common cause of symmetric calf pain in young athletes. These patients have a normal resting ABI, which may decrease with exercise; normal imaging of the popliteal fossa; and anterior lateral (72%), distal deep posterior (16%), and posterior superficial (12%) compartment pressures greater than or equal to 15 mm Hg.

Popliteal artery entrapment syndrome presents initially as calf and foot claudication during activity. The incidence is thought to be less than 0.2%. Functional entrapment presents in women twice as often as men at a mean age of 26 years and is bilateral in only 14% of cases. Patients are usually highly trained athletes, particularly runners. The resting ABIs are almost always normal in this group, but 40% note paraesthesias.

Anatomic popliteal artery entrapment tends to occur in males (70%) at a mean age of 35 (but sometimes as early as in the second decade), and causes more severe claudication at lower levels of

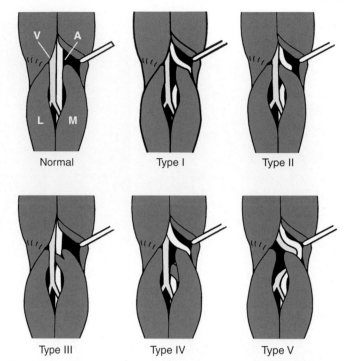

Figure 15-41. Schematic of popliteal artery entrapment (see Table 15-13). (V, Popliteal vein; A, popliteal artery; L, lateral head of gastrocnemius muscle; M, medial head of gastrocnemius muscle.) Type I: Medial deviation of popliteal artery around normal gastrocnemius muscle. Type II: Aberrant lateral insertion of the medial head of the gastrocnemius. Type III: Aberrant lateral slips of medial gastrocnemius muscle. Type IV: Entrapment by popliteus muscle or fibrous band. Artery shown medial to medial head of gastrocnemius muscle in this case. Type V: Entrapment of both popliteal artery and vein. (Adapted from Andrews RT. Diagnostic angiography of the pelvis and lower extremities. *Semin Interv Radiol.* 2000;17:71-111, with permission.)

Table 15-13 Types of Anatomic Entrapment Syndrome

Type	Characteristics
I	Medial deviation of popliteal artery around normal medial insertion of gastrocnemius muscle
II	Aberrant lateral insertion of the medial head of the gastrocnemius muscle causes medial deviation of popliteal artery
III	Aberrant lateral slips of medial gastrocnemius muscle entrap normally situated popliteal artery
IV	Popliteus muscle or fibrous band entraps popliteal artery; the artery may also pass medial to medial head of gastrocnemius muscle in some cases
V	Entrapment of both popliteal artery and vein by medial head of the gastrocnemius muscle

exertion than functional entrapment. Paraesthesias are reported by only 14% of patients. The anatomic abnormality causing entrapment is bilateral in about one third of affected patients but is not always symptomatic on both sides. Patients with anatomic popliteal artery entrapment are at risk for thrombosis (25%) with embolization to the tibial arteries. The resting ABI is abnormal in 30% of patients with anatomic entrapment, which is indicative of distal embolization. In 14% of patients with patent arteries, poststenotic dilatation or aneurysm formation is found.

Imaging with MRI and MRA provides excellent visualization of the aberrant relationship of the artery to the muscles in

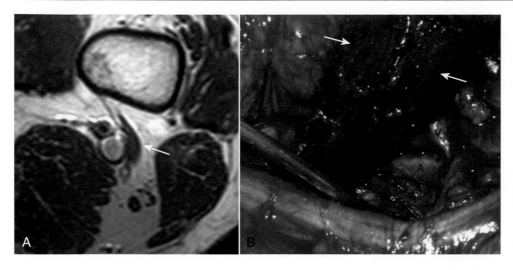

FIGURE 15-42. Anatomic popliteal artery entrapment in a young man with bilateral exercise-induced claudication, much worse on the right. **A,** Axial T1-weighted magnetic resonance image of the right knee shows an accessory slip of muscle *(arrow)* around the popliteal artery and vein. **B,** At surgery (approached from the posterior fossa), the slip of muscle *(arrows)* can be seen overlying the popliteal vein (V) and artery (A) (A variant of type III entrapment).

TABLE 15-14 Imaging Findings of Popliteal Artery Entrapment

Finding	Anatomic	Functional
Popliteal aneurysm (poststenotic)	+	–
Segmental occlusions (popliteal and/or tibial artery)	+	–
Medial deviation of the popliteal artery	+	–
Muscular anomalies in popliteal fossa	+	–
Compression of popliteal artery with stress maneuvers (active plantar flexion, dorsiflexion)	+	+
Hypertrophied normal muscles with normal popliteal artery	–	+

the popliteal fossa in patients with anatomic entrapment (Table 15-14 and Fig. 15-42). The tibial vessels should be included in the examination on the affected side. The contralateral popliteal artery should always be imaged to detect asymptomatic entrapment. Conventional angiography is rarely needed for diagnosis of entrapment, but should be performed with stress maneuvers when the artery is normal on initial images. In order to contract the gastrocnemius muscle, the foot is held in dorsiflexion while the patient tries to forcibly plantar flex (Fig. 15-43). Examination of both popliteal arteries in this fashion is mandatory in any young patient studied for claudication.

The treatment of confirmed functional popliteal artery entrapment involves detachment of the muscles from the medial tibia, partial resection of the plantaris muscle, and detachment of the anterior soleal fascia from the fibula. Anatomic popliteal artery entrapment is also treated surgically with release of the entrapped artery and reconstruction when necessary. Thrombolysis before surgery may recover some tibial arteries when occluded by emboli. Surgical treatment of chronic recurrent exertional compartment syndrome is fasciotomy of the affected compartment.

ADVENTITIAL CYSTIC DISEASE

Adventitial cystic disease is a rare disorder of the adventitia in which a focal accumulation of mucinous fluid compresses the arterial lumen. This entity should be considered in the differential diagnosis of patients presenting with unexplained popliteal artery occlusion, in that 82% of cases have been reported in the

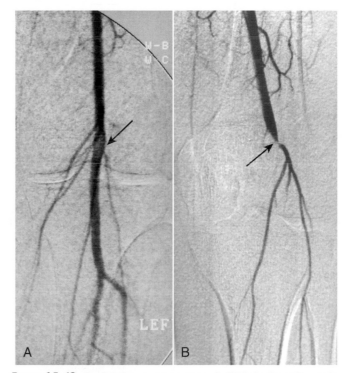

FIGURE 15-43. Popliteal artery entrapment. **A,** Digital subtraction angiogram with the knee extended showing subtle lateral deviation *(arrow)* of the left popliteal artery. **B,** Angiogram of the left popliteal artery with plantar flexion against resistance shows popliteal artery occlusion *(arrow)*. At surgery, type II entrapment was found.

popliteal artery (Box 15-11). Patients are typically men in their fourth or fifth decade who present with claudication. The imaging findings are characteristic, with extrinsic compression of the midportion of the popliteal arterial lumen by a cystic mass (see Fig. 1-41). Ultrasound, CTA, and MRI with MRA sequences are elegant techniques for imaging the cystic mass and the arterial compression. Surgical excision and bypass is the preferred treatment, because cyst aspiration always results in recurrence.

ERGOTISM

Ergot alkaloids are used for treatment of migraine headaches (ergotamine tartrate), for prophylaxis of deep vein thrombosis (dihydroergotamine), and for illicit recreation (lysergic acid diethylamide). An α-adrenergic blocking agent, ergotamine stimulates smooth muscle contraction. Excessive use of ergot alkaloids results in ergotism, with gastrointestinal, neurologic, and vascular symptoms. Patients tend to be younger than would be typical for atherosclerotic disease, with demographics that closely resemble those of the population with migraine headaches. Diffuse vasospasm, more commonly of the lower extremity than upper extremity arteries, results in symptoms of peripheral vascular disease. The aorta, carotid arteries, mesenteric vasculature, and retinal arteries may be affected as well. If left untreated, tissue loss and even gangrene may develop.

At conventional angiography, the stenoses are seen as long and smooth, and in unusual locations. The typical findings of atherosclerosis are usually absent. Remarkably, cessation of the ergot use may result in complete reversal of the occlusive lesions (see Fig. 1-32).

▰ RECONSTRUCTIVE SURGERY

Patients with nonhealing lesions of the extremity related to trauma or infection frequently undergo reconstructive surgical procedures that require tissue transfers. In addition, the proximal fibula is used in some patients as a vascularized bone graft. Preoperative vascular imaging is obtained in these patients to detect anatomic variants, exclude inflow occlusive lesions, and delineate donor or recipient vessels. This is particularly important in older patients in whom the inflow and tibial arteries may be abnormal. Determination of the dominant runoff artery to the foot is important when planning reconstructions.

Box 15-11. Etiologies of Popliteal Artery Occlusion

Atherosclerosis
Embolus
Thrombosis of degenerative aneurysm
Trauma
Popliteal artery entrapment
Adventitial cystic disease

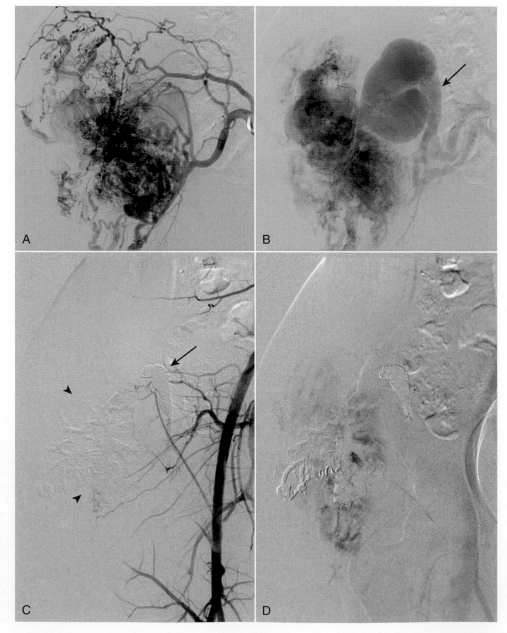

FIGURE 15-44. Arteriovenous malformation (AVM) of the lateral aspect of the right buttock symptomatic for pain and deformity. **A,** Superior gluteal artery digital subtraction angiogram (DSA) showing numerous enlarged feeding arteries and a diffuse arteriovenous malformation with early venous drainage. There was also blood supply from the iliac circumflex arteries and the profunda femoris artery. **B,** Later image from the same angiogram showing a large draining vein *(arrow)*. **C,** DSA with injection into the common iliac artery after staged treatments that included coil embolization of the outflow veins *(arrow)*, transarterial ethanol and glue injections *(arrowheads)*, and direct puncture embolization of the AVM with ethanol and glue. **D,** Very late image from the same injection showing residual nidus but no draining veins. The patient, who was asymptomatic at this point, elected to have the residual AVM resected.

The exact surgical plan should be understood in order to provide appropriate images. When the leg is the donor site, images of the recipient site may be required as well. MRA is used in many centers for this purpose, but conventional angiography remains important for this indication. Biplane views of the areas of interest are useful to fully delineate vascular anatomy.

ARTERIOVENOUS MALFORMATIONS

The lower extremities are a common location for congenital arteriovenous malformations (see Chapter 1). Arteriovenous malformations may be located in and involve any structure in the lower extremity, including skin, muscle, bone, and joints. In the pelvis, the bladder, reproductive organs, and bowel may be involved. Lesions that cause pain, deformity, bleeding, and high-output cardiac failure can sometimes be managed with transcatheter embolization techniques.

Cross-sectional imaging with MRI is useful to determine the extent of the lesion. Embolization of the nidus is essential for effective treatment, but sometimes these are multiple and inaccessible. When possible, occlusion of a dominant venous outflow, ideally temporarily with an occlusion balloon, can facilitate embolization of the arteriovenous malformation by slowing flow through the lesion (Fig. 15-44). Common embolization agents include glue, other polymers, and alcohol (see Chapter 4). Small particles should be avoided whenever large shunts are suspected. Coils placed in arterial inflow vessels have a high failure rate due to distal reconstitution around proximal occlusions. Pain control, antiinflammatory medications including steroids, and frequent neurologic examinations are important immediately after the procedure. Compartment syndrome, nerve dysfunction, skin and muscle necrosis, and pelvic organ dysfunction can occur with embolization. Patients should be carefully counseled that embolization controls, but does not cure, the lesion, and that multiple procedures may be necessary over their lifetime.

SUGGESTED READINGS

Adam DJ, Beard JD, Cleveland T, et al. Bypass versus angioplasty in severe ischaemia of the leg (BASIL): multicentre, randomised controlled trial. *Lancet*. 2005;366:1925-1934.

Ahmad F, Turner SA, Torrie P, Gibson M. Iatrogenic femoral artery pseudoaneurysms a review of current methods of diagnosis and treatment. *Clin Radiol*. 2008;63:1310-1136.

Ansel GM, Lumsden AB. Evolving modalities for femoropopliteal interventions. *J Endovasc Ther*. 2009;16:SII82-SII97.

Arain SA, White CJ. Endovascular therapy for critical limb ischemia. *Vasc Med*. 2008;13:267-279.

Attinger CE, Evans KK, Bulan E, et al. Angiosomes of the foot and ankle and clinical implications for limb salvage: reconstruction, incisions, and revascularization. *Plast Reconstr Surg*. 2006;117:S261-S293.

Balzer JO, Thalhammer A, Khan V, et al. Angioplasty of the pelvic and femoral arteries in PAOD: results and review of the literature. *Eur J Radiol*. 2010;75:48-56.

Bosiers M, Scheinert D, Peeters P, et al. Randomized comparison of everolimus-eluting versus bare-metal stents in patients with critical limb ischemia and infrapopliteal arterial occlusive disease. *J Vasc Surg*. 2012;55:390-398.

Brancaccio G, Celoria GM, Falco E. Ergotism. *J Vasc Surg*. 2008;48:754.

Chan D, Anderson ME, Dolmatch BL. Imaging evaluation of lower extremity infrainguinal disease: role of the noninvasive vascular laboratory, computed tomography angiography, and magnetic resonance angiography. *Tech Vasc Interv Radiol*. 2010;13:11-22.

Collins R, Cranny G, Burch J, et al. A systematic review of duplex ultrasound, magnetic resonance angiography and computed tomography angiography for the diagnosis and assessment of symptomatic, lower limb peripheral arterial disease. *Health Technol Assess*. 2007;11(20):iii-iv, xi-xiii, 1-184.

Conte MS. Bypass versus Angioplasty in Severe Ischaemia of the Leg (BASIL) and the (hoped for) dawn of evidence-based treatment for advanced limb ischemia. *J Vasc Surg*. 2010;51:S69-S75.

Conte MS, Geraghty PJ, Bradbury AW, et al. Suggested objective performance goals and clinical trial design for evaluating catheter-based treatment of critical limb ischemia. *J Vasc Surg*. 2009;50:1462-1473.

Creager MA, Belkin M, Bluth EI, et al. 2012 ACCF/AHA/ACR/SCAI/SIR/STS/SVM/SVN/SVS key data elements and definitions for peripheral atherosclerotic vascular disease. *Circulation*. 2012;125:395-467.

Creager MA, Kaufman JA, Conte MS. Acute limb ischemia. *N Engl J Med*. 2012;366:2198-2206.

Dake MD, Ansel GM, Jaff MR, et al. Paclitaxel-eluting stents show superiority to balloon angioplasty and bare metal stents in femoropopliteal disease: twelve-month Zilver PTX randomized study results. *Circ Cardiovasc Interv*. 2011;4:495-504.

Dake MD, Scheinert D, Tepe G, et al. Nitinol stents with polymer-free paclitaxel coating for lesions in the superficial femoral and popliteal arteries above the knee: twelve-month safety and effectiveness results from the Zilver PTX single-arm clinical study. *J Endovasc Ther*. 2011;18:613-623.

Frans FA, Bipat S, Reekers JA, et al. Systematic review of exercise training or percutaneous transluminal angioplasty for intermittent claudication. *Br J Surg*. 2012;99:16-28.

Foley WD, Stonely T. CT angiography of the lower extremities. *Radiol Clin North Am*. 2010;48:367-396.

Graziani L, Morelli L, Parini F, et al. Clinical outcome after extended endovascular recanalization in Buerger's disease in 20 consecutive cases. *Ann Vasc Surg*. 2012;26:387-395.

Hafez HM, Woolgar J, Robbs JV. Lower extremity arterial injury: results of 550 cases and review of risk factors associated with limb loss. *J Vasc Surg*. 2001;33:1212-1219.

Hirsch AT, Haskal ZJ, Hertzer NR, et al. ACC/AHA 2005 Practice Guidelines for the management of patients with peripheral arterial disease (lower extremity, renal, mesenteric, and abdominal aortic). *Circulation*. 2006;113:e463-e654.

Karnabatidis D, Spiliopoulos S, Tsetis D, Siablis D. Quality improvement guidelines for percutaneous catheter-directed intra-arterial thrombolysis and mechanical thrombectomy for acute lower-limb ischemia. *Cardiovasc Intervent Radiol*. 2011;34:1123-1136.

Kessel DO, Berridge DC, Robertson I. Infusion techniques for peripheral arterial thrombolysis. *Cochrane Database Syst Rev*. 2004(1):CD000985.

Kiernan TJ, Hynes BG, Ruggiero NJ, et al. Comprehensive evaluation and medical management of infrainguinal peripheral artery disease: "when to treat, when not to treat." *Tech Vasc Interv Radiol*. 2010;13:2-10.

Korngold EC, Jaff MR. Unusual causes of intermittent claudication: popliteal artery entrapment syndrome, cystic adventitial disease, fibromuscular dysplasia, and endofibrosis. *Curr Treat Options Cardiovasc Med*. 2009;11:156-166.

Kropman RH, Schrijver AM, Kelder JC, et al. Clinical outcome of acute leg ischaemia due to thrombosed popliteal artery aneurysm: systematic review of 895 cases. *Eur J Vasc Endovasc Surg*. 2010;39:452-457.

Menke J, Larsen J. Meta-analysis: accuracy of contrast-enhanced magnetic resonance angiography for assessing steno-occlusions in peripheral arterial disease. *Ann Intern Med*. 2010;153:325-334.

Met R, Bipat S, Legemate DA, et al. Diagnostic performance of computed tomography angiography in peripheral arterial disease: a systematic review and meta-analysis. *JAMA*. 2009;301:415-424.

Midy D, Berard X, Ferdani M, et al. A retrospective multicenter study of endovascular treatment of popliteal artery aneurysm. *J Vasc Surg*. 2010;51:850-856.

Mohler 3rd E, Giri J. Management of peripheral arterial disease patients: comparing the ACC/AHA and TASC-II guidelines. *Curr Med Res Opin*. 2008;24:2509-2522.

Napoli A, Anzidei M, Zaccagna F, et al. Peripheral arterial occlusive disease: diagnostic performance and effect on therapeutic management of 64-section CT angiography. *Radiology*. 2011;261:976-986.

Norgren L, Hiatt WR, Dormandy JA, et al. Inter-Society Consensus for the Management of Peripheral Arterial Disease (TASC II). *Eur J Vasc Endovasc Surg*. 2007;33:S1-75.

Olin JW, Allie DE, Belkin M, et al. ACCF/AHA/ACR/SCAI/SIR/SVM/SVN/SVS 2010 performance measures for adults with peripheral artery disease. *J Vasc Surg*. 2010;52:1616-1652.

Paravastu SC, Regi JM, Turner DR, et al. A contemporary review of cystic adventitial disease. *Vasc Endovascular Surg*. 2012;46:5-14.

Patterson BM, Agel J, Swiontkowski MF, et al. Knee dislocations with vascular injury: outcomes in the Lower Extremity Assessment Project (LEAP) Study. *J Trauma*. 2007;63:855-858.

Patterson BO, Holt PJ, Cleanthis M, et al. Imaging vascular trauma. *Br J Surg*. 2012;99:494-505.

Piazza G, Creager MA. Thromboangiitis obliterans. *Circulation*. 2010;27:1858-1861.

Rocha-Singh KJ, Jaff MR, Crabtree TR, et al. Performance goals and endpoint assessments for clinical trials of femoropopliteal bare nitinol stents in patients with symptomatic peripheral arterial disease. *Catheter Cardiovasc Interv*. 2007;69:910-919.

Rooke TW, Hirsch AT, Misra S, et al. 2011 ACCF/AHA focused update of the guideline for the management of patients with peripheral artery disease (updating the 2005 guideline). *Vasc Med*. 2011;16:452-476.

Saric M, Kronzon I. Cholesterol embolization syndrome. *Curr Opin Cardiol*. 2011;26:472-479.

Schillinger M, Sabeti S, Loewe C, et al. Balloon angioplasty versus implantation of nitinol stents in the superficial femoral artery. *N Engl J Med*. 2006;354:1879-1888.

Setacci C, De Donato G, Setacci F, Chisci E. Ischemic foot: definition, etiology and angiosome concept. *J Cardiovasc Surg*. 2010;51:223-231.

Sinha S, Houghton J, Holt PJ, et al. Popliteal entrapment syndrome. *J Vasc Surg*. 2012;55:252-262.

Spinosa DJ, Harthun NL, Bissonette EA, et al. Subintimal arterial flossing with antegrade-retrograde intervention (SAFARI) for subintimal recanalization to treat chronic critical limb ischemia. *J Vasc Interv Radiol*. 2005;16:37-44.

Tsilimparis N, Dayama A, Ricotta 2nd JJ. Open and endovascular repair of popliteal artery aneurysms: tabular review of the literature. *Ann Vasc Surg.* 2013;27:259-265.

Turnipseed WD. Functional popliteal artery entrapment syndrome: a poorly understood and often missed diagnosis that is frequently mistreated. *J Vasc Surg.* 2009;49:1189-1195.

Twine CP, Coulston J, Shandall A, McLain AD. Angioplasty versus stenting for superficial femoral artery lesions. *Cochrane Database Syst Rev.* 2009 Apr 15(2):CD006767.

van den Berg JC. Thrombolysis for acute arterial occlusion. *J Vasc Surg.* 2010;52:512-515.

Wain RA, Hines G. A contemporary review of popliteal artery aneurysms. *Cardiol Rev.* 2007;15:102-107.

Ward TJ, Lookstein RA. Drug-eluting stents for infrapopliteal arterial disease in the setting of critical limb ischemia. *Exp Rev Cardiovasc Ther.* 2011;9:1339-1346.

White C. Clinical practice. Intermittent claudication. *N Engl J Med.* 2007;356:1241-1250.

Wright LB, Matchett WJ, Cruz CP, James, et al. Popliteal artery disease: diagnosis and treatment. *Radiographics.* 2004;24:467-479.

Yamamoto H, Yamamoto F, Ishibashi K, et al. Intermediate and long-term outcomes after treating symptomatic persistent sciatic artery using different techniques. *Ann Vasc Surg.* 2011;25:837:e9-e15.

CHAPTER 16

Lower-Extremity Veins

John A. Kaufman, MD, MS, FSIR, FCIRSE

ANATOMY	CHRONIC VENOUS OBSTRUCTION AND POST-PHLEBITIC SYNDROME	KLIPPEL-TRENAUNAY AND PARKES-WEBER SYNDROMES
KEY COLLATERAL PATHWAYS		VENOUS MALFORMATIONS
IMAGING	CHRONIC VENOUS VALVULAR INSUFFICIENCY	VENOUS ANEURYSMS
ACUTE DEEP VEIN THROMBOSIS	SEPTIC THROMBOPHLEBITIS	

Venous pathology is eight times more common in the lower extremities than arterial disease. However, the range of clinically important venous pathology in the lower extremities is relatively narrow, with thrombotic disorders, chronic occlusion, and valvular insufficiency comprising more than 95% of cases. There are an estimated 2,000,000 new cases of deep venous thrombosis (DVT) each year in the United States. Complications of venous thromboembolism are thought to be responsible for 15% of in-hospital deaths. Severe chronic venous stasis with ulceration is believed to affect 3%-8% of the adult population and to cost the health care system more than $1 billion each year. Venous diseases are one of the most important areas of diagnosis and intervention in the current practice of interventional radiology.

ANATOMY

The pelvic veins consist of the external, internal, and common iliac veins. The external iliac vein begins at the inguinal ligament and ends at the merger with the internal iliac vein (Fig. 16-1). This vein is the direct continuation of the drainage of the lower-extremity blood, with small contributions from the anterior abdominal wall through the inferior epigastric veins, and from the pelvis through circumflex iliac and pubic veins. The right external iliac vein is initially located medial to the external iliac artery, but crosses posterior to this vessel before it is joined by the internal iliac vein. The left external iliac vein remains medial to the artery throughout its length. The external iliac vein may have a single valve.

The external and iliac veins join at roughly the level of the sacroiliac joints to form the common iliac veins. This occurs deep in the pelvis, so that the common iliac veins are angled both anteriorly and cranial. The common iliac veins do not have valves. The right common iliac vein has a vertical course posterior to the right common iliac artery. The left common iliac vein is located medial to the left common iliac artery. In order to join the inferior vena cava (IVC) on the right, the left common iliac vein passes underneath the right common iliac artery and anterior to the S1 or L5 vertebral body (see Fig. 13-11). This frequently results in broadening of the left common iliac vein and sometimes functional compression. The confluence of the common iliac veins forms the IVC.

The venous structures of the lower extremities are divided into superficial and deep systems, linked by perforating veins. The perforating veins direct blood from the superficial into the deep system (Fig. 16-2). All veins of the lower extremity normally have valves. In contrast to the upper extremities, the deep veins of the lower extremity are the dominant drainage pathway.

The common femoral vein (CFV) is formed by the confluence of the femoral vein (FV) and profunda femoris vein (PFV). The CFV lies within the femoral sheath medial to the common femoral artery (Fig. 16-3; see also Fig. 2-28). The smaller tributaries include the great saphenous vein (GSV), and the medial and lateral circumflex femoral veins.

The FV extends from the groin, where it is joined by the PFV, to the adductor canal. This vein is frequently referred to as the *superficial femoral vein*, or SFV, because of its anatomic proximity to the superficial femoral artery. However, this nomenclature can cause confusion when trying to distinguish between deep and superficial veins in the extremity, so the term *femoral vein*, or FV, is used in this text. The FV lies slightly deep and lateral to the superficial femoral artery in the thigh (see Figs. 15-3 and 16-3). This vein is duplicated or complex in up to 20% of patients (Fig. 16-4). The adductor canal in the thigh marks the transition of the FV to the popliteal vein. The PFV runs alongside the profunda femoris artery, draining the same muscles that are supplied by this artery. In approximately half of individuals, the PFV communicates directly with the popliteal vein at the level of the adductor canal.

The popliteal vein is formed from the confluence of the tibial veins in the upper third of the calf. In relation to the anterior surface of the leg, the popliteal vein lies posterior to the popliteal artery. In relation to the skin of the popliteal fossa (the posterior surface of the knee joint) it is more superficial (see Fig. 16-3). This vein is duplicated or complex in 35% of the population. In addition to the tibial veins, the gastrocnemius, soleal, and sural veins, and the small saphenous vein (SSV) all drain into the popliteal vein.

The deep veins of the calf are paired structures that parallel each of the three tibial arteries (see Figs. 16-1 and 16-3). The posterior tibial and peroneal veins are larger than the anterior tibial veins owing to the larger muscle mass of the posterior and medial compartments. The posterior tibial vein is a continuation of the venous structures of the plantar surface of the foot, whereas the anterior tibial veins drain the dorsal aspect of the foot. The peroneal vein originates at the level of the ankle. The posterior tibial and peroneal veins are joined by deep muscular branches from the soleus veins in the calf, and perforating branches from the superficial veins. The tibial veins reside in the same fascial compartments as their companion arteries.

The primary components of the superficial veins of the leg are the GSV and the SSV (see Figs. 16-1 and 16-2). These are sometimes referred to as the *long* and *short saphenous veins*, but this text uses GSV and SSV. Both vessels lie within the subcutaneous fat of the lower extremity superficial to the fascial layers of the muscles (Fig. 16-5). The location, toughness, and caliber of these veins contribute to their desirability as conduits for arterial bypass surgery. The GSV has its origins in the veins along the medial edge of the foot. At the ankle the vein becomes the GSV, which ascends along the medial aspect of the leg to join the CFV below the inguinal ligament. The GSV communicates with

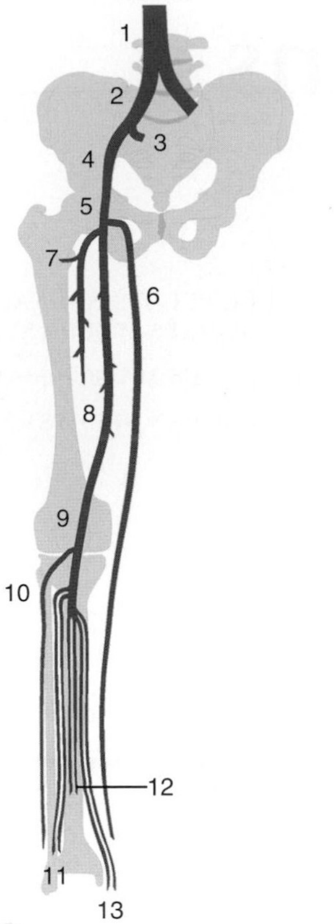

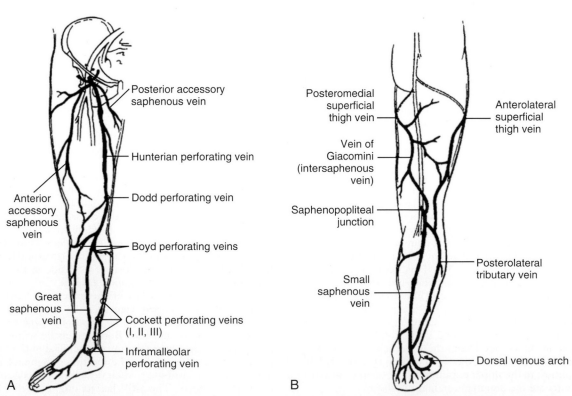

Figure 16-1. Drawing of lower-extremity veins. *1,* Inferior vena cava. *2,* Common iliac vein. *3,* Internal iliac vein. *4,* External iliac vein. *5,* Common femoral vein. *6,* Great saphenous vein. *7,* Profunda femoris vein. *8,* Femoral vein. *9,* Popliteal vein. *10,* Small saphenous vein. *11,* Anterior tibial veins. *12,* Peroneal veins. *13,* Posterior tibial veins.

the deep system along its entire length through small perforating veins. These veins are of great importance in that they drain the saphenous vein into the deep system, where venous return to the heart is assisted by the pumplike action of muscular contraction and relaxation around the veins. Disruption of the valves in the perforating veins allows blood to drain out of the deep into the superficial system, which contributes to varicose veins (dilated, tortuous superficial veins). The GSV receives tributaries from the anterior and posterior accessory GSVs, and variably from the inferior epigastric and external pudendal veins, just before joining the CFV.

The lateral edge of the foot drains into the SSV, a small vein that ascends along the posterior midline of the calf in a groove between the medial and lateral bodies of the gastrocnemius muscle (Fig. 16-6). The SSV joins the popliteal vein at or just below the knee joint. In some patients, the SSV also communicates with medial branches of the GSV through the vein of Giacomini, also known as the *intersaphenous* vein (see Fig. 16-2).

■ KEY COLLATERAL PATHWAYS

The deep venous system of the lower extremity provides collateral drainage for the superficial veins and vice versa. The drainage afforded by just one system alone is frequently sufficient to avoid swelling and discomfort in a prolonged upright posture. Obstruction of the CFV and external iliac vein results in drainage through the profunda femoral veins to the internal iliac veins via gluteal and other pelvic veins. In addition, drainage through the ipsilateral abdominal wall veins and across the perineum to the contralateral CFV can occur (Fig. 16-7).

Occlusion of one internal iliac vein results in drainage through the contralateral vessel. When both vessels are occluded, venous drainage through ascending lumbar, gonadal, and even inferior mesenteric veins can occur. Isolated occlusion of one common iliac vein results in retrograde flow in the ipsilateral internal iliac vein with cross-pelvic collateralization to the contralateral internal

Figure 16-2. Drawings of the superficial veins of the leg. **A,** The great saphenous vein with tributary and perforating veins. **B,** Posterior superficial veins. (Modified from Bergan JJ. Varicose veins: treatment by surgery and sclerotherapy. In Rutherford RB, ed. *Vascular Surgery,* 5th ed. Philadelphia: WB Saunders, 2000, with permission.)

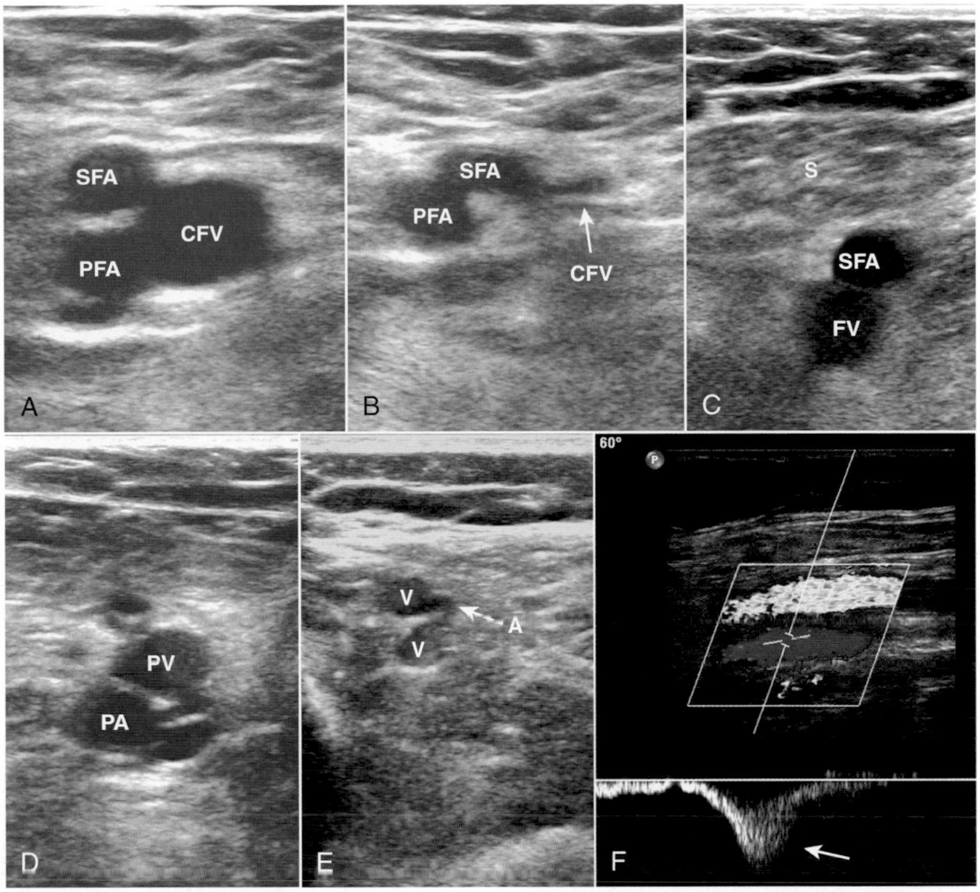

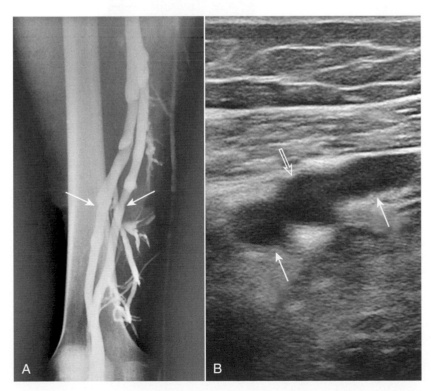

FIGURE 16-3. Anatomic relationships of the lower-extremity veins and arteries demonstrated on ultrasound. **A,** The right common femoral vein (CFV) lies medial to the right superficial femoral artery (SFA) and profunda femoral artery (PFA). **B,** When the ultrasound probe is used to apply pressure over the vein, the normal low-pressure vein collapses but the high-pressure arteries remain visible. **C,** In the thigh, the femoral vein (FV) travels lateral and deep to the SFA. Both structures lie below the sartorius muscle (S). **D,** The popliteal vein (PV) lies more superficial to the popliteal artery (PA) in relationship to the popliteal fossa (at the top of the image). Smaller arterial and venous branches are also visualized. **E,** The paired posterior tibial veins (V) bracket the single posterior tibial artery (A). **F,** Normal transient increased venous flow in the FV with calf compression (augmentation), indicating patency of the popliteal and femoral veins.

FIGURE 16-4. **A,** Contrast venogram showing duplicated popliteal and femoral veins *(arrows)*. **B,** Axial ultrasound image showing duplicated femoral vein in the thigh *(solid arrows)* bracketing the superficial femoral artery *(open arrow)*.

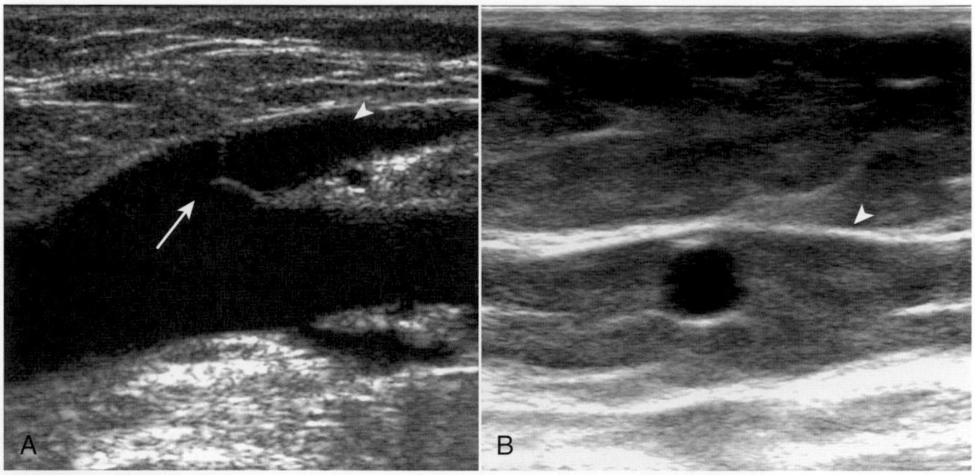

FIGURE 16-5. Ultrasound appearance of the normal great saphenous vein (GSV). **A,** Ultrasound showing valve leaflets *(arrow)* at the insertion of the GSV *(arrowhead)* into the common femoral vein, the saphenofemoral junction. **B,** The GSV in the distal thigh within the saphenous subcompartment bounded by the saphenous fascia anteriorly *(arrowhead)* and the deep fascia posteriorly. In the axial plane this compartment has a characteristic elliptical shape.

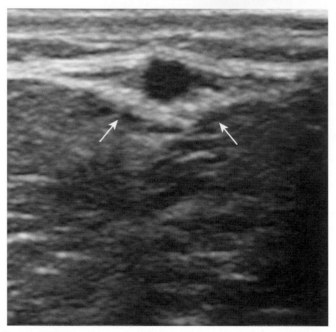

FIGURE 16-6. Ultrasound appearance of the normal small saphenous vein in the upper calf. In this thin patient, the vein lies within the groove *(arrows)* between the medial and lateral heads of the gastrocnemius muscle.

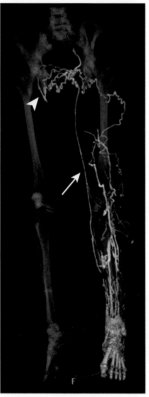

FIGURE 16-7. Digital computed tomography venogram showing chronic occlusions of the left popliteal, femoral, and iliac veins. Venous drainage of the lower extremity is via the left great saphenous vein *(arrow)* and unnamed collateral veins. At the pelvis the veins drain across the pubic region and lower abdomen to the right *(arrowhead)*. The scan was obtained by injecting dilute contrast (50-60 mg iodine/mL) through an intravenous catheter in the foot with a tourniquet around the ankle. The leg was scanned foot to pelvis after a 120-second delay. (Courtesy Constantino Pena MD, Miami, Fla.)

iliac vein. Occlusion of both the common and external iliac veins results in drainage through the pubic, inferior epigastric, and lumbar veins. Additional collateral drainage by lumbar, paraspinal, and other retroperitoneal veins can also occur. Occlusion of both common iliac veins is functionally identical to obstruction of the infrarenal IVC.

▬ IMAGING

Ultrasound is the primary imaging modality for the lower-extremity venous system. The procedure carries virtually no risk, can be successfully performed in most patients, and provides both anatomic and functional data. Massive obesity, severe edema, external orthopedic hardware, and large areas of abnormal skin can limit the study. The venous system from the tibial veins to the proximal CFV can be imaged with a 5- to 7.5-MHz linear transducer (see Fig. 16-3). Lower frequency transducers may be required in large patients and for the iliac veins. Superficial veins, such as the GSV, can be imaged with a 10-MHz transducer (see

Figs. 16-5 and 16-6). Imaging of the pelvic veins with ultrasound is inconsistent owing to the depth and tortuosity of the vessels.

A complete examination involves visualization of all portions of the venous system from the iliac veins to the ankle. The ultrasound transducer is used to compress the infrainguinal veins, which is not possible in the pelvis. Color-flow Doppler evaluation can determine patency and flow direction. The walls of the vein should coapt with gentle pressure (see Fig. 16-3A and **B**). Non-compressibility is diagnostic of an intraluminal abnormality, usually

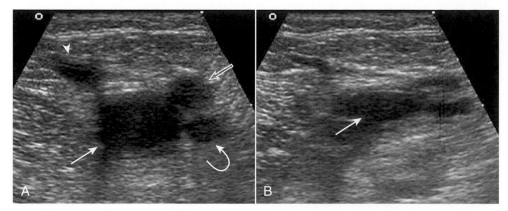

FIGURE 16-8. Noncompressible common femoral vein (CFV) due to acute deep vein thrombosis. **A,** Ultrasound image showing the hypoechoic CFV *(arrow)*. The great saphenous vein *(arrowhead)* is visible medially, and the superficial femoral artery (SFA; *open arrow*) and profunda femoral artery (PFA; *curved arrow*) laterally. **B,** With enough compression to collapse the SFA and PFA, the CFV is still noncompressed *(arrow)*, indicating acute deep venous thrombosis. Compare with Figure 16-3A and **B.**

TABLE **16-1** Ultrasound Appearance of Intraluminal Venous Filling Defects

Etiology	Ultrasound Appearance
Acute thrombus	Expanded vein, hypoechoic lumen, noncompressible vein Flow absent or around margins of filling defect
Chronic thrombus	Contracted vein, lumen partially or completely filled with hyperechoic material May have flow though center of lumen or small channels
Valve leaflet	Thin, linear, usually paired structure with mobile free margins in center of lumen

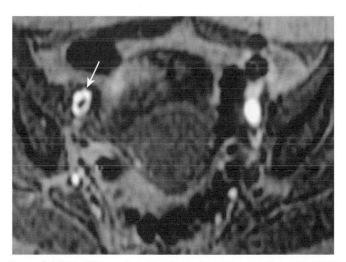

FIGURE 16-9. Axial image from a two-dimensional time-of-flight (2-D TOF) magnetic resonance venogram showing nonocclusive thrombus in the right external iliac vein *(arrow)*.

a thrombus (Fig. 16-8 and Table 16-1). The normal response to Valsalva maneuver is cessation of flow; a blunted response indicates proximal obstruction, and retrograde flow indicates valvular insufficiency (see Fig. 3-5). The patency of nonvisualized segments can be assessed indirectly by measuring the Doppler signal central to the area of interest while gently squeezing the calf ("augmentation") (see Fig. 16-3). A sudden increase in velocity or flow is the expected normal response.

The femoral and popliteal veins can be imaged with the patient supine or in slight reverse Trendelenburg (head up, foot down). A tourniquet at the knee or dangling the calf over the edge of the examination table may be required to optimally visualize the calf veins.

Diameter measurements and mapping of the superficial veins are frequently performed before harvest for surgical bypass. The course of the saphenous veins and the major branch points should be marked on the skin with indelible ink.

Magnetic resonance venography (MRV) of the lower-extremity veins using two-dimensional time-of-flight (2-D TOF) or contrast-enhanced three-dimensional (3-D) gradient-echo techniques can be used to image the lower-extremity and pelvic veins. When 2-D TOF sequences are used, a superior saturation band with slice thicknesses of 5-8 mm eliminates arterial signal (Fig. 16-9). Complex flow patterns in the pelvis frequently result in signal loss in the external iliac veins as they enter the pelvis and at the confluence with the internal iliac veins. Contrast-enhanced sequences are not susceptible to flow artifacts, although arterial signal can be confusing unless subtraction software is available. Blood-pool contrast agents are very useful

for venous imaging. Anatomic sequences are important when venous compression by an adjacent mass is suspected.

The low cost and ready availability of ultrasound limits the need for MRV in most patients with lower-extremity venous disease. Lower-extremity magnetic resonance imaging (MRI) with MRV sequences is useful in the evaluation of venous malformations, congenital abnormalities of venous anatomy, and suspected isolated pelvic deep vein thrombosis.

Lower-extremity CT venography (i.e., infusion of contrast via a foot vein) is feasible with multidetector row technology (see Fig. 16-7). In general, lower-extremity venous imaging with CT is performed by imaging during the venous phase of a conventional injection of contrast (Fig. 16-10). Venous phase imaging of the lower extremities and pelvis can be combined with pulmonary artery CTA in the evaluation of patients with suspected pulmonary embolism (PE). Arterial enhancement is always present, which can make identification of small and weakly opacified veins difficult. CT is an excellent choice when compression of iliac veins by a pelvic mass is suspected as the etiology of lower-extremity swelling.

Conventional contrast venography is rarely necessary. Ascending venography is performed with the patient on a tilting procedure table oriented for a reverse Trendelenburg position. A block is placed under the foot of the leg opposite the side under study. This allows the patients to support their weight on the normal leg

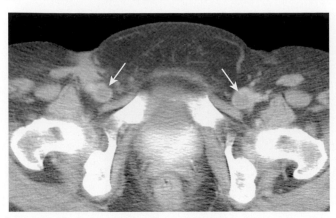

FIGURE 16-10. Axial image from contrast-enhanced computed tomography performed to look for a postoperative abscess, showing enlarged common femoral vein bilaterally *(arrows)* with low-attenuation centers and enhancement of the vein wall. These findings are diagnostic of acute thrombosis.

when the table is tilted. A 21-gauge or smaller butterfly needle or intravenous catheter is inserted into a vein on the dorsum of the foot and secured in place. Ideally, the tip of the needle should be oriented toward the toes, but most of the time one is satisfied with any usable access. Finding a vein can be a challenge in patients with edematous feet. Application of gentle pressure with a thumb or two fingers can displace the edema and reveal a usable vein in these patients.

Low osmolar contrast with 30% iodine should be used. The contrast is loaded into three or four 50-mL syringes. The table is tilted head-up 30-60 degrees with all weight-bearing on the leg opposite to the side of interest. A tourniquet is placed around the ankle to force contrast into the deep system. Hand injection is used to control the amount of contrast in the veins during the study. The initial injection of 5-10 mL of contrast is watched fluoroscopically as it exits the needle (Fig. 16-11). At the same time, the patient is questioned regarding pain at the injection site. The injection is stopped for obvious extravasation or persistent pain.

Filling of the venous system is monitored by intermittent fluoroscopy during continuous hand injection of contrast. The calf veins will be opacified in most patients with 50-80 mL of contrast. Images are obtained in three projections (anteroposterior and both obliques) using a large field of view coned side-to-side. Magnification views should be obtained of any area of question. Digital subtraction venography is usually not performed because contrast clears too slowly from the veins, resulting in poor image quality on subsequent images.

The contrast is followed as it ascends the leg. The saphenous vein, when opacified, should be included on the films. The iliac veins are filled by compressing the femoral vein, repositioning the table so that the patient is either flat or in mild Trendelenburg position, then releasing the femoral vein compression. The contrast-filled leg then empties into the iliac veins and proximal IVC.

When the study is completed, the foot is connected to an infusion of sterile saline or 5% dextrose solution. A minimum of 150-200 mL is infused to flush the contrast from the leg before removing the needle. Traditionally, an abdominal film is obtained after each venogram to evaluate renal excretion and contours.

Venography is a safe procedure, but requires 100-150 mL of contrast per limb and is time consuming. The overall complication rate is less than 5%.

◼ ACUTE DEEP VEIN THROMBOSIS

Thrombosis of the deep veins of the lower extremity is thought to occur in adults with a yearly incidence of 1 per 1000. The cumulative risk of developing venous thromboembolism by the age of 80 years may be as high as 11% in men. Acute DVT is rare

in children. The coagulation pathway is discussed in Chapter 1. A number of conditions are believed to or are known to predispose patients to development of DVT (Box 16-1). Nonocclusive thrombus is believed to form first in an area of slow flow in a valve cusp, followed by central propagation and occlusion.

DVT is left sided in 38% of cases, right sided in 32%, and bilateral in the remainder. The thrombus extends above the inguinal ligament in 8% of cases, between the knee and the inguinal ligament in 27%, and is isolated to the calf in almost 65%. Thrombosis limited to the iliac veins is unusual (<3%) and is often related to a pelvic mass, May-Thurner syndrome (see Chronic Venous Obstruction and Post-phlebitic Syndrome), or extension of internal iliac vein thrombus.

Asymptomatic PE is common in patients with proximal DVT, with up to 80% having abnormal results on pulmonary artery imaging. Conversely, DVT can be demonstrated in 80% of patients with symptomatic PE. Approximately 20%-30% of patients with symptomatic DVT also present with symptomatic PE. The risk of PE is higher with proximal thrombus (extending above the popliteal vein), but PE also occurs in approximately 10% of patients with isolated calf DVT. Post-thrombotic syndrome (see next section) occurs in 40%-60% of patients within 5 years of their first episode of thrombosis.

The clinical diagnosis of DVT is suggested by symptoms of leg swelling, pain, tenderness on deep palpation, erythema, and pain on dorsiflexion of the foot ("Homan sign"). The accuracy of these clinical clues as independent indicators of DVT, however, is widely accepted to be in the vicinity of only 50%. Assessment of patient risk factors improves the positive predictive value of the physical examination and serologic tests for DVT (Table 16-2). Many other common conditions can cause symptoms similar to acute DVT, such as heart failure, trauma, chronic venous insufficiency, and cellulitis. For these reasons, further diagnostic evaluation is necessary to establish the diagnosis.

Lower-extremity arterial insufficiency due to extensive DVT is a rare complication that can present in two forms (Table 16-3). Phlegmasia alba dolens, in which the limb is swollen, pale, with diminished pulses, is transient and believed to be due to arterial spasm in response to acute iliofemoral thrombosis. Phlegmasia cerulea dolens is characterized by sustained cyanosis, edema, and arterial insufficiency (Fig. 16-12). The mechanism of ischemia in these patients is arterial collapse due to massive tense edema in the presence of extensive venous thrombosis: in essence compartment syndrome involving the entire limb. Mortality rate is high (almost 25%), and venous gangrene and amputation complicates more than 25% of cases.

Measurement of serum fibrin D-dimer, a degradation product of fibrinolysis, can be used as an initial screening test for the presence of thrombus in patients with low risk for DVT. A normal D-dimer level (<500 µg/L) has greater than 95% sensitivity in this patient population. This test is less sensitive in hospitalized patients, those considered high risk, age older than 65 years, and pregnant women.

Imaging remains essential in the diagnosis of DVT. The most widely applied imaging modality for detection of lower-extremity DVT is ultrasound (Box 16-2). A noncompressible vein is the single most reliable criteria for the presence of thrombus, as long as the examination is adequate (see Fig. 16-8). The sensitivity and specificity for ultrasound are both greater than 95% for detection of thrombus in the popliteal vein and above in patients with symptoms of DVT. The sensitivity and specificity are both closer to 80% for calf DVT in asymptomatic patients. Small thrombi, particularly those limited to valve cusps or perforating veins, are easily missed by ultrasound. Great care must be taken to ensure that duplicated femoral or popliteal veins are not overlooked by ultrasound, because thrombus in one moiety of a duplicated vein segment can occur. Venous ultrasound for DVT is relatively inexpensive, with little risk, high sensitivity and specificity, and wide availability. As a result, both the threshold for ordering the study and the overall positive rates are low.

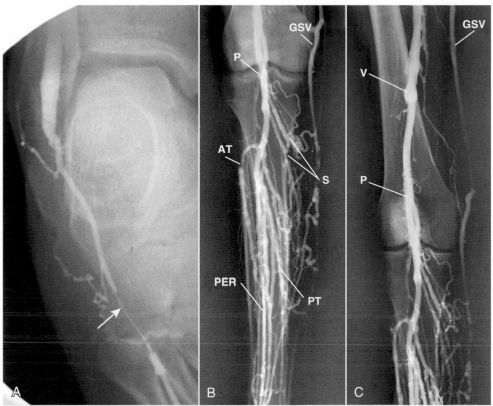

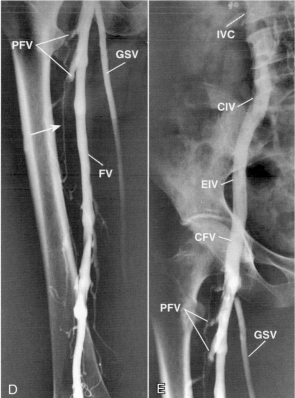

FIGURE 16-11. Conventional venogram performed with the patient tilted 50 degrees and bearing weight on the left leg. **A,** Initial image during injection of an intravenous catheter in a lateral foot vein *(arrow)* confirms absence of extravasation. **B,** Anterior view of the calf shows filling of the anterior tibial (AT), posterior tibial (PT), and peroneal (PER) veins. Sural (S) veins drain directly into the popliteal vein (P). The great saphenous vein is also filled. The complete study included two opposing oblique views of the calf. **C,** Anterior view of the popliteal vein. Note the large valve (V) in the above-knee portion of the vein. The GSV is also filled. **D,** Anterior view of the thigh showing the femoral vein (FV). Drainage of some deep muscular veins *(arrow)* faintly opacify the profunda femoris vein (PFV). **E,** Anterior view of the groin and pelvis showing the insertion of the GSV into the common femoral vein (CFV), known as the saphenofemoral junction. The valves at the origin of the PFV are competent, preventing retrograde opacification. The external iliac vein (EIV) and common iliac vein (CIV) are well visualized, but contrast in the inferior vena cava is attenuated by inflow from the left common iliac vein.

Detection of acute DVT by MRV has excellent sensitivity and specificity (both > 95%). The expense, length of the examination, and relatively limited availability (compared to ultrasound) have prevented routine use of this test. The introduction of blood-pool agents may substantially change the utilization of MRV for detection of DVT.

On CT images, venous thrombosis appears as either intra-luminal high density on noncontrast scans, or low density with enhancement in the vein wall on contrast studies. Thrombus in a lower-extremity vein is occasionally noted during the venous phase of pelvic CT obtained for other indications (see Fig. 16-10). The addition of a scan of the pelvis and legs following

Box 16-1. Risk Factors for Deep Venous Thrombosis

Previous episode of deep venous thrombosis
Immobilization
Malignancy
Trauma (especially spine and head)
Surgery (especially neurologic and orthopedic)
Central venous catheters
Antiphospholipid antibodies
Hyperhomocysteinemia
Protein C, S, and antithrombin deficiencies
Factor V Leiden
Oral contraceptives
Pregnancy
Iliac vein compression
  • Extrinsic mass
  • May-Thurner syndrome
Femoral vein puncture
Inflammatory bowel disease
Buerger disease
Atherosclerosis

TABLE 16-2 Modified Wells Score for Deep Vein Thrombosis

Feature	Points
Cancer	+1
Paralysis or recent limb immobilization	+1
Bed rest > 3 days or surgery < 4 weeks	+1
Pain on palpation of deep veins	+1
Swelling of entire leg	+1
Diameter difference affected calf > 3 cm	+1
Pitting edema (> on symptomatic side)	+1
Dilated superficial veins (not varicose, affected side)	+1
Prior deep vein thrombosis (DVT)	+1
Alternate diagnosis at least as probable as DVT	-2

Interpretation: Score ≤ 1 = DVT unlikely; ≥ 2 = DVT likely.
Adapted from Goldhaber SZ, Bounameaux H. Pulmonary embolism and deep vein thrombosis. *Lancet.* 2012;379:1835-1846.

pulmonary CT angiography (CTA) for PE reveals DVT in 8% of patients, half of whom do not have PE. The convenience of combined imaging of the lower-extremity veins and pulmonary arteries is balanced by the increased radiation exposure. Direct injection CT venography is not usually necessary for evaluation of lower-extremity DVT, but can be useful for evaluation of the pelvic veins.

Conventional venography is rarely performed for DVT. The small risk of complications, increased cost relative to ultrasound, and greater patient discomfort have made this an almost archaic examination. When performed, the most reliable venographic finding is an intraluminal filling defect outlined by contrast (Fig. 16-13).

Multidisciplinary guidelines on the treatment of DVT are available from both the American College of Chest Physicians (ACCP, updated every 4 years) and the American Heart Association (AHA). These guidelines should be consulted for the most current and specific treatment recommendations, but certain general principles are described herein. The primary treatment of acute proximal DVT is anticoagulation. In 2012, the ACCP recommended against anticoagulation of isolated calf DVT. The purpose of anticoagulation is to prevent formation of new thrombus while the existing thrombus undergoes thrombolysis by endogenous means.

TABLE 16-3 Clinical Presentation of Lower-Extremity Venous Thrombosis

Category	Findings
Superficial thrombophlebitis	Erythema, palpable cord in saphenous or other superficial vein, limited edema
Deep venous thrombosis	Edema, pain, distended superficial veins, warm extremity
Phlegmasia alba dolens	Pale, cool extremity with weak or absent pulses; usually transient
Phlegmasia cerulea dolens	Cyanotic, cool, painful, pulseless extremity; limb loss likely

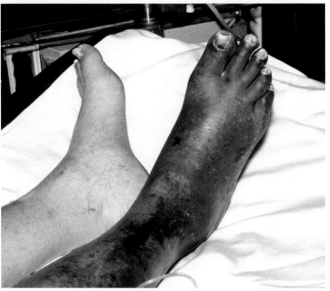

FIGURE 16-12. Photograph of a patient with phlegmasia cerulea dolens of the right foot. Note the edema and discoloration of the right foot. Subdermal bleeding and skin blisters are also common.

Box 16-2. Ultrasound Criteria of Acute Deep Venous Thrombosis

ABSOLUTE
Noncompressible, hypoechoic vein (frequently expanded)

ADJUNCTIVE
Intraluminal filling defect on color flow
Absent color-flow signal in lumen despite augmentation
Absent Doppler signal from lumen despite augmentation
Absent respiratory variation
Absent response to Valsalva

Heparin in either unfractionated or low-molecular-weight preparations is used to initiate therapy, followed by oral Coumadin or low-molecular-weight heparin for long-term therapy. New oral agents are undergoing evaluation for DVT treatment. The duration of therapy is 3-6 months with a target international normalized ratio (INR) of 2-3 (when Coumadin is used). The etiology of the DVT, the presence of comorbid conditions, and subsequent risk of new thromboembolic events all influence agent, intensity, and duration of anticoagulation. Compression stockings, 30-40 mm Hg (thigh-high initially and knee-high subsequently) should be used for acute control of edema and continued for at least 2 years to prevent post-thrombotic syndrome. Vena cava filters are

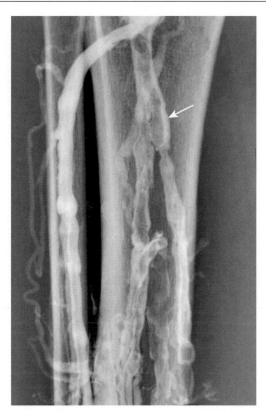

FIGURE 16-13. Classic venographic appearance of thrombosis, with contrast outlining a central filling defect *(arrow)*. There is thrombus in the posterior tibial and peroneal veins.

Box 16-3. Indications for Catheter Interventions in Deep Venous Thrombosis

Iliofemoral or femoral deep vein thrombosis
Recent onset of symptoms (within 21 days)
Threatened limb (phlegmasia cerulean dolens)
Inadequate response to initial anticoagulation
Low bleeding risk
Good physiologic reserve
Life expectancy greater than 6 months

Box 16-4. Principles of Venous Thrombolysis/Pharmacomechanical Thrombectomy

Fresh thrombus lyses quickest
Infuse agent over entire length of thrombus
Establish flow quickly: consider pharmacomechanical thrombectomy first, then thrombolysis
Anticoagulate during infusion (low dose with tissue plasminogen activators)
Platelet inhibitors (aspirin or glycoprotein IIB/IIIA agents)
Stents frequently required in patients with chronic disease
Long-term anticoagulation

not indicated in the treatment of uncomplicated DVT unless the patient cannot be anticoagulated, has sustained a massive PE, or lacks the cardiopulmonary reserve to tolerate a PE.

Some degree of patency of thrombosed venous segments is restored in more than 80% of patients by 6 weeks, with complete resolution of thrombus in up to 50% over time. The aggregate risk of a bleeding complication at an INR of 2-3 is 3%-5%. After completion of treatment, recurrent DVT occurs in 3%-10% overall, but with rates as high as 30% in patients with chronic risk factors.

The risk of symptomatic PE during initiation of therapy is approximately 2%-5%, and propagation of thrombus occurs in 6%-10%. Approximately 2% of patients receiving unfractionated heparin for more than 4 days experience a drop in platelets (heparin-induced thrombocytopenia, HIT); this complication is seen in only 0.2% of patients treated with low-molecular-weight heparin. In severe cases of HIT, widespread vascular occlusions due to platelet aggregation and hemorrhage (disseminated intravascular coagulation, DIC) develop.

Superficial thrombophlebitis (thrombus limited to the saphenous vein or its tributaries) makes up 4%-6% of all cases of acute lower-extremity venous thrombosis. This disorder is usually managed with elevation, compression stockings, and local heat when limited to short segments of vein. However, proximal DVT has been found in up to 10% of patients with long segment superficial thrombosis (>5 cm). Anticoagulation with fondaparinux or low-molecular-weight-heparin is recommended for 45 days when the thrombosed segment is 5 cm or more in length.

Surgical therapy for acute DVT is reserved for patients with impending or full-blown phlegmasia cerulea dolens. Iliofemoral thrombectomy, with or without creation of an arteriovenous fistula, has a 70%-80% patency rate at 5 years and reduces the severity of post-phlebitic syndrome. Fasciotomies are frequently necessary in patients with phlegmasia cerulea dolens. Despite these long-term results, surgical thrombectomy is infrequently performed in the United States.

Catheter-directed thrombolysis or pharmacomechanical thrombolysis for extensive lower-extremity DVT are very successful in rapidly restoring venous patency, and may reduce damage to venous valves. These techniques have essentially replaced surgical thrombectomy; many more patients currently undergo catheter-based interventions than would have been operated upon in the past. The indications for percutaneous intervention are patients with extensive, symptomatic or progressive iliofemoral or femoral DVT of less than 14-21 days' duration, low risk of bleeding complications, and a reasonable life expectancy (Box 16-3). Symptomatic isolated calf DVT should not be treated in this manner. Interventional therapy of DVT is the subject of a large randomized multicenter National Institutes of Health phase 3 study, the ATTRACT trial (Acute venous Thrombosis: Thrombus Removal with Adjunctive Catheter-directed Thrombolysis). The primary outcome of the trial is the presence of chronic venous insufficiency in the affected limb at 2 years after treatment.

Access for intervention can be achieved from a number of locations, but most interventionalists prefer to puncture a posterior tibial or popliteal vein on the affected side using ultrasound guidance. The thrombosed vein is easier to negotiate in an antegrade fashion; when accessed retrograde from a jugular vein or contralateral CFV the venous valves can impede catheter placement.

When catheter-based thrombolysis is used, multi-side-hole catheters must be placed across the entire length of the thrombus. A triaxial system can be assembled with infusion through a 5- or 6-French sheath at the access site, a 5-French infusion catheter in the middle segment, and a 3-French infusion catheter extending to the most central portion of the thrombus (Box 16-4 and Fig. 16-14). Patients receive systemic unfractionated heparin during the thrombolysis and should be maintained on chronic therapeutic anticoagulation afterward. Infusion for 2 and rarely 3 days may be required (Table 16-4). Symptomatic PE is uncommon during lysis, with fatal PE rarely reported. Nevertheless, the need for IVC filters during these procedures remains unclear, and many interventionalists place retrievable filters in these patients. Bleeding complications occur in 6%-25% of cases but usually consist of

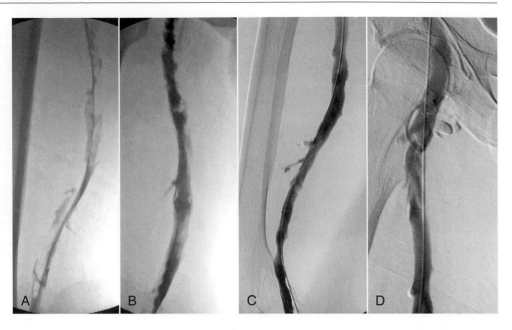

FIGURE 16-14. Lower-extremity venous intervention for acute deep venous thrombosis. **A,** Venogram of the thigh obtained after puncture of the posterior tibial vein using ultrasound guidance. There is extensive thrombus that was continuous from the tibial veins to the inferior vena cava (IVC). A guidewire has been advanced into the IVC. **B,** After passage of a mechanical thrombectomy device, there is substantial reduction in the volume of thrombus, but antegrade flow is still absent. **C,** After additional catheter-directed thrombolysis for 24 hours, there is excellent antegrade flow with only minimal filling defects in the femoral vein. **D,** View of the groin showing a patent common femoral vein.

TABLE 16-4 Thrombolytic Agents for Venous Thrombolysis

Agent	Total Hourly Dose	Heparin Hourly Dose	Duration
Urokinase	100,000-150,000 U	800-1200 U	48 hr
tPA	0.5-1 mg	500 U	24-48 hr
rtPA	0.5-1 U	500 U	24-48 hr
TNK	0.25-0.5 mg	500 U	24-48 hr

access-related hematomas. The risk of a major bleed is 2%-4%, with intracranial hemorrhage being rare.

Several pharmacomechanical thrombolysis devices are described in Chapter 4 (see Figs. 4-32 and 4-34). There is no clearly superior technique, but all offer rapid restoration of flow when compared to infusion techniques. In some instances the entire treatment can be completed in one session with these devices, but often a course of catheter-based infusion of a thrombolytic is required for optimal results. Access when using a pharmacomechanical device is similar to that used for catheter lysis. Patients should receive unfractionated heparin during the procedure, and adherence to device instructions for use greatly enhances outcomes.

Adjunctive techniques are commonly required during these procedures. Angioplasty and stent placement are required in the iliac veins in up to 70% of patients (Fig. 16-15). Patients with underlying May-Thurner syndrome (see Chronic Venous Obstruction and Post-phlebitic Syndrome) almost always require stent placement. Self-expanding stents should be sized at least 2-3 mm larger in diameter than the normal diameter of the vein (see Fig. 16-15). When stenting the common iliac veins it is optimal, but not always possible, to avoid extension too far into the IVC and "jailing" the opposite iliac vein. Stents that cross over the orifice of the contralateral iliac vein may increase the risk of contralateral lower-extremity thrombosis. In some instances, the IVC is also stenotic or occluded, and stents are purposively extended cephalad. A robust stent is necessary in the left common iliac vein to relieve the external compression from the right common iliac artery.

The management of the CFV in these situations can be challenging. Recently, there has been favorable experience with surgical removal of organized CFV thrombus alone or in combination with stenting of the iliac veins when necessary. This has been suggested as an alternative to extension of stents through the CFV into the leg. The long-term patency of these stents and fractures have not been an issue, but future femoral venous access can be compromised.

The initial results of randomized comparisons of aggressive interventions for acute symptomatic iliofemoral DVT are promising. In a randomized Norwegian trial comparing anticoagulation alone to anticoagulation plus catheter-based thrombolysis for iliofemoral DVT in 209 patients (the CaVenT study) there was an almost 15% reduction in post-thrombotic syndrome at 2 years ($P = 0.047$) in the treatment group. The ATTRACT trial will be substantially larger and address pharmacomechanical thrombolysis as well.

CHRONIC VENOUS OBSTRUCTION AND POST-PHLEBITIC SYNDROME

Venous obstruction, rather than valvular incompetence, is the underlying etiology of chronic lower-extremity swelling in almost 10% of patients. The most common cause of chronic obstruction is prior DVT (Box 16-5). Patients can present with edema, leg pain, varicose veins, and other manifestations of venous hypertension such as skin changes. The estimated prevalence of post-phlebitic syndrome is 5% of the U.S. adult population. When the extremity swelling and pain occur with exertion, it is termed "venous claudication." Patients may have abdominal and perineal venous distention, and a slightly dusky tinge to the leg.

Patients with May-Thurner syndrome (also called Cockett syndrome) may present with chronic symptoms of left leg edema and leg heaviness, or acute thrombosis as described previously. This entity may be a contributing factor to the increased incidence of left lower-extremity DVT compared to the right. The underlying abnormality is compression of the left common iliac vein between the right common iliac artery and the lumbosacral spine (Fig. 16-16). This anatomic compression is seen in up to one fourth of the asymptomatic adult population; patients should not be treated unless appropriate symptoms are present. The typical patient is in the second to fourth decade of life, with a female-to-male ratio of 3:1. Three venographic stages have been described: asymptomatic compression of the left common iliac vein with no filling of collaterals and a pressure gradient less than 2 mm Hg; intraluminal webs or "spurs"; and thrombosis.

The imaging of patients with chronic venous obstruction is directed at determining the level of occlusion and detecting

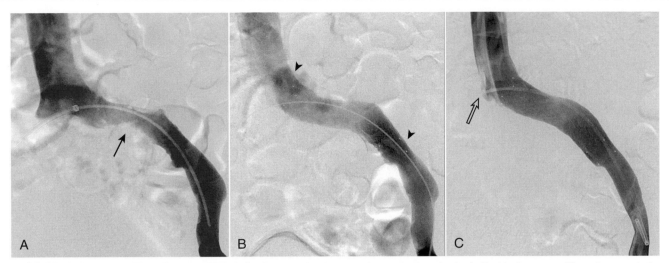

FIGURE 16-15. Left common iliac vein stent (CIV) during intervention for acute deep vein thrombosis. **A,** Residual common iliac vein stenosis *(arrow)* 36 hours after initiation of treatment that included pharmacomechanical thrombectomy, catheter thrombolysis, and angioplasty with a 14-mm diameter balloon. **B,** Venogram after placement of a 14-mm diameter by 60-mm long self-expanding nitinol stent *(arrowheads)* and repeat angioplasty shows improved luminal diameter. There is minimal protrusion of the stent into the inferior vena cava (IVC). **C,** Venogram obtained 1 week later during IVC filter removal shows excellent flow. There is unopacified blood *(open arrow)* entering the IVC from the right CIV.

Box 16-5. Etiologies of Chronic Obstruction of Lower-Extremity Veins

Deep venous thrombosis
Trauma
Irradiation
Retroperitoneal fibrosis
Neoplasm
Arterial aneurysms
Cysts (e.g., Baker cyst in popliteal fossa)
Muscular entrapment (e.g., type 5 popliteal artery entrapment)
May-Thurner syndrome

---

correctable underlying causes. Ultrasound is excellent for imaging the lower extremity, but less useful in the pelvis. Analysis of Doppler waveforms in response to respiratory maneuvers infers the status of the iliac veins. Both CT and MRI are excellent modalities for evaluating pelvic veins and surrounding soft tissues. Venous obstruction from extrinsic compression by lymph nodes, aneurysms, masses, and even the distended bladder can occur (Fig. 16-17). Diagnostic ascending venography, performed from either the foot (for obstruction of the extremity veins) or CFV (for obstruction in the iliac veins) is rarely required.

Several surgical procedures have been devised for iliac vein occlusion, including femoral-to-femoral venous bypass and CFV-to-IVC bypass with or without creation of a small arteriovenous fistula in the groin. The purpose of the fistula is to maintain high flow rates through the graft. Clinical improvement has been reported in about 75% of these patients, with similar graft patency rates. Results reported for May-Thurner syndrome have been better than those for chronic thrombosis. Surgical bypass for femoral and popliteal vein occlusion has poor results.

Endovascular reconstruction of occluded venous segments with metallic stents is preferred over surgical approaches due to the minimal morbidity and high technical and clinical success rates (Fig. 16-18). Both antegrade and retrograde approaches should be attempted. Jugular access provides excellent leverage for crossing common iliac vein occlusions. Antegrade recanalization may require access from below the CFV. A trial of thrombolysis can be beneficial in patients with suspected mixed acute and chronic thrombosis, but most interventionalists will angioplasty and then place stents. The principles of stent placement are the same as described in the preceding section.

Patients with central venous obstruction often have concomitant superficial venous reflux. Addition of endovenous ablation of abnormal GSVs (see Chronic Venous Valvular Insufficiency) can improve overall symptoms in these patients.

Patients should be anticoagulated for 3-6 months after successful recanalization. Antiplatelet therapy with aspirin is recommended indefinitely. The 1-year patency of iliac vein stents when the infrainguinal veins are patent is 90%. There is a paucity of data on femoral venous stents. Approximately 80% of patients reported improvement in pain, edema, and ulceration, with almost half of these reporting minimal symptoms. When the procedure can be performed safely, endovascular reconstruction should be attempted before surgery in most patients.

CHRONIC VENOUS VALVULAR INSUFFICIENCY

Incompetent valves in superficial, deep, and perforator veins result in venous hypertension in the lower extremity. Valvular incompetence in the GSV contributes to more than 75% of varicosities; SSV reflux is found in 10%-20% and nonsaphenous reflux (e.g., perforating veins, contribution from pelvic veins) in 10%-15%. Up to 30% of the adult population has a detectable abnormality related to this process, most often varicose veins or telangiectasias. Women and men are probably equally affected. In 3%-8% of the population, chronic venous insufficiency results in swelling, pain, hyperpigmentation, and dermatitis. Venous ulceration in patients older than 45 years occurs in 3.5 per 1000 and is recurrent in 75%. The cost of treatment of venous ulcers in the United States is estimated at $1 billion.

The pelvic veins may have a significant role in lower-extremity venous insufficiency. Iliac vein obstruction may contribute to reflux symptoms and should be excluded in patients with a history of iliofemoral DVT. Internal iliac vein reflux can contribute to perineal varicose veins, which can contribute in turn to lower-extremity varicose veins. In women, ovarian vein reflux that is transmitted through the perivaginal veins to the perineum and subsequently the leg can be the sole or contributing cause of lower-extremity varicose veins. A history or complaint of labial varices, or pelvic congestion symptoms should suggest this as a potential diagnosis.

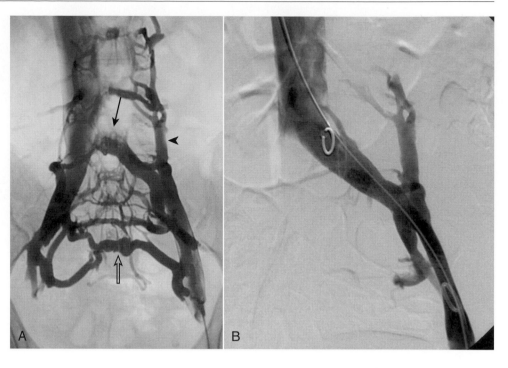

FIGURE 16-16. Venographic appearance of May-Thurner syndrome. The patient is a 21-year-old woman with chronic left leg swelling. **A,** Digital venogram obtained by injection of the left external iliac vein showing an attenuated left common iliac vein (CIV) *(closed arrow)*, with drainage via cross-pelvic collaterals *(open arrow)* to the right iliac system, and the ascending lumbar vein *(arrowhead)*. **B,** After angioplasty of the left CIV and placement of a 14-mm diameter self-expanding stent, there is excellent antegrade flow with diminished filling of collateral veins. The patient has a belly-button ring that is projected over the iliac vein.

The etiology of the valvular incompetence is multifactorial (Box 16-6). In evaluation of the patient with varicose veins it is important to identify prior DVT, which may indicate deep venous incompetence or obliteration and an increased risk of postintervention DVT. Patients with a history of an unprovoked DVT or a history suggestive of a hypercoagulable condition should undergo workup by a hematologist before proceeding with an intervention for varicose veins.

The organ at risk with venous insufficiency is the skin (Fig. 16-19). Although the initial abnormality is located at the venous valve, the most severe damage is to the skin and the subcutaneous tissues. The most extreme expression of this damage is ulceration. The pathophysiology of the skin changes is not completely understood, but it is linked to the high venous pressures. Venous pressures may rise to greater than 80 mm Hg at the ankle in patients with severe disease. The volume of refluxed blood is also important in development of symptoms.

A classification system has been developed to describe patients with chronic venous diseases (clinical class, etiology, anatomy, and pathology [CEAP], Box 16-7). The Venous Severity Scoring includes the degree of disability, severity of symptoms, and location and type of venous abnormality (Table 16-5).

Telangiectasias and reticular ("spider") veins (C1) are so common that they are considered by many to be normal manifestations of aging. Incompetent small perforator veins result in dilatation of the subdermal venous network. Telangiectasias are flat, red blemishes that blanch on pressure with slow return of color. When return of color is brisk or the lesion is pulsatile, an arteriovenous malformation should be suspected. Reticular veins are small, superficial, thin-walled veins that lie close to the surface of the skin.

Varicose veins (C2) are dilated, tortuous superficial veins that distend when the patient is upright and can cause aching. These veins can thrombose (superficial thrombophlebitis) and giant veins can rupture, resulting in major hemorrhage. The dilated veins collapse and symptoms improve with elevation of the extremity.

Edema (C3) due to chronic venous stasis indicates severe venous hypertension. Without intervention, there is a high likelihood of progression to permanent damage to the skin.

The characteristic skin changes of venous insufficiency (C4) are thickening, scaling, and/or brownish discoloration (see Fig. 16-19). This classification was recently subdivided into C4a

(pigmentation or eczema) and C4b (lipodermatosclerosis or atrophie blanche). There is almost always associated edema, and patients report itching and burning sensations. The color changes are largely irreversible.

Lower-extremity venous ulcers (C5, healed ulcers; C6, active ulcers) are the most severe manifestation of venous valvular insufficiency (see Fig. 16-19). These lesions must be distinguished from arterial, traumatic, and diabetic ulcers in order to initiate appropriate therapy. Venous ulcers are shallow, irregular, associated with characteristic skin changes, and located in the medial aspect of the supramalleolar region. Incompetence of the deep and perforating veins, with or without saphenous vein reflux, is present in more than 80% of these patients. Isolated saphenous vein reflux is unusual in patients with ulceration.

Imaging of patients with chronic venous insufficiency is aimed at determining the location and extent of reflux. Ultrasound with Doppler and color flow is highly sensitive and specific (both >95%) for valvular incompetence. This modality is less sensitive (80%) for identification of incompetent perforating veins but is highly specific. The examination is performed with the patient standing. Segmental evaluation is important to localize the abnormal veins. Both the great and small saphenous veins, the anterior and posterior accessory GSVs, and the deep veins should be studied. The limb below the vein is either briefly compressed manually or an automated cuff is rapidly deflated as the flow is interrogated with color or duplex US. Reversal of flow that lasts less than 0.5 second is normal, because time is needed for valve closure. Reversal of flow in the superficial veins for more than 0.5 second indicates valvular incompetence, while reversal for longer than 1 second is considered severe (Fig. 16-20). In the deep veins, reversal of flow for up to 1 second is acceptable. Dilated (≥3.5 mm diameter) incompetent (flow reversal ≥ 0.5 second) perforating veins underlying venous ulcers are considered pathologic. The physician assessing the patient and ultimately performing interventions should perform the ultrasound examination rather than rely upon a written report.

Contrast venography has an extremely limited role in the diagnostic evaluation of patients with chronic venous disease. When concomitant pelvic venous obstruction or gonadal vein reflux is suspected, CT or MRI of the pelvis and abdomen should be obtained.

The therapy of venous insufficiency varies with the clinical findings and the symptoms. There is currently no satisfactory

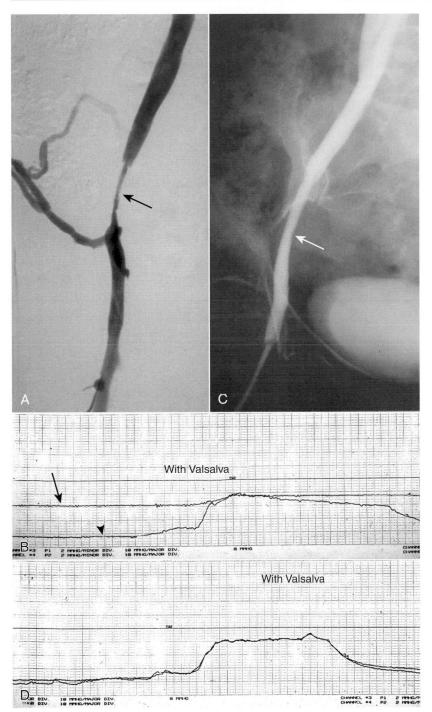

FIGURE 16-17. External iliac vein obstruction due to enlarged lymph nodes in a patient with metastatic cervical carcinoma. The patient had chronic right leg swelling. **A,** Digital venogram showing stenosis of the external iliac vein (EIV; *arrow*). **B,** Simultaneous pressures measured in the inferior vena cava (IVC; *arrowhead*) and right common femoral vein (CFV; *arrow*). There is elevated baseline pressure in the CFV. With Valsalva, the IVC pressure rises to meet the CFV pressure. **C,** Venogram after stent placement in the EIV *(arrow)*. **D,** Simultaneous pressure measurements from the IVC and right CFV now show identical, superimposed tracings.

method to reverse valvular incompetence. Many patients control their symptoms and limit skin changes by wearing compression stockings (20-30 mm Hg for mild symptoms; 30-40 mm Hg for moderate symptoms; 40-50 mm Hg for severe symptoms) and avoiding prolonged standing. Exercising the calf muscles (the "muscular pump") is important to reduce venous stasis.

Patients seek treatment of varicose veins for a variety of reasons (Box 16-8). Small veins are usually considered a cosmetic problem. Larger varicose veins can be painful, thrombose, or bleed when traumatized. Patients should undergo a trial of conservative management with compression stockings, frequent leg elevation, exercise of the calf muscles (the "muscular pump"), and nonsteroidal analgesics before considering intervention. When edema, skin pigmentation, or ulceration are present (C3 or higher),

intervention is medically indicated. Patients with ulcerations should be comanaged with a wound clinic or specialist.

Small varicose veins and telangiectasias can be treated with sclerotherapy. Larger varicosities can be either sclerosed or removed with mini-stab phlebectomy. The saphenous veins are usually treated with endovenous ablation, although traditional stripping is still performed in some patients. Perforating veins can be ligated, ablated with specialized probes, or injected under ultrasound guidance.

The traditional surgical interventions include surgical ligation of the saphenofemoral junction, saphenous vein stripping, division of incompetent perforating veins, and excision of abnormal vein clusters (phlebectomy). The complications of saphenous vein stripping include sensory nerve injury (15%, particularly when the stripping extends to the ankle), wound infection (3%), and deep

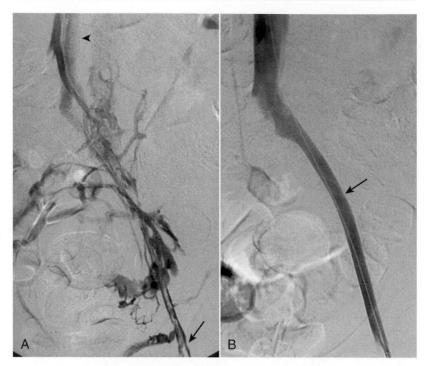

Figure 16-18. Recanalization of chronic left common iliac vein (CIV) and external iliac vein (EIV) occlusion. **A,** Digital venogram from injection into the left CFV shows a narrowed vein with an intraluminal filling defect consistent with chronic thrombosis *(arrow)*, no obvious EIV or CIV, and opacification of the IVC from collateral veins *(arrowhead, inferior vena cava)*. **B,** A hydrophilic guidewire and an angled catheter were used to negotiate through the occluded iliac veins, followed by angioplasty and self-expanding stent placement. There is now excellent flow through the stents *(arrow)*.

Box 16-6. Risk Factors for Lower-Extremity Venous Valvular Incompetence

Family history of varicose veins
Past history of deep or superficial venous thrombosis
Central venous obstruction
Multiple pregnancies
Prolonged standing
Prior intervention for varicose veins

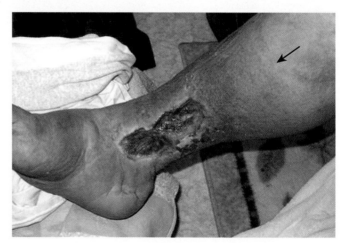

Figure 16-19. Chronic venous ulceration with associated skin changes extending halfway up the calf *(arrow)*.

vein thrombosis (<1%). Recurrence of varicosities after saphenous vein stripping has been reported to be as high as 25% at 5 years. Surgical reconstruction or transplant of venous valves has been unsuccessful unless performed in specialized centers.

Image-guided procedures have become the most common approach to interventions for chronic venous insufficiency due to superficial venous valvular incompetence. Catheter-based techniques for ablation of the saphenous veins offer an effective percutaneous alternative to venous stripping. Laser and radiofrequency (RF) ablation have been used with success for this purpose (Fig. 16-21). Newer technologies in development include catheter-based injection of sclerosants and steam. The common components of the endovenous ablation procedures are careful patient selection and evaluation. The patient history should be consistent with chronic venous disease, without suggestion of arterial, orthopedic, or neurologic causes of pain or swelling. Mapping of the superficial varicosities and interrogation of the deep system with ultrasound (by the treating physician) is essential. In addition, the extremity should be examined for evidence of arterial disease, infection, and other conditions that could impact treatment such as severe arthritis. Historical or clinical evidence of hypercoagulable syndromes, central venous obstruction, and occluded or absent deep veins should prompt reassessment of the need and type of intervention. A photographic record of the limb before treatment is useful to help assess treatment response.

Saphenous vein ablation with laser or RF share many similarities. These technologies can be applied to the great, small, and accessory saphenous veins. On the day of the procedure,

patients can apply a topical anesthetic cream to the leg over the vein to be treated. Immediately before treatment, the course of the saphenous vein is reconfirmed with ultrasound and marked on the skin. Veins of any depth can be treated, but very superficial veins (<5 mm below the dermis) may be both palpable and visible as a brownish stain for months after the treatment. The leg is sterilely prepared and draped, and percutaneous venous access is obtained with ultrasound guidance and a micropuncture needle. The usual site of entry is just below the lowest point of reflux. When access is below the knee for the GSV, there is an increased risk of injury to the cutaneous nerve branches, resulting in localized sensory loss over the medial calf. When treating the SSV, the access should not be lower than the lower border of the gastrocnemius muscle to avoid injury to the sural nerve. Either a long vascular sheath (laser) or the treatment probe is then inserted under ultrasound guidance. When treating the GSV, the ablation device is advanced to within 1 cm (laser) or 2 cm (RF) of the saphenofemoral junction, and when treating the SSV to just proximal to the junction of the small saphenous

Box 16-7. CEAP Classification of Chronic Venous Disease (2004 Revision)

BASIC

Clinical classification:
  C0: no visible or palpable signs of venous disease
  C1: telangiectasias or reticular veins
  C2: varicose veins
  C3: edema
  C4a: pigmentation or eczema
  C4b: lipodermatosclerosis or atrophie blanche
  C5: healed venous ulcer
  C6: active venous ulcer
  S: symptomatic, including ache, pain, tightness, skin irritation, heaviness, and muscle cramps, and other complaints attributable to venous dysfunction
  A: asymptomatic
Etiologic classification:
  Ec: congenital
  Ep: primary
  Es: secondary (postthrombotic)
  En: no venous cause identified
Anatomic classification:
  As: superficial veins
  Ap: perforator veins
  Ad: deep veins
  An: no venous location identified
Pathophysiologic classification:
  Pr: reflux
  Po: obstruction
  Pr,o: reflux and obstruction
  Pn: no venous pathophysiology identifiable

ADVANCED*
Superficial veins:
  Telangiectasies or reticular veins
  Great saphenous vein above knee
  Great saphenous vein below knee
  Small saphenous vein
  Nonsaphenous veins
Deep veins:
  Inferior vena cava
  Common iliac vein
  Internal iliac vein
  External iliac vein
  Pelvic: gonadal, broad ligament veins, other
  Common femoral vein
  Deep femoral vein
  Femoral vein
  Popliteal vein
  Crural: anterior tibial, posterior tibial, peroneal veins (all paired)
  Muscular: gastrocnemial, soleal veins, other
Perforating veins:
  Thigh
  Calf

*Same as basic CEAP, with addition that any of 18 named venous segments can be used as locators for venous pathology.
From Eklöf B, Rutherford RB, Bergan JJ, et al. Revision of the CEAP classification for chronic venous disorders: consensus statement. *J Vasc Surg.* 2004;40:1248-1252.

and gastrocnemius veins (Fig. 16-22). Dilute local anesthetic (20 ml 2% lidocaine with epinephrine, 20 ml bicatb in X mkl saline) (mixture of 50 mL of 1% lidocaine with epinephrine, 16 mL of 8.4% sodium bicarbonate, and 450 mL normal saline) is then infiltrated along the course of the saphenous vein using ultrasound guidance and multiple punctures. Termed "tumescent anesthesia," this critical step when using thermal ablation ensures patient comfort during the ablation, compresses the vein against the probe, and minimizes potential heat damage to surrounding structures by creating an insulating barrier of fluid (Fig. 16-23). When the vein to be treated is less than 1 cm deep to the skin, sufficient volume should be injected between the vein and the skin to create this distance.

Once adequate anesthesia has been achieved, the device is activated and withdrawn through the vein. Laser probes are withdrawn continuously, whereas the newer RF devices are moved in a stepwise fashion. The rate of withdrawal is manufacturer and device specific. The device should never be activated in the CFV. The device is turned off before withdrawing through the soft tissues and skin to avoid local burns and nerve damage. The common femoral or popliteal veins are then assessed with ultrasound for patency. A compression stocking and sometimes an Ace wrap is applied and the patient ambulates immediately.

Laser devices are available in different wavelengths, ranging from approximately 810 to 1470 nm. The higher wavelengths are more selective for water. Substantial efforts have been made to differentiate different laser wavelengths from each other, and laser from RF. The major difference is that postprocedure pain and bruising is reported less with higher wavelength lasers and RF. By 1 month, however, all outcome measures are identical. This procedure is performed on an outpatient basis, usually in clinics or private offices. The technical success rate is reported to be greater than 95%, with fewer than 10% recurrences at 2 years (Fig. 16-24). DVT occurs in fewer than 1% of patients, and nerve injury in fewer than 5%.

Localized small varicosities, telangiectasias, and reticular veins can be effectively treated with injection of dilute sclerosing agents (Box 16-9). When the GSV or SSV is incompetent, this should be treated first in order to achieve the most durable results with sclerotherapy. A small syringe is used to inject 0.5-1 mL of sclerosant directly into small veins through a 25-gauge or smaller needle. The small needle eliminates the need for local anesthetic. Entering the skin at an angle of about 30 degrees, slight negative pressure is applied to the syringe plunger. As soon as a flash of blood is seen, the sclerosant is gently injected. Blanching of the telangiectasias or reticular veins indicates an intravascular injection. Varices should be compressed proximal and distal to the injection site to retain the sclerosant in the target vessel. The injection is stopped immediately if the patient complains of pain or there is obvious local extravasation. The most commonly used agent worldwide is polidocanol 0.25%-0.5%, although sodium tetradecyl sulfate in similar concentrations is often used in the United States. Local ulceration, pain, and hyperpigmentation can occur, especially with concentrated sclerosants. Anaphylactic reactions have occurred with sodium morrhuate and sodium tetradecyl sulfate.

Detergent-based sclerosants can be foamed with room air or CO_2 for injection into larger veins (see Fig. 4-49). The typical ratio is 1 part sclerosant to 4 parts gas. This results in prolonged contact with the endothelium with a lower overall volume of sclerosant when compared to injection of liquid sclerosant. The foam is also highly visible on ultrasound, allowing monitoring depth and extent of penetration. Although some authors use up to 20 mL of foam in a single-session treatment of lower-extremity veins, we do not use more than 12 mL in total because there is risk of neurologic symptoms (migraine, visual disturbance, and transient ischemic attack) with large volumes due to right-to-left shunts. Elevation of the limb for 10-15 minutes after injection has been recommended. Foam can be used as an alternative or adjunct to treatment of the GSVs and SSVs. When used as a primary therapy, there is a higher rate of recanalization and retreatment than with thermal ablation, but the cost is lower.

Mini-stab phlebectomy is the extraction of superficial venous segments through small incisions using hooked tools and local

TABLE 16-5 Venous Clinical Severity Score

Attribute	0 (Absent)	1 (Mild)	2 (Moderate)	3 (Severe)
Pain	None	Occasional, not restricting activity or requiring analgesics	Daily, moderate activity limitation, occasional analgesics	Daily, severe limiting activities or requiring regular use of analgesics
Varicose veins	None	Few, scattered branch varicose veins	Multiple: GSV varicose veins confined to calf or thigh	Extensive: thigh and calf or GSV and SSV distribution
Venous edema	None	Evening ankle only	Afternoon edema, above ankle	Morning edema above ankle and requiring activity change, elevation
Skin pigmentation	None or focal, low intensity (tan)	Diffuse, but limited in area and old (brown)	Diffuse over most of gaiter distribution (lower one third) or recent pigmentation (purple)	Wider distribution (above lower third) and recent pigmentation
Inflammation	None	Mild cellulitis, limited to marginal area around ulcer	Moderate cellulitis, involves most of gaiter area (lower 2/3)	Severe cellulitis (lower third and above) or significant venous eczema
Induration	None	Focal, circum malleolar (<5 cm)	Medial or lateral, less than lower third of leg	Entire lower third of leg or more
Number of active ulcers	0	1	2	>2
Active ulceration duration	None	<3 mo	>3 mo, <1 yr	Not healed >1 yr
Active ulcer, size	None	<2 cm diameter	2-6 cm diameter	>6 cm diameter
Compressive therapy	Not used or not compliant	Intermittent use of stockings	Wears elastic stockings most days	Full compliance: stockings and elevation

GSV, Great saphenous vein; SSV, small saphenous vein.
Adapted from Kundu S, Grassi CJ, Khilnani NM, et al. Multi-disciplinary quality improvement guidelines for the treatment of lower-extremity superficial venous insufficiency with ambulatory phlebectomy from the Society of Interventional Radiology, Cardiovascular Interventional Radiological Society of Europe, American College of Phlebology and Canadian Interventional Radiology Association. *J Vasc Interv Radiol.* 2010;21:1-13.

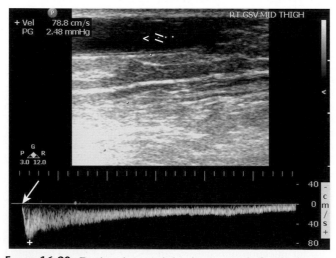

FIGURE 16-20. Duplex ultrasound showing retrograde flow in the great saphenous vein due to venous valvular insufficiency. Flow above the line is antegrade; flow below the line is retrograde. With release of an automated pressure cuff below the imaged level there is sudden brisk retrograde flow *(arrow)* in the great saphenous vein that is sustained for several seconds.

anesthetic. This outpatient procedure is an alternative to sclerotherapy for moderate and large varicosities, and even superficial segments of the GSV. The advantages of phlebectomy are related to removal of the abnormal vein segment, which reduces the pigmentation, palpable cords, and recanalization sometimes seen after sclerotherapy of large varices. The disadvantages are the need for multiple incisions, the higher risk of superficial nerve injury (especially around the ankle), and the greater time required to perform the procedure. Phlebectomy is generally not

Box 16-8. Indications for Intervention for Varicose Veins

General appearance
Aching pain
Leg heaviness
Leg fatigue
Superficial thrombophlebitis
External bleeding
Edema
Ankle hyperpigmentation
Skin changes
Venous ulcer

used to treat varicosities of the foot or those directly over the anterior surface of the tibia.

Phlebectomy is performed by first marking the veins to be removed with indelible ink (Fig. 16-25). After the extremity is prepped and draped, local anesthetic is administered by generous infiltration of dilute lidocaine in the subcutaneous tissues around the veins. The dilution is the same as used for tumescent anesthesia of saphenous veins. Direct injection into the veins should be avoided. A small incision is then made adjacent to the marked veins along natural fold lines. Either the tip of a #11 blade or a 16-gauge needle is used and the incision is tailored for the size of the vein to be removed—usually no more than 3-5 mm in length. A vein hook (there are numerous designs available, but sterilized Crochet hooks work as well) is then inserted through the incision, and using a combination of sweeping and probing maneuvers, the vein is engaged and withdrawn through the incision. The vein is secured with a small hemostat, and then gently pulled until the operator is able to visualize a loop of vein. Hemostats are placed on each side of the loop, the vein is divided between the

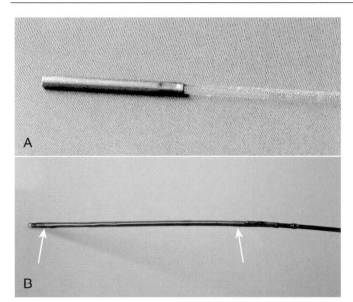

FIGURE 16-21. Endovenous thermal ablation probes. **A,** A 600-μ fiber with a gold jacket at the end to prevent contact between the tip of the laser and the vein wall. The laser is forward firing, and is withdrawn continuously during activation. This is a magnified view of the 4-French fiber. (Courtesy Angiodynamics Inc., Queensbury, N.Y.). **B,** A 7-French radiofrequency ablation catheter with a 7-cm treatment zone *(arrows)*. The vein is treated sequentially in 7-cm segments (Courtesy Covidien, Mansfield, Mass.).

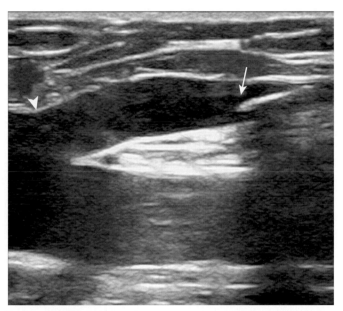

FIGURE 16-22. Ultrasound image showing a radiofrequency probe *(arrow)* in the great saphenous vein, approximately 2 cm distal to the saphenofemoral junction *(arrowhead).* The probe is never activated in the common femoral vein.

hemostats, and each end of the vein is gently pulled until it either breaks or the operator makes a new incision along the vein at an adjacent location and starts the process over again. Hemostasis is achieved with pressure or, for larger veins, ligation with absorbable suture of the residual vein stumps. When the extractions are complete, the incisions can be closed with Steri-strips or small 6-0 nylon sutures (we remove these after 48-72 hours to minimize scarring). A compression stocking and Ace wrap are applied, with the Ace wrap being removed when the patient goes to bed that evening. The patient should avoid lifting heavy objects (>25 lb) for a week and keep the incisions dry for 48 hours but otherwise

can continue with normal activity. The compression stockings are worn for 10 days.

Endovenous ablation, sclerotherapy, and phlebectomy are complimentary techniques. About two thirds of patients undergoing treatment of varicose veins require some combination of these techniques to achieve the best results. When ablation of a saphenous vein is combined with sclerotherapy or phlebectomy of a few varices, the procedures can be performed at the same time. When varices are extensive and there is also saphenous vein reflux, then endovenous ablation of the saphenous vein should be performed first, and the sclerotherapy/phlebectomy done about a month later. Waiting 3-4 weeks after saphenous vein ablation often results in a decrease in the size and number of the varices that subsequently need treatment.

Percutaneous replacement of venous valves is a promising experimental technique that may relieve reflux and venous hypertension in a nondestructive manner. A number of materials for construction of valves have been described. The valves are typically mounted in a metallic stent and delivered with imaging guidance.

▬ SEPTIC THROMBOPHLEBITIS

The definition of septic thrombophlebitis is pus and infected thrombus within the venous lumen. Almost all cases are acquired secondary to intravascular devices such as central venous catheters and pacemakers. The causative organism is *Staphylococcus aureus* in more than 50% of reported cases. The incidence is far lower than catheter or pacemaker pocket infections. Patients present with bacteremia, sepsis, pain over the affected vein, and sometimes purulence at the catheter insertion site. The finding of venous thrombosis, intraluminal gas, and extensive perivascular inflammatory changes are suggestive imaging findings. Removal of the device (with cultures of the intravascular portion), antibiotics, and rarely surgical thrombectomy are the standard treatment. Anecdotal cases of successful treatment with thrombolysis have been described.

▬ KLIPPEL-TRENAUNAY AND PARKES-WEBER SYNDROMES

Klippel-Trenaunay syndrome (KTS) is a congenital but not heritable syndrome involving combined vascular malformation (Table 16-6). The incidence of this rare syndrome (<1:10,000) is similar in males and females. In addition to the lower extremity, the pelvis, abdomen, and upper limb can be involved. Patients present with at least two of the following: cutaneous capillary malformations, atypical varicose veins or venous malformations, and limb hypertrophy (Fig. 16-26). The limb hypertrophy involves subcutaneous tissues and bone. There are two basic types: simple and complex. Simple KTS is characterized by less extensive cutaneous capillary malformations ("blotchy") and less extensive venous abnormalities. Patients with complex KTS have extensive ("geographic") cutaneous capillary malformations, absence or atresia of the deep venous system with extensive and anomalous (especially lateral) varicose veins, and lymphatic involvement in over 90% of cases. The lateral anomalous veins are termed *marginal veins*. Complex KTS is associated with a higher incidence of complications such as bleeding, skin ulceration, localized thrombophlebitis, cellulitis, PE, and Kasabach Merritt syndrome. The optimal imaging modality for the diagnosis of KTS and for planning intervention is MRI. Conventional venography is useful when other imaging studies are inconclusive.

Parkes-Weber syndrome (PWS) is related to but rarer than KTS. The cutaneous lesion in PWS is capillary arteriovenous malformation that is warm to the touch (unlike typical capillary cutaneous malformations) and may have a palpable or audible thrill (Fig. 16-27). The limb hypertrophy involves muscle and

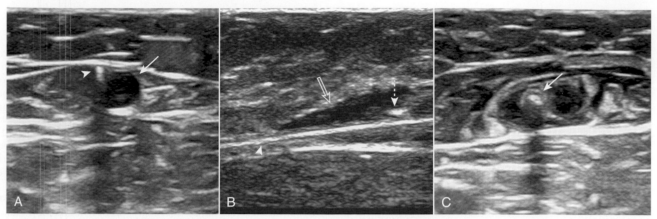

FIGURE **16-23**. Tumescent anesthesia. This is a critical step in the endovenous thermal ablation procedure. **A,** Axial ultrasound image of the great saphenous vein (GSV; *arrow*) with a probe in place *(arrowhead)*. **B,** Longitudinal image during injection of dilute anesthetic around the great saphenous vein. The *dashed arrow* is the 21-gauge needle used for injection. The anesthetic fluid *(open arrow)* dissects along the GSV compressing the vein around the probe *(arrowhead)*. The needle is continuously advanced within the perivenous space. Multiple punctures are required along the entire length of the vein to be treated. **C,** Axial image after infiltration of anesthetic around the GSV. The vein *(solid arrow)* is compressed around the catheter by the large volume of surrounding anesthetic fluid.

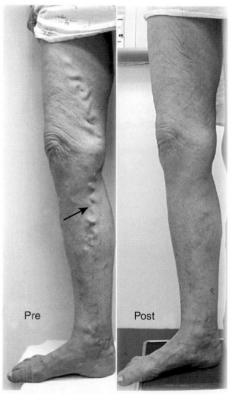

FIGURE **16-24**. Pretreatment and posttreatment images of a patient who underwent percutaneous endoluminal laser ablation of the greater saphenous vein (GSV) for varicosities. Distended, ropelike varicosities originating from the GSV *(arrow)* can be clearly seen on the pretreatment photograph (Pre). One month after ablation of the GSV, there is dramatic improvement (Post).

bone but can be less prominent than in KTS, and anomalous lateral varicose veins and lymphatic malformations are infrequent. About 77% of patients with PWS have unilateral lower limb involvement. The AVM can cause local complications such as bleeding and ulceration, as well as high-output cardiac failure.

Box 16-9. Sclerosing Agents

Sodium tetradecyl sulfate
Polidocanol
Sodium morrhuate
Hypertonic saline
Polyiodinated iodine

■ VENOUS MALFORMATIONS

Venous malformations are congenital lesions distinct from acquired varicosities (see Chapter 1). These lesions are most often isolated and sporadic, but can be associated with syndromes such as KTS. Venous malformations are soft, nonpulsatile, and decompress when the patient is prone. Superficial lesions can present with bleeding, limb discoloration, local thrombosis, and pain with ambulation. Deep lesions may present only as limb swelling without visible external abnormalities. The arterial pulse examination is normal. MRI is an excellent imaging modality for diagnosis and delineation of the extent of the lesion. Angiography demonstrates normal arteries with faint or absent opacification of the lesion; venography, especially with direct puncture of the malformation, allows diagnosis and treatment (Fig. 16-28). Sclerosis with alcohol, sodium tetradecyl sulfate, or polidocanol is effective in the management of these lesions. General anesthesia, injection of limited volumes of alcohol with fluoroscopic guidance, and multiple treatments are usually necessary. Skin necrosis, nerve and muscle dysfunction, and cardiac arrhythmia can occur.

■ VENOUS ANEURYSMS

True lower-extremity venous aneurysms are rare lesions, reported in all veins but most often in the popliteal vein (Fig. 16-29). Congenital venous aneurysms are focal dilatations of otherwise normal-diameter veins. Aneurysms can also develop in the outflow veins of patients with arteriovenous fistulas and malformations. Posttraumatic venous pseudoaneurysms have also been described. Complications of popliteal vein aneurysms include thrombosis and PE. Lower-extremity duplex ultrasound is an accurate diagnostic modality. Treatment with surgical excision has been recommended for symptomatic aneurysms.

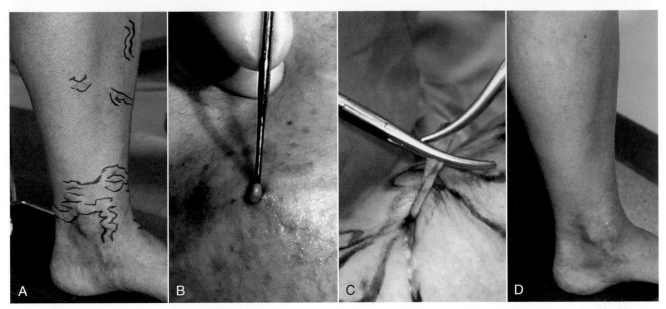

FIGURE 16-25. Phlebectomy of varicose veins. **A,** The veins to be removed have been marked with inedible ink while the patient is standing. Note the pigmentation around the ankle. The patient was then prepped and draped in the supine position, and generous amounts of dilute anesthetic solution were injected around the veins. **B,** Through a small incision, a vein hook was used to engage a loop of varicose vein. **C,** The loop of vein was clamped and divided, and gentle force was applied to each end of the vein to extract the segment. In this image, one end of the vein has already been removed. Force is applied until the vein segment breaks. **D,** Follow-up at 1 month. The incisions are barely perceptible, and all marked veins are now absent.

TABLE 16-6 Klippel-Trenaunay Syndrome

Feature	Incidence (%)
Capillary malformations ("port wine stain")	98
Atypical varicosities, hypoplasia or absence of deep veins	72
Bony and/or soft tissue hypertrophy	67
All three features	63
Two features	37
Unilateral lower limb	85
Bilateral lower limb	13
Upper and lower limb	10

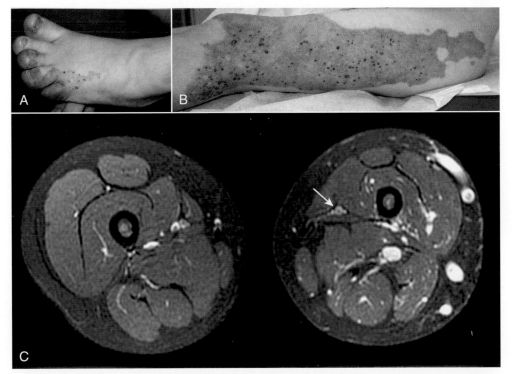

FIGURE 16-26. Complex Klippel-Trenaunay syndrome. **A,** Photograph of the patient's foot showing hypertrophy of toes 3, 4, and 5; the characteristic capillary cutaneous malformation; and a dilated superficial vein. **B,** Same patient, same leg. There is an extensive geographic capillary cutaneous malformation that is the same temperature as the surrounding normal skin. The dark papules are lymphangiectasias. **C,** Axial contrast-enhanced magnetic resonance image through the thighs. The right side is normal. On the left the muscles are smaller and the soft tissues increased; large anomalous veins are present; there is absence of the normal deep veins. The *arrow* identifies the left superficial femoral artery; note the absence of an accompanying femoral vein when compared to the right.

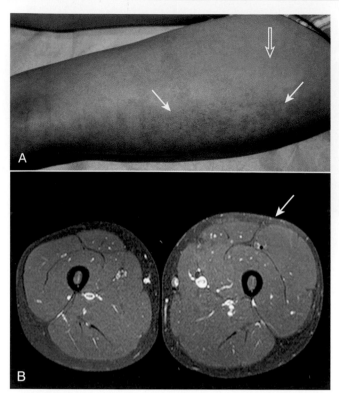

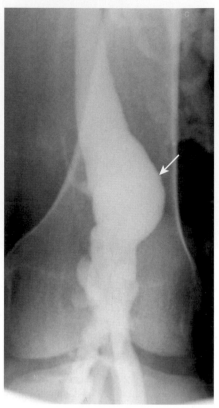

FIGURE 16-27. Parkes-Weber syndrome. **A,** Photograph of the left thigh showing the blotchy cutaneous lesion *(solid arrows)* that was warm to the touch compared to the surrounding skin, consistent with an arteriovenous malformation. The subcutaneous veins *(open arrow)* are prominent but not anomalous. **B,** Axial contrast-enhanced magnetic resonance imaging through the thighs. The left leg is symmetrically hypertrophied with enlarged but anatomically normal vascular structures. There are prominent subcutaneous veins beneath the capillary cutaneous malformation *(arrow).*

FIGURE 16-29. True popliteal vein aneurysm *(arrow).* There was no history of trauma or deep venous thrombosis.

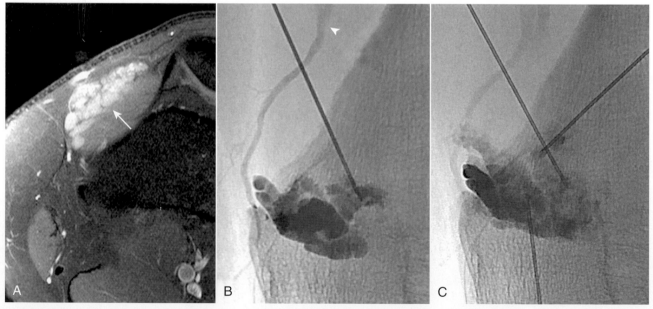

FIGURE 16-28. Venous malformation of the right leg symptomatic with pain and localized swelling. **A,** Contrast-enhanced axial magnetic resonance image showing the venous malformation *(arrow).* **B,** Digital venogram after direct puncture using ultrasound guidance. Contrast was slowly injected until a normal draining vein was identified *(arrowhead)* and the volume of contrast noted. **C,** Image obtained after access with two additional 21-gauge needles and injection of a combined total of 6 mL of dehydrated alcohol. Each alcohol injection matched the volume of contrast needed to opacify a draining vein.

SUGGESTED READINGS

Almeida JI, Raines JK. Ambulatory phlebectomy in the office. *Perspect Vasc Surg Endovasc Ther*. 2008;20:348-355.

Berry SA, Peterson C, Mize W, et al. Klippel-Trenaunay syndrome. *Am J Med Genet*. 1998;79:319-326.

Borsa JJ, Patel NH. The venous system: normal developmental anatomy and congenital anomalies. *Semin Interv Radiol*. 2001;18:69-82.

Chinsakchai K, Ten Duis K, Moll FL, et al. Trends in management of phlegmasia cerulea dolens. *Vasc Endovascular Surg*. 2011;45:5-14.

Ciccotosto C, Goodman LR, Washington L, et al. Indirect CT venography following CT pulmonary angiography: spectrum of CT findings. *J Thorac Imaging*. 2002;17:18-27.

Coleridge Smith P. Sclerotherapy and foam sclerotherapy for varicose veins. *Phlebology*. 2009;24:260-269.

Eklöf B, Rutherford RB, Bergan JJ, et al. Revision of the CEAP classification for chronic venous disorders: consensus statement. *J Vasc Surg*. 2004;40:1248-1252.

Enden T, Haig Y, Kløw NE, et al. Long-term outcome after additional catheter-directed thrombolysis versus standard treatment for acute iliofemoral deep vein thrombosis (the CaVenT study): a randomised controlled trial. *Lancet*. 2012;379:31-38.

Falagas ME, Vardakas KZ, Athanasiou S. Intravenous heparin in combination with antibiotics for the treatment of deep vein septic thrombophlebitis: a systematic review. *Eur J Pharmacol*. 2007;557:93-98.

Gillespie DL, Villavicencio JL, Gallagher C, et al. Presentation and management of venous aneurysms. *J Vasc Surg*. 1997;26:845-852.

Gillespie DL, Kistner B, Glass C, et al. Venous ulcer diagnosis, treatment, and prevention of recurrences. *J Vasc Surg*. 2010;52(5 Suppl):8S-14S.

Gloviczki P, Comerota AJ, Dalsing MC, et al. The care of patients with varicose veins and associated chronic venous diseases: clinical practice guidelines of the Society for Vascular Surgery and the American Venous Forum. *J Vasc Surg*. 2011;53(Suppl):2S-48S.

Goldhaber SZ, Bounameaux H. Pulmonary embolism and deep vein thrombosis. *Lancet*. 2012;379:1835-1846.

Jaff MR, McMurtry MS, Archer SL, et al. Management of massive and submassive pulmonary embolism, iliofemoral deep vein thrombosis, and chronic thromboembolic pulmonary hypertension: a scientific statement from the American Heart Association. *Circulation*. 2011;123:1788-1830.

Jeon UB, Chung JW, Jae HJ, et al. May-Thurner syndrome complicated by acute iliofemoral vein thrombosis: helical CT venography for evaluation of long-term stent patency and changes in the iliac vein. *AJR Am J Roentgenol*. 2010;195:751-757.

Kearon C, Akl EA, Comerota AJ, et al. Antithrombotic therapy for VTE disease: Antithrombotic Therapy and Prevention of Thrombosis, 9th ed: American College of Chest Physicians Evidence-Based Clinical Practice Guidelines. *Chest*. 2012;141(2 Suppl):419-494.

Khilnani NM, Grassi CJ, Kundu S, et al. Multi-society consensus quality improvement guidelines for the treatment of lower extremity superficial venous insufficiency with endovenous thermal ablation from the Society of Interventional Radiology, Cardiovascular Interventional Radiological Society of Europe, American College of Phlebology and Canadian Interventional Radiology Association. *J Vasc Interv Radiol*. 2010;21:14-31.

Kundu S, Grassi CJ, Khilnani NM, et al. Multi-disciplinary quality improvement guidelines for the treatment of lower extremity superficial venous insufficiency with ambulatory phlebectomy from the Society of Interventional Radiology, Cardiovascular Interventional Radiological Society of Europe, American College of Phlebology and Canadian Interventional Radiology Association. *J Vasc Interv Radiol*. 2010;21:1-13.

Leopardi D, Hoggan BL, Fitridge RA, et al. Systematic review of treatments for varicose veins. *Ann Vasc Surg*. 2009;23:264-276.

Mewissen MW, Seabrook GR, Meissner MH, et al. Catheter-directed thrombolysis for lower extremity deep venous thrombosis: report of a national multicenter registry. *Radiology*. 1999;211:39-49.

Nayak L, Hildebolt CF, Vedantham S. Postthrombotic syndrome: feasibility of a strategy of imaging-guided endovascular intervention. *J Vasc Interv Radiol*. 2012;23:1165-1173.

Nazir SA, Ganeshan A, Nazir S, et al. Endovascular treatment options in the management of lower limb deep venous thrombosis. *Cardiovasc Intervent Radiol*. 2009;32:861-876.

Nchimi A, Ghaye B, Noukoua CT, et al. Incidence and distribution of lower extremity deep venous thrombosis at indirect computed tomography venography in patients suspected of pulmonary embolism. *Thromb Haemost*. 2007;97:566-572.

Nesbitt C, Eifell RK, Coyne P, et al. Endovenous ablation (radiofrequency and laser) and foam sclerotherapy versus conventional surgery for great saphenous vein varices. *Cochrane Database Syst Rev*. 2011 Oct 5(10):CD005624.

Oklu R, Habito R, Mayr M, et al. Pathogenesis of varicose veins. *J Vasc Interv Radiol*. 2012;23:33-39.

Rasmussen LH, Lawaetz M, Bjoern L, et al. Randomized clinical trial comparing endovenous laser ablation, radiofrequency ablation, foam sclerotherapy and surgical stripping for great saphenous varicose veins. *Br J Surg*. 2011;98:1079-1087.

Redondo P, Aguado L, Martínez-Cuesta A. Diagnosis and management of extensive vascular malformations of the lower limb: part I. Clinical diagnosis. *J Am Acad Dermatol*. 2011;65:893-906.

Redondo P, Aguado L, Martínez-Cuesta A. Diagnosis and management of extensive vascular malformations of the lower limb: part II. Systemic repercussions, diagnosis, and treatment. *J Am Acad Dermatol*. 2011;65:909-923.

Shadid N, Ceulen R, Nelemans P, et al. Randomized clinical trial of ultrasound-guided foam sclerotherapy versus surgery for the incompetent great saphenous vein. *Br J Surg*. 2012;99:1062-1070.

Shingler S, Robertson L, Boghossian S, et al. Compression stockings for the initial treatment of varicose veins in patients without venous ulceration. *Cochrane Database Syst Rev*. 2011(11):CD008819.

Tellings SS, Ceulen RP, Sommer A. Surgery and endovenous techniques for the treatment of small saphenous varicose veins: a review of the literature. *Phlebology*. 2011;26:179-184.

Vedantham S. Interventional approaches to deep vein thrombosis. *Am J Hematol*. 2012;87(Suppl 1):S113-S118.

Wells PS, Anderson DR, Rodger M, et al. Evaluation of D-dimer in the diagnosis of suspected deep-vein thrombosis. *N Engl J Med*. 2003;349:1227-1235.

CHAPTER 17

Image-Guided Percutaneous Biopsy

Michael J. Lee, MSc, FRCPI, FRCR, FFR(RCSI), FSIR, EBIR

Percutaneous image-guided biopsy has gained wide popularity. It can be used to establish the identity of superficial or deep masses in many parts of the body. Advances in cytopathologic techniques, the ability to precisely guide needles to various locations in the body using computed tomography (CT) and sonography, and the safety of fine-needle biopsy have led to widespread acceptance of biopsy procedures by clinicians. The vast majority of biopsies are performed to confirm suspected malignancy, particularly in a patient with a known primary tumor. In addition, many biopsies are performed in oncologic patients with residual masses after therapy to determine whether such a mass represents residual viable tumor or necrotic tissue.

In the early years of image-guided percutaneous biopsy, most biopsies were obtained with thin needles (20-22 gauge). These needles obtain a cytologic aspirate that is sufficient to confirm or refute a diagnosis of malignancy, but that often is not able to provide a specific histologic diagnosis. More recently, there has been a tendency to use spring-activated cutting needles (biopsy guns) to obtain core biopsies. The advantage of core biopsy needles is that cores of tissues retain the organization of the lesion, often allowing precise histologic diagnosis of malignant tumor type or confidently allowing the diagnosis of benignity.

▬ PATIENT PREPARATION

The vast majority of image-guided biopsies can be performed on an outpatient basis. The clinician should obtain routine partial thromboplastin time (PTT), prothrombin time (PT), and platelet levels in all patients undergoing chest or abdominal biopsy or biopsy of any deep-seated lesion. If the lesion to be biopsied is superficial, such as in the neck, coagulation studies are not required, because direct pressure will achieve hemostasis if bleeding occurs. If the patient is receiving a nonsteroidal antiinflammatory drug such as aspirin, either defer the procedure for 10 days or, depending on the location of the lesion, perform a fine-needle biopsy, because the likelihood of bleeding (in the absence of any abnormality in PT, PTT, or platelet count) as a result of aspirin alone is very low. In some patients with drug-eluting stents, stopping therapy with clopidogrel would risk stent thrombosis. In these more difficult situations, the need for biopsy must be carefully weighed against the risk of bleeding; operators should use fine-gauge needles and minimize the number of passes made. Most biopsies can be performed with the patient under local anesthesia without the use of sedoanalgesia. Exceptions include biopsies in pediatric patients and biopsies of deep lesions such as pancreatic masses or retroperitoneal masses. In addition, if the patient is apprehensive, sedoanalgesia may be required. The combination of midazolam and fentanyl is the most advantageous for achieving conscious sedation. A loading dose of 1-2 mg of midazolam with 50-100 µg of fentanyl, given intravenously, is appropriate. Doses can then be titrated against the patient's level of anxiety throughout the procedure. Monitor patients with a pulse oximeter and VitaCuff for blood pressure measurements. A nurse should monitor the patient during the procedure so that the operator can concentrate solely on the biopsy.

▬ BIOPSY TECHNIQUE

Needle Choice

Fine-needle biopsies are obtained with 20- to 25-gauge needles (Table 17-1 and Fig. 17-1). There are a wide variety of needle types and needle tip designs on the market. Broadly, fine-gauge needles can be divided into those with a sharp beveled tip (e.g., Chiba or spinal needles for simple aspiration) or those with a modified, tissue cutting tip (see Table 17-1). The advantage of using a needle with a cutting tip is that a core of tissue may be obtainable with this needle type. The author's personal preference is the Turner needle for all fine-needle biopsies. Advantages of fine-needle biopsy include the ability to traverse bowel without ill effect, and the likelihood of inducing hemorrhage when sampling vascular lesions is minimal. In the author's practice, fine-needle biopsy is performed on virtually all lung biopsies, all neck biopsies, and in abdominal biopsies wherein the patient has a known primary with liver or other lesions that are thought to be metastases (Box 17-1). Large-gauge needle biopsies (14- to 19-gauge) are almost universally performed with a spring-activated, modified Tru-Cut system (Box 17-2). Many such systems of variable gauge, throw length, and design are available (Fig. 17-2). Most are disposable needle systems, although some, such as the Bard biopsy gun, can be used repeatedly with disposable needles. This is the least expensive option, in that, once the biopsy gun is obtained, only the needles

TABLE 17-1 Fine-Gauge Biopsy Needles

Name	Description	Company
Turner	45-degree bevel tip to provide cutting edge	Cook, Bloomington, Ind.
Franseen	Three-pronged needle tip like "teeth"	Cook, Bloomington, Ind.
Westcott	Slotted 2.2-mm opening, 3 mm from needle tip	Becton-Dickinson, Rutherford, N.J.
E-Z-EM	Trough cut in needle tip	E-Z-EM Inc., Westbury, N.Y.

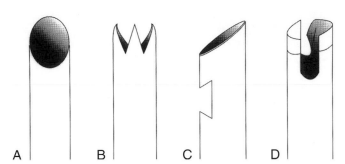

FIGURE 17-1. Turner (**A**), Franseen (**B**), Westcott (**C**), and E-Z-EM (**D**) needles. The Turner needle has a 45-degree bevel that provides a cutting edge. The Franseen needle has a three-pronged tip. The Westcott needle has a side-cutting trough near its end. The E-Z-EM needle has a trough cut in the tip of the needle. Despite the various appearances of these needles, there are no data to suggest any one needle yields consistently better samples. The author tends to predominantly use the Turner needle.

need be replaced. The author's preference is for a nondisposable biopsy gun and disposable 18- and 20-gauge needles. Advantages are (1) ease of use, (2) ability to hold the biopsy gun with one hand, which is particularly important when using ultrasound guidance, and (3) uniform consistency in size and amount of tissue obtained. This is a major advantage over non-automated large-gauge biopsy systems, wherein the consistency of the tissue obtained is directly related to the operator's skill. Using an automated system, the biopsy procedure is fast and the biopsy needle system does not remain in the patient for long. Anecdotally, patients appear to experience less pain than when conventional large-gauge biopsy systems are used. In general, large-gauge automated needle biopsies are performed in patients in whom there is no known primary tumor, when there is a possibility of lymphoma, or after fine-needle biopsy has failed (see Box 17-2).

In recent years, this distinction between large-gauge biopsy and fine-needle biopsy has become blurred because of the development of 20-gauge automated Tru-Cut needles. These 20-gauge needles are considered to be in the fine-needle category but obtain a core of tissue like any other Tru-Cut needle. These needles are now used more and more frequently, particularly when an experienced cytopathologist is not present for the biopsy procedure.

Image Guidance

CT and sonography are the two main image guidance modalities used for biopsy procedures. Although magnetic resonance interventional systems are used in clinical practice, their role in performing routine biopsies is limited by cost and lack of widespread availability. The choice between CT and sonography is largely guided by clinician preference and the nature, size,

Box 17-1. **Fine-Needle Biopsy (20- to 25-Gauge)**

Proper technique more important than needle type
Can traverse bowel if necessary
Computed tomography or sonographic guidance
Nonaspiration technique for vascular lesions
Coaxial or tandem technique can be used
Often sufficient when known primary neoplasm present

Box 17-2. **Large-Gauge Core Biopsy (14- to 19-Gauge)**

Spring-activated modified Tru-Cut needle preferable
Advantages: ease of use, consistent tissue obtained, decreased pain
Can be inserted in tandem with fine-gauge needle
Must not traverse bowel
Use if lymphoma suspected or failed fine-needle biopsy

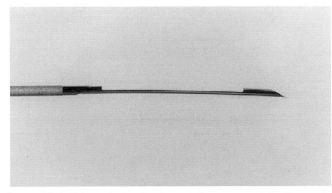

FIGURE 17-2. Schematic showing the end of an automated Tru-Cut needle. A trough is apparent in the end of the needle. A core of tissue that conforms to the length and depth of the trough is obtained when this needle is used. The core of tissue is cut by the outer needle sliding down over the trough and capturing the specimen.

TABLE 17-2 Image Guidance

Image Guidance Table	Computed Tomography	Sonography
Continuous needle visualization	No	Yes
Learning curve	Short	Long
Cost	Moderate	Low
Portable	No	Yes
Expediency	Slow	Fast
Ionizing radiation	Yes	No

location, and site of the lesion. All neck and soft tissue lesions, most liver lesions, large abdominal masses, and some pancreatic lesions can be biopsied under sonographic guidance. Mediastinal lesions, most pancreatic, retroperitoneal, adrenal and pelvic lesions, and some liver lesions are biopsied under CT guidance. The relative advantages and disadvantages of CT and sonography are listed in Table 17-2.

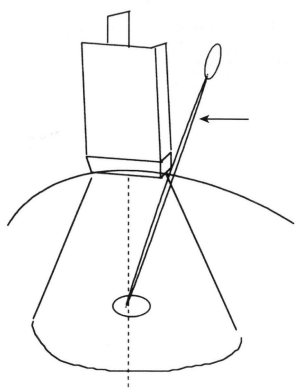

FIGURE 17-3. Schematic showing correct technique for freehand ultrasound-guided biopsy. The probe is maneuvered so that the lesion lies in the center of the ultrasound beam. The needle *(arrow)* is then inserted at the short end of the transducer, and with proper alignment in the ultrasound beam, the entire needle shaft should be visible at all times.

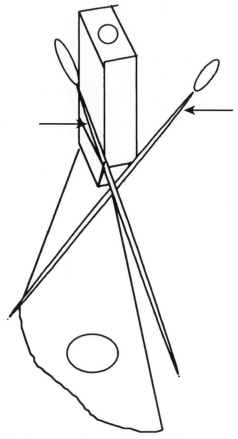

FIGURE 17-4. Schematic showing incorrect alignment. If the needle *(arrows)* is inserted at an angle to the direction of the ultrasound beam, the full length of the needle is not seen and the biopsy is difficult to perform. Proper alignment of the needle in the plane of the ultrasound beam is mandatory for correct visualization of the needle.

Sonography

Sonography should be used for image guidance because it provides continuous real-time needle visualization. There are many commercially available biopsy guides that can be fitted to existing ultrasound transducers that will direct the needle into the path of the ultrasound beam. The author prefers to use a freehand approach with the needle inserted through the skin into the plane of the ultrasound beam. The freehand technique offers more flexibility in that needle position and angle adjustments can be made as the biopsy is being performed to correct or realign the needle path if necessary.

The transducer can be covered with a sterile sheath using sterile K-Y Jelly as an acoustic coupling agent. Alternatively, the transducer can be sterilized by painting the surface with Betadine. The author's unit tends to use a sterile cover. The skin is cleansed with Betadine and the lesion located in the center of the ultrasound beam. The shortest and safest path to the lesion is chosen. The needle is aligned with the ultrasound beam and inserted through the anesthetized skin and subcutaneous tissues toward the lesion to be biopsied. With proper alignment of the needle within the plane of the ultrasound beam, the entire length of the needle shaft should be visualized at all times (Fig. 17-3). If the entire needle is not visible, some malalignment of the needle with the ultrasound beam exists (Fig. 17-4). This can be corrected by rechecking the alignment of the needle with the central beam of the transducer. A slight jiggling or in-and-out motion of the needle helps visualize the needle (Fig. 17-5). When experience is gained with sonographically guided freehand biopsy methods, this becomes a very rapid and reliable method of guiding biopsy needles to the target in question.

Sonographic guidance can be problematic in obese patients because the echogenic needle can be hard to visualize in the echogenic soft tissues. Lesions located within bones, or deep to bone or bowel, cannot be biopsied owing to lack of visualization of the lesion.

Computed Tomography

CT can be used to guide biopsy needles to virtually any area of the body. CT provides excellent visualization of the lesion to be biopsied and allows accurate identification of organs between the skin and the lesion. CT is particularly suited to guiding biopsy of deep lesions within the body such as retroperitoneal, pelvic, thoracic, and musculoskeletal lesions. The learning curve associated with CT-guided biopsies is generally shorter than that associated with sonographically guided biopsies, and it has therefore become a popular guidance modality. Scans through the region of interest are first performed with either a commercially available grid system (E-Z-EM, Westbury, N.Y.) or a homemade grid system placed on the patient's skin. Commercially available grid systems contain multiple lead lines constructed in a grid pattern. Alternatively, a homemade phantom can be constructed by taping together approximately ten 15-cm lengths of 4- or 5-French catheters at 1-cm intervals. The homemade grid fulfills the same function as the commercially available systems.

On the CT image that gives the best view of the lesion, a safe access route is chosen and the distance to the lesion marked on the image. The patient is then brought to the table position where the biopsy is to be performed and the skin site marked using the grid on the patient's skin and the centering laser light beam in the CT gantry. The needle is inserted to the predetermined

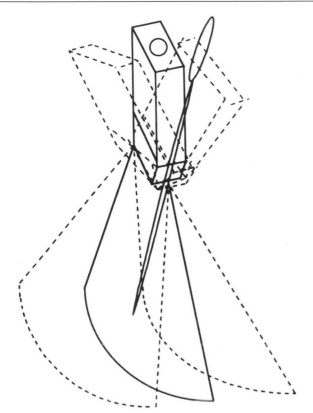

FIGURE 17-5. Visualization of the needle is aided by a gentle rocking movement of the transducer and a slight to-and-fro jiggling motion of the needle.

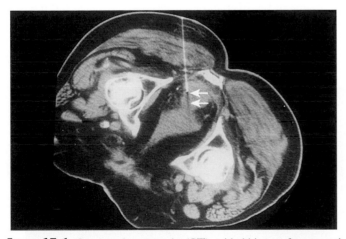

FIGURE 17-6. Computed tomography (CT)-guided biopsy of a presacral transgluteal mass illustrating the black streak artifact that occurs when the CT slice passes through the needle tip. A transgluteal approach has been used to biopsy this presacral mass. Streak artifact *(arrows)* can be seen at the tip of the needle. If this is not visualized, the CT slice has not passed through the needle tip.

depth and location. Scans are obtained at the level of the needle entry site to determine the location of the needle. The tip of the needle is readily recognized by a black streak artifact that occurs at the needle tip (Fig. 17-6). If the needle is not in an appropriate position, further needles can be inserted and scanned (using the first needle as a guide for adjusting the trajectory of further needles) until an appropriate position within the lesion is obtained.

Compared to sonography, the lack of real-time visualization with CT guidance is a limiting factor. The recent introduction of CT fluoroscopy with multislice CT scanners has attempted

to redress this balance. However, CT fluoroscopic units will undoubtedly make CT guidance a much more viable, albeit more expensive, option for biopsies.

Performing the Biopsy

Fine-Needle Aspiration Biopsy

A 10-mL syringe is applied to the hub of the needle that has been inserted into the lesion, and suction is applied. In general, 3-5 mL of suction is appropriate for most biopsies. If the lesion is vascular, such as a thyroid lesion or some liver lesions, minimal (1-2 mL) suction is appropriate. Larger amounts of suction may cause considerable quantities of blood to be aspirated into the syringe. For more scirrhous lesions such as pancreatic tumors, 5-10 mL of suction may be required. While suction is applied, the needle is moved quite firmly in a to-and-fro motion through the lesion for approximately 10-15 seconds or until blood appears in the hub of the needle. Suction is released while the needle is being removed to prevent aspiration of cells along the needle track that may confuse the cytologic interpretation of the sample. Ideally, a cytologic technician should be available to handle the specimen and a cytopathologist should be in attendance to render a preliminary report. The biopsy procedure can then be guided by the initial cytopathology report. If insufficient tissue is available for interpretation, more samples are obtained until a diagnosis is reached. If after four or five samples have been obtained a diagnosis is still not forthcoming, a large-gauge core biopsy sample should be obtained.

Nonaspiration Fine-Needle Biopsy

In some situations, it is more advantageous to perform a nonaspiration fine-needle biopsy. The nonaspiration technique is particularly valid for hemorrhagic organs such as the thyroid and occasionally hemorrhagic lesions within the liver. Using the nonaspiration technique, the needle is inserted into the lesion and again multiple to-and-fro motions through the lesion are performed until either blood appears in the hub of the needle or 15 seconds have elapsed. The needle is then removed. No syringe is used in the nonaspiration technique. The hypothesis is that cells advance into the needle lumen by capillary action.

This technique has not found widespread acceptance, although it is useful, in combination with aspiration cytology for biopsy of thyroid lesions.

Coaxial vs. Tandem Technique

Using the coaxial technique, a single needle is placed in the periphery of the lesion and a smaller, longer needle is placed through the initial needle to biopsy the lesion (Fig. 17-7). Using the Turner biopsy needle system, a 23-gauge needle will pass through a 20-gauge needle and a 22-gauge through a 19-gauge. The coaxial technique has several advantages in that only one puncture is made into the organ, reducing the propensity for hemorrhage or other complications. Multiple tissue samples can be obtained through the first needle. Lastly, precise needle placement is required only for the first needle.

Using the tandem technique, a 22-gauge needle is placed into the lesion and used as a reference needle (see Fig. 17-7). This reference needle then stays within the lesion until the end of the procedure. Further needles are inserted in tandem to the reference needle and are placed to the same depth and follow the same trajectory as the reference needle. This technique is useful for CT-guided biopsies wherein multiple fine-needle samples can be obtained without precisely localizing each subsequent needle that is passed.

In the main, the coaxial and tandem techniques are primarily used with CT guidance. With real-time sonographic guidance, the author's unit generally takes a sample with a single needle and guides subsequent needles into the lesion as required. Because of the flexibility of sonography and continuous real-time visualization, the tandem and coaxial techniques are rarely necessary. However, they are useful when using CT guidance so that further needle passes do not require precise CT monitoring, which is cumbersome and time consuming.

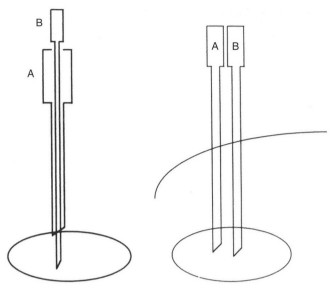

FIGURE 17-7. Schematic showing the coaxial *(left)* and the tandem *(right)* techniques. For the coaxial technique, a needle **(A)** is inserted down to the anterior edge of the lesion. A thinner, longer needle **(B)** is placed through the first needle and samples are obtained from the lesion using the insert needle. In this way multiple specimens can be obtained from the lesion without making separate punctures. Additionally, the larger needle can be manipulated at the skin so that it points in different directions for sampling different parts of the lesion. Using the tandem technique, a single needle **(A)** is first guided into the lesion and remains untouched throughout the biopsy. Other needles **(B)** are inserted in tandem to the first or reference needle **(A)** to obtain biopsies from the lesion. The subsequent needles do not have to be specifically guided into the lesion, when the first needle is used as a reference.

■ ABDOMINAL BIOPSY

Liver

CT or ultrasound can be used to guide liver biopsies, depending on clinician preference. The author prefers to use ultrasound, because it is less cumbersome, is faster, and employs real-time guidance (Fig. 17-8). In experienced hands, ultrasound can be used to biopsy the vast majority of liver lesions. For lesions that are high in the liver, near the diaphragm, the patient is placed in a right anterior oblique position. By scanning obliquely in the intercostal space, it is usually possible to visualize the lesion and guide needles in (Fig. 17-9). Occasionally, if a lesion near the dome of the diaphragm is not visible by sonography, a transpleural or transpulmonary route under CT guidance may be the only approach possible (Fig. 17-10). When biopsying peripheral lesions on the edge of the liver, it is best to try to traverse some normal liver before entering the lesion. This is particularly true when performing a large-gauge needle biopsy. By traversing normal liver first, there is a "safety zone" to tamponade any possible bleeding. In general, when biopsying a liver lesion, it is best to biopsy the edge of the lesion to avoid potentially necrotic areas in the center of the lesion (Fig. 17-11).

Liver biopsy for diffuse liver disease has become an increasing part of the service provided by interventional radiologists. Traditionally, these biopsies were performed by clinicians without any image guidance. Although generally a safe procedure, complications such as pneumothorax, hemothorax, and failure to obtain liver tissue occurred in patients with slightly abnormal anatomy. Many interventional radiologists are now performing these biopsies under ultrasound guidance. Most are performed on an outpatient basis. With the patient under suspended respiration, the author's unit uses ultrasound to locate the right lobe of the liver and obtain samples using an 18-gauge automated core biopsy needle. A point in the midaxillary line is chosen overlying the right lobe of the liver and local anesthetic is infiltrated into the skin. The liver capsule is also infiltrated with local anesthetic, which can be painful; the patient should be warned and asked not to move. Obtain two 18-gauge samples while the patient's breath is held in expiration. Patients should be told that, in about

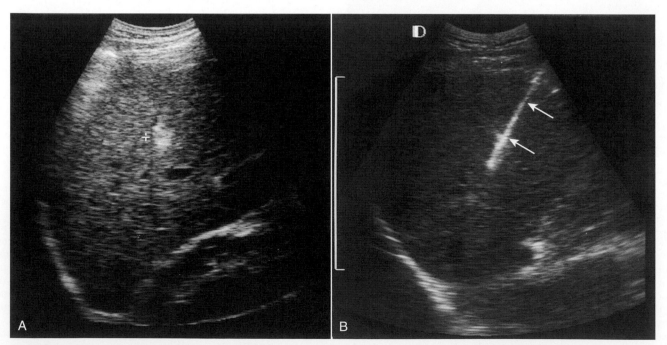

FIGURE 17-8. A patient with hepatitis B and a hyperechoic lesion seen on an annual screening ultrasound. **A,** Small (1.5-cm) hyperechoic lesion is seen in the right lobe of the liver. A magnetic resonance study excluded the presence of a hemangioma. **B,** Using freehand ultrasound technique, the lesion was biopsied using first fine needles and then an 18-gauge automated Tru-Cut needle. Note the full length of the needle *(arrows)* can be seen with appropriate ultrasound technique. This proved to be an area of fibrosis and did not represent hepatocellular carcinoma.

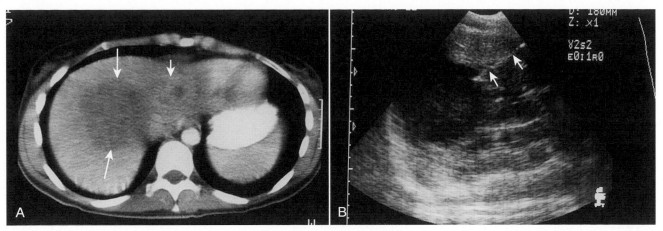

FIGURE 17-9. Patient with a previous history of melanoma and lesions present in the liver. **A,** Computed tomography scan showing a large lesion *(large arrows)* high near the dome of the diaphragm. A smaller lesion is noted in the left lobe *(small arrow)* of the liver. **B,** Using an intercostal approach with the patient in the right anterior oblique position, the lesion was easily sampled. A 22-gauge needle *(arrows)* can be seen entering the lesion. The biopsy confirmed a melanoma metastasis.

10%-20% of such biopsies, the patient experiences right shoulder tip pain after the procedure.

Pancreas

Pancreatic biopsy can be performed under ultrasound guidance if the lesion is visible. However, more often than not, the lesion is not optimally visualized under ultrasound, and CT guidance is used (Fig. 17-12). The stomach is avoided if possible, but if impossible, the stomach can be punctured with 20- or 22-gauge needles to access the pancreas. Many pancreatic cancers are associated with some surrounding pancreatitis, so that on a non-contrast CT scan the tumor may appear larger and biopsy of the area around the tumor may lead to a false-negative result. The accuracy of CT-guided pancreatic biopsy can be increased by performing a contrast-enhanced scan before the biopsy to precisely locate and map the tumor.

Pancreatic carcinomas are often very scirrhous and up to 10 mL of suction may have to be applied before cells are obtained. If appropriate specimens are not obtained after three or four passes, a large-gauge core biopsy may be required. This can be performed with the biopsy gun or other automated biopsy system. A useful alternative is to use a 20-gauge automated Tru-Cut needle, particularly when a cytologist is not in attendance for the biopsy. When a fluid-filled pancreatic lesion such as a cystic tumor is encountered, it is vitally important not to transgress the colon with a small-gauge needle en route to the lesion. This may convert a sterile mass into an abscess (Box 17-3).

Kidney

Renal biopsies are performed infrequently because most solid renal masses require surgical removal. Biopsies are performed if there is a suggestion of lymphoma or renal metastatic disease. Biopsy of renal lesions is also often performed before percutaneous ablation therapies. Complex renal cysts may also occasionally require aspiration. Renal lesions can be biopsied under ultrasound or CT guidance (Fig. 17-13). With ultrasound guidance, either a posterior or posterior oblique approach can be used. With CT guidance, a posterior approach is generally used. In general, core biopsies are needed for renal masses because sufficient tissue to differentiate metastases from primary tumors or to subtype lymphoma is required.

At many centers, nephrologic renal cortical biopsies are performed under ultrasound guidance. Ultrasound guidance is used to obtain core biopsies from both native and transplant kidneys.

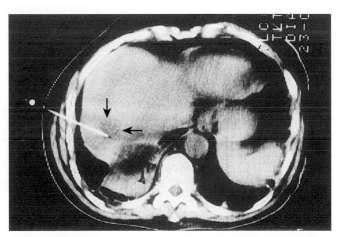

FIGURE 17-10. Transpulmonary biopsy of a small lesion near the dome of the diaphragm using computed tomography (CT) guidance. A solitary lesion *(arrows)* was seen in this patient with a previous history of cancer. The lesion measured 2.5 cm but could not be seen well with ultrasound. A transpulmonary CT-guided approach was therefore used to biopsy this lesion, which proved to be a colorectal metastasis. Although rarely used, this approach can be used if there is no other means of obtaining a biopsy specimen.

The lower pole is chosen for these biopsies and an 18-gauge automated core biopsy needle is guided into the lower pole. Biopsies are not performed in hydronephrotic systems, and it is important to avoid the renal hilum with the biopsy needle. Ultrasound guidance for nephrologic biopsy substantially reduces the complication rate when compared to blind biopsy.

Adrenal Glands

The need for adrenal biopsy has decreased dramatically with the recent introduction of lipid-sensitive imaging techniques for differentiating benign from malignant adrenal masses. Because of their position, high up in the retroperitoneum, the adrenal glands can pose problems for biopsy in that a direct posterior approach often passes through lung.

Adrenal lesions are predominately biopsied under CT guidance, although occasionally, if the adrenal mass is large, ultrasound guidance can be used (Fig. 17-14). There are a number of methods for performing the biopsy under CT guidance. These include the right lateral transhepatic approach (see Fig. 17-14)

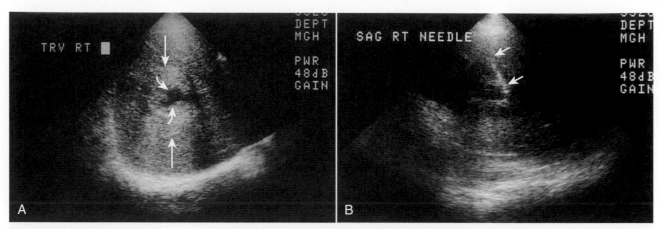

FIGURE 17-11. Biopsy of a necrotic liver lesion in a patient with colon cancer. **A,** Ultrasound shows a 4-cm lesion *(arrows)* in the right lobe of the liver. Central necrosis *(small arrows)* is seen in the center of the lesion. **B,** In this case, biopsy of the edge of the lesion is mandatory because a sample from the center of the lesion would be unrepresentative of the whole. The needle *(arrows)* can be seen in the edge of the lesion.

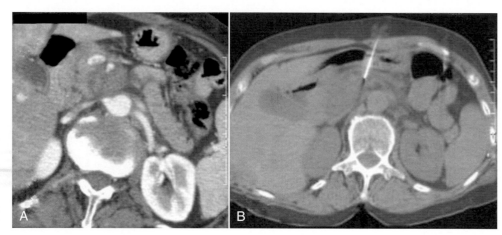

FIGURE 17-12. Patient presenting with mild jaundice and a 20-lb weight loss. **A,** Dynamic computed tomography through the head of the pancreas before biopsy reveals a small mass in the uncinate lobe of the pancreas. **B,** Using the tandem technique, a needle was placed into the abnormal area and biopsies were performed. The patient had pancreatic carcinoma.

Box 17-3. Pancreatic Biopsy

Computed tomography guidance often necessary
Stomach avoided if possible
Accuracy improved by giving intravenous contrast
Maximal suction often necessary
Do not traverse colon en route to a cystic lesion
20-gauge cutting needle is a useful addition

(right adrenal gland), the left anterior transhepatic approach (left adrenal), the angled posterior approach, and the lateral decubitus approach. The right transhepatic and left transhepatic approaches are direct routes to the right and left adrenal glands, respectively. The right transhepatic approach passes through the right lobe of the liver and into the right adrenal gland. The left transhepatic approach passes through the left lobe of the liver and into the left adrenal gland. The patient lies supine in both approaches. The angled prone approach takes advantage of Pythagoras' theorem to place a needle angled from a subcostal approach into the lesion (Fig. 17-15). The lateral decubitus approach works on the principle that when a patient is placed in the lateral decubitus position, the underlying lung expands less than the overlying lung. The patient is placed in a lateral decubitus position with the side containing the adrenal lesion placed nearest the table top (Fig. 17-16). A direct posterior approach can then be used, because the intervening lung is usually no longer present. The lateral decubitus approach is used predominantly in the author's unit such that a direct posterior approach can be used for adrenal biopsy.

Retroperitoneum

Retroperitoneal masses are generally biopsied under CT guidance. A posterior approach is usually used, passing either through or alongside the psoas muscle. If an anterior approach is used, thin-gauge needles are used because often many structures lie within the path of the needle (Fig. 17-17). Using a posterior approach, large-gauge needles can be used (Fig. 17-18). Occasionally in thin individuals retroperitoneal masses can be visualized with sonography using a posterior approach and the psoas muscle as an acoustic window. It is always worth checking whether the retroperitoneal mass can be seen with sonography. If it is visible, the biopsy can be performed under ultrasound guidance.

Prostate

There has been an explosion in the number of prostate biopsies performed since the introduction of the PSA (prostate-specific antigen) test in the late 1980s. Whereas a level of up to 4 ng/mL is considered within normal limits, a level greater than 4 ng/mL does not specifically imply cancer. The PSA level rises with benign prostatic hyperplasia (BPH) as well as with cancer, and many older men have abnormal PSA levels. However, it can be said that the higher the PSA, the greater the likelihood of cancer, particularly when the PSA level is greater than 10 ng/mL. To address the nonspecificity of a raised PSA level, PSA density testing has been introduced. This entails measuring gland volume and correlating gland volume with the PSA level. This latter measure reflects an attempt to correlate the PSA level with the amount of BPH. Measuring gland volume by

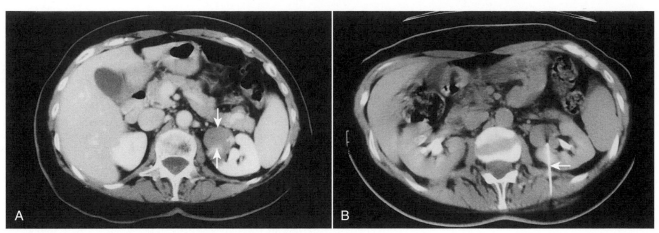

FIGURE 17-13. Patient with lymphoma and a renal mass discovered on a routine follow-up computed tomography (CT) scan. **A,** A nonenhancing mass *(arrows)* was noted on the dynamic CT. The patient was referred for biopsy rather than surgical removal because of the possibility that the mass represented recurrent lymphoma. **B,** A CT-guided biopsy was performed using a posterior approach. A 22-gauge needle *(arrow)* was inserted into the lesion and used as a reference. Multiple cores were then obtained from the lesion using 18-gauge automated biopsy needles. The lesion was recurrent lymphoma.

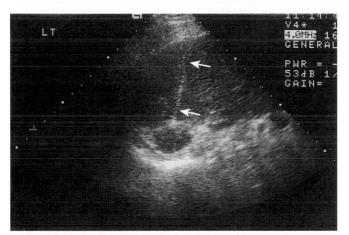

FIGURE 17-14. Right adrenal mass biopsy using a right lateral transhepatic approach. The adrenal mass was biopsied using a transhepatic approach under ultrasound guidance. The needle *(arrows)* can be seen entering the adrenal lesion. The adrenal mass was a small metastasis from a non-small-cell lung cancer.

transrectal ultrasound is also problematic, and many men ultimately undergo prostate biopsy.

There are two methods of performing prostate biopsy: transrectal (Fig. 17-19) and transperineal. Ultrasound guidance using a transrectal probe is used for both, but in the transperineal route, the needle is placed through the skin of the perineum, while in the transrectal route the needle is passed through the rectal wall. Proponents of the transperineal route claim a lower infection rate. However, the transperineal route is more cumbersome, requires local anesthesia, and takes more time. The author prefers the transrectal route because it is faster, requires no local anesthesia, and with appropriate antibiotic coverage, the infection rate is minimal.

Using the transrectal route, either 10 or 12 quadrant biopsies are performed with an 18-gauge automated needle system. The patient is placed in the decubitus position and the prostate is imaged. Hypoechoic lesions in the peripheral gland are biopsied if present, even though only 20%-30% of these are malignant. The author's unit uses an end-firing transrectal ultrasound probe. Many such probes are available, and most major ultrasound manufacturers offer transrectal ultrasound probes. It is important to biopsy the four quadrants of the prostate to reduce sampling error (in the author's unit, 10-12 samples are the norm). Samples are obtained in the axial plane, avoiding the midline area of the

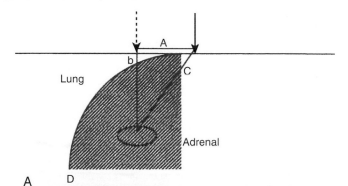

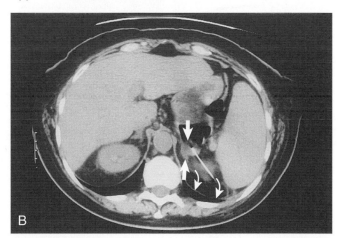

FIGURE 17-15. The angled prone approach to adrenal gland biopsy. **A,** Schematic showing the angled prone approach. *D* represents the diaphragm, the *shaded area* represents the abdominal cavity, and the *white area* above the diaphragm represents the lung. The *broken arrow* represents the direct posterior approach to the adrenal lesion, which would pass through lung parenchyma. The *solid arrow* represents the biopsy site to be used for the angled approach, which does not pass through lung parenchyma. Using the angled approach, the distance to the lesion can be calculated by using Pythagoras' theorem, which states that the square of the hypotenuse (C) is equal to the sum of the squares of the other two sides (A and B). This applies only for a right-angled triangle. Knowing distances A and B, the distance to the lesion using the angled approach can be calculated. The needle is inserted at a 45-degree angle. **B,** Example of an angled prone approach in this patient with a left adrenal lesion *(large arrows)*. An angled prone was used because there was intervening lung *(curved arrows)*. Note that scans through the lesion using this approach only show the distal half of the needle. Angling the CT gantry may help visualize the whole length of the needle.

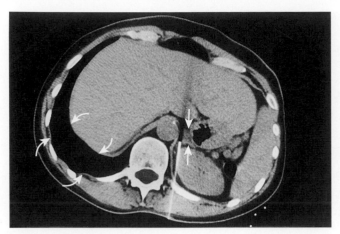

FIGURE 17-16. Lateral decubitus approach to the adrenal gland. In this patient, using a lateral decubitus position, a direct posterior approach was used to biopsy the adrenal lesion *(arrows)* because the intervening lung becomes hypovolemic and no longer is in the path of the needle. Note that the uppermost lung has hyperexpanded *(curved arrows)*.

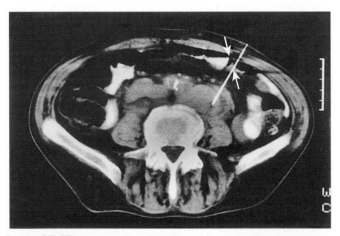

FIGURE 17-17. Computed tomography–guided anterior approach to the retroperitoneum. A lymph node mass was noted at the level of the aortic bifurcation in this patient with cervical cancer. A posterior approach was not possible because the iliac crest and transverse process denied a good access route. An anterior transabdominal approach was used with a 20-gauge needle placed into the lesion for sampling. The needle has passed through a loop of small bowel *(arrows)*. No complications were encountered and the biopsy was positive for metastatic spread from cervical cancer.

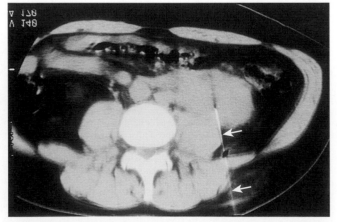

FIGURE 17-18. A posterior approach was used in this patient with a large retroperitoneal mass which proved to be metastatic cancer. A 20-gauge needle *(arrows)* is seen within the lesion. Using this needle as a guide, multiple large-gauge core samples were obtained for pathologic analysis.

prostate where the urethra lies. No local anesthesia is used but all patients receive antibiotic prophylaxis. The antibiotic regimen at the author's unit consists of oral ciprofloxacin 500 mg twice daily, starting the day before the procedure and continuing for 3 days after the procedure (i.e., 5 days in total); using this regimen, only three episodes of sepsis have occurred in more than 1000 prostate biopsies. To ensure that clot retention, which may lead to bladder obstruction, does not occur, the patient is asked to pass urine before leaving the department. The patient is told to expect hematuria and/or blood in the ejaculate for 24 hours and is instructed to return to the emergency department if he is unable to pass urine or fever develops.

Special Considerations

Biopsy of Pelvic Lesions

Masses in the pelvis can be approached using a variety of different access routes. The transrectal and transvaginal routes use ultrasound guidance, and the transgluteal approach through the greater sciatic notch and the presacral approach through the gluteal cleft use CT guidance. An anterior approach is occasionally possible (Fig. 17-20). The route chosen depends to a large extent on clinician preference. In general, practice at the author's unit has evolved such that we predominantly perform transvaginal and transrectal ultrasound-guided biopsy as opposed to transgluteal biopsy.

A transgluteal route was used extensively before transrectal and transvaginal ultrasound-guided biopsy became possible. The transgluteal route involves placing the patient prone on the CT table and passing a needle from the buttock through the greater sciatic foramen into the deep pelvis. Care is taken to avoid the sciatic nerve, which passes close to the ischial tuberosity. The needle is therefore passed as close as possible to the coccyx.

With the advent of endocavitary ultrasound probes, access to pelvic lesions is now possible via the transvaginal and transrectal routes. Most endocavitary probes have a needle guide through which a needle can be passed into the lesion. When using the transvaginal approach, the posterior fornix is infiltrated with local anesthetic and a 20- or 22-gauge needle passed into the lesion. Similarly, the rectal wall can be infiltrated with local anesthetic before passing a needle through the rectal wall. If needed, 18-gauge core samples can be obtained using an automated biopsy device. The access routes for pelvic biopsy are discussed in more detail in Chapter 18.

Celiac Ganglion Block

Celiac ganglion block has traditionally been performed by anesthetists using fluoroscopic guidance. It is a procedure that is ideally suited to CT guidance, because the precise location of the celiac axis, and therefore the celiac ganglia, can be determined. Either one or two 20-gauge needles are placed on either side of the celiac axis using an anterior or posterior approach. A test injection of air or contrast is performed to ensure that good diffusion of air or contrast occurs around the aorta and bathes the retroperitoneum between the celiac axis and superior mesenteric artery (Fig. 17-21). Twenty to 40 mL of 95% alcohol is then injected through the needle into the retroperitoneum.

Patients with pancreatic cancer or other malignancies in the upper abdomen respond well to celiac axis ablation (70%-80% response rate). Patients with chronic pancreatitis respond less well (50%-60% response rate; Box 17-4).

Lymphoma

Image-guided biopsy of suspected lymphoma deserves special mention. Not only is it necessary to differentiate lymphoma from carcinoma, but it is also necessary to differentiate Hodgkin from non-Hodgkin lymphoma and to subtype the Hodgkin or non-Hodgkin lymphoma. Treatment regimens may differ substantially depending on the lymphoma subtype. Although it may be possible to subtype lymphomas on fine-needle aspirates alone, it is prudent

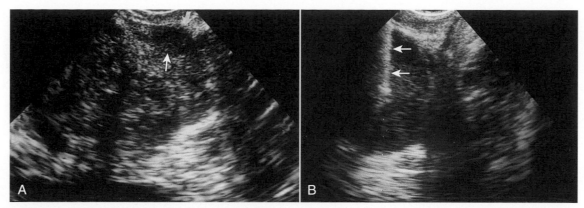

Figure 17-19. Transrectal ultrasound-guided prostate biopsy. **A,** Transrectal ultrasound of the prostate shows a focal hypoechoic nodule *(arrow)* in the peripheral gland in this patient with a raised PSA level. **B,** An 18-gauge core biopsy is obtained through the nodule using an automated Tru-Cut needle *(arrows)*. Random samples were also obtained from other parts of the prostate gland.

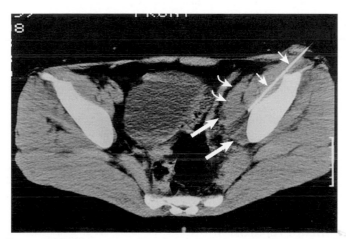

Figure 17-20. Anterior computed tomography–guided biopsy of a pelvic lymph node, using an anterior approach. The lymph node mass *(large arrows)* is seen adjacent to the external iliac vessels *(curved arrows)*. An anterior approach through the iliopsoas muscle was used to avoid the iliac vessels. A needle *(short arrows)* can be seen parallel with the iliac bone down to the lesion. The lesion was metastatic cancer.

to obtain some large-core biopsies if lymphoma is suspected. Two or three 18-gauge core biopsy samples generally ensure that the cytopathologist has enough tissue to render a diagnosis and to subtype.

Aftercare

Most abdominal biopsies are performed as outpatient procedures. After the procedure is finished, the patient is taken to a nursing observation area and vital signs are recorded every 15 minutes for 2 hours in patients who have had fine-needle biopsies and for 3-4 hours in patients who have had a large-gauge needle biopsy. After prostate biopsies, however, patients may leave as soon as they pass urine.

Patients are instructed to rest at home after the biopsy and are given information regarding the procedure that was performed, symptoms that may herald complications, and contact numbers for the interventional radiology department. If serious problems occur, patients are instructed to report to the nearest emergency department.

Complications of Abdominal Biopsy

Complications related to fine-needle abdominal biopsy are rare. Deaths have been reported: mortality rates reported in

three large studies of 66,397, 10,766, and 16,381 biopsies were 0.008%, 0.018%, and 0.031%, respectively. The first two studies were European; the third was North American. The majority of deaths were due to hemorrhage after liver biopsy, with the next major cause of death being pancreatitis after pancreatic biopsy. Anecdotally, it is apparent that biopsy of normal pancreatic tissue dramatically increases the risk for development of pancreatitis; therefore, it is imperative to be absolutely sure that a pancreatic mass exists before biopsying the pancreas (Fig. 17-22).

With liver biopsy, the complication rate can be reduced by avoiding the biopsy of a hemangioma. Hemangiomas can be characterized with either liver magnetic resonance imaging or nuclear scintigraphy, and the need for biopsy is thus avoided. In addition, superficial liver lesions should not be punctured directly; rather, the needle should be angled obliquely to pass through normal intervening liver tissue, which should tamponade any bleeding. Other measures to reduce the number of complications from liver biopsy include the correction of any bleeding diathesis and/or plugging the biopsy track with Gelfoam after performing the biopsy in patients with bleeding diathesis. Alternatively, in patients with a bleeding diathesis, a transjugular liver biopsy can be performed (Box 17-5).

Abdominal Biopsy Results

Image-guided biopsy has a reported accuracy of 70%-100%, depending on the abdominal location biopsied. Accuracy rates in the retroperitoneum tend to be a little lower than in the liver and other locations in the abdomen; biopsy of lymphomas in the retroperitoneum decreases accuracy.

▄ LUNG AND MEDIASTINAL BIOPSY

Percutaneous biopsy of the chest is often required for peripheral lung masses or for central masses that have had a negative bronchoscopy. In general, masses that involve lobar or segmental bronchi on chest radiography or CT suggest the presence of an endobronchial component, and these nodules are best approached and biopsied at bronchoscopy. Conversely, bronchoscopy is less likely to yield a specific cytologic diagnosis in peripheral nodules, which are best approached percutaneously. Possible metastatic lung lesions are also best approached percutaneously. Occasionally, sufficient tissue can be obtained from a suspected benign nodule to confirm benignity and avoid thoracotomy.

Similarly, mediastinal masses can be biopsied using percutaneous biopsy techniques. Contraindications to thoracic biopsy are relative and include severe chronic obstructive pulmonary

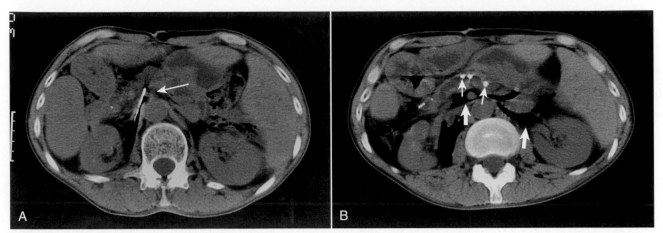

FIGURE 17-21. Computed tomography (CT)-guided celiac ganglion to block in a patient with chronic pancreatitis and severe intractable pain. **A,** A single 20-gauge needle was inserted from a posterior approach and placed close to the celiac axis *(arrow)*. Air was injected to ensure good diffusion throughout the retroperitoneum. **B,** CT section lower down shows the injected air *(large arrows)* bathing the retroperitoneum. Note the pancreas situated anteriorly with multiple areas of calcification *(small arrows)*. Thirty milliliters of 90% alcohol was injected into the retroperitoneum for celiac ganglion block. The patient had temporary relief of pain but the pain recurred 6 months later.

Box 17-4. **Celiac Ganglion Block**

Computed tomography guidance preferred
One or two needles placed adjacent to celiac axis
20-40 mL of alcohol injected
Patients with pancreatic cancers respond best
Patients with chronic pancreatitis respond less well

Box 17-5. **Steps to Reduce Complications**

Avoid biopsying liver hemangiomas
For superficial liver lesions, traverse normal liver parenchyma
Correct bleeding diathesis
Plug the biopsy track with Gelfoam if bleeding diathesis, or
    consider a transjugular liver biopsy
Do not biopsy "normal" pancreas

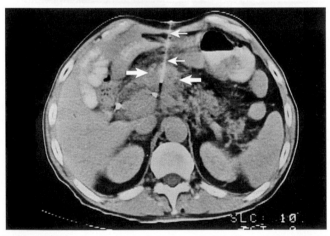

FIGURE 17-22. Computed tomography–guided pancreatic biopsy. This patient had two previous biopsies at another institution for a suspected pancreatic mass. Some peripancreatic inflammation was present at the time the patient underwent another pancreatic biopsy for possible pancreatic tumor. The needle *(small arrows)* can be seen entering the suspected mass *(large arrows)* in the pancreas. The biopsy revealed no malignant cells. Acute severe pancreatitis developed, and the patient remained in hospital for 35 days before eventually making a complete recovery. Follow-up imaging revealed no mass in the pancreatic head. Note also areas of calcification in the head of the pancreas. It is likely that the initial mass represented an area of focal pancreatitis.

disease wherein pneumothorax may not be well tolerated (forced expiratory volume less than 1 L), bleeding diathesis, and pulmonary hypertension. Patients should be cooperative. In general, the therapeutic and prognostic significance of obtaining a diagnosis must be weighed against the patient's condition. When contraindications are present, the biopsy technique can be modified to reduce possible complications.

Technique

Patient Preparation

Informed consent is obtained from the patient, and in particular the possible complication of a pneumothorax is discussed. For the vast majority of lung biopsies, intravenous sedation or analgesia is not required. The procedure can be performed safely and without causing patient discomfort under local anesthesia. Occasionally, if the patient is very restless or anxious, a small dose of intravenous midazolam can be given. It is important to enlist the patient's help for the procedure and careful explanation of breathing instructions should be performed and practiced.

Image Guidance

Large lung lesions can be biopsied quickly and inexpensively using fluoroscopic guidance. Preferably a fluoroscopic unit with a C-arm should be used so that needle position can be confirmed on both frontal and lateral projections. However, CT has largely superseded fluoroscopy as the guidance modality of choice.

Sonography can be used for pleural-based nodules, which are often easily visualized with high-frequency 5- or 7-MHz transducers (Fig. 17-23). Sonographically guided biopsy is then performed in a similar fashion to sonographically guided abdominal biopsy. CT is used for all mediastinal biopsies and the vast majority of lung biopsies. In particular, CT allows the operator to biopsy small lung lesions and large necrotic lesions for which biopsy of the wall is mandatory to obtain appropriate cytologic tissue (Fig. 17-24).

Needle Choice

Similar to abdominal biopsy, many of the same fine needles can be used for chest biopsy. The author's preference is the Turner

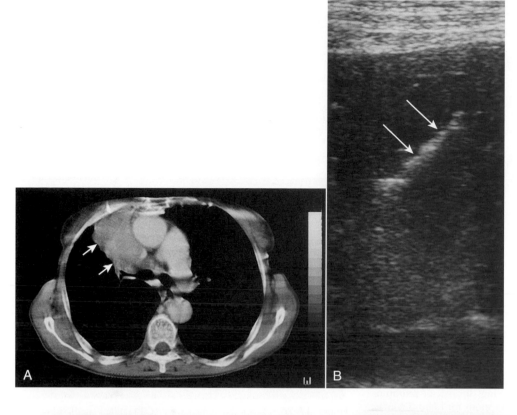

17-23. Ultrasound-guided biopsy of right upper lobe lung mass. **A,** Computed tomography scan shows a large right upper lobe lung mass *(arrows)* with some associated loss of volume. Because the mass abuts the pleural sur face, an ultrasound-guided biopsy was performed. **B,** An 18-gauge core biopsy needle was used to obtain a sample from the mass under ultrasound guidance. The needle *(arrows)* can be seen within the mass. This was a primary lung cancer.

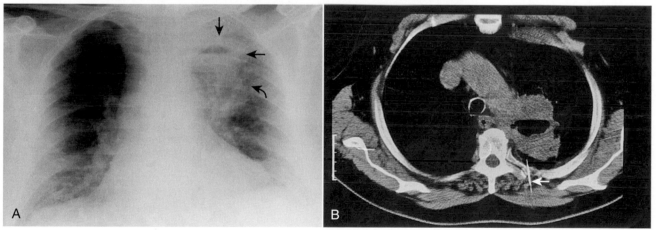

FIGURE 17-24. Computed tomography (CT)-guided biopsy of a necrotic lung lesion after two failed fluoroscopically guided biopsies. **A,** Plain chest radiograph showing a cavitating lesion in the left upper lobe *(arrows)* with associated hilar adenopathy *(curved arrows)*. Two previous fluoroscopic biopsies failed to obtain representative tissue because only necrotic cells were obtained. **B,** A CT-guided biopsy was performed using a coaxial technique. A 20-gauge needle *(arrow)* was placed in the periphery of the lesion and 23-gauge needles were used to obtain samples from the posterior wall of the lesion. The lesion was squamous cell carcinoma.

cutting needle (Cook, Bloomington, Ind.). Many authors prefer the Wescott side-cutting needle for chest biopsy, but there seems little to choose between these needles. For large pleural-based lesions or for mediastinal lesions (especially if lymphoma is suspected), a spring-activated modified Tru-Cut 18- or 20-gauge needle biopsy system should be used. The risk of pneumothorax is low for these lesions that abut the pleural surface. In addition, there has been a recent trend toward biopsying more deep-seated pulmonary lesions with 20-gauge spring-activated core biopsy needles. The 20-gauge caliber minimizes the risk of pneumothorax while maximizing tissue gain. At present, the author's unit reserves the option of using 20-gauge core biopsy needles for failed fine-needle biopsies. The 20-gauge spring-activated core biopsy needle is also useful for suspected benign lesions.

Performing the Biopsy

Computed Tomography Guidance

For CT-guided lung biopsies, the coaxial technique (see Fig. 17-7) is preferentially used if more than one sample is required. An advantage of CT guidance is that the lung parenchyma at the puncture site can be clearly visualized, and structures such as blebs and bullae can be avoided. Additionally, unaerated portions of lung abutting the pleural surface can be visualized and used as an access route to the lesion. This is particularly true of a collapsed or consolidated lung. If an area of unaerated lung is used as an access route to perform the biopsy, a pneumothorax will not occur. In most cases, it is best to use a direct approach to the lesion. The only exception is for small peripheral lesions. In this situation it

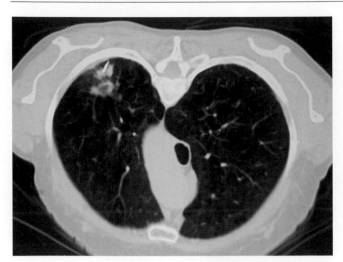

FIGURE 17-25. Coaxial biopsy for a small peripheral lung lesion. A 1.5-cm lung lesion with some cavitation is situated posterolaterally, covered by the scapula. A posteromedial approach was used to avoid the scapula. This tangential approach is often better for sampling small peripheral lung lesions than a direct approach. A 20-gauge needle was inserted into the lesion and 23-gauge needles were used to obtain multiple samples from the lesion. The lesion was a small primary non-small-cell cancer.

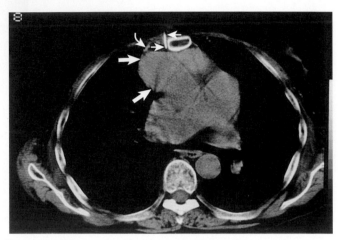

FIGURE 17-26. Computed tomography (CT)-guided mediastinal mass biopsy. A patient presented with an anterior mediastinal mass *(large arrows)* thought to be consistent with lymphoma. A dynamic CT scan was first performed to delineate the position of all vessels in the mediastinum. An anterior mediastinal approach was used. A 20-gauge needle was used as a reference *(small arrows)*. The internal mammary artery and vein *(curved arrow)* were avoided using this approach. Multiple 20-gauge core samples were obtained with an automated needle system placed in tandem to the initial 20-gauge reference. The mass was a non-Hodgkin lymphoma.

may be difficult to puncture the lesion directly and more than one puncture may be necessary, thus increasing the risk of pneumothorax. A tangential approach that allows room for needle course adjustment can be used in this situation (Fig. 17-25).

Lidocaine 1% is used to infiltrate the skin and subcutaneous tissues down close to the parietal pleura. The hypodermic needle used for lidocaine administration is then scanned to check needle course alignment with the lesion to be biopsied. The coaxial needle is introduced and inserted in increments of 2-3 cm with suspended respiration.

The needle course can be adjusted by withdrawing the needle to the periphery of the lung (taking care not to withdraw the needle outside the pleura) and adjusting the direction of the needle to puncture the lesion. Needle course adjustment can also be aided by patient inspiration or expiration, depending on the location of the needle in relation to the lesion. Additionally the bevel on the needle can be used to steer the needle somewhat toward the lesion, particularly when small adjustments are necessary. The outer coaxial needle is inserted 2-3 mm into the superficial edge of the lesion to be biopsied so that it has some purchase within the lesion during coaxial biopsies.

When the outer coaxial needle is in position, the insert needle is used to obtain multiple samples from the lesion. In the author's unit, a 10-mL syringe is attached to the insert needle and, with one hand holding the coaxial needle, a vigorous to-and-fro motion with the insert needle is used to obtain biopsy specimens (Box 17-6; see Fig. 17-25).

Mediastinal Biopsy

CT guidance is used for all mediastinal biopsies in the author's unit so that vascular structures can be avoided. It is important to perform a contrast-enhanced CT before performing any mediastinal biopsy to ensure that one is not dealing with an aneurysm or other vascular abnormality and to delineate the position of all mediastinal vessels. Anterior mediastinal masses are best approached using an anterior parasternal approach (Fig. 17-26). It is important, too, to avoid the internal mammary artery and vein, which course in a parasternal location approximately 1 cm lateral to the sternum. The needle is inserted lateral to the internal mammary artery and vein and angled medially, or occasionally

the needle is inserted medial to the internal mammary artery and vein. If necessary, the mediastinum may be widened by an injection of sterile saline. This is usually accomplished by first placing a 22-gauge needle into the anterior mediastinal fat and injecting saline to distend the anterior mediastinum. With the mediastinum distended, large-gauge cutting needles can be inserted into the anterior mediastinum without crossing adjacent lung parenchyma.

For masses in the posterior mediastinum and carinal area, a paravertebral approach can be used. The paravertebral space can be distended by inserting a 22-gauge needle into the paravertebral space and distending this with isotonic saline. In this way, large-gauge needles can be placed into the posterior mediastinum without crossing lung parenchyma.

Aftercare and Complications

Place the patient in the puncture-site-down position with the biopsied site dependent for 2 hours. The puncture-site-down position helps decrease the amount of air leakage at the biopsy site because the weight of the lung itself helps oppose the two pleural layers. After 2 hours, an erect chest x-ray study is obtained. If no pneumothorax is present, the patient is discharged. If a small pneumothorax is present at 2 hours and the patient is asymptomatic, another chest x-ray study is done at 4 hours. If the pneumothorax has resolved, the patient is discharged. If the pneumothorax is small and remains stable, the patient is discharged but must return the next day for another chest radiograph. If the pneumothorax is moderate or large, or if the patient is symptomatic, the patient is admitted to hospital and the pneumothorax treated. Depending on the size of the pneumothorax and the patient's symptoms, treatment can consist of simple aspiration, insertion of a small-gauge pneumothorax catheter and Heimlich valve, or insertion of a catheter with connection to an underwater seal. In the author's unit, simple aspiration with an 18-gauge cannula inserted into the second intercostal space is usually attempted first. If the pneumothorax recurs or symptoms deteriorate, a chest tube is inserted and connected to an underwater seal.

Pulmonary hemorrhage with or without hemoptysis rarely causes problems. For minor amounts of hemoptysis, patient reassurance is all that is necessary. If hemoptysis is moderate, the patient can be placed in the lateral decubitus position with the biopsied lung dependent to prevent aspiration of blood into the contralateral lung. The hemoptysis usually subsides within a few hours.

Air embolism is a rare complication of thoracic fine-needle aspiration biopsy (FNAB). Air embolism results when there is communication between a pulmonary vein and atmospheric air. Air embolism may be facilitated by leaving the needle open to the air while the needle is in the chest, or by deep breathing or coughing by the patient. Treatment includes administration of 100% oxygen, placing the patient in the left lateral decubitus position, with the head down (to prevent cerebral air embolism), and/or transfer to a hyperbaric unit.

Results

Sensitivity of FNAB for diagnosing neoplastic lung lesions ranges from 70% to 97%. A negative result often leads to a repeat biopsy, with positive results being obtained in as many as 35%-45% of patients undergoing repeat biopsies. The sensitivity of FNAB decreases with small lung lesions, necrotic lesions, and benign lesions. The reported accuracy of cutting needle biopsy is 95%, sensitivity of 93% and specificity of 98%.

In addition, the sensitivity of FNAB in determining cell type in primary bronchogenic carcinoma is high. Correlation between the FNAB, cytologic diagnosis, and eventual histologic diagnosis varies between 80% and 90%.

▬ NECK BIOPSY

Sonographically guided needle biopsy of thyroid nodules, cervical lymph nodes, and parathyroid glands is a highly accurate (90%-100% accuracy) and safe technique for differentiating benign from malignant conditions. High-frequency (7-10 MHz) transducers are required and biopsies are performed using 22- to 25-gauge hypodermic needles. The author finds that it is best to position the patient supine on a stretcher with the neck extended. The operator sits on a chair at the head of the patient's stretcher facing the ultrasound monitor, which is placed as near as possible to the operator (Fig. 17-27). Using this setup, one can perform the biopsy and watch the ultrasound monitor more easily than in other positions.

Hypodermic needles are preferred for neck biopsy as they pass through tissues easily and cause less patient discomfort in the neck. Because the thyroid is a vascular organ, minimal amounts of suction are applied to the needle to obtain samples. Alternatively,

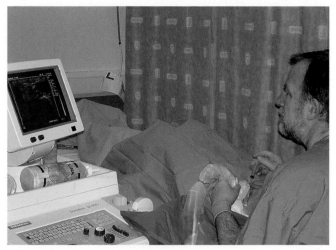

FIGURE 17-27. Room setup for neck biopsy. Room setup is important for facilitating appropriate ultrasound-guided neck biopsy. The patient lies supine on the stretcher with the neck hyperextended and feet toward the ultrasound machine. The operator sits at the patient's head facing the ultrasound monitor. An assistant is required to work the ultrasound machine. In this way, the biopsy procedure can be performed more easily than with other room arrangements.

samples can be taken without using any suction by using the non-suction technique. The author's practice is to obtain a sample with a 25-gauge needle (Becton-Dickinson, Rutherford, N.J.) using the suction technique and then to obtain a second sample using the nonsuction technique. Usually, core needles are not required for biopsying neck lesions. However, a 20-gauge Tru-Cut needle can be used with a "short" needle throw of 1-1.5 cm depending on the size of the lesion.

Cervical lymph nodes smaller than 1 cm can be biopsied using sonographic guidance (Fig. 17-28). In patients with previous thyroid cancer, it is useful to send samples for markers of thyroid cancer as well as for cytologic analysis. If the patient has a previous history of papillary or follicular cancer, a sample can be sent for thyroglobulin analysis. If the patient has a history of medullary cancer, a sample can be sent for calcitonin evaluation. The needle used to take the cytology sample is simply rinsed with 1 mL of saline into a sterile tube and sent to the endocrine laboratory for calcitonin or thyroglobulin analysis. In patients with metastatic lymph nodes, the thyroglobulin is dramatically elevated if the patient had a previous history of papillary or follicular cancer, and calcitonin is dramatically elevated in patients with prior histories of medullary carcinoma. This is a useful method of differentiating benign from malignant lymph nodes when cytology is unhelpful.

In patients with hyperparathyroidism secondary to a parathyroid adenoma, the adenoma can be ablated under ultrasound guidance using 95% alcohol. Depending on the size of the parathyroid adenoma, a small (1-2 mL) volume of absolute ethanol is injected into the gland under sonographic visualization. Parathyroid hormone and serum calcium levels are sequentially measured after ablation. This is a useful technique for managing hyperparathyroidism in patients who are unfit for surgery (Box 17-7).

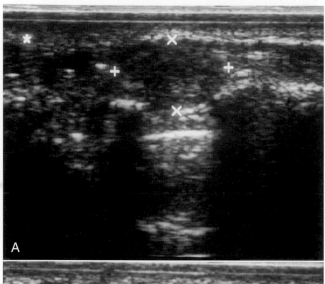

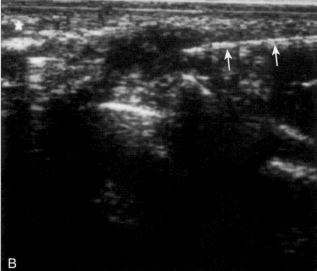

FIGURE 17-28. Ultrasound-guided neck lymph node biopsy in a patient with previous partial thyroidectomy for papillary thyroid cancer. **A,** Follow-up sonogram 2 years after surgery showed a 1-cm lymph node in the neck. **B,** Biopsy was performed using a 25-gauge hypodermic needle and ultrasound guidance with a 7-MHz probe. The needle *(arrows)* can be seen entering the lymph node and a diagnosis of recurrent papillary cancer was made.

Box 17-7. Neck Biopsy

22- to 25-gauge hypodermic needles used
Nonaspiration technique useful for thyroid lesions
Core biopsies may be helpful if fine-needle aspiration
  biopsy fails
Thyroid cancer markers useful for lymph node biopsy
Parathyroid adenoma ablation with alcohol can be
  performed

■ SUGGESTED READINGS

Ahrar K, Wallace M, Javadi S, et al. Mediastinal, Hilar and pleural image-guided biopsy: current practice and techniques. *Semin Respir Crit Care Med.* 2008;29(4):350-360.

Anderson JM, Murchison J, Patel D. CT-guided lung biopsy: factors influencing diagnostic yield and complication rate. *Clin Radiol.* 2003;58:791-797.

Bernardino ME. Automated biopsy devices: significance and safety. *Radiology.* 1990;176:615-616.

Bernardino ME. Percutaneous biopsy. *Am J Roentgenol.* 1984;142:41-45.

Brandt KR, Charboneau JW, Stephens DH, et al. CT- and US-guided biopsy of the pancreas. *Radiology.* 1993;187:99-104.

Bernardino ME, McClellan WM, Phillips VM, et al. CT-guided adrenal biopsy: accuracy, safety and indications. *Am J Roentgenol.* 1985;144:67-69.

Boland GW, Lee MJ, Mueller PR, et al. Efficacy of sonographically guided biopsy of thyroid masses and cervical lymph nodes. *Am J Roentgenol.* 1993;161:1053-1056.

Charboneau JW, Reading CC, Welch TJ. CT- and sonographically guided needle biopsy: current techniques and new innovations. *Am J Roentgenol.* 1990;154:1-10.

Fornari F, Civardi G, Cavanna L, et al. Complications of ultra sonically guided fine-needle abdominal biopsy: results of a multicenter Italian study and review of the literature. *Scand J Gastroenterol.* 1989;24:949-955.

Gupta S. Role of image-guided percutaneous needle biopsy in cancer staging. *Semin Roentgenol.* 2006;41(2):78-90.

Kattapuram SV, Rosenthal DI. Percutaneous biopsy of skeletal lesions. *Am J Roentgenol.* 1991;157:935-942.

Kinney TB, Lee MJ, Filomena CA, et al. Fine-needle biopsy: prospective comparison of aspiration versus nonaspiration techniques in the abdomen. *Radiology.* 1993;186:549-552.

Lee MJ, Hahn PF, Papanicolaou NP, et al. Benign and malignant adrenal masses: CT distinction with attenuation coefficients, size and observer analysis. *Radiology.* 1991;179:415-418.

Lee MJ, Mueller PR, vanSonnenberg E, et al. CT-guided celiac ganglion block with alcohol. *Am J Roentgenol.* 1993;161:633-636.

Lee MJ, Ross DS, Mueller PR, et al. Fine-needle biopsy of cervical lymph nodes in patients with thyroid cancer: a prospective comparison of cytopathologic and tissue marker analysis. *Radiology.* 1993;187:851-854.

Lee MJ, Mueller PR, Dawson SL, et al. Measurement of tissue carcinoembryonic antigen levels from fine-needle biopsy specimens: technique and clinical usefulness. *Radiology.* 1992;184:717-720.

Livraghi T, Damascelli B, Lombard C, Spagnoli I. Risk in fine needle abdominal biopsy. *J Clin Ultrasound.* 1983;11:77-81.

McNicholas MJ, Lee MJ, Mayo-Smith WW, et al. An imaging algorithm for the differential diagnosis of adrenal adenomas and metastases. *Am J Roentgenol.* 1995;165:1453-1459.

Moore EH. Technical aspects of needle aspiration lung biopsy: a personal perspective. *Radiology.* 1998;208:303-318.

Shepard JO. Complications of percutaneous needle aspiration biopsy of the chest: prevention and management. *Semin Interv Radiol.* 1994;11(3):181-186.

Silverman SG, Mueller PR, Pfister RC. Hemostatic evaluation before abdominal interventions: an overview and proposal. *Am J Roentgenol.* 1990:233-238.

Silverman SG, Mueller PR, Pinkney LP, et al. Predictive value of image-guided biopsy: analysis of results of 101 biopsies. *Radiology.* 1993;187:715-718.

Silverman SG, Lee BY, Mueller PR, Cibas ES, Seltzer SE. Impact of positive findings at image-guided biopsy of lymphoma on patient care: evaluation of clinical history, needle size and pathological findings on biopsy performance. *Radiology.* 1994;190:759-764.

Smith ED. Complications of percutaneous abdominal fine- needle biopsy. *Radiology.* 1991;178:253-258.

Weisbrod GL. Transthoracic percutaneous fine-needle aspiration biopsy in the chest and mediastinum. *Semin Interv.* 1991;8(1):114.

Weisbrod GL. Transthoracic percutaneous lung biopsy. *Radiol Clin N Am.* 1990;28:647-655.

Weiss H, Duntsch U, Weiss A. Risiken der feinnadelpunktion: ergebnisse einer umfrage in der BRD (DEGUM-Umfrage). *Ultraschall Med.* 1988;9:121-127.

Welch TJ, Sheedy PF, Johnson CD, et al. CT-guided biopsy: prospective analysis of 1000 procedures. *Radiology.* 1989;171:493-496.

Yeow KM, Tsay PK, Cheung YC, et al. Factors affecting diagnostic accuracy of CT-guided coaxial cutting needle lung biopsy: retrospective analysis of 631 procedures. *JVIR.* 2003;14:581-588.

CHAPTER 18

Percutaneous Abscess and Fluid Drainage

Michael J. Lee, MSc, FRCPI, FRCR, FFR(RCSI), FSIR, EBIR

Percutaneous drainage is now the accepted technique for draining abscesses in most body locations, especially since the evolution over the past 10-15 years of precise imaging localization of fluid collections, improved methods of percutaneous drainage, and improved antibiotic regimens. Initially, percutaneous abscess drainage (PAD) was reserved for those collections that were unilocular with a clear access route and without evidence of fistulous communication; now, however, it is the procedure of choice for drainage of a wide number of more complicated abscesses including multilocular collections, abscesses with fistulous communications, pancreatic abscesses, hematomas, enteric abscesses, splenic abscesses, and abscesses in difficult anatomic locations such as in the deep pelvis and subdiaphragmatic areas. Lung abscesses, mediastinal abscesses, and pleural empyemas are also amenable to percutaneous drainage.

Indeed, PAD is one of the major minimally invasive advances in patient management. When compared with surgical exploration, particularly in critically ill patients or in postoperative patients, the rapid imaging localization and percutaneous treatment of abscesses has played a major role in decreasing the morbidity and mortality associated with surgical exploration. Additionally, the role of the interventional radiologist in treating these patients is extremely gratifying, in that patients usually recover quickly as soon as the infected material has been drained.

ABDOMINAL FLUID COLLECTIONS

Patient Preparation

Any correctable abnormalities such as coagulopathies and fluid electrolyte imbalances should be corrected before abscess drainage. The patient should receive prophylactic intravenous antibiotics as determined by blood culture results. If blood cultures are negative, then an appropriate broad-spectrum antibiotic regimen such as gentamicin, ampicillin, and metronidazole (or other appropriate broad-spectrum coverage recommended by local infectious disease personnel) should be used.

Detection and Localization

Without doubt, computed tomography (CT) is the most appropriate modality for the detection and localization of intraabdominal fluid collections. Sonography may be helpful in detecting upper abdominal collections such as subdiaphragmatic collections, paracolic collections, or collections in solid viscera such as the liver and spleen. However, ultrasound suffers from its inability to penetrate gaseous interfaces. This is a particular problem in patients with intraabdominal abscesses, in that many have an associated ileus, which is particularly problematic in the postoperative patient. CT is therefore the preferred imaging modality for the identification of intraabdominal abscesses. Furthermore, because all adjacent organs can be visualized, an appropriate access route can be planned.

One of the disadvantages of CT is that loculation may be difficult to visualize, because often the septa are of the same density as the adjacent fluid and cannot be distinguished. Septation and loculation are much more easily identified by sonography. It is important also for patients to have appropriate bowel opacification with Gastrografin, when possible, because unopacified bowel may be difficult to differentiate from an abdominal abscess. Additionally, appropriate bowel opacification is necessary for planning the access route to ensure that small or large bowel is not traversed with a catheter when draining the abscess.

Neither sonography nor CT can determine whether a collection is infected or not (unless air is present). Gram stain and culture must be obtained to make this determination (Box 18-1).

For pleural space collections, plain films and sonography are often sufficient to demonstrate the entire fluid collection. With multiloculated empyemas, mediastinal abscesses, and lung abscesses, CT is necessary for full delineation of the abscess cavity.

Technique

Catheter Types

The various catheters available for drainage include sump designs and nonsump designs. Sump catheters have double lumens and are particularly suited for intraabdominal abscesses. The outer lumen in the sump catheter is designed to prevent side holes from becoming blocked when the catheter is adjacent to the wall of an abscess cavity. Twelve- to 14-French sump catheters are suitable for most intraabdominal abscesses (Boston Scientific, Natick, Mass.) (Fig. 18-1). However, sump catheters are not really necessary. Most pigtail catheters with reasonably large side holes work well in conjunction with adequate flushing. Larger (16- to 28-French) catheters are required in specific circumstances such as for pancreatic abscesses, hematomas, or when the abscess cavity contents are extremely viscous (see Fig. 18-1). Nonsump catheters are used in the chest. Generally these catheters have large side holes to permit appropriate drainage. Catheters inserted in the chest also tend to be larger (16- to 30-French) because kinking occurs commonly with smaller catheters because of respiratory excursion, which compresses the catheter against adjacent ribs. There is a vogue to place smaller pigtail catheters in the chest, which the author does occasionally for simple fluid collections, but for empyemas, the author prefers to place larger catheters.

Locking pigtail catheters (8- to 10-French) are used in specific circumstances such as when draining lymphoceles and seromas, or when draining deep pelvic abscesses transrectally or transvaginally. It is important to use locking catheters when using the transvaginal or transrectal route because any abdominal straining may dislodge a nonlocking catheter.

Image Guidance

The decision whether to drain an abscess under ultrasound or CT guidance is based largely on the location of the abscess, the size of the abscess, and operator preference. Most pleural fluid collections or empyemas can be drained under ultrasound guidance, as can hepatic abscesses, subphrenic abscesses, paracolic abscesses, and some of the larger, more central intraabdominal collections. However, from a practical point of view many abdominal abscesses are detected by CT scanning and therefore it is often easier to drain the abscess under CT guidance at the time of diagnosis. In addition, some abscesses absolutely require CT guidance, such as retroperitoneal and iliopsoas abscesses, deeply located abscesses, small abscesses, or abscesses that are not visible by ultrasound.

Box 18-1. Abscess Detection

Computed tomography is the preferred imaging modality
Appropriate bowel opacification is mandatory
Sonography can be useful for solid organ abscess detection
Sonography is best for identification of loculation
Imaging cannot determine whether a collection is infected or not

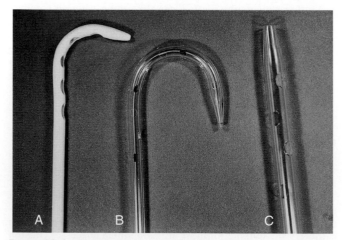

FIGURE 18-1. Various catheters used for abscess drainage. **A,** 14-French sump catheter (Boston Scientific, Natick, Mass.). **B,** 16-French nonsump catheter (Cook, Bloomington, Ill.). **C,** 24-French nonsump drainage catheter (Cook, Bloomington, Ill.). The sump catheter comes in 12- or 14-French sizes and is the predominant catheter used by the author for abdominal abscess drainage. The 16- and 24-French catheters are used for empyema drainage and for abscesses in the abdomen that need larger catheters placed.

Diagnostic Fluid Aspiration

Diagnostic fluid aspiration is often requested to determine whether a fluid collection detected by either CT or sonography is infected or uninfected. It is important to plan the access route carefully so that bowel is not transgressed en route to the collection. This is to ensure that a potentially sterile collection is not contaminated by a diagnostic aspiration. Generally a 20-gauge needle is used for diagnostic aspiration. This can be performed under ultrasound or CT guidance, provided a safe access route is visible. Two to 3 mL of fluid are aspirated and specimens sent for Gram stain and culture. If fluid cannot be obtained with a 20-gauge needle, an 18-gauge needle is placed in tandem to the 20-gauge needle into the fluid collection. Failure to aspirate fluid through this 18-guage needle usually means that the cavity contents are very viscous. Fluid can usually be aspirated in small amounts if rapid to-and-fro motions with the 18-gauge needle are performed. Alternatively, 1-2 mL of sterile saline can be injected into the cavity and reaspirated for the purpose of Gram stain and culture.

If the sample obtained is pus, a catheter should be placed straight away. If the specimen obtained is not pus and it is unclear whether it is infected or not, either wait for the result of the Gram stain or place a catheter. Some interventional radiologists prefer to wait for the result of the Gram stain. It is the practice in the author's unit to place a drain in the vast majority of abdominal collections, particularly if the patient is sick and has a high temperature. One can then await the result of the Gram stain and culture. If these are negative, the catheter can be removed after 48 hours (Box 18-2).

It is important for the interventional radiologist to be able to interpret Gram stain results because the result may directly affect decision making. A Gram stain that has abundant bacteria and white cells indicates an abscess. A stain that yields bacteria without white cells may be consistent with colonic contents. The CT scan should be reviewed to confirm that the suspected abnormality does represent an abscess and not unopacified colon and that the aspiration needle did not traverse the colon. Alternatively, bacteria without white cells may mean that the patient is immunocompromised and cannot mount a leukocyte response. It is not uncommon, with the modern use of antibiotics, that a Gram stain may show white cells without bacteria, indicating a so-called sterile abscess. These collections should, however, be drained (Box 18-3).

Drainage Procedure

It is now routine to perform the drainage procedure under either ultrasound or CT guidance at the initial time of localization of the intraabdominal fluid collection. An appropriate access route is chosen that allows a clear route to the collection without passing through adjacent structures.

There are two basic methods of draining an abscess or fluid collection: the Seldinger technique and the trocar technique.

Box 18-2. Diagnostic Fluid Aspiration

Do not transgress colon
18-gauge needle if no fluid obtained with 20-gauge
Inject and reaspirate saline if no fluid with 18-gauge needle
If pus obtained, place a catheter

Box 18-3. Gram Stain Interpretation

Abundant bacteria and white cells indicates an abscess
Bacteria without white cells indicates immunocompromise or needle through colon
White cells without bacteria indicates a sterile abscess

In the Seldinger technique, an 18-gauge long-dwell sheath is placed in the cavity and a 0.038-inch guidewire is coiled within the cavity. Alternatively, a one-stick system using a 22-gauge needle and 0.018-inch guidewire can be used (Neff set, Cook, Bloomington, Ind.). The track is dilated with fascial dilators to two French sizes larger than the catheter to be placed. The catheter is then inserted over a stiff guidewire into the collection. It is important to coil the catheter within the collection so that all of the side holes are within the collection. Initially, when using the Seldinger technique the needle, long-dwell sheath, and wire were placed into the abscess cavity under CT or ultrasound guidance and then the patient was moved to fluoroscopy to complete the procedure. When experience is gained, it is possible to perform the entire procedure under CT or ultrasound guidance. However, the Seldinger technique can be a relatively blind procedure without using fluoroscopy, and for this reason the author prefers to use the trocar technique where possible.

The trocar technique (Fig. 18-2) consists of placing a reference needle into the abscess cavity. A catheter with a sharp stylet is inserted alongside the localizing needle into the collection in a single stab. It is important to leave the reference needle in situ, because the catheter can be directed along the exact trajectory of the localizing needle. Adequate dissection of the skin and subcutaneous tissues with a standard surgical forceps is necessary for this procedure. A "give" is usually felt when the cavity is entered. Once the catheter is felt to be in place, the central stylet is removed and the catheter aspirated to confirm that the catheter is in the cavity. Once pus or fluid is aspirated, the catheter can be coiled in the cavity by disengaging and withdrawing the trocar and pushing the catheter forward (Fig. 18-3).

When the catheter is secure within the cavity, the cavity contents are completely aspirated. This is best performed using a closed system with a three-way stopcock and drainage bag. In this way the cavity contents can be completely aspirated and drained

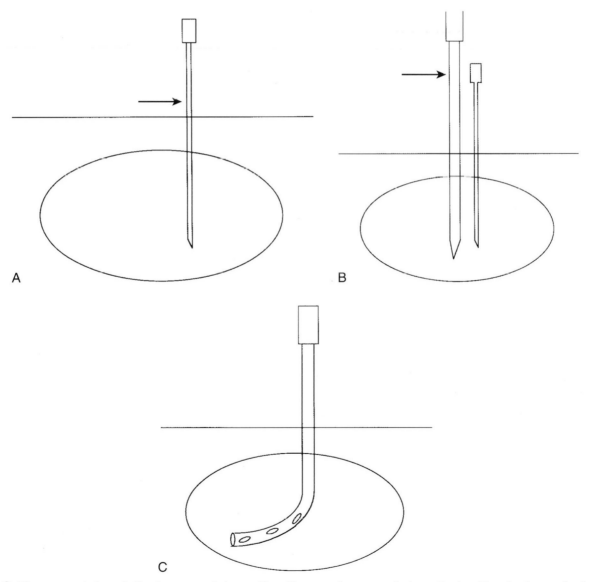

FIGURE 18-2. The trocar technique. **A,** For the trocar technique, a 20- or 22-gauge reference needle *(arrow)* is placed into the abscess after first planning an appropriate access route. The abscess is reimaged to confirm the location of the needle within the abscess cavity and fluid is aspirated for Gram stain and culture. **B,** The catheter to be placed *(arrow)* is then trocared into the cavity alongside the reference needle. Adequate skin dissection with a sterile forceps must be performed before catheter insertion. When the abscess cavity is entered, a "give" is felt. Confirmation that the catheter is in the abscess cavity can be obtained by withdrawing the stylet and aspirating pus. **C,** After confirming that the catheter is in the abscess cavity, the catheter is pushed forward into the cavity while withdrawing the trocar. The reference needle is then removed. The abscess cavity is completely aspirated and irrigated with normal saline until the aspirate comes back clear. At the end of the procedure the abscess cavity is reimaged to ensure that there are no undrained areas or loculations.

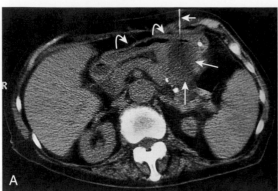
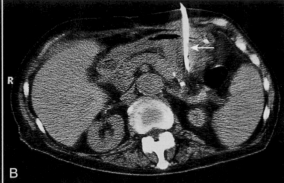
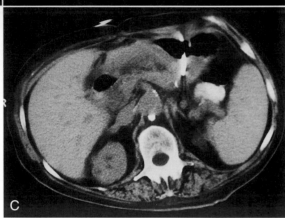

FIGURE 18-3. Trocar technique example. **A,** Patient with a pancreatic abscess *(large arrows)* referred for percutaneous drainage. The 20-gauge reference needle *(small arrow)* can be seen passing through the stomach *(curved arrows)* and into the abscess. Pus aspirated confirmed the location of the tip of the needle in the abscess. **B,** A 12-Fr sump catheter *(arrow)* was trocared into the abscess cavity alongside the needle and the needle then removed. This image was obtained after aspiration of the cavity contents. The cavity is now collapsed. **C,** Further computed tomography scan 4 days later shows no residual abscess cavity. The drainage through the catheter was less than 10 mL/day and the catheter was removed.

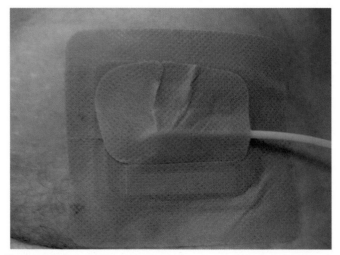

FIGURE 18-4. Catheter fixation. The "drain-fix" (Unomedical, Birkerod, Denmark) is specifically designed to stop migration, movement, and accidental removal of the catheter. Drain-Fix contains an absorbent wound-friendly hydrocolloid and tends to work quite well in preventing catheter migration.

into the drainage bag. When the cavity is completely aspirated, the cavity is irrigated with sterile saline until the aspirate returns clear to ensure that most of the debris and viscous contents, if present, are drained.

There are many methods for securing the catheter to the skin, ranging from simply suturing the catheter to the skin to using commercially available catheter fixation devices. The author's unit uses the "drain-fix" device (Unomedical, Birkerod, Denmark) (Fig. 18-4). A piece of tape is placed round the catheter and the tape is then sutured to the ostomy disk. This system works quite well for catheter fixation; the ostomy disk usually protects the surrounding skin if there is any pericatheter leakage.

Box 18-4. Draining an Abscess

Plan access route to avoid intervening organs
Seldinger or trocar technique used
Aspirate cavity and irrigate with saline until aspirate is clear
Repeat imaging to ensure no undrained locules

If ostomy disks are not available, the tape placed around the catheter can be sutured directly to the patient's skin or a fixation device can be used.

It is imperative to repeat imaging after evacuation of the cavity contents to ensure that the cavity is completely evacuated and that there is no loculation. If there is an undrained area, placement of a second or more catheters to completely drain the abscess cavity is required because the patient will not defervesce if pus is left behind (Box 18-4).

Aftercare

It is vitally important that the interventional radiologist be actively involved in patient management when a drainage catheter is placed. It is not acceptable to place a catheter and abdicate on the clinical responsibility of looking after the catheter and the patient's abscess. Respect by clinical colleagues is also gained by this approach and increased referrals to the interventional radiology service usually ensues. Interventional radiologists who have inserted the catheter know the abscess type, size, consistency of the fluid content, and loculation. It is mandatory that daily ward rounds be made on each patient with an indwelling catheter. During these ward rounds, the skin site, catheter and connections, the amount of drainage, clinical well-being, changes in white cell count, and fever are assessed. With daily ward rounds and careful observation, the interventional radiologist can decide whether follow-up imaging or intervention is required, and when the catheter should be removed.

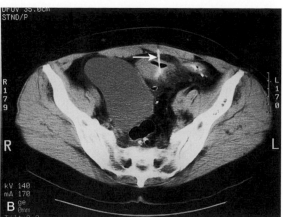

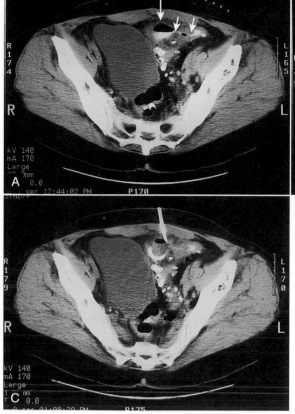

FIGURE 18-5. Patient with acute diverticulitis, high white cell count, fever, and marked tenderness in the left lower quadrant. **A,** Abdominal computed tomography scan shows pericolonic inflammatory stranding in the sigmoid colon consistent with acute diverticulitis and an abscess *(large arrow)* with a fistulous communication *(small arrows)* to the sigmoid colon. **B,** A reference needle *(arrow)* was placed into the abscess cavity and rescanned to document appropriate position. **C,** A 10-French catheter was trocared into the abscess cavity and coiled in the abscess. The catheter remained in situ for 10 days until drainage decreased to less than 10 mL/day. The small fistulous track closed spontaneously. The patient went on to have elective one stage surgery 2 months later.

Virtually all catheters are left to gravity drainage on the ward and fluid output is recorded. It is important that the catheter be irrigated three to four times daily with 10-mL aliquots of sterile saline to prevent clogging. This is usually performed by the nursing staff, but if there is any question of catheter patency, the catheter should be irrigated by the interventional radiologist on ward rounds to ensure patency.

The endpoint of catheter drainage is dependent on a number of factors. Primarily these are clinical factors such as clinical well-being, defervescence, reduction in white cell count, and decreased catheter drainage to less than 10-15 mL/day. It is not necessary to perform follow-up imaging on simple collections, particularly when the patient is recovering. Imaging endpoints include disappearance of the collection on repeat imaging and/ or a reduction in size of the cavity on a contrast abscessogram. In general, abscessograms are rarely performed unless the possibility of a fistulous communication exists. Resumption of appetite is another good clinical criterion for successful drainage. When some or all of these criteria are met, the catheter is withdrawn. Usually for simple collections that drain quickly and successfully, the catheter can be simply removed. For more complicated abscesses or those that take longer to resolve, the catheter is best withdrawn over a number of days, as with surgical drains, which is preferable to needing to redrain the abscess (Box 18-5).

Specific Abscess Drainages

Enteric Abscesses

Abscesses complicating appendicitis, diverticulitis, or Crohn disease are referred to as *enteric abscesses*. A complicating abscess in these conditions makes immediate surgery extremely difficult and may make multistage surgery, with its associated cost and discomfort, a reality for these patients. In these circumstances, percutaneous drainage, in combination with appropriate antibiotic therapy, can be used to effectively drain the abscess and

---

Box 18-5. Endpoints for Catheter Removal

Improvement in clinical well-being and resumption of appetite
Defervescence and normalization of white cell count
Catheter drainage (10-15 mL daily)
Disappearance or reduction in size of collection on repeat imaging

---

resolve sepsis. Elective one-stage surgery can then be performed at an appropriate interval after resolution of sepsis.

Drainage of diverticular abscesses can often avoid two- or three-stage surgery and convert the surgical procedure to an elective one-stage operation. The three-stage operation was in use before the general availability of antibiotics. The three-stage operation consisted of initial surgical abscess drainage and colostomy, a resection of the diseased colon and reanastomosis, and lastly a revision of the colostomy. In general, surgeons resect the diseased segment and any small associated abscess (less than 5 cm in diameter) and do a primary anastomosis. PAD is used for draining the larger abscesses to permit elective one-stage surgery (Fig. 18-5). Success rates between 80% and 90% have been quoted for PAD of diverticular abscesses, permitting single-stage surgery.

Periappendiceal abscesses result from a walled-off appendiceal perforation. Drainage of the periappendiceal abscess and appropriate antibiotic therapy usually permits elective appendicectomy in 4-6 weeks. Indeed, there is some debate in the surgical literature regarding whether interval appendicectomy is necessary. Success rates of 90%-100% have been quoted for PAD in periappendiceal abscesses.

Abscesses complicating Crohn disease occur in approximately 12%-25% of patients at some point in the disease course. Crohn abscesses are difficult to manage and PAD is useful in temporizing

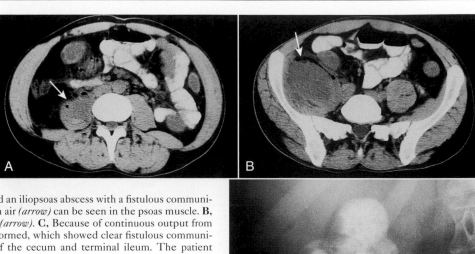

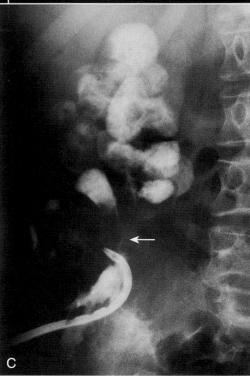

FIGURE 18-6. Patient with Crohn disease and an iliopsoas abscess with a fistulous communication to the cecum. **A,** Fluid collections with air *(arrow)* can be seen in the psoas muscle. **B,** Abscess also extends into the iliacus muscle *(arrow)*. **C,** Because of continuous output from the drain inserted, an abscessogram was performed, which showed clear fistulous communication *(arrow)* with the diseased segment of the cecum and terminal ileum. The patient improved with drainage but the fistulous communication did not heal. The patient eventually went to surgery for definitive resection of the terminal ileum and right hemicolectomy. The abscess drainage helped temporize the patient before surgery.

patients with enteric communication before definitive surgery (Fig. 18-6). Alternatively, PAD can be curative if there is no enteric communication. Enterocutaneous fistulas resulting from percutaneous drainage in patients with Crohn abscesses have not been reported to date. Success rates for abscess drainage in Crohn disease range from 70% to 90%.

It is important to use CT as both the diagnostic and therapeutic guiding modality in these patients with enteric abscesses. Good bowel opacification is necessary for secure diagnosis and for planning the access route for drainage. These abscesses occur in close proximity to bowel loops, and CT is mandatory to ensure that small or large bowel is not traversed by the catheter during drainage (Box 18-6).

Abscess-Fistula Complex

Fistulization to collections can occur from various structures including the pancreatic duct, bile duct, urinary system, and bowel. The most common abscess fistula complex is the enteric abscess with fistulous communication to the small or large bowel. Principles of treatment are the same for all abscesses associated with fistulas. Enteric abscesses associated with fistulous communication are discussed here representing the typical abscess-fistula complex.

The index of suspicion for fistulous communication should be high when managing enteric abscesses. Persistent high outputs (>100 mL/day) or an increase in output after 3-4 days of drainage

---

Box 18-6. Enteric Abscess Drainage

Abscesses associated with Crohn disease, diverticulitis, and appendicitis fall in this group
Abscess drainage generally allows elective one-stage surgery
Computed tomography best for abscess localization and access route planning
Good bowel opacification is mandatory

---

indicates the presence of a probable fistula. This can be confirmed with an abscessogram. Fistulas are designated as *high-output* when drainage is greater than 200 mL/day. In these high-output abscess-fistula complexes, the communication is usually with small bowel. Management principles include draining the abscess, proximal diversion of bowel contents, and bowel rest. Abscesses associated with fistulas also take longer to heal (often 3-6 weeks for high-output fistulas), which should be communicated to the referring physician and to the patient. Proximal diversion of bowel contents can be achieved by nasogastric suction and by placing a catheter through the fistulous track into the bowel (Figs. 18-7 and 18-8). The catheter placed in the fistulous track is left in situ for approximately 10-14 days to allow a mature fibrous track to form. When catheter output recedes to less than 30-40 mL/day the catheter

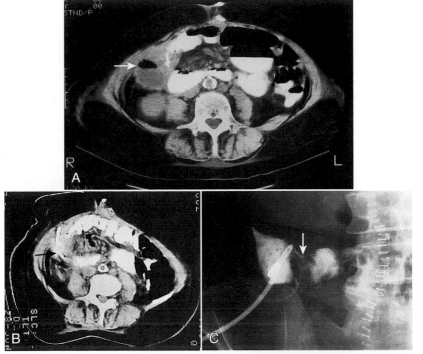

FIGURE 18-7. Abscess-fistula complex in a patient with fevers and a recent right hemicolectomy. **A,** Abdominal computed tomography scan shows an extraluminal collection with an air-fluid level *(arrow)* in the right paracolic gutter adjacent to the anastomotic site. **B,** A 14-French sump catheter *(arrows)* was placed into the abscess collection. It was noted on the day after insertion that the drainage had increased to greater than 100 mL/day and a fistulous communication was suspected. **C,** An abscessogram confirmed a fistulous communication *(arrow)* to the bowel. Because the fistulous communication was small, a catheter was not placed through the fistulous track. The fistulous track closed spontaneously after 9 days. During this time the patient had a nasogastric tube placed and was fed parenterally. The catheter was then removed.

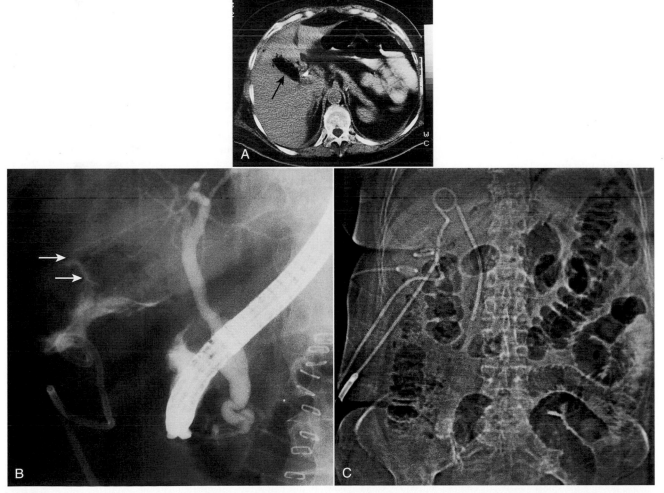

FIGURE 18-8. Patient with a biliary leak after laparoscopic cholecystectomy. **A,** Computed tomography scan showing an air collection *(arrow)* in the gallbladder fossa. Further air-fluid levels were noted around the liver and in the right paracolic gutter. **B,** Endoscopic retrograde cholangiopancreatography documented a fistulous communication *(arrows)* between a small right-sided bile duct with the gallbladder fossa and the abscess cavity, into which a catheter had been placed. A stent was placed in the bile duct to divert bile away from the fistula. **C,** A total of three catheters were placed to drain all of the abscesses in the right upper quadrant. A combination of stent insertion to divert bile and the abscess drainage allowed the fistula to heal spontaneously within 14 days. The abscess drainage catheters were removed. The stent was removed 2 months later.

can be slowly withdrawn. With high-output fistulas it is important to monitor and correct electrolyte and fluid losses from the small bowel to speed fistula healing. Patients with high-output fistulas are usually fed parenterally.

In patients with low-output fistulas from the colon, drainage of the associated abscess with bowel rest is often sufficient for complete healing of the fistula. As might be expected, low-output abscess-fistula complexes usually heal successfully with percutaneous drainage. High-output fistulas do less well. It is useful to clamp the abscess catheter before removing it for 2-3 days in patients with high-output fistulas. If a CT scan after 2-3 days of catheter clamping shows no evidence of recurrence, the catheter can be removed.

Other factors that influence successful drainage and fistula healing include the presence of distal obstruction, the health of the bowel at the fistula site, and the immune status of the patient. In the presence of distal obstruction, fistulas will not heal. Similarly, if the bowel at the fistula site is diseased (e.g., affected by Crohn disease or malignancy), the fistula is unlikely to heal. Additionally, if the patient is immunocompromised, fistula healing will be delayed. Quoted success rates for successful resolution of abscesses associated with fistulas vary from 66% to 82% (Box 18-7).

Subphrenic Abscess

The vast majority of subphrenic abscesses are postoperative, often resulting from pancreatic, gastric, or biliary surgery. Anatomically, they are located in a difficult position with the pleural attachment often making an extrapleural access route a technical challenge. The pleura is attached at the 12th rib posteriorly, 10th rib laterally, and eighth rib anteriorly. Traditionally, these abscesses were drained using a subpleural or extrapleural approach, which

involved angling an 18-gauge sheath needle or 22-gauge single-stick needle up under the rib cage and into the collection under ultrasound guidance and using fluoroscopic guidance to dilate a track over a stiff wire to place the catheter (Fig. 18-9).

It has become apparent that an intercostal approach can be used in selected cases without a major increase in the complication rate, and the author's unit now uses this route for the vast majority of subphrenic abscesses. It is likely that the two pleural surfaces are firmly adhesed by the time of drainage because of the adjacent abscess, making pneumothorax or empyema unlikely with an intercostal approach. However, it is prudent when draining these abscesses intercostally to go through the lowest intercostal space possible that gives access to the abscess (Fig. 18-10). Quoted success rates for PAD of subphrenic abscesses are between 80% and 90%.

Hepatic Abscess

Pyogenic hepatic abscess has become rare since antibiotic coverage of patients with abdominal sepsis has improved. In earlier days, most hepatic abscesses occurred secondary to bowel infections such as diverticulitis and appendicitis. Now, most hepatic abscesses are secondary to liver or biliary surgery. PAD of hepatic abscess is very successful and should be curative in more than 90% of cases. Many hepatic abscesses at presentation appear loculated with multiple septations; portions may even appear solid on imaging. However, it is worthwhile placing a catheter in all hepatic abscesses, in that almost all such abscesses respond dramatically to PAD (Fig. 18-11). Access can be intercostal or subcostal depending on the location of the abscess. Some interventionalists advocate needle aspiration alone for hepatic abscesses. The author prefers to place catheters for larger abscesses and use needle aspiration for smaller abscesses.

Renal Abscess

Renal abscesses can result from the liquefaction phase of focal bacterial nephritis or they can be hematogenous in origin. The hematogenous type is cortical in location, whereas those resulting from focal bacterial nephritis are medullary. Either type can break through into the perinephric space, resulting in perinephric extension. Small intrarenal abscesses often respond to appropriate antibiotics. Larger intrarenal abscesses, perinephric abscesses, or small intrarenal abscesses not responding to antibiotics require

---

Box 18-7. Abscess-Fistula Complex

Diagnosed by catheter outputs < 100 mL/day
High-output fistula > 200 mL/day
Managed by abscess drainage, proximal bowel diversion, and bowel rest
Fistula healing influenced by distal obstruction, integrity of bowel at fistula site, and immune status

---

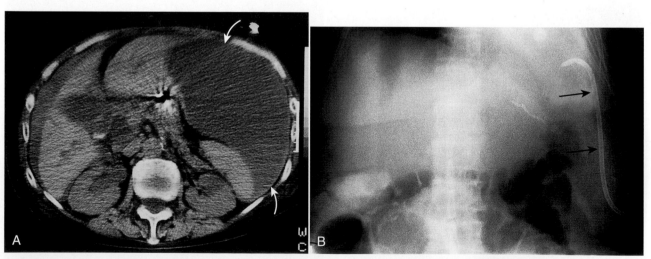

FIGURE 18-9. Patient with large left subphrenic abscess. **A,** An older patient presented with abdominal pain and fever and, on abdominal computed tomography examination, had a large *(arrows)* left subphrenic fluid collection that ultimately proved to be caused by a perforated colon. The subphrenic collection is pushing the spleen posteriorly and the collection extended down to just below the costal margin laterally. Note the patient also has gallstones. **B,** Plain film of the abdomen shows a sump catheter *(arrows)*, which was inserted from a lateral approach using ultrasound guidance and trocar technique. Because the abscess collection was so large and extended below the costal margin, it was relatively straightforward to use a subcostal approach. The collection ultimately proved to be fecal material and the patient eventually proceeded to surgery for a resection of the diseased colon after the patient's condition improved with abscess drainage.

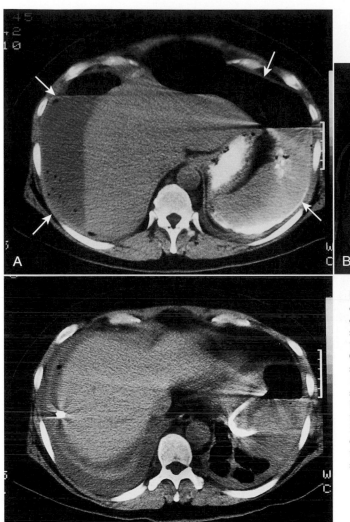

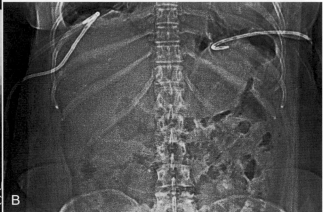

FIGURE 18-10. Patient with a leaking enterocolic anastomosis causing bilateral subphrenic abscesses. **A,** Computed tomography (CT) scan in the postoperative stage shows two large subphrenic abscesses *(arrows)*. The subphrenic abscess on the left contains Gastrografin. These were drained using 14-French sump catheters and trocar technique. **B,** Topogram from a CT examination performed 5 days later to assess the adequacy of drainage shows the right subphrenic abscess catheter placed between the ninth and 10th ribs, which was the lowest intercostal space available for puncture of the subphrenic abscess. On the left side, the drainage catheter is inserted between the eighth and ninth ribs. Undoubtedly, both of these catheters are transpleural but no complications developed from using this approach. It is important to use the lowest intercostal space possible to insert the catheter in order to reduce the complication rate. **C,** CT scan 5 days later shows catheters in situ with good drainage of both abscess cavities. The patient eventually made an uneventful recovery without recourse to surgery.

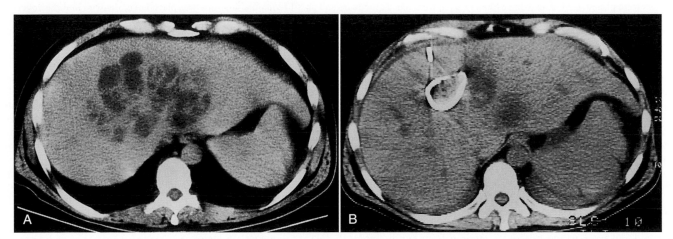

FIGURE 18-11. Patient with multilocular hepatic abscess. **A,** Computed tomography (CT) examination shows a multiloculated abscess in patient with high temperatures. **B,** Using ultrasound guidance, a 14-French sump catheter was trocared into the collection and, despite the loculation present, a dramatic response was achieved. Approximately 100-200 mL of pus was aspirated initially and the catheter was left in situ for 7 days. The combination of catheter drainage and appropriate antibiotic therapy resulted in a successful abscess drainage. A repeat CT examination after 5 days of drainage shows the abscess catheter in situ with marked diminution in size of the abscess cavity.

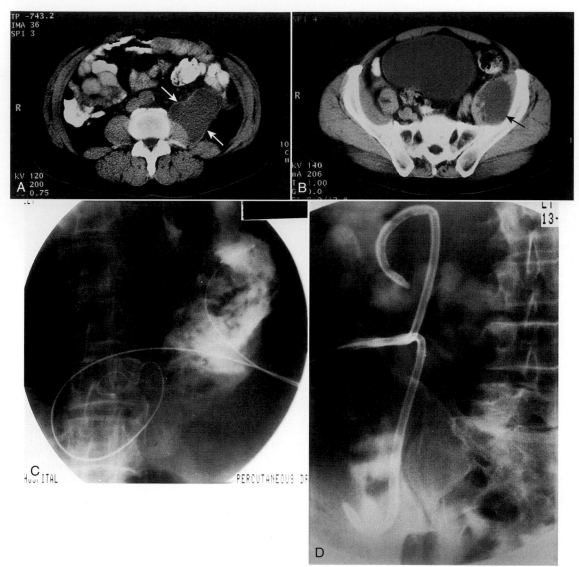

FIGURE 18-12. Patient with large iliopsoas abscess. **A,** Computed tomography (CT) examination just below the level of the kidney shows a large fluid collection *(arrows)* in or adjacent to the left psoas muscle. **B,** CT image of the pelvis shows the iliacus component *(arrow)*. A single catheter was placed but this was not sufficient to drain the abscess and the patient remained febrile. Two days later the patient returned to the radiology department and two catheters were placed. **C,** The existing catheter was moved over a guidewire and an 8-French feeding tube was placed over the wire into the collection. A second super-stiff 0.038-inch wire was then placed through the feeding tube. One wire was manipulated into the iliacus component of the collection and the second wire manipulated up into the psoas component. **D,** Two 14-French sump catheters were placed over each wire for adequate drainage. The patient settled after the second catheter was placed and the abscess drainage was ultimately successful.

drainage. Drainage can be performed under ultrasound or CT guidance. Locking catheters should be used if possible.

Infected urinomas are drained in a similar fashion. If there is a persistent communication with the urinary collecting system or obstructive uropathy, a percutaneous nephrostomy will be required to divert urine from the urinoma. If there is no communication, simply draining the urinoma should be sufficient.

Cure rates of 60%-94% have been reported for PAD of renal and perirenal abscesses.

Retroperitoneal Abscess

Retroperitoneal abscesses usually locate in the iliopsoas compartment and can have varied etiologies ranging from acute spinal osteomyelitis to Crohn disease or hematogenous spread. These abscesses require CT guidance for drainage because of their deep location. If the abscess involves the psoas muscle in the abdomen and the iliacus in the pelvis, it is often sufficient to place a catheter in the iliacus muscle because there is extensive communication between the iliacus and psoas muscles.

A catheter is first placed in the iliacus muscle and pus aspirated. If on the postprocedure CT scan the psoas component has also resolved, another catheter may not be necessary. If the psoas component has not fully resolved, another catheter will be necessary (Fig. 18-12). This is best done under fluoroscopic guidance, using the same puncture site as that used for the catheter in the iliacus abscess. The existing catheter is removed over a guidewire and a second guidewire inserted and manipulated up into the psoas muscle. Twelve- to 14-French catheters are then placed over each guidewire, one catheter in the iliacus abscess and the second in the psoas abscess.

Between 80% and 90% success rates have been reported for PAD of iliopsoas abscesses.

Splenic Abscess

There is a reluctance on the part of interventional radiologists to drain splenic abscesses, because the spleen is a highly vascular organ and there is a propensity for causing massive hemorrhage. However, over recent years the author's unit has drained

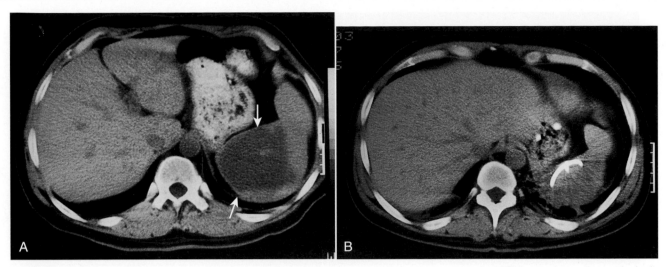

FIGURE 18-13. Immunocompromised patient with fever and high white cell count. **A,** Computed tomography (CT) image shows a large splenic abscess *(arrows).* **B,** A 10-French catheter was trocared into the abscess using ultrasound and fluoroscopic guidance, and 100 mL of pus was aspirated. A repeat CT scan shows the abscess catheter in situ with almost complete resolution of the abscess. The catheter remained in situ for 5 days until the abscess resolved. No complications were encountered.

a number of splenic abscesses. Careful attention to technique is important so that the catheter traverses the minimal amount of normal splenic tissue en route to the abscess. CT guidance is preferable for precise localization of the abscess and careful planning of the access route. Small 8- to 10-French catheters are used because of the vascular nature of the spleen (Fig. 18-13). Experience with splenic abscess drainage is limited, but it should no longer be a taboo organ for PAD (Box 18-8).

Pancreatic Collections

Pancreatic pseudocyst, abscess, and necrosis can be drained percutaneously, endoscopically, or surgically with varying results.

Pancreatic Pseudocyst

Not all pancreatic pseudocysts require drainage, and indications for percutaneous drainage are shown in Box 18-9. The most common reasons for drainage include pain or the possibility of infection. The access route is usually transperitoneal. CT guidance is preferable because the precise relationship of the pseudocyst with surrounding organs can be seen clearly. Usually an 8- or 10-French catheter suffices for drainage. This can be placed using the Seldinger or trocar technique. The author prefers to use a trocar technique and avoid intervening organs if possible (Fig. 18-14). If it is not possible to avoid the stomach, then a transgastric approach is used. Indeed, the approach is chosen for patients who seem unlikely to tolerate a tube for long periods of time or who have a pancreatic duct communication.

A catheter is placed for some days and the patient is then brought to the interventional suite. A nasogastric tube is inserted and the stomach inflated with air. The pseudocyst is filled with contrast and a 12-French vascular sheath is placed into the pseudocyst after removing the percutaneous catheter. Using lateral screening, a 10- or 12-French double biliary stent is placed between the pseudocyst and the stomach (Fig. 18-15). This internalizes drainage for patients who might not tolerate a percutaneous catheter for a long time. The author has been using this approach increasingly. The stent can be removed endoscopically after 3-4 months.

To a large extent, the relationship of the pseudocyst with the pancreatic duct determines the length of drainage. If there is communication with the pancreatic duct, the duration of drainage is prolonged for often up to 6-8 weeks. The duration of drainage can be decreased by the use of somatostatin or its analogue

Box 18-8. Miscellaneous Abscess Drainage

An intercostal approach can be used for many subphrenic abscesses
Multilocular liver abscesses are often cured by catheter placement
In iliopsoas abscesses, a single catheter in the iliacus component may drain the entire abscess
Splenic abscesses can be drained with small catheters (8-10 French)

Box 18-9. Indications for Pseudocyst Drainage

Size > 5 cm
Enlargement over time
Pain
Suspected infection
Biliary/gastrointestinal obstruction

octreotide. These peptides decrease the secretion of pancreatic juice and accelerate pseudocyst resolution. If there is communication and the downstream pancreatic duct is obstructed by a stricture or stone, pseudocyst drainage will not be successful unless the downstream obstruction is relieved (Fig. 18-16).

Modern percutaneous drainage should be successful in up to 90% of pancreatic pseudocysts (Table 18-1). The patient should be advised that drainage can take time, often up to 2-3 months (particularly if communication with the pancreatic duct exists) (Box 18-10).

Pancreatic Abscess

Drainage of pancreatic abscess is a challenge for interventional radiologists. Patients with pancreatic abscess have severe acute pancreatitis and usually have a severe systemic illness. In addition, pancreatic abscesses are often multilocular and the contents are usually very viscous, requiring large catheters (14- to 26-French) for drainage.

CT is the preferred guidance modality, because these patients have an associated ileus, making ultrasound guidance difficult. Catheters that are 16-French or smaller can be trocared

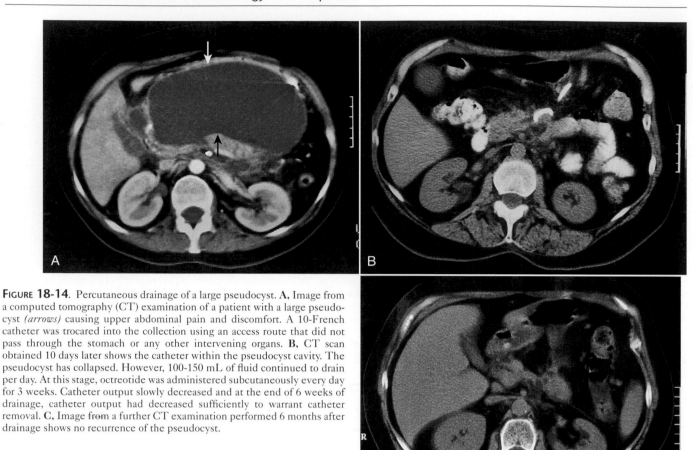

Figure 18-14. Percutaneous drainage of a large pseudocyst. **A,** Image from a computed tomography (CT) examination of a patient with a large pseudocyst *(arrows)* causing upper abdominal pain and discomfort. A 10-French catheter was trocared into the collection using an access route that did not pass through the stomach or any other intervening organs. **B,** CT scan obtained 10 days later shows the catheter within the pseudocyst cavity. The pseudocyst has collapsed. However, 100-150 mL of fluid continued to drain per day. At this stage, octreotide was administered subcutaneously every day for 3 weeks. Catheter output slowly decreased and at the end of 6 weeks of drainage, catheter output had decreased sufficiently to warrant catheter removal. **C,** Image from a further CT examination performed 6 months after drainage shows no recurrence of the pseudocyst.

into the collection under CT guidance. Catheters larger than 16-French ultimately require placement using the Seldinger technique and fluoroscopic guidance, after initial placement of the needle and guidewire under CT guidance. In many cases more than one catheter will be required because of very viscous cavity contents and/or multiloculation. Vigorous irrigation and careful monitoring of the patient is also necessary. Repeat CT scans should be performed if the patient is not defervescing or improving. It may be necessary to place larger catheters or multiple catheters depending on the size of residual collections. It is best to place large catheters (20- to 30-French) in patients with pancreatic abscess to achieve the best chance of success (Fig. 18-17).

There has been much confusion in the literature between pancreatic abscess and necrosis. Undoubtedly, in many series the lack of distinction between pancreatic abscess and infected necrosis has made the interpretation of pancreatic abscess results difficult. Success rates for drainage of pancreatic abscess vary from 32% to 80%. However, even if percutaneous drainage ultimately fails, a significant positive effect can be achieved, in that the patient may be temporized for surgery. In other words, the patient's condition may be considerably improved before surgery from the percutaneous drainage.

Pancreatic Necrosis

As opposed to pancreatic abscess, pancreatic necrosis occurs early in the course (<2 weeks) of severe acute pancreatitis (Table 18-2). It is diagnosed by dynamic contrast-enhanced CT as an area of absent perfusion in the pancreas. It is of critical importance to differentiate sterile from infected necrosis. This differentiation cannot be made clinically, because sepsis indicators can be raised in patients with both sterile and infected necrosis. Moreover, both groups of patients are usually critically ill. Patients with infected necrosis require immediate surgery (necrosectomy). The necrotic tissue usually requires scooping out by hand and has been likened to "dogmeat." Because of the nature of the contents in necrotic cavities, pancreatic necrosis is generally not suitable for percutaneous drainage. Occasionally, if the necrotic contents have liquefied, percutaneous drainage may be attempted. Large-bore 24- to 26-French catheters will be required for effective drainage. A number of authors have recently proposed "minimally invasive necrosectomy" as an alternative to open necrosectomy. This is similar to percutaneous nephrolithotomy, in that a 30-French sheath is placed into the area of necrosis using CT and fluoroscopic guidance. The patient is then brought to the operating room, where necrotic fragments are removed through the sheath with the aid of a rigid endoscope and graspers. The cavity is then irrigated. A large-bore catheter is left in place, so that more treatments can be performed if required.

The principal goal of interventional radiology in patients with pancreatic necrosis is to differentiate sterile from infected necrosis. This is done by percutaneous sampling of the necrotic area. Sampling is carried out with a 20-gauge needle under CT guidance (Fig. 18-18). It is of paramount importance not to introduce bacteria into a potentially sterile necrotic area. Therefore, it is

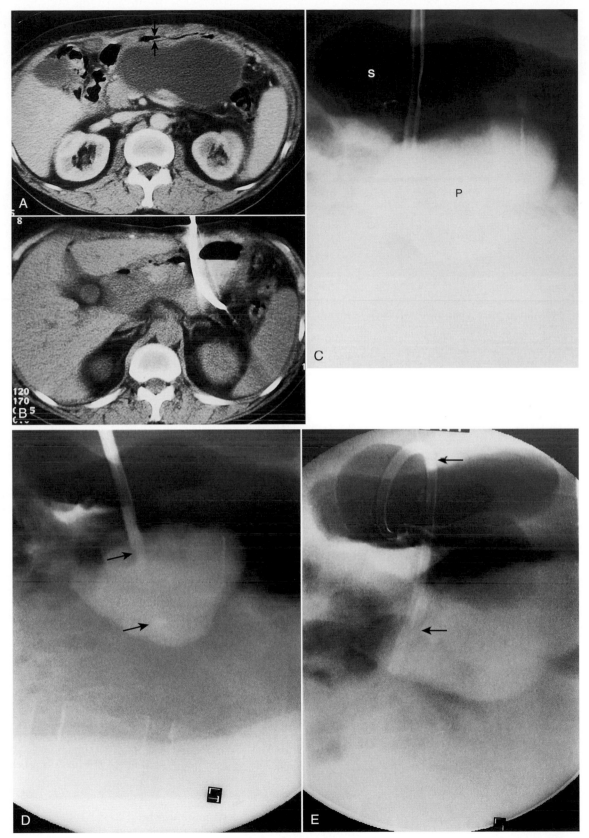

FIGURE 18-15. Transgastric stent placement for pseudocyst drainage. A 44-year-old man presented with a large pseudocyst 3 months after a bout of acute pancreatitis. The patient did not want an external tube. Endoscopic retrograde cholangiopancreatography had shown communication between the pancreatic duct and the pseudocyst. **A,** Computed tomography (CT) shows the large 10-cm pseudocyst in the lesser sac, behind the stomach *(arrows).* **B,** Using CT guidance, a 12-French catheter was trocared into the pseudocyst. **C,** A nasogastric tube was placed and the stomach (S) filled with air. Contrast material was injected into the pseudocyst (P). Lateral screening shows the catheter in the pseudocyst, which contains contrast material. **D,** The 12-French catheter was removed and a 12-French vascular sheath *(arrows)* was placed. **E,** A 5-cm 10-French double pigtail stent *(arrows)* was placed through the vascular sheath with its distal end in the pseudocyst and proximal end in the stomach. The stent was removed 3 months later, and follow-up imaging at 1 year shows no evidence of recurrence.

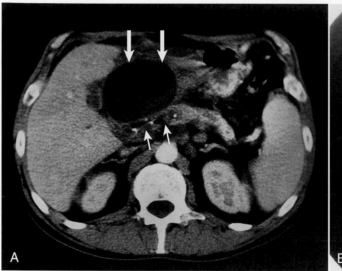
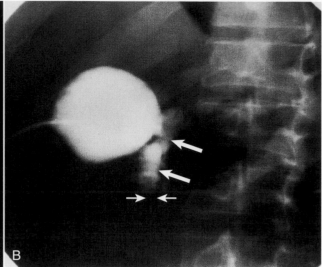

FIGURE 18-16. Failed pseudocyst drainage. **A,** Image from computed tomography (CT) examination in a patient with chronic pancreatitis and a pseudocyst. CT image shows a pseudocyst *(large arrows)* anterior to the head of the pancreas, a dilated pancreatic duct *(small arrows)*, and some areas of calcification within the pancreatic duct. The patient had upper abdominal pain and discomfort and was referred for drainage. **B,** It was decided to drain the pseudocyst under ultrasound and fluoroscopy. The initial needle inserted under ultrasound guidance was used to opacify the pseudocyst. This showed communication with a dilated pancreatic duct *(large arrows)*. The downstream duct near the ampulla contained a stone *(small arrows)*, which was causing the dilatation. Because of the downstream obstruction it was decided that percutaneous drainage was not feasible, and the patient was referred for a cystenterostomy. This procedure was successful and the patient had no further symptoms.

TABLE 18-1 Pseudocyst: Percutaneous Drainage Results

Author	Patients	Success (%)
Gerzof	11	90
Colhoun	10	100
Hancke	18	100
Torres	15	67
Matzinger	12	67
Grosso	43	76
vanSonnenberg	101	90
D'egidio	23	96
Sacks	7	88
Anderson	22	59
Burnweit	13	39
Lang	12	70

Box 18-10. **Pancreatic Pseudocyst Drainage**

Access route avoids stomach if possible
Communication with pancreatic duct prolongs drainage
Duration of drainage decreased by octreotide
Drainage may be unsuccessful if downstream pancreatic
    duct obstruction

---

vital to use CT to guide needle placement and to plan the access route so that the colon and intervening organs are avoided. If nothing can be aspirated with a 20-gauge needle, 2-3 mL of sterile saline can be injected and reaspirated. The aspirate is sent for Gram stain and for aerobic and anaerobic cultures.

Pelvic Abscess

Drainage of pelvic abscesses deserves special consideration because of the many different and evolving access routes available. Abscesses in the pelvis are surrounded by the pelvic bony ring and can be difficult to access. There are many different access routes: anterior transperitoneal, transgluteal, presacral, transvaginal, and transrectal. The anterior transperitoneal route is suitable for a minority of pelvic collections that tend to be located anteriorly underneath the anterior abdominal wall.

Transgluteal Access

The transgluteal route is the traditional method of draining deep pelvic abscesses. CT guidance is used, and with the patient placed prone on the CT table a 20-gauge needle is placed into the abscess. A CT scan confirms the position and ensures that the needle is close to the sacrum and not near the sciatic nerve, which exits behind the ischial tuberosity. A catheter is trocared alongside the 20-gauge needle, through the greater sciatic foramen, and into the abscess cavity. The access route should stay as close as possible to the sacrum to avoid the sciatic nerve, which exits through the greater sciatic foramen close to the ischial tuberosity (Fig. 18-19). This route requires adequate sedation as many fascial planes are crossed and there can be significant pain. If the catheter is close to the sacrum there are usually no sciatic nerve problems. Occasionally, temporary leg pain occurs but this usually resolves within 24-48 hours. The advantage of the transgluteal route is that large (12- to 16-French) catheters can be placed.

Presacral Access

The presacral route can be used for collections in the presacral space, but not for collections elsewhere in the pelvis. The patient lies prone on the CT table and a needle is placed into the presacral collection. The needle is placed through the gluteal cleft underneath the coccyx. The needle is then tracked parallel to the sacrum and angled up into the collection. Needle position can be confirmed by doing a scanogram and then scanning through the level of the needle tip as seen on the scanogram. This approach has limited applications but is useful for

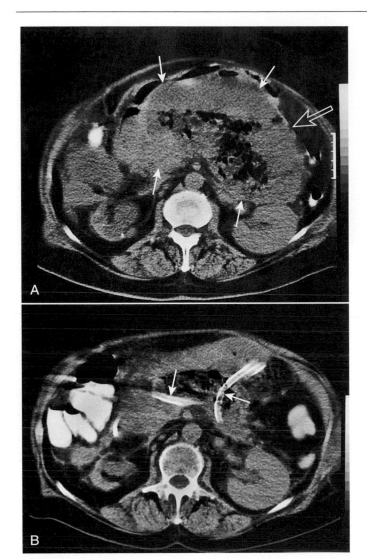

FIGURE 18-17. Percutaneous drainage of a pancreatic abscess. **A,** Patient with a large pancreatic abscess *(small arrows)* containing air. The patient was quite sick and required immediate drainage. An access route *(large arrow)* was available from an anterolateral approach, which avoided the bowel. Two 14-French catheters were trocared into the collection under computed tomography (CT) guidance using this approach. **B,** Because of the size of the collection, the 14-French catheters were upgraded to 20 French the next day to provide adequate drainage. This was done under fluoroscopic guidance using dilators to dilate up both tracts. A CT image obtained 5 days later shows almost complete collapse of the abscess cavity. Two 20-French abscess catheters *(arrows)* can be seen within the abscess cavity. Catheters remained in situ for 4 weeks and the patient made an uneventful recovery.

TABLE 18-2 Differentiation of Abscess from Infected Necrosis

	Abscess	Infected Necrosis
Onset	>4 weeks	1-2 weeks
Contents	Pus	Solid debris
Morbidity	++	++++
Mortality	10%-20%	15%-50%
Therapy	Percutaneous abscess drainage	Debridement

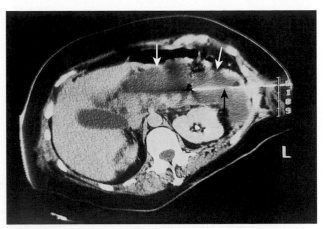

FIGURE 18-18. Computed tomography (CT)-guided aspiration of pancreatic necrosis. Image from a CT examination shows an extensive area of pancreatic necrosis *(white arrows)* in a sick patient with possible infected necrosis. A lateral approach was used for needle aspiration that avoided the colon. A 20-gauge needle *(black arrow)* was inserted into the collection and multiple areas sampled within the collection. Samples were sent for Gram stain and culture. There was no evidence of infection in this patient and the pancreatic necrosis was treated conservatively. This large area of pancreatic necrosis eventually evolved into a pseudocyst and the patient was treated by the surgical creation of a cystogastrostomy 6 months after the bout of acute pancreatitis.

presacral collections in patients who have had abdominoperineal resections.

Transvaginal and Transrectal Access

Transvaginal and transrectal routes have been gaining in popularity for draining abscesses in the rectouterine or rectovesical pouches. They are the most direct routes to abscesses in the deep pelvis and permit truly dependent drainage. The author's unit now tends to use the transvaginal route in women and the transrectal route in men.

Sonographic guidance is used for transvaginal catheter placement. The author uses an Acuson (Mountain View, Calif.) unit with a 7-MHz endocavitary probe. The endocavitary probe is fitted with a 9-French peel-away sheath (Cook), which is attached to the probe by rubber bands (Fig. 18-20). The probe with the attached sheath is placed into the vagina and the abscess localized. Local anesthetic is injected into the vaginal wall adjacent to the collection with a 20-gauge 20-cm needle (Chiba) and an 8-French pigtail catheter trocared into the cavity. Locking catheters should be used when using both the transvaginal and transrectal access routes, because nonlocking catheters can dislodge with straining, coughing, or any increase in abdominal pressure.

CT, fluoroscopy, or sonography can be used to place transrectal catheters. The author prefers to use sonography and a similar technique to that described for transvaginal drainage (Fig. 18-21). Advantages and disadvantages of transrectal and transvaginal drainage versus transgluteal are listed in Table 18-3.

Special Considerations

Hematoma

Drainage of hematoma is usually indicated only if the hematoma is infected. Most sterile hematomas resolve spontaneously and do not require therapy. Infected hematomas that have liquefied are relatively easy to drain. Acute organizing hematomas are almost impossible to drain percutaneously because they contain solid blood clot rather than fluid. It is therefore important to determine whether or not the collection is infected. Aspiration of the hematoma will yield the answer. It is usually necessary to use an

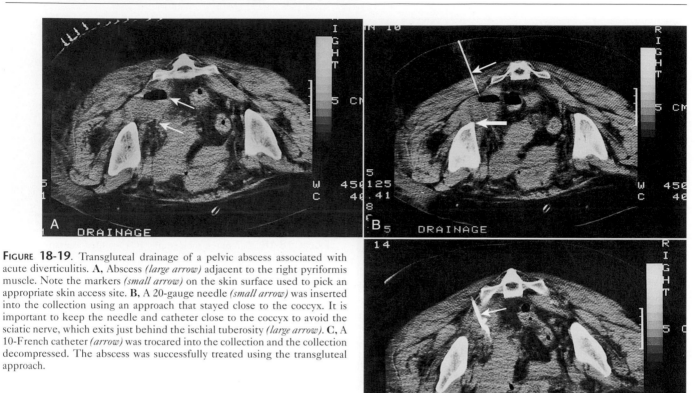

FIGURE 18-19. Transgluteal drainage of a pelvic abscess associated with acute diverticulitis. **A,** Abscess *(large arrow)* adjacent to the right pyriformis muscle. Note the markers *(small arrow)* on the skin surface used to pick an appropriate skin access site. **B,** A 20-gauge needle *(small arrow)* was inserted into the collection using an approach that stayed close to the coccyx. It is important to keep the needle and catheter close to the coccyx to avoid the sciatic nerve, which exits just behind the ischial tuberosity *(large arrow)*. **C,** A 10-French catheter *(arrow)* was trocared into the collection and the collection decompressed. The abscess was successfully treated using the transgluteal approach.

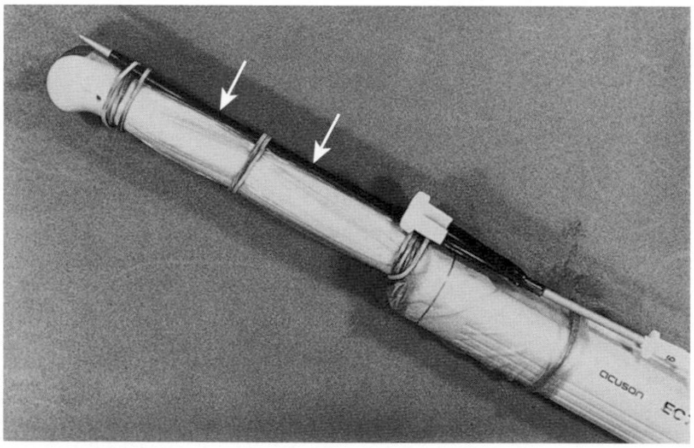

FIGURE 18-20. Endocavitary probe setup used for transrectal or transvaginal drainage. A 9-French peel-away sheath *(arrows)* is fitted to the probe in the same position as the probe's needle guide would be attached. It is attached to the probe by rubber bands and then covered further with a condom. The 9-French peel-away sheath is used to guide needles and catheters into pelvic collections for aspiration and drainage. An 8-French catheter can be trocared through the 9-French peel-away sheath into pelvic collections using either a transvaginal or transrectal approach.

18-gauge needle to retrieve some fluid for Gram stain and culture. If it is difficult to obtain fluid with an 18-gauge spinal needle, then the hematoma is usually not amenable to percutaneous drainage (Fig. 18-22). If the hematoma is organizing and infected, it is often not possible to drain percutaneously. If the hematoma is of mixed density, it may be possible to drain the fluid contents and then use a thrombolytic agent such as urokinase to lyse the clot. Early results with thrombolytic agents are promising in this regard.

Sclerosis

Occasionally, some collections (e.g., hepatic and renal cysts and lymphoceles) may require sclerosis because of recurrence or persistence despite long-term drainage. Lymphoceles are the classic example of collections that tend to recur and may take a long time to drain completely, because of persistent leakage from small lymphatics. Many different agents are available for sclerosis. The most common agents used are tetracycline, ethanol, bleomycin, and Betadine. The author's unit uses Betadine for sclerosing abdominal collections. It is important to delineate the cavity by injecting contrast through the catheter before starting sclerosis to ensure that there is no communication to bowel, ureter, or other organs. Betadine is instilled to a total of three-fourths the size of the cavity. The Betadine remains in the cavity for 1 hour, during which the patient turns every 15 minutes into supine, prone, and both decubitus positions. The Betadine is then reaspirated. If the collection is small (<5-10 cm) a single session may be sufficient. If the collection is large (>10 cm) or if the collection has recurred after a single-session injection of sclerosant, sclerosis is repeated on a daily basis for 7-10 days (Fig. 18-23). This can be performed on an outpatient basis. The collection decreases in size over this time period, necessitating a lesser volume of sclerosant. Finally, the catheter can be withdrawn when the collection has receded.

Thrombolysis-Assisted Drainage

When the contents of a collection are particularly viscous, thrombolysis with urokinase can help decrease the drainage duration and may help achieve a complete cure. Urokinase has been used successfully in drainage of pleural empyemas, abdominal abscesses, and hematomas. There is no significant deleterious effect on serum coagulation with the use of intracavitary

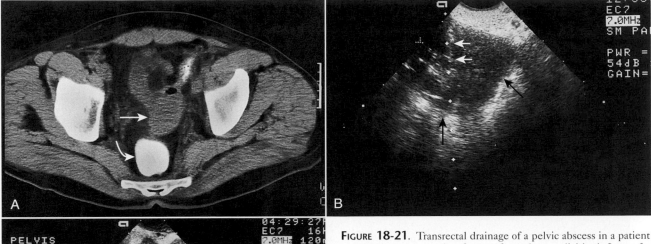

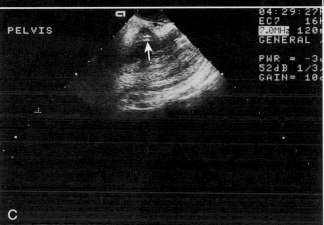

FIGURE 18-21. Transrectal drainage of a pelvic abscess in a patient who had recently been operated on for a perforated appendicitis. **A,** Image from a computed tomography (CT) examination shows the abscess cavity *(straight arrow)* anterior to the rectum *(curved arrow).* **B,** Transrectal drainage was performed. The collection *(black arrows)* can be seen adjacent to the endocavitary probe. After first infiltrating the wall with local anesthetic, the 20-guage needle *(white arrows)* has been inserted through the rectal wall to obtain a sample for microbiology study. **C,** An 8-French catheter was trocared through the rectal wall into the abscess cavity and the contents of the abscess cavity evacuated. The catheter *(arrow)* can be seen within the collapsed abscess. The catheter was left in situ for 3 days, after which time it was removed and the patient made an uneventful recovery.

TABLE 18-3 Endocavitary vs. Transgluteal Approach to Pelvic Abscess

	Transgluteal	Endocavitary
Catheter size	10-16 French	8-10 French
Catheter fixation	Good	Poor
Guiding modality	Computed tomography	Ultrasound
Procedural pain	High	Low
Sciatic nerve damage	Yes	No
Procedure time	Moderate	Short
Efficacy	>90%	>90%

urokinase. In the author's unit, the protocol consists of instilling 85,000 units of urokinase, followed by 10 mL of sterile saline into the collection. The catheter is clamped for 15 minutes and then unclamped. The process is repeated every 8 hours, up to a time limit of 48 hours.

Amebic Abscess and Echinococcal Cyst Drainage

Amebic abscesses are treated medically and usually do not require percutaneous drainage. In some circumstances PAD may be necessary particularly if the abscess fails to respond to medical therapy. Some authors have also advocated PAD for abscesses greater than 8-10 cm, abscesses with signs of pleural or peritoneal leakage, and abscesses that occur in the left lobe of the liver which have a greater likelihood of intrathoracic rupture with potentially serious consequences. PAD is usually curative within a few days.

Echinococcal cysts or abscesses were traditionally considered unsuitable for percutaneous drainage because any leakage of cyst contents into the peritoneal cavity could potentially cause anaphylactic shock. However, there are now many reports of successful PAD in these patients without the development of anaphylaxis. The cysts can also be sclerosed with alcohol to prevent recurrence.

Complications

Complications during PAD are rare and can be minimized with appropriate planning of the access route and daily supervision of the catheter after insertion. Total complication rates are reported between none and 10%. Minor complications such as pain can be avoided by routine use of sedoanalgesia and adequate local anesthesia during catheter placement. It is not unusual for catheter drainage of an abscess to induce a bacteremia because abscess walls are highly vascular. It is important to ensure that the patient has appropriate broad-spectrum antibiotic coverage before performing the abscess drainage. If the patient does not, then start the patient on intravenous ampicillin, gentamicin, and metronidazole before the procedure. When Gram stain and culture results become available, the antibiotic regimen may be changed according to sensitivities. Two deaths have been reported due to septicemia and disseminated intravascular coagulation after catheter placement for abscess drainage, and although this is not a common occurrence, it can be prevented by appropriate antibiotic coverage.

As with all interventional procedures, bleeding can occur but its frequency can be reduced by correction of any coagulopathy before the procedure. Bleeding may also be more likely when draining abscesses in vascular organs such as the liver or spleen (Fig. 18-24). Use of a small sized catheter may help minimize bleeding problems, particularly in the spleen. Vascular laceration

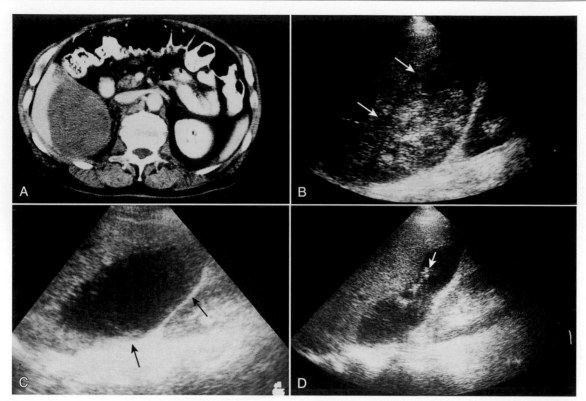

FIGURE 18-22. Drainage of an infected hematoma in a patient with signs of abdominal sepsis after a cholecystectomy. **A,** Computed tomography (CT) examination shows a collection of high density in the Morrison pouch. This was thought to be consistent with a hematoma. **B,** Ultrasound at the same time showed the collection *(arrows)* to be of mixed echogenicity. An 18-gauge needle inserted into the collection yielded some clot but no free flowing fluid. At this time it was decided that the collection was not amenable to percutaneous drainage. The patient was placed on antibiotics but low-grade fevers continued. **C,** Five days later the patient returned for ultrasound examination, at which time the fluid collection *(arrows)* had liquefied. A 14-French catheter was trocared into the collection for decompression. **D,** The catheter *(arrow)* was inserted and the cavity decompressed. The patient defervesced and the hematoma was completely evacuated over a period of 5 days.

may also occur from needles or catheters used to access abscesses. If the vessel is small, the bleeding will usually stop spontaneously. Occasionally, a larger catheter may have to be inserted to tamponade the bleeding. If this does not work, angiographic embolization may be required.

PAD may be complicated by bowel perforation from being transfixed by a needle or catheter. If the bowel has been transfixed by a needle only, there will usually be no sequelae. However, if a catheter has been placed through the bowel en route to the abscess, the situation is slightly more complex. Recognition of enteric communication is usually evident after the catheter has been in place, in that small bowel contents usually drain through the catheter. The catheter can be left in place for 10 days, after which a mature fibrous track should form around the catheter. By this time, the abscess should have healed and the catheter can be removed. Any leakage from the bowel can then pass into the fibrous track and there will not be free communication with the peritoneal cavity. The percutaneous track will usually close over within 12-24 hours, provided there is no distal obstruction. However, if the patient develops signs of peritonitis after catheter transfixation of bowel, then surgical intervention may be required immediately. This complication can usually be prevented by careful planning of access routes and ensuring adequate opacification of the bowel when draining abscesses under CT guidance.

Most complications occurring during PAD can be managed conservatively by the interventional radiologist. However, it is also true that most complications that do occur can be prevented by close attention to the technique of abscess drainage. The anatomic location of the abscess, preprocedural broad-spectrum antibiotic coverage, careful planning of the access route, sedoanalgesia, and careful postprocedural catheter care should all

help reduce abscess drainage complications. Delayed catheter problems such as kinking, blockage, and dislodgement can be managed expeditiously by performing daily ward rounds and anticipating or dealing with problems as they arise (Box 18-11).

Thoracic Fluid Collections

Aspiration and drainage of thoracic fluid collections follow similar principles to those for abdominal collections. Ultrasound guidance is used for guiding needles and catheters into the majority of pleural fluid collections. CT is required as the guidance modality for draining mediastinal and lung abscesses.

■ PLEURAL FLUID COLLECTIONS

Diagnostic Thoracentesis

Pleural effusions are divided into transudates and exudates based on aspirated fluid characteristics (Table 18-4). Common causes of transudates and exudates are shown in Box 18-12. Transudates result from decreased oncotic pressure or from changes in hydrostatic pressure with congestive heart failure being the most common cause. Exudative effusions are most commonly malignant or infective in nature with other causes being less frequent.

The two main indications for diagnostic thoracentesis are to exclude malignancy or infection in the pleural space. The evaluation of parapneumonic effusions is an important use of diagnostic thoracentesis because some of these parapneumonic effusions will progress to form empyemas and require drainage.

There are three stages in the formation of empyemas described by Light and associates. The first, or exudative, stage occurs when a focus of infection contiguous to the pleura promotes a

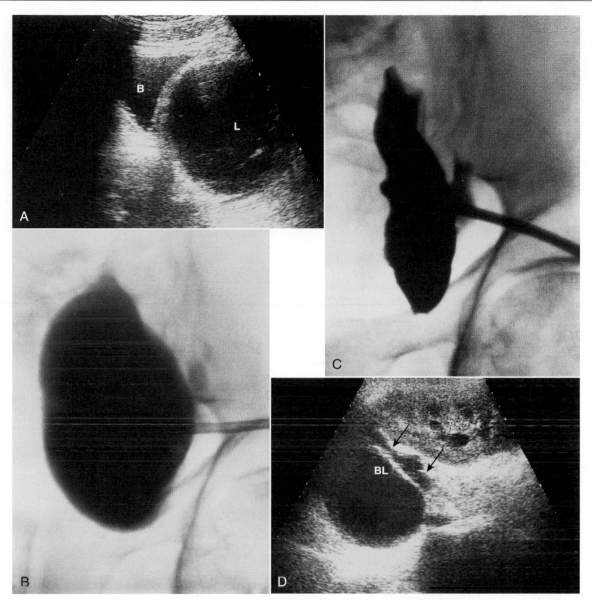

FIGURE 18-23. Patient with a lymphocele after renal transplantation. The lymphocele was marsupialized into the peritoneal cavity but recurred. **A,** Axial ultrasound image through the pelvis shows the bladder (B), which is pushed to the right by a large fluid collection (L) consistent with a lymphocele. This lymphocele was also causing ureteric compression and hydronephrosis. **B,** The lymphocele was drained percutaneously using ultrasound guidance, and a 12-French catheter was inserted into the collection. On this contrast study no communication was noted between the lymphocele and the ureteric system. The volume of the cavity was 200 mL, so 150 mL of Betadine was instilled into the cavity on a daily basis for 7 days. **C,** Contrast material injected on the eighth day shows that the cavity has markedly reduced in size and the catheter was removed at this stage. **D,** Follow-up ultrasound examination performed 2 months after sclerosis shows the bladder (BL) and transplant kidney with a small residual collection *(arrows)* between the two. Note that the hydronephrosis is now resolved in the transplant kidney. The sclerosis was ultimately successful and the graft was not compromised.

pleural effusion. Lactate dehydrogenase (LDH) levels are raised above 200 IU/L, but pH, glucose, and polymorphonuclear leukocytes levels are normal. Appropriate antibiotic therapy is usually all that is required to treat this exudative stage. The second, or fibrinopurulent, stage occurs when the effusion is colonized by bacteria. Glucose and pH levels fall (glucose ≤ 40 mg/dL or 2.2 mmol/L, pH ≤ 7) and catheter drainage is required to prevent progression to the third stage. In the third stage, fibrin is deposited in the form of a pleural peel, which is usually not amenable to percutaneous therapy. Surgical drainage and decortication are usually required for this stage (Box 18-13).

Technique

Patients are placed sitting on the side of a stretcher facing away from the operator. Ultrasound is used to locate the pleural effusion and a 22-gauge needle is inserted into the pleural fluid collection immediately above the adjacent rib. Needle entry should be performed above the rib to avoid the neurovascular bundle. Thirty to 50 mL of fluid are aspirated and routinely sent for Gram stain and culture, total protein, LDH, glucose, and cytology. If there is any indication of infection, fluid is also sent for pH assessment. Ultrasound-guided thoracentesis is a highly effective procedure. Difficulties may arise in patients with small amounts of fluid or in ventilated patients in whom access may be limited.

Pleural Biopsy

Not infrequently, diagnostic aspiration may not yield a diagnosis and pleural biopsy is required. This can be performed percutaneously or thoracoscopically. The advantage of thoracoscopic biopsy is that the pleura can be visualized and areas

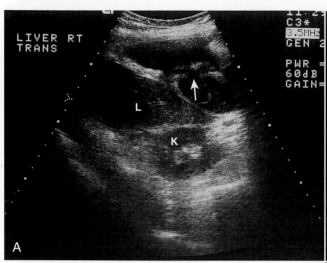

FIGURE 18-24. Older patient presented with a perforated gallbladder and a right subphrenic abscess. This patient developed a large hepatic hematoma after catheter drainage. **A,** Initial ultrasound examination shows a perforated gallbladder *(arrow)* with a collection anterior to the gallbladder. A further collection was noted in the right subphrenic space. Liver (L) and kidney (K) can also be seen. **B,** A 10-French catheter was inserted into the collection anterior to the gallbladder and a 12-French catheter trocared into the right subphrenic collection. Computed tomography (CT) image 3 days later shows the 12-French catheter *(arrows)* in the right subphrenic space with almost complete drainage of the right subphrenic collection. On the fourth day the patient developed acute respiratory distress and a pulmonary embolus was suspected. The patient was started on anticoagulation therapy but became over-anticoagulated. Two days after starting anticoagulant therapy the patient became acutely hypotensive and had a large drop in hematocrit. **C,** A repeat CT scan on the sixth day showed a large intrahepatic hematoma in the right lobe of the liver *(arrows)*, presumably related to anticoagulation and percutaneous catheter drainage of the right subphrenic abscess. The patient settled with conservative management and stabilized. The patient died 12 days later from acute respiratory distress syndrome.

Box 18-11. Minimizing Complications of Percutaneous Abscess Drainage

Ensure appropriate broad-spectrum antibiotic coverage before percutaneous abscess drainage (PAD)
Use adequate sedoanalgesia
Correct any coagulopathy
Use adequate bowel opacification for computed tomography
Perform daily rounds on the patient after PAD

TABLE 18-4 Differentiation of Transudates from Exudates

	Exudates	Transudates
Pleural fluid protein	>3 q/dL	<3 q/dL
Pleural: serum protein	>0.5	<0.5
Pleural fluid LDH	>200 IU	<200 IU
Pleural: serum LDH	>0.6	<0.6

Box 18-12. Common Causes of Transudates and Exudates

TRANSUDATES
Congestive cardiac failure
Cirrhosis
Nephrotic syndrome
Peritoneal dialysis
Constrictive pericarditis

EXUDATES
Malignancy
Infected parapneumonic effusion/empyema
Tuberculous effusion
Pulmonary infection
Systemic lupus erythematosus
Rheumatoid
Dressler syndrome
Pancreatitis
Trauma

Box 18-13. Empyema Stages

In the exudative stage (LDH > 100 IU/L, normal pH, glucose, and WBC count), antibiotics are usually curative
In the fibrinopurulent stage (glucose ≤40 mg/dL, pH ≤7.0) catheter drainage is required
In the third stage, a pleural peel forms which requires surgical decortication

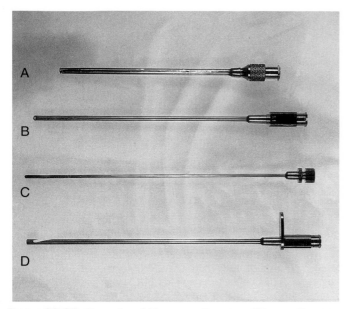

FIGURE **18-25** Cope pleural biopsy needle system. The needle system consists of four components: a short, open-ended outer cannula (**A**), an open-ended trocar with a 45-degree angle tip (**B**), a solid stylet (**C**), and the Cope needle itself (**D**), which has a reverse-bevel cutting edge.

of abnormality specifically biopsied. Percutaneous biopsy, although less invasive, is more often negative owing to sampling errors. Percutaneous biopsy with a large-gauge cutting needle is the procedure of choice when a pleural mass or thickening is present. However, institutional preferences may dictate whether percutaneous or thorascopic biopsy is performed in patients with pleural effusions and a negative diagnostic thoracentesis.

Technique

Cope or Abrams needles can be used to biopsy the pleura. The author prefers the Cope needle system, which consists of (1) a short, blunt, open-ended cannula; (2) an open-ended trocar sharpened at a 45-degree angle; (3) a solid stylet, also at a 45-degree angle, that fits into the cannula; (4) a reverse-bevel cutting-edge needle (Fig. 18-25). The first three parts are inserted as a unit into the pleural fluid and the stylet and trocar removed (Fig. 18-26). The cutting needle is inserted beyond the tip of the short outer cannula and the needle is then withdrawn at a steep angle, using the rib as a fulcrum until resistance is encountered. Resistance indicates engagement of the pleura. The outer cannula is inserted over the needle to shear the core sample within the cutting needle, which is then withdrawn. The outer cannula is left in situ and the stylet and trocar are reinserted to seal the pleural space. Specimens are sent for both microbiologic and cytologic examination.

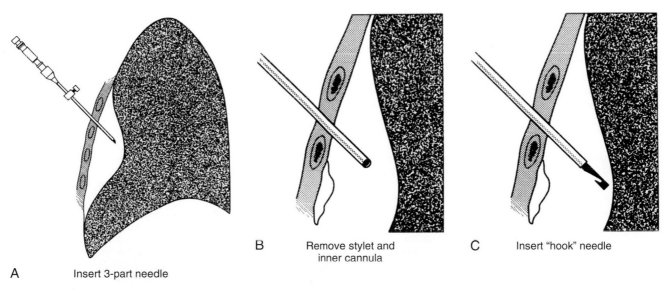

A   Insert 3-part needle

B   Remove stylet and inner cannula

C   Insert "hook" needle

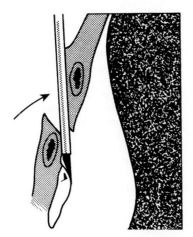

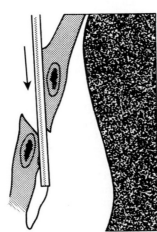

D   "Hook" pleura

E   Cut pleura with outer cannula

FIGURE **18-26.** Schematic illustrating a pleural biopsy. **A,** The cannula, trocar, and stylet are fitted together and inserted into the pleural space. **B,** The stylet and trocar are removed. **C,** The Cope needle is inserted. **D,** The Cope needle and outer cannula are maneuvered using the rib as a fulcrum so that the Cope needle is adjacent to the pleura. The needle system is then withdrawn until the hook engages the pleura. **E,** Once the pleura is engaged, the outer cannula is advanced over the Cope needle to capture the piece of pleura. The Cope needle is then withdrawn and the trocar and stylet placed back through the outer cannula in case other pleural biopsies are required. (From Mueller PR, Saini S, Simeone JF, et al. Image-guided pleural biopsies: indications, technique, and results in 23 patients. *Radiology.* 1988;169:1-4.)

Therapeutic Thoracentesis

The principal indication for therapeutic thoracentesis is to relieve chest discomfort and dyspnea in patients with malignant pleural effusions. This procedure can be performed on an outpatient basis in the vast majority of patients.

Technique

There are many different methods used to perform therapeutic thoracentesis, including using a large-gauge needle, an intravenous cannula, or a small catheter. The author prefers the catheter technique using a 7-French catheter (Electro-catheter Corp., Rahway, N.J.) with multiple side holes, which is trocared into the pleural space. It is connected by a three-way stopcock and tubing to a sterile 1-L vacuum bottle, which drains fluid from the chest. This can be changed when full. Usually a total of 2-3 L is removed during any one procedure. If severe coughing, dyspnea, or chest pain develop, the rate of fluid removal can be slowed and titrated in accordance with the patient's symptoms. If symptoms persist, the catheter is clamped and a chest radiograph obtained to check for a pneumothorax.

In patients with malignant pleural effusions, occasionally the lung does not expand when fluid is removed; the underlying lung appears to be noncompliant. The cause of this is uncertain but it may be related to lymphangitis carcinomatosa, which is microscopic in nature. This phenomenon ("vacuthorax") does not have any clinical symptoms and does not require treatment even when large. If treated with chest tube insertion, the lung usually does not reexpand.

Pleurodesis

Malignant effusions often recur following therapeutic thoracentesis and may require pleurodesis for effective palliation. The sclerosing agent is injected into the pleural space and is designed to irritate the pleura so that the visceral and parietal pleura become fixed and prevent the reaccumulation of fluid. A number of sclerosing agents are available, with the most commonly used being doxycycline, bleomycin, or talc. Talc is generally instilled into the pleural space by surgeons in the operating room with the patient under general anesthesia. Doxycycline and bleomycin can be administered percutaneously. Tetracycline was originally used for pleurodesis but is no longer made by the manufacturer; doxycycline has been substituted. Doxycycline is administered in doses of 1-2 g dissolved in 100 mL of normal saline on 3 consecutive days. Bleomycin pleurodesis is performed in one session using 60 IU dissolved in 50 mL of 5% dextrose as a single dose. It has been shown by Belani and associates that bleomycin is the most cost-effective therapy for pleurodesis, even though initially more expensive than doxycycline.

Technique

Before pleurodesis, the pleural effusion needs to be drained almost dry for maximal sclerosant effect. Small catheters tend to kink in the pleural space and therefore larger (16- to 24-French) catheters are preferred. The catheter is connected to 20-cm negative wall suction using an underwater-seal pleural drainage system. Although the aim is to drain the effusion completely, this is frequently not possible with most malignant effusions. Therefore a compromise position is reached such that, when the chest tube output has fallen below 100 mL/day, sclerotherapy is performed. If sclerotherapy is performed with chest tube drainage greater than 100 mL/day, the pleurodesis is more likely to fail.

After the agent is injected, the catheter is clamped for 1 hour and the patient is rolled every 15 minutes from supine to right lateral decubitus to prone to left lateral decubitus positions. This ensures efficient distribution of the sclerosing agent throughout the pleural space. The chest tube is then unclamped and the

Box 18-14. Pleurodesis

Agents used include talc, doxycycline, and bleomycin
Bleomycin is most cost-effective
Pleurodesis performed when chest tube drainage is less than 100 mL/day
After pleurodesis the chest tube is placed on underwater seal for 24 hours and then removed

sclerosant allowed to drain through the chest tube. The tube is then placed on underwater seal drainage for 24 hours, and if a chest radiograph performed at that time shows no pneumothorax, the tube is removed (Box 18-14).

Empyema Drainage

Parapneumonic effusions that are complicated based on Light's criteria (described previously) require drainage. In addition, any diagnostic thoracentesis that yields pus or has a positive Gram stain or culture requires drainage.

It is logical to use image-guided catheter drainage for loculated empyemas as opposed to blind surgical techniques, which are based on the chest radiograph as a reference. Not infrequently, blind empyema drainage results in a tube being placed in the pleural space outside the loculated empyema. Precise catheter placement with image guidance should be the first choice for loculated empyema drainage.

Technique

Ultrasound is the preferred image guidance modality in that it is fast, efficient, and portable. The patient is positioned in a similar position to either a diagnostic or therapeutic thoracentesis. The skin position is marked over the mid-point of the loculated fluid collection. The skin is infiltrated with local anesthetic and incised with a #11 scalpel blade. Deep blunt dissection with a forceps considerably helps with tube placement and should be performed routinely. Large catheters are mandatory for empyema drainage to prevent tube clogging and kinking; 16- to 24-French catheters can be used, but the author prefers catheters larger than 20-French, particularly to reduce the effect of kinking, which often happens with smaller catheters because of the effect of respiratory excursions pressing the catheter against the adjacent rib. The smaller catheters can usually be inserted using a trocar technique, while larger catheters are best inserted using the Seldinger technique (Fig. 18-27). The larger catheters can be inserted solely under ultrasound guidance by the Seldinger technique, but if the operator is uncomfortable with this, the patient can be brought to fluoroscopy and a combination of ultrasound and fluoroscopy used. After catheter insertion, the catheter is stitched to the skin and connected to an underwater-seal pleural drainage system. Close daily supervision of the patient and catheter should be performed by the interventional team.

Although the patient may be followed up by chest radiography, the author prefers CT scanning to evaluate the adequacy of drainage, particularly if the collection has been loculated. The catheter can be removed if the patient is afebrile and drainage has decreased to less than 10-15 mL/day. Loculated empyemas or more complex collections may require multiple catheters for complete drainage and/or the use of intrapleural urokinase to lyse fibrinous septae and hemorrhagic components. The author's unit routinely uses urokinase if the patient remains febrile and there is residual fluid identified on follow-up imaging. Eighty-five thousand units are injected through the indwelling catheter, which is clamped for 1-2 hours and then restored to suction. This is repeated every 8 hours for a total of 4-6 treatments. If

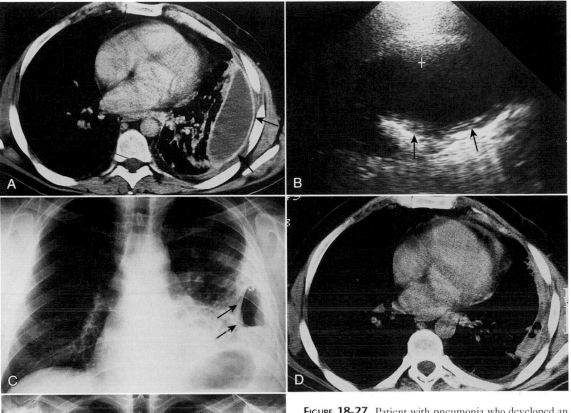

FIGURE 18-27. Patient with pneumonia who developed an empyema. **A,** A computed tomography (CT) scan was performed because of persisting sepsis despite a surgical chest tube having been placed for a presumed empyema. CT showed the loculated empyema *(arrows).* The surgical chest tube was anterior to the loculated empyema. **B,** Under ultrasound guidance, a 20-French chest tube was inserted into the loculated empyema, which is clearly visualized on ultrasound *(arrows).* The chest tube was inserted using the Seldinger technique. **C,** Chest radiograph obtained after the procedure shows the 20-French chest tube *(arrows)* sited within the loculated empyema. **D,** Follow-up CT scan 5 days after initial chest tube insertion shows that the empyema has virtually resolved. The chest tube was removed. **E,** Follow-up chest radiograph 2 months later shows some pleural thickening along the left costal margin and some blunting of the left costophrenic angle, but otherwise no sequelae of the empyema are seen.

urokinase treatment fails then open surgical drainage is usually indicated.

Results

Ultrasound-guided diagnostic thoracentesis is a low-risk procedure that can be successfully performed in up to 97% of patients. In patients with proven malignant effusions, the yield from cytologic examination of aspirated pleural fluid is approximately 50%. In exudative effusions remaining undiagnosed after thoracentesis, a pleural biopsy may be performed. Pleural biopsy is highly specific for either tuberculosis or malignancy, with sensitivities of 90% and 68%, respectively. Pleural biopsy is particularly useful when tuberculosis is suspected, but less useful when malignancy is suspected.

Belani and associates, in a metaanalysis of the literature, reported overall success rates for pleurodesis with tetracycline, bleomycin, and talc of 68.1%, 74.9%, and 94.1%, respectively. However, bleomycin proved to be the most cost-effective treatment overall.

The overall success rate for percutaneous drainage of empyema from reported series is 77%, which compares favorably to the 32%-71% success rates reported for conventional surgical

tube placement. It is likely that the overall success rate can be increased by the use of urokinase in selected patients.

Complications

Complications are uncommon with image-guided pleural intervention. Pneumothorax rates for ultrasound-guided thoracentesis vary from none to 3%, which compares favorably with the pneumothorax rates of 3%-20% associated with blind aspiration. The author's unit has reported a pneumothorax rate of 7.5% in 350 consecutive patients who underwent therapeutic thoracentesis, with approximately 3% of these patients requiring chest tube placement. Reexpansion pulmonary edema has been reported by others as a result of rapid evacuation of pleural fluid, but in practice this is an extremely infrequent occurrence and the author's unit routinely aspirates 2-3 L of fluid in one treatment session. Complications reported with image-guided drainage of empyemas are uncommon, less than 2%.

Pneumothorax is a common complication with all of the various pleural and lung interventions. Interventional radiologists should be familiar with the techniques of image-guided treatment of pneumothorax as detailed in Chapter 17.

Lung and Mediastinal Abscesses

Primary lung abscesses are rare. When they do occur, they are most commonly due to aspiration or as a consequence of primary specific pneumonias due to organisms such as *Klebsiella, Pseudomonas,* or *Staphylococcus.* Secondary lung abscesses may result from septic emboli or obstructing bronchogenic neoplasms. Percutaneous drainage of lung abscesses is rarely required, in that about 80%-90% of patients respond to antibiotic therapy. For those lung abscesses that do not respond to antibiotic therapy, PAD is a valuable procedure both for abscess decompression and the avoidance of surgical lobectomy.

Although percutaneous drainage of lung abscesses can be performed under fluoroscopy, the author prefers to use CT guidance for placement of the initial needle into the abscess cavity. Small 8- or 10-French locking catheters are used for drainage. These can be placed either by trocar or Seldinger technique. It is important to repeat the CT scan after drainage to ensure that there are no undrained locules, and careful monitoring of the catheter after the procedure is necessary. The abscess contents are aspirated after the catheter has been inserted and the catheter is connected to an underwater seal pleural drainage system. As with pleural empyema, CT is best used to evaluate the adequacy of drainage. When drainage has decreased to less than 10 mL/day and CT shows effective resolution of the abscess, the catheter can be removed. Success rates of 80%-90% have been described for percutaneous drainage of lung abscesses.

Mediastinal abscesses are very uncommon, but may occur after cardiothoracic operations. Drainage of these abscesses follows the same principles as for mediastinal biopsy. Because of the proximity of vascular and mediastinal structures, these abscesses require very precise guidance and are best drained under CT control with the Seldinger technique. After the initial needle is placed, the patient is brought to fluoroscopy for track dilatation and catheter insertion. As with mediastinal biopsy, careful planning of the access route to avoid the internal mammary artery and vein and distension of the mediastinum with sterile saline may be necessary to avoid pneumothorax.

▬ SUGGESTED READINGS

Acunas B, Rozanes I, Celik L, et al. Purely cystic hydatid disease of the liver: treatment with percutaneous aspiration and injection of hypertonic saline. *Radiology.* 1992;182:541-543.

Balthazar EJ, Freeny PC, vanSonnenberg E. Imaging and intervention in acute pancreatitis. *Radiology.* 1994;193:297-306.

Beland MD, Gervais DA, Levis DA, et al. Complex abdominal and pelvic abscesses: efficacy of adjunctive tissue-type plasminogen activator for drainage. *Radiology.* 2008;247(2):567-573.

Belani CP, Eiranson TR, Arikan SR, et al. Cost-effectiveness analysis of pleurodesis in the management of malignant pleural effusion. *J Oncol Manag.* Jan/Feb. 1995:24-34.

Bennett JD, Kozak RI, Taylor MB. Deep pelvic abscesses: transrectal drainage with radiologic guidance. *Radiology.* 1992;185:825-828.

Boland GW, Lee MJ, Dawson SL, et al. Percutaneous abscess drainage: complications. *Semin Interv Radiol.* 1994;11:267-275.

Boland G, Lee MJ, Silverman S, et al. Review: interventional radiology of the pleural space. *Clin Radiol.* 1995;50:205-214.

Bucher P, Pugin F, Morel P. Minimally invasive necrosectomy for infected necrotizing pancreatitis. *Pancreas.* 2008;36(2):113-119.

Casola G, vanSonnenberg E, Neff CC. Abscesses in Crohn disease: percutaneous drainage. *Radiology.* 1987;163:19-22.

Casola G, vanSonnenberg E, D'Agostino HB, et al. Percutaneous drainage of tubo-ovarian abscesses. *Radiology.* 1992;182:399-402.

Eisenberg PJ, Lee MJ, Boland GW, et al. Percutaneous drainage of a subphrenic abscess with gastric fistula. *Am J Roentgenol.* 1994;162:1233-1237.

Gazelle GS, Haaga JR, Stellato TA, et al. Pelvic abscesses: CT-guided transrectal drainage. *Radiology.* 1991;181:49-51.

Hovsepian DM. Transrectal and transvaginal abscess drainage. *J Vasc Interv Radiol.* 1997;8:501-515.

Keeling AN, Leong S, Logan PM, Lee MJ. Empyema and effusion: outcome of image-guided small-bore catheter drainage. *Cardiovasc Intervent Radiol.* 2008;31(1):135-141.

Kerlan RK, Jeffrey RB, Pogany AC, Ring EI. Abdominal abscess with low-output fistula: successful percutaneous drainage. *Radiology.* 1985;155:73-75.

Lahorra JM, Haaga JR, Stellato T, et al. Safety of intracavitary urokinase with percutaneous abscess drainage. *Am J Roentgenol.* 1993;160:171-174.

Lambiase RE, Deyoe L, Cronan JJ, et al. Percutaneous drainage of 335 consecutive abscesses: results of primary drainage with 1-year follow-up. *Radiology.* 1992;184:167-179.

Lambiase RE. Percutaneous abscess and fluid drainage: a critical review. *Cardiovasc Interv Radiol.* 1991;14:143-157.

Lambiase RE, Cronan JJ, Dorfman GS, et al. Postoperative abscesses with enteric communication: percutaneous treatment. *Radiology.* 1989;171:497-500.

Lee MJ. Non-traumatic abdominal emergencies: imaging and intervention in sepsis. *Eur Radiol.* 2002;12:2172-2179.

Lee KS, IM JG, Kim YH, et al. Treatment of thoracic multiloculated empyemas with intercavitary urokinase: a prospective study. *Radiology.* 1991;179:771-775.

Lee MJ, Saini S, Brink JA, et al. Interventional radiology of the pleural space: diagnostic thoracentesis, therapeutic thoracentesis, pleural biopsy, and pleural sclerosis. *Semin Interv Radiol.* 1991;8:23-28.

Lee MJ, Saini S, Brink JA, et al. Interventional radiology of the pleural space: management of thoracic empyema with image-guided catheter drainage. *Semin Interv Radiol.* 1991;8:29-35.

Lee MJ, Rattner DW, Legemate DA, et al. Acute complicated pancreatitis: redefining the role of interventional radiology. *Radiology.* 1992;183:171-174.

Lee MJ, Wittich GR, Mueller PR. Percutaneous intervention in acute pancreatitis. *RadioGraphics.* 1998;18:711-724.

Light RW. Parapneumonic effusions and empyemas. *Clin Chest Med.* 1985;6:55-61.

Light RW, Macgregor ML, Luchsinger PC, et al. Pleural effusions: the diagnostic separation of transudates from exudates. *Ann Intern Med.* 1972;77:507-513.

Light RW, Erozan YS, Ball WC. Cells in the pleural fluid: their value in differential diagnosis. *Arch Intern Med.* 1973;132:854-860.

Loveday BP, Mittal A, Phillips A, Windsor JA. Minimally invasive management of pancreatic abscess, pseudocyst, and necrosis: a systematic review of current guidelines. *World J Surg.* 2008;32(11):2383-2394.

Martin EC, Karlson KB, Fankuchen EI, et al. Percutaneous drainage of postoperative intraabdominal abscesses. *Am J Roentgenol.* 1982;138:13-15.

Moore AV, Zuger JH, Kelley MJ. Lung abscess: an interventional radiology perspective. *Semin Interv Radiol.* 1991;8:36-43.

Moulton JS, Moore PT, Mencini RA. Treatment of loculated pleural effusions with transcatheter intracavitary urokinase. *Am J Roentgenol.* 1989;153:941-945.

Mueller PR, Saini S, Wittenbeurg J, et al. Sigmoid diverticular abscesses: percutaneous drainage as an adjunct to surgical resection in 24 cases. *Radiology.* 1987;164:321-325.

Neff CC, vanSonnenberg E, Casola G, et al. Diverticular abscesses: percutaneous drainage. *Radiology.* 1987;163:15-18.

Position Paper of the American Thoracic Society adopted by the ATS Board of Directors, June 1988. Guidelines for thoracentesis and needle biopsy of the pleura. *Am Rev Respir Dis.* 1989;140:257-258.

Position Paper, Health and Public Policy Committee, American College of Physicians. Diagnostic thoracentesis and pleural biopsy in pleural effusions. *Ann Intern Med.* 1985;103:799-802.

Rattner DW, Legemate DA, Lee MJ, et al. Early surgical debridement of symptomatic pancreatic necrosis is beneficial irrespective of infection. *Am J Surg.* 1992;163:105-111.

Rivera-Sanfeliz G. Percutaneous abdominal abscess drainage: a historical perspective. *AJR Am J Roentgenol.* 2008;191(3):642-643.

SCVIR Standards of Practice Committee. Quality improvement guidelines for adult percutaneous abscess and fluid drainage. *J Vasc Interv Radiol.* 1995;6:68-70.

Shepard JO. Complications of percutaneous needle aspiration biopsy of the chest: prevention and management. *Semin Interv Radiol.* 1994;11:181-186.

vanSonnenberg E, Mueller PR, Ferrucci JT. Percutaneous drainage of 250 abdominal abscesses and fluid collections: I. Results, failures, and complications. *Radiology.* 1984;151:337-341.

vanSonnenberg E, Mueller PR, Ferrucci JT. Percutaneous drainage of 250 abdominal abscesses and fluid collections: II. Current procedural concepts. *Radiology.* 1984;151:343-347.

vanSonnenberg E, Wittich GR, Casola G, et al. Periappendiceal abscesses: percutaneous drainage. *Radiology.* 1987;163:23-26.

vanSonnenberg E, D'Agostino HB, Casola G, et al. US-guided transvaginal drainage of pelvic abscesses and fluid collections. *Radiology.* 1991;181:53-56.

vanSonnenberg E, D'Agostino HB, Casola G, et al. Percutaneous abscess drainage: current concepts. *Radiology.* 1991;181:617-626.

vanSonnenberg E, Wroblicka JT, D'Agostina HB, et al. Symptomatic hepatic cysts: percutaneous drainage and sclerosis. *Radiology.* 1994;190:387-392.

Walters R, Herman CM, Neff R, et al. Percutaneous drainage of abscesses in the postoperative abdomen that is difficult to explore. *Am J Surg.* 1985;149:623-626.

Watkinson AE, Adam A. Complications of abdominal and retroperitoneal biopsy. *Semin Interv Radiol.* 1994;11:254-266.

Weisbrod GL. Transthoracic percutaneous fine-needle aspiration biopsy in the chest and mediastinum. *Semin Interv Radiol.* 1991;8:1-14.

Westcott JL. Percutaneous catheter drainage of pleural effusion and empyema. *Am J Roentgenol.* 1985;144:1189-1193.

Zerbey AL, Dawson SL, Mueller PR. Pleural interventions and complications. *Semin Interv Radiol.* 1994;11:187-197.

CHAPTER 19

Gastrointestinal Tract Intervention

Michael J. Lee, MSc, FRCPI, FRCR, FFR(RCSI), FSIR, EBIR

The role of the radiologist in gastrointestinal tract intervention has mushroomed with the advent of percutaneous gastrostomy and more recently esophageal and colorectal stenting. These new procedures, coupled with the older procedures of gastrointestinal stricture dilatation, have made gastrointestinal tract intervention an important area of visceral intervention. Additionally, these procedures are predominantly performed under fluoroscopic guidance so that they can be performed in almost all radiology departments.

PERCUTANEOUS GASTROSTOMY

Surgical gastrostomy was first proposed in 1837 and successfully performed in 1876. It was not until almost a century later that Gauderer reported the endoscopic placement of a gastrostomy tube with the patient under local anesthesia. The technique of radiologic gastrostomy was established in 1983, and numerous papers describing and refining the technique have followed.

Indications

Percutaneous gastrostomy is predominantly performed in patients who need prolonged nutritional support, such as patients with neurologic disease (degenerative central nervous system disease, cerebral vascular accidents); head, neck, and esophageal carcinoma; swallowing disorders; and esophageal strictures. Chronic conditions such as cystic fibrosis and congenital heart disease may also require a percutaneous gastrostomy. Occasionally, a percutaneous gastrostomy or gastrojejunostomy may be placed for bowel decompression. Indications include malignant small bowel obstruction or patients with prolonged ileus following major abdominal operations.

Contraindications

Box 19-1 lists absolute and relative contraindications. Absolute contraindications include colonic interposition, total gastrectomy or severe uncorrectable coagulopathy, and extensive gastric varices. In patients with relative contraindications, the procedure may be technically more demanding and require more careful planning but is usually possible.

Technique

Patient Preparation (Box 19-2)

Informed consent is obtained before the procedure, usually from a relative or from the patient, if possible. The referring team should be asked to place an intravenous cannula for sedoanalgesia and to fast the patient from midnight of the evening before the procedure. The referring team is also asked to pass a nasogastric tube on the evening before the procedure and administer 300 mL of an oral barium suspension. The barium serves to delineate the relationship of the transverse colon to the stomach on the day of the procedure (Fig. 19-1). When commencing placement of gastrostomy tubes, it is reasonable to give barium beforehand. However, with experience, the barium can be omitted because the colon can be adequately visualized on fluoroscopy without barium labeling. Additionally, when the stomach is distended, it tends to push the transverse colon inferiorly and out of the way. If, however, you are not happy that the colon is visible, air can be insufflated via a rectal tube to demonstrate the colon. Alternatively, if lateral fluoroscopy is available the stomach is distended and a forceps is placed at the skin entry site and the location of the skin entry site vis-à-vis the stomach is ascertained. Usually the stomach is directly underneath the anterior abdominal wall with no intervening bowel loops. When the position of the colon

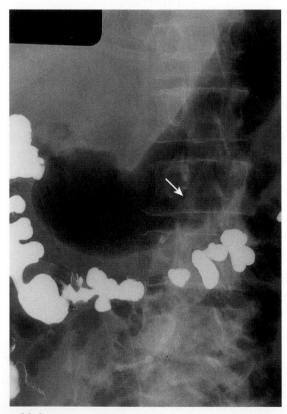

Figure 19-1. Patient referred for percutaneous gastrostomy. Barium given the night before delineates the colon, which can be seen clearly separated from the stomach. The stomach is distended with air via the nasogastric tube *(arrow)*. Colonic opacification is important so that it can be avoided during pregastrostomy gastrostomy.

is ascertained, the stomach is distended with air via the nasogastric tube.

Occasionally, in patients with esophageal strictures it may not be possible for the referring team to place a nasogastric tube. In this situation, in the author's unit, the nasogastric tube is placed under direct fluoroscopic visualization at the time of the percutaneous gastrostomy. It is usually possible to place a nasogastric tube even through tight strictures by first using a 5-French angiographic catheter and a hydrophilic wire. Once the stricture is crossed, the hydrophilic wire can be exchanged for a superstiff wire and a nasogastric tube placed in the stomach.

In the author's unit, a paralytic agent such as glucagon or n-hyoscine butyl bromide is routinely used to induce gastric paralysis. Antibiotic prophylaxis is not routinely given unless a percutaneous endoscopic gastrostomy (PEG) tube will be placed through the mouth under fluoroscopic guidance. Some authors mark the position of the left lobe of the liver using ultrasound. This is not done in the author's unit, and there have been no hepatic complications in over more than 500 procedures. Once the stomach is fully distended, the entry site is usually well below the left lobe of the liver. In general, the puncture site should be lateral to the rectus sheath to avoid the superior epigastric artery. If orientation and size of the stomach prevents use of a puncture site lateral to the rectus sheath, then a midline puncture is chosen. A combination of midazolam and fentanyl are used in small amounts for sedoanalgesia.

Gastropexy

The author's unit performs a gastropexy routinely in all patients. Advantages and disadvantages are discussed later. Gastropexy fixes the anterior wall of the stomach to the anterior abdominal wall and prevents guidewire buckling into the peritoneal cavity and early or late intraperitoneal leakage. Gastropexy is performed using T-fasteners (Kimberly Clark, Draper, Utah, or Balt, Montmorency, France) (Fig. 19-2). With the stomach maximally inflated, the puncture site into the stomach is chosen midway between the superior and inferior margins of the inflated stomach just proximal to the incisura. The puncture site is marked on the skin and subcutaneous injections of local anesthesia are given at the puncture site and at the four corners of a 2.5-cm square around the puncture site. A slotted 18-gauge needle is used to insert four T-fasteners at the corner of this square. The T-fasteners consist of a metal T-bar attached to a nylon suture, which is attached to a cotton wool pledget. The nylon suture runs through the cotton wool pledget, and between the cotton wool pledget and the distal end of the suture there are two small metal cylinders that are freely mobile on the suture (see Fig. 19-2).

The T-fasteners are loaded on the slotted 18-gauge needle. The 18-gauge needle is attached to a partially saline-filled syringe and the stomach is punctured at the four corners of the 2.5-cm square. When air is aspirated, the tip of the slotted 18-gauge needle lies in the stomach. The syringe is removed and the stylet is used to push the T-fastener out of the needle and into the stomach. The stylet and needle are removed and gentle tension on the external nylon suture opposes the stomach wall to the anterior abdominal wall (Fig. 19-3). The stomach is fixed in position by crimping the metal cylinders around the suture using a sterile forceps. When all four T-fasteners are in situ, the gastrostomy tube is placed (Fig. 19-4).

Gastrostomy Tube Placement (Box 19-3)

The proposed site of entry for the gastrostomy tube (in the center of the T-fastener square) is anesthetized, and a 3- to 4-mm transverse incision is made and dissected with a blunt forceps. The slotted needle that was used for the gastropexy is used to puncture the stomach, and a 0.035-inch superstiff guidewire inserted so that it coils in the stomach lumen. The author tends to angle the puncture site toward the pyloric canal or antrum, so that the angle of the track will facilitate the conversion from gastrostomy to percutaneous gastrojejunostomy if it becomes necessary (Fig. 19-5). It is important to keep the stomach inflated during gastropexy and gastrostomy tube placement. Complications are more likely to be encountered if the stomach is not maximally inflated at all times. Successive fascial dilators can be

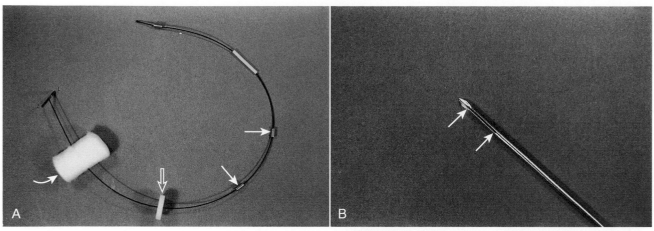

FIGURE 19-2. T-fastener gastropexy device. **A,** The T-fastener consists of a metal "bar" (T) attached to a nylon suture, which has a dental pledget *(curved arrow)*, plastic ring washer *(straight arrow)*, and two small metal cylinders *(small arrows)*. The T-fastener is inserted into the end of the slotted needle, which is inserted into the stomach. The T-fastener is dislodged using the stylet that comes with the set. The cotton wool pledget lies on the anterior abdominal wall and the metal cylinders are crimped on the nylon suture using a surgical forceps while maintaining tension on the suture. This helps fix the stomach to the anterior wall. **B,** Close-up of the end of the slot of the slotted needle showing the slot *(arrows)* in the end of the needle into which the T-fastener fits.

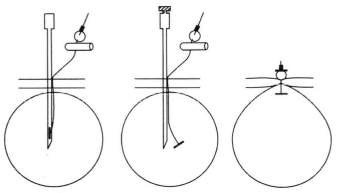

FIGURE 19-3. Illustration showing T-fastener gastropexy. The slotted needle containing the T-fastener is inserted into the stomach, and the T-fastener is pushed out of the needle using the stylet. Tension on the suture then opposes the T-fastener against the anterior abdominal wall, which pulls the stomach up to the anterior abdominal wall. By crimping the metal cylinder on the suture, the stomach is fixed to the anterior abdominal wall.

used to dilate the percutaneous track. The track is dilated to a size that is 1- to 2-French larger than the catheter to be inserted. A 14- to 18-French gastrostomy catheter is placed through a peel-away sheath into the stomach. The peel-away sheath is usually provided with the gastrostomy tube. The guidewire is removed and contrast injected to confirm the intraluminal position of the gastrostomy tube. Although the percutaneous track may be angled toward the antrum, the gastrostomy tube usually ends in the fundus of the stomach, because the fundus is more posterior and more capacious than the gastric antrum (Fig. 19-6). The nasogastric tube is removed at the end of the procedure and the patient returned to the ward.

Aftercare

Begin tube feeding after 12-24 hours. Gastrostomy tubes should be flushed thoroughly after each feeding to prevent clogging. This is particularly important after administration of crushed tablets through the tube. If clogging occurs, it can be treated by gentle flushing with hot water to dissolve impacted material. The T-fasteners are cut at 2-5 days and allowed to fall into the stomach. This is simply performed by cutting the

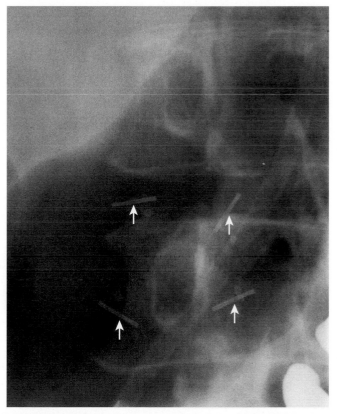

FIGURE 19-4. T-fastener gastropexy. Four T-fasteners *(arrows)* have been inserted at the corners of a 2.5-cm square to fix the stomach to the anterior abdominal wall. The gastrostomy tube can now be inserted.

nylon suture underneath the cotton wool pledget on the anterior abdominal wall. A new T-fastener device made by Kimberly Clark has a biodegradable suture that does not have to be cut.

In the author's unit, gastrostomy catheters are not fixed to the skin because there is usually an internal fixation device on the catheter that prevents catheter dislodgment. The catheter entry site is simply covered with a sterile dressing. Suturing of the catheter to the skin may cause skin irritation and skin breakdown particularly, if there is any leakage around the tube.

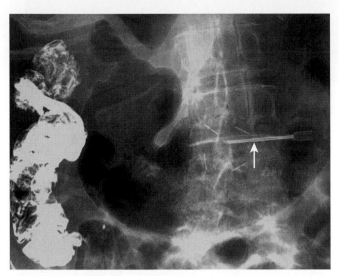

FIGURE 19-5. Gastrostomy tube angle of entry. The hypodermic needle *(arrow)* shows the approximate angle of entry of the gastrostomy tube into the stomach. The needle is inserted toward the pylorus at a 45-degree angle; if conversion of the tube to a gastrojejunostomy is required at a later date, the track will be angled toward the pylorus.

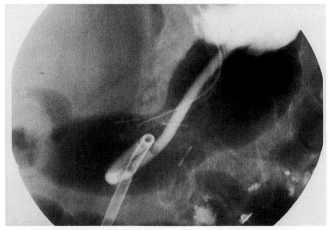

FIGURE 19-6. Gastrostomy tube insertion. After tract dilatation, the catheter is inserted through a peel-away sheath and then locked in position. The catheter placed has a pigtail retention device (Cook, Bloomington, Ind.), which keeps the catheter in place. Even though the gastrostomy track is angled toward the pylorus, the tip of the tube usually ends in the most dependent portion of the stomach—the fundus.

Special Considerations

Is Gastropexy Necessary?

Many authors do not routinely perform a gastropexy when a percutaneous gastrostomy tube is being placed. Gastropexy was devised to emulate surgical gastropexy, which is used before placing surgical gastrostomy tubes. There is a lot of debate as to whether routine use of gastropexy devices is necessary. The

literature indicates that routine use is probably not necessary. There are many large series in the literature that describe percutaneous gastrostomy without gastropexy without any increase in complications. The theoretical advantages of using gastropexy are that larger catheters can be placed de novo, catheters and guidewires do not buckle into the peritoneal cavity, peritoneal leakage of gastric contents is less likely, and the catheter can be replaced if it is inadvertently pulled out soon after the procedure.

We recently performed a prospective randomized study involving 90 consecutive patients referred for percutaneous radiologic gastrostomy (PRG) placement. Forty-eight patients underwent T-fastener gastropexy, while 42 underwent PRG without gastropexy. In four of the 42 patients (9%) from the nongastropexy group, serious technical difficulties were encountered with misplacement of the gastrostomy tube in the peritoneal cavity in two patients. This was discovered on injecting contrast material at the end of the procedure. T-fastener gastropexy was performed, and the procedure completed radiologically in two patients. In another patient the procedure was completed successfully without T-fastener gastropexy. In the remaining patient, it was decided to repeat the procedure on the following day. However, the patient underwent endoscopic placement of a gastrostomy tube the following day. In the gastropexy group, five patients experienced pain at the gastrostomy site, which was relieved by removing the T-fasteners. This would suggest that the placement of large-bore gastrostomy tubes (greater than 14-French) may cause problems without performing gastropexy. However, it is very much up to the operator's preference whether or not gastropexy is performed.

There are some situations in which use of a gastropexy device is important, including patients with ascites in whom gastropexy combined with regular paracentesis is necessary to prevent tube dislodgment from the stomach.

Computed Tomography Guidance

The author occasionally uses CT guidance for percutaneous gastrostomy in patients with no safe percutaneous access route to the stomach by means of standard fluoroscopic guidance, in patients in whom a nasogastric tube cannot be placed owing to esophageal obstruction, and in patients with very scaphoid abdomen in which the stomach is tucked up underneath the rib cage. In addition, CT is often used in patients who have failed PEG because of poor transillumination from the stomach to the anterior abdominal wall. In the latter situation, use of CT is often prudent to outline the relationships of the stomach to the anterior abdominal wall. Also, in patients who have undergone previous gastric surgery, CT guidance may be necessary to place the tube. CT guidance is used in a minority of patients and the routine use of CT is unwarranted.

If CT guidance is used, the patient is placed supine on the CT table and a radiopaque grid placed on the anterior abdominal wall overlying the stomach. When the stomach is located, a safe path is chosen to place the initial needle. If a nasogastric tube has not been placed in the stomach and the stomach is not distended, it may be possible to distend the stomach somewhat by giving carbonated granules to the patient before the CT procedure. If nasogastric tube placement is not possible or if carbonated granules cannot be given, a 22-gauge Chiba needle is placed into the stomach and contrast injected to confirm an intraluminal position. Air is then injected through the 22-gauge needle to distend the stomach. A 0.018-inch guidewire is placed through the needle into the stomach and a 5-French introducer sheath is placed over the guidewire with a final exchange made for a 0.038-inch J-guidewire. The patient is then moved so that fluoroscopy may be used for the remainder of the procedure (Fig. 19-7).

Although CT guidance is necessary only in a minority of patients, it solves the anatomic or other impediments that make patients unsuitable for fluoroscopically guided gastrostomy.

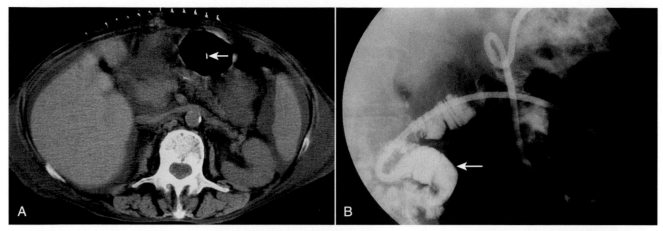

FIGURE 19-7. Computed tomography (CT)-guided gastrostomy tube placement in a patient with a previous Billroth II gastrectomy. **A,** CT was used to guide the initial needle placement because of the small stomach remnant. The stomach was distended with air using a nasogastric tube with the aid of glucagon to decrease peristalsis. A needle *(arrow)* was placed into the stomach under CT guidance and the patient moved to undergo fluoroscopy. **B,** After track dilatation, the gastrostomy tube was placed into the efferent limb of the gastroenteric anastomosis. Contrast injection at the end of the procedure shows the catheter tip *(arrow)* located distally in the efferent limb.

The Postoperative Stomach

A previous subtotal gastrectomy is considered a relative contraindication to percutaneous gastrostomy. However, a number of techniques have been described to place gastrostomy tubes percutaneously in these patients. One of the problems with patients who have Billroth II procedures or gastrojejunostomies is that air insufflated into the stomach almost immediately passes into the small bowel. In these patients it is useful to give glucagon or hyoscine butyl bromide to paralyze the stomach and small bowel. In general, the procedure can be performed under fluoroscopy. Lateral fluoroscopy is helpful to assess the position of the stomach remnant vis-à-vis the anterior abdominal wall. Giving barium before the procedure helps localize the colon. If a safe access is visualized, then the procedure is carried out under fluoroscopy. If not, CT guidance is used (see Fig. 19-7). Some authors have described the placement of a large balloon into the stomach remnant, wherein the balloon is inflated and direct puncture of the balloon is used to obtain initial percutaneous access. In the author's unit, we use a technique similar to that used for a standard gastrostomy. Cephalocaudal angulation of the x-ray tube can help substantially in accessing a small stomach that lies subcostally. Sometimes the body of the stomach can be entered directly with a needle; on other occasions the efferent small bowel loop is punctured and the catheter tip ultimately positioned in the gastric remnant.

In general, gastric remnants that have previously been operated on are relatively fixed in the abdomen owing to postoperative fibrosis and adhesions. T-fasteners are therefore not generally used. Once access to the stomach is gained with a one-stick needle system, the track is dilated and a 12- to 14-French nephrostomy type catheter is placed in the gastric remnant.

Results

Technical success rates of 98%-100% have been reported in several large series describing percutaneous gastrostomy (Table 19-1). In one metaanalysis of the literature by Wollman and associates, the average success rate of percutaneous gastrostomy tube placement was 99.2% in a combined series of 837 patients (Table 19-2). This compares favorably with a 95.7% success rate for placement of PEG tubes and 100% for surgical gastrostomy tube placement. By and large, percutaneous gastrostomy has become a widely accepted technique for gastrostomy tube placement and compares favorably with the endoscopic technique. The advantage of percutaneous

TABLE 19-1 Technical Success and Complications Associated with Percutaneous Gastrostomy in Adults

Author	Year	Patients	Technical Success (%)	Complications (%) Major	Minor	Procedure-Related Mortality (%)
O'Keefe	1989	100	100	0	15	0
Saini	1990	125	99	1.6	9.5	0
Halkier	1990	252	99	1.6	4.4	0.8
Hicks	1990	158	100	6	12	2
Bell	1995	519	95	1.3	2.9	0.4
Ryan	1997	316	99	1.9	3.2	0.3
Kim	2008	248	99	5.1	14.4	0
Perona	2010	254	100	1.3	4.5	0.2
Power	2012	260	99	1.2	12.8	0.4

TABLE 19-2 Comparison of Radiologic, Endoscopic and Surgical Gastrostomy

Gastrostomy Method	Patients	Technical Success (%)	Complications (%) Major	Minor	Procedure-Related Mortality (%)
Radiologic	837	99.2	5.9	7.8	0.3
Endoscopic	4194	95.7	9.4	5.9	0.5
Surgical	721	100	19.9	9.0	2.5

Data from Wollman BD, Agostino HB, Walus Wigle, et al. Radiologic, endoscopic, and surgical gastrostomy: an institutional evaluation and meta-analysis of the literature. *Radiology.* 1995;197:699-704.

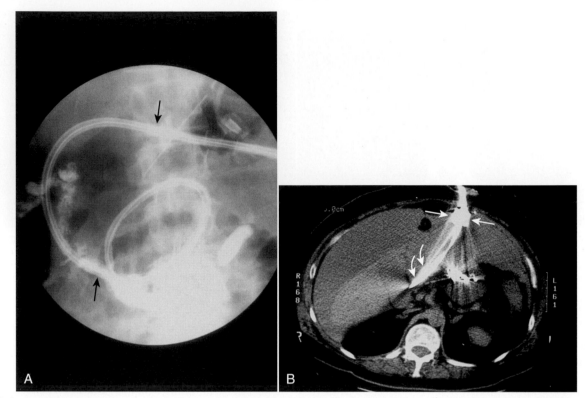

FIGURE 19-8. Gastric tube dislodgment with leakage of gastric contents into the peritoneal cavity in a patient with malignant ascites. **A,** A gastrojejunostomy tube *(arrows)* was placed for drainage of the small bowel, which was partially obstructed. **B,** Twenty-four hours later the patient complained of severe abdominal pain and had peritoneal signs. A computed tomography scan shows a moderate amount of ascites within the peritoneal cavity. Note the retention balloon device *(straight arrows)* on the gastric catheter lying underneath the anterior abdominal wall. The retention device of the gastrostomy catheter had pulled out of the stomach because of the weight of the ascites pressing on the stomach wall. The remainder of the gastrostomy catheter *(curved arrows)* remains within the stomach. It is important when performing percutaneous gastrostomy in a patient with ascites to drain the ascites on a regular basis to prevent this from happening. This patient was brought to the operating theater where it was noted that the four T-tacks had pulled through the stomach wall and were lying under the anterior abdominal wall. There was a 2-cm necrotic area in the anterior wall of the stomach, which was repaired. (From McFarland EG, Lee MJ, Boland GW, et al. Gastropexy breakdown and peritonitis after percutaneous gastrojejunostomy in a patient with ascites. *Am J Roentgenol.* 1995;164:189-193.)

gastrostomy over other techniques includes the ability to perform a percutaneous gastrojejunostomy at the time of initial tube placement, conversion of existing gastrostomy tubes to gastrojejunostomy tubes, and the ability to perform a gastrostomy in those patients with esophageal strictures through which an endoscope cannot pass.

Complications

Complications are described as major or minor as in the surgical literature. Minor complications include dislodged or leaking tubes and superficial wound infections requiring skin care. Major complications include wound-related problems (e.g., major infection, septicemia), aspiration, peritonitis, other gastrointestinal complications (perforation, hemorrhage), and dislodgment of the tube (Fig. 19-8) requiring a repeat procedure. From Wollman's metaanalysis of the literature, the complication rate for percutaneous gastrostomy is quite low in these categories. The complication rates are listed in Table 19-2. Additionally, complication rates in two of the largest series in the radiologic literature are also quite low. In the series by Bell and associates, a major complication rate of 1.3% was seen in a total of 519 gastrostomy procedures; the minor complication rate was 2.9% (see Table 19-1). The major complication rate included four patients with peritonitis, two with hemorrhage requiring blood transfusion, and one with external leakage of gastric contents. In a second series by Ryan and associates, a major complication rate of 1.9% was seen in 316 consecutive patients with a minor complication rate of 3.2% (see Table 19-1).

Procedure-related complications can be minimized by careful attention to detail. Prior opacification of the colon and avoiding the location of the superficial epigastric artery can help avoid colonic perforation and hemorrhage, respectively. Adequate gastric distention at all times is mandatory to avoid losing access to the stomach during the procedure. Performing a gastropexy may help decrease the incidence of guidewire buckling and dislodgement of the gastrostomy tube into the peritoneal cavity. Postprocedural complications such as tube clogging and dislodgement generally can be managed conservatively. Adequate grinding of pills and tablets before administration helps decrease the incidence of tube clogging. Clogged tubes can be opened with either high-pressure syringes, heated water, or carbonated beverages. If the tube remains clogged, often the tube can be opened up by passing a guidewire down through the tube.

If the tube becomes dislodged it is important to have the patient return to the interventional suite as soon as possible. The percutaneous track will often close over within 24-48 hours depending on the maturity of the track. If the patient comes to the interventional suite soon after catheter dislodgment, it is usually possible to regain access to the stomach using a combination of a Kumpe catheter and hydrophilic wire. A new catheter can then be placed. The referring clinician should be advised to replace the tube if it does fall out at night or over a weekend so that the percutaneous track is kept open until a new tube can be placed the following morning. The patient is not fed through the replaced tube until it is checked or replaced.

Wound infection may occur with any percutaneous procedure. Management depends on the extent. Minor edema can be treated

Box 19-4. **Avoiding Complications**

Prior colonic opacification
Regular paracentesis if ascites present
Optimal gastric distention during procedure
T-fastener gastropexy allows a more controlled procedure
Avoid superficial epigastric artery

with frequent dressing changes and wound cleansing. More significant cellulitis requires antibiotic therapy.

Leak of gastric contents around the tube is a rare phenomenon. However, when it does occur it may lead to marked skin irritation, infection, and skin breakdown. The combination of wound toilet, application of an antacid solution around the stoma, and upsizing the tube all help to control the skin irritation and breakdown. Occasionally, none of these procedures work and the tube may have to be removed, particularly if the skin breakdown is severe (Box 19-4).

■ NEW DEPARTURES IN PERCUTANEOUS GASTROSTOMY

Placement of Endoscopic Catheters

Recently, modifications of the percutaneous gastrostomy technique have been employed. Unfortunately, existing gastrostomy catheters are derived from either "abscess drainage" catheters or "Foley"-type balloon catheters. Both are associated with the long-term complications of catheter clogging or dislodgment. Consequently, some authors have embarked upon the placement of the more robust endoscopic gastrostomy tubes using a percutaneous approach. In general, the "pull" type endoscopic gastrostomy catheters are used. The stomach is punctured and a guidewire is placed in the stomach. A 5-French angiographic catheter is placed over the guidewire and used to cannulate the esophagus. The catheter and guidewire are brought out through the mouth. If the esophagus cannot be cannulated from below, a snare can be used to pull the guidewire out of the stomach, into the esophagus, and out through the mouth. The pull type endoscopic gastrostomy catheter is then pulled from the mouth down through the esophagus and out through the anterior abdominal wall. A pull type gastrostomy tube is more secure and durable, and is less likely to occlude than radiologic counterparts. Disadvantages include seeding of metastases from oropharyngeal or esophageal tumors, potential risk of infection, and the need for two operators to perform the procedure.

Primary Button Gastrostomy Placement

Button gastrostomy catheters have been widely used in the pediatric population where the low-profile nature makes them esthetically pleasing. A major disadvantage of the "button"-type catheter is the fact that a mature track of at least 3 months is advised before insertion of a gastrostomy button. The author's unit has recently embarked upon primary button gastrostomy catheter placement using a percutaneous technique.

There are two types of retaining devices used in button gastrostomy catheters. One uses a "mushroom"-retaining device (Abbott Laboratories, Abbott Park, Ill.) while the other uses a "balloon" (Cubby, Corpak, Wheeling, Ill.; and Mic-Key, Ballard Medical Products, Draper, Utah) (Fig. 19-9). We have not been able to place the mushroom-type button without having a mature track; we have placed the balloon retention gastrostomy button in more than 100 patients.

Fourteen-, 16-, or 18-French gastrostomy button catheters can be placed radiologically. The patient preparation is similar to that for standard gastrostomy catheter insertion. T-fastener gastropexy

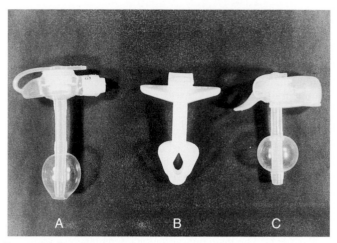

FIGURE 19-9. Image showing three different button gastrostomy catheters. **A** and **C** are examples of the balloon-retention type gastrostomy button, while **B** is a mushroom-type retention gastrostomy button. Traditionally, these buttons were placed in mature tracks; that is, tracks that were in place for at least 6 weeks. The balloon-retention type buttons can be placed de novo by percutaneous means using a gastropexy. We have not been able to place the mushroom-type button de novo. (**A,** Mic-Key gastrostomy button, Ballard Medical Products, Draper, Utah; **B,** Abbott Laboratories, Abbott Park, Ill.; **C,** Cubby button, Corpak, Wheeling, Ill.)

is mandatory for primary button gastrostomy catheter insertion. Accurate measurement of the track length is essential for button placement. When the stomach has been punctured and a superstiff guidewire placed, the track length can be measured by using an angioplasty balloon catheter, which is inflated within the stomach and pulled back until it abuts the anterior abdominal wall. The operator then holds the shaft of the catheter between the thumb and forefinger at skin level. The balloon catheter is then deflated and the balloon is withdrawn over the guidewire until it is fully visible. The balloon is then reinflated and the distance between the proximal end of the balloon and the operator's thumb and forefinger is measured to give the track length. In general, a button is chosen that is 5 mm longer than the track length measured (buttons vary in length from 2 to 5 cm). The slightly longer button accounts for changes in patient position, which may require extra adjustment of catheter length.

Alternatively, the track can be measured using the guidewire technique. The latter involves placing an angiographic catheter over the guidewire and into the stomach. Lateral screening is necessary to measure the track length using this method. The guidewire is pulled back until the end of the guidewire is flush with the anterior wall of the stomach. A kink is made in the guidewire at the catheter hub. The guidewire is then pulled back until the distal end of the guidewire is at the skin site. Another kink is made in the guidewire at the hub of the catheter. The distance between the two kinks in the guidewire equates to the track length.

The track can be dilated using either the balloon catheter or serial fascial dilators. To place a 14-French button, the track is dilated to 18 French; to place a 16-French button, the track is dilated to 20 French; to place an 18-French button, the track is dilated to 22 French. When the track is dilated, a small fascial dilator is placed through the button and loaded on the guidewire (6-French dilator for a 14-French button; 7-French dilator for a 16-French button; 8-French dilator for an 18-French button). Abundant sterile jelly is used to lubricate the button, which is then pushed through the track into the stomach. The balloon is inflated with 5 mL of saline, the guidewire is removed, and the dilator is pulled back into the button before contrast material is injected to confirm an intragastric position (Fig. 19-10). Kimberly Clark has recently produced a kit for primary button insertion containing T-fasteners with bioabsorbable sutures, a telescoping dilator, and a short balloon catheter for track measurement.

The advantages of button catheters are many, with the most significant being the avoidance of catheter clogging due to the short tube length. Also, the low-profile nature means that confused patients cannot grip the catheter sufficiently to remove it. The main disadvantage is that because it is a balloon retention device the balloon eventually bursts. On average the balloon lasts 3-6 months. The button devices can be simply replaced at the patient's bedside with a similar balloon retention button device. Alternatively, a mushroom-type button can be placed because the track is mature (Box 19-5).

PERCUTANEOUS GASTROJEJUNOSTOMY

There is some debate as to whether percutaneous gastrojejunostomy rather than a percutaneous gastrostomy should be performed in all patients. The main indication for a percutaneous gastrojejunostomy is a previous history of reflux or aspiration. In one study comparing percutaneous gastrostomy to percutaneous gastrojejunostomy, scintigraphy was used to detect gastroesophageal reflux and determine whether gastrostomy tubes caused reflux. Patients were evaluated over 2 years with scintigraphic studies immediately before and 1 week after percutaneous gastrostomy. In almost half the patients, at least one scintigraphic study was positive for reflux. No causal relationship was noted between the presence of the gastrostomy tube and reflux. This would indicate that the gastrostomy tubes per se do not appear to incite reflux. The interesting point from this study was that a large number of patients (46%) referred for percutaneous gastrostomy had evidence of reflux, supporting the theory that gastrojejunostomy tubes should be placed de novo in many patients. However, it is difficult to determine from this study whether the reflux was significant or not. Some authors do prefer to insert percutaneous gastrojejunostomy tubes de novo. The author prefers to place gastrostomy tubes initially unless there is a history of aspiration, if there is a large hiatus hernia, or if the patient's pulmonary status is such that an episode of aspiration could not be tolerated. If any of the above situations exist, a gastrojejunostomy tube is placed de novo.

Percutaneous gastrojejunostomy can be more technically challenging and tedious because the gastrostomy catheter has to be negotiated past the pylorus and duodenum into the jejunum. While this is often straightforward, it can be difficult in some patients. Additionally, a totally different feeding regimen is used for jejunal than for gastric tubes. With gastric tubes feedings are usually of the bolus variety. For nursing staff, bolus tube feedings are more convenient because less time is spent monitoring feeding. In addition, for the patient who is active, bolus feeding intrudes minimally on a patient's lifestyle. Bolus feeding cannot be used for jejunal tubes because severe diarrhea will ensue. A slower drip feeding is used for jejunal tubes, which leads to more prolonged feeding times and increased nursing care. Jejunal feeding is also more of an intrusion on the patient's lifestyle. Indeed, some nursing homes are slow to accept patients on continuous feeding as opposed to bolus feeding. For these reasons, the author's unit tends not to place percutaneous gastrojejunostomy tubes de novo. However, once the decision is made to place a percutaneous gastrojejunostomy tube, the procedure is not dissimilar to percutaneous gastrostomy tube placement.

Technique

One of the prerequisites for performing a percutaneous gastrojejunostomy tube placement is the angulation of the percutaneous track. It is vitally important to angle the track toward the pylorus to facilitate passage of a guidewire and eventual passage of the tube toward the pyloric canal. Failure to do this may result

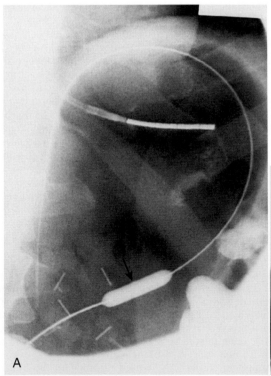
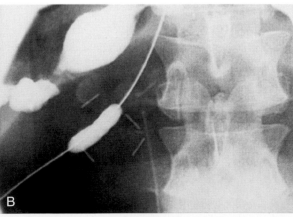

FIGURE 19-10. Gastrostomy button placement in a patient with neurologic disease. **A,** T-fastener gastropexy has been performed. A 6-mm balloon *(arrow)* was used to measure track length by inflating the balloon in the stomach and pulling it back against the stomach wall. The balloon catheter is gripped between the operator's thumb and forefinger at the skin, the balloon is deflated, removed from the stomach, and reinflated. The distance between the operator's thumb and forefinger on the shaft and the proximal end of the inflated balloon yields the rack length. **B,** The balloon catheter is then used to dilate the percutaneous track.

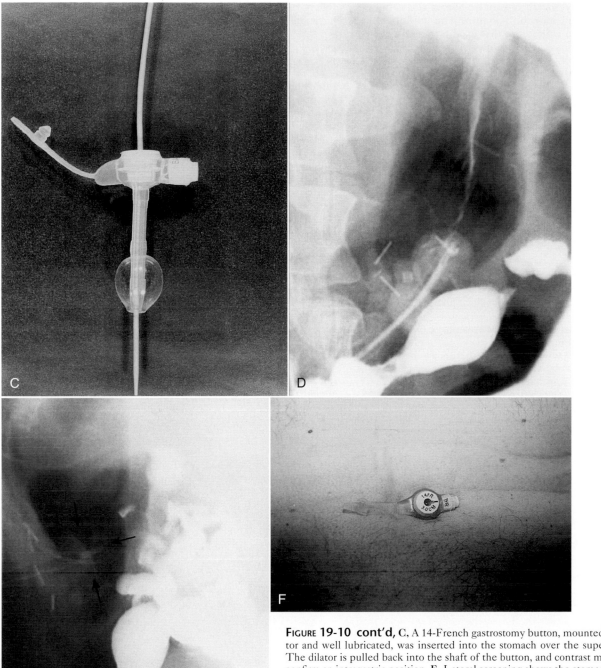

FIGURE 19-10 cont'd, C, A 14-French gastrostomy button, mounted on a 6-French dilator and well lubricated, was inserted into the stomach over the superstiff guidewire. **D,** The dilator is pulled back into the shaft of the button, and contrast material is injected to confirm an intragastric position. **E,** Lateral screening shows the stomach filled with air and the button balloon *(arrows)* present within the stomach lumen. **F,** The low-profile nature of the inserted button can be seen in this image of the patient's abdomen after removal of T-fasteners.

in catheter and guidewire buckling up into the fundus of the stomach.

The procedure followed is similar to that of percutaneous gastrostomy initially. The stomach is distended and a gastropexy performed. The needle is then inserted through the chosen point of entry into the stomach and angled toward the pylorus. At this stage a 0.035-inch J-guidewire is passed through the needle toward the pylorus. A Kumpe catheter is placed over the guidewire and the guidewire removed. A small amount

of contrast is injected through the Kumpe catheter to outline the pyloric canal, duodenal cap, and descending duodenum. A 0.035-inch hydrophilic guidewire is then used in conjunction with the Kumpe catheter to negotiate the pyloric canal and duodenum. The guidewire and Kumpe catheter are placed beyond the ligament of Treitz in the proximal jejunum, and the hydrophilic guidewire is exchanged for a 0.035-inch superstiff guidewire (Meditech, Watertown, Mass.). The track is dilated and a peel-away sheath is loaded over the guidewire down toward the pylorus. The peel-away sheath also helps direct the catheter through the pylorus and into the jejunum. The author's unit uses a similar but longer catheter to that used for percutaneous gastrostomy; it has a similar self-retaining proximal pigtail (Cook Inc., Bloomington, Ind.). When the catheter is placed, contrast is injected to confirm the jejunal location, and the peel-away sheath is removed (Fig. 19-11).

Results and Complications

Percutaneous gastrojejunostomy is associated with a high technical success rate similar to that of percutaneous gastrostomy. However, the success rate is slightly lower because of occasional technical problems in cannulating the pylorus. Bell and associates, in a large series, reported a 2.8% failure rate because of inability to catheterize the pylorus.

The complications associated with percutaneous gastrojejunostomy are similar to those reported for percutaneous gastrostomy.

> **Box 19-5. Percutaneous Gastrostomy Modifications**
>
> Standard radiologic gastrostomy tubes have poor long-term patency
> Pull-type percutaneous endoscopic gastrostomy tubes can be placed percutaneously
> Balloon retention button gastrostomy catheters can be placed de novo
> T-fastener gastropexy required for button gastrostomy

Rarely, duodenal perforation has been reported as a distinct complication of percutaneous gastrojejunostomy.

Conversion of Percutaneous Gastrostomy to Gastrojejunostomy

More and more frequently, the author's unit is asked to convert existing gastrostomy tubes to gastrojejunostomy tubes in patients who aspirate or who are not able to tolerate gastric feeding. There are a number of factors to consider before converting one of these tubes.

The first consideration is whether the existing tube was inserted radiologically, endoscopically, or surgically. The second consideration is the length of time between initial tube placement and the request for conversion. For some radiologic and endoscopic tubes, a mature track may not have had time to form between the stomach and the anterior abdominal wall. In this situation, there is a risk of disrupting the track or losing access during attempts at conversion to a percutaneous gastrojejunostomy tube. A further consideration is the size of the existing tube. Generally, surgically and endoscopically placed gastrostomy tubes may be larger than radiologically placed tubes. The catheter that is intended to be placed must be of a size that will take up most of the percutaneous track; otherwise leakage of gastric contents may be a problem.

Radiologic Gastrostomy Tube Conversion

When we place percutaneous gastrostomy tubes at our institution, we place T-fasteners and the percutaneous track is usually angled toward the pylorus to facilitate easy conversion of the

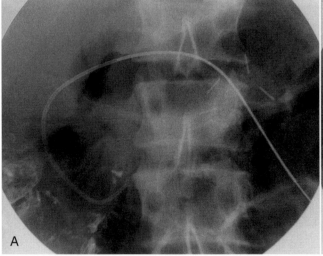
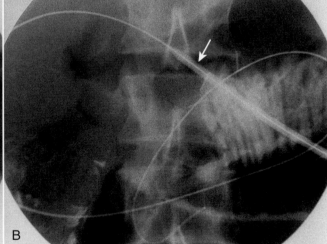
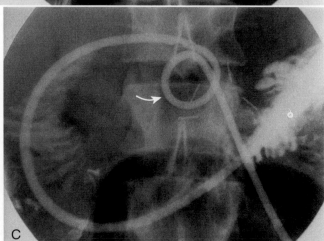

FIGURE 19-11. Placement of a percutaneous gastrojejunostomy tube in a patient with a history of reflux and aspiration. **A,** A Kumpe catheter (Cook, Bloomington, Ind.) is used to cannulate the pylorus with the aid of a 0.035- or 0.038-inch guidewire. Track angulation toward the pylorus is important to facilitate this maneuver. When the Kumpe catheter is in the jejunum, the guidewire is exchanged for a 0.038-inch superstiff guidewire (Boston Scientific, Nadick, Mass.) and the percutaneous track dilated. **B,** The gastrostomy catheter *(arrow)* is inserted through a peel away sheath over the guide wire and into the jejunum. **C,** An injection of contrast medium at the end of the procedure shows the retention loop of the catheter *(curved arrow)* in the stomach with the catheter tip in the jejunum distal to the ligament of Treitz.

gastrostomy tube to a percutaneous gastrojejunostomy tube. By using T-fasteners, even if the track is immature, the conversion can still be performed because access to the stomach is not lost.

Endoscopic Gastrostomy Tube Conversion

Most PEG tubes have inner bumpers designed to hold the tube in place. It is not usually possible to pull these bumpers through the percutaneous track. One may cut the endoscopic tube flush with the skin and allow the inner portion with the bumper to fall into the stomach. Alternatively, the PEG tube can be left in situ and a new percutaneous gastrojejunostomy tube inserted through a new track. The author prefers to cut the PEG tube at the skin and allow the inner bumper to fall into the stomach. One of the downsides in using this approach is that occasionally the inner bumper may cause symptoms of gastrointestinal obstruction. In the author's experience this happens rarely, but this complication has been reported in the literature. Another problem with use of PEG tubes is that the percutaneous track is often angled toward the fundus of the stomach, making it difficult to redirect the track toward the antrum. The use of a large 15- or 16-French peel-away sheath and dilator has been helpful in this regard (Fig. 19-12). Over a wire placed in the stomach, the 16-French peel-away sheath is placed and the track angled toward the antrum by applying pressure to the peel-away sheath. The guidewire is then redirected toward the pyloric antrum. Once this is done, the dilator is removed, leaving the peel-away sheath and guidewire in situ. A Kumpe catheter and glidewire are then used to negotiate the pyloric canal, and the

procedure is then performed in a similar fashion to percutaneous gastrojejunostomy.

Surgical Conversion to Percutaneous Gastrojejunostomy

The success of surgical gastrostomy conversion to percutaneous gastrojejunostomy depends on the type of surgical procedure used to place the gastrostomy tube. The common procedure is the Stamm procedure in which, through a laparotomy incision, a portion of the midgastric body is opened and a Malecot or Foley-type catheter is placed. Concentric pursestring sutures are placed around the catheter and tightened around the gastrostomy tube. The tube is then delivered externally through a separate stab incision in the anterior abdominal wall. The stomach is pulled up to the anterior abdominal wall and sutured to it with a number of interrupted sutures. The other technique described is that of a Witzel gastrostomy. In this procedure a long subcutaneous tunnel is fashioned around the external portion of the tube. This tunnel is directed toward the fundus of the stomach. In the author's experience, if a Witzel gastrostomy has been performed, it is virtually impossible to convert to a percutaneous gastrojejunostomy. In this situation, it is best to start de novo and perform a separate percutaneous gastrojejunostomy.

It is usually possible to convert surgical gastrostomy tubes to percutaneous gastrojejunostomy tubes if the Stamm technique has been used. Again, similar to PEG tube conversion, a

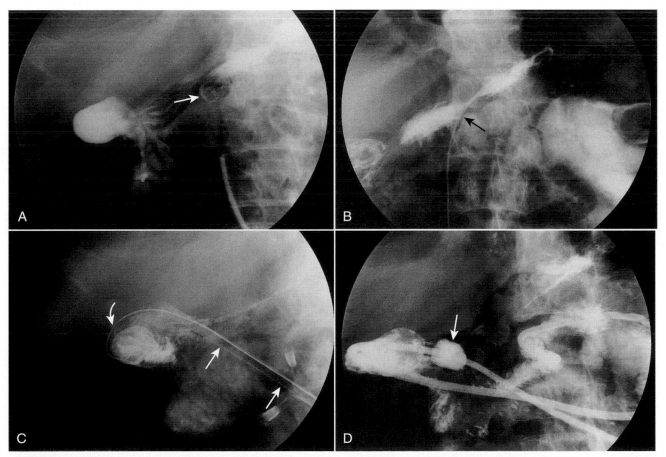

FIGURE 19-12. Conversion of an endoscopically placed gastrostomy tube to a gastrojejunostomy tube. **A,** Contrast injection through the endoscopically placed gastrostomy tube shows the tube and balloon retention device *(arrow)* present within the stomach lumen. **B,** The tube was removed and a Kumpe catheter inserted into the stomach. Note the track angulation *(arrow)* toward the fundus of the stomach. **C,** A 16-French peel-away sheath *(straight arrows)* was placed into the stomach and used to redirect the percutaneous tract toward the pylorus. A Kumpe catheter *(curved arrow)* was used to cannulate the pylorus and a 0.038-inch superstiff guidewire was manipulated into the proximal jejunum. **D,** A gastrojejunostomy catheter was placed through the peel-away sheath with the tip placed into the proximal jejunum. Note the balloon retention device *(arrow)* on this catheter.

16-French sheath is used to reangle the track toward the antrum. When this is done the gastrojejunostomy tube is placed as with the PEG conversion (Box 19-6).

Results

In a study of 63 patients by Lu and associates, conversion of surgical gastrostomy to percutaneous gastrojejunostomy was successful in 83%. The success rate for conversion of PEG tubes to percutaneous gastrojejunostomy tubes was slightly lower at 78%, while conversion of percutaneous gastrostomy tubes to percutaneous gastrojejunostomy tubes had a success rate of 100%. Failures with surgical tubes and PEG tubes were related to the inability to redirect the percutaneous track toward the pyloric antrum. Recoil of the guidewire into the fundus of the stomach invariably occurred in these patients and pyloric cannulation was not possible. In these patients a de novo percutaneous gastrojejunostomy tube had to be placed. The 100% success rate for conversion of percutaneous gastrostomy tubes to percutaneous gastrojejunostomy tubes reflects the fact that T-fasteners are used at the author's institution and that the percutaneous track is angled toward the pylorus on initially placing gastrostomy tubes.

▬ COMPARISON OF PERCUTANEOUS, ENDOSCOPIC, AND SURGICAL GASTROSTOMY

Percutaneous gastrostomy performed radiologically has the lowest rate of major complications as well as the lowest procedural mortality when compared with PEG and surgical gastrostomy. However, it has been estimated that percutaneous gastrostomy accounts for 35% of all gastrostomies in academic institutions, decreasing to 18% in community practices. This is partially due to the fact that percutaneous gastrostomy was described after the PEG technique, but it also reflects the lack of access to patients by interventional radiologists.

In a metaanalysis of 5752 patients (837 percutaneous gastrostomy procedures, 4194 PEG procedures, and 721 surgical procedures), significant differences in rates of successful tube placement between PEG and percutaneous gastrostomy techniques were seen (95% vs 99.2%, $P < 0.01$). A smaller difference was seen between percutaneous gastrostomy and surgical gastrostomy. Significant differences ($P < 0.01$) in the procedural mortality rate between all three techniques were also seen, with percutaneous gastrostomy having the lowest procedural mortality rate (percutaneous gastrostomy, 0.3%; PEG, 0.53%; surgical gastrostomy, 2.5%). The 30-day mortality rate was similar for all three gastrostomy techniques and ranged from 7% to 14%. This reflects the underlying debility of many of these patients referred for gastrostomy procedures rather than the efficacy of the procedure itself. Major complications occurred less frequently after percutaneous gastrostomy (5.9%) than in PEG (9.4%) and surgical gastrostomy (19.9%).

Other points to consider are that PEG offers diagnostic capabilities that are not available with percutaneous gastrostomy. In other words, the stomach can be inspected endoscopically during the PEG procedure and abnormalities recorded and/or treated. The rate of abnormal findings seen during PEG procedures has varied from 10% to 70.1% in the literature. The most common are inflammation or ulceration of varying degrees of severity. However, almost none of the abnormalities are as serious as an unexpected cancer.

It seems that percutaneous gastrostomy and PEG are both viable, minimally invasive techniques for performing gastrostomy and both should be preferred over surgical gastrostomy. They are both quick and easy to perform and associated with fewer complications than surgical gastrostomy. However, percutaneous gastrostomy is associated with significantly fewer major complications, lower rates of tube complications, and slightly higher rates of successful tube placement. The advantage of percutaneous gastrostomy over other techniques includes the ability to perform gastrojejunostomy at the time of initial tube placement, conversion of existing gastrostomy tubes to gastrojejunostomy tubes, and the ability to perform gastrostomy in those patients who are unsuitable for PEG tube placement (Box 19-7).

▬ DIRECT PERCUTANEOUS JEJUNOSTOMY

Direct percutaneous jejunostomy is infrequently performed but has some well-recognized indications. The most common indication is when gastrojejunostomy tube conversion is not appropriate or has failed in a patient who is aspirating. A unique indication for direct percutaneous jejunostomy is the replacement of a prematurely dislodged surgical jejunostomy tube.

Technique

Direct percutaneous jejunostomy can be performed under fluoroscopic or CT guidance. Hallisey and Pollard reported on the first large series of patients. In their technique, a jejunal loop in the left upper quadrant is identified by air insufflation through a nasogastric tube. A direct puncture of the distended loop is then performed with a 17-gauge needle under fluoroscopic guidance. Contrast material is injected once the needle is in position, and when intraluminal position is confirmed a 0.035-inch hydrophilic guidewire is introduced along with a 5-French hydrophilic catheter. An anchoring procedure with Cope sutures or T-fasteners is then performed to hold the jejunum up to the anterior abdominal wall. Dilatation of the tract is performed followed by placement of a 14-French locking pigtail catheter.

Ultrasound or CT guidance can also be used for jejunal catheter placement. Using ultrasound or CT, a safe path to a proximal jejunal loop can be chosen and in particular the colon can be avoided. Additionally, it is important not to traverse more than one jejunal loop. The author tends to place a 0.018-inch wire in the jejunal loop after first puncturing the jejunal loop with a 22-gauge needle. The patient is then transferred to fluoroscopy and T-fasteners are inserted followed by tract dilatation and tube placement.

Results and Complications

The total number of patients in whom direct percutaneous jejunostomy has been performed is small and the reported technical success rates have varied from 60% to 100%. In a recent study of 51 patients, Hu and colleagues had a 100% technical success rate using the single anchor technique. Complications are similar to those described for percutaneous gastrostomy.

▬ PERCUTANEOUS CECOSTOMY

Cecostomy has been a standard surgical technique since 1710 when it was first described. It is usually performed through an open surgical procedure but more recently it has been performed laparoscopically. Percutaneous cecostomy is a novel alternative to the surgical technique. The method used is similar to that for percutaneous gastrostomy. Percutaneous cecostomy can be performed under local anesthesia and intravenous sedoanalgesia as opposed to the surgical technique which is usually performed under general anesthesia.

Indications

Cecal dilatation of greater than 10 cm is associated with a significant risk of perforation. If perforation occurs, there is an associated mortality of up to 50%. Therefore, it is prudent to decompress the at-risk cecum quickly and effectively. The main indication for colonic decompression is colonic pseudo-obstruction or the so-called Ogilvie's syndrome. Colonoscopic decompression has been used for this condition and can be successful in up to 70% of cases. However, patients who do not respond to colonoscopic decompression will require cecostomy. Other indications for percutaneous cecostomy include cecal dilatation proximal to a distal large bowel obstruction and cecal volvulus.

Before a percutaneous cecostomy is planned, it is important to make sure that there is no evidence of bowel necrosis or perforation. If there are clinical signs of perforation or bowel necrosis, then surgical exploration and appropriate surgical therapy is warranted.

Technique

Access Route

The author's unit uses an anterior transabdominal approach to the cecum. This is an intraperitoneal approach, as might be expected. An extraperitoneal approach has been described, which involves using a posterior access route and CT guidance. The potential advantage of this approach is that any leak is extraperitoneal. However, the right peritoneal reflection often extends in a deep posteromedial direction behind the cecum, which leaves only a small portion of the cecum that is extraperitoneal. It can be difficult to be sure that a catheter inserted from a posterior approach is in fact extraperitoneal. For this reason and because the anterior approach is more straightforward, the anterior approach is preferred.

Cecopexy

The author uses T-fasteners to perform a cecopexy that fixes the anterior wall of the cecum to the anterior abdominal wall and helps prevent leakage into the peritoneal cavity. This is an important part of percutaneous cecostomy and, even though it may be optional for the percutaneous gastrostomy technique, it should be performed during percutaneous cecostomy. The patient is placed in a supine position on the table and the midpoint of the distended cecum is chosen as the needle entry site. T-fasteners are inserted at the corners of a 2-cm square around the needle entry site as previously described for percutaneous gastrostomy.

When the T-fasteners are in situ, they are fixed with gentle traction on the suture (Fig. 19-13).

Cecostomy Catheter Insertion

Using a 14- to 16-French gastrostomy catheter (Cook, Bloomington, Ind.), the cecum is punctured at the needle entry site with the slotted needle used for T-fastener insertion. A 0.038-inch superstiff wire is inserted into the cecum and manipulated up the ascending colon. The percutaneous track is dilated with serial fascial dilators and a 14- to 16-French gastrostomy catheter is placed through a peel-away sheath (see Fig. 19-13).

Aftercare

The catheter is left to gravity drainage and attached to a bag. Frequent flushing with 50-100 mL of normal saline every 2-4 hours helps break down solid fecal material and prevent catheter blockage. Cecostomy catheters require close supervision from the interventional radiology team and daily rounds are required to detect any catheter malfunction, pericatheter leakage, or intraperitoneal leak (Box 19-8).

Results

Limited numbers of percutaneous cecostomy procedures have been reported with good technical success. Chait and colleagues recently reported a 100% technical success in 163 patients with an 89% response rate in children with fecal incontinence. The main indication for cecostomy was Ogilvie's syndrome. In all cases, the catheters have functioned well with good cecal decompression. Catheters have remained in situ for between 24 hours and 1 month. Most authors have used fluoroscopy for guidance, with occasional use of CT. One author used no imaging guidance, which is not recommended (Table 19-3).

Complications

Complications reported in the literature are few and include one patient with a pericatheter leak of fecal material, another patient with a septicemia postprocedure, and a third patient with abdominal wall sepsis. In this latter patient, multiloculated abscesses formed in the anterior abdominal wall due to fecal contamination along the catheter track. This patient eventually died of sepsis and multiorgan failure. Potential complications are many and include catheter dysfunction, pericatheter leakage, fecal peritonitis, sepsis, and cecal trauma during the procedure (see Table 19-3). With close attention to detail, many of these complications can be minimized. The use of T-fasteners should theoretically help prevent fecal peritonitis and pericatheter leakage. Placement of large-bore catheters (>12-French) and frequent irrigation with normal saline should reduce the incidence of catheter blockage.

Overall percutaneous cecostomy is an effective method for decompression of the cecum and is associated with a low complication rate as long as close attention is paid to technique.

▬ RADIOLOGIC MANAGEMENT OF GASTROINTESTINAL TRACT STRICTURES

Benign Gastrointestinal Strictures

Strictures of the gastrointestinal tract have traditionally been treated by surgical techniques that have been associated with unacceptably high morbidity and mortality. More recently, endoscopic and interventional radiologic procedures are rapidly becoming accepted as an effective method for dealing with this frustrating clinical problem. Esophageal stenoses are the most

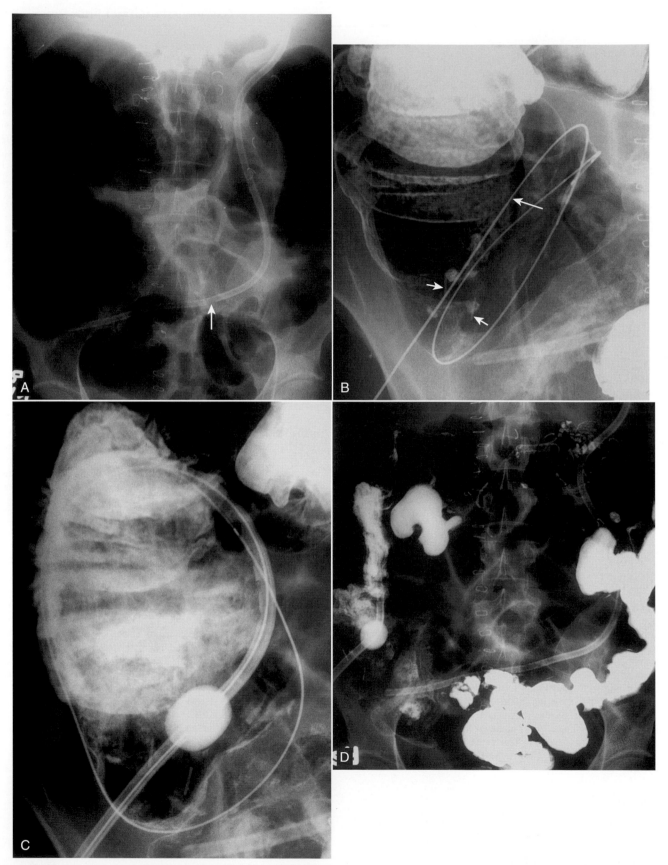

FIGURE 19-13. Percutaneous cecostomy in a patient with ovarian cancer and encasement of the sigmoid colon causing colonic obstruction. The patient was debilitated and a poor surgical risk. **A,** Plain film of the abdomen shows considerable colonic distention with the cecum measuring 15 cm. One staple line is noted on the anterior abdominal wall and a long nasogastric decompression tube *(arrow)* is noted within the small bowel. However, this did not decompress the colon. **B,** Using an anterior approach, two T-fasteners *(small arrows)* were placed into the cecum, the T-fastener needle was used to puncture the cecum, and a 0.038-inch Ring guidewire was placed *(large arrow)*. **C,** A 14-French gastrostomy catheter with retention balloon was then placed into the cecum through a peel-away sheath. **D,** Plain film of the abdomen obtained 2 days later shows decompression of the colon from the cecostomy tube. Regular irrigation with 50 mL of saline was performed every 4-6 hours to facilitate drainage of cecal contents. After a week of cecostomy tube drainage, the patient returned to theater for a colostomy.

common strictures that present for treatment. However, gastric, duodenal, and colorectal strictures may also be amenable to balloon dilatation.

Balloon Dilatation of Esophageal Strictures

Bougienage has been performed for centuries for esophageal stricture dilatation. This involves the use of an instrument with a round, oval tip, which is inserted through the stricture and progressively stretches the stricture to achieve the desired lumen. This procedure is now performed endoscopically and most of the bougies used can now be passed over a guidewire. These devices have one major disadvantage compared with balloon dilatation: They produce significant longitudinal shear forces on the stricture and on the normal esophagus (Fig. 19-14). These shear forces can lead to perforation or mucosal tears. On the other hand, balloon dilatation, which involves passing a small balloon catheter over a guidewire, produces radial stretch forces only without any element of longitudinal shear. Theoretically, this should decrease the risk of mucosal tear or perforation.

Technique

If a recent barium swallow study is not available, then a barium swallow study should be performed to assess the size and location of the stricture. The author's unit generally performs this on the day before the procedure. On the day of the procedure, the patient is placed in a decubitus position and a mouthpiece placed in the mouth. A transoral route is preferred for this procedure. A topical anesthetic spray is applied to the back of the throat to reduce the gag reflex. We then use a 5-French angiographic catheter and a hydrophilic guidewire to enter the esophagus under fluoroscopic control. The guidewire and catheter are manipulated down to a level just above the stricture. A small amount of contrast is injected at this stage to outline the proximal end of the stricture. The guidewire and catheter are then manipulated through the stricture and down into the stomach. The guidewire is then changed for an exchange length stiff wire (180 or 260 cm).

Depending on the stricture, start with a 10- or 12-mm diameter balloon. The goal is a luminal diameter of 20 mm. However, it is prudent to start with a smaller balloon and, if this is well tolerated, then a 15-mm diameter balloon followed by a 20-mm diameter balloon can be used. However, if the patient experiences

significant discomfort with a 10- or 12-mm balloon, the session is terminated for that day. The balloon is left inflated for 1-2 minutes until the waist disappears (Fig. 19-15).

The author's unit does not do an immediate esophagogram after the procedure but prefers to wait for 6-12 hours. If the patient experiences significant pain during the procedure, we inject some non-ionic contrast material to make sure there is no mucosal tear or frank perforation. Otherwise the patient returns to the ward and is kept fasting until the esophagogram is performed 4-6 hours later. If the esophagogram is performed immediately after dilatation, the stricture often appears similar to the predilatation stricture. This is because of acute muscular spasm induced by the dilatation. A technical success rate of 90%-95% should be expected with appropriate dilatation. Approximately 70% of patients remain asymptomatic for 2 years following dilatation.

Some authors have developed retrievable metallic stents particularly for use in patients with benign strictures. The stents have hooks at the proximal end which can be grasped using an

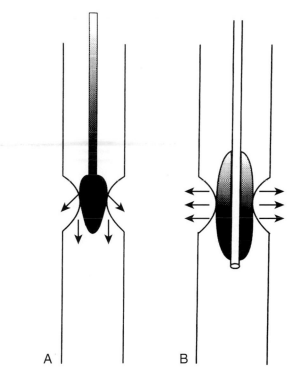

FIGURE 19-14. Schematic showing the difference between a bougie dilatation and balloon dilatation. **A,** Bougie dilatation produces longitudinal sheer stress as shown by the arrows. This is more likely to perforate the esophagus. **B,** Balloon dilatation on the other hand produces radial forces, which are less likely to perforate the esophagus.

Box 19-8. Percutaneous Cecostomy: Key Points

Do not perform if signs of bowel ischemia/perforation
Anterior transabdominal approach and fluoroscopic guidance
T-fastener cecopexy mandatory
14- to 16-French catheter placed
Frequent catheter irrigation with 50-100 mL of saline
Close catheter supervision mandatory

TABLE 19-3 Literature Experience with Percutaneous Cecostomy

First Author	Year	Patients	Indication	Guidance Modality	Approach	Major Complications (Number)
VanSonnenberg	1990	5	Ogilvie's	CT	IP	1
Morrison	1990	2	Miscellaneous	Fl	IP	0
Salim	1991	28	Distal bowel obstruction	Fl	IP	0
Chait	2003	163	Fecal incontinence	Fl	IP	8
Sierre	2007	21	Fecal incontinence	Fl	IP	0

CT, Computed tomography; Fl, fluoroscopy; IP, intraperitoneal.

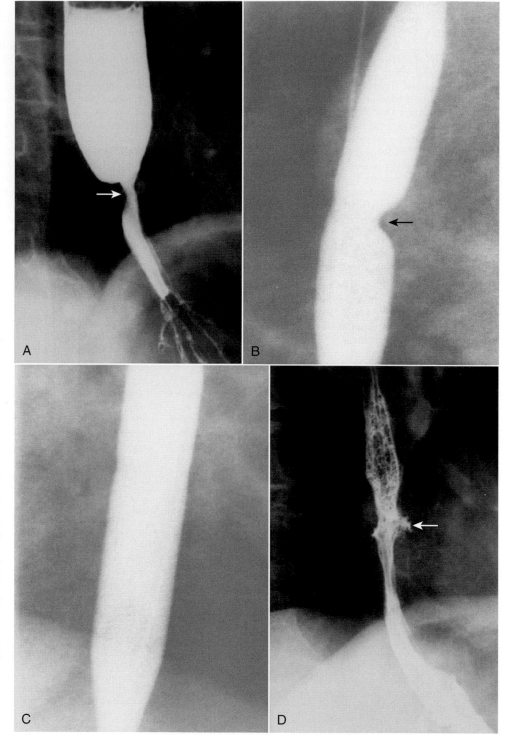

FIGURE 19-15. Patient with a recurrent benign esophageal reflux stricture referred for balloon dilatation. **A,** Esophagogram performed before the procedure shows a tight stricture *(arrow)* in the distal esophagus. **B,** The stricture was negotiated with a 5-French angiographic catheter and guidewire. Initially, 12- and 15-mm balloons were used to dilate the stricture. Minimal effect was noted. A 20-mm balloon was placed and a waist *(arrow)* was clearly seen on the balloon. **C,** The balloon was inflated until the waist had disappeared and the balloon remained inflated for 2 minutes. **D,** Esophagogram the following day shows a good result with decompression of the esophagus. There was a little intramural tear and contrast present in the esophageal wall *(arrow)*. The patient was asymptomatic and remained fasting for a further 2 days, at which time the small intramural tear had healed.

endoscope and the stent removed. In general, the stent can be removed only within 3 months after insertion. These stent designs may have a limited role to play in patients with benign esophageal strictures in whom recurring problems are common (Box 19-9).

Gastric and Duodenal Strictures
Strictures of the gastric antrum, pylorus, and duodenum can also be dilated. Twenty- to 30-mm balloons are usually necessary for successful dilatation in these locations. The balloon used in the author's unit is the Rigiflex balloon (Boston Scientific, Natick, Mass.). These strictures are often more technically challenging than esophageal strictures. The stomach may be distended and

---

Box 19-9. Benign Esophageal Stricture Dilatation

Esophagogram before procedure
Start with 10- to 12-mm balloon
Eventual goal is 20-mm balloon
Keep fasting after procedure
Esophagogram next morning
Metal stents—caution!

filled with food, making negotiation of the stricture difficult. Although a long 5-French angiographic catheter can be tried initially, it may be necessary to use stiffer catheters such as those used for duodenal intubation.

Colorectal Strictures

The vast majority of colorectal strictures are anastomotic strictures after colorectal surgery. A limited barium enema is necessary beforehand to identify the location of the stricture. This is best done on the day before stricture dilatation. For stricture dilatation, the patient is placed in the decubitus position and a Kumpe catheter and hydrophilic guidewire used to traverse the stricture. The hydrophilic guidewire is exchanged for a 0.035-inch superstiff guidewire, which is placed proximally in the sigmoid colon. Dilatation is performed with a 20- or 30-mm Rigiflex balloon (Boston Scientific, Natick, Mass.). The balloon is inflated until the waist disappears and is left inflated for 2-3 minutes (Fig. 19-16). At the end of the procedure a plain film of the abdomen is obtained to rule out any free air. A limited Gastrografin enema is performed 4-6 hours after the procedure. If there is no mucosal tear or perforation, the patient can go home.

Malignant Gastrointestinal Strictures (Metallic Stent Placement)

Esophageal Carcinoma

Most patients with malignant esophageal strictures have locally advanced or metastatic disease that is often incurable. The object of palliation is to restore oral feeding and improve the quality of life for the patient. Rigid plastic endoprostheses have been used in the past but are difficult to insert and are associated with a high complication rate (Fig. 19-17). Complications are associated with rigid plastic endoprosthesis in 36% of patients, with esophageal perforation (5%-11%), tube dislodgment (11%-15%), hemorrhage (1%-5%), pressure necrosis (1%-3%), and aspiration pneumonia being the most common. In published series, the procedural mortality rate is 2%-4%, but in one study the rate was as high as 16%. Similarly, laser therapy has been used and offers effective palliation, but the palliation is usually short-lived and it has to be repeated every 4-6 weeks. Also, it is a high-cost procedure. Self-expanding metal stents have recently emerged as an attractive alternative for palliating patients with esophageal carcinoma.

Metal Stent Types and Design

Current esophageal stent designs have changed considerably from earlier stainless steel uncovered varieties. Many different dedicated stent designs are now on the market. Almost all are totally covered or partially covered stents made from nitinol or similar flexible material. They come in various lengths and may have antireflux valves (Dostent, MI Tech, Korea; Gianturco-Rosch Z-Stent, Cook, Denmark; FerX-ella stent, Ella CS, Czech Republic) or retrievable design for endoscopic removal (Choo stent, MI Tech, Korea; Song stent, Sooho Medical, Korea; FerX-ella, Ella CS, Czech Republic) (Fig. 19-18). Other stent types include the Ultraflex stent and Wallflex stents (Boston Scientific, Galway, Ireland), EsophaCoil (IntraTherapeutic, St. Paul, Minn.) and the Memotherm (Bard, Covington, Ga.). A new plastic stent made of silicone with an encapsulated monofilament braid of polyester (Boston Scientific, Ireland) is now available. This stent is retrievable and flexible, producing less radial force than metal stents (Fig. 19-19).

The stent to use is an individual choice but there are some broad guidelines to be remembered. In the past, uncovered stents were used at the GE junction because of the migration risk with covered stents. Now, however, most covered stents have the covering on the inside and have flared proximal, distal, or proximal and distal ends to prevent migration. Stents with antireflux valves can be considered for use at the gastroesophageal junction. We tend to use the Choo stent or Do stent for the latter indication.

Covered stents should always be used for patients with esophageal fistulas. Care must be taken in choosing a stent for patients with benign esophageal strictures. The retrievable metal stents such as the Song, Choo, and FerX-Ella can be used or, alternatively, the Polyflex plastic stent can be used. The Polyflex or Ultraflex stents are also recommended for the upper esophagus to decrease the pain associated with the stiffer metal stents in this area.

Technique

Like for esophageal stricture dilatation, a barium swallow should be obtained before the procedure to document the location and length of the stricture. The patient is sedated and placed in the decubitus position with an oral mouthpiece. The author uses a 5-French angiographic catheter and hydrophilic guidewire to access the esophagus after first anesthetizing the oropharynx with a local anesthetic spray. The catheter is manipulated into the esophagus under screening control and brought to a level just above the stricture (Fig. 19-20). A small amount of contrast is injected to outline the stricture and the guidewire and catheter are then manipulated through the stricture. The hydrophilic wire is then replaced with an exchange length 0.035- or 0.038-inch superstiff wire. The stent is then ready to be placed.

The stent is loaded on to the guidewire and inserted down through the stricture. The stent is placed so that there is sufficient overlap above and below the stricture. The delivery mechanism is simple in that the stent is covered by a sheath on the distal end of the delivery catheter. The stent can be released by pulling back the sheath on the delivery catheter outside the patient. The stent delivers from distal to proximal and the stent can be recaptured up to a point where as much as 50% of the stent has been deployed. In some cases, if the esophageal stricture is very tight, it may be necessary to dilate the stricture beforehand. Once the stent is released, the delivery system is removed and the stent dilated in place with a 12- or 15-mm balloon. An esophagogram is performed the following day to assess stent location and the level of dilatation. The patient remains on a sloppy diet for 1-2 weeks after stent placement, after which solid food is gradually introduced.

Gastroesophageal Junction Strictures

Palliation of strictures at the gastroesophageal junction deserves special mention. Because this proportion of the stent has to be placed in the stomach, and is therefore not in contact with the esophageal wall, there is a high propensity for stents in this region to migrate. It is therefore vitally important to choose an appropriate stent. Initially the author's unit used uncovered Wallstents in this location because the covered variety was prone to migrate. More recently, we have begun to use the conical wall stent (Flamingo) with good results (Fig. 19-21). When performing the procedure it is important to coil the super-stiff guidewire in the stomach. The stomach is often collapsed, and injection of air through the initial 5-French angiographic catheter is helpful to distend the stomach so that the guidewire can be coiled into the stomach. The conical stent is placed such that the minimum amount of stent necessary to cover the stricture is placed in the stomach. The larger the length of stent in the fundus of the stomach, the more likely the stent is to migrate.

Malignant Tracheoesophageal Fistulas

Malignant fistulas occurring between the esophagus and the trachea or main bronchi are a devastating complication of esophageal malignancy. Patients are often unable to swallow their own saliva without aspirating. Without treatment most patients die within a month because of malnutrition or thoracic sepsis.

Perforation of the esophagus may also occur in the treatment of patients with esophageal carcinoma. It occurs in approximately 4%-6% of patients during laser treatment and in 5%-8% treated with plastic endoprostheses. Again, perforation may lead

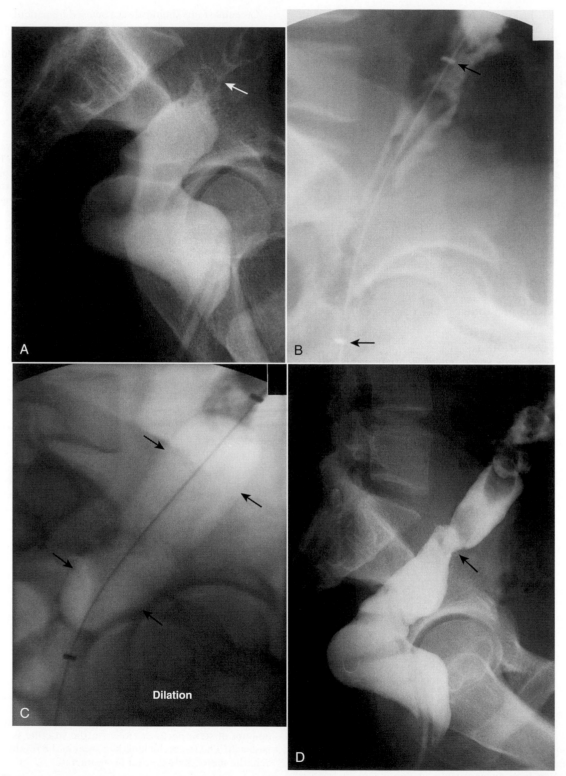

FIGURE 19-16. Anastomotic rectosigmoid stricture dilatation in a patient who underwent a sigmoid resection for diverticulitis complicated by the development of a stricture at the anastomosis. **A,** The patient presented with constipation and partial colonic obstruction and had a barium enema performed. The barium enema showed a tight stricture *(arrow)* at the rectosigmoid anastomosis. **B,** Using a combination of midazolam and fentanyl for sedoanalgesia, a balloon dilatation was performed. The stricture was negotiated using a Kumpe catheter and a 0.035-inch guidewire. The guidewire was exchanged for a 0.035-inch superstiff wire and a 30-mm Rigiflex balloon placed across the stricture *(arrows)*. **C,** The 30-mm Rigiflex balloon was dilated with air *(arrows)* and remained inflated for 2 minutes. It is important to use air to dilate the balloon as contrast or fluid cannot be aspirated fully from the balloon so that balloon decompression is difficult. **D,** Gastrografin enema performed the following day shows a good result at the anastomosis *(arrow)*. The patient has been asymptomatic for 10 years since balloon dilatation.

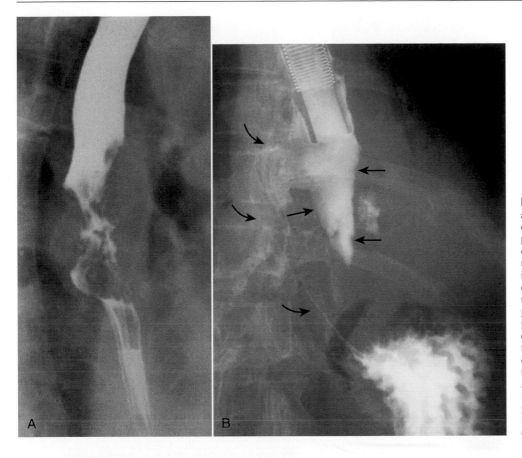

FIGURE 19-17. Esophageal perforation associated with insertion of a rigid plastic endoprosthesis. **A,** The 34-year-old patient with breast cancer presented with dysphagia secondary to esophageal wall metastases. Barium swallow shows an irregular stricture in the mid to lower esophagus. **B,** The patient was brought to the operating theater and, with the patient under general anesthesia, a rigid plastic endoprosthesis was placed. This caused a perforation *(straight arrows)* in the esophagus. Note the distal end of the endoprosthesis is actually lying outside the esophageal lumen *(curved arrows).* Associated collapse of the left lower lobe is seen. The tube was removed and the patient was managed conservatively for a number of weeks but eventually an esophagectomy was performed.

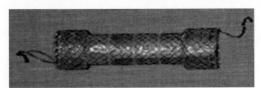

FIGURE 19-18. The Choo stent (MI Tech, Korea). Note the flared distal and proximal ends to prevent migration and the proximal string for endoscopic retrieval if necessary. (From Laasch H-U, Martin DF. Antireflux stents. *Tech Gastrointest Endosc.* 2010;12:216-224.)

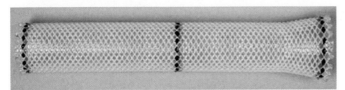

FIGURE 19-19. The Polyflex stent (Boston Scientific, Natick, Mass.). The completely covered Polyflex stent is a silicone device with an encapsulated monofilament braid made of polyester. This material has been suggested to reduce nontumoral tissue overgrowth, which is commonly seen with metal stents, particularly in patients surviving 20 weeks or longer. Radiopaque markers are seen at both ends of the stents. (From Repici A, Rando G. Expandable stents for malignant dysphagia. *Tech Gastrointest Endosc.* 2008;10:175-183.)

to mediastinal abscess, which has a high mortality, and survival is short without appropriate treatment. A number of reports in the literature have indicated that placement of covered metallic endoprostheses is a highly effective means of treating these patients (Fig. 19-22). Success rates vary from 90% to 100% in excluding the fistula or perforation. It is important to place the covered portion of the stent over the perforation or fistulous site.

An esophagogram is performed the next day and, if there is any persistent evidence of perforation or fistula, a second overlapping stent is placed. It is not advisable to place a stent above the upper esophageal sphincter because it causes pain and inability to swallow saliva. It may then be necessary to place a covered metal stent in the trachea. This is usually done as a joint procedure with the respiratory physician (Box 19-10).

Results

The first report of successful treatment of a malignant esophageal stricture with a metal stent was made by Domschke and associates in 1990. Since then, there have been many studies in variable numbers of patients describing the placement of covered and uncovered metallic stents of different designs. Overall success rates vary from 90% to 100%, and experience at the author's institution reflects that of the literature in that it is a safe procedure that can be simply performed under fluoroscopic guidance without the need for endoscopic control. For appropriately placed stents, there is almost always an improvement in the patient's dysphagia. Results are listed in Table 19-4. Comparison of metallic endoprosthesis with other therapies for palliation of malignant esophageal strictures shows that metallic endoprostheses deserve to be the first-choice treatment in palliation of patients with inoperable malignant esophageal strictures. Although similar dysphagia scores have been achieved in a comparative study between plastic and metallic stents, the use of plastic stents is associated with a much greater morbidity and mortality than that associated with metallic stents.

In yet a further study comparing palliation with metallic stents versus palliation with laser therapy, laser therapy was associated with an unsatisfactory level of dysphagia relief compared with metallic endoprostheses. In addition, laser therapy was associated with perforation rates of 6%-9%.

In patients with malignant esophageal fistulas or perforations, insertion of covered metallic endoprostheses is associated with

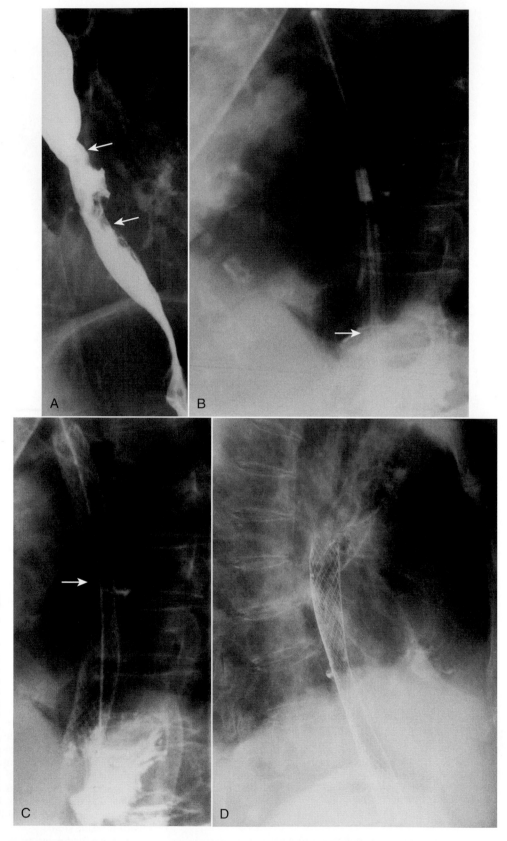

FIGURE 19-20. Metal stent placement in a patient with squamous cell cancer of the esophagus and considerable dysphagia. The patient was unfit for surgery. **A,** Barium swallow obtained before esophageal stent insertion shows an irregular, ulcerated stricture *(arrows)* in the distal esophagus. **B,** After manipulating a wire down through the stricture, a conventional covered Wallstent was placed. The distal end of the stent is partially deployed *(arrow)* and can be seen springing away from the distal end of the catheter. **C,** After full deployment, a slight waist *(arrow)* is noted in the region of the stricture. This was dilated with a 15-mm balloon. **D,** Lateral chest x-ray radiograph obtained 2 months later shows the stent in good position and the patient was eating a normal diet at this time.

a success rate of more than 95%. In one of the largest studies reported of 39 patients with esophageal respiratory fistulas or perforations, covered Wallstents were used in 36 patients and covered Gianturco stents in three. Nineteen perforations and 18 of 20 fistulas were successfully closed, leading to a success rate of 95%. In three patients, fistulas recurred and were treated with an additional esophageal stent in one patient and tracheal stents in two patients. The other advantage of using metallic endoprostheses for treating these patients is that the dysphagia as well as the fistula is treated by the placement of the covered metallic stent. The author prefers to use covered Wallstents for the treatment of patients with esophageal respiratory fistulas but covered Gianturco stents can

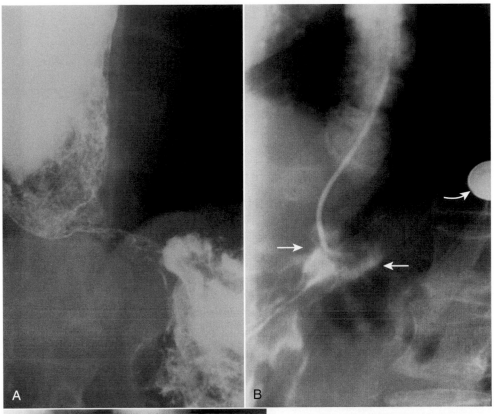

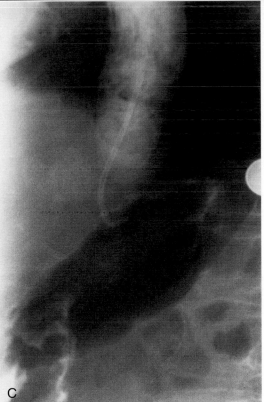

FIGURE 19-21. Patient with adenocarcinoma of the esophagus and marked dysphagia who required stenting before undergoing neoadjuvant radiotherapy and chemotherapy before esophageal resection. **A,** Barium swallow shows a tight stricture at the gastroesophageal junction with marked dilatation of the proximal esophagus. **B,** A 5-French angiographic catheter and 0.035-inch guidewire were used to negotiate the stricture and gain purchase in the stomach. Note that the fundus of the stomach *(straight arrows)* is collapsed, making coiling of a guidewire in the fundus of the stomach impossible. A coin *(curved arrow)* taped to the patient's skin marks the position of the stricture. **C,** The stomach was inflated with air through the 5-French angiographic catheter to facilitate coiling of a guidewire in the stomach for better purchase.

FIGURE 19-21. cont'd, D, A 0.038-inch superstiff guidewire is inserted for stent deployment. **E,** A 24/16-mm conical Wall-stent was placed across the stricture as shown. Note the waist in the region of the stricture. This was dilated using a 15-mm balloon. The patient was started on 20 mg of omeprazole daily. The patient underwent esophageal resection after neoadjuvant therapy and the stent was removed at the same time as the esophagus.

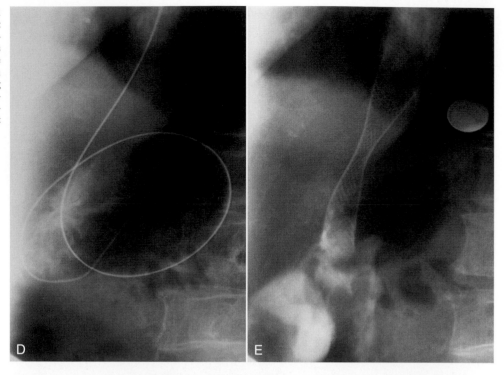

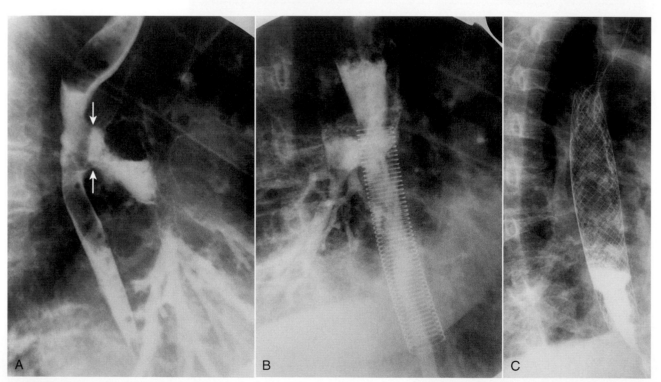

FIGURE 19-22. Esophagobronchial fistula treated with a covered Wallstent in a patient with lung cancer that had invaded the esophagus and caused the fistula. **A,** Barium swallow shows a fistula *(arrows)* between the esophagus and bronchial tree. **B,** The patient was brought to the operating theater and, with the patient under general anesthesia, a rigid plastic stent was deployed. This however did not exclude the fistula. There is contrast present within the bronchial tree on this Gastrografin swallow performed after the rigid plastic tube was inserted. **C,** The rigid plastic tube was removed and a covered Wallstent was placed. Barium swallow after Wallstent placement shows that the bronchial fistula has been excluded.

also be used. A synopsis of the reported literature can be seen in Table 19-5.

Metallic stents have also been placed in patients with benign esophageal strictures. However, the results have not been encouraging. In one study, 14 metallic stents were placed in 12 patients with benign esophageal strictures. Delayed complications occurred in all patients with new strictures forming in five patients above, below, or within the lumen of the stent. Stent migration occurred in six patients while formation of a new stricture occurred in one patient. Later studies with retrievable stent designs and with the Polyflex plastic stent are more optimistic and these latter stents would be the stents of choice for this indication.

Complications

The main complications associated with metallic endoprostheses include stent migration, tumor ingrowth, perforation, food impaction, chest pain, and hemorrhage. Tumor ingrowth was reported to occur in up to 20%-30% of patients who had uncovered metallic stents in place. This problem has now largely been abolished by the use of covered metallic stents. Stent migration occurred more frequently with covered stent designs, particularly where the polyurethane cover is placed on the outside of the stent (Fig. 19-23). Migration is considerably less with newer stent designs where the proximal, distal, or both ends of the stents are flared. However, variable migration rates of 10%-30% are quoted in the literature depending on the type of covered stent. Other complications reported with esophageal metal stent placement include food impaction, which occasionally occurs. Patients should be instructed to drink carbonated beverages after eating to help clear the stent of residual debris. Transient chest pain related to stent deployment has been reported and may be severe enough to require narcotic analgesia. The reasons for this are unclear. Tumor overgrowth has been reported in some series and can occur in up to 6.2% of patients. This can be treated by placement of a further metal stent.

Hemorrhage has been reported in 3%-8% of patients. This is mostly mild and self-limiting. In some patients, it is not clear where the hemorrhage originates; some of these patients receive radiotherapy, but it is unclear whether this increases the risk for bleeding complications. The mortality rate for metallic stent insertion is low, up to 1.4%

Colorectal Cancer

Metallic stents have been placed in patients with colonic neoplasms who present with acute large bowel obstruction. The stents are placed as a temporizing measure to allow colonic decompression and permit elective surgery rather than emergency surgery. The mortality rate for elective surgery varies from 0.9% to 6%, compared with 22% for patients undergoing emergency surgical treatment for acute colorectal obstruction. Additionally, patients with acute large bowel obstruction are often in a poor general state of health because of the underlying disease, dehydration, and electrolyte imbalance. Placing a stent across the colonic tumor to alleviate the obstruction also allows time for correction of any electrolyte imbalance and allows time for the clinical condition of the patient to be optimized for elective surgery. Some patients with colorectal cancer and distal metastases can be palliated by colonic stenting, particularly if they are unfit for surgical palliation.

Technique

A preprocedure-limited barium enema is performed to delineate the site of the stricture. If there is total colonic obstruction, no attempt is made to place barium through the lesion. Endoscopic

---

Box 19-10. Esophageal Stent Placement

Uncovered stents or conical stents with internal covering for gastroesophageal junction strictures
Covered stents for non-gastroesophageal junction strictures
Covered stents for tracheoesophageal fistulas
Predilatation necessary if stricture is tight
Omeprazole 20 mg daily for gastroesophageal junction stent patients

---

TABLE 19-4 Recent Esophageal Stent Results for Palliation of Esophageal Cancer

Stent	No. of Studies	Year	Patient Numbers	Recurrent Dysphagia		Complications	
				Tumor Overgrowth (%)	Migration (%)	Major Complications (%)	Hemorrhage (%)
Ultraflex	8	2001-2008	539	3-26	4-23	6-25	0-15
Polyflex	5	2003-2008	249	10-30	5-29	0-20	0-20
Wallflex	1	2010	37	11	6	8	-
Niti-S	3	2006-2009	102	5-24	7-12	12	5
Z-stent ++	3	2001-2007	192	12-18	6-12	22-25	15-18

Modified from Gray RT, O'Donnell ME, Scott RD, et al. Self-expanding metal stent insertion for inoperable esophageal carcinoma in Belfast: an audit of outcomes and literature review. *Dis Esophagus.* 2011;24:569-574.

TABLE 19-5 Esophagorespiratory Fistulas or Perforation: Covered Metal Stent Results

First Author	Year	Patients	Stent Type	Success (%)	Complications
Watkinson	1995	6	Wallstent-4 Gianturco-2	100	2
Saxon	1995	12	Gianturco	100	3
Weigert	1995	8	Gianturco	87.5	2
Mintlan	1996	10	Gianturco	100	4
Han	1996	10	Gianturco	100	4
Morgan	1997	39	Wallstent-36 Gianturco-3	95	8
Shin	2004	61	Homemade Gianturco/Nitinol	80	13
Lee	2009	9	Retrievable Nitinol	100	5

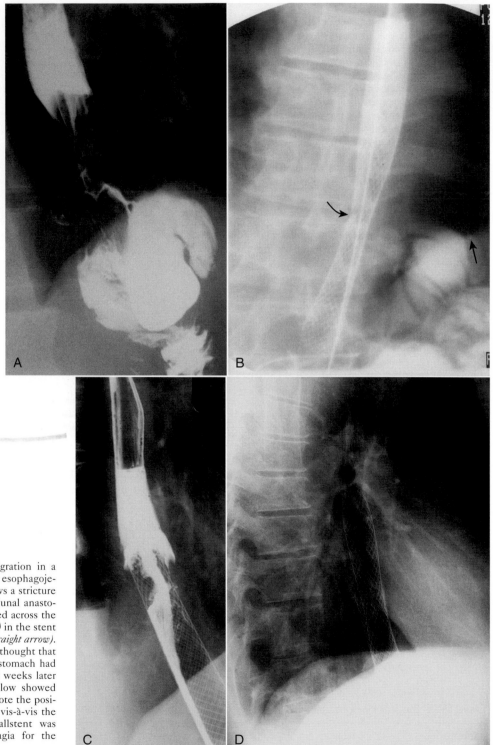

FIGURE 19-23. Esophageal Wallstent migration in a patient with recurrent gastric cancer and an esophagojejunal anastomosis. **A,** Barium swallow shows a stricture in the distal esophagus at the esophagojejunal anastomosis. **B,** A covered Wallstent was deployed across the stricture. Note that the waist *(curved arrow)* in the stent is present at the level of the diaphragm *(straight arrow).* A covered stent was placed because it was thought that the stent would not migrate because the stomach had been removed. **C,** The patient returned 6 weeks later with recurrent dysphagia. A barium swallow showed that the Wallstent had migrated distally. Note the position of the proximal end of the Wallstent vis-à-vis the diaphragm. **D,** A second uncovered Wallstent was placed which provided relief of dysphagia for the patient's remaining life.

confirmation of the malignant nature of the stricture is also usually performed. Patients are sedated with midazolam and placed in a decubitus position on the fluoroscopy table. Approximately 75% of colonic neoplasms occur on the left side of the colon and it is predominantly these that are amenable to radiologic techniques. In general, lesions in the rectosigmoid can usually be accessed and stented radiologically. Lesions in the descending colon or transverse colon require combined endoscopic and radiologic guidance for stent placement.

A 5-French angiographic catheter and a hydrophilic wire are used to cross the stricture. Both ends of the stricture are

delineated with contrast material and the length of the stricture is measured. A stent that provides 2-3 cm of overlap on both sides of the stricture is chosen for placement. The author uses the WallFlex stent (Boston Scientific, Watertown, Mass.), which varies in diameter from 22 to 25 mm and can vary in length from 60 to 120 mm. Once the lesion is crossed, a superstiff 0.035-inch wire is placed across the lesion and manipulated proximally into the colon. The stent is then delivered to the site of the tumor and placed so that overlap is obtained above and below the tumor. The stent is delivered and the stent delivery system removed. The stent is dilated in position with a 12- to 15-mm balloon to

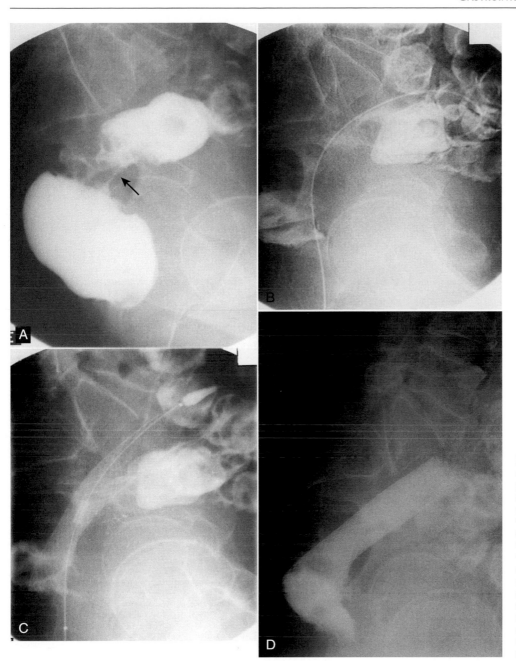

FIGURE 19-24. Patient with a rectal carcinoma and partial obstruction. The patient was unfit for surgery. **A,** A barium enema shows a stricture *(arrow)* in the midrectum. **B,** The stricture was traversed using a 5-French Kumpe catheter and a hydrophilic guidewire. **C,** A conventional covered esophageal Wallstent was deployed across the stricture. The esophageal Wallstent was placed because the newer enteral stent was not available at that time. **D,** A limited barium enema study shows the Wallstent in situ with free flow of contrast both proximally and distally. The Wallstent provided effective palliation and the patient did not require a colostomy.

initiate the self-expanding process and to promote immediate colonic decompression (Fig. 19-24). A plain film of the abdomen is obtained to assess the position and degree of dilatation of the stent before sending the patient back to the ward. The plain radiograph is used as a marker for future comparisons. A follow-up film is obtained at 24-48 hours to assess the degree of colonic decompression and the degree of dilatation and location of the stent.

Results and Complications
Results have shown metallic stents to be safe and effective in relieving acute colonic obstruction and avoiding emergency surgery. In a metaanalysis of colorectal stents used for colonic decompression as an alternative to emergency surgery, Sebastian and colleagues tabulated data from 54 studies on 1198 patients. The median technical and clinical success rates were 94% and 91%, respectively. The success rate when used as a bridge to surgery was 71.7%. Perforation occurred in 3.7%, stent migration in 11.8%, and reobstruction in 7.3%. This procedure is effective in

palliation of colorectal cancer and is a useful alternative to emergency colostomy in patients with colorectal obstruction, allowing single-stage surgery in most of these patients.

SUGGESTED READINGS

Acunas B, Rozanes I, Akpinar S, et al. Palliation of malignant esophageal strictures with self-expanding nitinol stents: drawbacks and complications. *Radiology.* 1996;199:648-652.

Adam A, Ellul J, Watkinson A, et al. Palliation of inoperable esophageal carcinoma: a prospective randomized trial of laser therapy and stent placement. *Radiology.* 1997;202:344-348.

Adam A, Morgan R, Ellul J, Mason RC. A new design of the esophageal Wallstent endoprosthesis resistant to distal migration. *Am J Roentgenol.* 1998;170:1477-1481.

Adam A, Watkinson AF, Dussek J. Boerhaave syndrome: to treat or not to treat by means of insertion of a metallic stent. *J Vasc Interv Radiol.* 1995;6:741-743: discussion 744–746.

Bell SD, Carmody EA, Yeung EY, et al. Percutaneous gastrostomy and gastrojejunostomy: additional experience in 519 procedures. *Radiology.* 1995;194:817-820.

Binkert CA, Ledermann H, Jost R, et al. Acute colonic obstruction: clinical aspects and cost-effectiveness of preoperative and palliative treatment with self-expanding metallic stents: preliminary report. *Radiology.* 1998;206:199-204.

Canon CL, Baron TH, Morgan DE, Dean PA, Keebler RE. Treatment of colonic obstruction with expandable metal stents: radiologic features. *Am J Roentgenol.* 1997;168:199-205.

Choo IW, Do YS, Suh SW, et al. Malignant colorectal obstruction: treatment with a flexible covered stent. *Radiology.* 1998;206:415-421.

Clark JA, Pugash RA, Pantalone RR. Radiologic peroral gastrostomy. *J Vasc Interv Radiol.* 1999;10:927-932.

Cwikiel W, Stridbeck H, Tranberg KG, et al. Malignant esophageal strictures: treatment with a self-expanding nitinol stent. *Radiology.* 1993;187:661-665.

Cwikiel W, Tranberg KG, Cwikiel M, Lillo-Gil R. Malignant dysphagia: palliation with esophageal stents: long-term results in 100 patients. *Radiology.* 1998;297:513-518.

Dawson SL, Mueller PR, Ferrucci JT, et al. Severe esophageal strictures indications for balloon catheter dilatation. *Radiology.* 1984;153:631-635.

Ellul JP, Watkinson A, Khan RJ, Adam A, Mason RC. Self-expanding metal stents for the palliation of dysphagia due to inoperable oesophageal carcinoma. *Br J Surg.* 1995;82:1678-1681.

Given MF, Hanson J, Lee MJ. Interventional radiology techniques for provision of enteral feeding. *CVIR.* 2005;28:692-703.

Given MF, Lyon SM, Lee MJ. The role of the interventional radiologist in enteral alimentation. *European Radiology.* 2004;14:38-47.

Hallisey MJ, Pollard JC. Direct percutaneous jejunostomy. *J Vasc Interv Radiol.* 1984;5:625-632.

Han YM, Song HY, Lee JM, et al. Esophagorespiratory fistula due to esophageal carcinoma: palliation with a covered Gianturco stent. *Radiology.* 1996;199:65-70.

Hill J. Stenting in colorectal cancer. *Br J Surg.* 2008;95(10):1195-1196.

Ho CS, Yeung EY. Percutaneous gastrostomy and transgastric jejunostomy. *Am J Roentgenol.* 1992;158:251-257.

Hoffer EK, Cosgrove JM, Levin DQ, Herskowitz MM, Sclafani SJ. Radiologic gastrojejunostomy and percutaneous endoscopic gastrostomy: a prospective, randomized comparison. *J Vasc Interv Radiol.* 1999;10:413-420.

Knyrim K, Wagner HJ, Bethge N, Keymling M, Vakil N. A controlled trial of an expansile metal stent for palliation of esophageal obstruction due to inoperable cancer. *N Engl J Med.* 1993;28(329):1302-1307.

Kuo YC, Shlansky-Goldberg RD, Mondschein JI, et al. Large or small bore, push or pull: a comparison of three classes of percutaneous fluoroscopic gastrostomy catheters. *J Vasc Interv Radiol.* 2008;19(4):557-563.

Kwak S, Leef JA, Rosenblum JD. Percutaneous balloon catheter dilatation of benign ureteral strictures: effect of multiple dilatation procedures on long-term patency. *Am J Roentgenol.* 1995;165:97-100.

Lee MJ, Kiely P. Percutaneous radiological gastrostomy and gastrojejunostomy. *J ICPS.* 1998;27:13-16.

Lopera JE, Ferral H, Wholey M, et al. Treatment of colonic obstructions with metallic stents: indications, technique and complications. *Am J Roentgenol.* 1997;169:1285-1290.

Lu DS, Mueller PR, Lee MJ, et al. Gastrostomy conversion to transgastric jejunostomy: technical problems, causes of failure and proposed solutions in 63 patients. *Radiology.* 1993;197:679-683.

Mainar A, Tejero E, Maynar M, Ferral H, Castaneda-Zuniga W. Colorectal obstruction: treatment with metallic stents. *Radiology.* 1996;198:761-764.

Miyayama S, Matsui O, Kadoya M, et al. Malignant esophageal stricture and fistula: palliative treatment with polyurethane- covered Gianturco stent. *J Vasc Interv Radiol.* 1995;6:243-248.

Morgan RA, Ellul JPM, Denton ERE, et al. Malignant esophageal fistulas and perforations: management with plastic-covered metallic endoprostheses. *Radiology.* 1997;204:527-532.

Olson DL, Krubsack AJ, Steward ET. Percutaneous enteral alimentation: gastrostomy versus gastrojejunostomy. *Radiology.* 1993;187:105-108.

Pocek M, Maspes F, Masala S, et al. Palliative treatment of neoplastic strictures by self-expanding nitinol Strecker stent. *Eur Radiol.* 1996;6:230-235.

Ragunath K. Refractory benign esophageal strictures: extending the role of expandable stents. *Am J Gastroenterol.* 2008;103:2995-2996.

Ryan JM, Hahn PF, Boland GW, et al. Percutaneous gastrostomy with T-fastener gastropexy: results of 316 consecutive procedures. *Radiology.* 1997;203:496-500.

Sabharwal T, Cowling M, Dussek J, Owen W, Adam A. Balloon dilation for achalasia of the cardia: experience in 76 patients. *Radiology.* 2002;224:719-724.

Sabharwal T, Morales JP, Irani FG, Adam A. Quality improvement guidelines for placement of esophageal stents. *CVIR.* 2005;28:284-288.

Saini S, Mueller PR, Gaa J, et al. Percutaneous gastrostomy with gastropexy: experience in 125 patients. *Am J Roentgenol.* 1990;154:1003-1006.

Sawada S, Tanigawa N, Okuda Y, Mishima K, Ohmura N. Clinical value of combined stents in esophageal cancer: combined use of Ultraflex and self-expanding zigzag metallic stents. *Am J Roentgenol.* 1997;169:493-494.

Saxon RR, Barton RE, Katon RM, et al. Treatment of malignant esophagorespiratory fistulas with silicone-covered metallic Z stents. *J Vasc Interv Radiol.* 1995;6:237-242.

Saxon RR, Barton RE, Katon RM, et al. Treatment of malignant esophageal obstructions with covered metallic Z stents: long-term results in 52 Patients. *J Vasc Interv Radiol.* 1995;6:747-754.

Saxon RR, Morrison KE, Lakin PC, et al. Malignant esophageal obstruction and esophagorespiratory fistula: palliation with a polyethylene-covered Z-stent. *Radiology.* 1997;202:349–254.

Sebastian S, Johnston S, Geoghegan T, et al. Pooled analysis of the efficacy and safety of self-expanding metal stenting in malignant colorectal obstruction. *Am J Gastroenterol.* 2004;99(10):2051-2057.

Silas AM, Pearce LF, Lestina LS, et al. Percutaneous radiologic gastrostomy versus percutaneous endoscopic gastrostomy: a comparison of indications, complications and outcomes in 370 patients. *Eur J Radiol.* 2005;56(1):84-90.

Song HY, Park SI, Do YS, et al. Expandable metallic stent placement in patients with benign esophageal strictures: results of long-term follow-up. *Radiology.* 1997;203:131-136.

Song HY, Park SI, Jung HY, et al. Benign and malignant esophageal strictures: treatment with a polyurethane-covered retrievable expandable metallic stent. *Radiology.* 1997;203:747-752.

Szymski GX, Albazzaz AN, Funaki B, et al. Radiologically guided placement of pull-type gastrostomy tubes. *Radiology.* 1997;205:669-673.

Tan BS, Kennedy C, Morgan R, Owen W. Adam A: Using uncovered metallic endoprostheses to treat recurrent benign esophageal strictures. *Am J Radiol.* 1997;169:1281-1284.

Thomson A, Baron TH. Esophageal stents: one size does not fit all. *J Gastroenterol Hepatol.* 2009;24:2-4.

Thornton FJ, Fotheringham T, Alexander M, et al. Enteral nutrition provision in amyotrophic lateral sclerosis (ALS): endoscopic or radiologic gastrostomy? *Radiology.* 2002;224:713-717.

Thornton FJ, Fotheringham T, Haslam, et al. Percutaneous radiological gastrostomy (PRG) with and without T-fastener gastropexy: a randomised comparison. *Cardiovasc Interv Radiol.* 2002;25:467-471.

Thornton FJ, Varghese JC, Haslam PJ, et al. Percutaneous gastrostomy in patients who fail or are unsuitable for endoscopic gastrostomy. *Cardiovasc Interv Radiol.* 2000;23:279-284.

Tsukuda T, Fujita T, Ito K, et al. Percutaneous radiologic gastrostomy using push-type gastrostomy tubes with CT and fluoroscopic guidance. *AJR Am J Roentgenol.* 2006;186(2):574-576.

Varghese JC, Lee MJ. Percutaneous cecostomy. *Semin Interv Radiol.* 1996;13: 351-354.

Watkinson AF, Ellul J, Entwisle K, et al. Plastic-covered metallic endoprostheses in the management of oesophageal perforation in patients with oesophageal carcinoma. *Clin Radiol.* 1995;50:304-309.

Watkinson AF, Ellul J, Entwisle K, Mason RC, Adam A. Esophageal carcinoma: initial results of palliative treatment with covered self-expanding endoprostheses. *Radiology.* 1995;195:821-827.

Weigert N, Neuhaus H, Rosch T. Treatment of esophagorespiratory fistulas with silicone-coated self-expanding metal stents. *Gastrointest Endosc.* 1995;41:490-496.

Winkelbauer F, Schofl R, Niederle B, et al. Palliative treatment of obstructing esophageal cancer with nitinol stents: value, safety, and long-term results. *Am J Roentgenol.* 1996;166:79-84.

Wollman BD, Agostino HB, Walus Wigle J, Easter DW, Beale A. Radiologic, endoscopic, and surgical gastrostomy: an institutional evaluation and meta-analysis of the literature. *Radiology.* 1995;197:699-704.

CHAPTER 20

Biliary Intervention

Michael J. Lee, MSc, FRCPI, FRCR, FFR(RCSI), FSIR, EBIR

Percutaneous transhepatic cholangiography (PTC) and percutaneous biliary drainage (PBD) techniques gained widespread popularity in the late 1970s and early 1980s after they were first described. However, the use of both PTC and PBD has declined with the development of diagnostic and therapeutic endoscopic retrograde cholangiopancreatography (ERCP). PTC and PBD remain an important part of interventional radiology and are performed on a regular basis at many institutions. The indications for biliary intervention are less numerous; even so, they are widely accepted and well defined.

INTRAHEPATIC DUCTAL ANATOMY

Intrahepatic ductal anatomy is modeled on the segmental anatomy of the liver as described by Couinaud. At the hilum there are two main hepatic ducts, the right and left, which join to form the common hepatic duct. The right hepatic duct drains segments 5-8 and is formed by the right posterior duct (RPD) and the right anterior duct (RAD). The RAD drains segments 5 and 8 while the RPD drains segments 6 and 7. The RPD has a more horizontal course on anteroposterior cholangiographic images of the liver while the RAD has a more vertical course. Normally, the RPD passes behind the RAD and joins the RAD on its medial side to form the right hepatic duct. The left hepatic duct is usually horizontally orientated in the left lobe of the liver and drains segments 2-4. It joins with the right hepatic duct to form the common hepatic duct and exits the liver at the biliary hilum in conjunction with the portal vein and hepatic artery. The common hepatic duct is joined by the cystic duct, which drains the gallbladder, to form the common bile duct.

This standard anatomy is present in approximately 57% of patients (Fig. 20-1). There are a wide number of variations in bile duct anatomy which can have a profound effect on planning a biliary drainage. The variations that most affect biliary drainage procedures are those involving anomalous drainage of the RPD and the RAD (see Fig. 20-1). The RPD may drain into the left hepatic duct (Fig. 20-2A) or alternatively into the common hepatic duct. The RAD can also drain into the left hepatic duct

but not as frequently as the RPD. In addition, occasionally the RAD, RPD, and left hepatic duct form a triple confluence so that there is no right hepatic duct (see Fig. 20-2B).

Knowledge of the anatomic relationships of the intrahepatic bile ducts is important to know before planning biliary drainage procedures, particularly in patients with obstructions at the level of the biliary hilum. If a patient with a hilar obstruction has anomalous drainage of the RPD into the left hepatic duct, then a left hepatic drainage is the appropriate drainage procedure, in that most of the liver is drained by a single drainage procedure. Conversely, if a right-sided biliary drainage is performed, only a small amount of liver is drained (that drained by the RAD), which may not be enough to provide adequate hepatic function to relieve jaundice and pruritus. The RPD is said to drain into the left hepatic duct in 23% of patients and the RAD in 5%. It is also important to be aware of anomalous drainage of right-sided ducts into the left hepatic duct when performing biliary drainages from the right side. Often, if the RPD drains anomalously into the left hepatic duct, a very acute angle may be formed by the junction of the RPD with the left hepatic duct. This may make it impossible to pass catheters or guidewires from the right side into the left hepatic duct and then down the common hepatic duct. Indeed, trying to do so may increase the risk of complications such as hemorrhage. In the author's unit, we now perform magnetic resonance cholangiography (MRC) on all patients before biliary drainage to fully assess intrahepatic bile duct anatomy and assess any variations so that appropriate biliary drainage can be planned.

Patient Preparation

Patient preparation is similar for all transhepatic biliary interventional procedures. Antibiotic prophylaxis is mandatory before any biliary interventional procedure. Common antibiotic regimens include gentamicin 80 mg intravenously (IV) and ampicillin 1 g IV before the procedure. The author's unit used to use this regimen but has changed to using piperacillin/tazobactam 4.5 g IV before the procedure. Piperacillin/tazobactam consists of a penicillin

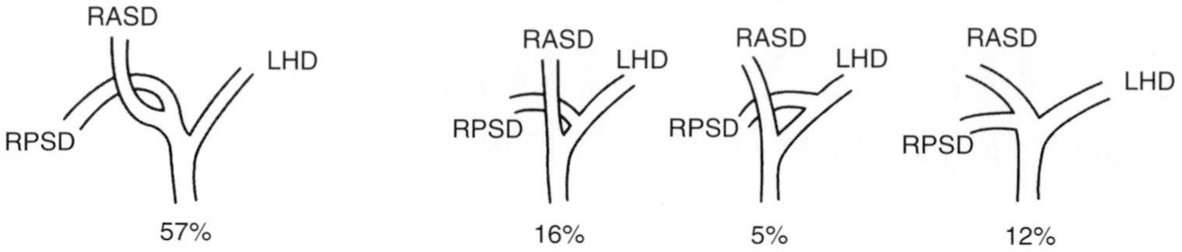

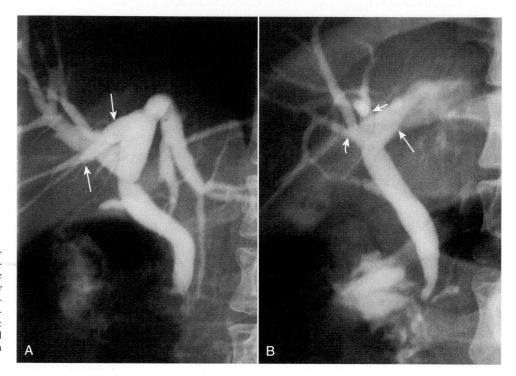

FIGURE 20-1. Normal bile duct anatomy and its variants. Note that in approximately 21% of patients the right posterior sectoral duct (RPSD) joins the left hepatic duct (LHD). In 16%, the RPSD joins the left LHD close to the hilum, while in the other 5% it joins the LHD at some distance from the hilum. In patients with hilar strictures and aberrant drainage of the RPSD to the LHD, left-sided drainage drains a large amount of liver and provides excellent liver function. RASD, right anterior sectoral duct.

FIGURE 20-2. **A,** Aberrant biliary anatomy. Endoscopic retrograde cholangiopancreatography film showing drainage of the right posterior sectoral duct *(large arrows)* into the left hepatic duct. **B,** Trifurcation bile duct. Note the right anterior sectoral duct *(curved arrow),* right posterior sectoral duct *(short arrow),* and left hepatic duct *(long arrow)* forming a trifurcation at the hilar confluence.

(piperacillin) and a β-lactamase inhibitor (tazobactam). Piperacillin is a broad-spectrum antibiotic with activity against gram-positive, gram-negative, and aerobic infections. High levels are found in bile when administered IV; and the addition of the β-lactamase inhibitor protects piperacillin against β-lactamase–producing anaerobes. Piperacillin/tazobactam is an ideal monotherapy for biliary drainage procedures, but gentamicin and ampicillin can be used when piperacillin/tazobactam is not available. For PTC, a single dose is given before the procedure. For biliary drainage, we now continue piperacillin/tazobactam 4.5 g IV t.i.d. for 2 days.

Coagulation parameters must be checked carefully and any bleeding tendency corrected with fresh frozen plasma and/or vitamin K. In jaundiced patients who are undergoing biliary drainage for relief of malignant biliary obstruction, we place the patients on intravenous fluids as soon as they are referred for biliary drainage. We use 2½ L of Hartman's solution daily for 3-4 days around the time of the drainage procedure. Fluid replacement is important in these patients in the periprocedural time period to prevent hepatorenal failure. Many jaundiced patients have not been eating or drinking appropriately before coming to the hospital, and when they do reach hospital they are fasted for different tests, such as ERCP, computed tomography (CT) scans, and ultrasound. Usually by the time they are referred for biliary drainage they are quite dehydrated, which increases the risk of hepatorenal failure developing. Informed consent is obtained from all patients before the procedure by a member of the interventional team.

PERCUTANEOUS TRANSHEPATIC CHOLANGIOGRAPHY

The indications for PTC have fallen dramatically since the introduction of ERCP and more recently MRC. We occasionally are asked to perform a diagnostic PTC in patients who have had a laparoscopic bile duct injury, in patients with sclerosing cholangitis, and in patients in whom ERCP is not possible because of altered upper gastrointestinal anatomy. Contraindications are rare but would include an uncorrectable coagulopathy.

Technique

PTC is performed predominantly from the right side for diagnostic purposes. The patient is placed supine on the fluoroscopy table and the right flank is sterilely prepared. A combination of midazolam and fentanyl is used for sedoanalgesia. Under fluoroscopic control, the patient is asked to take a deep breath and the position of maximal lung descent is marked. A point is chosen one or two interspaces below this point for needle access. The needle access point should also lie in the midaxillary line. Once the point is marked on the skin, the skin is infiltrated with local anesthetic and a small incision made with a #11 scalpel blade. A 22-gauge Chiba needle (15 cm in length) is used for PTC. The needle is inserted under fluoroscopic guidance from the right flank toward the 12th vertebral body. The needle is

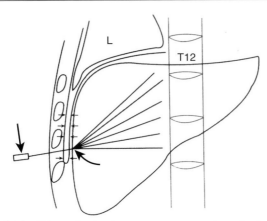

FIGURE 20-3. Schematic showing percutaneous transhepatic cholangiography technique. The patient is asked to take a deep inspiration and the point of maximal lung descent marked. An interspace below is chosen for puncture. The 22-gauge needle *(long arrow)* is aimed toward the T12 vertebral body and withdrawn slowly while injecting dilute contrast medium until a biliary duct is entered. The procedure is repeated in a fan shape inferiorly if a bile duct is not entered. It is important not to take the needle fully out of the liver so that only one hole in the liver capsule *(curved arrow)* is made. Note that invariably the needle passes through the pleura *(small arrows)* but should not pass through the lung (L).

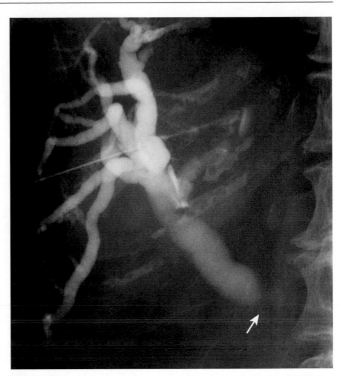

FIGURE 20-4. Percutaneous transhepatic cholangiography (PTC) in a patient with failed endoscopic retrograde cholangiopancreatography. A 22-gauge needle inserted into the liver toward the T12 vertebral body was withdrawn slowly with small pulses of contrast material injected until the right anterior sectoral duct was entered. The contrast injected shows a dilated biliary system with an obstruction at the lower end of the bile duct *(arrow)*. Note the left duct is often not seen with a right-sided PTC. Trendelenburg positioning may help fill the left duct.

inserted parallel to the tabletop in one smooth motion. The stylet is withdrawn and a syringe containing dilute contrast material is attached to the hub of the needle via an extension tube. The needle is slowly withdrawn and small aliquots of contrast material are injected every 1-2 mm until a bile duct is entered. When a bile duct is entered, contrast material flows away from the tip of the needle, slowly, akin to wax flowing down a candlestick. This is a characteristic phenomenon and is easily differentiated from hepatic vein or portal vein branches wherein contrast washes quickly away either toward the heart if a hepatic vein is entered or toward the periphery of the liver if a portal vein branch is entered. If a bile duct is not entered on the first pass, successive passes are made in a fan shape down through the liver toward the biliary hilum (Fig. 20-3). It is important, however, not to withdraw the needle fully outside the liver capsule so that only one hole in the liver capsule is made. This helps reduce bleeding complications.

When a bile duct is entered, contrast is injected to outline the biliary system (Fig. 20-4). With low bile duct obstructions, it is often advantageous to have a table that can tilt. In the supine position, the injected contrast material may not reach the level of the obstruction. By tilting the patient to a semierect position, the heavier contrast material falls and displaces the lighter bile so that the level of obstruction can be accurately depicted. Radiographs are obtained in anteroposterior (AP) and both oblique projections, and the needle is withdrawn if a biliary drainage is not planned.

Results and Complications

Success rates for PTC are between 97% and 100% in experienced hands. Technical difficulties can be experienced in patients without biliary dilatation. As many as 15-20 passes can be safely made, but thereafter, if a bile duct has not been entered, the procedure is best terminated. Alternatively, one can place a needle into the gallbladder and inject contrast material through the gallbladder to outline the biliary system. This is possible only if the biliary obstruction is below the junction of the cystic duct and common hepatic duct. Placing the patient in Trendelenburg position aids filling of the intrahepatic ducts if a gallbladder access is used.

Complications are minimal and occur in about 1%-2% of patients. Possible complications include hemorrhage, sepsis, and

Box 20-1. Indications for Biliary Intervention

Failed endoscopic drainage
Hilar obstruction
Biliary problems after biliary enteric anastomoses
Injury after laparoscopic cholecystectomy

bile leak leading to biliary peritonitis. The incidence of hemorrhage can be decreased by correction of any abnormal coagulation parameters beforehand and by making only one hole in the liver capsule. If the blood coagulation parameters are abnormal, the percutaneous track can be embolized with Gelfoam or autologous blood clot as the needle is withdrawn though the track. This helps further decrease the incidence of hemorrhage and/or bile leak. Bile leakage is rare after PTC but occurs more frequently after biliary drainage. Appropriate antibiotic coverage can help minimize the significance of bacteremia and prevent sepsis.

BILIARY DRAINAGE

PBD was first described by Molnar and Stockholm in the late 1970s and enjoyed a preeminent position in biliary intervention until the advent of therapeutic ERCP. Now, management of patients with biliary obstruction depends to a large extent on the expertise available in any given institution. However, most patients are managed by endoscopic techniques such as stone extraction or stent placement for common bile duct (CBD) stones and stent placement for malignant biliary obstruction. At the author's institution, the indications for biliary drainage are limited but remain important; they are shown in Box 20-1. The main

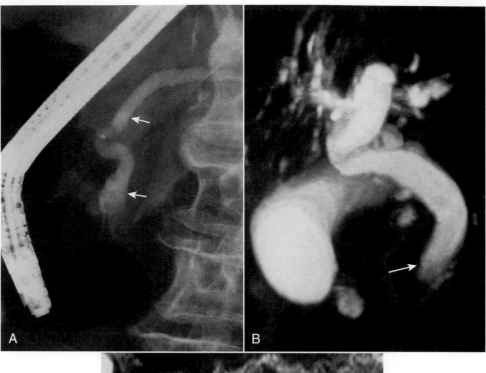

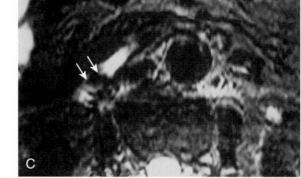

FIGURE 20-5. Magnetic resonance cholangiography in a patient with failed endoscopic retrograde cholangiopancreatography (ERCP). **A,** ERCP shows a dilated pancreatic duct *(arrows)*. However, the bile duct could not be cannulated at ERCP. **B,** MR cholangiopancreatography shows a dilated bile duct *(large arrow)* down to the level of the ampulla. **C,** Axial images through the region of the ampulla show a small periampullary tumor *(arrows)*, which is causing the obstruction. Note the dilated pancreatic duct proximal to the periampullary tumor. This appearance was confirmed at percutaneous transhepatic cholangiography. The patient was 83 years of age and unfit for surgery. A biliary drainage was performed with metal stent placement.

indication for PBD is when ERCP fails or is not possible due to altered upper gastrointestinal anatomy.

Preprocedure Imaging

It is important before embarking upon a biliary drainage that all relevant information regarding the probable cause of the biliary obstruction, the level of obstruction, and details of relevant biliary anatomy are obtained. If the ERCP has failed, the endoscopists may not have injected contrast material into the biliary system. Often, even if contrast material is injected into the biliary system, it may not have outlined the whole biliary system so that bile duct anatomy cannot be ascertained. An ultrasound of the liver is important to confirm intrahepatic biliary duct dilatation, to eliminate metastatic disease, to determine the level of obstruction, and to rule out the presence of ascites. Usually an ultrasound has been performed before the ERCP; if not, it should be performed. A CT scan can also be helpful to check for evidence of a pancreatic tumor and again to look for liver metastases. More recently, in the author's unit we have tended to perform MRC in conjunction with ultrasound in all patients referred for biliary drainage (Fig. 20-5). We perform MRC using a torso coil and heavily T2-weighted fast spin echo pulse sequences. Coronal and axial acquisitions are obtained using breath-hold techniques if possible. MRC is particularly useful for evaluating biliary anatomy and planning the appropriate biliary drainage procedure in patients with hilar obstruction (Box 20-2).

Box 20-2. Patient Preparation for Biliary Drainage Procedure

Appropriate antibiotic prophylaxis
2½ L of intravenous fluids daily
Sonography and magnetic resonance
   cholangiopancreatography beforehand
Define level of obstruction
Define any aberrant biliary anatomy

Right-Sided Biliary Drainage

This is the most common approach for biliary drainage. We use a one-stick needle system (Cook, Bloomington, Ind.) for biliary access (Fig. 20-6). A right-sided PTC is performed as described previously. When a bile duct is entered, contrast material is injected to opacify the biliary system. If the patient is septic, the minimum amount of contrast material is injected to allow safe performance of the biliary drainage, without overdistending the biliary system. If a favorable duct is entered by the initial needle puncture, a 0.018-inch guidewire is placed through the needle and manipulated toward the hepatic hilum and common bile duct (Fig. 20-7). If a favorable duct has not been entered by the initial needle, a second 22-gauge Chiba needle is used to puncture

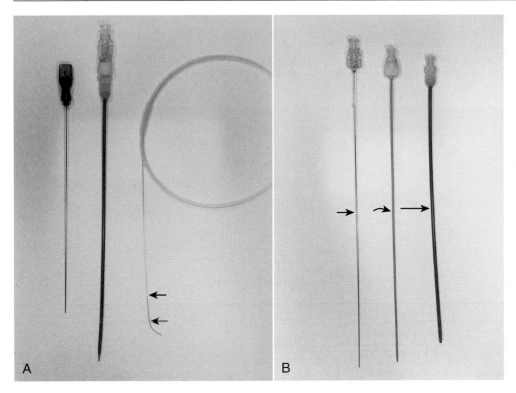

Figure 20-6. One-stick system (Neff, Cook, Bloomington, Ind.) used for biliary access. **A,** A 22-gauge needle, 5-French sheath system and 0.018-inch guidewire form the components of the system. The guidewire has a floppy platinum curved tip *(arrows).* **B,** The 5-French sheath system consists of a metal trocar *(small arrow),* a plastic trocar *(curved arrow),* and an outer 5-French sheath *(large arrow).* When the 0.018-inch guidewire enters the bile duct, the sheath assembly is placed over the guidewire as a unit. When the sheath assembly enters the bile duct, the metal trocar is unhooked from the plastic trocar and the 5-French sheath fed over the guidewire into the bile duct. The metal trocar is too stiff to maneuver around acute angles in the biliary tree and should be withdrawn when the bile duct is entered or else it will kink the guidewire.

a duct with a more favorable orientation to bring the guidewire to the biliary hilum. It is important, when draining patients with hilar obstruction, to gain entry into a peripheral duct, particularly if a stent will be placed. Occasionally the 0.018-inch guidewire does not run appropriately down the duct toward the hepatic hilum. This can be remedied by turning the bevel of the needle in 90-degree aliquots and probing with the wire (Fig. 20-8). Alternatively, the needle may have to be pulled back slightly if the needle is up against the medial wall of the bile duct entered. Once the 0.018-inch guidewire has gained reasonable purchase within the bile duct and is at the level of the common hepatic duct or more distally, the needle is withdrawn and the 5-French sheath assembly placed over the 0.018-inch guidewire into the bile duct.

Problems can be encountered when a vertical bile duct has been entered, in that the 5-French sheath assembly may not follow the guidewire down toward the biliary hilum. It is important to withdraw the metal stiffening cannula when the 5-French sheath assembly reaches the bile duct. The metal trocar is too stiff to follow the 0.018-inch guidewire around a 90-degree curve down into the bile duct. By withdrawing the metal trocar, the more flexible 4-French plastic cannula and 5-French sheath should follow the guidewire down toward the hepatic hilum.

Occasionally, despite appropriate technique, the plastic 5-French sheath and 4-French cannula will not follow the 0.018-inch guidewire down to the biliary hilum. In this situation, the author places the sheath assembly into the vertically orientated duct punctured, removes the 4-French plastic cannula, and places a 0.035-inch hydrophilic guidewire or 1.5-mm J-guidewire through the 5-French sheath and manipulates these down the duct. The 0.018-inch guidewire can be left in place during this maneuver because there is enough room in the 5-French sheath for both guidewires. The 5-French sheath virtually always follows the larger 0.035-inch guidewire.

Once good purchase is obtained, the 4-French inner plastic cannula and 0.018-inch guidewire are removed and a 0.035- or 0.038-inch J-guidewire placed through the 5-French sheath into the biliary tree. At this stage, the 5-French plastic sheath is removed and a hockey-stick type catheter is placed over the J-guidewire. The J-guidewire is then removed and exchanged

for a 0.035-inch hydrophilic guidewire with a straight tip. The hockey-stick catheter and hydrophilic guidewire are manipulated down to a level just above the stricture. The guidewire is removed and contrast material is injected just above the stricture because often there is a small nipple of compressed duct above the stricture which points the way for guidewire manipulation. The hockey-stick catheter and hydrophilic guidewire are manipulated into the area where the nipple of contrast material was seen and the stricture probed with the hydrophilic guidewire until the stricture is crossed. The hockey-stick catheter is advanced through the stricture over the hydrophilic guidewire and both are manipulated into the proximal jejunum. The hydrophilic guidewire is exchanged for a 0.035-inch superstiff guidewire and the percutaneous track is ready for dilatation.

The percutaneous track through the liver is dilated with a 7-French dilator and a 9-French peel-away sheath placed through the percutaneous track. If the obstructing lesion is not appropriate for stenting, an internal/external biliary drainage catheter is placed to drain the biliary system. The catheter we use is an 8.3-French Ring catheter (Cook, Bloomington, Ind.) with either 32 or 42 side holes (Fig. 20-9). The 32–side-hole catheter is used for patients with low CBD obstruction while the 42–side-hole catheter is used for patients with hilar obstruction. The tapered tip on the Ring catheter helps the catheter pass through the strictured area. The peel-away sheath protects the liver parenchyma, prevents buckling of the guidewire and catheter in the perihepatic space, and helps direct the pushing force applied to the catheter down the bile duct. The Ring catheter is placed well into the duodenum and the guidewire is removed. Contrast material is injected and the catheter withdrawn until contrast material is seen to opacify the biliary tree proximal to the obstruction. This implies that there are catheter side-holes above and below the level of obstruction. The catheter is placed to gravity drainage and attached to a bag.

Left-Sided Biliary Drainage

In the author's unit we generally perform left-sided biliary drainages only when the patient has a hilar stricture. However, some authors prefer to use the left side for most, if not all, biliary drainages. A left-sided biliary drainage can be technically more challenging than using the right side, depending on the size of the left lobe, the anatomic configuration of the xiphisternum and costal margins, and the relationship of the left lobe to the costal margins and xiphisternum. There is a limited window of access to the left lobe through the inverted "V" formed by the xiphisternum and medial edges of the right and left costal margins. Depending on the size and position of the left lobe of the liver, the angle of entry into the left lobe may be shallow and within the

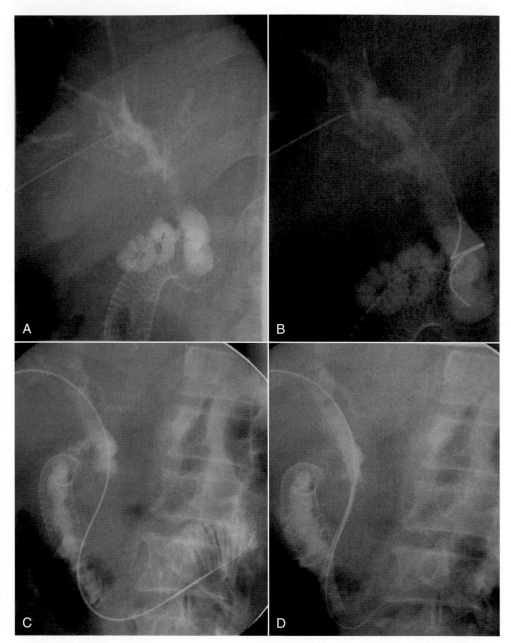

FIGURE 20-7. A patient with pancreatic cancer invading the duodenum, which required placement of a duodenal stent. **A,** A right-sided puncture with a 22-gauge Chiba needle was performed outlining the right hepatic ducts. **B,** Through this Chiba needle, a 0.018-inch guidewire was manipulated into the bile duct and passed to the level of the obstruction. **C,** A hockey-stick catheter and 0.035-inch Terumo guidewire were used to negotiate the stricture and access the duodenum. The Terumo guidewire was exchanged for a 0.035-inch superstiff guidewire. Note: The ampulla is just distal to the duodenal stent. **D,** After dilating the percutaneous track to 8French, an 8-French peel-away sheath was placed, and through this a 10- × 90-mm Wallstent was placed across the stricture in the bile duct. Note: The waist in the Wallstent shows the position of the tumor. A safety catheter was left in situ for 2 days. The Wallstent is self-expanding and expands to its full diameter over approximately 7 days.

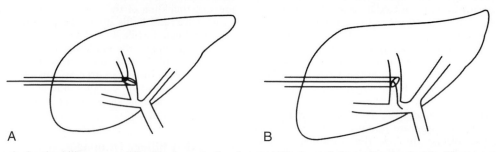

FIGURE 20-8. Schematic showing biliary access difficulties in vertically orientated bile ducts. **A,** Access is gained with a 22-gauge needle into a vertically orientated bile duct in the right lobe of the liver. When the bevel on the needle tip is pointing superiorly, the 0.018-inch guidewire tends to travel superiorly within the bile duct. **B,** By turning the bevel, it is often possible to manipulate the guidewire in an inferior direction toward the common bile duct.

inverted "V" formed by the bony landmarks of the upper abdomen; or indeed if the left lobe is small, it may be quite steep and angled up underneath the right costal margin (Fig. 20-10).

We use ultrasound to locate the left lobe of the liver, assess the angle of approach into the bile duct, and indeed guide the needle into a bile duct. In general, the segment-3 bile duct, which courses inferiorly toward the inferior margin of the left lobe, is

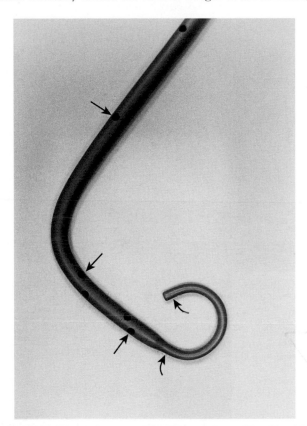

FIGURE 20-9. Ring catheter used for biliary drainage. The Ring biliary drainage catheter (Cook, Bloomington, Ind.) is 8.3-French, is made from polyethylene, and has 32 side holes *(straight arrows)* (zoomed view of catheter tip). The catheter is stiff and has a tapered tip *(curved arrows)* that passes through biliary strictures with minimal difficulty. This catheter is preferentially used for biliary drainages. It is not suitable for long-term internal/external biliary drainage: a larger, softer catheter is used for this.

chosen for entry. Depending on the size of the left lobe, a segment-2 duct, which has a more horizontal course in the left lobe, can be entered if the left lobe is large enough to permit access to segment 2. The advantage of using the segment-2 duct is that there is a more gentle curve with a less acute angle for manipulating guidewires and catheters down into the common bile duct. For patients with hilar obstruction, it is important to gain access to the left lobe biliary system in as peripheral a location as the anatomy allows.

A 22-gauge Chiba needle is used to access the segment-2 or -3 duct and contrast material is injected to outline the biliary system. A 0.018-inch guidewire is manipulated toward the biliary hilum followed by the 5-French sheath system as on the right side. The hydrophilic guidewire and Kumpe catheter are used to negotiate the stricture and are placed in the proximal jejunum. The percutaneous track is dilated over a 0.035-inch superstiff guidewire and a 9-French peel-away sheath is placed. The 9-French peel-away sheath is important particularly when access is gained through a segment-3 duct because it helps direct the pushing force applied to the catheter down the common bile duct and makes placement of the catheter significantly easier. The 8.3-French Ring catheter is placed through the peel-away sheath and over the guidewire so that side holes are left above and below the stricture (Fig. 20-11 and Box 20-3).

▬ PALLIATION OF MALIGNANT BILIARY OBSTRUCTION WITH METAL STENTS

The introduction of metal stents for palliation of malignant biliary strictures has revolutionized percutaneous treatment in these cases. The metallic biliary stents require significantly less track dilatation than do plastic stents (7-French versus 10- to 12-French), they can be placed at the same time as the initial biliary drainage procedure, they are associated with shorter hospital stays, and they are overall more cost-effective than plastic stents (Fig. 20-12). For these reasons, in the author's unit, metallic endoprostheses exclusively are placed for palliation of patients with malignant bile duct obstruction.

Hilar Obstruction

Patients with hilar obstruction form a subset of patients with biliary obstruction who are technically challenging to treat and who are usually best palliated by percutaneous methods if the obstruction is not surgically resectable. Knowledge of liver and

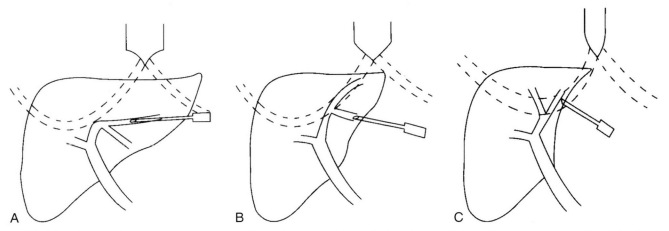

FIGURE 20-10. Schematic showing the various approaches to left lobe drainage; choice of approach depends on the anatomy of the left lobe. **A,** In patients with a large left lobe it may be possible to enter the segment-2 bile duct, which generally has a horizontal course in the left lobe and allows easy access into the common hepatic duct. **B,** In patients with smaller left lobes, the segment-3 duct is usually accessible, but there is a more acute angle for entry down the bile duct. A peel-away sheath is important in this situation to ensure that the pushing force applied to catheters is directed toward the common bile duct. **C,** In patients with very small left lobes, a left-sided biliary drainage is difficult with a very acute angle of entry into the segment-3 duct, making guidewire purchase and other manipulations difficult.

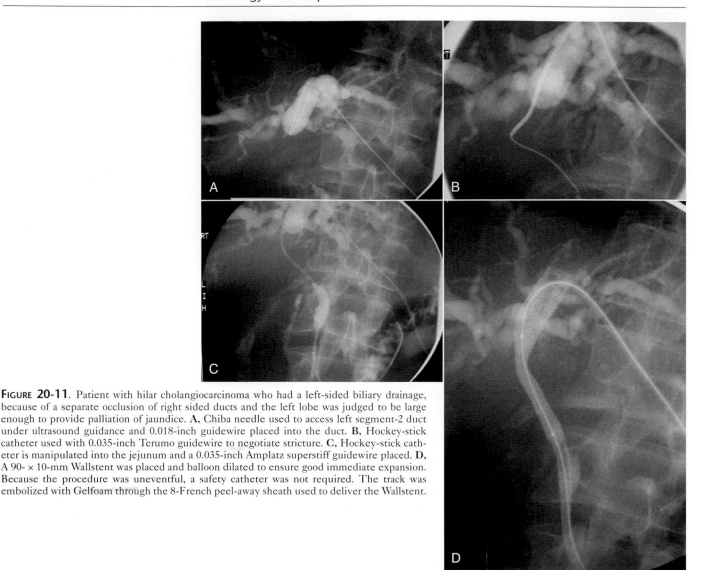

FIGURE 20-11. Patient with hilar cholangiocarcinoma who had a left-sided biliary drainage, because of a separate occlusion of right sided ducts and the left lobe was judged to be large enough to provide palliation of jaundice. **A,** Chiba needle used to access left segment-2 duct under ultrasound guidance and 0.018-inch guidewire placed into the duct. **B,** Hockey-stick catheter used with 0.035-inch Terumo guidewire to negotiate stricture. **C,** Hockey-stick catheter is manipulated into the jejunum and a 0.035-inch Amplatz superstiff guidewire placed. **D,** A 90- × 10-mm Wallstent was placed and balloon dilated to ensure good immediate expansion. Because the procedure was uneventful, a safety catheter was not required. The track was embolized with Gelfoam through the 8-French peel-away sheath used to deliver the Wallstent.

Box 20-3. Biliary Drainage: Key Points

One-stick needle system used for access
Stricture negotiated with short catheter and hydrophilic wire
9-French peel-away sheath placed
8.3-French Ring catheter inserted
Allow 2-3 cm of "slack" when fixing the catheter

---

biliary anatomy is important before planning biliary drainage and/or stent placement. If there is anomalous drainage of the RPD into the left hepatic duct, draining the left lobe alone may be sufficient. If not, the author's practice is to drain both right and left lobes and stent both sides. The other significant factor that influences the approach taken is the Bismuth classification of the lesion (Fig. 20-13). If there is separate occlusion of the RAD and RPD (stage 3a), then draining the right side is of little benefit to the patient. In this situation, it is often best to drain the left side by itself as long as the left lobe is of adequate size and there is no second-order bile duct involvement on the left side. When there is multisegmental involvement on both sides, there is very little that any drainage procedure can offer the patient.

Magnetic resonance cholangiography is a very useful preprocedure imaging test to assess both the anatomy of the biliary system and the Bismuth classification of the hilar tumor (Fig. 20-14). Most hilar malignancies are due to cholangiocarcinoma of the bile duct or the so-called Klatskin tumor. The natural history of this tumor is to grow centrally into the liver along the bile ducts. Eventually, this leads to segmental and subsegmental obstruction. With this in mind, the principle of palliation is to drain as much functioning liver as possible. Although some operators drain one side only, we have found over the years that optimal palliation is achieved when both sides are stented. Even though our reasons for doing this are anecdotal, given the progressive nature of the disease, it seems appropriate to drain both sides. In addition, there is a faster resolution of jaundice and pruritus. Draining both sides also means that there are no undrained segments that may become infected at a later date and require a further drainage procedure. However, it is not always feasible to drain both lobes in every patient.

There are a number of metal stents used in the biliary tree, with the most popular being the Wallstent (Boston Scientific, Natick, Mass.) and the Gianturco (Cook, Bloomington, Ind.). We prefer the Wallstent, which is a self-expanding stainless steel mesh (see Fig. 20-12). It can have many differing lengths but the preferred length for the biliary tree is 9 cm and the preferred diameter is 1 cm. The Wallstent has a small delivery catheter (7-French), the delivery system is flexible, and the stent has a large luminal diameter (1 cm).

The Wallstent is loaded by the manufacturer on the end of the 7-French delivery catheter. The Wallstent is compressed on the

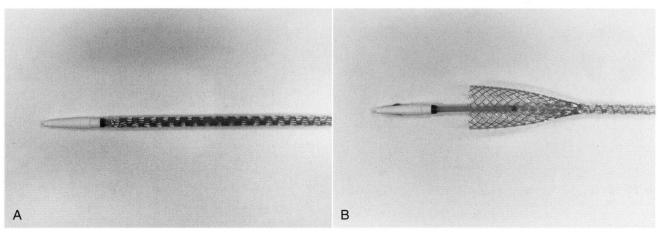

FIGURE 20-12. Wallstent endoprosthesis used for biliary drainage. **A,** Close-up view of the end of the 7-French Wallstent delivery catheter. The Wall-stent is compressed on the end of the delivery catheter by a plastic sheath. **B,** The stent is deployed by pulling back the sheath on the delivery catheter. The stent deploys from distal to proximal but tends to move a little forward as it is deployed. It is important to readjust the position of the stent as it is being deployed. The author's unit generally uses a 90 × 10 mm Wallstent.

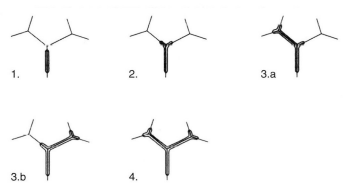

FIGURE 20-13. Bismuth classification used to stage biliary hilar tumors. In stage 1, the tumor involves the common hepatic duct and is driven 2 cm from the biliary hilum. In stage 2, the tumor involves the biliary hilum and the right and left hepatic duct. In stage 3a, the tumor grows out along the right hepatic duct with involvement of the segmental ducts on the right. In stage 3b, the tumor encases the left hepatic duct and involves the segmental ducts on the left. In stage 4, there is segmental duct involvement in both right and left lobes of the liver.

end of the delivery catheter by a sheath, which is withdrawn by the operator to deliver the stent. The stent deploys from distal to proximal and tends to move a little forward as it deploys. It is important to reposition the delivery catheter during stent deployment for this reason.

Covered stents have also been used for palliation of malignant biliary obstruction (Viabil, Gore Medical, Flagstaff, Ariz.). These are best used in the lower CBD rather than the biliary hilum so that side branches are not covered.

There are a number of different approaches to stenting right and left lobes. In one approach, a single right- or left-sided biliary drainage is performed and two Wallstents are placed across the biliary hilum in a T-configuration. A stent is initially placed across the biliary hilum from right to left side to form the top of the "T" (Fig. 20-15). A guidewire is placed through the metal mesh of this initial stent, down into the duodenum, and an 8-mm balloon is used to make a hole in the mesh of this stent. A second stent is placed through the hole in this initial stent to complete the "T." We have used this approach in some patients, but have abandoned this approach because the junction of the right and left ducts are almost never horizontal and this procedure does not provide optimal drainage.

The approach that we currently use is based on bilateral deployment of Wallstents in a Y-configuration (see Fig. 20-15).

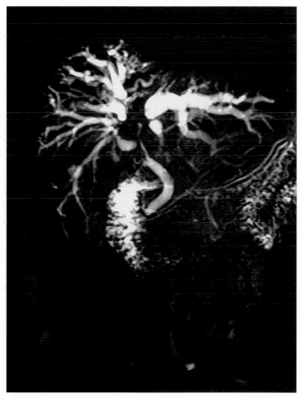

FIGURE 20-14. Magnetic resonance cholangiography in a patient with hilar cholangiocarcinoma. Thick slab single shot fast spin echo (SSFSE) coronal sequence shows dilatation of the intrahepatic ducts with a stricture at the hilar confluence, and separate occlusion of the right-sided ducts indicates a Bismuth 3A lesion.

This means that bilateral biliary drainages are performed for stent placement.

The principles of effective palliation for hilar strictures are:
- Peripheral purchase within the biliary tree
- Overstenting

Overstenting means that the proximal end of the stent is situated at least 2-3 cm above the proximal edge of the tumor. To facilitate this procedure, peripheral access into the biliary tree is mandatory when performing the initial biliary drainage.

To deploy the stents, two 0.035-inch superstiff guidewires are placed across the stricture into the duodenum. The stents are

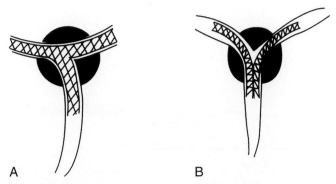

A B

Figure 20-15. Schematic showing "T" and "Y" stenting. **A,** In patients with a horizontally orientated hilar confluence, it may be possible to perform T-stenting from a single biliary drainage. The first stent is laid between the right and left hepatic ducts. A hole is made in the first stent with a balloon and the second stent is placed through the first stent into the common bile duct. However, the vast majority of patients do not have a horizontally orientated hepatic hilum, so T-stenting is not suitable for the majority of patients. **B,** For Y-stenting, bilateral biliary drainages are performed with metal stents inserted. This is the author's preferred method for stenting patients with hilar lesions.

Box 20-4. Hilar Strictures and Metal Stents

Double-Y stenting best where possible
10- × 90-mm Wallstent used
Peripheral biliary purchase necessary
Proximal stent position 2-3 cm above tumor
Y-stents placed simultaneously and deployed sequentially

---

loaded on each wire in turn and placed across the stricture from right and left sides. The stents are positioned so that there is an approximate 2-3 cm of stent above the tumor. The stents are then deployed, one at a time, by simply pulling back the sheath that covers the stent on the delivery catheter (Fig. 20-16).

If the procedure has gone smoothly without evidence of hemobilia, and if the patient is not septic, we generally do not leave a safety catheter. We do decompress the biliary system if not leaving a safety catheter. We also embolize the track with either Gelfoam or a mixture of glue and lipiodol. However, if there is any doubt about the patient's condition, or if there is significant hemobilia, a safety catheter is left through both sides. An 8.3-French Ring catheter is generally used for this purpose and left for 2-3 days on gravity drainage, at which time the patient is brought back for a further cholangiogram. If at this time the biliary system is clear and the patient's condition has normalized, the catheter is removed.

We generally do not dilate the stents in situ unless we are not leaving a safety catheter. If we are not leaving a safety catheter, then we dilate the stent in the area of the stricture with an 8-mm balloon to speed up the self-expanding process. The Wallstent is a self-expanding stent and tends to expand and shorten over time. It is an easy stent to deploy, but correct positioning is important or else the proximal end of the stent may shorten to lie within the tumor (Box 20-4).

Low Common Bile Duct Obstruction

The majority of patients with low CBD obstruction have pancreatic carcinoma. These patients are most often palliated endoscopically, but occasionally endoscopic stent insertion fails and the patient is referred for biliary drainage and stent placement. It is important not to place a metal stent if the patient is an operative candidate, so this information should be obtained by consultation

with the referring clinician or surgeon before the biliary drainage (Fig. 20-17). If the patient is not a candidate for surgery, then a stent can be placed at the time of initial biliary drainage. For patients with low CBD obstruction, it is not as important to gain peripheral access into the biliary tree, but it is again important to overstent and to ensure that there is no duodenal encasement by the pancreatic tumor. This can be done by injecting contrast material into the duodenal loop using the hockey-stick catheter when the tumor has been crossed. It is very important to do this before stenting. Obviously, if there is duodenal encasement, the stent will not provide effective palliation and the patient may need a gastro-jejunostomy or other form of surgical decompression. Occasionally, if the patient is not fit for surgery, a duodenal stent can be placed or a long-term internal/external drainage catheter can be placed with its tip placed in the proximal jejunum (Fig. 20-18).

The stent is placed in a similar fashion as for hilar stenting. Approximately 3-4 cm of the stent is placed above the proximal edge of the tumor and the distal end of the stent is left in the duodenum. Again, a safety catheter is not left in place if the procedure has been uneventful, but the stent is balloon dilated if a safety catheter is not left in situ (Box 20-5).

Aftercare

Correct catheter fixation to the skin is important for biliary drainage catheters because they are subject to the effects of liver movement during breathing, movement which can be significant. This is particularly true of right-sided biliary drainage catheters. If the catheter is tied tightly at the skin entry site, the catheter is not free to move with the liver as the patient breathes. If the catheter cannot move in and out because it is tied tightly at the skin, it tends to back out of the liver as the patient breathes and forms a loop between the liver capsule and the abdominal wall (Fig. 20-19). This can lead to drainage problems such as backbleeding through the catheter if a side hole migrates back into the liver and communicates with a vein (Fig. 20-20). Or, a side hole may migrate outside the liver and communicate with either the pleural space or abdominal cavity, leading to a bile leak. To avoid these problems, allow approximately 2 cm of slack in the catheter when suturing the catheter to the skin.

Daily rounds by a member of the interventional team are important to monitor these patients. The catheter is usually irrigated with 5 mL of saline every 6 hours for the first 48 hours. The patient is maintained on piperacillin/ tazobactam 4.5 g three times per day for 2-3 days after the procedure and is also maintained on intravenous fluids (2-2½ L of Hartman's solution daily for 48-72 hours). Intravenous fluids are important to correct choleresis, which is often marked in these patients and which may precipitate hepatorenal failure. The skin site should be inspected to make sure that the catheter has not backed out. The bag should also be inspected to ensure that there is no backbleeding into the bag. If problems are encountered with the catheter, the patient should be brought to the interventional suite for a cholangiogram and appropriate action taken.

Results

PBD should be technically successful achieving either internal drainage, external drainage, or stent placement in 95%-100% of patients with malignant bile duct obstruction. Similarly, effective palliation by catheter or stent placement should be possible in approximately 90% of patients. The success rates for metal stent placement are listed in Table 20-1. A recent study in 80 patients with low CBD obstruction who had Viabil-covered stents placed showed stent patency rates of 95.5%, 92.6%, and 85.7% at 3, 6, and 12 months, respectively. Complications occurred in 6.4%, including acute cholecystitis in three patients resulting from covering of the cystic duct.

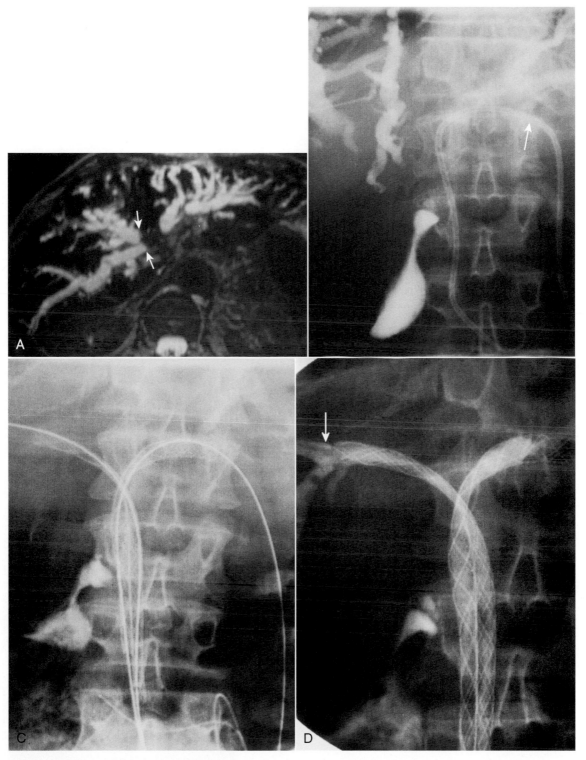

FIGURE 20-16. A 59-year-old patient with hilar cholangiocarcinoma unsuitable for surgery (Bismuth stage 3a). **A,** Axial reformatted view from magnetic res nce cholangiography shows separation of the anterior and posterior sectoral ducts on the right *(arrows)* with no segmental duct encasement on the left (Bismuth stage 3a). Because of the patient's young age, bilateral Y-stenting was performed. **B,** Peripheral access into the left segment-3 duct *(arrow)* was achieved with similar peripheral access on the right. **C,** 90- ×10-mm Wallstents were deployed over 0.035-inch superstiff guidewires. Both stents were dilated with an 8-mm balloon and a safety Ring catheter was left through the right-sided stent. **D,** Two days later the safety catheter was removed over a guidewire and injection was made through a 4-French dilator *(arrow)* at the proximal end of the right-sided stent. Good flow of contrast is seen in both stents. Note the peripheral access on both right and left lobes, which permits overstenting of the tumor. The patient survived for 18 months after the procedure without further jaundice or cholangitis.

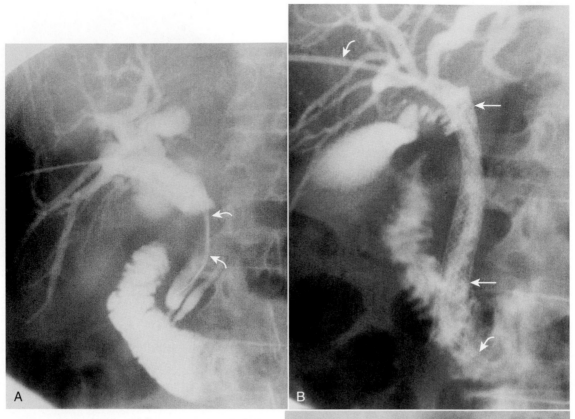

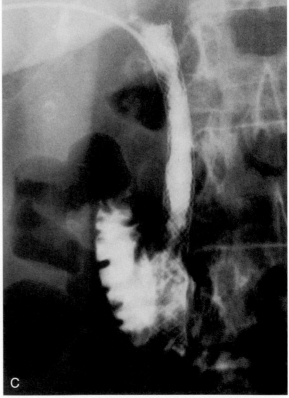

FIGURE 20-17. Metal stent placement in a patient with pancreatic cancer who had a failed endoscopic retrograde cholangiopancreatography. The patient had a low platelet count of 35,000 and received 6 units of platelets before the biliary drainage. **A,** Biliary drainage was performed and the stricture *(curved arrows)* was traversed with a hockey-stick catheter and hydrophilic guidewire. Note the normal duodenum without evidence of encasement. **B,** A 70- ×10-mm Wallstent was placed across the stricture *(straight arrows)* and a safety catheter was left in situ for 3 days *(curved arrows)* because of some bleeding at the time of the biliary drainage. **C,** The patient returned for a tube injection 3 days later. The stent was in good position and there was good flow of contrast into the duodenum. The safety catheter was removed.

Complications

Major complications related to PBD include hemorrhage, bile leak with potential biliary peritonitis, and sepsis. Major complications have been reported in approximately 5%-10% of patients (see Table 20-1). Death has also been reported with PBD in 1%-2.5% of patients. Most of these series describing PBD were from the early 1980s; with newer techniques the mortality rate should be less than 1%.

Hemobilia frequently occurs after biliary drainage but is almost always transient. Transgression of vascular structures with guidewires and catheters is to be expected during a biliary drainage,

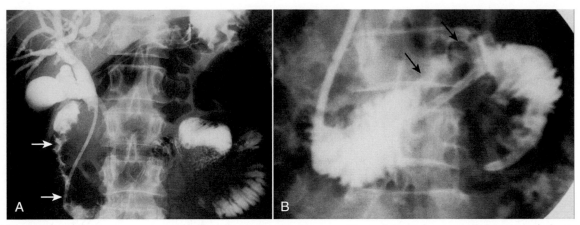

FIGURE 20-18. A patient with pancreatic cancer and encasement of the duodenum. **A,** During initial biliary drainage it was noted that the second part of the duodenum *(arrows)* and the fourth part of the duodenum (not shown) were encased. It was not practical to place a metal stent. The patient had a gastrojejunostomy to decompress the stomach. **B,** A long 14-French biliary Cope catheter (Cook, Bloomington, Ind.) was placed into the proximal jejunum and extra side holes cut in the catheter to provide appropriate biliary drainage. The catheter was clamped at the skin and provided adequate internal drainage for 3 months until the patient died. Note the stricture *(arrows)* in the fourth part of the duodenum also. An alternative approach in patients with a single stricture in the duodenum is to place a metal stent across the stricture.

Box 20-5. Low Common Bile Duct Obstruction and Metal Stents

Metal stent placed during biliary drainage if not an operative candidate and diagnosis known
Check for duodenal encasement
If no safety catheter, then stent is balloon-dilated

---

but bleeding usually settles over 2-3 days. Backbleeding through the catheter can occur if a catheter side hole is left in the hepatic parenchyma where it may communicate with a hepatic vein (Fig. 20-21). This can be remedied by repositioning the catheter during catheter cholangiography so that there is no venous communication. Serious hemorrhage is usually evidenced by a fall in the hematocrit, abdominal pain, and obvious hemobilia. Although hemobilia is frequent, severe or prolonged hemobilia occurs in fewer than 4% of patients. It is important before embarking on a PBD to correct any coagulation abnormality with fresh frozen plasma. It is also best to give the fresh frozen plasma before the procedure, during the procedure, and after the procedure because the half-life of fresh frozen plasma is short. In the author's unit, we generally administer 2 units of fresh frozen plasma before the procedure, 2 units during the procedure, and 2 units immediately after the procedure.

Hemobilia that presents after several days of drainage is usually more serious and requires immediate intervention. It may be due to either pseudoaneurysm formation or tumor bleeding. Replacing the catheter with a larger catheter often tamponades bleeding from a pseudoaneurysm. If bleeding continues, embolization should resolve the problem.

Tumor bleeding occurs in patients with hilar tumors that are managed by long-term internal/external drainage catheters. We generally do not see this problem because most patients with hilar cholangiocarcinomas are managed by indwelling metal stents. Tumor bleeding, if it does occur, is difficult to deal with and may not respond to embolization or to placement of a larger catheter.

Patients undergoing percutaneous biliary interventional procedures are prone to development of septicemia because the obstructed biliary system may be infected in as many as 25%-50% of patients with malignant obstruction. Bacteremia almost invariably occurs in these patients with infected and obstructed biliary systems. For these reasons, appropriate antibiotic coverage is

mandatory before undertaking biliary interventional procedures. Despite appropriate antibiotic coverage, septicemia may occur in these patients. A number of patients have developed septicemic shock after biliary drainage despite adequate coverage with ampicillin and gentamicin. In the author's unit, we have therefore changed our antibiotic regimen to piperacillin/tazobactam 4.5 g three times per day. The antibiotic is started either on the morning of the PBD, or the day before, if the procedure is anticipated. We also continue the antibiotic regimen for 2 days after the biliary drainage because we have seen septic shock develop within 24 hours after biliary drainage.

In patients, who are septicemic before the procedure with high temperature and white cell count, it is best to perform the minimum intervention necessary. The biliary tree should not be overdistended with contrast material, and it may be appropriate to simply place an external biliary drainage catheter rather than place an internal/external catheter. After appropriate antibiotic therapy and drainage, the patient can return to the interventional suite in 2-3 days for further definitive drainage.

Bile leak and biliary peritonitis can cause severe abdominal pain and tenderness. For unknown reasons, the presence of even small amounts of bile in the peritoneal cavity can cause a severe chemical peritonitis in some patients, while the presence of large amounts of bile in the peritoneal cavity in other patients does not appear to cause any symptoms. Bile leaks can be avoided with careful technique and experience. It is important when performing a biliary drainage that dilators and catheters not be removed from the liver until the next dilator or catheter is ready to be placed. This minimizes the amount of time that the guidewire is present in the percutaneous track by itself. If the track has been dilated and only the guidewire is present in the track, then bile can flow out along the guidewire into the peritoneal cavity. Similarly, the use of a 9-French peel-away sheath helps protect the peritoneal cavity from biliary leaks because the bile leaks externally through the 9-French peel-away sheath during catheter manipulations. In addition, proper fixation of the catheter and proper siting of the catheter within the biliary tree is important to prevent the catheter from backing out of the biliary tree and possibly having side-hole communication with the peritoneal cavity. Lastly, embolizing the percutaneous track with Gelfoam or glue when removing catheters helps prevent bile leakage or bleeding through the track.

Other complications that have been reported with PBD, such as pneumothorax, empyema, or bilious pleural effusion, may occur due to the use of a transpleural approach, which is necessitated by the location of the liver. It is important that the catheter is sited properly so that a side hole does not communicate with the pleural space (Box 20-6).

Immediate complications related to metal stent insertion are usually similar to those for PBD techniques. Careful positioning of the metal stent is important to allow for stent shortening so that adequate coverage of the stricture is obtained. Migration is rare with metallic stents. Late complications of metallic stent insertion include occlusion and tumor ingrowth. The relative frequency of these is shown in Table 20-2. The incidence of occlusion and/or cholangitis requiring intervention varies between 7% and 20% in reported series.

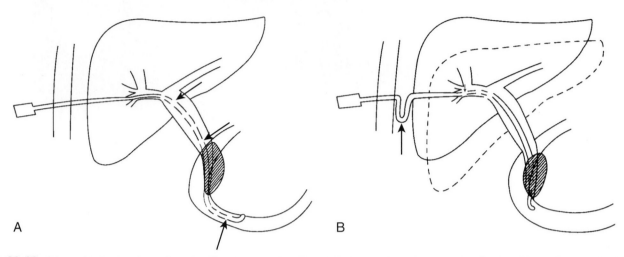

FIGURE 20-19. Schematic showing the catheter buckling between the skin and the liver owing to inappropriate fixation of the catheter at the skin entry site. **A,** Biliary catheter appropriately placed with side holes *(arrows)* above and below the stricture in the lower bile duct. **B,** If the catheter is fixed tightly at the skin entry site, ascent and descent of the liver during respiration cause the catheter to back slowly out of the liver and form a loop *(arrow)* between the abdominal wall and the liver. This may result in a catheter side hole *(small arrow)* lying close to or within the hepatic parenchyma and possibly communicating with a hepatic or portal vein. If this happens, back bleeding can occur. In addition, it can be technically difficult to straighten this loop if it is large, because any guidewire inserted may cause the loop to enlarge and the catheter may flip completely out of the liver.

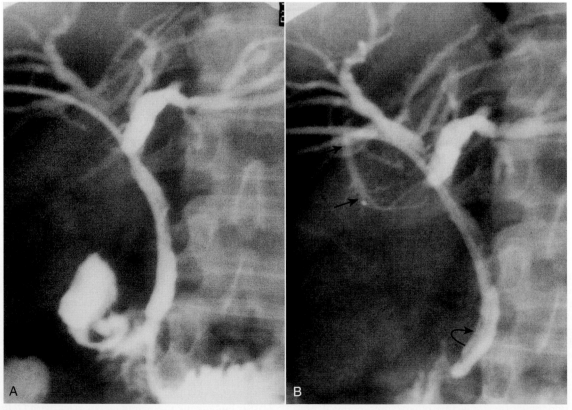

FIGURE 20-20. Example of backbleeding in a patient with hilar cholangiocarcinoma. **A,** A catheter inserted from the right at the time of initial biliary drainage shows good flow of contrast both proximally in the bile duct and distally in the duodenum at the end of the procedure. **B,** The next day the patient had dark blood appearing through the catheter in the drainage bag. The patient returned to the radiology department for catheter injection. Catheter injection shows communication with a hepatic vein branch *(straight arrows)*. Note also the catheter has migrated proximally *(curved arrow)*, with the tip of the catheter now lying in the distal bile duct rather than in the duodenum. This was rectified by inserting the catheter more distally into the duodenum using a guidewire.

Special Considerations

External Biliary Drainage

External biliary drainage is rarely performed. It involves leaving a catheter in the biliary tree above the level of obstruction. In general, with hydrophilic guidewires it is usually straightforward to cross most biliary obstructions at the first sitting. However, before the advent of hydrophilic guidewires it was not unusual to perform an external biliary drainage and 1-2 days later convert the external drainage to internal/external biliary drainage. The indications for performing external biliary drainage now include a patient with septicemic shock due to cholangitis in whom the minimum intervention necessary to drain the patient is appropriate (Fig. 20-22).

Other indications would include a patient with a bile duct stricture or transection at laparoscopic cholecystectomy. Drainage of the intrahepatic biliary tree by an external biliary drainage catheter helps temporize the patient before definitive surgery.

When performing an external biliary drainage, the catheter used is important. The catheter needs to have a relatively small pigtail with relatively large side holes to promote biliary drainage. A 5- or 7-French angiographic pigtail catheter is not appropriate because it does not drain well and tends to fall out. The catheter the author uses is an 8-French locking pigtail catheter designed for percutaneous cholecystostomy (Cook, Bloomington, Ind.). This catheter has a small pigtail with relatively large side holes; it is easy to place and provides good drainage.

TABLE 20-1 Metal Stent Results

Author	Patients	Tech Success (%)	Complications (%)	Occlusion Rate(%)
Lee (1992)	34	100	0	12
Becker (1993)	58	100	24	26
Rossi (1994)	240	-	8	22
Lee (1997)	100	-	-	21
Oikarinen (1999)	39	97	30	-
Inal (2003)	154	-	28	-

Box 20-6. Preventing Complications

Appropriate antibiotic prophylaxis for biliary sepsis
Intravenous fluids to prevent hepatorenal failure
Backbleeding prevented by appropriate catheter positioning
Fresh frozen plasma to correct coagulopathy
If cholangitis present, minimum intervention to drain the biliary tree
9-French peel-away minimizes bile leak and protects liver parenchyma
Catheter fixation allowing "slack" in the catheter

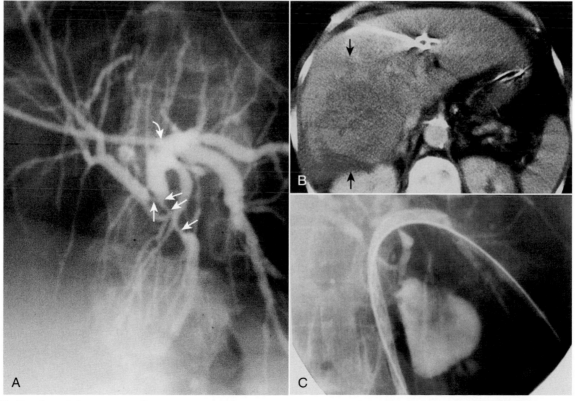

FIGURE 20-21. Intrahepatic hemorrhage after biliary drainage in a patient referred from another hospital. **A,** Right-sided access shows the catheter tip in the left hepatic duct *(curved arrow)*. A cholangiocarcinoma with stricture *(small arrows)* involving the origin of the right and left hepatic ducts is noted in the common hepatic duct. Attempts to manipulate guidewires from the left hepatic duct into the common hepatic duct were unsuccessful. The patient's hematocrit fell and pain developed. An external catheter was left in situ and the patient returned to the ward. Attempts to manipulate catheters and guidewires from the left hepatic duct into the common hepatic duct from a right-sided access is not advised because of the acute angulation involved. **B,** A computed tomography scan performed shortly afterward revealed a large right intrahepatic hemorrhage *(arrows)*. **C,** After a 7-day interval during which the patient's symptoms subsided, a left-sided biliary drainage was performed and a 90- ×10-mm Wallstent was placed from the left side across the stricture. The intrahepatic hematoma spontaneously resolved over the ensuing months.

Long-Term Internal/External Biliary Drainage

As with external biliary drainage, the long-term use of internal/external biliary drainage catheters is no longer common. The advent of metallic stents has proved a much more effective and more comfortable method for palliating malignant biliary obstruction. Long-term internal/external biliary drainage catheters may be used after balloon dilatation of anastomotic strictures and in

TABLE 20-2 Benign Biliary Strictures

Author	Patients	Success (%)	Follow-Up (Months)
Mueller	73	67	24
Williams	74	78	30
Russell	23	100	?
Citron	17	70.5	32
Gallacher	13	77	8-30
Lee	14	93	38
Pitta	25	88	60
Davids*	35	83	50
Bezzi	180	82	68
Kocher	21	94	12
Bonnel	110	90	59

*Surgical series.

patients with duodenal encasement from pancreatic carcinoma where a metal stent cannot be placed.

The catheter used for long-term internal/external biliary drainage is usually a 10- or 12-French catheter rather than the 8.3-French Ring catheter placed at initial biliary drainage. The larger bore catheters are more difficult to place initially and an 8.3-French catheter is appropriate at the time of initial biliary drainage. The track can then be dilated over the ensuing week to 12-French and a 12-French Cope (Cook, Bloomington, Ind.) or Flexima (Boston Scientific, Natick, Mass.) catheter placed. When the 12-French catheter is placed, it is left to free drainage for 1-2 days and then clamped, as long as the patient has no fever. If the patient tolerates catheter clamping, the patient can be discharged. The idea is that bile will drain through the side holes above the obstruction, through the catheter, and out the side holes below the obstruction into the duodenum. The patient is given a bag to take home and if fever develops, the patient is instructed to attach the bag to the catheter for free drainage and to return to the interventional radiology department for further management. These catheters need replacement every 2-3 months, or sooner if catheter occlusion or fever occurs.

■ TISSUE DIAGNOSIS OF MALIGNANT BILIARY OBSTRUCTION

Obtaining a tissue diagnosis for patients with biliary obstruction is important, particularly if radiotherapy or other forms of nonsurgical therapy are being considered. The simplest way of obtaining cells for cytologic evaluation is to send a sample of bile obtained

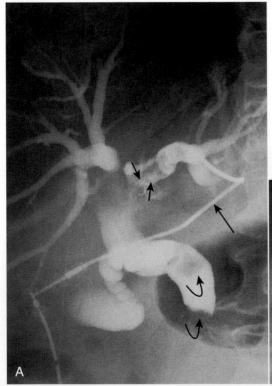
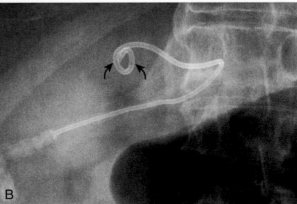

FIGURE 20-22. External biliary drainage performed in a 75-year-old patient with ascending cholangitis secondary to choledocholithiasis. The patient was profoundly hypotensive, in respiratory distress, and with a platelet count of 43,000. The patient was given 8 units of platelets and an external biliary drainage was performed. **A,** A left-sided external biliary drainage was performed instead of a right-sided biliary drainage so that splinting of the diaphragm and further respiratory distress would not occur. A cholangiogram performed 3 days after the procedure shows a catheter *(large arrow)* sited in the left hepatic duct with stones *(curved arrows)* in the lower bile duct causing the obstruction. Some blood *(small arrows)* is present within the bile duct resulting from the biliary drainage procedure. The patient settled with external biliary drainage, and because of the patient's age, a double pigtail stent was placed percutaneously after 5 days. **B,** Note the small size of the pigtail *(curved arrows)* on this catheter (Cook, Bloomington, Ind.). The catheter is 8.5-French and is ideally suited for external biliary drainage.

during the initial biliary drainage to the histopathology laboratory. The bile is best collected after the stricture has been traversed and before the final internal/external biliary drainage catheter is placed. Collecting the bile sample at this time helps increase the diagnostic yield from bile cytology, in that malignant cells may be shed into the biliary tree after manipulation of guidewires, for example, through the malignant stricture. Just before placing the internal/external biliary drainage catheter, the hockey-stick catheter is placed through the 9-French peel-away sheath to a level just above the stricture and a sample of bile obtained for bile cytology. Bile cytology is successfully used to establish a diagnosis in approximately 40%-60% of cases.

If bile cytology is negative or inconclusive, biliary brushing can be performed. For this procedure a small brush, similar to that used for bronchoscopic brushing of strictured bronchi, is placed through a 9-French peel-away sheath and vigorous brushing of the internal lumen of the stricture is performed. The brush is then removed through the 9-French sheath and a sample spread on a glass slide. This can be repeated a number of times until sufficient samples are obtained. Some operators have also used atherectomy catheters to obtain cells for diagnosis. The author has not done this because biliary brushing usually suffices.

Brushing is only appropriate for malignant strictures primarily originating in the bile duct. For patients with pancreatic carcinoma, the mass can be biopsied percutaneously.

■ PERCUTANEOUS BILIARY DRAINAGE AFTER FAILED ENDOSCOPIC RETROGRADE CHOLANGIOPANCREATOGRAPHY

The author's unit is often asked to perform a PBD after a failed ERCP in patients with malignant biliary obstruction. Some interventional radiologists perform the PBD immediately after the failed ERCP, but, unless the patient is febrile or requires immediate drainage, we prefer to wait a few hours when resedation is less difficult. Patients are usually given a significant amount of sedoanalgesia for the endoscopic procedure and may even be given reversal agents at the end of the procedure, making it difficult to resedate the patient for the PBD. We have found that patients are often very uncomfortable during the PBD, making PBD technically difficult and perhaps more prone to complications.

The other determining factor with regard to how soon the PBD should be performed after the ERCP is whether contrast material has been injected above the level of obstruction. If not, the PBD can be postponed for a number of days as long as the patient does not have signs of sepsis. If, however, contrast material has been injected above the level of obstruction, the biliary drainage should be performed relatively soon after the ERCP. If the ERCP has been performed in the morning with contrast material injected above the obstruction, the biliary drainage is performed in the afternoon. If the ERCP is performed in the evening and contrast material has not been injected above the level of obstruction, then the biliary drainage is performed the following day. If the ERCP is performed in the afternoon or the evening and contrast material has been injected above the level of obstruction, we generally place the patient on intravenous fluids and antibiotics and perform the biliary drainage early the next morning (Box 20-7).

■ INTERVENTIONAL MANAGEMENT OF LAPAROSCOPIC CHOLECYSTECTOMY COMPLICATIONS

The advent of laparoscopic cholecystectomy has dramatically changed the treatment of gallstone disease. Most patients prefer a laparoscopic cholecystectomy rather than an open cholecystectomy because of shorter hospital stay, less pain, and a quicker return to work. Bile duct injuries with laparoscopic cholecystectomy have been reported to occur up to 10 times more frequently than with open cholecystectomy. However, with experience, the complication rate declines and in most large series the complication rate is less than 1%.

The most frequent complication is bile leakage. This usually occurs when surgical clips slip from the cystic duct or occasionally small ducts that drain the gallbladder directly into the liver may leak after the gallbladder is laparoscopically removed. Bile tends to collect in the gallbladder fossa, subhepatic space, subphrenic space, or paracolic gutter. Bile accumulation can be managed by one or more percutaneous drains placed under ultrasound or CT guidance. If there is a leak from the cystic duct stump, then endoscopic stenting of the bile duct helps decrease the amount of leakage. The more serious complications include bile duct injury and ligation. Bile duct injury or ligation may result from aberrant biliary anatomy such as a left-sided entry of the cystic duct into the common bile duct, or indeed mistaking the common bile duct for the cystic duct.

Key points in the management of these patients include delineation of the anatomy, defining the site and nature of the bile duct injury, and diverting bile away from the site of biliary leakage. If the bile duct is intact and there is leakage only from the cystic duct stump, then retrograde stenting by ERCP is appropriate. However, if the bile duct has been injured and there is associated leakage, then drainage and stenting is best performed percutaneously. With ligation, the intrahepatic bile ducts can be drained percutaneously by leaving an external biliary drainage catheter above the level of the ligation. Any associated bile leakage can be drained percutaneously. After a number of weeks of drainage, the patient returns to theater for a definitive reconstructive procedure. By allowing time for the inflammation and effects of the first surgery to settle, the reconstructive surgery is made easier (Box 20-8).

■ REINTERVENTION FOR METAL STENT OCCLUSION

The average patency rate for metallic stents in the biliary tree is approximately 6 months. Metallic stents do occlude and may require further reintervention. Occlusion is usually manifested by recurrent jaundice or cholangitis. These patients can be managed by percutaneous reintervention or endoscopic intervention. The causes of occlusion are either tumor overgrowth at the upper or lower end of the stent, tumor ingrowth through the wire mesh of the stent, or occlusive debris clogging the stent. Tumor overgrowth can be prevented by overstenting of the stricture.

Box 20-7. Biliary Drainage After Failed Endoscopic Retrograde Cholangiopancreatography

If no contrast material injected and patient not septic, percutaneous biliary drainage (PBD) within 2 days
If septic, drain immediately
If contrast material injected above obstruction, start intravenous fluids and antibiotics and do PBD within 8-12 hours

---

Box 20-8. Laparoscopic Cholecystectomy and Bile Duct Injury

Delineate anatomy by percutaneous transhepatic cholangiography (PTC)
Define site and nature of bile duct injury: PTC/endoscopic retrograde cholangiopancreatography
Divert bile from site of biliary leakage: external biliary drainage and/or endoscopic stent placement
Drain intraabdominal collections: percutaneous abscess drainage

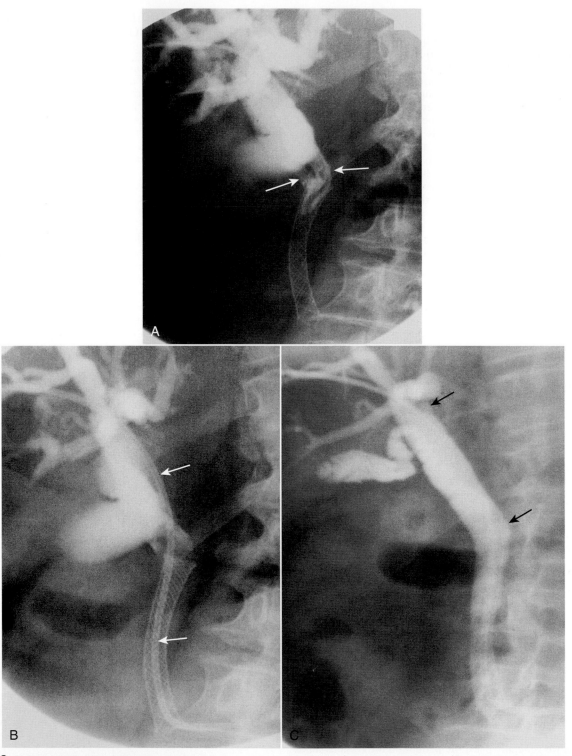

FIGURE 20-23. Reintervention for metal stent occlusion. A patient with pancreatic cancer who had a metal stent placed 5 months earlier returned to the hospital with recurrent jaundice and cholangitis. **A,** A percutaneous transhepatic cholangiography showed tumor overgrowth above the stent *(arrows)*. **B,** A guidewire was manipulated down through the stent and a Ring catheter *(arrows)* placed into the duodenum. **C,** A second metal stent was placed through the first with an appropriate overlap above the tumor *(arrows)*.

Tumor ingrowth cannot be prevented but occurs less commonly. For patients with tumor overgrowth above the stent, a PBD can be performed and a guidewire manipulated down through the stent into the duodenum. The tumor above the stent can then be dilated and a second Wallstent inserted in a sleeved fashion through the first Wallstent (Fig. 20-23). Similarly, patients with tumor ingrowth can be managed with balloon dilatation of the first stent in the region of the tumor ingrowth and placement of a

second stent. Lastly, patients with stent occlusion by inspissated debris or sludge can be managed by manipulating a guidewire down through the lumen of the occluded stent and using a balloon catheter to sweep the occluded metal stent clear of debris. As with patients for primary biliary drainage, these patients need intravenous antibiotic coverage as well as intravenous fluids.

Another approach to metal stent occlusion is the endoscopic or retrograde approach. Depending on the operator's level of expertise, the referral pattern, and the clinical state of the patient, it may be appropriate to place a plastic stent through the existing metal stent at ERCP to reinstate drainage.

PERCUTANEOUS MANAGEMENT OF BENIGN BILIARY STRICTURE

Percutaneous balloon dilatation of benign biliary stricture has been in use since early reports first described the technique in the 1970s. It is a procedure associated with low morbidity and may avoid the necessity of complex hepatobiliary operations.

Indications

Percutaneous balloon dilatation of biliary strictures is most often performed in patients with anastomotic strictures such as choledochojejunal or hepaticojejunal anastomoses. Patients with iatrogenic strictures of the bile duct are also suitable candidates for percutaneous biliary dilatation. Patients with sclerosing cholangitis may benefit from balloon dilatation as long as there is a dominant stricture. Biliary strictures due to pancreatitis or biliary calculi can be balloon-dilated, but these are usually dilated at ERCP rather than by the percutaneous route.

Preprocedure Evaluation

In patients with anastomotic strictures, imaging findings may be misleading. CT and ultrasound may show no dilated intrahepatic bile ducts. However, patients with anastomotic strictures often have episodes of cholangitis with rigors requiring oral and/ or intravenous antibiotics. The patient is usually asymptomatic between attacks and often may not present for evaluation until a number of attacks have occurred. The most sensitive indicator of anastomotic stricture formation is the serum alkaline phosphatase level, which is almost invariably elevated. The role of MRC in imaging these patients is unclear. It is, however, an attractive noninvasive method of obtaining cholangiogram-like images to look at the hepaticojejunal anastomosis and intrahepatic biliary tree.

Patients with iatrogenic strictures usually present either immediately or soon after the initial surgical procedure. Usually, ERCP is first performed in these patients and MR cholangiopancreatography or PTC may be necessary to give full anatomic delineation of the abnormality.

Technique

Patient Preparation

As with other biliary procedures, broad-spectrum antibiotic coverage is mandatory for biliary dilatation. Sedoanalgesia is even more important because many patients experience considerable pain during the balloon inflation process. Indeed, in the author's unit we performed this procedure with the patient under general anesthesia in earlier years, but now with appropriate use of sedoanalgesia this is not necessary. The combination of midazolam and fentanyl works extremely well to control patient pain. A loading dose followed by regular aliquots of both drugs should be administered throughout the procedure. When planning a retrograde access through a jejunal Roux loop, then a CT scan of the abdomen is useful before embarking upon the procedure to confirm the location of the Roux loop and to ascertain the position of the colon vis-à-vis the loop (Box 20-9).

Biliary Access

The traditional method of access is transhepatic with dilatation of a track through the liver parenchyma and placement of a balloon catheter across the stricture site. A less traumatic access is the use of a retrograde access through the Roux loop. Some surgeons

---

Box 20-9. Biliary Stricture Dilatation: Patient Preparation

Appropriate broad-spectrum antibiotic prophylaxis
Baseline serum alkaline phosphatase level performed
Magnetic resonance cholangiography performed
Computed tomography to assess position of Roux loop
Liberal sedoanalgesia

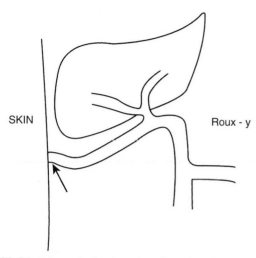

FIGURE 20-24. Schematic showing a long Roux loop brought out to the skin after creation of a biliary enteric anastomosis. A long limb on the Roux loop *(arrow)* can be brought out to the skin and sutured underneath the skin. The position of the loop can be marked with metal clips or a metal ring, providing access for any future percutaneous biliary intervention.

when fashioning the Roux loop for the hepaticojejunostomy or choledochojejunostomy fix a portion of the Roux loop anteriorly underneath the abdominal wall (Fig. 20-24). The loop is then marked with either a metallic suture or a circular metallic ring. By marking the Roux loop and fixing the loop underneath the anterior abdominal wall, the loop can be accessed under fluoroscopic guidance and guidewires and catheters placed retrogradely through the loop up into the intrahepatic biliary tree. This avoids the necessity for transhepatic access. Even if the surgeon has not fixed the Roux loop underneath the anterior abdominal wall, the loop can still be used for retrograde access (Fig. 20-25). A transhepatic cholangiogram is first performed and contrast is injected into the intrahepatic biliary tree. When contrast enters the Roux loop, the loop can be punctured under fluoroscopic guidance and used for biliary access. When performing this procedure it is important to first perform a CT scan to ascertain where the colon is in relation to the Roux loop. Lateral screening also helps to identify the most anterior portion of the Roux loop for puncture.

Performing the Dilatation

It can occasionally be difficult to determine whether there is some evidence of narrowing at the anastomotic site. Some operators have used biliary manometry to help decide whether there is a real obstruction present or not. However, in the author's unit we have found this cumbersome and difficult to interpret. Instead, we place a 10-mm balloon across the anastomosis and inflate the balloon. Presence of a stricture is determined by the presence of a waist in the balloon. The balloon is inflated until the waist disappears (see Fig. 20-25). The number of balloon dilatations per session, the length of time the balloon remains inflated, and the number of sessions vary widely between different operators. Some authors inflate the balloon for variable

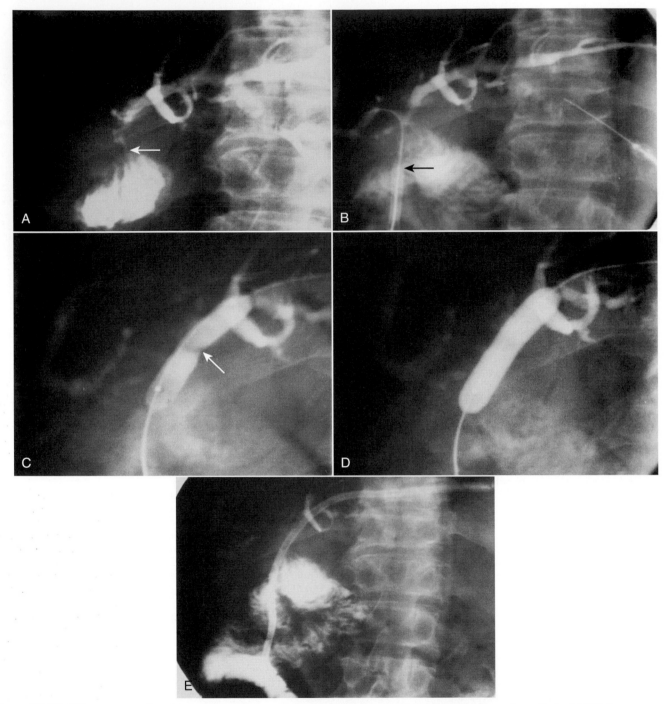

FIGURE 20-25. Biliary anastomotic stricture dilatation in a patient with multiple previous biliary operative procedures. **A,** An initial left percutaneous transhepatic cholangiography was performed to outline the biliary tree and define the Roux loop. Note the stricture *(arrow)* at the biliary enteric anastomosis. **B,** Using the contrast material in the Roux loop as a guide, the Roux loop was punctured percutaneously from the anterior abdominal wall using a one-stick needle system. A hockey-stick catheter was used to access the biliary tree and a peel-away sheath *(arrow)* placed within the Roux loop. **C,** A 12-mm balloon was placed across the strictured anastomotic site. A waist *(arrow)* can be seen in the center of the lumen. **D,** The balloon was inflated until the waist disappeared and for a total time of 2 minutes. **E,** Finally, a 12-French biliary Cope catheter was placed across the stricture into the left hepatic ducts. A catheter injection performed 3 weeks later showed a patent anastomosis and the catheter was removed.

periods from 30 seconds to 15-20 minutes and repeat until the waist on the balloon disappears. Others leave the balloon inflated for up to 2 hours. We inflate the balloon for 2-3 minutes and repeat the procedure until the waist disappears. In many instances the waist on the 10-mm balloon is minimal, so a 12-mm balloon is used.

The role of long-term stenting of the dilated stricture is also controversial. Some authors advocate leaving a long-term stent across the anastomosis for 6-12 months. We prefer to leave the

catheter across the stricture for 3-4 weeks. Normally a 10- to 12-French soft catheter (Cope Loop, Cook, Bloomington, Ind.) is left across the anastomosis. The catheter can be clamped and the patient discharged with the catheter in situ. After 3-4 weeks, the patient returns as an outpatient for a cholangiogram. If the anastomosis appears widely patent, then the catheter is removed. If the anastomosis is not patent, the balloon dilatation is repeated and the catheter left for another 3-4 weeks (Box 20-10).

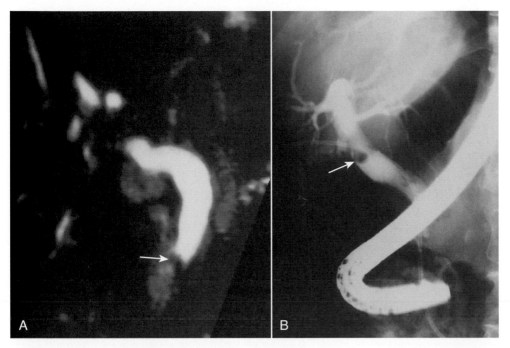

FIGURE 20-26. Rendezvous procedure in a patient with failed endoscopic retrograde cholangiopancreatography (ERCP). **A,** Coronal image from magnetic resonance cholangiopancreatography examination shows a stone *(arrow)* at the lower end of the bile duct in this patient who failed ERCP. **B,** A transhepatic biliary drainage was performed and a Ring catheter manipulated across the bile duct into the duodenum. Note the stone *(arrow)* in the common bile duct. At ERCP the next day, a guidewire passed through the percutaneous catheter was snared by the endoscopist and pulled out through the mouth. Access to the bile duct was then assured for further biliary manipulation. In this case, a sphincterotomy was performed and the stone removed.

Box 20-10. Biliary Stricture Dilatation: Key Points

Percutaneous transhepatic cholangiography to delineate anatomy and identify Roux loop
Puncture Roux loop and negotiate anastomosis
10-mm balloon followed by 12-mm balloon
14-French biliary catheter inserted through Roux loop
Catheter removed after 3 weeks if open anastomosis

Metallic Stents for Benign Biliary Stricture

The use of metallic stents for benign biliary strictures has been reported in the literature. In general, it is used as a last resort when benign biliary strictures fail to respond to balloon dilatation. In the author's unit, our practice is to perform at least three separate balloon dilatations before resorting to metallic stenting. Additionally, the age and condition of the patient is important. If the patient is young, surgical revision may be the best option if balloon dilatation fails. If the patient is older, then perhaps metallic stenting is appropriate. The procedure should first be discussed with the referring surgeon or clinician. If it is decided to place the metallic stent, then a Gianturco-Rosch stent should be placed rather than a Wallstent. The Gianturco-Rosch stent exerts a stronger radial force and presents a lesser surface area for the development of intimal hyperplasia. It is therefore the preferred stent for dealing with recalcitrant biliary strictures.

Results

The success rate of balloon dilatation for benign biliary strictures is listed in Table 20-2. In earlier reports the success rate varied from 50% to 90%. One of the criticisms of earlier reports was the fact that follow-up tended to be short, with a maximum follow-up of approximately 3 years. Two newer studies report longer-term follow-up with patency rates of 80%-90% over 9 years. This compares very favorably with reports from surgical series.

Surgical repair of benign biliary strictures has a long-term (5-year follow-up) success rate which varies between 70% and 80% at the first attempt, but decreases exponentially after each unsuccessful attempt at surgical repair. The success rate of a third operation is approximately 60%. It would seem that surgery is the best initial option for patients with iatrogenic strictures, but percutaneous balloon dilatation should be used for the management of patients who present with anastomotic strictures. Anastomotic strictures develop in approximately 15%-25% of patients who undergo surgical repair of iatrogenic strictures. A surgical policy of fixing the Roux loop underneath the anterior abdominal wall would facilitate the further management of patients in whom anastomotic strictures develop.

Balloon dilatation of strictures in patients with sclerosing cholangitis has a lower success rate, varying between 42% and 59%. However, for patients with sclerosing cholangitis, balloon dilatation may represent the only form of treatment available, particularly for intrahepatic ductal strictures. It is worthwhile to dilate dominant strictures in patients with sclerosing cholangitis because significant improvement of patient well-being may occur. Indeed, the last resort for these patients is liver transplantation if multiple complex strictures are present.

Complications associated with this procedure are those associated with biliary drainage (discussed previously).

▬ PERCUTANEOUS MANAGEMENT OF COMMON BILE DUCT STONES

Most common bile duct stones are removed endoscopically, which is the best option for most patients. In some situations, endoscopic removal is not possible. ERCP may be unsuccessful because of previous gastric surgery, because of a large diverticulum at the ampulla of Vater, or because of other technical problems.

If ERCP is unsuccessful, a number of methods can be used to remove or manage common bile duct stones. The preferred method in the author's unit is the rendezvous procedure (Fig. 20-26). Standard biliary drainage is performed and an internal/external biliary drainage catheter left in the duodenum. After 1-2 days, an ERCP is performed. An exchange length guidewire is passed through the internal/external biliary drainage catheter and used by the endoscopist to facilitate bile duct cannulation. In this way, the stones can be removed endoscopically.

If the rendezvous procedure is not possible because of altered upper gastrointestinal anatomy, alternatives include open surgical removal of the common bile duct stones or transhepatic stone removal. Depending on the size of the stones present, the transhepatic approach can be used to perform a sphincteroplasty by inflating a 10-mm balloon across the sphincter Oddi and pushing any small stones into the duodenum with a semiinflated balloon.

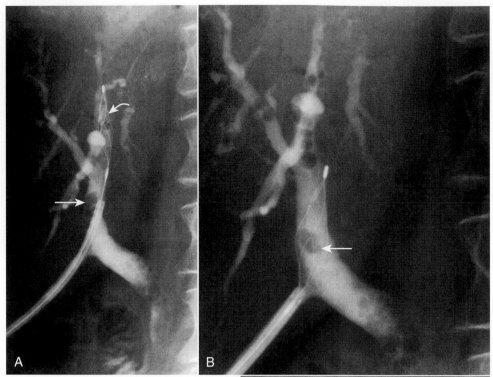

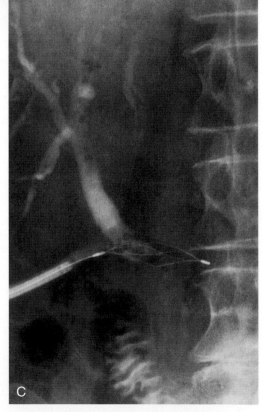

Figure 20-27. Percutaneous extraction of a retained common bile duct stone through a T-tube track. **A,** The T-tube has been removed and a steerable Burhenne catheter placed through the percutaneous track into the bile duct to the level of the stone *(small arrow)*. A basket *(curved arrow)* has been placed distal to the stone. **B,** The basket is pulled back and manipulated so that the stone *(arrow)* is engaged within the basket and the basket is then pulled back against the end of the Burhenne catheter. Basket, stone, and Burhenne catheter are then removed through the percutaneous track. **C,** There is some air present in the lower bile duct. The basket was traversed through the lower bile duct but no further stones were present. Contrast injection at the end of the procedure showed a clear bile duct.

Transhepatic stone removal is rarely performed, but if it is to be performed, a mature tract through the liver is required. This involves initial PBD and sequential tract dilatation up to 14- to 16-French size, followed by basket extraction of the stones. If the stones are larger, mechanical lithotripsy can be performed to crush the stones before removal.

Percutaneous Extraction of Common Bile Duct Stones Through T-Tube Tract

If the patient has a postoperative T-tube in place, then ERCP is inappropriate because any retained stones can be removed easily through the percutaneous tract (Fig. 20-27). If stone removal through the T-tube tract is planned, the T-tube is left in situ for 4-6 weeks until a mature tract develops. Patients return to the hospital for stone removal and are given standard antibiotic prophylaxis. A T-tube cholangiogram is performed to confirm that the stones are still present. In many instances, the stones may have passed in the interval. If a stone is not present, the T-tube can be removed.

If a stone is still present, extraction is required. The T-tube is removed over a guidewire and access to the duodenum is achieved using a combination of a hydrophilic wire and Kumpe catheter. A superstiff wire is placed in the duodenum and left as a safety wire. A steerable catheter (Burhenne) is placed in the bile duct through the percutaneous T-tube tract. The handle of the Burhenne is used to deflect the tip of the catheter so that the catheter can be manipulated either up or down the bile duct, depending upon where the stone is located. The Burhenne catheter is placed a little distal to the stone and a basket placed through the Burhenne catheter. The basket is opened distal to the stone, and the Burhenne catheter and basket are slowly withdrawn until the stone is reached. The Burhenne catheter and basket are then jiggled so that the stone falls within the basket. The basket is then pulled back against the end of the Burhenne catheter to grip the stone, and the Burhenne catheter and basket are removed as a unit from the bile duct through the percutaneous tract. If the stone is too large to be removed through the percutaneous tract, the stone can be fragmented by electrohydraulic, laser, or mechanical lithotripsy. (See the section on percutaneous cholecystolithotomy in Chapter 21.) After the procedure, a 12-French catheter is left in the duodenum for 2-3 days if significant edema is present at the ampulla. If the procedure has been atraumatic then no catheter need be left.

▓▓▓ SUGGESTED READINGS

Bezzi M, Bonomo G, Salvatori FM, et al. Ten years follow-up percutaneous management if benign biliary strictures: how successful are we? *RSNA 1995. Radiol Suppl.* 1995;197:241.

Diamond T, Parks RW. Perioperative management of obstructive jaundice. *Br J Surg.* 1997;84:147-149.

Fanelli F, Orgera G, Bezzi M, et al. Management of malignant biliary obstruction: Technical and clinical results using an expanded polytetrafluoroethylene fluorinated ethylene propylene (ePTFE/FEP)-covered metallic stent after 6 year experience. *Eur Radiol.* 2008;18:911-919.

Gazelle GS, Lee MJ, Mueller PR. Cholangiographic segmental anatomy of the liver: implications for interventional radiology. *Semin Interv Radiol.* 1995;12(2):119-125.

Hausegger KA, Kugler C, Uggowitzer M, et al. Benign biliary obstruction: is treatment with the Wallstent advisable? *Radiology.* 1996;200:437-441.

Lammer J, Hausegger KA, Fluckiger F, et al. Common bile duct obstruction due to malignancy: treatment with plastic versus metal stents. *Radiology.* 1996;201:167-172.

Lee MJ, Mueller PR, Saini S, Hahn PF, Dawson SL. Percutaneous dilatation of benign biliary strictures: single-session therapy with general anesthesia. *Am J Roentgenol.* 1991;157:1263-1266.

Lee MJ, Dawson SL, Mueller PR, et al. Palliation of malignant bile duct obstruction with metallic biliary endoprostheses: technique, results, and complications. *J Vasc Interv Radiol.* 1992;3:665-671.

Lee MJ, Dawson SL, Mueller PR, et al. Percutaneous management of hilar biliary malignancies with metallic endoprostheses: results, technical problems, and causes of failure. *Radiographics.* 1993;13:1249-1263.

Lee MJ, Dawson SL, Mueller PR, et al. Failed metallic biliary stents: causes and management of delayed complications. *Clin Radiol.* 1994;49:857-862.

Mathisen O, Bergan A, Flatmark A. Iatrogenic bile duct injuries. *World J Surg.* 1987;11:392-397.

McNicholas MMJ, Lee MJ, Dawson SL, Mueller PR. Complications of percutaneous biliary drainage and stricture dilatation. *Semin Interv Radiol.* 1994;11(3):242-253.

Morrison MC, Lee MJ, Saini A, Brink JA, Meuller PR. Percutaneous balloon dilatation of benign biliary strictures. *Radiol Clin N Am.* 1990;28:1191-1201.

Mueller PR, vanSonnenberg E, Ferrucci JT, et al. Biliary stricture dilatation: multicenter review of clinical management in 73 patients. *Radiology.* 1986;160:17-22.

Rossi P, Bezzi M, Salvatori FM, Maccioni F, Porcaro M. Recurrent benign biliary strictures: management with self-expanding metallic stents. *Radiology.* 1990;175:661-665.

Russell E, Yrizarry JM, Huber JS, et al. Percutaneous transjejunal biliary dilatation: alternate management for benign strictures. *Radiology.* 1986;159:209-214.

Schima W, Prokesch R, Österreicher C, et al. Biliary Wallstent endoprosthesis in malignant hilar obstruction: long-term results with regard to the type of obstruction. *Clin Radiol.* 1997;52:213-219.

Warren KW, Jefferson MF. Prevention of repair of strictures of the extrahepatic bile ducts. *Surg Clin N Am.* 1973;53:1169-1190.

Yee ACN, Ho CS. Complications of percutaneous biliary drainage: benign vs malignant diseases. *Am J Roentgenol.* 1997;148:1207-1209.

CHAPTER 21

Gallbladder Intervention

Michael J. Lee, MSc, FRCPI, FRCR, FFR(RCSI), FSIR, EBIR

DIAGNOSTIC GALLBLADDER INTERVENTION
Gallbladder Aspiration
Diagnostic Cholecystocholangiography
Gallbladder Biopsy

THERAPEUTIC GALLBLADDER INTERVENTION: PERCUTANEOUS CHOLECYSTOSTOMY

Technique
Results
Catheter Care
Complications
Patient Outcomes
Treatment of Gallbladder Perforation and Bile Leakage

NONSURGICAL GALLSTONE THERAPIES
Percutaneous Cholecystolithotomy
Gallbladder Ablation

Gallbladder intervention in the form of gallbladder decompression was first proposed as a definite technique in the second half of the last century. However, percutaneous gallbladder intervention did not gain widespread acceptance because of the fear of bile leakage and life-threatening vagal reactions. It was not until the 1980s that percutaneous drainage of the gallbladder and other percutaneous therapies for gallstones became popular.

Percutaneous gallbladder intervention can be divided into diagnostic and therapeutic techniques. Diagnostic techniques include gallbladder aspiration, biopsy, and diagnostic cholecystocholangiography. Therapeutic techniques include percutaneous cholecystostomy, biliary drainage and stent placement via the gallbladder, MTBE (methyl-tert-butyl ether) dissolution therapy, percutaneous cholecystolithotomy, and gallbladder ablation. Apart from percutaneous cholecystostomy, many of these techniques are infrequently performed. The advent of laparoscopic cholecystectomy, to a large extent, has meant the demise of percutaneous techniques to treat gallstones such as percutaneous cholecystolithotomy and MTBE dissolution therapy.

▬ DIAGNOSTIC GALLBLADDER INTERVENTION

Gallbladder Aspiration

Aspiration of bile for Gram stain gained some popularity in the 1980s in intensive care units (ICUs) or in critically ill patients with suspected acute calculous or acalculous cholecystitis. The lack of an accurate noninvasive test to diagnose cholecystitis in these patients led to the practice of gallbladder aspiration for Gram stain and culture of bile. Using ultrasound guidance, a 20- to 22-gauge needle was placed in the gallbladder and bile aspirated for microbiologic analysis. However, the accuracy of gallbladder aspiration in this clinical situation is approximately 50%, which is equivalent to tossing a coin. Additionally, one has to wait several days for culture results. A major reason for the lack of sensitivity is that patients are often on broad-spectrum antibiotics before gallbladder aspiration so that Gram stains may be negative even in the presence of acute cholecystitis. This procedure has largely been abandoned because of the low sensitivity.

Diagnostic Cholecystocholangiography

In limited clinical situations, diagnostic cholecystocholangiography may be performed instead of percutaneous transhepatic cholangiography. In patients with minimally sized intrahepatic bile ducts, who only require a diagnostic study, a gallbladder puncture can be used. In the author's unit we usually perform transhepatic cholangiography first, and only if this fails do we resort to a gallbladder puncture. A 22-gauge needle is placed in the gallbladder under ultrasound guidance and contrast material injected under fluoroscopy. If the cystic duct is open, contrast material flows into the common bile duct and common hepatic duct. It may be necessary to place the patient in Trendelenburg position for contrast medium to fill the intrahepatic ducts fully. If the patient requires therapeutic procedures with biliary drainage or stent placement, it is best to use a transhepatic route, because it may be difficult to manipulate stents and catheters through the cystic duct into the common bile duct (Box 21-1).

Gallbladder Biopsy

The gallbladder wall can be biopsied successfully using small (20- or 22-gauge) needles, if there is a gallbladder mass (Fig. 21-1). Gallbladder masses are usually due to either primary gallbladder adenocarcinoma or metastatic disease. The procedure is usually performed under ultrasound guidance and has a success rate of more than 90% in obtaining a diagnosis. It is best to use small needles to prevent bile leakage. However, if the mass is large and the gallbladder lumen is totally replaced, then cutting needles (e.g., Tru-Cut) can be used.

▬ THERAPEUTIC GALLBLADDER INTERVENTION: PERCUTANEOUS CHOLECYSTOSTOMY

Percutaneous cholecystostomy is a valuable technique for the management of patients with either calculous or acalculous cholecystitis who are critically ill and unfit for surgery. In these patients, percutaneous cholecystostomy is performed as a temporizing measure, with definitive surgery carried out at a later date when the patient has recovered from the acute illness. In acalculous cholecystitis, percutaneous cholecystostomy may be curative in that once the inflammation resolves the patient may not need a cholecystectomy. Percutaneous cholecystostomy is also useful in the management of empyema and hydrops of the gallbladder.

Percutaneous cholecystostomy has also been used for drainage of the biliary tree in patients whose cystic duct is patent and the biliary obstruction lies below the insertion of the cystic duct into the common bile duct. Transhepatic biliary drainage is usually a better alternative for long-term drainage of the biliary tree, but in selected cases percutaneous cholecystostomy may be of benefit. Selected clinical situations include pancreatitis wherein short-term decompression of an obstructive biliary tree may be necessary, and biliary cholangitis and distal obstruction of the common bile duct for which endoscopic retrograde cholangiopancreatography (ERCP) has failed to provide drainage. For long-term palliation of patients with obstructive jaundice, the transhepatic route is preferred because stenting can be performed easily through the transhepatic tract. It can be difficult to manipulate a wire through the cystic duct and into the common bile duct using a gallbladder approach. Additionally, long-term catheter drainage of the biliary tree via the gallbladder in patients with distal malignant obstruction is not optimal because both pancreatic cancer and cholangiocarcinoma eventually grow to obstruct the origin of the cystic duct. For these reasons, percutaneous cholecystostomy for decompression of the biliary tree is only performed for temporary decompression and only in selected patients (Fig. 21-2).

Technique

There are a number of technique variations to consider before performing a percutaneous cholecystostomy. The access route used can be either transhepatic or transperitoneal, while the catheter can be placed using either a Seldinger or trocar technique. The access route and method of catheter insertion chosen is a matter of personal preference. The author's unit has tended to place cholecystostomy catheters using ultrasound guidance and trocar technique in ICU patients, while patients who can travel to the department may have the procedure performed using a Seldinger or trocar technique.

Box 21-1. Diagnostic Cholecystocholangiography

Use only if intrahepatic ducts minimally dilated and if transhepatic approach fails
Biliary obstruction must be at a level below junction of cystic duct and common hepatic duct
Ultrasound guidance and a 22-gauge needle are used
Trendelenburg positioning may be necessary to fill intrahepatic ducts

Transperitoneal vs. Transhepatic Access

Use of a transhepatic or transperitoneal approach is largely a matter of personal preference. Many authors prefer the transperitoneal approach because it is more direct and avoids the necessity of going through the liver. Additionally, if percutaneous cholecystectolithotomy (PCCL) is being considered, a track can safely be dilated if a transperitoneal approach has been used. One of the main problems with the transperitoneal approach is that catheters and guidewires often buckle outside of the gallbladder, particularly when using the Seldinger technique. This is due to gallbladder mobility. The closer the entry site to the fundus of the gallbladder, the more mobile the gallbladder is and the more likely this is to happen (Fig. 21-3). The Seldinger technique also increases the likelihood of this happening. Additionally, the transverse colon may occasionally overlie the fundus of the gallbladder and may result in perforation of the transverse colon if the transperitoneal approach is used (Fig. 21-4).

The author prefers the transhepatic approach because entry of the catheter into the gallbladder is closer to the attachment of the gallbladder to the liver (the bare area) where the gallbladder is relatively fixed in position compared to the fundus. The bare area represents the attachment of the gallbladder to the liver and also represents the extraperitoneal surface of the gallbladder. The bare area is situated superolaterally in the gallbladder fossa and, in an ideal world, it would be best to place catheters through the bare area into the gallbladder. Thus, any bile leakage would be extraperitoneal and tamponaded by the liver. However, in practice it is very difficult to traverse the bare area because its precise location cannot be determined by any imaging method. In the author's unit we therefore insert the catheter vertically into the gallbladder, making sure that the catheter passes through a portion of the liver en route to the gallbladder (Fig. 21-5). One of the potential disadvantages of using the transhepatic approach is that if a PCCL is required at a later stage, a large track through

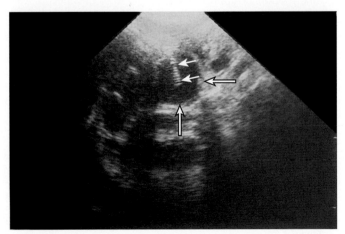

FIGURE 21-1. Gallbladder biopsy. Transverse image from an ultrasound of the right upper quadrant showing the gallbladder *(large arrows)* containing predominantly solid material. The patient was suspected to have a gallbladder cancer. A fine-needle biopsy was performed under ultrasound guidance and the needle *(small arrows)* can be seen within the mass. Gallbladder cancer was confirmed upon pathologic examination of the biopsy specimen.

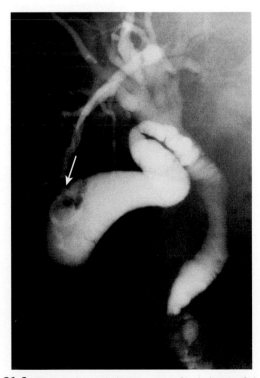

FIGURE 21-2. Percutaneous cholecystostomy for drainage of the biliary tree in a patient with severe cholangitis and hypotension. A percutaneous cholecystostomy catheter *(arrow)* was placed in the gallbladder using the Seldinger technique. A stricture can be seen in the lower bile duct, caused by a small pancreatic tumor. The catheter remained in situ until the patient went to surgery for a Whipple procedure.

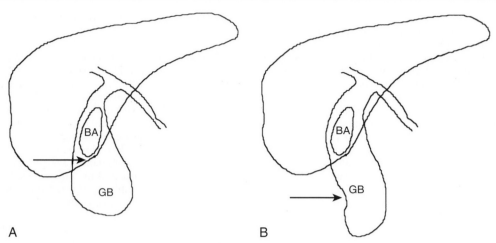

A   B

FIGURE 21-3. Transhepatic versus transperitoneal insertion of gallbladder catheters. **A,** Schematic diagram showing the gallbladder (GB) with bare area (BA) shown near the neck of the gallbladder. The bare area represents the extraperitoneal surface of the gallbladder or the attachment of the gallbladder to the liver. A transhepatic insertion *(large arrow)* will be nearer the bare area and thus the gallbladder will be less mobile in this location than if a transperitoneal access route is chosen. **B,** A transperitoneal insertion is nearer the fundus of the gallbladder, which is also the most mobile portion of the gallbladder. The gallbladder wall may indent and move away from the needle or catheter using a transperitoneal approach. In addition, dilators or even the catheter may catch in the wall of the gallbladder and cause the guidewire to buckle outside the lumen of the gallbladder. (From Stafford-Johnson D, Mueller PR, Varghese J, et al. Percutaneous cholecystostomy: a review. *J Interv Radiol.* 1996;11:1-8.)

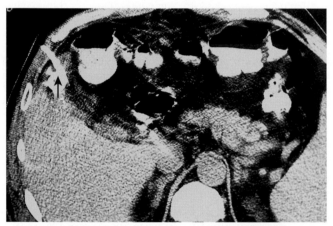

FIGURE 21-4. Clinical example showing a transperitoneal insertion of a percutaneous cholecystostomy catheter. The catheter can be seen *(arrow)* entering the gallbladder through the peritoneum. Note the position of the colon more anterior, indicating that an anterior approach was not possible in this patient.

> **BOX 21-2.** **Advantages and Disadvantages of Transhepatic Approach for Percutaneous Cholecystostomy**
>
> Catheter entry site closer to the bare area of the gallbladder
> Bile leaks potentially tamponaded by liver
> Gallbladder less mobile closer to bare area
> If large tracks required for percutaneous cholecystectolithotomy, risk of hemorrhage increased

> **BOX 21-3.** **Advantages and Disadvantages of Transperitoneal Approach**
>
> Gallbladder more mobile near the fundus and may be more difficult to puncture
> Transverse colon may overlie fundus of gallbladder
> Seldinger technique prone to guidewire buckling when transperitoneal approach used
> Large tracks can be easily dilated for percutaneous cholecystolithotomy, if required

the liver will have to be created. Some operators are reluctant to dilate a 1-cm tract through the liver into the gallbladder. We have done this on a considerable number of patients without mishap (Boxes 21-2 and 21-3).

Trocar vs. Seldinger Technique

The Seldinger technique requires fluoroscopic and sonographic guidance and is unsuitable for placement of cholecystostomy catheters in the ICU or at the bedside. For the Seldinger technique the gallbladder is first located with ultrasound and a 22-gauge needle from a one-stick needle system (Cook, Bloomington, Ind.) is inserted into the gallbladder under ultrasound guidance.

The gallbladder is opacified with dilute contrast material and a 0.018-inch guidewire inserted through the 22-gauge needle into the gallbladder using fluoroscopic guidance. The 5-French sheath system is placed over the 0.018-inch guidewire into the gallbladder. A 0.035-inch J-shaped guidewire is then placed through the 5-French sheath into the gallbladder. As much as possible of the

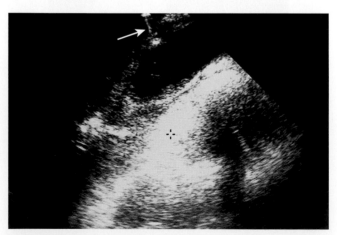

FIGURE 21-5. Example of a transhepatic catheter insertion into the gallbladder in a patient with acalculous cholecystitis. The catheter *(arrow)* is inserted through the liver into the gallbladder. Although the catheter almost certainly does not traverse the bare area, the gallbladder is less mobile with a transhepatic route.

0.035-inch J-guidewire should be coiled into the gallbladder to achieve adequate purchase. Once this is done the percutaneous track is ready for dilatation.

The track is dilated using 7- and 9-French dilators and finally an 8-French pigtail with a small pigtail is placed (Cook, Bloomington, Ind.). Care must be taken during track dilatation such that the guidewire does not kink at the gallbladder entry site. If this happens and is not recognized, further dilatation or catheter placement may cause the guidewire to buckle at this site, resulting in the guidewire flipping into the peritoneal cavity. This is more likely to happen with a transperitoneal approach (Fig. 21-6). If the guidewire kinks during track dilatation, the guidewire should be replaced by removing the kinked wire using the 5-French sheath and inserting a new 0.038-inch J-guidewire or indeed a stiffer guidewire such as a 0.038-inch Ring guidewire (Cook, Bloomington, Ind.).

The trocar technique is the author's preferred method of accessing the gallbladder (Table 21-1). The trocar technique is particularly suited to those patients who cannot travel to the radiology department. Ultrasound is used to locate the gallbladder and an access route is chosen that passes through the liver. Local anesthetic is administered to the skin at the puncture site, an incision is made with a #11 scalpel, and the superficial tissues are dissected with a surgical forceps. Under ultrasound guidance, insert a 22-gauge spinal needle into the gallbladder as a reference needle. Bile aspiration confirms the needle to lie within the gallbladder cavity. An 8-French pigtail catheter (Cook, Bloomington, Ind.) is inserted into the gallbladder in tandem to the reference needle. Importantly, a quick thrust is required when inserting the catheter into the gallbladder rather than a gradual approach. With a gradual or incremental advance, the gallbladder may move ahead of the catheter and make entry of the catheter into the gallbladder difficult or impossible. With a quick thrust, the catheter usually pierces the anterior wall of the gallbladder. This can be confirmed with ultrasound and/or by aspirating bile from the catheter. When the catheter is in the gallbladder, the catheter is advanced off the cannula, which is withdrawn, and the catheter tip is coiled in the gallbladder. A locking pigtail catheter is necessary to prevent dislodgment.

Results

Technically, the success rate for percutaneous cholecystectomy should be 100% in experienced hands. In patients with calculous cholecystitis who are too ill to undergo formal surgery, percutaneous cholecystostomy acts as a temporizing measure until the patient is fit enough for surgery. In the patient with acalculous cholecystitis, percutaneous cholecystostomy may be curative and no further intervention such as cholecystectomy may be required. In ICU patients, acalculous cholecystitis is a frequent and often underdiagnosed cause of sepsis. The author's unit has used percutaneous cholecystostomy as a therapeutic trial in ICU patients with persisting sepsis of unknown origin. A percutaneous cholecystostomy is performed only when other causes of sepsis have been excluded. In a series of 82 such patients, Boland and associates showed a dramatic response in 48 patients (59%). The response usually occurs within 24-48 hours and is evidenced by a decrease in white cell count, normalization of body temperature, and reduced dependence on vasopressor support (Box 21-4).

Catheter Care

When a percutaneous cholecystectomy catheter is inserted, daily rounds by the interventional team are important to ensure that catheter kinking or dislodgment does not occur. Catheters also need to be irrigated two to three times per day because many of these patients have biliary sludge that tends to clog the 8-French catheters that are placed.

Percutaneous cholecystostomy catheters must be left in place for a minimum of 2 weeks before removal to ensure that a mature track develops between the gallbladder and skin surface. If the catheter is removed before a mature tract develops, bile contamination of the peritoneal cavity may result. Before removing the cholecystostomy catheter, the author's unit performs a cholecystocholangiogram to ensure patency of the cystic duct and to exclude the presence of gallstones in the cystic duct, gallbladder, or bile duct. If stones are present in the gallbladder, the patient may require cholecystectomy, or percutaneous cholecystolithotomy if the patient is unfit for surgery. If an occluding gallstone is present in the cystic duct, the catheter should not be removed until the stone is dealt with either surgically or percutaneously. Lastly, if there is a stone in the common bile duct, the patient will require ERCP and stone removal, or the stone can be removed percutaneously.

If the catheter is to be removed, it is withdrawn over a guidewire and a Kumpe catheter or a 5-French dilator is placed over the guidewire into the opening of the percutaneous track. Using a Tuohy-Borst adapter, contrast material is injected into the percutaneous track. If the track is mature, contrast material will outline the track all the way to the gallbladder (Fig. 21-7). If the track is immature, contrast material will spill into the peritoneal cavity (Fig. 21-8). If this happens, the catheter is reinserted over the guidewire into the gallbladder. The procedure is repeated at weekly intervals until the track is mature (Box 21-5).

Complications

The complication rate for percutaneous cholecystostomy is low compared to surgical cholecystostomy. The rate of complications for surgical cholecystostomy is approximately 24% compared with rates of up to 8% reported for percutaneous cholecystostomy. The major complications reported include bleeding, bradycardia and hypotension (which is vagally mediated), and biliary peritonitis. Locking catheters reduce the risk of catheter dislodgment and subsequent biliary peritonitis. If bile leakage is suspected, antibiotic administration is started and close supervision of the patient is mandatory. Laparoscopy or laparotomy may be required if the patient does not settle. Some authors advocate the use of atropine before percutaneous cholecystostomy because of the risk of vagally mediated bradycardia and hypotension. However, the author's unit has not encountered a single episode of hypotension or bradycardia in more than 250 percutaneous cholecystostomies. Therefore, we do not give prophylactic atropine but we do make sure that it is at hand, if required.

Patient Outcomes

In patients who recover from a bout of acute acalculous cholecystitis, percutaneous cholecystostomy usually allows the cystic duct obstruction to resolve so that the likelihood of a repeat attack occurring is low and the catheter can be removed at the appropriate time. There is usually no need for surgical cholecystectomy in these patients. In patients with calculous cholecystitis, the situation is different in that the gallstones remain in the gallbladder and future bouts of acute cholecystitis are probable. In older patients with severe intercurrent illnesses, the situation is compounded in that further bouts of acute cholecystitis may be the terminal event for some patients. Nonsurgical gallstone therapy has a role in treating gallstones in this subgroup of patients. In a recent study, Boland and associates reported the clinical outcome in 26 older patients with severe intercurrent illness who underwent percutaneous cholecystostomy for acute calculous cholecystitis. Of the 26 patients, seven died, seven recovered from the acute illness and underwent surgical cholecystectomy at a later date, and 12 underwent nonsurgical gallstone therapies. Nonsurgical therapies

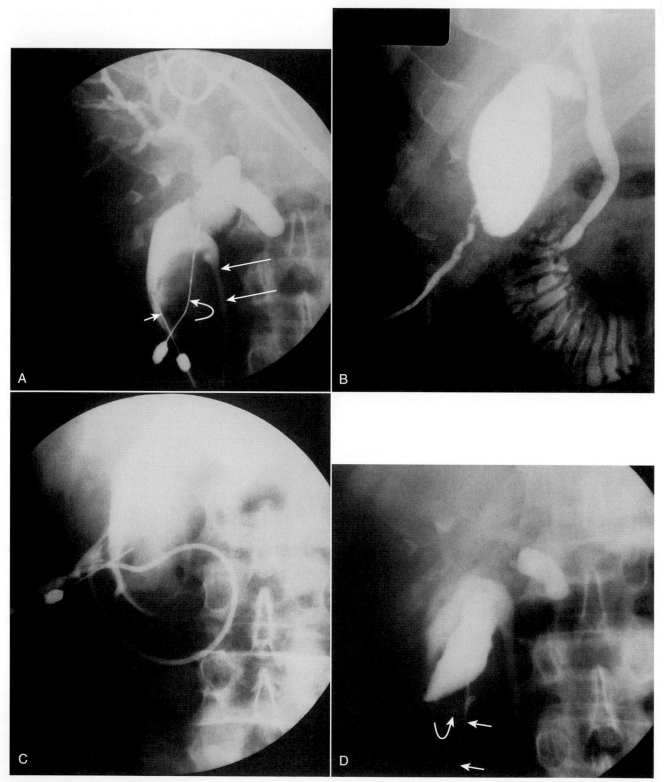

FIGURE 21-6. Example of the Seldinger technique and the transperitoneal approach causing buckling of the guidewire and catheter out of the gallbladder. **A,** Patient with a pancreatic carcinoma who was scheduled for a Whipple procedure had markedly elevated liver function tests. The surgeon requested a biliary decompression before surgery. Attempts at percutaneous biliary drainage were unsuccessful and the gallbladder was accessed with a 22-gauge spinal needle with a view to doing a cholangiogram. Note the spinal needle *(small arrow)* for injecting contrast material into the gallbladder. A second 18-gauge needle *(curved arrow)* was used to place a 0.038-inch Ring guidewire into the gallbladder. Contrast material can be seen in the pelvicalyceal system *(long arrows)* from the repeated attempts at percutaneous transhepatic cholangiography. **B,** During dilatation of the percutaneous track, a large guidewire loop formed outside the gallbladder because of buckling of the guidewire. **C,** The catheter was placed but proved to be outside the gallbladder. **D,** Using ultrasound guidance, a second 8-French catheter *(straight arrows)* was trocared into the gallbladder to provide decompression. The first catheter *(curved arrow)* was left in situ to drain the contrast and bile from around the gallbladder. The patient did not experience any pain or evidence of biliary peritonitis and proceeded to surgery for a Whipple resection 1 week later. (From Stafford-Johnson D, Mueller PR, Varghese J, et al. Percutaneous cholecystostomy: a review. *J Interv Radiol.* 1996;11:1-8.)

TABLE 21-1 Trocar vs. Seldinger Technique

	Trocar	Seldinger
Ultrasound guidance	Yes	No
Portable	Yes	No
Fluoroscopic guidance	No	Yes
Speed of performance	Fast	Slower
Guidewire and catheter buckling into peritoneal cavity	No	Yes

---

Box 21-4. **Acalculous Cholecystitis**

Frequently occurs in intensive care unit patients
No accurate noninvasive diagnostic test
Gallbladder aspiration has 50% accuracy
Percutaneous cholecystostomy can be used as a therapeutic trial if other causes of sepsis excluded

---

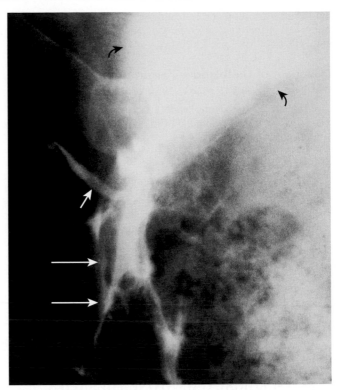

FIGURE 21-8. Patient with an immature track after percutaneous cholecystostomy catheter removal. The patient developed pain after removal of the gallbladder catheter. The percutaneous track was not documented to be mature before catheter removal. An injection of contrast material through the track *(small arrow)* after percutaneous cholecystostomy catheter removal shows wide extravasation of contrast material *(large arrows)* into the peritoneal cavity because of an immature track. The gallbladder itself *(curved arrows)* can be seen at the top of the image. (From Stafford-Johnson D, Mueller PR, Varghese J, et al. Percutaneous cholecystostomy: a review. *J Interv Radiol.* 1996;11:1-8.)

Box 21-5. **Catheter Care**

Percutaneous cholecystostomy catheters should be left in place for 2-3 weeks before removal
A catheter cholecystogram is performed to ensure no stones in the common bile duct
A mature track must be demonstrated before catheter removal
If acalculous cholecystitis, the catheter can be removed and cholecystectomy is not required

---

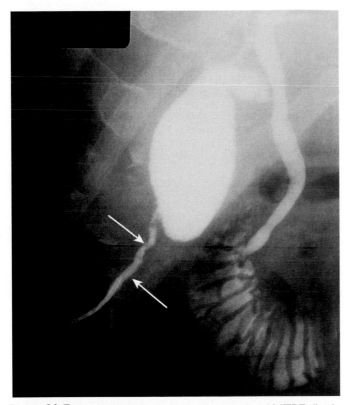

FIGURE 21-7. Mature track in a patient who completed MTBE dissolution therapy for gallstones. Contrast injected while the catheter was in the gallbladder shows a patent cystic duct and clear common bile duct. The catheter was then removed and a small dilator placed in the percutaneous track. Contrast injected in the track shows a mature track *(arrows)* with no evidence of any peritoneal extravasation of contrast material. The gallbladder catheter is safe to take out at this stage. It usually takes a track 2-3 weeks to develop around the catheter. (From Mueller PR, Lee MJ, Saini S, et al. Percutaneous contrast dissolution of gallstones; complexity of radiological care. *Radiographics.* 1991;11:759-764.)

---

included MTBE dissolution therapy in three patients, percutaneous cholecystolithotomy in two patients, ERCP removal of a stone which passed from the gallbladder into the common bile duct in one patient, and long-term catheter drainage of the gallbladder in six patients who were terminally ill. These results emphasize the need for nonsurgical gallstone therapy options because many of these patients with severe medical illnesses are unfit for surgery.

In a review of national trends of percutaneous cholecystostomy between 1994 and 2009, Duszak and Behram identified from Medicare claims patients who had percutaneous cholecystostomy performed. During the time period, annual PC procedures increased by 567% (from 1085 to 7239 cases). In a study by Hsieh and colleagues, 166 patients with high surgical risk were treated by percutaneous cholecystostomy for acute cholecystitis. The overall in-hospital mortality rate was 15.1%. Of the 126 patients who recovered, 11 experienced recurrent cholecystitis within 2 months. Fifty-three patients underwent cholecystectomy. In yet another study, Joseph and colleagues had a 68% clinical improvement in 106 patients after percutaneous cholecystostomy for acute cholecystitis.

Treatment of Gallbladder Perforation and Bile Leakage

In older patients with complicated medical illnesses, acute cholecystitis, when it occurs, can result in perforation that occasionally can be life-threatening. The author's unit has treated a number of patients with gallbladder perforation by performing percutaneous cholecystostomy and draining any localized abscesses in the abdominal cavity using percutaneous abscess drainage (Fig. 21-9). In this high-risk patient group, the patient can be temporized for future surgery. Perforation of the gallbladder usually implies gangrenous change with necrosis, and surgical principles suggest that emergent removal of the gallbladder should be performed. However, this is not always possible in older patients with severe intercurrent illnesses. In this situation, percutaneous cholecystostomy can decompress a gallbladder and prevent the escape of more infected bile as well as allow the gallbladder perforation to seal over. Imaging of the peritoneal cavity by CT or ultrasound can then help identify any loculated pockets of pus that can be drained separately. This combination of percutaneous cholecystostomy and percutaneous drainage is potentially life- saving in these special circumstances.

▬ NONSURGICAL GALLSTONE THERAPIES

Percutaneous Cholecystolithotomy

In a patient with acute cholecystitis and severe intercurrent illness, the mortality rate for cholecystectomy ranges from 10% to 30%. In fact, the patient may never be fit for surgery. In this high-risk group, PCCL can be used to remove gallstones from the gallbladder to prevent further attacks of acute cholecystitis. PCCL can be performed regardless of the number, size, and composition of stones.

Technique

Using the existing percutaneous cholecystostomy track, a larger track is dilated into the gallbladder. The track needs to be dilated to between 26- and 30-French. Track dilatation can be achieved by using either an 8- to 10-mm balloon or using fascial dilators. The author prefers to use a balloon for track dilatation. When the track has been dilated, a large 26- to 30-cm sheath is placed into the gallbladder (Cook, Bloomington, Ind.). The transperitoneal approach is preferable when large tracks are to be dilated. However, the transhepatic approach has been used in many patients without complication. In general, symptoms of acute cholecystitis should subside before performing track dilatation and stone removal. The time interval between percutaneous cholecystostomy and PCCL is usually 4-6 weeks in most patients.

If stones are small, they can be removed from the gallbladder using standard basket techniques (Fig. 21-10) or using graspers or alligator forceps. Larger stones usually require some form of lithotripsy to make them small enough to remove through the percutaneous track. There are a number of ways of breaking up larger stones, including electrohydraulic, laser, ultrasonic, and mechanical lithotripsy. The first three all require the insertion of an endoscope into the gallbladder. Mechanical lithotripsy involves using a basket to capture the stone and then the wires on the basket are tightened to crush the stone. This does not require direct vision and it can be performed under fluoroscopy. In the author's unit, we usually perform mechanical lithotripsy first; if this fails then ultrasonic lithotripsy is performed. Ultrasonic lithotripsy is performed in the operating room using a rigid nephroscope and the same equipment that is used for ultrasonic lithotripsy of renal stones. No matter which technique is used,

there are usually small stone fragments remaining at the end of the procedure which can be removed under fluoroscopy using a basket. At the end of the procedure, a large catheter is inserted into the gallbladder; we usually place a 26- to 28-French Malecot catheter to maintain the track and prevent bile leakage. The catheter remains in place for another 2-3 days and then the patient returns for a final check cholecystogram. If this is clear and there is good flow of contrast material into the bile duct and duodenum, the catheter is removed.

Results

There are a number of papers in the radiology literature describing the results from PCCL. Gillams and associates achieved complete stone clearance in 100 of 113 patients with 73.4% of patients requiring a single-stage procedure in a mean time of 64 minutes. Picus and associates were successful in removing all of the stones in 56 of 58 patients. These stones ranged from 3 to 40 mm in diameter. Intracorporeal electrohydraulic lithotripsy was used to fragment large stones in 31 patients, with one stone removal session required in 32 patients, two sessions in 15 patients, three sessions in 8 patients, and four sessions in two patients. Cope and associates were successful in removing all gallstones from 17 of 20 patients using PCCL. Stone sizes varied from 2 to 22 mm and were removed in one session in 11 of 17 patients and in two consecutive sessions in six patients. However, in a long-term follow-up of 439 patients over a 10-year period, Zou and colleagues showed a gallstone recurrence rate of 41.46% (182 of 439 PCCL patients). Ninety-four of the 182 patients with recurrent gallstones were asymptomatic, 80 suffered from non-specific upper GI symptoms, and eight had abdominal pain and biliary colic. Thirty-eight of the 182 patients underwent cholecystectomy. It would appear from the latter study that the recurrence rate of gallstones after PCCL is high, but patients are often asymptomatic.

Complications

Complications are mainly those reported for percutaneous cholecystostomy. Picus and associates reported major complications in five of 58 patients (9%). Four of these major complications were related to bile leakage after the cholecystostomy tube was removed. One patient died of extensive bowel infarction secondary to hypotension. These complications emphasize the need for careful tube handling and delayed tube removal in this patient group (Box 21-6).

Gallbladder Ablation

It is well known that the risk of symptomatic gallstones recurring in patients after surgical cholecystolithotomy is high. Unfortunately, all forms of nonsurgical gallstone therapies leave a diseased gallbladder in place which has the potential for stone recurrence. Symptoms of biliary tract disease reoccur in 20%-50% of patients 2-5 years after the initial nonsurgical gallstone therapy. In patients in whom nonsurgical gallstone therapies are performed, the high recurrence rate of systematic gallstones is problematic. Therefore, the idea of ablating the gallbladder so that stones cannot recur was proposed.

Technique

Gallbladder ablation was popularized in the late 1980s and early 1990s with experimental animal studies and one human study. However, again with the advent of laparoscopic cholecystectomy, the need for gallbladder ablation has decreased enormously and is now rarely performed.

Complete gallbladder ablation to prevent stone recurrence can be achieved only by ablating both the gallbladder and cystic duct mucosa. The cystic duct is usually first ablated using either a laser fiber or radiofrequency ablation. In general, access will already have been gained and some form of nonsurgical therapy will have been used to remove the gallstones. A laser fiber or a

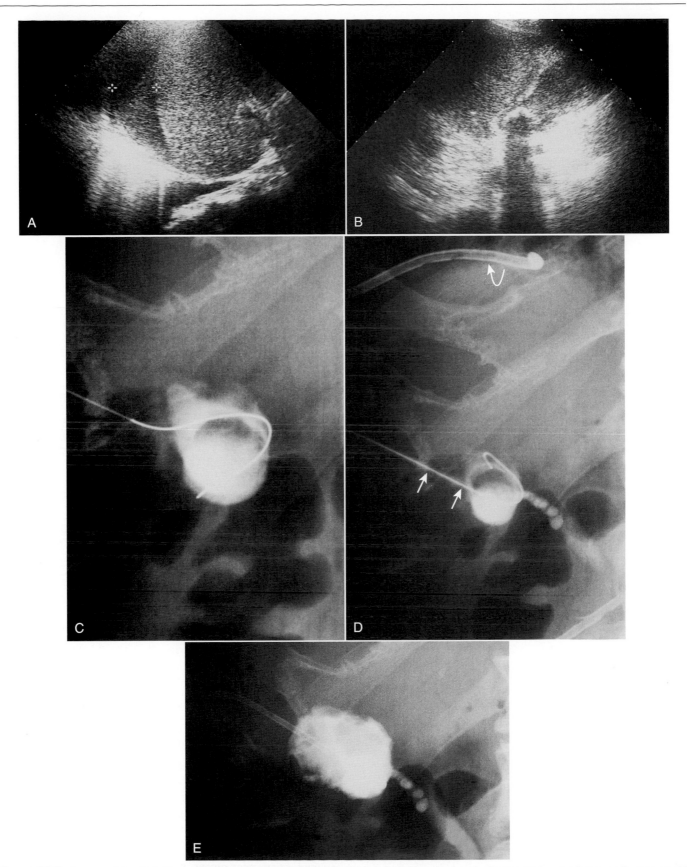

FIGURE 21-9. Patient with gallbladder perforation and a right subphrenic abscess. **A,** A right subphrenic abscess can be seen between the cursors with some echogenic material in the inferior half. **B,** A longitudinal image of the gallbladder shows a stone in the neck of the gallbladder with echogenic material throughout the gallbladder. **C,** The patient was obtunded and a percutaneous cholecystostomy and drainage of the subphrenic abscess was performed. A one-stick needle system (Cook, Bloomington, Ind.) was used to access the gallbladder, and the platinum-tipped 0.018-inch guidewire can be seen coiled in the gallbladder. **D,** A larger 0.035-inch J-guidewire was coiled in the gallbladder and track dilatation was performed. A dilator can be seen *(straight arrows)* over the guidewire dilating the track. Note the sump catheter in the right subphrenic abscess *(curved arrows)*. **E,** An 8-French catheter was placed in the gallbladder for decompression. The patient recovered sufficiently in 10-14 days to have a cholecystectomy. At cholecystectomy the gallbladder was gangrenous with a perforation that had been spontaneously sealed by some omentum.

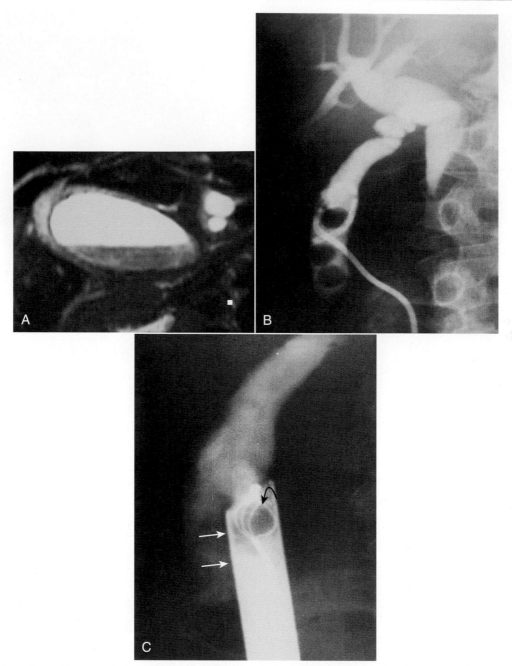

Figure 21-10. Older patient with acute calculous cholecystitis who was unfit for surgical cholecystectomy. The patient did not settle on conservative management with intravenous antibiotics and a percutaneous cholecystostomy was performed. **A,** Axial magnetic resonance cholangiopancreatography image through the gallbladder shows a rim of hyperintense signal around the gallbladder and a fluid-sludge level within the gallbladder consistent with acute cholecystitis. **B,** An 8-French pigtail catheter was placed into the gallbladder using a trocar technique. A catheter cholecystogram was performed when the patient's symptoms had settled. This showed three stones within the gallbladder. Note the common bile duct is moderately dilated, but this was presumed to be secondary to loss of elasticity through the normal aging process. The liver function tests were normal. **C,** Six weeks after the initial percutaneous drainage, track dilatation was performed using a 1-cm diameter balloon and a 30-French sheath *(straight arrows)* was placed into the gallbladder. A Wittich basket (Cook, Bloomington, Ind.) is shown extracting one of the stones *(curved arrows)* through the sheath.

radiofrequency catheter is then negotiated into the cystic duct and energy is delivered to the gallbladder mucosa while the laser fiber or radiofrequency catheter is slowly pulled backward into the gallbladder. This destroys the mucosa of the cystic duct, with eventual scar formation.

The second step is to ablate the gallbladder, which is usually achieved by chemical sclerotherapy using sodium tetradecyl sulfate (STS) and 95% ethanol. The volume of the gallbladder is first determined and an equal volume of each sclerosant is then given. Ethanol is instilled first and left in place for 30 minutes

followed by STS, which is left in place for 30 minutes. The cholecystostomy tube is removed after sclerotherapy when the drainage from the gallbladder is less than 20 mL per day. Repeat sclerotherapy may be necessary if the gallbladder fails to obliterate and a persistent mucus discharge occurs through the cholecystostomy tube track.

Results

Animal results reported by Girard and Becker and associates have demonstrated successful obliteration of the cystic duct

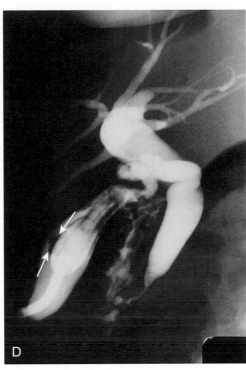

FIGURE 21-10, cont'd. **D,** A 24-French Foley catheter was placed in the gallbladder after the procedure and 2 days later the patient returned for a catheter cholecystogram. The gallbladder is clear with some residual clot *(arrows)*. The catheter, however, was removed. The patient had no further symptoms.

Box 21-6. Percutaneous Cholecystectolithotomy

Can be performed regardless of stone composition
26- to 30-French track required
Stones removed by basket or, if large, lithotripsy performed
Performed only in those patients with symptomatic gallstones who are unfit for surgery

---

and gallbladder. Girard's team used laser ablation of the cystic duct, while Becker's team used radiofrequency ablation. Although animal studies were successful in ablating gallbladder mucosa and cystic duct mucosa, human studies have not been as successful. Becker's team reported successful gallbladder ablation in five of eight patients. However, in three patients mucus discharge persisted, and forceps biopsy of the gallbladder in these three patients showed evidence of gallbladder mucosa regeneration.

It is likely that the extensive regenerative capability of the gallbladder mucosa makes complete ablation of the human gallbladder less likely to succeed than in the animal model. The author's unit rarely performs gallbladder ablation, anticipating that the short life expectancy of many of the older patients who are unfit for surgery or cholecystectomy will usually not be sufficient to make recurrent stone formation a major concern.

■ SUGGESTED READINGS

Beardsley SL, Shlansky-Goldberg RD, Patel A, et al. Predicting infected bile among patients undergoing percutaneous cholecystostomy. *Cardiovasc Intervent Radiol.* 2005 May-Jun;28(3):319-325.

Becker CD, Quenville NF, Burhenne HJ. Gallbladder ablation through radiologic intervention: an experimental alternative to cholecystectomy. *Radiology.* 1989;171:235-240.

Becker CD, Fache JS, Malone DE, Stoller JL, Burhenne HJ. Ablation of the cystic duct and gallbladder: clinical observations. *Radiology.* 1990;176:687-690.

Boland GW, Lee MJ, Mueller PR, et al. Gallstones in critically ill patients with acute calculous cholecystitis treated by percutaneous cholecystostomy: nonsurgical therapeutic options. *Am J Roentgenol.* 1994;162:1101-1103.

Boland GW, Lee MJ, Leung J, Mueller PR. Percutaneous cholecystostomy in critically ill patients: early response and final outcome in 82 patients. *Am J Roentgenol.* 1994;163:339-342.

Cope C, Burke DR, Meranze SG. Percutaneous extraction of gallstones in 20 patients. *Radiology.* 1990;176:19-24.

Duszak R Jr, Behram SW. National trends in percutaneous cholecystostomy between 1994 and 2009: perspectives from Medicare provider claims. *J Am Coll Radiol.* 2012;9:474-479.

Gillams A, Curtis S, Donald J, et al. Technical considerations in 113 percutaneous cholecystolithotomies. *Radiology.* 1992;183:163-166.

Girard MJ, Saini S, Mueller PR, et al. Percutaneous chemical gallbladder sclerosis after laser-induced cystic duct oblivation: results in an experimental model. *Am J Roentgenol.* 1992;159:997-1000.

Griniatsos J, Petrou A, Pappas P, et al. Percutaneous cholecystostomy without interval cholecystectomy as definitive treatment of acute cholecystitis in elderly and critically ill patients. *South Med J.* 2008 Jun;101(6):586-590.

Ha JP, Tsui KK, Tang CN, et al. Cholecystectomy or not after percutaneous cholecystostomy for acute cholecystitis in high risk patients. *Hepatogastroenterology.* 2008 Sep-Oct;55(86-87):1497-1502.

Hsieh YC, Chen CK, Su CW, et al. Outcome after percutaneous cholecystostomy for acute cholecystitis: a single-center experience. *J Gastrointest Surg.* 2012;16:1860-1868.

Joseph T, Unver K, Hwang GL, et al. Percutaneous cholecystostomy for acute cholecystitis: ten-year experience. *J Vasc Interv Radiol.* 2012;23:83-8.

Lee MJ, Saini S, Brink J, et al. Treatment of critically ill patients with sepsis of unknown cause: value of percutaneous cholecystostomy. *Am J Roentgenol.* 1991;156:1163-1166.

Leveau P, Andersson E, Carlgren I, et al. Percutaneous cholecystostomy: a bridge to surgery or definite management of acute cholecystitis in high risk patients? *Scand J Gastroenterol.* 2008;43(5):593-596.

McGahan JP, Lindfors KK. Percutaneous cholecystostomy: an alternative to surgical cholecystostomy for acute cholecystitis. *Radiology.* 1989;173:481-485.

Mirvis SE, Wainright JR, Nelson AW. The diagnosis of acute acalculous cholecystitis: a comparison of sonography, scintigraphy and CT. *Am J Roentgenol.* 1986;147:1171-1175.

Mueller PR, Lee MJ, Saini S, et al. Percutaneous contrast dissolution of gallstones; complexity of radiological care. *Radiographics.* 1991;11:759-764.

Nemcek AA, Bernstein JE, Vogelzang RL. Percutaneous cholecystostomy: does transhepatic puncture preclude a transperitoneal catheter route? *J Vasc Interv Radiol.* 1991;2:543-547.

Picus D. Percutaneous gallbladder intervention. *Radiology.* 1990;176:5-6.

Picus D, Hicks MR, Darcy MD, et al. Percutaneous cholecystolithotomy: analysis of results and complications in 58 consecutive patients. *Radiology.* 1992;183:779-784.

Picus D, Marx MV, Hicks ME, Larg EV, Edmundowiez SA. Percutaneous cholecystolithotomy: preliminary experience and technical considerations. *Radiology*. 1989;173:487-491.

Stafford-Johnson D, Mueller PR, Varghese J, Lee MJ. Percutaneous cholecystostomy: a review. *J Interv Radiol*. 1996;11:1-8.

Thistle JL, May GR, Bender CE, et al. Dissolution of cholesterol gallbladder stones by MTBE administered by percutaneous transhepatic catheter. *N Engl J Med*. 1989;320:663–639.

Valff V, Froelich JW, Lloyd R, et al. Predictive value of an abnormal hepatobiliary scan in patients with severe inter- current illness. *Radiology*. 1983;146:191-194.

vanSonnenberg E, Casola G, Zakko SF, et al. Gallbladder and bile duct stones: percutaneous therapy with primary MTBE dissolution and mechanical methods. *Radiology*. 1988;169:505-509.

vanSonnenberg E, D'agostino HB, Casola G, et al. Benefits of percutaneous cholecystostomy for decompression of selected cases of obstructive jaundice. *Radiology*. 1990;176:15-17.

vanSonnenberg E, D'Agostino HB, Casola G, et al. Gallbladder perforation and bile leakage: percutaneous treatment. *Radiology*. 1991;178:687-689.

vanSonnenberg E, D'Agostino HB, Casola G, Varney RR, Ainge GD. Interventional radiology in the gallbladder: diagnosis, drainage, dissolution and management of stones. *Radiology*. 1990;174:1-6.

Zou YP, Du JD, Li WM, et al. Gallstone recurrence after successful percutaneous cholecystolithotomy: a 10-year follow-up of 439 cases. *Hepatobiliary Pancreat Dis Int*. 2007;6:199-203.

CHAPTER 22

Percutaneous Genitourinary Intervention

Michael J. Lee, MSc, FRCPI, FRCR, FFR(RCSI), FSIR, EBIR

Although the first percutaneous genitourinary procedure was a renal cyst puncture reported in 1867, it wasn't until approximately 100 years later that the first percutaneous nephrostomy using the Seldinger technique was described. Since then, percutaneous access to the kidney has been employed for a wide variety of renal and ureteric pathology. Relief of acute urinary obstruction remains the most common procedure of the genitourinary track performed by interventional radiologists. However, percutaneous access to the kidney has also been used to remove ureteric or renal calculi, dissolve certain types of renal calculi, place ureteric stents, biopsy pelvicaliceal lesions, perform endopyelotomy for ureteropelvic junction (UPJ) obstruction, and remove foreign bodies from the collecting system.

Many of these procedures gained widespread popularity during the 1980s, but the development of extracorporeal lithotripsy and ureteroscopy has limited the number and variety of percutaneous procedures of the genitourinary track that are performed. However, depending on the clinical circumstances, interventional radiologists may be called upon to perform many or all of these techniques.

ANATOMY RELEVANT TO PERCUTANEOUS GENITOURINARY INTERVENTION

Kidney

The kidneys are paired organs located in the retroperitoneum surrounded by fat. They are usually located between the level of the 11th or 12th thoracic to the second or third lumbar vertebral bodies. The left kidney usually lies 1-2 cm higher than the right. The pleura is attached to the 10th rib laterally and the 12th rib posteriorly. Normally the 12th rib crosses over the upper pole of the right kidney, whereas on the left side the upper renal pole is often covered by the 11th and 12th ribs. Because of this anatomy, percutaneous intervention through the upper pole will almost certainly be transpleural, so the risk of pneumothorax or hydro-pneumothorax is increased. The lower poles of both kidneys are located more anteriorly than the upper poles, such that, when

performing percutaneous nephrostomy, it is important to remember that the lower poles are further away from the skin than the mid and upper poles when the patient is in the prone position.

At the renal hilum, the renal vein is situated anteriorly. The renal artery lies posterior to the renal vein and the renal pelvis lies posterior to both. Therefore, in the prone position, the renal pelvis is the most posterior structure of the renal pedicle and nearest the skin. The renal artery separates into anterior and posterior divisions as it approaches the renal hilum, with the anterior division dividing into three or four segmental branches and the posterior division giving rise to one segmental branch. The segmental renal arteries become interlobar arteries in the renal sinus, cross through the septum of Bertin, course along the medullary pyramid, and arch around the distal end of the pyramids to divide into arcuate arteries. The arcuate arteries are located at the base of the pyramids and give rise to interlobular arteries, which supply the peripheral renal cortex.

The Brödel line is a relatively avascular plane in the posterolateral aspect of the kidney between the posterior and anterior intrapolar vascular territories. Because of the absence of large arterial branches, this avascular plane is theoretically safer for placing catheters into the renal pelvicaliceal system. However, in practice this plane cannot be routinely identified and placement of a catheter into a calyceal fornix is usually adequate and safe for percutaneous nephrostomy (Fig. 22-1).

Percutaneous puncture and placement of a catheter directly into the renal pelvis is not recommended because of the proximity of the renal vascular pedicle and the propensity to cause arterial damage and major hemorrhage. Placement of a catheter through the peripheral cortex of the kidney is the recommended route for percutaneous access because of the proximity to the avascular plane of Brödel and the presence of smaller blood vessels in this region (see Fig. 22-1).

Renal calyceal anatomy is also important for planning percutaneous nephrostomy. Because percutaneous nephrostomy is performed with the patient in the prone position, gaining access to a posterior calyx is the preferred entry point into the renal pelvicaliceal system. Because the posterior calyces are closer to the

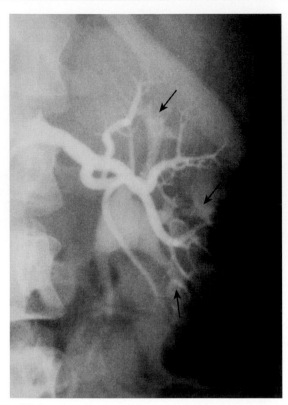

FIGURE 22-1. Arterial anatomy of the kidney. Selective angiographic image of the left kidney shows the arterial anatomy overlying the pelvicaliceal system. Arrows denote the calyces. Nephrostomy access is best gained through peripheral calyces where adjacent arteries tend to be smaller, rather than more centrally where the arteries are larger.

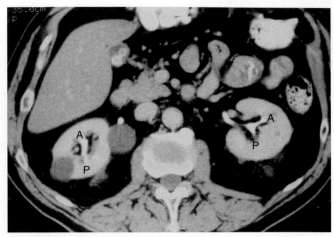

FIGURE 22-3. Contrast-enhanced computed tomography scan showing the relationship of the anterior (A) and posterior (P) calyces. In the majority of patients, the anterior calyces in the right kidney are situated medially and the posterior calyces are situated laterally. The opposite is true in the left kidney. In this example, the anterior and posterior calyces are in the same plane on the right, while on the left the anterior calyces are situated laterally and the posterior calyces are situated medially.

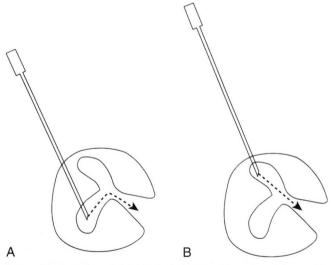

FIGURE 22-2. Schematic showing the difference between a posterior calyceal puncture and an anterior calyceal puncture. **A,** Puncture of an anterior calyx may pose problems for guidewire access into the renal pelvis because of the more acute angle between the calyx and the renal pelvis. **B,** Puncture of a posterior calyx allows easy access of guidewires and catheters into the pelvis.

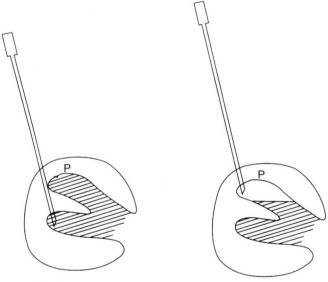

FIGURE 22-4. Schematic showing how the use of air can help identify posterior calyces during percutaneous nephrostomy. The air rises into posterior (P) calyces making them easier to identify.

skin surface in the prone position, the angle of entry from a posterior calyx into the renal pelvis is more direct and less acute than that associated with an anterior calyx (Fig. 22-2). The location of anterior and posterior calyces in relation to the lateral contour of the kidney is not constant. Brödel proposed that anterior calyces are located medially and posterior calyces laterally, while Hodson proposed the opposite; that is, anterior calyces are located laterally and posterior calyces medially. However, more recently Kaye and Reinke studied calyceal location using computed tomography imaging. They found that the Brödel description is far more common on the right, whereas the Hodson calyceal description is more often present on the left (Fig. 22-3).

Because of the variation in the anterior and posterior calyces, in the author's unit we tend to use either carbon dioxide or air to outline the posterior calyces (Fig. 22-4). When there is marked hydronephrosis, differentiation of anterior from posterior calyces is usually not of any technical advantage. However, in renal collecting systems that are moderately or minimally dilated, delineation of the posterior calyces with air or CO_2 may make placement of the percutaneous nephrostomy catheter technically easier.

The colon is occasionally positioned laterally or even posterior to the kidney. Posterior colonic location is rare and if present may well result in colonic transgression (Fig. 22-5). However, it

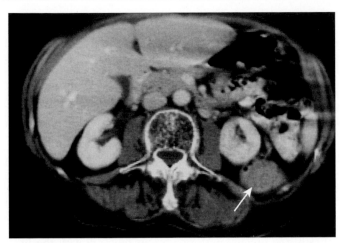

FIGURE 22-5. Computed tomography scan showing the colon *(arrow)* situated posterior to the left kidney. This is an unusual occurrence but ultrasound is recommended before percutaneous nephrostomy to ensure that there is no colon posterior to the kidney.

Box 22-1. Renal Anatomy

Renal vein, artery, and ureter run anterior to posterior in this order

The Brödel plane is theoretical, not practical

Anterior and posterior calyces may have different mediolateral orientations in right and left kidneys

The colon is rarely found posterior to the kidney

---

is so rare that routine pre-nephrostomy imaging with computed tomography (CT) or barium studies is not warranted. Lateral colonic location is more frequent and mitigates against using a lateral access route for percutaneous nephrostomy. Therefore, in practice, a posterolateral route is chosen for gaining access to the kidney so that if the colon is located laterally it will be avoided (Box 22-1).

Ureter

The ureter descends from the renal hilum on the anteromedial surfaces of the psoas muscle. As it passes over the common iliac artery, a slightly more medial course is assumed, followed by a posterolateral course in the pelvis. Finally, as the ureter approaches the bladder, the ureter turns medially and enters the bladder at the ureterovesical junction. There are three areas of physiologic narrowing in the ureter. These are located at the UPJ, the common iliac artery, and the ureterovesical junction.

Bladder

The urinary bladder is located behind the symphysis pubis. The superior wall or dome of the bladder is the only portion of the bladder covered by peritoneum. The neck is fixed in position and as the bladder fills and distends it becomes elevated well above the symphysis pubis. As the bladder fills, all bowel loops are pushed superiorly out of the pelvis, allowing for safe percutaneous access. The vascular supply of the bladder enters through the posterior and lateral aspects of the bladder wall, which also makes for safe percutaneous access through the anterior wall. When planning a percutaneous suprapubic cystostomy, it is important to remember that the inferior epigastric vessels run down the anterior abdominal wall on each side of the rectus muscles and are avoided by selecting an entry site close to the midline.

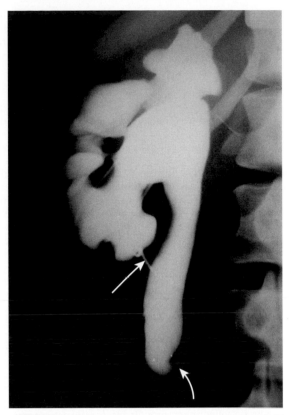

FIGURE 22-6. Antegrade pyelogram in a patient with right-sided hydronephrosis and pain. The needle *(straight arrow)* was inserted into the lower pole calyx. Contrast material injected showed a dilated collecting system with clubbed calyces and characteristic medial deviation of the upper ureter *(curved arrow)*, indicating a retrocaval ureter.

■ PATIENT PREPARATION

As for other interventional procedures, a coagulation profile and informed consent are obtained before the procedure. Coagulation abnormalities are corrected if necessary. Intravenous sedoanalgesia with fentanyl and midazolam is given before and during the procedure for adequate pain relief. The patient is placed prone on the fluoroscopy table. Patients with a recent anterior abdominal wall surgical scar may need sedation and analgesia before being turned prone.

Preprocedure antibiotics are given if there is a suspicion of pyonephrosis or an infected collecting system. The antibiotic regimen chosen depends on operator preference. The author uses gentamicin 80 mg IV and ampicillin 1 g IV.

■ RENAL INTERVENTION

Antegrade Pyelography

Antegrade pyelography refers to the insertion of a needle into the pelvicaliceal system and the injection of contrast material to delineate the anatomy of the pelvicaliceal system and ureter (Fig. 22-6). It currently forms a starting point for many percutaneous genitourinary interventions. It was widely used in the 1980s as a diagnostic technique when intravenous urography failed to adequately opacify the pelvicaliceal system or ureter. However, with the advent of cystoscopy and retrograde injection of contrast medium into the ureter, its popularity has declined. Moreover, with the more extensive use of modalities such as ultrasound, computed tomography, and magnetic resonance imaging (MRI), many renal and ureteric abnormalities can be fully evaluated without recourse to either antegrade pyelography or retrograde pyelography. However, it still remains the mainstay for performance of the Whittaker test and for delineating the anatomy and cause of obstruction before percutaneous nephrostomy.

Technique

The patient is positioned prone on the fluoroscopy table and the kidney is located with ultrasound. Because only a single needle is being placed, the renal pelvis or a calyx can be chosen as a target. It is easier to access the renal pelvis in most instances and in the author's unit we generally choose the renal pelvis as a target. The needle can be directed into the renal pelvis using fluoroscopy alone. The commonly chosen landmark is approximately 2-3 cm lateral to the transverse process of L2. Alternatively, some authors prefer to use ultrasound alone to direct the needle into the renal pelvis or renal calyx using a freehand technique. We prefer to use ultrasound to mark the location and if there is marked dilatation of the pelvicaliceal system the needle is inserted into the renal pelvis without ultrasound guidance. If there is mild or moderate hydronephrosis, ultrasound guidance is used. A 20- or 22-gauge needle can be used, but a 20-gauge needle is preferred because it is a little stiffer and can be directed through the muscles and perinephric tissues without the tip becoming deflected as can happen with 22-gauge needles. Once urine is aspirated from the needle, the needle hub is connected to extension tubing and contrast material is injected. If there is high-grade obstruction, it is important to remove adequate amounts of urine before injecting contrast material to avoid overdistention of the collecting system. A tilting table may help delineate the lower level of the obstruction, particularly in the severely hydronephrotic collecting system. By placing the patient semierect, the heavier contrast material will gravitate toward the lower end of the ureter and delineate the level of the obstruction.

Complications

Complications encountered with antegrade pyelography are rare. Bacteremia can be induced by injecting contrast material into a high-pressure collecting system particularly if the urine is infected. If the urine is cloudy on visual inspection, it is important to decompress and remove an adequate amount of urine before contrast material is injected.

Whittaker Test

The Whittaker or ureteral perfusion test is used to determine whether or not a dilated urinary system is obstructed. It has been regarded as the gold standard for this determination but is performed rarely. Lasix renography can often determine the presence or absence of an obstruction but does have a 10%-15% false-positive rate, particularly in patients with dilated collecting systems. The Whittaker perfusion test was devised to evaluate the presence or absence of obstruction to flow in the presence of a dilated but nonrefluxing upper urinary track. It is more commonly used in pediatric patients where dilated nonrefluxing ureters can pose a diagnostic dilemma. Its most common use in adults is to determine whether pelvicaliceal dilatation due to pelviureteric junction (PUJ) dysfunction is causing obstruction. Similarly, it can be used in adults to evaluate the adequacy of pyeloplasty for the treatment of PUJ obstruction.

The Whittaker test is basically a ureteral stress test. The ureter is perfused with known volumes of fluid at known flow rates. An antegrade needle is placed in the pelvicaliceal system and a Foley catheter placed in the bladder. Manometers are attached to both the antegrade needle and the bladder catheter, and contrast material is infused through the antegrade needle using a pump at known flow rates.

On placement of the antegrade needle, a sample of urine is aspirated for bacteriologic assessment. If the urine appears cloudy, it is

best to delay the procedure until the Gram stain can be obtained. An opening pressure is recorded by connecting a water manometer to the antegrade needle. A water manometer is also connected to the bladder catheter (Fig. 22-7). An opening pressure from the bladder is recorded. It is important to have the base of the manometers at the same level as the tip of the antegrade needle. Water manometers are usually strapped to drip infusion stands and can be set to a similar level as the tip of the antegrade needle by calculating the amount of needle length within the patient. The ureter is then perfused with contrast material diluted to a 20% concentration at a flow rate of 10 mL/min for 5 minutes. Then the perfusion is halted and pressures are again taken from the kidney and bladder. If no evidence of obstruction is present the ureter can be further stressed at a higher flow rate of 15-20 mL/min for another 5 minutes. The subtraction of the recorded bladder pressure from the renal pressure provides the differential pressure. Normal and abnormal pressure differentials are listed in Table 22-1.

Lastly, the ureteral perfusion test is repeated with the bladder full to evaluate the effect of increased bladder pressure on the urinary track. This is important in situations where the bladder pressure is high owing to either outlet obstruction or neurogenic disease. Intermittent or continuous high bladder pressures greater than 20 cm H_2O places the kidney at risk even in the absence of ureteral obstruction.

The ureteral perfusion test is abandoned if the opening pressure in the kidney is greater than 35 cm H_2O or if the patient develops pain during the procedure.

Percutaneous Nephrostomy

Percutaneous nephrostomy remains the most common procedure performed on the kidney by the interventional radiologist. The most common indications for percutaneous nephrostomy include obstruction from ureteric stones and malignant obstruction from carcinomas of the bladder and prostate. The ureters may also be involved by secondary malignant deposits from cancers of the uterus, colon, breast, and abdominal lymphoma. Other indications for percutaneous nephrostomy include postsurgical damage to the ureter, ureteral fistulas, and idiopathic retroperitoneal fibrosis.

Nephron damage and parenchymal atrophy can begin as early as a few days to a week following the onset of obstruction. Undoubtedly, nephron damage occurs much earlier if the urine is infected. Information on how long the kidney can tolerate high-grade obstruction is incomplete, but nephron damage is influenced by whether the obstruction is unilateral or bilateral, whether there is superimposed infection, and whether there is preexisting renal or vascular disease. Because of the uncertainty as to when irreversible nephron damage begins, an obstructed urinary system should be drained as soon as possible after diagnosis.

Technique

Pelvicaliceal Access
The patient is placed prone on the fluoroscopy table and the obstructed kidney is imaged with ultrasound to determine its location and the degree of hydronephrosis. An antegrade pyelogram is performed as previously described and contrast material injected to outline the pelvicaliceal system. During antegrade pyelography, the level and cause of obstruction is determined, if not known already. The only exception is when a pyonephrosis is encountered. If a pyonephrosis is encountered, the minimum amount of contrast material is injected and minimal manipulation of the pelvicaliceal system is carried out. Once the pelvicaliceal system is outlined by contrast material, a calyx is chosen for puncture. The calyx chosen depends on the anatomy of the kidney and on the likelihood of any future procedures such as antegrade ureteral stent insertion. If antegrade stent insertion is likely, then a midpole calyx is preferable; if not, a lower pole calyx can be chosen.

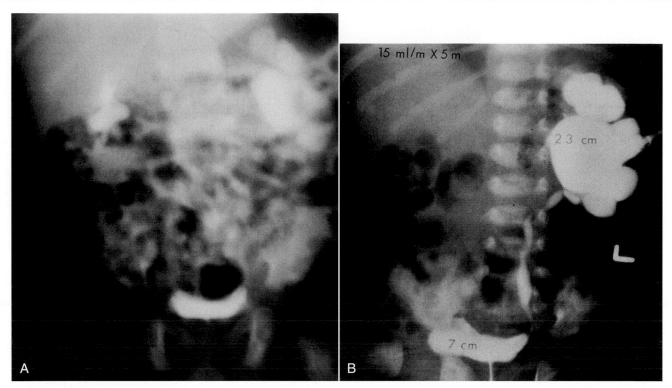

FIGURE 22-7. Whittaker ureteral perfusion test in a 2-month-old baby with left-sided hydronephrosis. The hydronephrosis was noted on an antenatal ultrasound scan and was thought to represent an ureteropelvic junction obstruction. **A,** An intravenous pyelogram performed at 2 months shows a dilated collecting system on the left with no visualized ureter. **B,** A ureteral perfusion test was performed with the patient under general anesthesia by inserting an antegrade needle into the left collecting system and a small catheter into the bladder. Pressure differential after perfusion of the collecting system with 15 mL/min of contrast material for 5 minutes was 16 cm H_2O, which is equivalent to a mild obstruction. Because of the minimal nature of the obstruction it was decided not to perform surgery at this time but to adopt a conservative approach with regular follow-up.

TABLE 22-1 Normal and Abnormal Pressure Differentials Associated with the Whittaker Test

Flow Rate (mL/min)	Pressure Differential (cm H_2O)	Grade of Obstruction
10	<13	Normal
10	14-22	Mild or equivocal
10	23-35	Moderate
10	>35	Severe

Having decided on the calyx of choice, the next step is to decide whether the calyx seen is an anterior or posterior calyx. The best way to do this is to inject either carbon dioxide or air via the antegrade needle into the pelvicaliceal system (Fig. 22-8). If CO_2 is not available, 10-15 cc of air can be injected through the antegrade needle. It is important to ensure that the antegrade needle is not in communication with a vein, so that air embolus is avoided. The air or CO_2 will rise into the posterior calyces, which can then be readily identified. At this stage, some operators like to turn the patient into the prone oblique position, which theoretically makes the angle from the calyx into the infundibulum and renal pelvis more shallow and easier to negotiate. In the author's unit we prefer to leave the patient in the prone position because usually there is little or no difficulty in negotiating a wire from a posterior calyx into the pelvis.

A single-stick needle access system (Neff Set, Cook, Bloomington, Ind.; Acustick, Meditech, Watertown, Mass.) is used to gain access into the calyx. These needle access sets are composed of a 22-gauge, 15-cm needle, a 0.018-inch guidewire, a metal cannula, a 4-French plastic cannula, and a 5-French sheath. A skin position is marked using fluoroscopy 1.5-2.0 cm lateral to the calyx chosen. The skin is infiltrated with local anesthetic, an incision is made with a #11 scalpel, and the needle is inserted under fluoroscopic guidance into the calyx. The depth of insertion can usually be gauged by the depth of the antegrade needle inserted to gain access to the renal pelvis; because the lower pole of the kidney is more anterior, the second needle is inserted a little deeper than the antegrade needle to gain access to the collecting system. A 10-mL syringe with 2 mL of saline is placed on the hub of the needle. The stylet is removed and the needle is slowly withdrawn until urine or air bubbles appear in the syringe. The 0.018-inch guidewire is then manipulated down through the needle into the calyx and into the renal pelvis. Occasionally, difficulty is encountered in advancing the guidewire from the tip of the needle, even though urine has been aspirated through the needle. Often this is because the needle tip is up against the wall of the calyx. Withdrawing the needle slightly and turning the needle so that the bevel points in different directions may aid in negotiating the guidewire into the renal pelvis. When the 0.018-inch guidewire is in the renal pelvis, the needle is removed over the guidewire and the 5-French sheath assembly is placed over the wire into the pelvicaliceal system. It is important to detach the metal stiffening cannula when the sheath system has entered the calyx. The metal cannula is too stiff to traverse the angle between the calyx and renal pelvis. Once the metal cannula is withdrawn, the 5-French sheath and inner plastic cannula are flexible enough to follow the guidewire into the renal pelvis. If the metal cannula is left in place, attempts to force the sheath system into the renal pelvis result in guidewire kinking in the calyx and further pushing may cause the guidewire to slip out of the kidney altogether. Once the 5-French sheath is in the renal pelvis, a 0.035-inch J-guidewire is inserted through the 5-French sheath and is coiled in the renal pelvis, placed in the upper pole calyx, or manipulated down the ureter (Fig. 22-9).

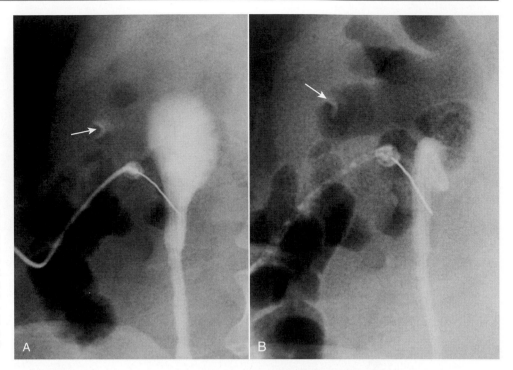

FIGURE 22-8. A patient with a ureteral stent that was calcified and was not possible to remove cystoscopically. **A,** An antegrade needle was placed near the apex of the proximal end of the stent and contrast material injected. Because of the low access, contrast material did not opacify the calyceal system apart from one anterior calyx *(arrow)*. **B,** Air was injected, which helped outline the posterior calyces for puncture. Note the small amount of contrast material remaining in the anterior calyx *(arrow)* in the lower pole of the kidney.

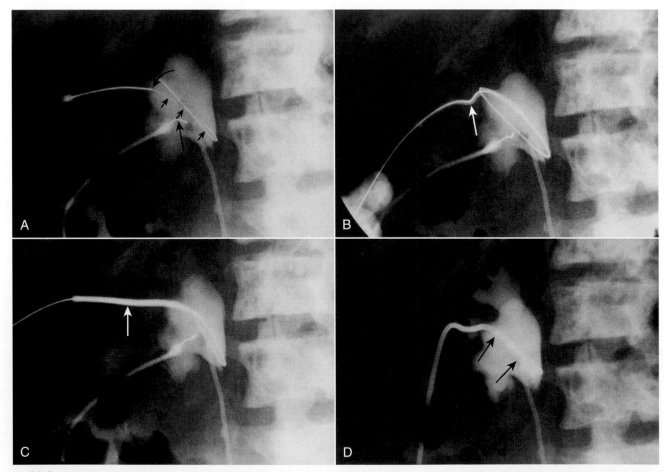

FIGURE 22-9. Percutaneous nephrostomy in a patient with a blocked ureteral stent and fever. **A,** An antegrade needle *(straight arrow)* was inserted to outline the pelvicaliceal system. A second 22-gauge needle *(curved arrow)* was used to puncture a midpole calyx and a 0.018-inch guidewire *(small arrows)* coiled in the renal pelvis. **B,** The sheath system *(arrow)* can be seen inserted over the 0.018-inch wire into the renal pelvis. The guidewire was removed and a 0.35-inch J-guidewire inserted. **C,** Track dilatation was performed with 8- and 10-French dilators. The 10-French dilator *(arrow)* is seen dilating the percutaneous track. **D,** Finally, an 8-French nephrostomy catheter *(arrows)* was inserted and coiled in the renal pelvis.

Placing the Nephrostomy Catheter

When the 0.035-inch J-guidewire is present in the renal pelvis, the track is dilated. Some others prefer using a stiffer guidewire such as a 0.035-inch Ring-Lunderquist (Cook, Bloomington, Ind.) guidewire, but with experience the J-guidewire is usually adequate. If an 8-French catheter is being placed, the track is dilated with 8- and 10-French dilators. If a 10-French catheter is being placed the percutaneous track is dilated with 8-, 10-, and 12-French dilators and so on. An 8-French nephrostomy catheter is placed for the vast majority of percutaneous nephrostomies. Only if one encounters a pyonephrosis should a 10- or 12-French catheter be placed. It is important to fluoroscopically monitor the guidewire while dilating the track to ensure that kinking of the guidewire does not take place. When the track is dilated the nephrostomy catheter (Cook, Bloomington, Ind.; Meditech, Watertown, Mass.) is passed over the guidewire into the renal pelvis. The nephrostomy catheters usually come with a metal stiffening cannula, which is used to provide stability for the catheter as it passes through the subcutaneous tissues, muscles, and retroperitoneal tissues on the way to the kidney. Once the catheter has entered the kidney, it is important again to detach the metal stiffening cannula and withdraw it slightly while sliding the catheter forward over the guidewire. Failure to do this will result in kinking of the wire and/or loss of purchase within the kidney.

Depending on where the guidewire is coiled, the catheter is placed in the upper pole calyx, coiled in the pelvis, or placed down the ureter over the wire. The string on the end of the catheter is then pulled to form the pigtail loop. If the catheter is down the ureter, pulling the catheter back until the tip is approximately 4-5 cm from the PUJ ensures that, when the string is pulled, the catheter flipped back into the renal pelvis, forming a nice pigtail (Fig. 22-10 and Box 22-2).

Aftercare

Catheter fixation to the skin is important and can be done in a number of ways. The author uses a Hollister ostomy disk, which is placed on the patient's skin with the catheter threaded through the opening in the center of the Hollister disk. Adhesive tape is placed around the catheter and the adhesive tape is then sutured to the ostomy disc. Alternatively, the adhesive tape that is first placed around the catheter can be sutured directly to the patient's skin. Unless there has been a lot of bleeding and clot formation, it is usually not necessary to irrigate a nephrostomy catheter. Urine contains proteolytic enzymes that will tend to break down any clot forming in the catheter and keep the catheter patent. The author's unit tends to use irrigation only when there is thick pus in the collecting system or when there is significant clot formation after the procedure.

Results

The success rate for percutaneous nephrostomy approaches 100% in experienced hands. Difficulties may be encountered with the nondilated collecting system, but these are surmountable by appropriate placement of an antegrade needle and adequate distention.

Complications

Complications resulting from percutaneous nephrostomy are infrequent and have been estimated to be around 4%. Hemorrhage (Figs. 22-11 and 22-12) and infection are the two most frequent complications requiring therapy. Some bleeding is

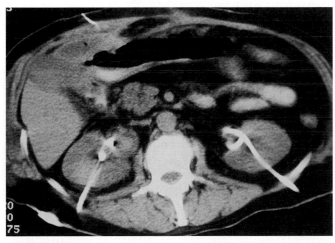

FIGURE 22-10. Computed tomography scan showing appropriately placed nephrostomy catheters. The catheters are placed from a posterolateral approach through the renal cortex into both collecting systems. Catheters are placed through the renal cortex with the intention of tamponading any potential bleeding.

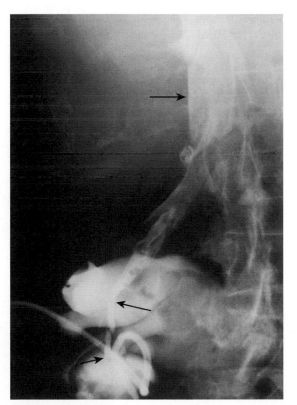

FIGURE 22-11. Backbleeding through a percutaneous nephrostomy catheter placed in a ptotic and obstructed right kidney. A nephrostogram performed through the nephrostomy catheter shows communication with the renal vein and inferior vena cava *(straight arrows)*. The catheter had pulled back into the percutaneous track such that one of the side holes was communicating with a renal vein branch *(small arrow)*, which was corrected by inserting the catheter more medially into the renal pelvis over a guidewire.

BOX *22-2.* Percutaneous Nephrostomy

20-gauge antegrade needle first placed in renal pelvis
CO_2 or air injected to identify posterior calyces
Single-stick needle system used to access chosen calyx
Nephrostomy catheter metal stiffener withdrawn at calyceal level
Minimal contrast injection and manipulation in infected system

not infrequent after most percutaneous nephrostomies. However, severe bleeding may indicate arterial damage such as a pseudoaneurysm or arteriovenous fistula. If there is significant backbleeding through the catheter with an associated decrease in hematocrit, then an arteriogram may be indicated with embolization at any bleeding site. This is a rare occurrence, and the author's unit has had only one major bleeding complication in the past 10 years. Bleeding can be prevented to a large extent by correcting any coagulopathy beforehand and placing the catheter

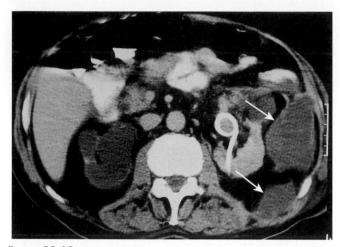

FIGURE 22-12. CT scan performed after a percutaneous nephrostomy in a patient who became hypotensive. Note the nonfunctioning kidney on the right side. The nephrostomy catheter is in good position but there is extensive retroperitoneal hemorrhage *(arrows)* around the kidney. The kidney is also displaced forward by the hemorrhage. The patient settled with conservative management and no operative or other percutaneous intervention was required. The reason for the bleeding was unclear as the percutaneous nephrostomy was uncomplicated and the patient did not have a coagulation disorder.

peripherally through the cortex into a calyx rather than placing the catheter directly into the renal pelvis (Fig. 22-13).

Sepsis is the other major complication that can complicate percutaneous nephrostomy. Sepsis almost invariably occurs in patients with a pyonephrosis, infected stone, or infected urine. During the percutaneous nephrostomy, bacteria and endotoxins from the collecting system invariably enter the bloodstream, which may cause septicemia in some patients, despite appropriate antibiotic coverage. It is important not to overdistend the collecting system in these patients and to use the minimum amount of manipulation necessary to place the catheter.

Catheter-related problems such as dislodgment and occlusion do occur. With modern pigtail catheters, it is rare for catheters to become dislodged. However, if dislodgment does occur, it is important to bring the patient to the interventional suite as soon as possible. Depending on the maturity of the track, it may be possible to probe the track and reinsert a nephrostomy catheter. Generally, in the author's unit we use an angled hydrophilic guidewire and Kumpe catheter to probe the track. If access to the pelvicaliceal system is gained, it is usually a straightforward task to place a new nephrostomy catheter. If access cannot be gained, a new percutaneous nephrostomy procedure is performed.

Catheter occlusion is more likely to occur the longer the catheter is left in situ. It may be possible to open the existing catheter by using a guidewire. If this is not possible, the catheter can be exchanged by using a 9-French peel-away sheath. The hub of the catheter is cut and the peel-away sheath inserted over the catheter into the collecting system. The catheter is then removed and a new catheter inserted into the pelvicaliceal system. A guidewire is not used for this procedure.

Special Circumstances

Transplant Kidney

Occasionally, an interventional radiologist may be called upon to place a nephrostomy catheter in a patient with a transplant kidney

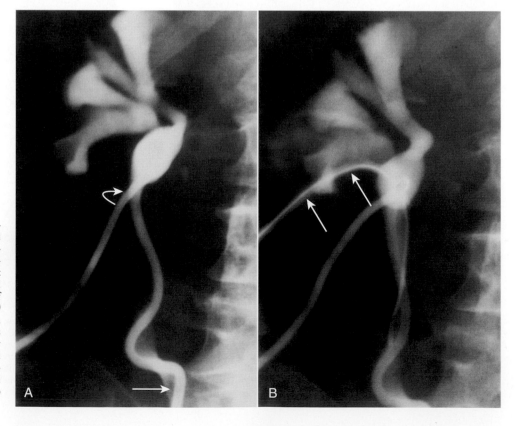

FIGURE 22-13. Example of a percutaneous nephrostomy catheter inserted directly into the renal pelvis. **A,** Nephrostomy catheter *(curved arrow)* insertion performed at an outside hospital shows that the nephrostomy catheter was inserted directly into the renal pelvis. The tip of the nephrostomy catheter *(straight arrow)* is in the proximal ureter and not coiled in the renal pelvis. **B,** The patient was referred for antegrade stenting, and a new access into a lower pole calyx was obtained *(arrows)* for the purpose. Direct manipulation of the renal pelvis is not advised because of the potential for damage to arterial or venous structures.

(Fig. 22-14). Often, the cause of obstruction may be edema at the ureterovesical junction. The nephrostomy drainage may therefore be of a temporary nature. Rarely, the obstruction may be due to ureteric torsion or ureteric ischemia leading to a stricture.

Because the transplant kidney is superficially placed in the right or left flank, the procedure is more easily performed than in a native kidney. For percutaneous nephrostomy in the transplant kidney, a single needle puncture suffices for both antegrade pyelography and access to the pelvicaliceal system. Ultrasound is used to place a 22-gauge needle in a calyx. This needle is then used to inject contrast material for antegrade pyelography and a 0.018-inch guidewire can be inserted through the needle for access into the pelvicaliceal system. Any calyx can be chosen for access. However, if a ureteric stent is to be placed, a midpole calyx or upper pole calyx is preferable. Track dilatation is usually easier than in the native kidney because of the decreased amount of tissue between the skin and the transplant kidney. However, in patients who have had more than one transplant kidney placed in the same area, extensive fibrotic tissue may make dilatation difficult. In some cases, it may not be possible to pass the sheath system over the 0.018-inch guidance. In these situations the author has used a 19-gauge long-dwell needle to make the initial puncture and inserted a superstiff guidewire to aid track dilatation. An 8-French nephrostomy tube is placed in a similar fashion to that described for percutaneous nephrostomy in a native kidney.

Retrograde Nephrostomy Drainage Via Ileal Loop

In the patient with an ileal loop who presents with obstructive uropathy, a retrograde approach to the ileal loop is worth considering for nephrostomy drainage (Fig. 22-15). The obstruction is usually due to recurrent tumor or stricture at the anastomotic site between the ureter and ileal loop. It is prudent to perform a loopogram first to document that there is no reflux of contrast medium from the ileal loop into the ureter. This helps confirm the presence of obstruction. Additionally, if there is bulky tumor in the ileal loop, it is best to perform the nephrostomy drainage from an antegrade approach.

The ostomy site is cannulated with a Kumpe catheter and straight or angled 0.035-inch hydrophilic guidewire. The Kumpe catheter and hydrophilic guidewire are manipulated to the end of the ileal loop. When the Kumpe catheter has reached the end of the ileal loop, the guidewire is removed and exchanged for a

0.035-inch superstiff or extra stiff wire. A 9-French peel-away sheath is placed over the superstiff wire. The peel-away sheath usually reaches the end of the ileal loop. This is the key step in the retrograde procedure. The 9-French peel-away sheath straightens out any tortuosity of the ileal loop and protects the guidewire and Kumpe catheter from peristalsis, which may cause the guidewire and Kumpe catheter to be extruded from the ileal loop. The Kumpe catheter is again placed over the superstiff wire and the latter is exchanged for a hydrophilic guidewire. The ureteric orifice is then sought using the Kumpe catheter and hydrophilic guidewire. It is helpful to inject contrast material because often a small nipple can be seen where the ureteric orifice arises. It is also helpful to review previous intravenous pyelograms or loopograms, which may guide the operator to the appropriate place to search for the ureteric orifice. Once the ureteric orifice is negotiated, the hydrophilic guidewire and Kumpe catheter are manipulated up the ureter into the kidney. The hydrophilic guidewire is removed and the superstiff or extra stiff guidewire is placed up into the kidney.

Depending on the distance from the ostomy site to the renal pelvis, a nephrostomy catheter, an internal/external ureteral stent, or an internal ureteral stent can be placed. A rough estimate of the distance to be traversed can be gained by using the Kumpe catheter as a marker. An 8-French nephrostomy catheter can be placed, or if the distance is longer, either internal or internal/external ureteral stents can be placed. Whichever catheter is placed, it is important to leave the end of the catheter in the patient's ostomy bag and not in the ileal loop. The distal end of the catheter tends to clog rapidly if left in the ileal loop, because the ileal loop sheds mucosal cells on a regular basis and the catheter side holes become clogged with silt.

If it is not possible to negotiate the ureteric orifice, then the patient can be turned prone and an antegrade nephrostomy performed (Box 22-3).

Nondilated Collecting System

Percutaneous nephrostomy in the nondilated collecting system is technically difficult. This situation is most commonly encountered in patients with ureteric leaks after surgery. Percutaneous nephrostomy and/or stent placement is the preferred treatment but the collecting system will be decompressed because of the ureteric leak. On ultrasound the collecting system is usually decompressed and ultrasound guidance is not usually helpful. In this situation, the author's unit gives 50-75 mL of a 300%

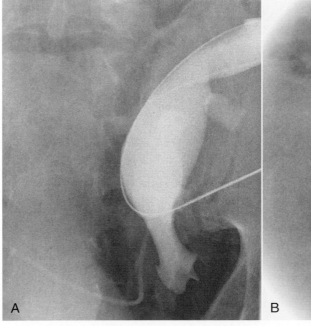

A

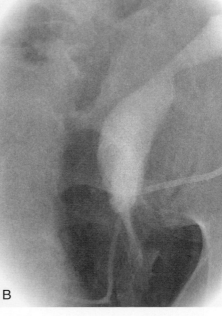

B

FIGURE 22-14. Percutaneous nephrostomy in a patient with a transplant kidney who had a stent placed that malfunctioned. The patient was noted to have a raised serum creatinine with hydronephrosis detected on ultrasound. **A,** A stent can be seen in situ. Ultrasound determined that a midpole calyx was the largest calyx and ultrasound guidance was used to place a 22-gauge needle. After placing the 5-French sheath over the 0.018-inch guidewire, a 0.35-inch J-wire was coiled in the upper pole calyx. **B,** After track dilatation, an 8-French nephrostomy catheter was placed in the upper pole calyx. The hydronephrosis was due to ureteric ischemia.

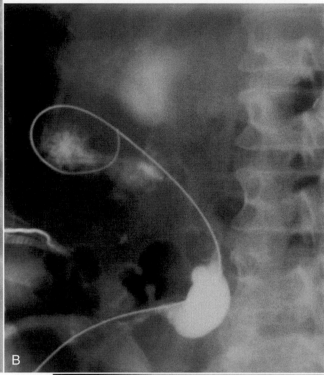

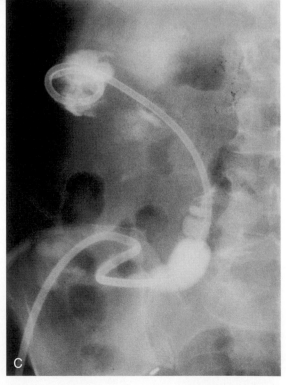

FIGURE 22-15. Retrograde nephrostomy catheter placement in a patient with an ileal loop. This patient had a solitary kidney with recurrent transitional cell cancer (TCC). **A,** A loopogram shows recurrent TCC at the anastomosis between the ileal conduit and the upper ureter *(arrows)*. **B,** After manipulating a Kumpe catheter and a hydrophilic guidewire down the ileal loop toward the kidney, a superstiff guidewire was placed into the kidney, which helped straighten out the ileal conduit for future catheter placement. A 9-French peel-away sheath was placed into the loop for added rigidity. **C,** An 8-French nephrostomy catheter was placed retrograde into the kidney through the peel-away sheath and the end left in the ostomy bag for drainage. The patient survived for almost a year with this catheter in place.

contrast material to opacify the pelvicaliceal system. When the pelvicaliceal system is opacified, an antegrade needle is inserted into the renal pelvis under fluoroscopic guidance. This needle is then used to distend the pelvicaliceal system and a calyx is chosen for nephrostomy access. Because many of these patients will be having antegrade stents placed, a midpole calyx is preferable. A 22-gauge needle is placed into the midpole calyx and a 0.018-inch guidewire manipulated into the renal pelvis. It is important to keep the pelvicaliceal system distended by having an assistant maintain a steady injection of dilute contrast material into the pelvicaliceal system using the antegrade needle. This often aids the passage of the 0.018-inch guidewire into the renal pelvis. The pelvicaliceal system is collapsed in these patients and optimal distention is important to facilitate the passage of a guidewire from the calyx to the renal pelvis. Once access is gained, the procedure can be performed in the traditional fashion.

Computed Tomography–Guided Nephrostomy Drainage

Rarely, CT guidance is necessary to gain access to the kidney. This almost exclusively occurs in patients with severe scoliosis who require a nephrostomy drainage (Fig. 22-16). It can be very difficult to assess the relationship of the kidney to adjacent organs in the severely scoliotic patient. Particularly, it is important to assess the relationship of the colon with the obstructed kidney in these patients. In addition, obstructed kidneys in the severely scoliotic patients can be difficult to identify with ultrasound and it can be extremely difficult to work out the relationships of the kidney with adjacent organs on ultrasound.

The patient is placed supine or prone on the CT table and a noncontrast CT scan through the kidneys is performed. The patient is then placed in the position that best facilitates access

---

Box 22-3. **Retrograde Ileal Loop Nephrostomy**

Loopogram first to confirm obstruction
9-French peel-away sheath important to straighten out loop
Kumpe catheter and hydrophilic guidewire used to negotiate ureteric orifice
Leave distal end of catheter or stent in ostomy bag and not in ileal loop

---

to the kidney. Under CT guidance, either a 22-gauge needle can be placed into the renal pelvis as an antegrade needle for opacifying the pelvicaliceal system, or a 22-gauge needle can be placed directly into a calyx and the patient transferred to undergo fluoroscopy for the completion of the procedure. Either way, the anatomic relationship of the kidney with adjacent organs can be ascertained and a safe access route to the pelvicaliceal system planned.

Percutaneous Lithotripsy and Nephrolithotomy

Traditionally, staghorn calculi were removed surgically. However, from about 1980 on, percutaneous nephrolithotomy became the procedure of choice for the removal of large staghorn calculi and indeed for the removal of upper urinary track calculi in many institutions. The subsequent introduction of extracorporeal shockwave lithotripsy (ESWL) reduced the number of indications for percutaneous nephrolithotomy but these are now well defined and commonly accepted. These include complete staghorn calculi and partial staghorn calculi or smaller renal calculi refractory to ESWL. In some institutions, renal stones in calyceal diverticula may also be managed by percutaneous nephrolithotomy. In many instances, both techniques are used together for the larger staghorn calculi; if clearance is incomplete after percutaneous nephrolithotomy, ESWL is performed.

Technique

Percutaneous nephrolithotomy consists of placing a large-bore track or tracks (up to 30-French) into the kidney for stone fragmentation (Fig. 22-17). Stone fragmentation is usually achieved

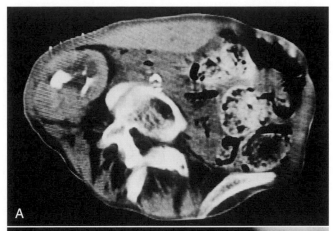
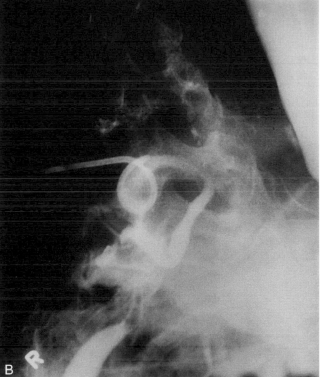

FIGURE 22-16. Computed tomography (CT)-guided nephrostomy drainage in a patient with severe scoliosis, renal stones, and fever. **A,** CT guidance was used because of the severe scoliosis. A noncontrast CT scan was performed and a 22-gauge needle placed into the midpole calyx. Note the radiopaque stones in the kidney. **B,** The patient was then moved to a fluoroscopic suite and an 8-French nephrostomy catheter was placed. CT was useful to guide the initial needle puncture and ensure that there were no intervening organs between the skin and the kidney.

with a rigid 24- to 26-French nephroscope. Because of the inflexibility of the nephroscope, it is vitally important to access the kidney proximal to the stone to be fragmented. In other words, peripheral access into a calyx is vital. The nephroscope looks straight ahead and can only fragment stones in front of it. Although smaller flexible scopes can be used to enter individual calyces, this is a more tedious procedure. Close cooperation between the urologist and interventional radiologist is mandatory for appropriate track placement. In patients with large staghorn calculi, it may be necessary to place as many as two to three large-bore tracks into the kidney. In some centers the track is created and a 24-French catheter left in situ for 1-2 days, after which the patient is brought to the operating room for stone removal. The advantage of using this technique is that any bleeding that occurs during track preparation has usually cleared after 1-2 days and a clear view of the stone will be available at the time of stone fragmentation. Others prefer to perform the whole procedure in one sitting in which track preparation is performed and a large 30-French sheath inserted into the kidney. The patient is then transferred to the operating room where a nephroscope is inserted and the stone fragmented. Although we initially used the two-stage procedure, we now prefer a one-stage procedure. The disadvantage of the two-stage procedure is that the large 24-French catheter in the kidney is quite painful over the intervening days until surgical removal of the stone.

In general, the procedure can be performed almost entirely under fluoroscopic guidance. A 22-gauge antegrade needle is placed directly down on top of the stone in the renal pelvis. After the antegrade needle is placed, urine is aspirated. If the urine appears cloudy or infected, then a simple nephrostomy tube is placed to allow drainage and appropriate antibiotic therapy started. It is imperative not to proceed with large track formation into the kidney in the presence of infection. This can lead to profound septic shock and occasionally disseminated intravascular coagulation. If the urine is clear, track preparation is performed. An appropriate calyx is chosen that will yield the maximum stone clearance from the pelvicaliceal system. In some instances, two or even three tracks may be required for this purpose.

A one-stick system (Neff Set, Cook, Bloomington, Ind.; Acustick, Meditech, Watertown, Mass.) is inserted into the peripheral portion of the calyx chosen. The 0.018-inch wire is then manipulated into the renal pelvis. To aid passage of the 0.018-inch wire into the renal pelvis, it is invaluable to have an assistant inject dilute contrast material through the antegrade needle to distend the collecting system and allow some space to develop between the stone and the surrounding uroepithelium. This facilitates passage of the guidewire into the renal pelvis. If the 0.018-inch guidewire cannot be manipulated into the renal pelvis, access to the calyx is maintained and a Kumpe catheter and hydrophilic guidewire used to gain access to the renal pelvis. Once access to the renal pelvis is gained, the Kumpe catheter and hydrophilic guidewire are used to access the ureter. The Kumpe catheter is placed down the ureter as far as the ureterovesical junction or into the bladder. The hydrophilic guidewire is then exchanged for a 0.035-inch superstiff guidewire (Meditech, Watertown, Mass.). The percutaneous track is then ready to be dilated.

The track can be dilated in two ways: with serial fascial dilators from 8- to 30-French or with a balloon catheter (10 mm × 10 cm). The author prefers to use the balloon catheter for track dilatation because it is faster and one is less likely to kink the guidewire. Usually a waist is seen in the balloon at the renal capsule and it is important to inflate the balloon until this waist disappears. During balloon dilatation, any persistent waist that does not disappear despite increased inflation pressure implies that the percutaneous track will need to be dilated with larger fascial dilators such as 26- and 28-French for complete track dilatation. After balloon dilatation, a 30-French Amplatz sheath (Cook, Bloomington, Ind.) is placed over the guidewire into the renal pelvis. A second safety wire is placed down the ureter and a small balloon catheter (4-6 mm diameter) inflated in the upper ureter to prevent stone migration. Alternatively, the balloon catheter can be inserted retrograde at cystoscopy into the upper ureter. The patient is transferred to the operating room and the stones fragmented using ultrasonic lithotripsy, electrohydraulic lithotripsy, or laser lithotripsy.

In the author's unit we use ultrasonic lithotripsy under direct endoscopic visualization. Stone fragments are washed back out through the sheath using a high-flow irrigation system that is

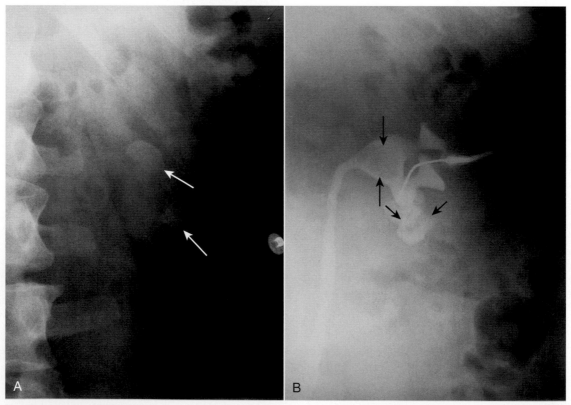

FIGURE 22-17. Percutaneous nephrolithotomy in a patient with uric acid stones in the left kidney. **A,** The plain film shows two stones *(arrows)* in the left kidney, one in the renal pelvis and one in a lower-pole calyx. **B,** An antegrade nephrostogram was performed where stones can be seen *(arrows)* as filling defects in the contrast medium column.

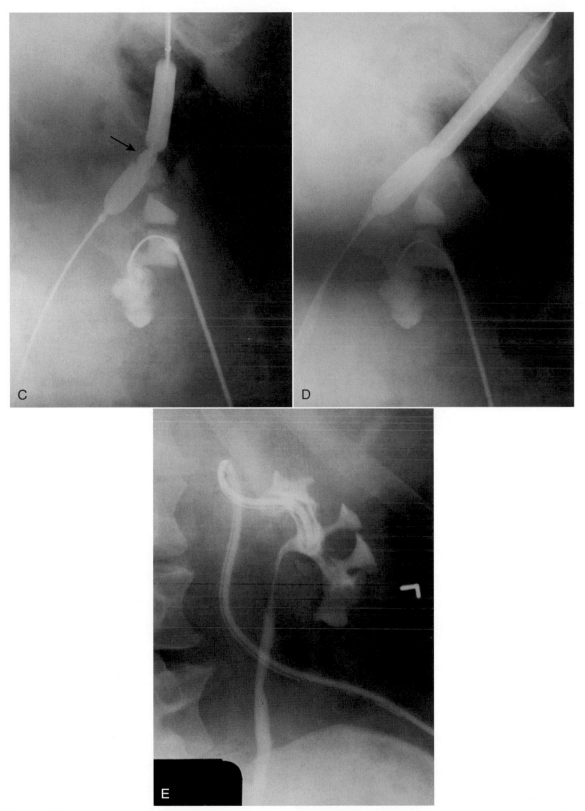

FIGURE 22-17, cont'd C, An upper pole access was chosen to ensure complete removal of both stones. After access was gained down the ureter, a 1-cm balloon was used to dilate the percutaneous track. Note the waist in the balloon at the level of the renal cortex *(arrow)*. D, The balloon was further inflated and the waist disappeared. After the balloon was removed, a 30-French Amplatz sheath and dilator were inserted over the superstiff wire. We usually place a second safety guidewire down the ureter and place a small balloon catheter in the upper ureter to prevent stone fragments from going down the ureter. E, Nephrostogram performed 24 hours after nephrolithotomy in the operating room shows that the stones have been completely removed. There is a little narrowing of the upper ureter due to edema. This settled spontaneously and the catheter was removed after 2 weeks.

connected to the nephroscope. At the end of the procedure, a 26-French Foley balloon catheter or Malecot catheter is placed in the renal pelvis for 2-3 weeks after the procedure. If there are remaining stone fragments, ESWL can be performed. Two to three days after the procedure, a nephrostogram is done to help identify remaining stone fragments and assess pelvicaliceal or ureteral damage. Stone fragments identified in the ureter may require further retrograde intervention. Remaining stones in the kidney can be shattered by ESWL. Renal pelvis perforation usually heals rapidly with a nephrostomy tube in place (Box 22-4).

Results

Percutaneous nephrolithotomy has proven very effective in the management of renal stones with low complication rates and results approaching those of open lithotomy. For large staghorn calculi, success rates for complete stone removal vary from 70% to approximately 90% in experienced hands. Success rates for complete removal of smaller pelvicaliceal stones are as high as 98%, with the size of the stone, location, the sitting of the percutaneous track, and the experience of the operators influencing results. The main advantage of this technique over open lithotomy is that

patients can return to their normal lifestyle and activities within a few days after the procedure.

Complications

The published complication rates for percutaneous nephrolithotomy approach 4%. The main complications are bleeding and sepsis. Bleeding may occur due to injury or laceration of a small segmental artery during track dilatation. This can be remedied by tamponading the track with a large nephrostomy catheter, or it may require angiographic embolization. Additionally, arteriovenous fistulas or arterial pseudoaneurysms may rarely occur and may require angiographic embolization.

Postprocedure sepsis occurs in up to 1% of patients. Patients with infected stones are more prone to develop sepsis and it is important to look for indications of infection before the procedure. This includes ensuring that the patient does not have a fever before the procedure and that the white cell count and erythrocyte sedimentation rate are normal. Sepsis can occur even in patients who are adequately covered by antibiotics. In the author's experience, the subset of patients that can often have undetected infection are those with spina bifida. It is vitally important to aspirate and inspect the urine after antegrade needle placement. If there is any doubt as to whether the urine is infected, an immediate Gram stain should be performed before proceeding to track dilatation. If the urine is infected, then an 8-French nephrostomy catheter is placed and the patient placed on appropriate antibiotic therapy. When the urine is clear, track dilatation can commence.

Pneumothorax or hemothorax may rarely occur after percutaneous nephrolithotomy (Fig. 22-18). This complication is predisposed to by an upper pole renal access. If an upper pole renal

---

Box 22-4. Percutaneous Nephrolithotomy

Access to the peripheral part of the calyx is vital
Many large tracks may be necessary depending on stone size
Do not proceed if infected urine is found
A 10 mm × 10 cm balloon is used for track dilatation
The entire procedure is performed in one sitting

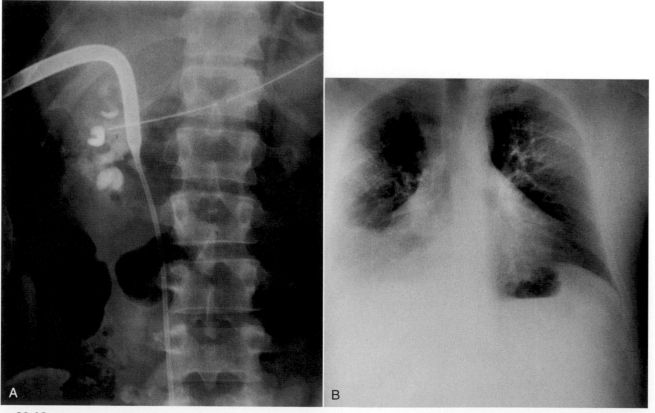

FIGURE 22-18. Hemothorax which occurred after placement of a percutaneous nephrolithotomy track. **A,** A two-stage procedure was performed on this patient with the placement of a large pyeloureteral stent using an upper pole access. The patient was brought to the operating room the next day. **B,** In the recovery room after nephrolithotomy the patient became hypotensive and a chest radiograph performed showed a pleural effusion that was not seen preoperatively. This was tapped and proved to be a hemothorax, which is a known complication of upper pole track formation. This was drained and the patient settled with conservative management.

access is performed, this complication should be anticipated and the appropriate catheters should be readily available for treatment.

Rarely, strictures of the UPJ occur from injury at the time of ultrasonic, laser, or electrohydraulic lithotripsy. If this is recognized on the nephrostogram immediately after stone fragmentation, early antegrade stent placement helps prevent formation of a stricture.

Occasionally, foreign bodies may remain in the collecting system after percutaneous nephrolithotomy. They may include pieces of guidewires, baskets, or graspers. These are best removed endoscopically through the percutaneous track.

Percutaneous Stent Extraction

Rarely, ureteric stents cannot be removed at cystoscopy, owing either to marked encrustation or migration of the distal pigtail of the stent proximally up into the ureter. Access to the pelvicaliceal system is gained in the manner previously described for percutaneous nephrostomy and, depending on the size of the stent retained in the ureter, an appropriate peel-away sheath is placed into the pelvicaliceal system (Fig. 22-19). If the ureteric stent is 6-French, then a 12- to 14-French peel-away sheath is placed; if the ureteric stent is 8-French, then a 14- to 16-French peel-away sheath is placed. It is useful to cut a 45-degree bevel in the end of the peel-away sheath as this will greatly aid stent engagement within the peel-away sheath. The peel-away sheath is placed into the renal pelvis as close as possible to the stent. Either a three-pronged grasper or a long alligator forceps are used to grasp the stent. The stent is then pulled through the peel-away sheath and delivered externally. It is not always possible to grasp the end of the stent and often the proximal portion of the stent is grasped. The stent then folds on itself while being pulled through the peel-away sheath. If insertion of another stent is required this can be performed through the peel-away sheath by placing a guidewire down into the bladder and placing an antegrade stent.

In a similar fashion, biopsy of suspected pelvicaliceal tumors can be performed through a peel-away sheath. A biopsy forceps can be placed through the peel-away sheath to biopsy pelvicaliceal lesions. This is rarely necessary as most patients with suspected urothelial tumors undergo retrograde biopsy or cell sampling of urine from the affected side.

■ URETERIC INTERVENTION

Antegrade Stent Placement

Antegrade stent placement is a well-established percutaneous technique that evolved from the placement of percutaneous nephrostomy tubes. An interventional radiologist may be called upon to place an antegrade ureteric stent when retrograde stenting by the urologist fails. The usual indications are for malignant obstruction or occasionally benign disease such as strictures, stones, and ureteric leaks or fistulas.

Technique

The two key points in the procedure are:
- Getting appropriate access to the pelvicaliceal system
- The use of a peel-away sheath

A midpole access is the preferred access point for antegrade stent placement because there is a more direct route to the ureter. The peel-away sheath helps direct the pushing force applied to the stent down the ureter rather than toward the medial wall of the renal pelvis (Fig. 22-20).

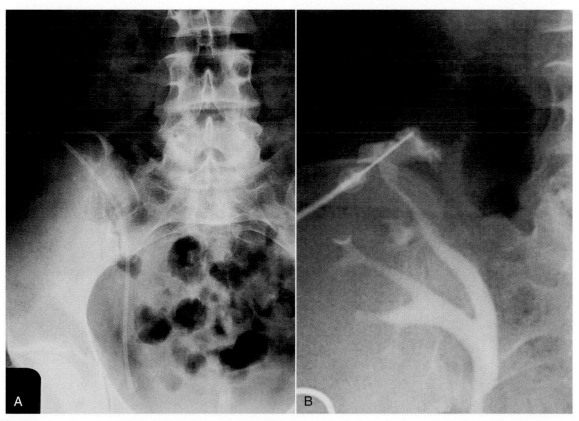

FIGURE 22-19. Percutaneous stent extraction in a patient with a transplant kidney in whom a ureteric stent was placed. The distal end of the stent was cut before placement because the stent was too long. The stent migrated proximally in the ureter and could not be retrieved retrograde. **A,** Plain radiograph showing the stent in situ. Note the distal pigtail has been cut. **B,** Antegrade needle placed in upper-pole calyx under ultrasound guidance.

Continued

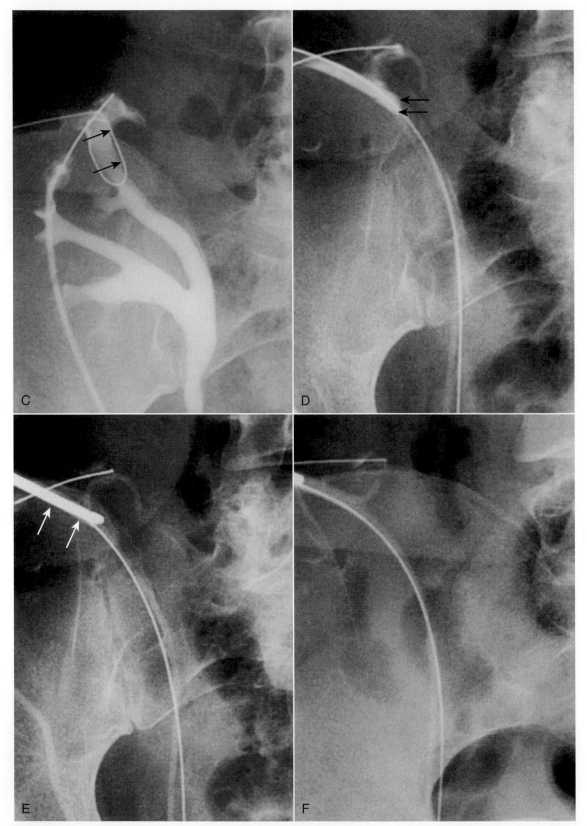

FIGURE 22-19, cont'd **C,** Upper pole access gained using a 22-gauge needle and 0.018-inch guidewire *(arrows)*. Note the antegrade needle is used to distend this unobstructed collecting system for guidewire manipulations. **D,** A track was dilated and a 12-French peel-away sheath inserted with a 45-degree bevel cut at its distal end *(arrows)*. **E,** A small alligator forceps *(arrows)* was used to grasp the 6-French stent near its proximal end. **F,** The stent was doubled over on itself and removed. A nephrostomy catheter was left in situ for 2 days.

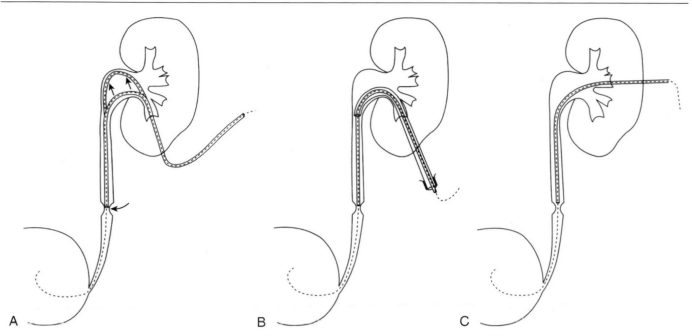

FIGURE 22-20. Schematics showing how the use of a peel-away sheath aids the process of stent insertion. **A,** During stent insertion, the stent is pushed through a fixed obstruction *(curved arrow).* When a lower pole access is used, the stent tend to loop *(small arrows)* in the renal pelvis as the force vector applied to the stent is directed toward the patient's head. **B,** Placement of a peel-away sheath in the upper ureter redirects the force vector down the ureter and aids in the eventual placement of the stent. **C,** Use of midpole access also helps convey pushing forces applied to the stent down the ureter.

TABLE 22-2 Length of Ureteric Stent Required for Various Patient Heights

Height (cm)	Stent Length (cm)
<178	22
178-193	24
>193	26

Modified from Seymour H, Patel U. Ureteric stenting: current status. *Semin Interv Radiol.* 2000;17(4):361.

Access is gained to the kidney in the manner described for percutaneous nephrostomy. An antegrade needle is first placed and access to a midpole calyx is preferably achieved. Once the 5-French sheath from the one-stick system is in the renal pelvis, a J-guidewire is placed in the renal pelvis and a Kumpe catheter placed over the guidewire. A straight or angled hydrophilic guidewire is then placed through the Kumpe catheter and directed down the ureter into the bladder. Once the Kumpe catheter is in the bladder, the hydrophilic guidewire is exchanged for a 0.035-inch Amplatz superstiff guidewire, which is coiled in the bladder. The percutaneous track is dilated with 6- and 8-French dilators and the 9-French peel-away sheath is placed into the pelvicaliceal system with the tip of the peel-away sheath placed at the UPJ or just into the upper ureter. In the author's unit, we use an 8-French stent (Meditech, Watertown, Mass.), which comes in 22-, 24-, 26-, and 28-cm lengths for patients with malignant ureteric obstruction. We tend to place a 6-French stent in patients with benign ureteric obstruction; a 22- or 24-cm length is suitable for the vast majority of average sized people. In general we place 22-cm stents in women and 24-cm stents in men of average height. Table 22-2 correlates stent length with patient height.

The stent system consists of an inner plastic cannula, a pusher catheter, and the stent (Fig. 22-21). A nylon suture is attached to the proximal end of the stent. The stent is loaded over the inner plastic cannula so that the proximal end of the stent lies alongside the distal end of the pusher catheter. The pusher catheter is usually loaded onto the inner plastic cannula by the manufacturer. The distal end of the pusher catheter has a metallic marker which marks the proximal end of the stent for stent placement. The whole assembly is placed over the superstiff guidewire and inserted down the ureter into the bladder. The stent is placed in the bladder until the marker on the distal end of the pusher catheter is in the renal pelvis. The guidewire and plastic inner cannula are removed, leaving the pusher catheter and the stent through the peel-away sheath. The nylon suture in the proximal stent is pulled to form the proximal loop. The distal loop forms automatically once the guidewire and plastic inner cannula are removed. With a little to-and-fro motion and gentle tugging on the nylon suture, the proximal pigtail loop forms in the renal pelvis (Figs. 22-22 and 22-23).

If there has been bleeding and there is clot in the collecting system, leave a nephrostomy catheter in situ. This is simply placed through the peel-away sheath into the renal pelvis without using a guidewire. The nephrostomy catheter can be removed after 24-48 hours when the clot has cleared from the pelvicaliceal system. If, on the other hand, the procedure has been relatively atraumatic, the peel-away sheath can simply be removed without placing a nephrostomy catheter. If the stents are for long-term drainage, they are usually changed cystoscopically at 3-6 monthly intervals depending on the referring urologist (Box 22-5).

Commonly Encountered Problems

Inappropriate Pelvicaliceal Access
Occasionally a nephrostomy catheter is already in situ when placement of an antegrade stent is requested. The nephrostomy catheter may have been placed at another institution and is often placed through a lower pole calyx. Lower pole calyceal access usually results in a more difficult angle of entry toward the upper ureter. It also means that any pushing force applied to the stent will tend to be directed toward the roof of the renal pelvis rather than down the ureter (see Fig. 22-20). An extra stiff or superstiff guidewire and a 9-French peel-away sheath placed into the upper ureter makes stent insertion much easier. However,

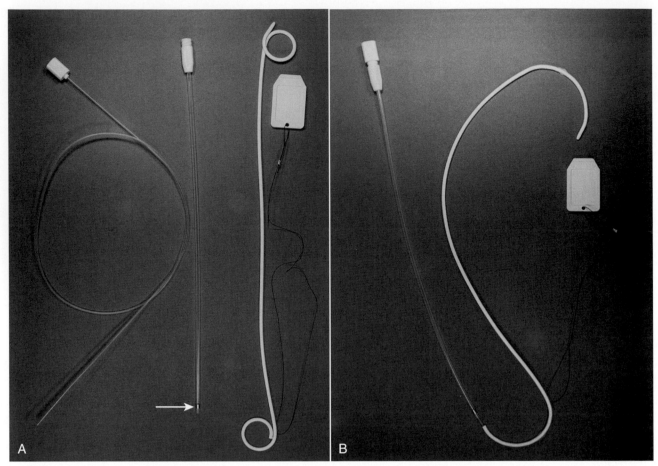

Figure 22-21. An 8-French ureteral stent. **A,** The stent assembly comprises a stent *(right)*, a pusher catheter *(middle)*, and a plastic stiffening cannula *(left)*. The inner plastic stiffening cannula and pusher catheter are inserted through the proximal end of the stent. Note the metallic marker *(arrow)* on the end of the pusher catheter, which marks the proximal end of the stent. The strings on the proximal end of the stent are used to form the proximal pigtail and/or reposition the proximal end of the stent if needed. (Note the 6-French stent does not have a plastic stiffening cannula). In general, we place the 8-French stent for malignant ureteric obstructions and the 6-French stent for patients with stone disease. **B,** The 8-French stent assembly is fitted together by placing the plastic stiffening cannula through the pusher catheter and stent.

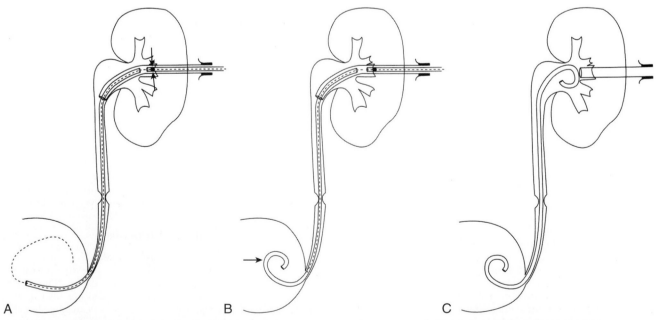

Figure 22-22. Schematics showing an antegrade ureteric stent insertion. **A,** A 0.035-inch superstiff guidewire is placed across the ureteric stricture into the bladder. A 9-French peel-away sheath is placed in the renal pelvis and the stent is placed over the guidewire and into the bladder. Note the metallic marker *(small arrows)* on the end of the pusher catheter, which denotes the proximal end of the stent. The stent is inserted so that its proximal end lies in the renal pelvis. **B,** By withdrawing the guidewire and inner plastic stiffener (for an 8-French stent), the distal pigtail *(arrow)* forms. The proximal pigtail is formed by withdrawing the guidewire completely and by pulling the string on the proximal end of the stent. **C,** The peel-away sheath remains in situ and can be used to place a nephrostomy catheter if required.

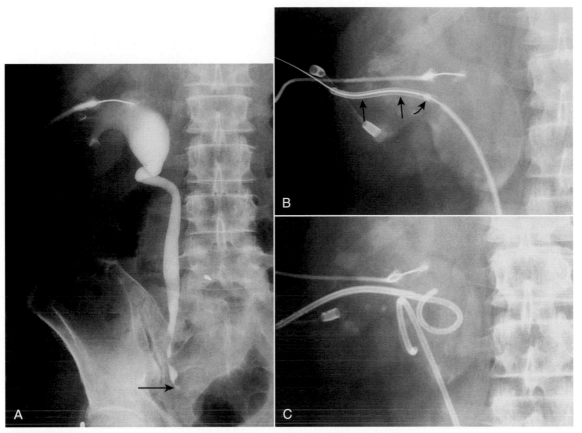

FIGURE 22-23. Antegrade ureteral stent insertion in a patient with an obstructing stone in the lower ureter and a failed attempt at retrograde stent insertion because the ureter had been reimplanted some years earlier. **A,** Antegrade pyelography shows a tortuous ureter with a dilated collecting system down to the level of the stone *(arrow)* in the lower ureter. **B,** Using midpole calyceal access, an antegrade stent was inserted through a peel-away sheath *(straight arrows).* The metallic marker *(curved arrow)* on the pusher catheter denotes the proximal end of the stent. **C,** With withdrawal of the guidewire, the distal pigtail forms in the bladder. Withdrawing the guidewire further and pulling on the string attached to the stent forms the proximal pigtail. Because of the hemorrhage in the collecting system, a pigtail nephrostomy catheter was left in situ for 2 days. The pigtail catheter was simply inserted through the peel-away sheath without using a guidewire.

> **Box 22-5. Antegrade Stent Insertion**
>
> Access via a midpole calyx is best
> A 9-French peel-away sheath helps direct the stent down the ureter
> Tight obstructions are crossed with a Kumpe catheter and hydrophilic guidewire
> Occasionally, a microcatheter and microwire are useful to traverse very tight strictures
> Van Andel catheter can be used to dilate tight obstructions before stent placement
> Nephrostomy is left in situ for 48 hours only if the procedure is traumatic

the problem can be avoided altogether by using a midpole access when possible.

Tortuous Ureter

Many pelviureteric systems that are obstructed have kinks or tortuousities in the mid or upper ureter. These can be difficult to negotiate, but the use of a Kumpe catheter and guidewire greatly facilitates negotiation of these kinks (Fig. 22-24). If it is not possible to negotiate ureteric kinks using a Kumpe catheter and hydrophilic guidewire, then draining the system for 2-3 days reduces the amount of dilatation and often helps in the successful negotiation of these ureteric kinks.

Stent Assembly Malfunction

Initially the author's unit had problems with the proximal end of the stent becoming engaged in the distal end of the pusher catheter. This happens particularly with stent systems that do not have a metallic marker on the end of the pusher catheter. Particularly in patients with tight obstructions, considerable force may be necessary to pass the stent through the obstruction. This sometimes results in the pusher catheter becoming engaged in the proximal end of the stent. Using a peel-away sheath helps avoid this problem, and passing a Van Andel catheter through the stricture beforehand also facilitates passage of the stent. Using stent systems with a metallic marker on the distal end of the pusher system is important; not only does it facilitate ready identification of the proximal end of the stent, but also it helps prevent engagement of the pusher catheter with the proximal end of the stent.

Difficulty Forming the Proximal Pigtail Loop

Occasionally, the proximal pigtail may be released from the inner plastic cannula and pusher catheter in the proximal ureter rather than in the renal pelvis where the proximal pigtail cannot form because of insufficient space. The stent can be pulled back into the renal pelvis by using the nylon suture attached to the proximal end of the stent. To prevent the proximal end of the stent from flipping into a mid or lower pole calyx when the nylon suture is used, the peel-away sheath may be used as an anchor to fix the proximal end of the stent while traction is applied to the nylon suture.

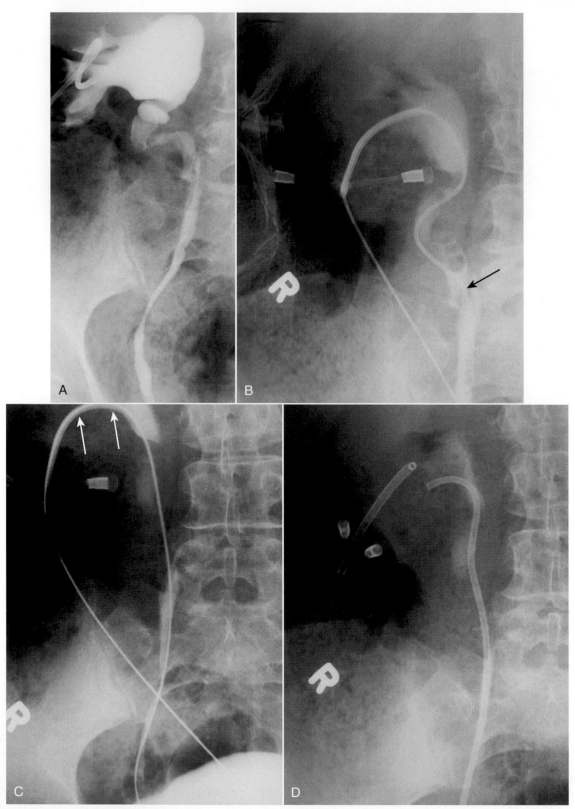

FIGURE 22-24. Tortuous ureter. **A,** A tortuous upper ureter was noted in this patient who required an antegrade stent because of pelvic malignancy. **B,** Using a Kumpe catheter *(arrow)* and hydrophilic guidewire, the upper ureter was negotiated without difficulty. **C,** Placement of a superstiff guidewire into the bladder straightened the tortuosity for eventual stent placement. Note the peel-away sheath bridging the percutaneous track into the upper ureter *(arrows)*. **D,** An 8-French antegrade stent was inserted without difficulty. A nephrostomy catheter was not left in situ because of the relatively atraumatic nature of the stent placement.

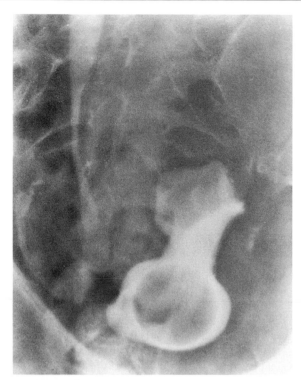

FIGURE 22-25. The empty bladder. Many patients referred for antegrade ureteric stent placement will have bladder catheters in situ as in this patient. It is important to clamp the Foley catheter and fill the bladder either antegrade or retrograde with dilute contrast material to allow room for guidewires and the like to coil within the bladder.

Tight Ureteric Obstruction

If the ureteric obstruction is felt to be tight, difficulty may be encountered in negotiating the ureteric obstruction with a hydrophilic guidewire or Kumpe catheter. The author's unit has found that the vast majority of obstructions can be bypassed by using a Kumpe catheter and hydrophilic guidewire in the first sitting. Occasionally, a microwire and microcatheter is required to negotiate a tight stricture with a 5-French catheter railroaded over the microcatheter. Rarely, we may leave the patient to decompress for 1-2 days and reattempt negotiation of the ureteric obstruction. A more significant problem is the passage of the 8-French stent through the tight ureteric obstruction. This can be facilitated by passing a Van Andel catheter to predilate a track through the ureteric obstruction. The Van Andel catheter has a long tapered distal end that facilitates this process. Use of the peel-away sheath also helps direct the force applied to the pusher catheter and stent down the ureter so that more leverage is obtained. Rarely is predilatation of the stricture with a balloon catheter necessary. If the stricture is very tight, a 6-French stent can be used.

Empty Bladder

Many patients referred for antegrade stent insertion will have bladder catheters in situ. Manipulation of guidewires and catheters in the empty bladder is difficult for the surgeon and painful for the patient. Clamping the bladder catheter before the procedure or putting 100 mL of dilute contrast into the bladder via the Kumpe catheter helps ameliorate this problem (Fig. 22-25).

Results

Use of an appropriate midpole access and a peel-away sheath results in a success rate approaching 100% for antegrade stent placement. In a study by Lu and associates, use of the peel-away sheath resulted in a 96% success rate compared to 81% when

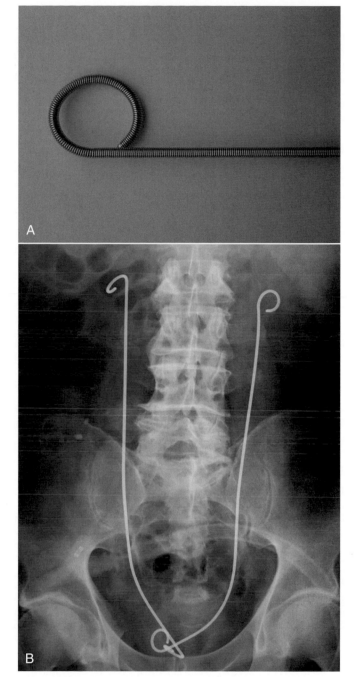

FIGURE 22-26. The Resonance stent (Cook, Bloomington, Ind.). **A**, Close-up view of the Resonance stent consisting of tightly coiled spiral of metal alloy without end holes. Urine drains around the stent and through the stent if pressure is high in the urinary system. **B**, Patient with inoperable bladder cancer who had bilateral hydronephrosis and bilateral resonance stents placed. They can remain in situ for up to 1 year.

a peel-away sheath was not used. The 3-month and 6-month patency rates in this study were 95% and 54%, respectively. Newer stents are now available with hydrophilic coating which should make negotiation of tighter strictures easier and should increase the technical success rate. New metal stents are also available which can be used in patients with malignancies. The author uses the Resonance stent (Cook, Bloomington, Ind.), which is a long metal spring shaped like a double pigtail stent. Urine drains both through and around the stent. This stent can be left in situ for up to 12 months. It is deployed through a long sheath that is negotiated into the bladder (Fig. 22-26).

Complications

Complications are similar to those seen with percutaneous nephrostomy. The author's unit has encountered a number of cases of renal pelvic perforation particularly without the use of the peel-away sheath when the force applied to the stent may be directed toward the medial wall of the renal pelvis and not down the ureter. This usually resolves with percutaneous drainage and has not posed a significant problem.

Balloon Dilatation of Ureteric Strictures

Usually benign ureteric strictures occur after instrumentation for stone disease. Ureteric strictures can be dilated antegrade or retrograde. If the retrograde route is not possible or has failed, dilation of the ureteric stricture may need to be done from an antegrade approach. First, a percutaneous nephrostomy is performed as described previously. Using a Kumpe catheter and hydrophilic guidewire, access through the stricture is gained and the catheter manipulated into the bladder. The hydrophilic guidewire is exchanged for a 0.035-inch superstiff guidewire and a 6- or 8-mm balloon manipulated over the guidewire and across the stricture (Fig. 22-27). The balloon is inflated until the waist disappears on the balloon, and is left inflated for approximately 2 minutes. It is then deflated and removed. A 9-French peel-away sheath is placed down as far as the UPJ and an 8-French stent placed antegrade across the stricture into the bladder, as described previously.

Results of balloon dilatation of ureteric strictures have shown a limited success rate. Long-term success rates vary from approximately 50% to 70%. The procedure is worth considering first because the alternative may involve ureteric reimplantation or some other urologic operation.

Ureteral Occlusion

Ureteral occlusion is occasionally performed in patients with malignant strictures of the ureter associated with severe ureteric bleeding episodes, or occlusion may be indicated in patients with underlying malignancy and ureteral or vesical fistulas. Percutaneous nephrostomy is performed in the usual fashion and a Kumpe catheter and hydrophilic guidewire manipulated down the ureter. The catheter is positioned just above the malignant stricture. Many different agents have been used for ureteral occlusion, including coils, Gelfoam, and glue. In the author's unit, we use a combination of coils and glue. The ureter can be packed with coils and glue through the Kumpe catheter, which is an end-hole type catheter (Fig. 22-28). In this manner, the ureter can be completely occluded. Patients do have an indwelling nephrostomy catheter for the remainder of their lives.

Endopyelotomy

Traditionally, the gold standard for treatment of UPJ obstruction has been open pyeloplasty. Success rates for this procedure are approximately 90%. With more widespread use and interest in minimally invasive techniques, antegrade and retrograde methods have been described for treating UPJ obstruction without the need for open surgery (Fig. 22-29). These techniques consist of either antegrade or retrograde balloon dilatation, or more recently, antegrade or retrograde techniques that produce a longitudinal full-thickness cut in the ureter. It is well known that such a cut in the ureter causes regeneration of normal uroepithelium to bridge the defect while minimizing damage to the ureteral blood supply.

If antegrade balloon dilatation is performed, a percutaneous nephrostomy is undertaken, as described previously. Access is gained to the renal pelvis and a short Cobra catheter is used to cross the UPJ with the help of a hydrophilic guidewire. The Kumpe catheter does not have enough rigidity for use in the capacious renal pelvis. An oversized balloon catheter is then placed across the UPJ and inflated until extravasation of contrast material occurs. The idea behind balloon dilatation is that disruption of the ureter and extravasation of contrast material must be seen before the procedure is terminated. An antegrade stent is then placed in the bladder. The particular stent placed has a 14-French proximal end which lies across the UPJ and an 8-French terminal portion which resides in the bladder. The stent is left in situ for 3 months, after which it is removed.

More recently ureteral cutting balloons have been developed which result in simultaneous balloon dilatation and incision of the UPJ. Again, this technique can be performed either retrograde or antegrade. It is important before using a cutting balloon to ensure that there are no crossing blood vessels adjacent to the UPJ. This is usually accomplished by performing a preprocedure CT scan. After access to the ureter is gained in either retrograde or antegrade fashion, the cutting balloon catheter is placed across the UPJ, the cutting wire is placed in a posterolateral position, and an endopyelotomy is performed by simultaneously inflating the balloon and activating the cutting wire. The current is continuously applied to the cutting wire until the waist on the balloon disappears. The balloon is then left inflated for 1-2 minutes before removal. Again, it is important to leave a 14-/8-French internal stent across the UPJ.

Overall results using cutting balloon catheters approach those of open pyeloplasty. While this technique is still in its infancy, it shows great promise for the treatment of this condition.

▄ BLADDER INTERVENTION

Suprapubic Cystostomy

Suprapubic cystostomy is often used for providing bladder decompression in patients with acute urinary retention. Small-bore 10-French catheters are usually placed by trocar technique and are very effective for the relief of urinary retention where transurethral catheterization has failed or is contraindicated. Long-term bladder drainage can also be achieved by the use of suprapubic catheters. Large-bore catheters (16-French or greater) are necessary for long-term drainage because the small-bore catheters tend to block easily. Traditionally, suprapubic bladder catheters for long-term drainage have been placed in the operating room under general or regional anesthesia. More recently, radiologic suprapubic placement of bladder catheters has been described as an effective alternative to the operative procedure (Fig. 22-30).

Indication

The most common patients referred for long-term suprapubic cystostomy include those with bladder neck outflow obstruction from prostatic hypertrophy or prostatic cancer, where surgery is either not possible or contraindicated. Patients with neurogenic bladders form the second largest patient referral group. In the author's unit we have rarely performed percutaneous suprapubic cystostomy for patients with urethral trauma, radiation cystitis, vesicocolonic or vesicovaginal fistula, urinary incontinence, and pyocystis.

Technique

The procedure is performed in the radiology department on a standard fluoroscopy table. Local anesthesia and intravenous sedoanalgesia (midazolam and fentanyl) are used. The patient is placed supine on the fluoroscopy table and the bladder filled with dilute contrast medium. Bladder filling can be achieved either by a transurethral Foley if present, or by placing a 20-gauge spinal needle into the bladder under ultrasound guidance if a transurethral Foley catheter cannot be placed. The bladder needs to be

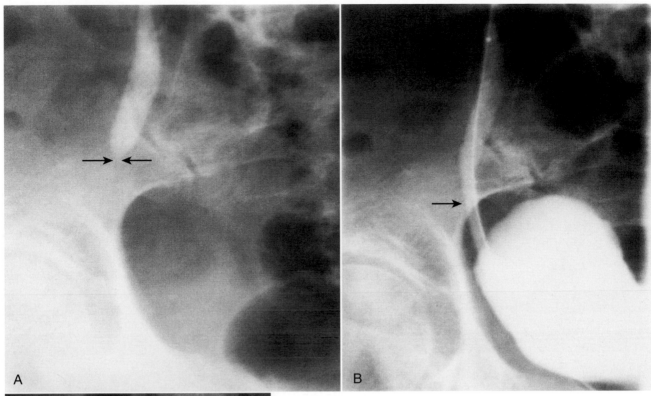

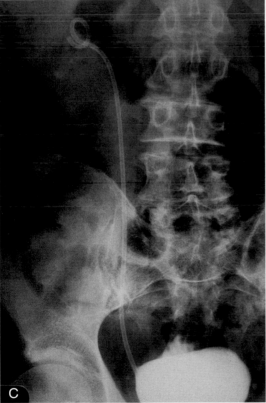

FIGURE 22-27. Ureteric stricture dilatation. **A,** This patient had ureteric instrumentation for removal of a ureteric stone and developed a stricture *(arrows)* in the lower ureter. This was approximately 8 cm in length. **B,** A percutaneous nephrostomy was performed and a 6-mm × 8-cm balloon *(arrows)* was used to dilate the stricture in the lower ureter. **C,** An 8-French stent was placed at the end of the procedure and left in situ for 3 months. The patient made an uneventful recovery and did not require surgery.

filled almost to capacity to displace loops of small bowel out of the pelvis.

An 18-gauge sheath needle or a one-stick needle is placed into the bladder in a vertical, paramedian position, approximately 2-3 cm above the pubic symphysis. It is important to use ultrasound to guide the needle into the bladder to make sure that no small bowel loops lie between the bladder and the needle puncture site on the anterior abdominal wall. This is particularly important for patients with small-capacity bladders that may not distend very well. A 0.035-inch superstiff guidewire is then coiled in the bladder and the percutaneous track is dilated. The percutaneous track can be dilated with sequential fascial dilators, but the author prefers to use a balloon catheter for dilatation. The advantage of using the balloon catheter is that it is a single-stage

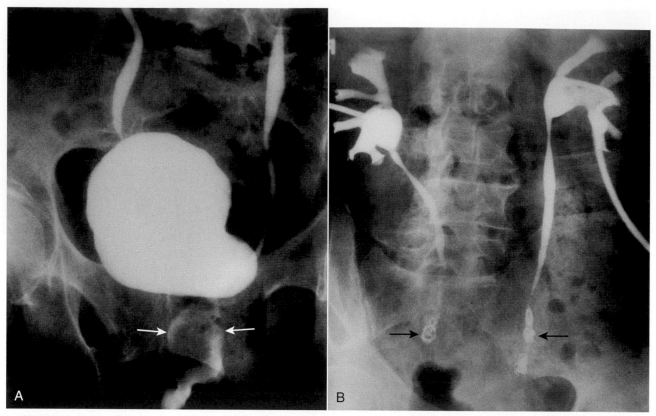

FIGURE 22-28. Ureteral occlusion in a patient with an inoperable pelvic malignancy and a vesicovaginal fistula. The patient was uncomfortable because of a constant urine leak. **A,** Intravenous pyelogram shows the leak *(arrows)* from the bladder into the vagina. **B,** Bilateral nephrostomy catheters were placed and both ureters occluded with a mixture of coils and glue *(arrows).* This completely dried up the vesicovaginal fistula and the patient had bilateral nephrostomy catheters for her remaining days. The patient died 2 months after the procedure.

dilatation and is less painful than using the sequential dilators. Additionally, the guidewire is less likely to kink during dilatation. The balloon catheter used is 7 cm × 7 mm (Meditech, Watertown, Mass.). The balloon is inflated until the waist disappears and is left inflated for 3 minutes. The balloon catheter is then removed and a peel-away sheath placed over the superstiff guidewire into the bladder. The peel-away sheath should be two French sizes larger than the proposed Foley catheter to be placed (Box 22-6). Foley catheters between 16- and 20-French are appropriate for long-term bladder drainage and these are placed over the guidewire, through the peel-away sheath and into the bladder. Because the Foley catheter has no end-hole either, the tip of the Foley catheter can be cut or a 15-gauge needle can be inserted through one of the distal side holes and out through the tip of the Foley catheter, through which the guidewire can be loaded retrograde through the Foley catheter. The Foley balloon is inflated with 5 mL of saline and the peel-away sheath finally removed. The catheter is pulled snugly against the anterior abdominal wall for catheter fixation. There is no need for skin fixation devices or sutures.

Results

In the author's unit we have found that a single-stage suprapubic catheter insertion is not possible in two groups of patients. In obese patients or patients with extensive midline scarring, it is difficult to dilate an appropriate track in a one-stage procedure. In these patients, we place a 10- or 12-French nephrostomy catheter into the bladder after initially dilating the track with fascial dilators. Two or 3 weeks later when the existing track is mature, we bring the patient back for track dilatation with a 7-mm diameter balloon. At this stage the track is usually

easily dilated and an 18- or 20-French Foley catheter can be placed.

The success rate for percutaneous suprapubic cystostomy approaches 100%, comparing very favorably with surgical cystostomy. Two-stage procedures may be required for some patients as described above. Long-term efficacy is also excellent with appropriate catheter care. Percutaneous suprapubic cystostomy can be performed on an outpatient basis, but follow-up care is important. Long-term bladder catheters are associated with an increased risk of infection and stone formation. Patients should therefore remain on low-dose trimethoprim/sulfamethoxazole to prevent bladder infection. Catheter exchange is performed every 2-3 months. This can be performed at the bedside or in the physician's office once the percutaneous track is mature. The existing Foley balloon is deflated, the catheter removed, and a new catheter inserted through the existing track. This can be performed without the use of a guidewire.

Complications

Complications associated with percutaneous suprapubic cystostomy are minimal. Minor complications such as hematuria are extremely common but this is usually not significant and resolves spontaneously. Localized cellulitis at the skin site may occur but again is rare with good hygiene. Occasionally, treatment with systemic antibiotics may be required. One of the most feared complications is traversal of a small bowel loop by the catheter en route to the bladder. Attention to technique is important to prevent this complication. Adequate distension of the bladder and ultrasound evaluation of the proposed needle puncture site will ensure that small bowel loops are not present between the anterior abdominal wall and the bladder. Catheter problems such as occlusion do occur but can be rectified by simple catheter exchange.

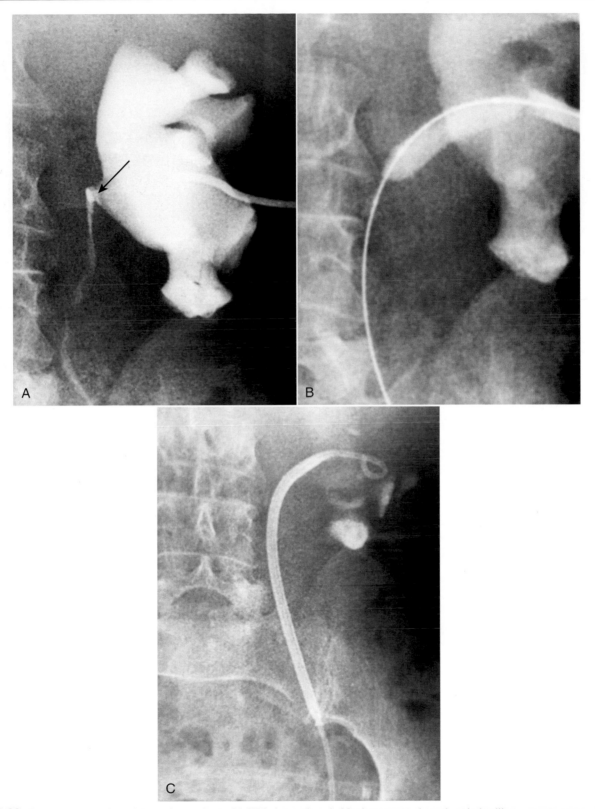

FIGURE 22-29. Percutaneous endopyelotomy in a patient with UPJ obstruction. **A,** Nephrostogram through an indwelling percutaneous nephrostomy catheter shows the ureteropelvic junction *(arrow)* obstruction. **B,** A 10-mm × 4-cm balloon was placed across the UPJ and inflated until the waist disappeared. **C,** A stent was inserted across the UPJ, after dilatation. The stent used tapered from 14-French in its upper end to 8-French in its lower end. The stent was removed after 3 months. Follow-up at 1 year shows no evidence of recurrence.

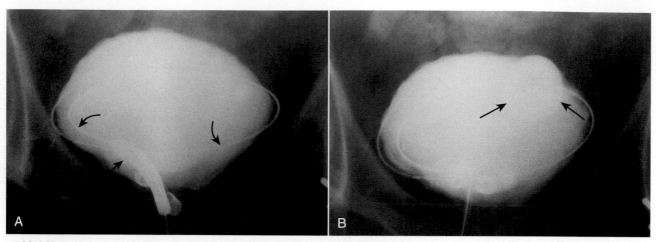

FIGURE 22-30. Suprapubic cystostomy in a patient who required a long-term bladder catheter. **A,** After gaining access to the bladder using a right paramedian needle puncture, a 0.038-inch superstiff wire *(curved arrows)* was inserted into the bladder and coiled. Track dilatation was performed with a 7-mm balloon catheter, after which a 22-French peel-away sheath *(straight arrow)* was placed into the bladder. **B,** A 24-French Foley catheter was inserted over the guidewire through the peel-away sheath and into the bladder. Contrast material *(arrows)* can be seen in the Foley balloon. This is only for the purpose of documenting that the catheter is in the bladder. The balloon is emptied of contrast material and refilled with saline.

Box 22-6. Suprapubic Cystostomy

Distend the bladder well and use ultrasound to make sure no bowel loops are adjacent to puncture site

A balloon catheter (7 mm × 70 mm) is used for track dilatation

The peel-away sheath used should be two French sizes larger than the chosen Foley catheter

Patients are placed on long-term trimethoprim and sulfamethoxazole

---

SUGGESTED READINGS

Banner MP, Amendola MA, Pollack HM. Anastomosed ureters: fluoroscopically guided transconduit retrograde catheterization. *Radiology.* 1989;170:45-49.

Bing KT, Hicks ME, Picus D, Darcy MD. Percutaneous ureteral occlusion with use of Gianturco coils and gelatin sponge: II. Clinical experience. *Semin Vasc Interv Radiol.* 1992;3:319-321.

De la Toille A, et al. Treatment of ureteral stenosis using high pressure dilation catheters. *Prog Virol.* 1997;7:408-414.

Faerber GJ, Richardson TD, Farah N, Ohl DA. Retrograde treatment of ureteropelvic junction obstruction using the ureteral cutting balloon catheter. *J Urol.* 1997;157:454-458.

Krebs TL, Papanicolaou N, Yoder IC, Tung GA, Pfister RC. Antegrade pyelography and ureteral perfusion in children with urinary tract dilatation. *Semin Interv Radiol.* 1991;8(3):161-169.

Lee MJ, Papanicolaou N: Extracorporeal lithotripsy and percutaneous interventions in symptomatic urinary tract lithiasis. *Postgrad Radiol.* 11:27–44 (see also Editors' comments, 25-26).

Lee WJ, Smith AD, Cubelli V, Vernace FM. Percutaneous nephrolithotomy: analysis of 500 consecutive cases. *Urol Radiol.* 1986;8:61-66.

Lee WJ, Smith AD, Cubelli V, et al. Complications of percutaneous nephrolithotomy. *Am J Roentgenol.* 1987;148:177-180.

Lee MJ, Papanicolaou N, Nocks BN, Valdez JA, Yoder IC. Fluoroscopically guided percutaneous suprapubic cystostomy for long-term bladder drainage: an alternative to surgical cystostomy. *Radiology.* 1993;188:787-789.

LeRoy AJ, May GR, Bender CE, et al. Percutaneous nephrostomy for stone removal. *Radiology.* 1984;151:607-612.

Lu DSK, Papanicolaou N, Girard M, Lee MJ, Yoder IC. Percutaneous internal ureteral stent placement: review of technical issues and solutions in 50 consecutive cases. *Clin Radiol.* 1994;49:256-261.

Maher MM, Fotheringham T, Lee MJ. Percutaneous nephrostomy. *Semin Interv Radiol.* 2000;17:329-339.

Pender SM, Lee MJ. Percutaneous suprapubic cystostomy for long-term bladder drainage. *Semin Interv Radiol.* 1996;13(2):93-99.

Pfister RC, Newhouse JH, Hendren WH. Percutaneous pyeloureteral urodynamics. *Urol Clin N Am.* 1982;9:41-49.

Reznek RH, Talner LB. Percutaneous nephrostomy. *Radiol Clin N Am.* 1984;22:393-406.

Segura JW, Patterson DE, LeRoy A, et al. Percutaneous removal of kidney stones: review of 1000 cases. *J Urol.* 1985;134:1077-1081.

Seymour H, Patel U. Ureteric stenting: current status. *Semin Interv Radiol.* 2000;17(4):351-365.

CHAPTER 23

Image-Guided Breast Intervention

Niamh Hambly, MBBChBAO, MRCPI, FFR(RCSI)

Breast cancer is the most common non–skin cancer in women in the developed world, with one in eight women expected to develop breast cancer in their lifetime. However, the vast majority of women presenting to breast clinics have benign disease. Breast imaging is generally performed in (1) asymptomatic women in age groups most at risk for cancer and (2) for diagnostic purposes in women who present with symptoms such as breast lumps, mastalgia, or nipple discharge. Image-guided intervention plays a pivotal role in the investigation and management of women with breast disease. In symptomatic women with breast cysts or abscesses, therapeutic fine-needle aspiration (FNA) may be performed to alleviate symptoms. Minimally invasive image-guided percutaneous breast biopsy is performed to differentiate benign from malignant disease in symptomatic women with abnormalities on imaging as well as in women with screen-detected abnormalities. Image-guided localization is necessary to guide accurate surgical excision of impalpable invasive or in situ carcinoma and high-risk lesions. Finally, minimally invasive image-guided techniques are under investigation as an alternative to surgery in the management of benign and malignant breast disease.

■ IMAGE-GUIDED BREAST BIOPSY

Indications

Minimally invasive image-guided breast biopsy is now the standard of care for the diagnosis of palpable breast lumps and for nonpalpable radiologically detected abnormalities. The diagnostic accuracy of needle biopsy is comparable to open surgical excision, and compared to surgical excision, imaged-guided biopsy has many advantages (Box 23-1). In patients with a benign diagnosis, image-guided biopsy negates the need for surgery, and in patients with malignancy, preoperative diagnosis allows the patient to have one definitive surgery.

Before biopsy, the lesion should be fully worked up (which may include mammographic additional views and ultrasound), and all relevant imaging should be interpreted by a breast radiologist. Correlation should also be made with clinical examination to ensure the lesion being targeted corresponds to any palpable abnormality. The lesion should be assigned a BI-RADS category (or RCR category in the United Kingdom and Ireland) to determine the level of suspicion for malignancy (Box 23-2). In general, BI-RADS lesions 4 and 5 warrant a biopsy (RCR

lesions 3-5 are biopsied). For suspicious lesions, the radiologist should look for multifocal, multicentric, and contralateral disease. If the imaging appearances are suggestive of multifocal or multicentric disease, a second site of disease should be biopsied.

Contraindications

Before biopsy, patients are asked if they are taking anticoagulant or antiplatelet therapy. If taking warfarin, the latest international normalized ratio (INR) should be obtained (preferably within 5 days). All patients are then informed of the potential risk for bleeding, bruising, and hematoma formation and that this risk is greater for patients on antiplatelet or anticoagulant medication. However, due to the easy compressibility of the breast, most radiologists now perform biopsies in patients on aspirin and warfarin if the INR is less than 2.5 (some institutions use an INR of 4.0 as a cutoff for core biopsies and 2.5 for vacuum-assisted biopsies). Studies have shown that there are no significant complications in patients undergoing core needle biopsy on aspirin or warfarin. For patients on Plavix, the risk of discontinuing the drug must be balanced against the risk of hematoma formation, which is greater than in patients on aspirin.

Contraindications specific to each imaging modality are discussed in subsequent sections.

Complications

Significant complications (hematomas requiring drainage or infection requiring drainage or antibiotic therapy) have been reported in fewer than 1% of breast biopsies. The most significant risk related to bleeding during needle biopsy is related to obscuring the lesion, thus leading to possible sampling error.

For ultrasound-guided biopsies, there is a theoretical risk of pneumothorax if too vertical an approach is used. However, this should never occur if an appropriate technique is adopted and the needle is kept parallel to the chest wall at all times.

The postbiopsy care and instructions are the same for all biopsies, although the risk of bruising is increased with larger gauge vacuum-assisted biopsies and in patients on anticoagulants. Manual pressure is applied to the biopsy site and skin incision for 5-10 minutes or until hemostasis is achieved. A compression dressing and ice pack may be applied in patients with large hematomas or those on anticoagulants.

Box 23-1. Advantages of Image-Guided Breast Biopsy Over Open Surgical Biopsy

Comparable diagnostic accuracy
Quick
Relatively inexpensive
Minimally invasive
Less hospital time
Reduced morbidity with shorter recovery time
Does not require sedation or general anesthesia
Better cosmetic results
Less scarring on future breast imaging
Negates the need for surgery in patients with a benign diagnosis
Allows for scheduling of one definitive surgery in patients with malignant diagnosis

Box 23-2. BI-RADS Categories

1-Normal
2-Benign findings
3-Probably benign (<2% rate malignancy)
4-Suspicious for malignancy
5-Highly suggestive of malignancy (≥95% chance malignancy)

Box 23-3. Indications for Clip Placement

Small lesions
Lesions with subtle appearance
Complete excision of the target at biopsy
Correlation across imaging modalities
Patients undergoing neoadjuvant chemotherapy
Magnetic resonance imaging–guided biopsies

General Principles

Clip Placement

Metallic biopsy marker clips are increasingly being placed at the time of image-guided biopsy to mark the biopsy site (Box 23-3). In general a clip is placed if the biopsied lesion may be difficult to visualize on repeat imaging due to small size or subtle appearance, or when the target is completely excised at biopsy. A clip may also be placed for correlation across imaging modalities, that is, to confirm that a lesion biopsied at ultrasound corresponds to a mammographic abnormality (Fig. 23-1). Clips should also be placed in patients undergoing neoadjuvant chemotherapy in case the tumor shrinks and cannot be subsequently visualized for needle localization (Fig. 23-2). In these patients, clip placement is also helpful to identify the tumor bed at histopathology. Finally, clips should be placed at magnetic resonance imaging (MRI)-guided biopsy to allow for wire-guided localization and excision in case of an abnormal result.

Most clips are made of titanium or stainless steel and are preloaded in a sterile disposable introducer, which is inserted under image guidance to the target location. When the needle is in satisfactory position, the marker clip is deployed by depressing a plunger; most introducers have a safety switch to prevent inadvertent deployment. For ultrasound-guided clip placement, the introducer needle is introduced under direct sonographic guidance using the same technique as for core biopsy so that the tip of the introducer lies centrally within the targeted lesion. Most vacuum-assisted biopsy devices have compatible preloaded clip introducers that are inserted through the biopsy device or coaxial sheath.

Many clips now available are embedded in cylindrical plugs of polymer material or collagen to inhibit clip migration and can be easily visualized under ultrasound, thus facilitating ultrasound localization. Clips are available in a variety of shapes and if multiple lesions are present, placement of markers of different shapes should be performed to distinguish between biopsy sites. MRI compatible clips are also available.

Needle Selection

There are two main categories of core biopsy needle used for breast biopsies: automated spring-loaded core biopsy needles

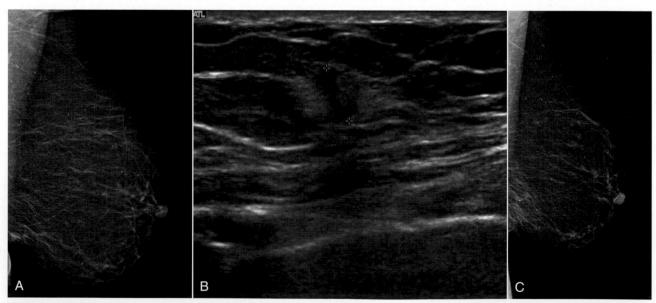

FIGURE 23-1. Clip placement after ultrasound-guided biopsy of an incidental 7-mm mass in a 75-year-old woman confirming correlation between the mammographic and sonographic abnormalities. **A,** Standard left mammographic views showing a focal asymmetry in the lower inner quadrant of the left breast. **B,** Ultrasound demonstrated a 7-mm hypoechoic mass that was thought to represent a correlate for the mammographic finding. Ultrasound-guided biopsy yielded invasive ductal carcinoma. A biopsy clip was placed at the time of biopsy. **C,** Postbiopsy mammogram confirming clip deployment in the area of mammographic concern confirming correlation between mammographic and sonographic findings. (This was subsequently localized under mammographic guidance; see Fig. 23-13.)

and vacuum-assisted biopsy devices. Breast lesion excision systems which remove small sections of intact tissue are sometimes used for complete excision of small lesions but are currently not in widespread use for routine diagnosis (see Breast Lesion Excision Systems).

Automated Spring Loaded Core Biopsy Devices

Automated spring loaded core biopsy devices are the needle of choice for ultrasound-guided procedures. In general, the larger the gauge, the greater the diagnostic accuracy and needles smaller than 14 gauge should not be used. These needles consist of an inner stylet with a trough that collects the sample and an outer cutting cannula (Fig. 23-3). They ideally produce a core of tissue 1-2 cm in length and 1-2 mm in width. When deployed the inner stylet moves forward at high velocity, the tissue falls into the trough, and the cutting cannula then moves forward at

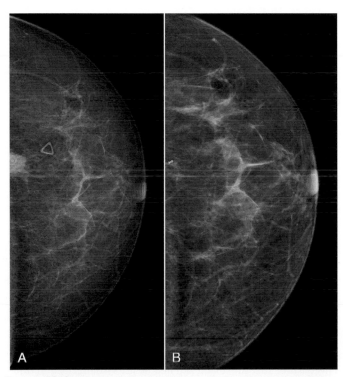

FIGURE 23-2. Illustrates the importance of clip placement in women undergoing neoadjuvant chemotherapy. **A,** Standard craniocaudal view of the left breast showing an ill-defined mass in the deep central breast. This was biopsied under ultrasound guidance, which yielded invasive ductal carcinoma. A clip was placed at the time of biopsy before commencing neoadjuvant chemotherapy. **B,** A repeat left mammogram following neoadjuvant chemotherapy demonstrates complete resolution of the mammographic abnormality. The biopsy marker clip marks the site of the previously biopsied mass and was used as the target for wire-guided localization.

high speed to cover the trough (Fig. 23-4). The needle can then be withdrawn. The tissue sample is retrieved by retracting the outer cutting cannula and exposing the trough containing the tissue sample.

Vacuum-Assisted Biopsy Devices

Vacuum-assisted biopsy needles use vacuum suction to pull the target tissue into the central aperture, which collects the samples. They remove larger volumes of tissue, leading to improved diagnostic accuracy and lower rates of underestimation of atypical ductal hyperplasia (ADH) and ductal carcinoma in situ (DCIS), and are the needle of choice for stereotactic-guided and MRI-guided biopsies (Tables 23-1 and 23-2). Handheld vacuum-assisted devices may also be used under sonographic guidance but do not confer any diagnostic benefit. However, these devices do generate larger core samples and some operators use these devices to excise small benign lesions under sonographic guidance (see Breast Lesion Excision Systems).

A number of high-quality vacuum-assisted devices are approved for clinical use, many of which are MRI compatible. These include Mammotome (Johnson and Johnson Ethicon Endo-Surgery Inc, Cincinnati, Ohio), Encor (C.R. Bard, New York, N.Y.), and Suros ATEC and Eviva (Suros Surgical Systems Inc, Indianapolis, Ind.). Vacuum-assisted biopsy devices are available in 8-14 gauge, and while diagnostic accuracy improves when changing from an automated spring-loaded core biopsy needle to a vacuum-assisted device, there is no significant decrease in underestimation rates with increasing needle gauge.

Selection of which needle to use depends on operator and institution preference. Some of these needles adopt a coaxial approach whereby an introducer sheath and stylet are first inserted and the biopsy needle is subsequently placed through the introducer. Other biopsy devices allow for a single direct insertion of the biopsy probe. Most devices are available with a variety of probe lengths and in both standard and petite (shorter biopsy chamber) sizes to allow for biopsy of lesions in smaller breasts. The needle is positioned in the breast so that the aperture is at the center of the target lesion. When vacuum suction is applied, the tissue is aspirated into the aperture and a rotating cutter is then advanced forward and the sample captured. Most vacuum-assisted devices have a built-in sample collection chamber that allows for capture of multiple samples without withdrawing the needle. Different parts of the same lesion are sampled by rotating the direction of the aperture through 360 degrees. If the biopsy device lies to one side of the lesion, sampling can be concentrated in the direction of the lesion. When sampling is complete, saline lavage can be performed to irrigate the biopsy cavity to minimize hematoma formation. Most devices also allow for direct instillation of local anesthesia through the device during tissue sampling to minimize pain during the procedure. Vacuum-assisted devices allow for direct clip placement through the biopsy device or coaxial introducer sheath for accurate clip positioning in the biopsy bed.

See Box 23-4 for advantages of vacuum-assisted devices.

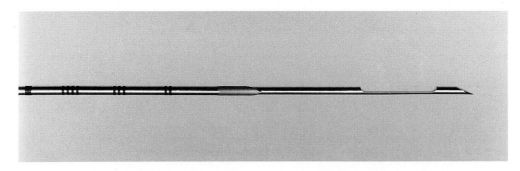

FIGURE 23-3. Fourteen-gauge core biopsy needle. The outer needle is pulled back to show the inner needle with tissue notch at the distal end.

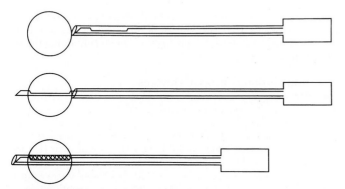

FIGURE 23-4. Core biopsy. The diagram at the top shows the needle position before firing. The center diagram demonstrates the position of the inner needle when it has been fired. The lower diagram shows the final position as the outer needle moves forward to cover the notch containing the tissue sample.

TABLE 23-1 Atypical Ductal Hyperplasia Underestimation Rates at Stereotactic Biopsy

Type of Biopsy	Type of Needle	Underestimation Rate
Stereotactic	14-G Automated needle	50% (Range 20%-56%)
Stereotactic	11-G Vacuum-assisted device	20% (Range 10%-27%)

TABLE 23-2 Comparison of Sample Weight for Different Biopsy Devices

Biopsy Device	Specimen Weight (Approximate Value)
14-G Automated spring loaded device	17 mg
14-G Vacuum-assisted biopsy device	37 mg
11-G Vacuum-assisted biopsy device	95 mg
8-G Vacuum-assisted biopsy device	190 mg
10-mm Breast lesion excision system	800 mg
20-mm Breast lesion excision system	3000 mg

Box 23-4. Advantages of Vacuum-Assisted Biopsy Devices

Larger samples
More accurate characterization of complex histologic findings
Lower atypical ductal hyperplasia underestimation rate
Decreased rebiopsy rate for nonsampling of calcifications
Allows for accurate clip placement through the needle at biopsy site
Complete percutaneous removal of small lesions possible
Multiple samples obtained with single probe insertion
Local anesthesia can be instilled through the device for optimal anesthesia at the biopsy site
Saline lavage of the biopsy site may reduce hematoma formation

---

Breast Biopsy Reports

Box 23-5 highlights the pertinent information to include in breast biopsy reports.

Selection of Imaging Modality

Biopsy may be performed under sonographic, stereotactic, or MRI guidance. Recently systems to biopsy lesions under positron emission mammography (PEM) and breast-specific gamma imaging (BSGI) guidance has become commercially available.

In general, breast lesions should be biopsied using the modality with which they are best visualized. Before biopsy, the radiologist should review all of the relevant imaging to ensure that the most appropriate modality is used. However, selection of imaging modality also depends on patient factors such as comfort and mobility, on operator preference and experience, and on cost and equipment availability.

Ultrasound-Guided Biopsy

Patient Selection and Preparation

In general, if a lesion can be visualized using ultrasound, then ultrasound is the modality of choice. However, ultrasound-guided biopsy is technically difficult and has a longer learning curve than stereotactic biopsy (Table 23-3). There are no specific contraindications to ultrasound-guided biopsy.

Before commencing the biopsy, a complete ultrasound examination of the mass should be performed and representative images recorded. Informed consent is obtained as for all biopsies.

For most lesions amenable to ultrasound-guided biopsy, 14-gauge spring-loaded automated core biopsy needles provide adequate samples. There is no proven benefit to using larger vacuum-assisted devices.

Technique

A high-frequency linear array transducer of at least 10 MHz should be used for the procedure. The patient is positioned supine in a slightly oblique position with the side to be biopsied slightly elevated and the ipsilateral arm over her head. A wedge cushion can be placed behind the patient's shoulder to support her in this position. If possible the patient and ultrasound machine should be positioned so that the patient lies between the operator and the ultrasound screen so the breast lesion, needle, transducer, and screen are all in the operator's direct line of vision. This ensures that the lesion and needle are visualized at all times and avoids the need for the operator to perform uncomfortable twisting movements.

The biopsy needle should be inserted into the breast, keeping the needle parallel to the chest wall and transducer at all times to avoid the potential for pneumothorax. Firm pressure should be maintained on the lesion with the transducer to stop it from moving. This is especially important in the case of fibroadenomas,

---

Box 23-5. Breast Biopsy Reports

Type of procedure performed
Side, location, and type of abnormality
Type and amount of anesthesia administered
Gauge and type of needle used (automated or vacuum-assisted device)
Number of samples obtained
If specimen radiograph was performed
Presence or absence of calcifications on specimen radiograph
If a clip was placed
Location of clip with respect to the biopsied lesion
Complications and associated treatment

which can be very mobile. The long axis of the needle and especially its tip should be visible along the long axis of the transducer during the entire procedure. Before firing the automated needle, the operator should be satisfied with the position. After firing, an image of the needle within the lesion should be recorded to document accurate sampling. If necessary, an orthogonal view can be obtained by rotating the transducer 90 degrees to confirm needle placement in the lesion by visualizing the echogenic dot of the needle (Figs. 23-5 and 23-6). The number of cores obtained depends on the adequacy of the samples but in general two or three good samples should suffice. If the targeted lesion contains calcifications, then a specimen radiograph may be obtained. See Figure 23-3.

Postbiopsy care is as standard for all breast biopsies.

Troubleshooting at Ultrasound-Guided Biopsy

Biopsy of deep lesions, especially in large or dense breasts, may be technically challenging. For deep lesions close to the chest wall, a bolus of local anesthetic or sterile saline can be given deep to the lesion to raise the lesion off the chest wall. For deep lesions, in order to stay parallel to the chest wall, the skin incision

TABLE 23-3 Comparison of Ultrasound-Guided and Stereotactic-Guided Biopsy

Ultrasound Guided	Stereotactic Guided
Patient supine—more comfortable	Patient is prone or upright Breast held in compression for duration of biopsy— uncomfortable
Quick to perform	Longer to perform
Does not involve ionizing radiation	Involves ionizing radiation
Lesion and biopsy needle visualized in real-time, confirming sampling accuracy	
No weight limitations	Weight limitation for prone units
Access to all areas of breast	Access to axillary and posterior lesions more limited
Less expensive	More expensive
Small breasts are not a limitation	Difficult to perform in small breasts
Visualization of calcification and some architectural distortion is more limited	Calcifications, architectural distortion easily targeted
Biopsy of small masses in large mobile breasts can be technically difficult	Small masses in larges breasts easier to target as breast is immobilized
Longer learning curve	Shorter learning curve

should be made further from the transducer. Downward pressure should be applied after the tip of the needle is inserted into the skin, ensuring the needle is advanced parallel to the chest wall and not angled vertically.

Stereotactic-Guided Biopsy

Patient Selection and Preparation

The main indication for stereotactic biopsy is mammographic calcifications. However, stereotactic-guided biopsy can also be performed for areas of architectural distortion, focal asymmetries, and masses with no sonographic correlate. Sometimes in very large mobile breasts with small deeply located masses, stereotactic biopsy is technically easier than ultrasound-guided biopsy.

There are no absolute contraindications to stereotactic biopsy. Relative contraindications to stereotactic biopsy include an inability of the patient to remain still, limited mobility (especially of the neck and shoulders), weight greater than 300 lb for prone tables, and small breasts (Box 23-6). Traditionally stereotactic biopsy was not possible in breasts compressing to less than 25-30 mm. However, with modern petite biopsy vacuum-assisted devices, biopsy is possible in breasts compressing to as little as 22 mm.

Most centers now use vacuum-assisted biopsy devices for stereotactic biopsy due to the improved diagnostic accuracy and lower rates of ADH underestimation. However, 14-gauge automated spring-loaded core biopsy devices can also be used.

Types of Stereotactic Unit

Two types of stereotactic units are available: (1) dedicated prone biopsy tables and (2) upright add-on devices, which are attached to diagnostic mammography units (Fig. 23-7). With the prone unit, the patient is positioned prone on the biopsy table and her breast is placed through an aperture in the table and positioned against the image receptor. The radiologist operates from underneath the table, out of the patient's line of vision. Using the prone table, a lesion can be targeted from any approach.

With the upright device, the patient is either seated or positioned in the lateral decubitus position. With lateral arm attachments for upright units, 360-degree access to either breast can be achieved. Table 23-4 compares the two types of unit.

Most units now use digital imaging to allow real-time visualization of images and computerized targeting of the abnormality.

Technique

Before biopsy, both prone and upright units must be calibrated in accordance with manufacturer instructions. The radiologist reviews all available imaging and determines the optimal approach for biopsy. This is usually the shortest distance to the target but patient positioning and comfort is also taken into account. Informed consent is obtained as standard.

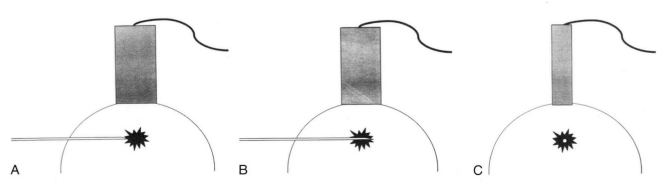

FIGURE 23-5. Technique for ultrasound-guided breast biopsy. **A,** Pre-fire position. If the needle is kept parallel to the long axis of the transducer, the entire needle length will be visualized as it is advanced and the needle tip can be optimally positioned. **B,** Postfire position. The needle tip has passed through the lesion. **C,** Postfire position. The orthogonal view demonstrates that the needle has passed through the center of the lesion and not to one side.

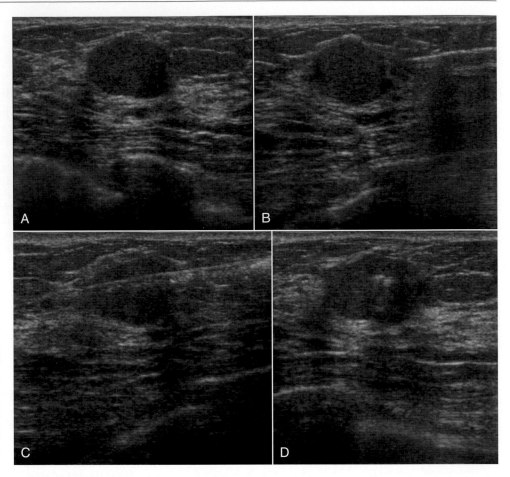

FIGURE 23-6. Ultrasound-guided biopsy of a mass in a 35-year-old woman. **A**, A 22-mm well-circumscribed hypoechoic mass with imaging features suggestive of a fibroadenoma. **B**, Pre-fire position with the needle parallel to the chest wall. **C**, Postfire position. The needle passes through the lesion but remains parallel to the chest wall. **D**, The probe is rotated through 90 degrees to confirm that the needle has passed through the lesion and not to one side.

Box 23-6. Relative Contraindications to Stereotactic Biopsy

Inability of the patient to remain still
Limited mobility (especially of the neck and shoulders)
Weight greater than 300 lb for prone tables
Small breasts
Very posterior lesions
Very superficial lesions
Lesions very close to the nipple

After the approach is chosen, the patient is positioned with the breast against the image receptor. A compression paddle with an aperture to allow access to the breast is used. A scout image (zero degrees) is obtained to ensure target visualization within the aperture of the compression paddle (Fig. 23-8). The skin is usually marked when a satisfactory position is achieved to determine if there is any subsequent movement of the breast. Next two stereotactic images are acquired by angling the tube 15 degrees to the right and the left of the upright (the stereo pair). The radiologist views the images on the monitor and targets the calcifications (or mass, area of distortion or asymmetry) on both images by placing an "x" at the desired target on both images. The computer software then calculates the x, y, and z (depth) coordinates of the lesion in the breast relative to reference points on the scout image. The apparent movement of the lesion between one stereotactic image and the other is used to calculate its depth within the breast. If an automated needle device is being used, multiple targets must be picked, but for modern vacuum-assisted devices, a single central target is sufficient.

The needle holder is then moved to the target (zeroed). The skin is cleaned in the usual manner, and local anesthetic is administered for superficial and deep anesthesia. Many of the newer vacuum-assisted biopsy devices allow for further instillation of local anesthesia through the device during the biopsy. A small skin incision is made using a scalpel to facilitate insertion of the biopsy needle. The biopsy needle is then inserted to the appropriate z-depth. Most needles are inserted in a pre-fired state and then "fired" within the breast. Although this is not necessary with most vacuum-assisted devices, firing can assist with more accurate targeting because it prevents the target from being pushed away from the needle. Most operators repeat the stereo pair in the pre-fire position to ensure that the target has not moved significantly. If there has been significant movement, then retargeting can be performed by withdrawing the needle to just below the skin surface and then repositioning to avoid repeated skin incisions. If the targeting is satisfactory, the needle is fired. Another set of postfire images is usually obtained before sampling. Most vacuum-assisted devices allow for multiple samples to be acquired without removing the needle, and the aperture of the needle can be rotated through 360 degrees, obtaining a sample at every 1-2 clock positions. If the target lies to one side of the needle, the samples can be concentrated in that direction (e.g., from 12 to 3 o'clock or 2 to 4 o'clock). It is standard to acquire a minimum of six samples, with many radiologists acquiring 10-12. Most radiologists agree that the diagnostic yield increases and ADH and DCIS underestimation rates decrease with increasing the number of core samples obtained, although improvement is probably not increased with more than 12 specimens.

Specimen Radiograph

After samples are obtained, a specimen radiograph is acquired (only for calcifications; not for masses, architectural distortion, or asymmetries). This may be performed in a dedicated specimen radiography unit or by using magnification on a standard unit. If the specimen radiograph confirms the presence of calcifications,

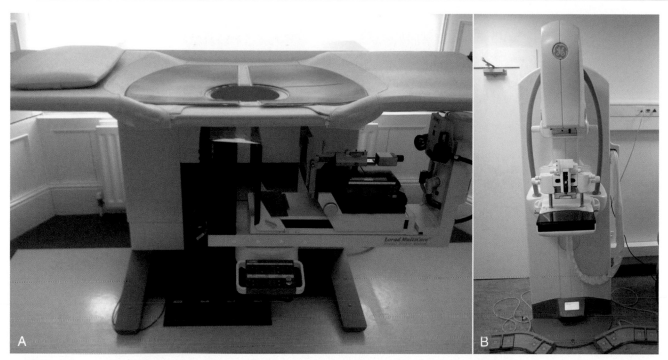

Figure 23-7. **A**, Prone stereotactic unit. The patient is positioned prone on the table. The breast is passed through the aperture in the table and positioned against the image receptor, which lies under the table. **B**, Upright add-on stereotactic unit.

Table 23-4 Comparison of Prone Table and Add-on Stereotactic Unit

Upright Add-On Unit	Prone Table
Patient seated upright or in lateral decubitus position	Patient prone
Vasovagal reactions more common	Vasovagal reactions reduced
Patient can easily visualize the needle	Patient unable to visualize the needle
Targeting of inferior lesions more difficult but improved with lateral arm	Breast can be easily approached from any angle
Unaffected breast may interfere with image acquisition, especially for a medial approach in lateral decubitus position	Unaffected breast can be easily positioned away from the image receptor
Less expensive	More expensive
Compact, requiring little storage or floor space	Large floor space needed, usually a dedicated room
The unit can be used for both diagnostic mammograms and biopsies	Can only be used for biopsies
Posterior/axillary tail lesions more accessible	Access to posterior/axillary tail lesions limited
Weight and body habitus less important	Manufacturer recommended weight limitation (usually 300 lb)
Easier for patients with limited mobility	Patients with medical comorbidities may have problems climbing onto the table or lying prone

then no further sampling is necessary. If calcifications are identified, the specimens containing calcifications may be marked with ink or submitted separately to assist the pathologist. If the pathologist is unable to locate the calcifications, then a radiograph of the tissue block may be helpful in determining the presence or absence of calcifications.

If calcifications are not demonstrated on specimen radiograph, then more samples should be acquired. The stereo pair should be repeated and retargeting performed if necessary. If calcifications are still not demonstrated despite resampling, or if further sampling is not possible due to patient discomfort or obscuration of the target by postbiopsy change and hematoma, then the samples are still sent for pathologic evaluation because a diagnosis may

be obtained. However, a benign diagnosis without calcifications demonstrated on specimen radiograph should be considered discordant and a repeat biopsy scheduled.

See Box 23-7 for causes of sampling errors at stereotactic biopsy.

If all or most of the target lesion has been removed, a biopsy marker clip should be placed at the time of biopsy. Clip migration at stereotactic biopsy is most common in the z-axis (i.e., in the plane orthogonal to the compression plane used). This occurs when the clip deploys adjacent to rather than in the biopsy site. This distance may be small when the breast is compressed, but when compression is released the breast springs up, increasing the distance between the clip and the biopsy site and magnifying the discrepancy (called the accordion effect) (Fig. 23-9).

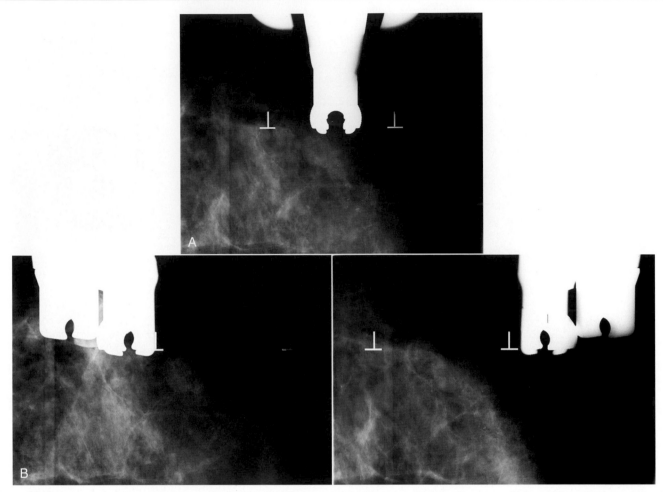

Figure 23-8. Stereotactic biopsy of microcalcifications in the upper outer right breast in a 50-year-old woman. **A**, Scout image (0 degrees) showing satisfactory positioning with the calcifications in the aperture of the compression paddle. **B**, Stereotactic pair taken at 15 degrees to the right and left of the upright and used to target the calcifications.

Magnetic Resonance Imaging–Guided Biopsy

Patient Selection

Breast MRI is increasingly used (1) for preoperative evaluation of extent of disease in biopsy-proven carcinoma (especially lobular carcinoma), (2) for high-risk screening, (3) in patients undergoing neoadjuvant chemotherapy, and (4) for the investigation of axillary metastases with no primary site evident on mammography or ultrasound. Whereas MRI is very sensitive, the specificity is more varied, and suspicious lesions identified on MRI require a tissue diagnosis. If a suspicious abnormality requiring biopsy (BI-RADS 4 or 5) is seen, the radiologist may choose to use ultrasound to look for a correlate to target under sonographic guidance. A sonographic correlate is more likely to be identified for masslike lesions, larger lesions, and BI-RADS 5 abnormalities. If no definite sonographic correlate is seen or if the MRI and sonographic findings are discordant, an MRI-guided biopsy is recommended. MRI-guided biopsies are frequently recommended, such that all institutions performing breast MRI should have MRI-guided biopsy capability.

Limitations and Contraindications

There are a number of limitations inherent to MRI-guided biopsies that are not encountered in ultrasound- or stereotactic-guided biopsies (Boxes 23-8 and 23-9).

First, the nature of MRI imposes physical limitations and requires the movement of the patient in and out of the magnet during the procedure, which is cumbersome and time consuming. MRI-guided biopsy cannot be performed in patients with contraindications to MRI (e.g., cardiac pacemakers) or to intravenous

gadolinium administration. All equipment used must be MR compatible and a number of MR-compatible vacuum-assisted devices are now available.

MRI-guided biopsy cannot be performed if the patient is unable to remain still in a prone position for 30-60 minutes. Claustrophobic patients may find MRI-guided biopsy challenging, and oral sedation may be required. As with stereotactic biopsy, very posterior lesions that are close to the chest wall and small breasts may pose a problem (see Troubleshooting at Magnetic Resonance Imaging–Guided Biopsy).

Accessibility to the magnet can be limited in busy institutions with a high demand for table time. Procedure time (from acquisition of the first to the last MR image) is approximately 35 minutes but total MRI suite occupation time may be up to 1 hour.

The target at MRI is a vanishing one; that is, identification is based on gadolinium enhancement, and once the gadolinium washes out, the target is no longer visible. Unlike in ultrasound where real-time evidence of sampling accuracy can be obtained, the lesion may not be visible by the end of the biopsy procedure, which can make it difficult to confirm accurate sampling. Therefore speed and accuracy are very important. In addition, unlike in stereotactic biopsy, specimen mammography is not helpful to confirm sampling accuracy. Therefore, ensuring concordance between imaging and pathology is paramount.

Concordance

Due to the limitations of confirming accurate target sampling, if biopsy yields a benign pathologic result, the radiologist must be

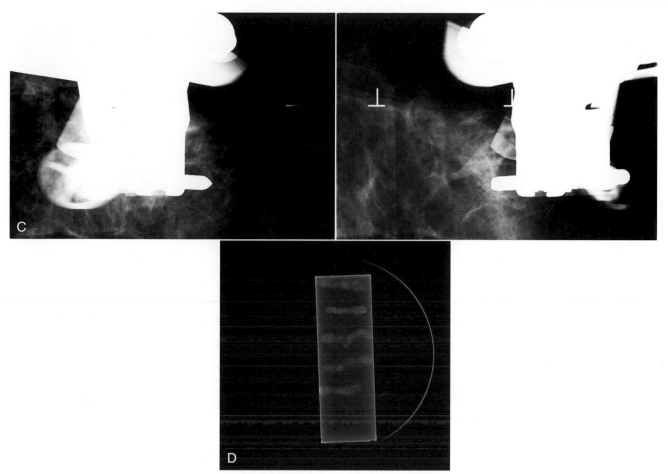

FIGURE 23-8, cont'd C, A repeat stereotactic pair is performed following needle insertion, confirming satisfactory position. **D,** Specimen radiograph confirms satisfactory sampling of the calcifications. (Usually a minimum of six samples is acquired but the procedure was terminated prematurely in this patient due to a vasovagal reaction.) Due to the extent of the calcifications on mammography, a biopsy marker clip was not placed in this case.

Box 23-7. Causes of Sampling Errors at Stereotactic Biopsy

Incorrect calibration of biopsy unit
Patient movement
Inaccurate lesion targeting by radiologist
Vague target (subtle architectural distortion)
Displacement of lesion by local anesthetic/hematoma
Obscuration of lesion by local anesthetic/hematoma
Malfunction of biopsy device

---

confident that the results are concordant. If there is any discordance (e.g., benign pathology but suspicious MRI appearances), then an immediate repeat biopsy should be performed. If there is a specific diagnosis to account for the MRI appearance (e.g., a fibroadenoma) and if immediate postbiopsy imaging shows a biopsy cavity that includes the area of suspicion, then routine follow-up may not be necessary. However, even in cases of presumed concordance, a short interval follow-up MRI is generally recommended to confirm that the target was sampled and to exclude any lesion growth. The optimal time for first follow-up MRI or the duration of follow-up has not been determined but many authors suggest performing a follow-up MRI at 6 months and, as for other modalities, stability for 2 years should confirm benign nature. As with stereotactic biopsies, there is a significant rate of ADH underestimation (up to 50% in some studies) and a biopsy result yielding a high-risk lesion warrants surgical excision.

Patient Preparation

Oral sedation is not routinely necessary but can be given on patient request, especially in claustrophobic patients. Standard informed consent should be obtained before biopsy. In addition to the usual risks, it should be explained to the patient that there is a possibility that the lesion will not be visualized, in which case biopsy cannot be performed (see Troubleshooting at Magnetic Resonance Imaging–Guided Biopsy).

Technique

The patient is positioned prone and the breast placed in a dedicated surface breast coil. The breast is compressed gently in the breast biopsy device (Fig. 23-10). The radiologist must ensure that the breast is taut but not so compressed as to prevent lesion enhancement. Because patient repositioning prolongs procedure time, optimizing patient position within the coil at the start of the procedure is very important and the radiologist should confirm satisfactory patient position before commencing image acquisition.

There are two types of biopsy devices available: (1) the grid system and (2) the pillar-and-post system. The description that follows is for the grid system in which the breast is compressed between two sterile perforated localization grids. The general principles are the same for both methods, but the pillar-and-post method allows for angulation of the needle. Most current coils allow for both a medial and a lateral approach.

Once the patient is in satisfactory position, fiducial markers are placed in the grid. The patient is then moved into the magnet and localization images acquired, ensuring that the entire breast

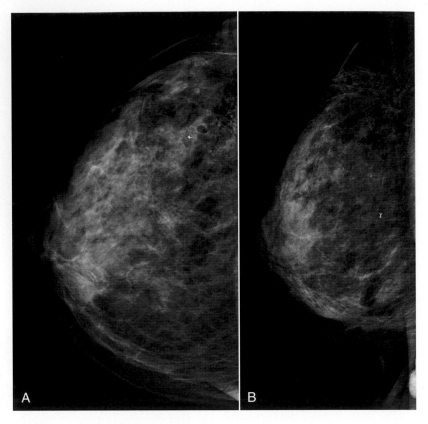

FIGURE 23-9. Postbiopsy mammogram in a 40-year-old woman who underwent stereotactic biopsy of a cluster of calcifications on an upright unit in the craniocaudal position. **A,** Postbiopsy CC view shows postbiopsy change and apparent satisfactory clip position adjacent to residual calcifications. **B,** On the straight lateral view, the clip is displaced 2 cm inferior to the biopsied cluster of calcifications. This occurred due to the accordion effect. If the lesion is targeted in the CC position, then clip displacement is usually greatest on the lateral view and vice versa.

Box 23-8. Limitations of Magnetic Resonance Imaging–Guided Biopsy

Vanishing target
Specimen radiograph not possible
More difficult to confirm accurate lesion sampling
Patient must be moved in and out of magnet during the biopsy
Equipment must be magnetic resonance imaging (MRI) compatible
Expensive
Limited access to MRI suite
Time consuming

Box 23-9. Contraindications to Magnetic Resonance Imaging–Guided Biopsy

General contraindications to magnetic resonance imaging (e.g., cardiac pacemaker)
Contraindications to gadolinium administration
Severe claustrophobia
Inability of patient to lie prone for 30-60 minutes
Very posterior lesions close to chest wall

(to include the estimated site of the lesion to be targeted) and the fiducial markers are in the field of view. Standard fat-suppressed three-dimensional spoiled gradient echo sequences are acquired before and after gadolinium administration at a dose of 0.1 mmol/L per kg of body weight, injected as a rapid bolus through an intravenous catheter. It is the author's preference to acquire these images in the sagittal plane.

Lesion targeting is then performed. The patient can be removed from the magnet for this but her breast remains in compression in the breast coil. The radiologist must first identify the target lesion. It is helpful to perform image subtraction in the setting of subtle enhancing lesions. Once the lesion is identified, use of computer-aided detection (CAD) programs determines the lesion position within the breast and provides the operator with the appropriate fenestration on the grid, the appropriate guide hole, and the needle insertion depth. However, it is important for the radiologist to be able to perform this manually in the absence of CAD. The z-position (depth) is calculated by subtracting the skin position (usually taken to be the image where indentations from the cross lines of the grid are visualized as low signal intensity lines on the skin) from the lesion position. The x- and y-positions are determined by correlating the position of the lesion relative to the fiducial on the grid image.

Once the position has been calculated, the skin is cleaned in the usual manner, 1% lidocaine is administered for superficial and deep anesthesia, and a skin incision made.

There are a number of MR-compatible vacuum-assisted devices commercially available that are compatible with both the grid and the pillar-and-post systems. These are coaxial systems and most use a needle guide that stabilizes the biopsy device and prevents needle angulation. The introducer sheath and stylet are first inserted to the predetermined z-depth through the needle guide. Once in position, the sharp stylet is replaced with an MR-compatible obturator and a repeat set of images in the sagittal and axial plane are obtained to confirm satisfactory position. For most biopsy devices, the ideal location is for the tip of the obturator to lie just at the lesion, which should correlate with the center of the biopsy chamber.

If the obturator position is satisfactory, the patient is removed from the magnet again and sampling is performed. The obturator is removed and replaced by the handheld biopsy device. Usually 10-12 samples are acquired in a 360-degree rotation. Unlike stereotactic biopsy, a specimen radiograph cannot be performed to confirm sampling accuracy so in general more samples are acquired. If the obturator is positioned eccentrically within the lesion on presampling images, the direction of tissue sampling

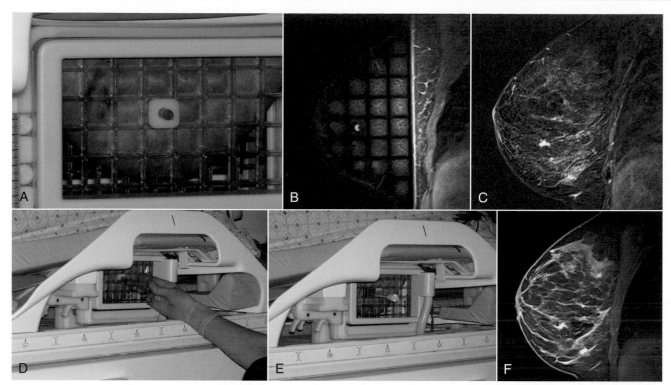

FIGURE 23-10. Magnetic resonance imaging–guided biopsy in a 35-year-old BRCA-1 carrier with a 10-mm area of masslike enhancement in the right breast. **A,** Photograph showing the right breast positioned in the dedicated breast surface coil with sterile compression grid containing a fiducial. **B,** Sagittal T1-weighted fat-saturated spoiled gradient recalled echo (SPGR) image showing the skin and compression grid. The fiducial appears as a T1 bright spot. **C,** Sagittal T1-weighted fat-saturated SPGR image showing the 10-mm area of masslike enhancement. **D,** The target position has been determined and the skin cleaned using Betadine; 1% lidocaine is administered for superficial and deep anesthesia before making a skin incision. **E,** Photograph shows the introducer sheath with MRI-compatible inner obturator in position in the needle guide. **F,** Sagittal T1-weighted SPGR image showing the tip of the obturator as a low signal intensity dot lying adjacent to the targeted lesion. Because the obturator lies eccentrically in the lesion, sampling was directed toward the inferior breast.

can be adjusted accordingly. If there is any concern over needle position, a postbiopsy set of images can be obtained to confirm satisfactory sampling, although the presence of air and high T1 signal intensity blood can make visualization of any residual enhancing lesion difficult. Alternatively, the operator may proceed directly to clip placement. Before clip placement, the biopsy cavity should be lavaged with saline to remove excess blood, which makes postbiopsy change easier to see and should make clip deployment more accurate. A final set of images is usually acquired to confirm clip deployment and to confirm satisfactory position of the postbiopsy hematoma. Standard postbiopsy care is employed.

Postbiopsy two-view mammogram is necessary to confirm clip position relative to postbiopsy change. As with stereotactic biopsy, clip displacement is largely due to distortion of the breast by compression during the biopsy (the accordion effect) and significant clip displacement should be documented in the report.

Troubleshooting at Magnetic Resonance Imaging–Guided Biopsy

Posterior lesions that lie close to the chest wall may be positioned outside the breast coil. If the lesion is known to be close to the chest wall, then time should be spent on optimal positioning to pull as much tissue into the coil as possible. If the lesion lies just outside the coil and close to the grid, then placement of the probe just inferior to the lesion and sampling toward the chest wall (in the 12-o'clock axis) may allow satisfactory sampling. Alternatively, MRI wire-guided localization and surgical excision with placement of the wire as close to the lesion as possible is recommended.

Very small breasts may pose a problem because it can be difficult to compress and immobilize them adequately within the coil. Also, as for stereotactic biopsy, the thickness of the compressed breast must be large enough to accommodate the entire aperture and tip of the biopsy needle. Again, a generous skin wheal of local anesthesia can increase depth and extrinsic circumferential pressure (bolstering) on the breast can increase thickness. As for stereotactic biopsy, petite devices should be used for small breasts.

In some cases, the target may disappear (fail to enhance) at the time of biopsy, which has been described in up to 14% of cases. Nonenhancement of the target may be due to biopsy being recommended for hormonal/background enhancement at initial MRI. If the rate of target disappearance is too high this may suggest that too many biopsies are being recommended for benign background enhancement. Sometimes enhancement can be delayed or absent due to breast compression limiting blood flow to the tissue. In the case of nonvisualization of the lesion, the operator should first confirm that intravenous gadolinium was administered and the intravenous cannula did not become dislodged. If necessary a repeat dose can be injected. Releasing breast compression slightly may help by allowing more blood flow to the breast. If the enhancing lesion is still not visualized, then a follow-up MRI scan should be performed in 2-3 months.

■ BREAST LESION EXCISION SYSTEMS

Vacuum-assisted biopsy devices can be used to excise small biopsy-proven benign lesions as an alternative to open surgical excision. This can be used in young women requesting removal of fibroadenomas in whom optimal cosmesis is desired and documentation of complete lesion excision is not paramount due to benign nature. Compared to open surgical excision, this minimally invasive technique is quick, performed under local anesthesia with minimal complication rates, and associated with just a small scar. However, with vacuum-assisted biopsy devices, lesions are removed piecemeal, rendering assessment of margins impossible, which is undesirable when documentation of complete lesion excision and margin status is necessary.

Breast Lesion Excision System

The Intact breast lesion excision system (BLES) (Intact Medical Corporation, Natick, Mass.) is a novel vacuum-assisted device that uses radiofrequency (RF) cautery to excise small intact breast lesions with a rim of normal tissue. This has the advantage of allowing for histologic evaluation of lesion architecture and assessment of margins. BLES has been shown to be a viable alternative to surgical excision for complete removal of small benign lesions. Initial studies on the use of BLES for stereotactic breast biopsy have shown a trend toward lower rates of DCIS and ADH underestimation with fewer sampling errors. It is under investigation for the complete removal of high-risk lesions, and a potential role in the management of small in situ or invasive malignancies is being evaluated. It can be used under both sonographic and stereotactic guidance for masses, architectural distortion, calcifications, and focal asymmetries.

The Intact breast lesion excision device gained FDA approval for sampling biopsy in 2001 and for complete removal of an imaged abnormality in 2005. It consists of an approximately 6-gauge biopsy "wand" with a basket retrieval device on the distal end. The device comes in a variety of sizes and can obtain ovoid samples with a diameter of up to 20 mm and weighing up to 3 g. The device is inserted under local anesthetic through a small skin incision using sonographic or stereotactic guidance, employing the same general technique as for image-guided biopsy as described earlier. A rigorous local anesthetic protocol must be implemented to ensure complete anesthesia because the sampling acquisition takes 8-10 seconds and unlike in other image-guided biopsies more lidocaine cannot be instilled once sampling commences. Once the wand is in position, metallic prongs with their tips connected by a cutting RF wire pass from the wand and encircle the target area of tissue. RF waves are passed into the tissue to excise the target and achieve hemostasis. Correct wand placement is paramount because once the RF probes are deployed, repositioning is not possible. A retrieval basket is deployed to circumscribe the lesion; once the lesion is captured, the wand and the excised sample in the basket are removed from the skin. A sample radiograph is obtained to confirm inclusion of the targeted lesion and a marker clip placed in the excision bed.

Contraindications

Due to the use of RF waves, BLES is not suitable in patients with implanted electronic devices such as cardiac pacemakers. The manufacturers also do not recommend its use in pregnant women. The use of RF waves is associated with a risk of thermal burns and skin necrosis, so it is not suitable for use in small breasts or in lesions close to the skin, chest wall, or axilla.

Complications

In general, BLES is well tolerated with a side-effect profile similar to that for vacuum-assisted biopsy. Most patients report minor to moderate discomfort during sample acquisition, and there is a risk of bleeding, infection, and skin burns. Studies have reported more delayed healing at the biopsy site in comparison to vacuum-assisted devices, and this is thought to be due to hemostasis associated with the RF cautery, which inhibits migration of fibrins and fibrinogens to the wound site. The samples excised by BLES show diathermy artifact measuring less than 1 mm at the edge of the sections, which

TABLE 23-5 Comparison of Vacuum-Assisted Core Needle Biopsy and Breast Excision System

Vacuum-Assisted Core Needle Device	Breast Lesion Excision System
Piecemeal excision of lesion	Excision of complete lesion
Margin assessment not possible	Margin assessment possible
Lesion architecture may be disrupted	Intact lesion architecture
Quicker	More time consuming
Smaller skin incision	Larger skin incision
Quicker healing	Delayed healing
Higher rate ADH/DCIS underestimation	Lower rate ADH/DCIS underestimation
Can be performed in patients with cardiac pacemakers, pregnancy	Contraindicated in patients with cardiac pacemakers, pregnancy
Most lesions are suitable	Not suitable in all lesions—small breasts, superficial or deep lesions
Can reposition at any time	Cannot reposition once sampling commenced
Local anesthetic important but can instill more during the procedure	Rigorous local anesthesia essential

ADH, Atypical ductal hyperplasia; DCIS, ductal carcinoma in situ.

was concerning in the past for pathologists. However, studies have shown that this is not of clinical significance.

Table 23-5 compares vacuum-assisted biopsy to breast lesion excision systems.

Axillary Lymph Node Sampling

Staging of the axilla is a crucial part of breast cancer workup and management, and the presence and extent of lymph node involvement is an important prognostic indicator of outcome. Sentinel lymph node biopsy has generally replaced axillary lymph node dissection as the primary staging surgical procedure. However, a positive sentinel node biopsy necessitates a second surgical procedure for completion of axillary clearance.

Axillary ultrasound and image-guided sampling of abnormal nodes has become increasingly used in most oncology centers for preoperative staging of the axilla. The specificity of axillary biopsy is 100% and patients with positive results at biopsy proceed directly to axillary clearance, thus avoiding sentinel lymph node biopsy. In addition, the diagnosis of axillary metastases before surgery allows the patient to undergo staging workup, usually with CT scan of the thorax, abdomen, and pelvis, and a bone scan. However, the sensitivity of biopsy is more variable and the false-negative rate of axillary sampling is such that a negative biopsy result does not negate the need for sentinel lymph node sampling.

In general, axillary ultrasound is performed at the time of initial assessment in patients with lesions that are highly suspicious for breast cancer and in all patients with newly diagnosed invasive carcinoma or extensive DCIS, if not already performed. Suspicious features at imaging include diffuse or nodular cortical thickening (>3 mm), loss of the fatty hilum, and nonhilar cortical blood flow. The thickened cortex is the target for biopsy. The most suspicious node should be selected when there are multiple abnormal nodes.

Axillary lymph node sampling can be performed by either FNA or core needle biopsy. In general, the selection of one method over the other depends on institution practice and operator preference because the sensitivity of both options is similar and there is no clear advantage of either technique.

Axillary Fine-Needle Aspiration

Axillary FNA is inexpensive and is generally perceived to be a less invasive, safer procedure with fewer complications compared to core biopsy. However, in addition to requiring a skilled radiologist for FNA, a skilled cytologist with significant experience is also needed.

Technique

Informed consent is obtained. The patient is positioned as for a breast biopsy in the oblique position with the ipsilateral arm over her head. The skin is cleaned in the usual manner and 1% lidocaine given for local anesthetic. A 22- to 25-gauge needle attached to a 5-10 mL syringe is inserted into the cortex of the abnormal node under sonographic guidance. Applying gentle suction, the needle is passed in and out of the cortex in a rapid movement. This is repeated a number of times. Ideally, a cytologist should be on site to confirm specimen adequacy. The sample is sent to the lab in CytoLyt solution.

■ WIRE-GUIDED LOCALIZATION

Since the introduction of screening mammography, increasing numbers of small impalpable in situ and invasive carcinomas are being detected. Wire-guided localization is necessary for accurate localization of impalpable lesions to ensure complete excision of the target lesion with negative margins while ensuring avoidance of unnecessarily large excisions to obtain good cosmesis. Wire-guided localization and surgical excision is generally performed for therapeutic purposes in patients with a known pathologic diagnosis of malignancy following image-guided biopsy. In addition, patients with a high-risk lesion diagnosed at image-guided biopsy require image-guided localization and surgical excision. When image-guided biopsy is not technically possible, wire-guided localization and excisional biopsy may be performed for diagnostic purposes, but open biopsies should be kept to a minimum.

Selection of Image Modality

As with imaged-guided biopsy, image-guided wire localization is performed using the imaging modality with which the lesion is best visualized, taking into account operator preference and availability (Box 23-10 compares modalities). In general, if the lesion can be seen on ultrasound, ultrasound-guided wire placement is performed. The advantages of sonographic guidance include patient comfort and avoidance of ionizing radiation. In addition vasovagal reactions which are quite common during mammographic guidance are rare at ultrasound. Another advantage is that the needle is placed with the patient lying supine in the same orientation as she will be during surgery and this generally means that the surgeon dissects through a smaller volume of tissue during surgery to get to the target.

Mammographic guidance is the modality of choice for localizing calcifications and some biopsy marker clips. (Many newer clips are embedded in echogenic polymers, allowing for accurate sonographic localization). Before localization of a clip, it is necessary to review both the prebiopsy and postbiopsy images to ensure accurate clip position. If the clip deployed at a location remote from the biopsy site, it is usually prudent to excise both the biopsy site with any residual abnormality and the clip. As previously stated, in these cases it is helpful to place the wire and the patient in the same orientation as at the time of biopsy, because clip displacement is usually maximal in the z-position due to the accordion

---

---

effect. By placing the wire in the same orientation, the biopsy site and clip usually lie along the same trajectory and can usually both be localized by the same wire.

MRI-guided wire localization is infrequently performed since the advent of MRI-guided biopsy. However, it may be necessary in very posterior lesions detected on MRI in which tissue biopsy is not possible. In this case, the wire can be deployed immediately adjacent to the area of concern and the surgeon informed to excise the wire and the tissue posterior to it (i.e., between the wire and the pectoral muscle). MRI localization can also be performed for lesions previously biopsied under MRI guidance if the clip failed to deploy or deployed too distant from the abnormality to allow for accurate localization of the lesion.

Needles

There are a variety of wire-needle systems available for needle localization, including the spring hook-wire, modified spring hook-wire, J-wire, and "barbed" wire systems. some of which are MRI compatible. In general, these systems consist of a wire with a hook or barb on the distal end, which is passed through a needle and anchored in the breast to mark the location of the abnormality requiring excision for the surgeon (Fig. 23-11).

The inner wire must be sufficiently strong to resist breakage or cutting by a scalpel during surgery. The outer needles are 19 or 20 gauge, come in various lengths of 3-15 cm, and are scored with 1-cm marks on the needle shaft, which are used to adjust needle position. Until the wire is deployed, the needle can be positioned and repositioned. There is a burnished mark or deployment bead near the proximal end of the wire to show the operator when the distal hook is deployed from the needle (usually when the deployment bead is flush with the hub of the needle). By withdrawing the needle back over the wire, the hook or barb is released and engages in the tissue. Some varieties of wire have multiple barbs on the distal end to minimize migration. With most hook-wire systems repositioning is not possible once the wire is deployed. However, some systems available allow the operator to readvance the needle over the wire for repositioning. In these systems, the wire cannot be retracted without first readvancing the needle, thus providing resistance against migration. Once the needle has been removed, the wire projecting from the skin is flexible and can be taped to the skin to avoid pulling.

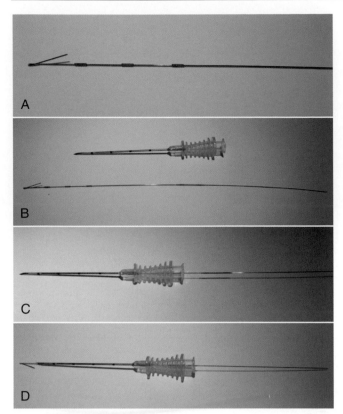

FIGURE 23-11. Photographs of a typical hook-wire system (Ghiatas Beaded Breast Localization Wire, Bard, Ariz.). **A**, A typical localization wire showing the distal barb and proximal marking beads. **B**, Note the 1-cm depth reference marks on the outer 5-cm introducer needle. Also note the deployment bead on the proximal end of the wire. **C**, The wire has been inserted into the introducer needle but the barb has not been deployed. **D**, The wire has been advanced until the deployment bead is flush with the hub of the needle. The distal barb has deployed from the needle.

Most wires have a distal reinforced segment, usually 2 cm in length, which provides a reference point for describing the location of the lesion to the surgeon. The reinforced segment should ideally lie within or directly adjacent to the lesion.

Technique

Sonographic Localization

The patient is positioned as for biopsy in a slightly oblique position with the ipsilateral arm elevated over her head. The skin is cleaned and lidocaine used for superficial and deep anesthesia. As for biopsy, a skin entry point is selected that will allow the needle to be inserted parallel to the chest wall and transducer. A needle length long enough to extend 1 cm distal to the lesion is selected. Using direct sonographic guidance, the needle is advanced parallel to the chest wall and passed through the lesion so the tip lies 1 cm distal to it. When the needle is in an appropriate position, the wire is deployed through the needle and the needle removed, ensuring not to advance or withdraw the wire in the process. Sonographic images of the lesion with the wire in place are obtained. The distance from the skin to the lesion is measured on the final ultrasound image and an "X" is marked on the skin directly overlying the targeted lesion. A mammogram may be obtained for the surgeon to document wire position but is usually not necessary. A dressing is then applied to secure the wire against the patient's skin.

Mammographic-Guided Localization

The radiologist performing the procedure must first review previous imaging to determine the optimal approach. The straight

lateral and craniocaudal (CC) views permit the most accurate estimate of target location and the needle should be inserted using the approach with the shortest distance from skin to target (i.e., if the lesion is closest to the superior surface of the breast, the needle will be inserted in the CC position from above and if the lesion is closest to the inferior surface of the breast it will be inserted in the CC position from below by rotating the gantry). For a lesion closest to the lateral surface, a lateromedial approach is used; for the lesion closest to the medial surface, a mediolateral approach is used. Once the approach is chosen, an appropriate needle length is selected by measuring the distance from the skin to the target and adding 1 cm.

The patient is positioned by the radiographer using special compression paddles for wire localizations. These vary somewhat but usually have a single fenestration with calibration markers along the sides of the fenestration. Alternatively, some radiologists prefer compression plates that contain multiple small fenestrations at regular intervals. However, if the lesion to be targeted does not lie within one of these fenestrations, the paddle must be repositioned, which can be cumbersome.

The radiographer acquires an image to ensure that the target lies within the fenestration on the paddle (Fig. 23-12). It is helpful to mark the skin of the breast at the corners of the fenestration to determine whether the patient moves during the procedure. The radiologist locates the position of the target on the monitor and records the coordinates. Digital systems have electronic crosshairs that are used to determine the coordinates accurately.

The corresponding location on the patient's skin is then determined by aligning the crosshairs/laser lights in the tube collimator with the coordinates on the sides of the fenestration. The skin is cleaned and 1% lidocaine administered for superficial anesthesia. Deeper anesthesia is usually not necessary and can move the target. The needle is placed at the target position on the skin. The needle is then lined up parallel to the x-ray beam (perpendicular to the skin) by ensuring that the shadow of the hub of the needle projects directly over the skin entry point when the centering light is on. The needle is inserted quickly in one straight movement. The needle should be inserted to its hub or as far as possible because it is easy to withdraw the needle at subsequent steps but once the position of the breast has been changed the needle should not be advanced. A repeat image is obtained to ensure satisfactory position of the needle relative to the target. Ideally the needle and hub of the needle should project directly over the target. If the position is not satisfactory, the needle should be withdrawn and reinserted.

If the position is satisfactory, compression is slowly released by the radiographer while the radiologist stabilizes the needle. The patient is repositioned and an image obtained in the orthogonal view to document needle depth relative to the target. If necessary, the needle should be withdrawn so that the tip of the needle lies 1 cm beyond the target. This ensures that the wire deploys with the reinforced portion at the level of the target. If the needle is short of the lesion, it should not be advanced because the needle may be advanced in a different plane to the target and localization will be inaccurate. Therefore, if the needle is short of the lesion, the needle must be removed and the procedure started again.

Once the needle is in a satisfactory position, the wire is deployed through the needle so that the deployment bead on the wire is at the hub of the needle. The wire is then stabilized while the needle is withdrawn over it, taking care not to advance or withdraw the wire. A final image is obtained to document wire position relative to the target. Ideally the wire should lie within 5 mm of the target. A dressing is then applied to secure the wire against the patient's skin. Finally, the films should be labeled and orientated for the surgeon.

For patients with multiple lesions, two or more wires can be placed. For patients with a larger lesion (e.g., a large group of

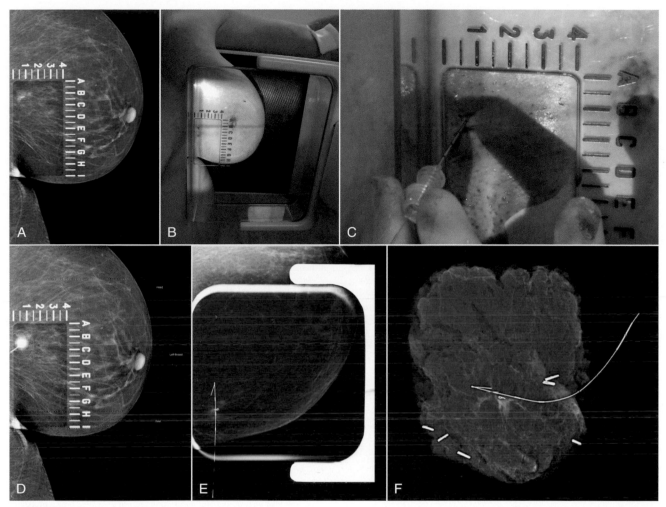

FIGURE 23-12. Mammographic-guided wire localization of a biopsy-proven invasive ductal carcinoma with biopsy marker clip in situ. **A,** Scout mediolateral view confirms satisfactory positioning with the target in the fenestration of the paddle. The target coordinates are determined. **B,** The corresponding location on the patient's skin is determined. **C,** After cleaning the skin and administering lidocaine for superficial anesthesia, the needle is inserted parallel to the x-ray beam, ensuring that the shadow of the hub of the needle projects over the skin entry point. **D,** Repeat mediolateral view confirms satisfactory positioning of the needle relative to the targeted clip. **E,** After the depth position of the needle in the CC position is determined, the wire is deployed and the needle withdrawn. A final CC image is acquired to show final wire position with the beaded section lying at the level of the target. **F,** Specimen radiograph demonstrates inclusion of the targeted density and clip. Histopathology confirmed complete excision of a 10-mm invasive ductal carcinoma with negative margins.

calcifications), bracket localization can be performed whereby a wire is placed at either end of the area to be excised and the surgeon excises the tissue in between.

Magnetic Resonance Imaging–Guided Localization

MRI-guided localization is performed using the same general technique as for MRI-guided biopsy. However, for MRI localization, a different needle guide—which contains multiple small apertures to fit 18- or 20-gauge needles—is used. The aim of the needle guide is to stabilize the needle and ensure insertion in a straight line perpendicular to the skin. However, some radiologists prefer to perform needle localization without the needle guide.

Patient positioning and lesion targeting is performed using the same technique as for MRI-guided biopsy. The needle guide is placed into the appropriate grid position and the MRI-compatible needle/hook-wire system inserted through the appropriate aperture to the appropriate depth. As for ultrasound- and mammographic-guided localization, the needle is placed so the tip lies approximately 1 cm deep to the target. (If a needle guide is used, the depth of the guide must be added to the target depth.)

A repeat set of MRI scans is acquired, usually in the sagittal and axial plane to confirm satisfactory needle position before deploying the wire. When the patient is removed from the magnet, a set of orthogonal mammographic images is acquired to guide the surgeon.

Specimen Radiograph

Following wire-guided localization and surgical excision, a specimen radiograph must be obtained and reviewed by the radiologist performing the procedure to document satisfactory inclusion of the target and the wire in the excised specimen. This also serves to document the position of the target within the specimen for the pathologist and can suggest whether the lesion is close to or abuts the margins. If sonographic localization was performed and the lesion is not visible mammographically, then ultrasound of the specimen can be performed by placing a protective sheath over the transducer. For MRI localization, specimen radiography is performed to document retrieval of the wire but the targeted lesion is often not seen. Radiologic and histologic correlation is very important in this situation. Postoperative MRI can be performed if there is any suspicion that the lesion may have been missed.

Complications

Needle localization is a very safe procedure. There is a risk of bruising and infection but this is extremely rare. When the procedure is performed under sonographic guidance, there is a theoretical risk of pneumothorax, but this should not occur if correct technique is used. Vasovagal reactions may occur during mammographic localization, often because the patient is fasting. Sometimes intravenous fluid replacement is necessary, but usually the patient responds after lying flat.

Radio-Guided Occult Lesion Localization

Radio-guided occult lesion localization (ROLL) is a technique used largely in Europe, whereby instead of placing a wire, a radio-active tracer (Tc-99) is injected into the tumor under image guidance on the day before surgery. A handheld gamma probe guides intraoperative identification of the tumor and surgical resection. This is performed using the same technique as described for wire-guided localization under sonographic or mammographic guidance. This procedure can be performed simultaneously with sentinel node identification—a procedure known as SNOLL. A number of European studies have shown a significantly lower percentage of margin reexcisions and wider surgical margins with ROLL. Studies have also reported smaller surgical specimens and better centering of the tumor. A final advantage is that lesion localization and sentinel node detection can be performed with a single injection.

■ SUGGESTED READINGS

Abe H, Schmidt RA, Sennett CA. US-guided core needle biopsy of axillary lymph nodes in patients with breast cancer: why and how to do it. *Radiographics*. 2007;27(suppl 1):S91-S99.

Abe H, Schmidt RA, Kulkarni K, et al. Axillary lymph nodes suspicious for breast cancer metastasis: sampling with US-guided 14 gauge core needle biopsy - clinical experience in 100 patients. *Radiology*. 2009;250:41-49.

Allen SD, Nerurkar A, Della Rovere GUQ. The breast lesions excision system (BLES): a novel technique in the diagnostic and therapeutic management of small indeterminate breast lesions? *Eur Radiol*. 2011;21:919-924.

American College of Radiology. *ACR practice guideline for the performance of ultrasound-guided percutaneous breast interventional procedures*. Reston, VA: American College of Radiology; 2009.

American College of Radiology. *ACR practice guideline for the performance of stereotactically guided percutaneous breast interventional procedures*. Reston, VA: American College of Radiology; 2009.

Brennan SB, Sung JS, Dershaw DD, et al. Cancellation of MR imaging-guided breast biopsy due to lesion nonvisualization: frequency and follow-up. *Radiology*. 2011;261:92-99.

Cardenosa G. *Breast Imaging—The Core Curriculum*. Baltimore: Lippincott Williams and Wilkins; 2004.

Dershaw DD. *Imaging-guided interventional breast techniques*. New York: Springer-Verlag; 2002.

Georgian-Smith D, Lawton TJ. Variations in physician recommendations for surgery after diagnosis of a high-risk lesion on breast core needle biopsy. *AJR Am J Roentgen*. 2013;198:256-263.

Giacalone PL, Bourdon A, Trinh PD, et al. Radioguided occult lesion localization plus sentinel node biopsy (SNOLL) versus wire-guided localization plus sentinel node detection: a case control study of 129 unifocal pure invasive non-palpable breast cancers. *EJSO*. 2012;38:220-229.

Heller SL, Moy L. Imaging features and management of high risk lesions on contrast enhanced dynamic breast MRI. *AJR Am J Roentgen*. 2012;198:249-255.

Jackman RJ, Marzoni FA, Rosenberg J. False-negative diagnoses at stereotactic vacuum-assisted needle breast biopsy: long-term follow-up of 1,280 lesions and review of the literature. *AJR Am J Roentgen*. 2009;192:341-351.

Kalinyak JE, Schilling K, Berg WA, et al. PET-guided breast biopsy. *Breast J*. 2011;17:143-151.

Killebrew LK, Oneson RH. Comparison of the diagnostic accuracy of a vacuum-assisted percutaneous intact specimen sampling device to a vacuum-assisted core needle sampling device for breast biopsy: initial experience. *Breast J*. 2006;12:302-308.

Kiluk JV, Acs G, Hoover SJ. High-risk benign breast lesions: current strategies in management. *Cancer Control*. 2007;14:321-329.

Kohr JR, Eby PR, Allison KH, et al. Risk of upgrade of atypical ductal hyperplasia after stereotactic breast biopsy: effects of number of foci and complete removal of calcifications. *Radiology*. 2010;255:723-730.

Kopans DB. *Breast Imaging*. 3rd ed. Baltimore: Lippincott Williams and Wilkins; 2007.

Lehman CD, Deperi ER, Peacock S, et al. clinical experience with MRI-guided vacuum-assisted breast biopsy. *AJR Am J Roentgen*. 2005;184:1782-1787.

Liberman L, Morris EA. *Breast MRI-Diagnosis and Intervention*. New York: Springer; 2005.

Liberman L, Kaplan JB, Morris EA, et al. To excise or to sample the mammographic target: what is the goal of stereotactic 11 gauge vacuum-assisted breast biopsy? *AJR Am J Roentgen*. 2002;179:670-683.

Liberman L. Percutaneous image-guided core breast biopsy. *Radiol Clin North Am*. 2002;40:483-500.

Liberman L, Morris EA, Dershaw DD, et al. Fast MRI-guided vacuum-assisted breast biopsy: initial experience. *AJR Am J Roentgen*. 2003;181:1283-1293.

Liberman L, Holland AE, Marjan D, et al. Underestimation of atypical ductal hyperplasia at MRI guided 9 gauge vacuum-assisted breast biopsy. *AJR Am J Roentgen*. 2007;188:684-690.

Li J, Dershaw DD, Lee CH, et al. MRI Follow-up after concordant, histologically benign diagnosis of breast lesions sampled by MRI guided biopsy. *AJR Am J Roentgen*. 2009;193:850-855.

Lomoschitz FM, Helbich TH, Rudas M, et al. Stereotactic 11 gauge vacuum-assisted breast biopsy: influence of number of specimens on diagnostic accuracy. *Radiology*. 2004;232:897-903.

Mainiero MB, Cinelli CM, Koelliker SL. Axillary ultrasound and fine-needle aspiration in the preoperative evaluation of the breast cancer patient: an algorithm based on tumor size and lymph node appearance. *AJR Am J Roentgen*. 2010;195:1261-1267.

Melotti MK, Berg WA, et al. Core needle breast biopsy in patients undergoing anticoagulation therapy. *AJR Am J Roentgen*. 2000;174:245-249.

Noroozian M, Gombos EV, Chikarmane S, et al. Factors that impact the duration of MRI guided core needle biopsy. *AJR Am J Roentgen*. 2010;194:150-157.

Orel SG, Rosen M, Mies C, et al. MR imaging guided 9 gauge vacuum-assisted core needle breast biopsy: initial experience. *Radiology*. 2006;238:54-61.

Pritchard MG, Townend JN, Lester WA, et al. Management of patients taking antiplatelet or anticoagulant medication requiring invasive breast procedures: United Kingdom survey of radiologists' and surgeon's current practice. *Clin Radiol*. 2008;63:305-311.

Rao R, Lilley L, Andrews V, et al. Axillary staging by percutaneous biopsy: sensitivity of fine-needle aspiration versus core needle biopsy. *Ann Surg Oncol*. 2009;16:1170-1175.

Rauch GM, Dogan BE, Smith TB. Outcome analysis of 9 gauge MRI guided vacuum-assisted core needle breast biopsies. *AJR Am J Roentgen*. 2012;198:292-299.

Rosen EL, Vo TT. Metallic clip deployment during stereotactic breast biopsy: retrospective analysis. *Radiology*. 2001;218:510-516.

Sie A, Bryan DC, Gaines V. Multicenter evaluation of the breast lesion excision system, a percutaneous, vacuum-assisted, intact-specimen breast biopsy device. *Cancer*. 2006;107:945-949.

Somerville P, Seifert PJ, Destounis SV, et al. Anticoagulation and bleeding risk after core biopsy. *AJR Am J Roentgen*. 2008;191(4):1194-1197.

Vilar VS, Goldman SM, Ricci MD, et al. Analysis by MRI of residual tumor after radiofrequency ablation for early stage breast cancer. *AJR Am J Roentgen*. 2012;198:285-291.

Whitworth PW, Simpson JF, Poller WR, et al. Definitive diagnosis for high-risk breast lesions without open surgical excision: the intact percutaneous excision trial (IPET). *Ann Surg Oncol*. 2011;18:3027-3052.

CHAPTER 24

Musculoskeletal Intervention

Farah G. Irani, MD, Xavier Buy, MD, and Afshin Gangi, MD, PhD

Musculoskeletal interventional procedures are a fast growing area for interventional radiology. The most commonly performed techniques and the most promising new techniques are described in this chapter.

IMAGE GUIDANCE

Percutaneous musculoskeletal interventions, like other interventional procedures, are usually performed with a single imaging technique: ultrasound, fluoroscopy, computed tomography (CT), or magnetic resonance imaging (MRI). Fluoroscopy and CT are the most frequently used guidance techniques.

Fluoroscopy offers multiple planes and direct real-time imaging but suffers from poor soft tissue contrast and radiation exposure for both patient and operator. CT is well suited for precise interventional needle guidance because it provides good visualization of bone and surrounding soft tissues. This helps avoid damage to adjacent vascular, neurological, and visceral structures. CT guidance seems to be more appropriate for interventions at difficult locations.

FluoroCT, with acquisition of eight to 12 images per second, is helpful if the region of interest moves during the procedure (e.g., breathing). FluoroCT is not used routinely, but it is used in difficult cases when accurate positioning of the needle is required or to view the distribution of cement during vertebroplasty. However, the radiation dose to the operator and the patient is quite high when using this technique.

A combination of CT and fluoroscopy for interventional procedures has been recommended for complex procedures. For fluoroscopy, a mobile C-arm is positioned in front of the CT gantry.

MRI offers excellent soft tissue contrast and three-dimensional acquisition techniques, as well as rapid multiplanar image acquisition and reconstruction. Another attractive quality of MRI is the absence of radiation exposure to the interventionist and the patient. Despite these advantages, MR-guided interventions are challenging owing to limited access to the patient, strong magnetic and radiofrequency (RF) fields that require special interventional devices, inferior image frame rates and spatial resolution, and MRI scanner noise.

In the musculoskeletal system, MR guidance is advantageous if the lesion is not visible by other modalities, for regions adjacent to hardware and implants, subselective targeting, intraarticular locations, and periarticular cyst aspiration. MR guidance has also been used for a host of spine injections and pain management.

Interventional procedures can be performed using a vertically open 0.5-T MR unit equipped with in-room display monitors using fast spin echo and gradient echo sequences. However, with the rapid evolution of technology, 1.5-T interventional MR scanners have been developed, which have a larger and shorter bore for easier access to the patient. Imaging in real-time is possible with radial or spiral k-space filling as with MR-guided vascular interventional procedures.

However, interventional MRI is not widely available and the expense limits accessibility.

■ BIOPSIES OF THE MUSCULOSKELETAL SYSTEM

Histopathologic and bacteriologic analysis is often required on musculoskeletal lesions to establish a definitive diagnosis and guide treatment. Percutaneous musculoskeletal biopsy (PMSB) has become a routine procedure, performed by interventional radiologists, and has in many instances done away with the need for open biopsy. PMSB is a safe and cost-effective technique, which can be performed on an outpatient basis with the patient under local anesthesia and resulting in minimal complications (Box 24-1).

Indications

The objective of PMSB is to obtain a sufficient volume of tissue, representative of the underlying disease, with minimum risk to the patient.

Percutaneous bone biopsy is performed whenever pathologic, bacteriologic, or biologic examinations are required for definitive diagnosis or treatment.

Determination of whether a metastasis is present is the most frequent indication for which a bone biopsy is performed. Positron emission tomography (PET) CT is able to establish the presence of hypermetabolic lesions suggestive of metastasis with increasing accuracy, often obviating the need for biopsy. However, in certain equivocal cases, tissue diagnosis is essential to prove the metastatic origin of the lesion before commencement of treatment or to identify the primary tumor. In certain situations, such as breast cancer, a biopsy may provide information regarding the hormonal sensitivity of the lesion, which has direct therapeutic implications. For primary bone tumors, biopsy is not indicated if complete surgical excision is planned. However, a biopsy can be performed if doubt persists as to the nature of the lesion or if the histology will change therapy.

Infectious lesions (osteitis, septic arthritis, and discitis) are another indication for PMSB, which is used to discover the causative organism.

Box 24-1. Percutaneous Musculosketal Biopsy

Determination of metastatic disease is the most frequent indication

Positron emission tomography can help obviate the need for biopsy

Tumor seeding should be considered for primary bone tumors and the procedure planned so that the track can be excised

Lesions with mild ossification can be biopsied with a 14-gauge Ostycut needle; drilling is necessary for lesions that are densely ossified

---

Contraindications

Bleeding diatheses, biopsies of inaccessible sites (e.g., odontoid process, anterior arch of C1), and soft tissue infection with high risk of contamination of bone are known contraindications for PMSB.

All diagnostic imaging modalities should be reviewed before proceeding to biopsy to avoid unnecessary procedures and afford maximum safety benefit to the patient. The risk of tumor seeding should be considered, especially for sarcomas, and the biopsy trajectory should be planned with the surgeon so that the biopsy tract can be resected with the tumor.

Tools

Soft tissue and lytic lesions without ossification are directly biopsied using a 14- to 18-gauge coaxial biopsy gun. We use the semi-automated side notch cutting Temno needle, which allows for manual advancement of the trocar, followed by automated firing of the outer cannula. We perform a CT scan after the deployment of the trocar but before firing of the outer cannula to allow for accurate positioning of the needle and to prevent complications caused by inadvertent biopsy of nearby structures.

In cases of mild ossification, lesions surrounded by minimal cortex, and spinal biopsies, we use a 14-gauge Ostycut bone biopsy needle (Ostycut, Angiomed/Bard, Karlsruhe, Germany). Penetration of the cortex is performed using a surgical hammer. For primary bone tumors or lymphoma with mild sclerosis, we use an 8-gauge trephine needle (Laredo type).

In cases of dense ossification or osteoblastic metastasis, or if dense cortical bone needs to be penetrated, drilling is necessary. We use a 2-mm diameter hand drill or a 14-gauge Bonopty Penetration set (Radi Medical Systems, Uppsala, Sweden).

Technique

A CT scan is performed to localize the lesion precisely. The entry point and the pathway are determined by CT, such that the shortest route from skin to tumor is selected, avoiding neural, vascular, and visceral structures. The patient is positioned prone, supine, or oblique. In cases of spine and disc biopsy, a combination of CT and fluoroscopy is used.

Bone biopsy is usually performed under local anesthesia. Neuroleptanalgesia may be necessary for painful lesions. General anesthesia is used for children.

After sterile draping, the biopsy trajectory is anesthetized with 1% lidocaine from skin to periosteum using a 22-gauge spinal needle. This needle is then repositioned at the soft tissue tumor interface and a confirmatory scan performed. The biopsy needle is then inserted parallel to the spinal needle using the tandem needle technique. In cases of bone biopsy wherein cortical penetration is required, a surgical hammer may be required to tap the needle into position. Frequent scans are performed to check for correct needle trajectory because once the needle has entered the bone it is very difficult to change direction. The use of fluoroscopy allows for real-time monitoring of needle progression. A combination of CT and fluoroscopy allows for rapid and safe performance of the procedure. Once the needle is within the lesion and the position is confirmed with CT, sampling is performed.

For histopathologic examination, the specimen is fixed in 10% formalin. If bacteriologic analysis is necessary, the specimens are not fixed and are sent for culture in normal saline. Single-use needles are preferred for biopsies.

On completion of the biopsy, the needle is removed and compression applied. A completion CT through the biopsy site is done to rule out hemorrhage.

- Peripheral long bone: The approach has to be orthogonal to the bone cortex, which avoids the needle tip slipping off the cortex. The approach must avoid tendons as well as nerves, vessels, and visceral and articular structures.

- Flat bones (scapula, ribs, sternum, and skull): An oblique approach using a 30- to 60-degree angle is recommended. This approach is a compromise between the tangential approach, which avoids damage to underlying structures, and the orthogonal approach, which avoids slippage of the needle tip (Fig. 24-1).
- Pelvic girdle: A posterior approach is used to avoid the sacral canal and nerves.
- Vertebral body biopsy: Different approach routes can be selected depending on the vertebral level biopsied: the anterolateral route is used for the cervical level; the transpedicular or intercostovertebral route for the thoracic level; and the posterolateral or transpedicular route for the lumbar level (Box 24-2).

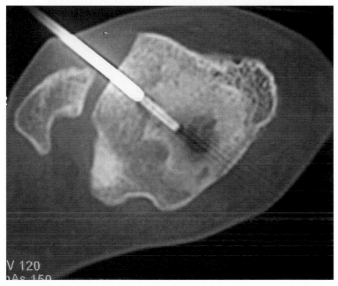

FIGURE 24-1. Computed tomography guided biopsy of the talus using a Laredo needle and an orthogonal approach.

Box 24-2. Percutaneous Musculoskeletal Biopsy

An orthogonal approach is used for peripheral long bones
An oblique (30- to 60-degree) approach is used for flat bones
An anterolateral approach is used for the cervical vertebrae
A transpendicular or intercostovertebral approach is used for the thoracic vertebrae
A posterolateral or transpendicular approach is used for the lumbar vertebrae
Overall accuracy of computed tomography–guided PMSB varies from 74% to 96%

- For the neural posterior arch, a tangential approach is used to avoid damage to underlying neural structures.
- Vertebral disc biopsy: As for vertebral biopsies, the approach changes depending on the level where the biopsy is performed. For the lumbar level, a transforaminal route using the "Scotty dog" technique is used to gain access to the disc (Fig. 24-2). At the thoracic level, the intercostotransverse route is used with the needle advanced in the direction of the fluoroscopic beam, which is directed 35 degrees from the patient's sagittal plane (Fig. 24-3).

Complications

Complications are rare following image-guided bone biopsies with an incidence of up to 2%.

The major complication is infection. Strict sterility should be maintained throughout the intervention. In immunocompromised patients, the biopsy should be done under antibiotic coverage. Other reported complications are hematoma, reflex sympathetic dystrophy, neural and vascular injuries, and pneumothorax following biopsies in the thorax. The risk of tumor seeding is rare but real. Hence, it is absolutely necessary in patients with primary bone tumors to choose the needle trajectory in consultation with the surgeon.

Murphy and colleagues, in a large review of 9500 percutaneous skeletal biopsies, identified 22 complications (0.2%). They reported nine pneumothoraces, three cases of meningitis, and five spinal cord injuries. Serious neurologic injury occurred in 0.08% of procedures. Death occurred in 0.02%.

In our experience, we observed only three complications, all paravertebral hematomas: Two cases resolved spontaneously; the other was caused by needle tip breakage in cortical bone. We believe that the low complication rate is related to the systematic use of CT and/or dual guidance.

Results

The overall diagnostic accuracy of CT-guided biopsies ranges from 74% to 96%. However, diagnostic accuracy of CT-guided biopsies for spinal lesions and for infectious etiology is much lower.

In our department, 620 percutaneous musculoskeletal biopsies were performed on an outpatient basis. There were 63% female and 37% male patients, with a mean age of 58 years (range 2-87 years). The distribution of lesions was vertebral 68%, pelvic girdle 17%, and peripheral long bones 15%. Of the biopsied lesions, 55% were lytic, 24% were sclerotic or mixed, and 21% were vertebral compression fractures. In the spine the distribution of lesions was as follows: cervical 5%, thoracic 28%, lumbar 55%, and sacrum 12%.

We found a specificity of 100%, sensitivity of 93.9%, positive predictive value of 100%, and negative predictive value of 87.5%.

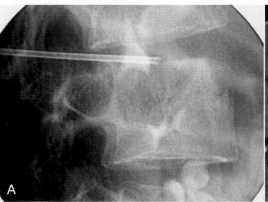
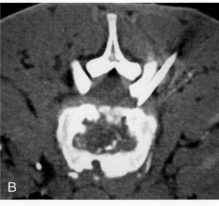

FIGURE 24-2. Infective lumbar discitis. **A,** Fluoroscopic view showing the transforaminal approach to the disc and endplate with the 14-gauge Ostycut needle within the disc. **B,** Computed tomography image demonstrating the pathologic disc with the biopsy needle passing close to the articular process and through the lower part of the foramen.

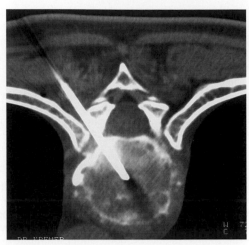

FIGURE 24-3. Computed tomography guided biopsy of thoracic disc using the intercostopedicular approach.

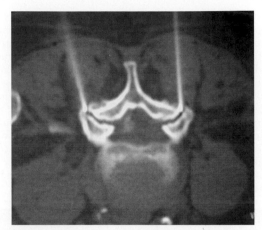

FIGURE 24-4. Bilateral facet joint infiltration: Precise positioning of the tip of the 22-gauge spinal needles in the facet articulation using computed tomography guidance.

FACET JOINT INFILTRATION

The annual incidence of back pain has been estimated at 5% with recent studies showing that chronicity and recurrence occurs in 35% to 79% of these patients. Chronic low back pain presents a major medical, social, and economic burden for society.

Lumbar zygapophysial joints (facet) have been implicated as one of the causes of chronic low back pain.

The term *facet syndrome* was introduced by Ghormeley. Facet joint pain is attributed to segmental instability, synovitis, and degenerative arthritis. The signs of facet syndrome are local paralumbar tenderness, pain relieved by recumbency, pain on hyperextension, absence of root tension signs and neurologic deficit, and absence of hip, buttock, or back pain when the straight leg is raised. In the absence of precise diagnostic clinical features or criteria, the diagnosis of facet syndrome relies exclusively on the results of diagnostic blocks. The differentiation between disc disease and facet syndrome can be difficult. The diagnosis is often arrived at by exclusion.

Local anesthetic agents act on the nociceptive fibers within the synovium, whereas intraarticular corticosteroids reduce inflammation of the synovium and thus ameliorate pain. The choice of injection levels is based on the location of focal tenderness over the joints or the presence of osteoarthritis involving the joints. The "block test" with intraarticular injection of local anesthetics into the facet joint must produce complete pain relief to support the presumptive diagnosis. When considering facet joint syndrome, another test is done which consists of injecting 0.5 mL of 5% hypertonic saline into the joints to provoke the usual back pain.

Indications

Intraarticular injection of steroids is performed in patients in whom "diagnostic blocks" prove that the facet joints are the source of back pain.

Technique

Facet joint injection in the lumbar spine is a simple and safe procedure that can be performed on an outpatient basis under CT or fluoroscopic control. Facet joint degenerative disease usually affects multiple levels on both sides, and thus multilevel facet joint injections (L3-L4, L4-L5, and L5-S1) may be necessary.

The patient is placed in a prone position on the CT or fluoroscopy table. A CT scan of the affected level is used to

> **Box 24-3. Facet Joint Infiltration**
>
> Facet joints have been implicated in many cases of chronic low back pain
>
> Differentiation of disc disease from facet disease can be difficult
>
> Injection level is based on location of tenderness and/or facet joint degeneration
>
> A block test with local anesthetic must produce complete pain relief to confirm the diagnosis
>
> Immediate pain relief varies from 59% to 94% and long-term relief varies from 27% to 54%

determine the needle pathway and the entry point. A 22-gauge needle is advanced vertically into each joint (Fig. 24-4). Once the needle is in the joint, a solution of cortivazol and lidocaine 1% is injected into the joint. Cortivazol is provided in 1.5 mL of solution (containing 3.75 mg of long-acting steroid) and with the addition of 1.5 mL of lidocaine 1%, a 3-mL solution is obtained. Usually the injection is performed bilaterally and 1.5 mL of this solution is injected into each side. The global dose of 3.75 mg of cortivazol per session should not be exceeded.

Complications

The complications of lumbar facet joint injections with precise needle positioning are rare. Severe allergic reactions to local anesthetic are uncommon. Steroid injections can produce local reactions, which occur most often immediately after the injection. These reactions last 24-48 hours, and they can be relieved by the application of ice. The most serious complication is septic arthritis, which is avoided by adherence to strict aseptic technique. The only serious complication we have observed is a temporary episode of agitation in a patient as a reaction to the steroid injected. Other complications are rare if the usual contraindications to steroid use are respected.

Results

The value of steroid injection into the facet joint remains controversial. In the literature, immediate relief of pain occurs in 59%-94% of cases, and long-term relief occurs in 27%-54%. In our experience with 166 facet blocks, immediate pain relief was obtained in 62% of patients but long-term relief (persistence of relief for at least 6 months) in only 31% (Box 24-3).

RHYZOLYSIS: RADIOFREQUENCY NEUROTOMY OF THE ZYGAPOPHYSIAL JOINTS

The zygapophysial joints are a potent source of low back pain impairing quality of life.

The lumbar zygapophysial joints are innervated by the medial branch of the dorsal rami from L1 to L4 and the L5 dorsal ramus for the L5/S1 joint. The medial branch of the dorsal rami have a fixed course across the base of the superior articular process between their origin from the dorsal ramus at the superior aspect of the transverse process and their passage under the mamilloaccessory ligament at the caudal edge of the superior articular process. At the L5 level, the dorsal ramus passes over the ala of the sacrum in the bony groove formed by the base of the superior articular process and ala of the sacrum. The caudal origin of the medial branch at this level is not accessible by a percutaneous approach; therefore the target nerve at L5 is the dorsal ramus.

The zygapophysial joints have dual nerve supply. The superior portion of each joint is innervated by the medial branch originating one level above, while the inferior portion of the joint is supplied by the medial branch originating at that level. Hence for complete denervation of the joint, coagulation of both nerves needs to be performed.

Indication

Patients in whom the block test is positive, who have undergone successful facet joint block using a mixture of steroid and local anesthetic, and in whom pain relief is complete but very short lasting may benefit from RF neurotomy of the zygapophysial joints.

Technique

The procedure is performed on an outpatient basis (Box 24-4). We use dual CT and fluoroscopic guidance. The patient is positioned prone.

A perfect anteroposterior (AP) projection of the involved vertebral body is obtained, which may require craniocaudal angulation of the fluoroscopic tube so that there is perfect alignment of the vertebral endplates. Dispersive ground pads are placed on the medial aspect of the patient's thigh.

After sterile draping, local anesthesia is infiltrated superficially in the skin and the subcutaneous tissues. We do not advocate deep anesthesia or conscious sedation, because these can interfere with the patient's perception of pain, which is important for correct positioning of the electrode.

An 18-gauge insulated needle with an active 5-mm tip is then advanced under fluoroscopic guidance so that the tip is positioned in the groove formed by the junction of the superior articular process and the transverse process. If fluoroscopy alone is used, a lateral view is obtained to confirm the ideal position of the needle; it should not be too deep within the soft tissues for risk of damage

to the dorsal nerve root. With dual guidance, a CT scan ensures correct positioning of the needle. Maintaining contact with bone ensures a safe positioning of the needle. At the L5 level, the tip of the needle should rest in the groove between the superior articular process and the sacral ala.

Once correct positioning of the needle is obtained, the electrode is inserted and connected to the generator (Smith and Nephew). Electrode impedance should be less than 500 ohms, which indicates good position of the electrode. The generator is put in stimulation mode and sensory stimulation is performed by gradually increasing the voltage to reproduce the pain that the patient normally feels in the back. It is important for the patient to only feel pain in the back and not radiating down the leg. Radiation of pain down the leg indicates that the electrode is in contact with the dorsal ramus and needs to be repositioned. Following sensory stimulation, motor stimulation is performed with gradual augmentation of the voltage, such that there is local contraction of the muscles of the back without any contraction of the muscles of the buttocks, thigh, or leg.

The generator is switched to the RF mode and coagulation is obtained by gradually increasing the RF current to achieve a temperature of 80°C, which is maintained for 90 seconds. If during the RF ablation (RFA) of the targeted nerve the patient experiences pain, injection of local anesthesia through the needle can be performed and the procedure continued to complete treatment.

Multiple levels can be treated at one visit. The patient is maintained in recumbent position for 1 hour and then discharged home.

Complications

The procedure is safe. The most serious complication is damage to the dorsal nerve root due to incorrect positioning of the electrode. This is avoided by fluoroscopic and CT-guided placement of the electrode and the use of the stimulation mode before commencing the ablation.

Results

Dreyfuss and colleagues in a prospective audit of 15 patients who were selected for rhyzolysis following a positive bloc test reported that 60% of the patients obtained at least 90% relief of pain at 12 months, and 87% obtained at least 60% relief. Relief was associated with denervation of the multifidus in those segments in which the medial branches had been coagulated.

In a randomized controlled trial of 31 patients, Van Kleef and colleagues reported success in 10 of 15 patients treated with RF compared with six of 16 in the sham group. The adjusted odds ratio was 4.8 ($P < 0.05$, significant). The differences in effect on the visual analog scale scores, global perceived effect, and the Oswestry disability scale were statistically significant. Three, 6, and 12 months after treatment, there were significantly more success patients in the RF group than in the sham group.

Leclaire and colleagues in a randomized controlled trial of 70 patients undertaken to assess the clinical effectiveness of RF facet joint denervation concluded that the procedure provided some short-term improvement in functional disability among patients with chronic low back pain, but could not establish the efficacy of the treatment modality. However, the main drawback of their study was the patient selection criteria. All patients with chronic nonspecific low back pain were eligible for intraarticular zygapophysial joint injection, which was performed and reported by 30 different referring physicians. Furthermore, only one block test was performed and the levels infiltrated were not reported.

In our experience, rhyzolysis is effective in the management of pain in patients with pure axial back pain attributed to facet syndrome. However, the durability of pain relief is limited to 1 year with many patients experiencing recurrence of pain. Our results are similar to those of Schofferman and colleagues. They reported that RF neurotomy is effective but temporary in the management of lumbar facet pain. Repeated RF neurotomies are effective in long-term palliative management of lumbar facet pain. Each RF neurotomy has a mean duration of relief of 10.5 months and is successful in more than 85% patients.

■ PERCUTANEOUS EPIDURAL AND NERVE ROOT BLOCK

Back pain has a diverse etiology and causes pain, suffering, and disability, which have a great social and economic impact. Disc herniation, defined as the rupture of the fibrocartilaginous annulus fibrosus with extrusion of the central gelatinous nucleus pulposus, is the most common cause of back pain presenting as axial spinal pain and or radicular (arm, intercostals, or leg) pain.

There is no clear, single explanation as to why a disc rupture causes back pain or sciatica. Some disc ruptures remain asymptomatic. Physical pressure on a peripheral nerve alone does not produce pain; it produces paresthesia. It is postulated that biochemical factors such as inflammatory cytokines, prostaglandins, nitrous oxide (NO), and cyclooxygenase-2 (COX-2) may be involved in the pathogenesis of radiculitis caused by mechanical discoradicular compression.

Pain management in disc herniation relies mainly on conservative care, combining rest, physiotherapy, and oral medication (analgesics and antiinflammatory drugs). Open discectomy remains a major surgical procedure and the long-term outcome, complications, and suboptimal results associated with surgery have led to the development of minimally invasive percutaneous techniques that avoid opening the spinal canal.

Percutaneous periradicular infiltration (PPRI) consists of injecting a mixture of long-acting steroid and anesthetic into the epidural space at the level of the pathologic disc. It is ideally performed under image guidance to ensure the proper deposition of steroid. It aims to stop the inflammatory reaction around the nerve root.

Indications

- Treatment of radicular pain of discogenic origin (without nerve paralysis) resistant to conventional medical therapy
- Postdiscectomy syndrome

Contraindications

- Patients with diabetes or gastric ulceration and pregnant patients in whom steroid use is contraindicated
- Bleeding diathesis (anticoagulant therapy): Epidural puncture is contraindicated for fear of producing an epidural hematoma, resulting in thecal sac compression; foraminal injection should be performed carefully
- Spinal canal stenosis: Long-acting synthetic steroids are avoided due to their hyperosmotic effect

Technique

The procedure is performed on an outpatient basis. CT or MRI guidance can be used. There is limited accessibility to MR interventional suites and special MR-compatible needles must be used. CT with its easy accessibility is presently the imaging modality of choice because it allows for accurate needle positioning within the epidural space close to the discoradicular interface.

Lumbar Infiltrations

The patient is placed prone on the CT table and a short CT acquisition through the level of interest is performed without gantry tilt with a maximum scan thickness of 3 mm. The entry point and the needle pathway are determined from the axial slices and the position marked on the skin.

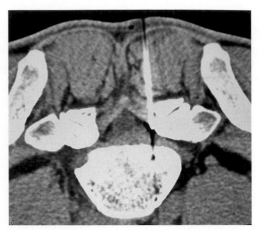

FIGURE 24-5. Epidural lumbar infiltration: Air epidurogram confirming the epidural position of the needle tip close to the discoradicular interface before steroid injection.

Epidural Lateral Infiltration (Fig. 24-5)

Epidural lateral infiltration is used for posteromedial and posterolateral disc herniation. After sterile painting and draping, the skin entry point is anesthetized. A 22-gauge spinal needle is then introduced via a posterior approach, using CT guidance so that the tip is positioned close to the painful nerve root. A sterile flexible connecting tube is attached to the needle to avoid inadvertent displacement of the tip during injection. The extradural position of the needle is determined by negative aspiration of cerebrospinal fluid and gas epidurography by injection of CO_2 or injection of iodinated contrast material. A mixture of 1.5 mL cortivazol (3.75 mg) and 1 mL of 1% lidocaine is then injected. During injection, the patient may experience a spontaneous recurrence of pain lasting a few seconds, brought on by stretching of the dura.

If the dura is punctured due to adhesions or an incorrect maneuver, the needle should be withdrawn into the epidural space and a natural steroid like hydrocortancyl (prednisolone acetate) injected without lidocaine. Long-acting synthetic steroids should never be injected intrathecally because they may precipitate in the cerebrospinal fluid and produce a chemical arachnoiditis. In spinal canal stenosis, only natural steroids such as hydrocortancyl (prednisolone acetate) should be used to avoid worsening of the symptoms due to the hyperosmolar effect of long-acting steroids.

Foraminal Infiltration

This approach is used for foraminal and extraforaminal herniations. The procedure is similar but the entry point is more lateral. The needle is positioned under CT guidance so that it glides across the articular process, with the tip being positioned just behind the emerging nerve root. If the nerve root is touched, the patient experiences a sharp electric sensation down the lower limb and the needle tip should be withdrawn a few millimeters before injection of the steroid-anesthetic mixture.

Cervical Infiltration (Fig. 24-6)

The patient is positioned supine with the neck hyperextended and the head turned to the opposite side. The painful nerve root is infiltrated as it exits its foramen. The entry point is determined by a CT scan (2-mm slice thickness) through the relevant level. After sterile draping, local anesthesia is infiltrated only into the subcutaneous tissues. A 22-gauge spinal needle is positioned using a lateral approach, in contact with the anterior side of the facet joint, behind the nerve root, avoiding the anteriorly situated vertebral artery. One- to 2-mL of iodinated contrast is then injected through a connecting tube after aspiration for blood, to check for

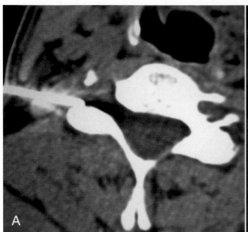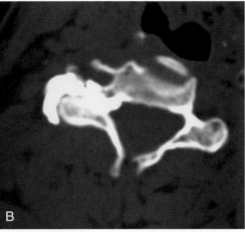

FIGURE 24-6. Cervical infiltration. **A,** Computed tomography image of the tip of the 22-gauge spinal needle in the posterior part of the cervical foramen, in contact with the posteriorly located facet joint, away from the anteriorly situated vertebral artery. **B,** Good diffusion of contrast within the foramen and canal.

correct position of the needle tip and to exclude intravascular injection. Then 1.5 mL (3.75 mg) cortivazol is injected. Lidocaine is never injected in the cervical region to avoid diffusion via the foramen around the cord, which would result in transient paralysis.

Postprocedure Care

The patient can stand up immediately and return to work. The sterile dressing can be removed after 36 hours. Restriction of dietary sodium is advocated for 2 weeks following the injection to reduce the hyperosmolar effect of the steroid medication.

Complications

It is rare to have complications from percutaneous steroid injections. The reported incidence is less than 0.05%, mostly for cervical infiltrations.

- Infectious complications (e.g., meningitis, spondylodiscitis, and epidural abscess) leading to neurologic insult (e.g., paraplegia, quadriplegia, multiple cranial nerve palsies, nystagmus) have been reported following epidural or intrathecal administration of steroids. Strict sterility should be maintained during the procedure.
- Vascular complications such as intravascular injection and puncture of the vertebral artery have been reported at the cervical level. Medullary infarction following percutaneous steroid injection (PSI) has been reported. It is thought to have occurred due to damage to a low arising artery of Adamkiewicz. Hence, careful observation of the distribution of contrast material is mandatory before injection of steroid. Epidural hematomas have been observed both in the lumbar and the cervical levels but these rarely need surgical decompression.
- Symptomatic epidural lipomatosis is extremely rare and is seen following local injection of steroid. The maximum of four infiltrations per year should be respected.
- Thecal calcifications can be seen following the use of triamcinolone hexacetonide. Hence we do not advocate the use of this steroid. Intrathecal injection of cortivazol can cause chemical arachnoiditis and thecal calcifications. Hence strict epidural positioning of the needle is mandatory before injection.
- Immediate transient anesthesia in the distribution of the treated nerve root is possible in lidocaine-sensitive individuals. Full neurologic recovery is observed in an hour and the patient can be discharged.

Results

Nonrandomized studies on PSI report success in 33%-72% of patients. The short-term benefit of percutaneous nerve root

Box 24-5. Percutaneous Disc Decompression

The principle consists of ablating a small amount of nucleus pulposus to decrease intradiscal pressure

Chemical ablation using chemopapain ozone or alchohol are no longer advocated

Patients who fail 6 weeks of conservative therapy are candidates for percutaneous disc decompression

Laser, Coblation, or intradiscal electrothermal therapy can be used

block is quite high, with good pain relief especially in irritative radiculopathy, but the benefit seems to be less helpful for more chronic radicular pain. Steroids speed the rate of recovery and return to function, allowing a reduction of medication while awaiting the natural improvement expected in most spinal disorders.

Riew and colleagues suggest that patients suffering from lumbar radicular pain due to disc herniation should be considered for selective infiltrations before being considered for operative intervention.

Combining the results of several nonrandomized studies, it is suggested that at long-term follow-up, no difference is noted between the steroid-treated groups and the control groups. However, a beneficial effect is seen in patients with radicular pain syndromes at intermediate-term follow-up.

In our experience of more than 5000 periradicular steroid infiltrations performed under CT guidance, short-term benefit was quite high with good pain relief in 78% of extraforaminal herniations and 72% for other locations. We had no major complications. The use of image guidance for periradicular infiltrations significantly increases accuracy and decreases complication rates.

▄ PERCUTANEOUS DISC DECOMPRESSION (BOX 24-5)

Disc herniation is an important cause of back pain. Failure of 6 weeks of conservative treatment with selective image-guided periradicular steroid injection for control of radicular pain results in the treatment being directed to the disc.

Open disc surgery is a major procedure and is associated with suboptimal results: nonnegligible morbidity and failed back syndrome.

Percutaneous minimally invasive techniques for disc decompression are based on the principle that the intervertebral disc is a closed hydraulic space and that ablation of a small volume of nucleus pulposus results in a significant decrease in intradiscal pressure, thus inducing reduction of disc herniation.

Chemical nucleolysis can be performed using chymopapain, oxygen-ozone, and alcohol. However, chemical nucleolysis is no longer advocated due to the unpredictable and uncontrolled ablation of the disc.

Percutaneous thermal nucleotomy techniques are minimally invasive, can be performed under local anesthesia on an outpatient basis, protect the surrounding soft tissues, leave no scar, and are cost effective. However, the limitation is that they can only be used for contained disc herniations.

Indications

Patients who have a contained disc herniation as visualized on CT or MRI, with symptoms of radicular pain (leg/arm pain of greater intensity than back pain, positive straight leg raising test, abnormal and/or decreased sensation but with normal motor and tendon reflex) and who have failed 6 weeks of conservative therapy and selective steroid injection are best suited for percutaneous techniques. The decompression is effective if symptoms are reproduced by maneuvers that increase pressure on the posterior spinal ligament: positive cough sign and positive memory pain on provocative discography.

Contraindications

Nerve paralysis, hemorrhagic diathesis, spondylolisthesis, free fragment, spinal stenosis, significant psychological disorders, severe degenerative disc with collapse greater than 50%, workplace injuries with future prospects of monetary gain, and local infection of the skin, subcutaneous, or muscular layers are the few contraindications to performing the procedure.

Previous surgery at the same level is considered a relative contraindication. An extruded disc is generally considered a contraindication, but according to Choy, patients with extruded but nonsequestrated disc herniations may also be included in the group selected for percutaneous laser disc decompression (PLDD).

Percutaneous Laser Disc Decompression

PLDD was pioneered by Choy and colleagues in the late 1980s.

The principle of laser disc decompression is based on the principle of conversion of light energy into thermal energy. The light energy is transmitted into the disc via a thin optical fiber and the thermal energy produced causes vaporization of a small volume of disc, resulting in reduced intradiscal pressure and hence reduction of the contained hernia. In addition, heating results in the destruction of nerve transmitter production sites and denervation of the pain receptors of the annulus fibrosus and spinal ligaments.

Material

For disc treatment, laser energy in the near infrared or visible green region can be used with wavelengths varying from 514 to 2150 nm. We use the diode laser 805 nm wavelength (Diomed, Cambridge, UK) with a quartz optical fiber of 400 μm.

Technique (Fig. 24-7)

PLDD can be performed under fluoroscopy guidance only; however, the nucleus vaporization can be visualized only with CT. A standard posterolateral approach (Scotty dog technique for discography) is used, avoiding the nerve root and visceral structures. Continuous neurologic assessment is required during the procedure to avoid damage to the nerve root and spinal cord, and hence the procedure is performed under local anesthesia, avoiding sedation and deep anesthesia of the nerve root. Strict asepsis should be maintained throughout.

Through a skin incision, an 18-gauge spinal needle is inserted into the pathologic disc. The patient must be monitored for pain

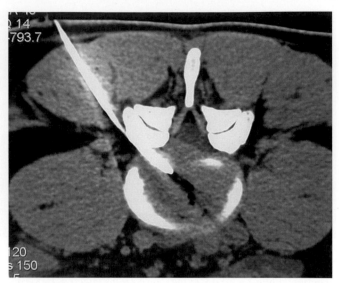

FIGURE 24-7. Percutaneous laser disc decompression. Axial computed tomography image showing gas due to vaporization within the disc following placement of the laser fiber through a curved 18-gauge spinal needle.

during the whole intervention and the needle repositioned if radicular pain occurs. To confirm contained disc herniation, or if any doubt persists, a discogram can be performed just before PLDD.

The fiber is then inserted into the disc through the 18-gauge spinal needle, using a side-arm connector. The distal end of the fiber should not extend more than 5 mm from the needle tip.

Recommended laser doses for PLDD range from 1200 to 1500 J for L1-L2, L2-L3, L3-L4, and L5-S1 levels, and from 1500 to 2000 J for L4-L5. Commonly the volume of vaporization ranges from 1 to 1.5 cm³.

Vaporization depends on the color of the disc. If no vaporization is visible after 400 J on CT, the fiber should be removed and the tip dipped in iodine or in the patient's blood to achieve a photothermal effect.

Postoperative Care

The patient is discharged 3 hours after the procedure, with strict instructions to rest for 1 week. Analgesics, antiinflammatory, and muscle relaxant drugs are prescribed for a couple of days postprocedure. Sitting, bending, and stooping are restricted for 2 weeks after intervention. Athletic activities are banned for a minimum of 6 weeks. Physiotherapy is commenced on the third postoperative week to stretch the trunk area.

Follow-up relies mainly on clinical symptoms. CT or MRI of the lumbosacral spine is only performed if any complication is suspected. The shrinkage of the herniation is generally modest to moderate and only visible after several months.

Complications

Overall complication rate at the lumbar level is 0.4%-0.5% and 0.6%-1% at the cervical level.

The major complication of PLDD is septic spondylodiscitis, which is avoided by maintaining strict sterility throughout the procedure.

Aseptic thermal spondylitis of the adjacent vertebral endplates has been reported. Treatment is with nonsteroidal antiinflammatory drugs, but symptoms can last up to 6 months.

Recurrence of disc herniation or free fragment extrusion has been reported in about 5% of patients. They often occur within the first month following the PLDD procedure and are usually due to reinjury. Strict adherence to postoperative instructions

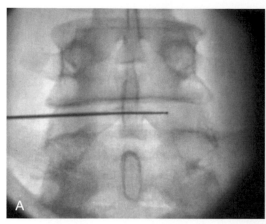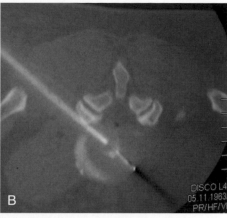

FIGURE **24-8**. Radiofrequency nucleoplasty lumbar level. Fluoroscopy (**A**) and computed tomography (**B**) images of the RF electrode (SpineWand) positioned in the disc coaxially through the 17-gauge introducer needle.

is mandatory to avoid excessive stress on the disc before its complete healing.

In our practice we have encountered the following complications: septic discitis in one patient, two cases of thermal spondylitis, and expulsion of nuclear free fragment into the canal in one patient, without the need for surgery.

Results

The reported success rate of PLDD for radicular pain is 70%-89%. Immediate pain relief is reported in 60% of patients with an initial rapid reduction in pain, which stabilizes after 6 weeks. Black and colleagues reported good or fair results in 88% of patients treated with PLDD for pure low back pain with positive discograms. Half of the patients treated with PLDD at lumbar level return to work by postoperative week 4.

In our institution, 458 patients with herniated lumbar disc and radicular pain were treated by PLDD from 1991 to 2000. The mean age was 42 years, with average follow-up of 22 months. MacNab's criteria and visual analogue scales (VAS) were used to grade response to treatment. The overall success rate was 76% with good results in 55.6% and fair results in 20.2%. In four cases, the PLDD was performed at two levels. Immediate relief of leg pain was achieved in 63% of patients. Thirty-six patients with poor results or recurrence were treated surgically. After 6-12 months, a reduction of disc herniation was observed with CT or MRI. At 3-year follow-up, the results remained stable, with 71% of patients reporting no recurrence of radicular pain. These data provide encouraging information substantiating the validity of percutaneous laser nucleotomy for contained lumbar disc herniation.

The three most critical elements for successful PLDD are proper patient selection, correct needle placement, and effective vaporization.

▬ BIPOLAR RADIOFREQUENCY NUCLEOPLASTY

RF nucleoplasty (RFN) relies on Coblation (ArthroCare, Sunnyvale, Calif.) technology to ablate soft tissue. Coblation technology removes tissue by using a low-energy bipolar RF wave to create an ionic plasma field from sodium atoms within the nucleus. This ionic plasma field disintegrates the intramolecular bonds in the nucleus, transforming complex tissue molecules into gases, which are evacuated though the introducer cannula. Unlike other RF systems, which are temperature driven, this technology does not rely on heat energy to remove tissue, so thermal damage and tissue necrosis is avoided. This transmission of energy via a plasma field is called *Coblation*, a mixture of the words *cold* and *ablation*.

This technique, initially used for arthroscopic surgery, was introduced for disc decompression in the year 2000. It uses a special electrode SpineWand Perc-DLR in the thoracic and lumbar discs and SpineWand Perc-DC, which has a looped tip in the cervical region.

Using the Coblation mode, as the electrode is advanced, several channels are dug to remove the desired amount of nucleus to achieve disc decompression. These channels have sharp margins, with no signs of thermal injury and without modification of the fibrocartilage cells and the collagen matrix. As the electrode is withdrawn, each channel is thermally treated (coagulated) using a lower range of energy below the threshold that activates the plasma field. Coagulation induces higher temperatures, with potential for shrinkage of the disc (fusion of collagen fibers in the annulus). Furthermore, the low temperature ionized plasma field also induces biochemical modifications in the disc, which may play an additional therapeutic role.

Because Coblation technology operates in a lower temperature range, this method appears safer for decompression in the smaller discs of the thoracic and cervical regions, as compared to PLDD. In our department, all thoracic and cervical disc decompressions are performed using this technique.

Technique

The material for RFN consists of an introducer needle, a bipolar RF probe (SpineWand), and an RF generator, in which both the Coblation and coagulation modes are directly controlled by the operator via foot pedals.

The procedure is performed on an outpatient basis with the patient under local anesthesia. Fluoroscopic guidance alone is sufficient, but dual guidance using CT and fluoroscopy allows for precise positioning of the needle and visualization of gas after Coblation.

Lumbar Level (Fig. 24-8)

The approach is similar to discography. A 17-gauge introducer needle is advanced under fluoroscopic control using the standard extrapedicular posterolateral approach so that the tip is positioned at the posterior annular-nuclear junction. Patients must be monitored for pain during the intervention; therefore, it is strongly advised not to use sedation.

The electrode is then advanced coaxially through the introducer needle into the disc with the Coblation mode activated so that tissue along the path of the device is disintegrated. Using a rapid smooth action, the electrode is withdrawn to the starting position using the coagulation mode so that the ablation channels are thermally treated.

After the first channel is created, the SpineWand is rotated clockwise. Because the device is curved, each rotation changes its direction and creates a new channel inside the nucleus. Approximately 6 to 12 channels are created in total, depending on the desired amount of tissue reduction.

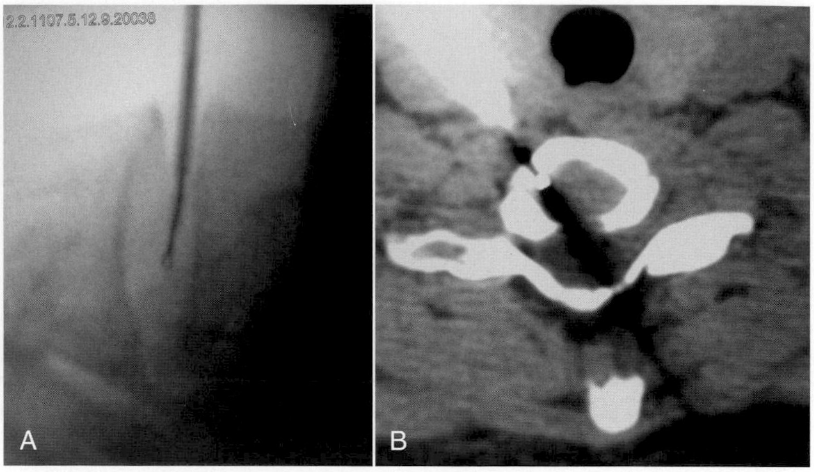

Figure 24-9. Radiofrequency nucleoplasty cervical level. **A,** Fluoroscopic positioning of the looped tip of the Perc-DC SpineWand in the midportion of the disc through the 19-gauge introducer needle. **B,** Computed tomography image showing the electrode tip within the disc and the trajectory between the caroticojugular complex laterally and the thyroid medially.

Thoracic Level

The intercostotransverse route is used to gain access to the disc. After obtaining an anteroposterior view of the involved disc such that the vertebral endplates are exactly parallel to each other, the C-arm is rotated 35 degrees from the patient's sagittal plane. The disc is punctured using the 17-gauge introducer needle. Due to the smaller size of the disc and its reduced height, only six Cobla-tion channels are produced: three on the right and three on the left, with no channel created with the electrode tip facing the endplates.

Cervical Level (Fig. 24-9)

The patient is positioned supine with the neck hyperextended. A right-sided approach is used so as to avoid the esophagus. Strict sterility is maintained, because the proximity of oropharyngeal structures increases the risk of infection. The carotid artery is pal-pated and the carotid sheath pulled laterally and posteriorly so that the operator's fingers are in direct contact with the vertebral body and the carotid pulsations are felt behind the palpating fin-gers. The 19-gauge introducer needle is introduced in front of the operator's fingers into the disc. The needle trajectory is between the carotid artery laterally and the thyroid gland medially.

The Perc-DC SpineWand specially designed for the cervical level is introduced coaxially and fastened to the introducer needle hub. Under anteroposterior and lateral fluoroscopic control, the tip of the electrode is advanced to the midpart of the disc, but never beyond the mid-third/posterior-third junction to avoid dam-age to the spinal cord or nerve roots. After checking for absence of neurologic stimulation using the coagulation mode, Coblation is performed, rotating the electrode through 180 degrees over approximately 5 seconds. The device is withdrawn 1-2 mm with-out coagulation mode and Coblation is repeated to make a series of three spherical voids.

Postoperative Instructions

These are the same as for percutaneous laser disc decompression.

Following cervical disc decompression the patient is pre-scribed a neck collar for 1 week and neck rotation and bending is restricted for 2 weeks.

Complications

The literature reports transient minor side effects with RFN, namely numbness, tingling, or soreness at the puncture site. Potential complications include discitis, hematoma, neural and vascular injuries, and pneumothorax for low cervical and thoracic levels. Fulminant fatal mucormycosis spondylodiscitis has been

reported following a nucleoplasty procedure. Most complications can be avoided by maintaining strict asepsis and respecting the technique.

The risk of thermal damage to the vertebral endplates is sig-nificantly less than for PLDD, because Coblation uses a low-temperature, high-energy ionic field. However, the use of the coagulation mode results in diffusion of heat to the adjacent structures and hence must be used prudently.

In our experience, two patients developed endplate damage. This could have resulted from the wand coming in contact with the cartilage.

Extrusion of a large free fragment causing cauda equina syn-drome and requiring surgery was seen in one patient as a result of heavy weight-bearing on postoperative day 4. Strict adherence to postoperative instructions is mandatory during the early phases of disc healing.

Results

Nucleoplasty is a relatively new technique and there have been only a few published studies.

Sharps and colleagues reported on 49 patients with a follow-up of 12 months and a success rate of 79%. Reddy reported a reduc-tion in medication and functional improvement after nucleoplasty, with significant reduction in work and leisure impairment. At cer-vical level, Nardi obtained 80% complete resolution of pain with nucleoplasty, with a faster return to work than with conservative care. Several authors report a 75%-80% efficacy for nucleoplasty with significant improvement in the patient's quality of life.

In our series, the overall success rate was 81% according to MacNab's criteria, with a good outcome in 50% and a fair out-come in 31%. The mean VAS score decreased from 76 to 16 mm. The clinical outcome was fixed after 4-6 weeks and generally remained stable during the following months.

Conclusion

Nucleoplasty allows for a fast, safe and effective disc decompres-sion when conservative therapies fail. It can be safely performed under local anesthesia, on an outpatient basis, without any scar or risk of epidural fibrosis. Moreover, due to the low range of tem-peratures, the risk of thermal damage to the vertebral endplates is reduced.

■ TARGETED DISC DECOMPRESSION

Targeted disc decompression (TDD) uses a flexible thermal bipo-lar RF catheter (Acutherm, Smith and Nephew) to treat symptom-atic disc herniation. TDD stems from intradiscal electrothermal

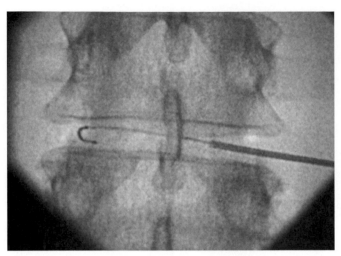

FIGURE 24-10. Targeted disc decompression. Fluoroscopic image showing the electrode winding around the disc with the active 1.5-cm tip marked by the two radiopaque markers, facing the herniation.

therapy (IDET) but the range of temperature applied is higher and the energy more focused. IDET is indicated for treatment of pure discogenic pain due to annular tears, while TDD is used to decompress disc herniations.

TDD has the same indications and contraindications as other percutaneous decompression devices (PLDD, RFN). However, TDD can be potentially used for the treatment of foraminal herniations.

The device is inserted through a 17-gauge needle into the disc, via a standard posterolateral approach. It winds around the nucleus so that its 1.5-cm active tip directly faces the herniation (Fig. 24-10). This deployment may be difficult with kinking of the electrode in 10% of cases.

Once in position, the temperature is gradually increased over 6 minutes to reach a plateau of 90°C, which is maintained for 6 minutes. This achieves focal thermal treatment of the contained herniated disc with shrinkage.

In foraminal herniations, the annulus is thicker and standard operative treatment is more difficult. Use of TDD allows for targeted thermal treatment of the herniation, with potential annulus shrinkage. One drawback of this technique is the proximity of the nerve root to the electrode. For this reason, the procedure should only be performed under local anesthesia to have complete neurologic control of the patient. In addition, in about 10% of patients, it may be difficult to position the electrode due to multiple annular tears.

This technique seems to be promising, but no study on TDD has been published yet.

THERMAL ABLATION OF BONE TUMORS

Metastatic cancer is the most common neoplasm of the skeletal system. Of approximately 965,000 new cancer cases each year in the United States, 30%-70% will develop skeletal metastasis. Bone metastases are a cause of significant morbidity, adversely affecting quality of life and reducing performance status as a result of pain, pathologic fractures, and decreased mobility.

Metastatic bone pain is extremely debilitating and difficult to treat. The possible mechanisms are thought to be stretching of the periosteum secondary to tumor growth, fracture (micro and macro), cytokine-mediated osteoclastic bone destruction resulting in local release of bradykinin, prostaglandin, histamine, and substance P, which irritate the endosteal nerves, and tumor growth into the surrounding nerves and tissues.

Treatment is mainly palliative and conventional therapies in the form of external beam radiation, surgery, systemic chemotherapy,

---

Box 24-6. Thermal Ablation of Bone Tumors

Ablation techniques used to control local bone pain
Percutaneous cementoplasty can be used as an adjuvant to provide mechanical stablization
Radiofrequency ablation and cryoablation are mainly used
Key site of ablation is bone tumor interface where nerve endings reside
95% reduction in pain scores have been reported

---

hormonal therapy, bisphosphonates, and analgesics show partial response and high relapse rates.

Percutaneous ablative techniques are proving very useful in the management of metastatic bone pain and can be combined with percutaneous cementoplasty to provide mechanical stabilization in weight-bearing areas, resulting in an effective local therapy that can be performed in a single setting, improving quality of life in these patients with limited life expectancy (Box 24-6).

Percutaneous Alcohol Ablation of Bone Metastases

This percutaneous technique involves instillation of 95% ethanol under CT guidance into the lesion. In our small series, satisfactory results were obtained in 71% of cases. Even though it is cost effective, we do not advocate this method any more due to the unpredictable diffusion of alcohol resulting in uncontrolled ablation.

Percutaneous Radiofrequency Ablation and Cryoablation

RFA is an image-guided procedure using thermal energy to produce tumor ablation. A closed loop circuit is produced by placing a generator, a large dispersive electrode (ground pad), a patient, and an electrode needle in series. High-frequency alternating electric current (200-1200 kHz) is conducted into the tissue using a shielded electrode, resulting in local ionic agitation and subsequent frictional heat, leading to localized coagulation necrosis.

Effective ablation needs optimized heat production and minimized heat loss.

Irreversible cellular damage with protein coagulation occurs between 60°C and 100°C. Below this temperature (40°C-60°C), more time is required to achieve the cytotoxic effect, while above 100°C, carbonization and vaporization of tissue is seen.

Cryoablation refers to the application of extreme cold to destroy diseased tissue, including cancer cells. Research in the field of cryobiology has demonstrated that the critical temperature to achieve cell death is between –20°C and –40°C with temperatures higher than this resulting in supercooling of the tissues, but no intracellular ice formation. Since the 1960s, cryoablation has been used to destroy skin lesions. With improvement in imaging techniques and the development of percutaneous cryoprobes, physicians have begun to perform cryoablation for prostate, liver, bone, kidney, and cervical cancer. First generation devices were limited to intraoperative use. The use of liquid nitrogen for tissue cooling using large diameter and poorly insulated probes required laparoscopic interventions. Percutaneous cryoprobes are based on delivery of argon gas through a segmentally insulated probe with rapid expansion of the gas in the sealed probe tip, resulting in rapid cooling that reaches –100°C within a few seconds. Active thawing of the ice ball is achieved by instilling helium gas instead of argon into the cryoprobes.

Indications

- Painful osteolytic and osteoblastic bone metastasis
- Metastasis with risk of impending or pathologic fracture, in conjunction with cementoplasty

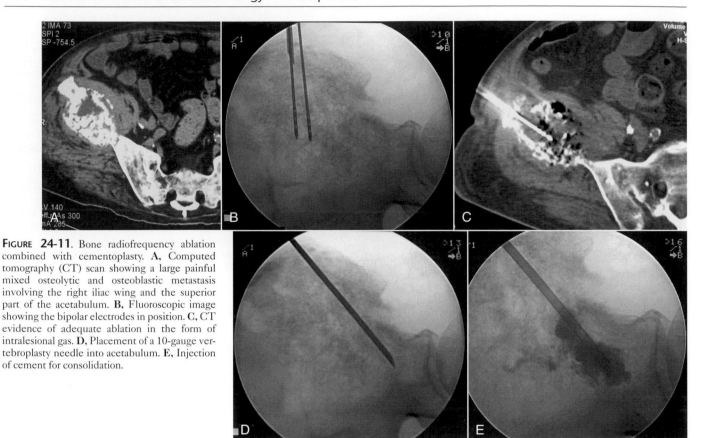

Figure 24-11. Bone radiofrequency ablation combined with cementoplasty. **A,** Computed tomography (CT) scan showing a large painful mixed osteolytic and osteoblastic metastasis involving the right iliac wing and the superior part of the acetabulum. **B,** Fluoroscopic image showing the bipolar electrodes in position. **C,** CT evidence of adequate ablation in the form of intralesional gas. **D,** Placement of a 10-gauge vertebroplasty needle into acetabulum. **E,** Injection of cement for consolidation.

- If conventional anticancer therapy is ineffective and high doses of opiates are necessary to control pain
- When rapid pain relief is needed (radiation and chemotherapy usually require 2-4 weeks for onset of action)
- The main aim of bone RFA is palliation of the patient's pain, but in rare cases with solitary bone metastasis curative treatment may be achieved.
- Thyroid cancer metastasis, where RFA is used to reduce the bulk of the tumor while the remaining metastases are treated by iodine-131 therapy.

The indications for and the procedure of cryoablation is very similar to RFA. The planning of the procedure is the same. However, up to 25 cryoprobes can be inserted simultaneously. The learning curve is shorter but the danger of surrounding tissue damage still exists.

We mainly use thermal ablation for the treatment of vertebral, acetabular, sacral, and iliac metastasis. Because these are weight-bearing regions, we usually combine thermal ablation with cementoplasty to achieve mechanical consolidation in these areas (Fig. 24-11). This association increases the cost of the procedure and needs to be performed with the patient under general anesthesia, especially with RFA. Therefore, it is used only in cases when consolidation or RFA alone is insufficient to manage the symptoms of the patient. Furthermore, thermal ablation alone can be used in patients with large paraspinal tumors with minimal bone destruction and in metastasis to the ribs for control of local pain.

Bone thermal ablation differs from hepatic or renal thermal ablation in that cancellous bone shows poor heat transmission and cortical bone has an insulative effect.

Technique

The procedure is performed under CT or MR guidance. We use dual CT and fluoroscopy guidance, with fluoroscopy providing real-time imaging and CT allowing accurate placement of electrodes, avoiding sensitive adjacent structures like the nerves, vessels, and bowel.

New MR sequences allow for visualization of the thermal lesion size and shape during RFA, thus potentially ensuring more complete lesion ablation.

The procedure is performed with the patient under general anesthesia but good neurolept analgesia controlled by the anesthetist can be used.

The needle is positioned in the lesion so that the long axis of the lesion is along the long axis of the active tip. If cortical bone is to be perforated a larger metallic needle is used as a coaxial introducer. The 16- to 18-gauge infused electrode is inserted coaxially inside the tumor. The active tip of the electrode should not be in contact with the coaxial needle because this would result in conduction of current and heat along the coaxial needle path, resulting in nontarget ablation of the surrounding tissues. The end point of ablation is when there is a high rise in impedance or a control CT shows presence of gas within the tumor.

The major limitation of the monopolar RF technique is the limited size of the ablation zone. For large lesions (>4 cm), the procedure should be repeated after repositioning the needle electrode to achieve complete tumor coagulation. Multiple overlapping applications are necessary, which can result in incomplete ablation of the tumor cells and result in high recurrence rates, risking damage to adjacent structures (e.g., bowel, nerve root, thecal sac).

The bipolar RF technique, uses two perfused needle electrodes (Integra, Tuttlingen, Germany), which can be applied in sequential, simultaneous, alternating, and bipolar modes. The bipolar method creates large, well-defined oval areas of coagulative necrosis and is less dependent on local tissue inhomogeneities.

We have used bipolar RFA for the treatment of vertebral metastases that have destroyed the posterior vertebral wall and are within 1 cm of the spinal cord without thermal damage to the cord.

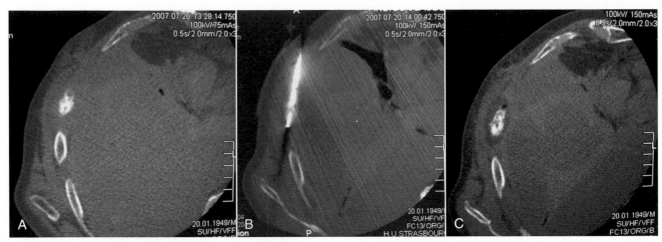

FIGURE 24-12. Bone cryoablation. **A,** Axial computed tomography scan showing painful right 10th rib metastasis from breast carcinoma. **B,** Insertion of a cryoprobe into the metastatic rib lesion using CT guidance. **C,** Hypodensity surrounding the rib metastasis indicative of the ice ball and hence the cryoablative zone.

During RFA of bone lesions, the key site of electrode deployment is the bone tumor interface to destroy the nerve endings that are likely to cause pain.

Postprocedural pain is controlled by injectable analgesics and nonsteroid antiinflammatory drugs in the first hours after the procedure. Strict sterility should be maintained during the procedure to avoid septic complications. Neurologic complications are avoided by precise needle positioning, use of a thermocouple, and good anatomic knowledge of the treated region.

Cryoablation is performed under sedation or general anesthesia. Percutaneous cryoablation appears to require less analgesia than RFA. For complete necrosis of the tumor, it is important to extend the margins of the ice ball a minimum of 5 mm beyond the tumor margins in order to ensure complete cell death. The ice ball can be visualized by various imaging techniques, including ultrasound, CT, and MRI. Insulation and protection of surrounding organs is best achieved with carbon dioxide and fluid should be avoided (Fig. 24-12).

Results

Callstrom and colleagues reported a 95% (59/62 patients) reduction in pain following RFA for painful bone metastases. Highly significant reductions in worst pain, average pain, and pain interference were noted. Significant decreases were seen for all pain parameters beginning week 1 and extending to week 24. They also reported a significant reduction in opioid usage by weeks 8 and 12. There was a 6.5% incidence of major complication after treatment, mainly in the form of worsening of tumor—cutaneous fistulas in patients treated for presacral metastases abutting the sacrum. They also reported the development of second-degree skin burn at the grounding pad site, a minor complication (1.6%).

In our series, 92% of patients (69/75) had a significant (minimum 3 points) and durable decrease of pain. The mean decrease in the pain score using the visual analogue scale was 5.1 mm. Twenty-seven patients died within 2 months following the procedure due to advanced systemic disease. The remaining patients had stable results in the treated area. We did not observe any major complication due to RFA, but had two minor asymptomatic cement leakages into the soft tissues. Compared with other forms of percutaneous ablation, cryoablation offers the additional advantages of direct visualization of the ice ball and less postprocedural pain. Cryoablation is also efficient in painful sclerotic bone metastases.

▬ PERCUTANEOUS VERTEBROPLASTY

Percutaneous vertebroplasty is a therapeutic, image-guided procedure that involves injection of radiopaque cement into a painful, partially collapsed vertebral body to internally splint it, in an effort to relieve pain and provide stability.

Vertebral compression fracture (VCF) is an important cause of severe debilitating back pain, adversely affecting quality of life, physical function, psychosocial performance, mental health, and survival. Osteoporotic fractures affect one in two women and one in five men older than age 50 years, resulting in an annual estimated cost to the health service of around €30 billion in all of Europe. Patients with VCFs have a 23% increased risk of mortality compared with age-matched controls without VCFs. This is primarily related to compromised pulmonary function as a result of thoracic as well as lumbar fractures.

Percutaneous vertebroplasty was originally described by Deramond and colleagues in 1987 for the treatment of an aggressive vertebral hemangioma. Over the past decade, this technique has evolved to become a standard of care for VCFs.

Indications

- Painful osteoporotic vertebral compression fractures. PVP has become the standard of care for painful osteoporotic fractures. It is performed early in the course of the disease in combination with the medical treatment for osteoporosis especially in older patients. The advantages of early treatment are stabilization of the fracture and restoration of vertebral body strength, resulting in pain relief without use of narcotic dosage of analgesics; early mobilization, thus preventing decubitus complications such as deep venous thrombosis, pneumonia, decubitus ulcers, and thrombophlebitis; and prevention of further collapse of the vertebral body, resulting in abnormal mechanics of the spine. Patients with chronic osteoporotic fractures for more than 1 year without sclerosis and treated with vertebroplasty have benefited from the procedure.
- Painful vertebrae due to aggressive primary bone tumors such as hemangiomas, for which treatment is aimed at pain relief, strengthening of bone, and devascularization. It can be used alone or in combination with sclerotherapy, especially in cases of epidural extension causing spinal cord compression.
- Painful vertebrae with extensive osteolysis due to malignant infiltration by multiple myeloma, lymphoma, and metastasis. Only painful metastasis and lesions affecting the stability of the spine should be treated. The procedure is palliative and does not address tumor progression and hence is used

as a complement to other anticancer treatments. In patients with destruction of the vertebral body with paravertebral tumor extension, vertebroplasty can be combined with RFA for reduction of tumor mass and consolidation of the vertebral body.
- Painful fracture associated with osteonecrosis (Kummel disease)·
- Conditions in which reinforcement of the vertebral body or pedicle is desired before or after posterior surgical stabilization.

Absolute Contraindications

- Asymptomatic vertebral body tumors without fracture
- Cord compression
- Osteomyelitis, discitis, or active systemic infection
- Uncorrectable coagulopathy
- Allergy to bone cement or opacification agents
- Prophylaxis in osteoporotic patients

Relative Contraindications

- Fracture of the posterior vertebral body wall—increased risk of cement leak and bone fragment displacement
- Vertebral collapse greater than 70% of body height—needle placement may be difficult
- Patients with more than five or diffuse metastases and diffuse pain
- Osteoblastic lesions
- Severe pulmonary insufficiency: use of the prone position can further compromise the pulmonary function and can produce adverse clinical outcome
- Lack of surgical backup and monitoring facilities

Patient Selection

A multidisciplinary team consisting of an interventional radiologist, rheumatologist, endocrinologist, oncologist, and spine surgeon must decide which patients should undergo the procedure.

All patients must have an office visit with the treating interventional radiologist before the procedure to discuss the procedure, intended benefits, complications, and success rate. Written and informed consent must be obtained. A detailed clinical examination in conjunction with the imaging findings must be carried out to determine the level/levels to be treated and rule out other causes of back pain such as radiculopathy, degenerative spondylosis, and neurologic compromise. Imaging findings must be given precedence over clinical examination and absence of pain over the involved spinous process with positive features on MRI should not exclude patients from treatment with PVP.

Imaging

Imaging is the prerequisite for preoperative planning and helps exclude other causes of back pain like facet arthropathy, spinal canal stenosis, and disc herniation.

All patients undergoing percutaneous vertebroplasty should have an MRI scan. Our protocol consists of T1-weighted, T2-weighted STIR sagittal images of the entire spine with T2-weighted axial images through the relevant levels. Gadolinium-enhanced scans are reserved for patients with hemangiomas and tumors to delineate epidural and paravertebral extension compromising adjacent structures. Acute, subacute, and nonhealed fractures are hypointense on T1-weighted images and hyperintense on T2-weighted and STIR sequences because of marrow edema (Fig. 24-13). MRI helps in localizing the exact levels that need to be treated. No treatment is provided for a collapsed vertebral body without marrow edema. Further MRI helps differentiate benign from malignant causes of vertebral body collapse and rules out infection. In addition, presence of a retropulsed fragment causing cord compression or abnormal cord signal can be visualized on MRI.

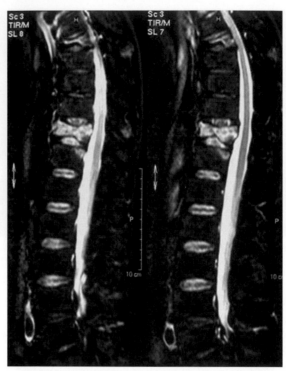

FIGURE 24-13. Vertebroplasty. Sagittal T2-weighted STIR magnetic resonance image showing high signal within the fractured vertebral body, indicative of marrow edema.

Box 24-7. Vertebroplasty

Patients with vertebral compression fractures (VCFs) have a 29% increased risk of mortality from pulmonary compromise

All patients should have a magnetic resonance imaging scan before vertebroplasty

VCFs without marrow edema do not warrant treatment with PVP

The transpendicular route is used in the thoracic and lumbar levels and an anterolateral approach in the cervical area

Polymethylmethacrylate is the cement of choice

Cement leakage is the most frequent complication

Ninety percent of patients have complete pain relief after vertebroplasty for acute fractures

---

Thin-section CT (1 mm) through the affected spinal region with multiplanar reconstruction in the sagittal and coronal planes allows for accurate delineation of the fracture, presence of posterior free fragments, and any compromise of the posterior vertebral wall. In malignant cases, it provides information regarding the location and extent of the lytic process, the visibility and degree of involvement of the pedicles, the presence of epidural or foraminal stenosis caused by tumor extension, or retropulsed bone fragments, which can increase the likelihood of complications. CT detects osteoblastic metastases, which are very difficult to treat with vertebroplasty, and delineates sclerosis in the vertebral body, which may necessitate a bipedicular rather than a unipedicular approach. With multiplanar reconstruction, CT provides an accurate overview of the spine, with assessment of the degree of vertebral collapse.

Bone scanning is only used in equivocal cases. Presence of tracer uptake is an indication for performing vertebroplasty and is a predictor of positive clinical outcome after the procedure (Box 24-7).

Procedure

The procedure is performed under sedoanalgesia or general anesthesia administered by the anesthesiologist with continuous patient monitoring with ECG, pulse oximetry, and blood pressure. A recent normal complete blood count, coagulation profile, and inflammatory marker (C-reactive protein) screen is essential. Intraprocedural antibiotic cover (Cefazolin 1 gm IV) is recommended in immunocompromised patients, but there is no clear consensus for what to use in other patient groups. Strict asepsis must be maintained throughout the procedure.

The patient is positioned prone for the lumbar and thoracic levels and supine for the cervical level. The classic transpedicular route is employed for the lumbar and thoracic levels because it is inherently safe. In the thoracic vertebrae, the intercostovertebral route can be used, especially when the pedicles are small or destroyed. In the cervical vertebrae, an anterolateral approach is used. The needle path should avoid the carotid jugular complex.

Biplane Fluoroscopy

The appropriate radiographic profile for a transpedicular approach is a straight anteroposterior view with 5- to 10-degree angulation, in which the pedicle appears oval. For an optimal approach, the entry point and its distance from the midline can be measured on axial CT or MR images. Using AP screening, the beveled needle is advanced through the upper and lateral aspect of the pedicle, making sure that the needle tip remains within the pedicular ring until the posterior vertebral wall is breached to avoid injury to the spinal cord or nerve root. Using lateral screening with the bevel facing laterally, the needle tip is positioned in the anterior part of the vertebral body, such that the tip lies in the midline. This allows for bilateral filling of the vertebral body, obviating the need for a bipedicular approach.

Dual Guidance

The combination of CT and fluoroscopy allows for precise needle placement, reduces complications, and increases the comfort of the operator. This association is particularly useful in difficult cases or in case of destruction of anatomic landmarks. Fluoroscopy is provided by placing a mobile C-arm in front of the CT gantry.

Venography is reserved only for highly vascular lesions such as hemangiomas and vascular metastases to check for large vascular spaces with rapid shunting of blood.

Cement Injection

Polymethylmethacrylate (PMMA) is the cement of choice for percutaneous vertebroplasty. New generation cements are intrinsically radiopaque, allowing good visualization at the time of injection and early detection of leaks.

Cement is prepared once the needle is in position. It is injected in its pasty polymerization phase to reduce the risk of venous intravasation.

Injection should be performed either using a dedicated injection set (e.g., Optimed, Allegiance, Cook, or Stryker) or a 2-mL Luer lock syringe. The injection sets allow aspiration and direct injection of cement in continuous flow, with minimal effort and without the need for multiple syringe changes during the procedure. Although the use of the injection sets increases the expense of the procedure, it is safer than freehand injection and allows the operator to focus on the fluoroscopic image.

Injection of cement is done under continuous lateral fluoroscopic control with intermittent AP screening. The lateral projection allows for early detection of an epidural leak, while AP screening rules out lateral leaks. With biplane fluoroscopy, both planes are viewed simultaneously during injection.

The risk of cement leakage is particularly high at the beginning of cement injection. If a leak is detected, the injection is immediately stopped, and the pressure reversed. Waiting for 30 to 60 seconds allows the cement to harden and seal the leak. If on further injection the leak persists, the needle position and/or the bevel direction should be modified. If the leak continues, the injection is terminated and the needle removed. If incomplete fill of the vertebral body is obtained, the contralateral pedicle is accessed and completion of fill achieved.

The cement injection is stopped when the anterior two thirds of the vertebral body is filled and the cement is homogenously distributed on both sides and between both endplates. The mandrel of the needle is replaced under fluoroscopy control, before the cement begins to set and the needle is then carefully removed.

The effective working time with the Osteopal V cement is 8-10 minutes after mixing (room temperature 20°C), following which it begins to set. However, some new cements have longer setting times.

In patients with osteoporosis, approximately 2.5 to 5 mL of cement provides optimal filling of the vertebra to provide consolidation and pain relief.

There is no significant association between the volume of cement injected and the clinical outcomes of postprocedure pain and medication use, and operators should strive to achieve the maximal safe filling of individual vertebral bodies.

Postprocedural Care

The patient is removed from the operating table only after the cement in the mixing bowl has set. The patient is maintained in recumbent position for 2 hours. Vital signs and neurologic evaluation focused on the extremities are monitored every 15 minutes for the first hour and then half hourly for the next 2 hours. The patient can be mobilized the same evening of the procedure and discharged home the next day.

In cases of epidural or foraminal leaks, strict neurologic surveillance is maintained. In case of clinically significant neurologic compromise or neurologic deterioration, urgent neurosurgical decompression must be carried out.

Complications

Published data has placed the occurrence of complications in PVP for osteoporotic fractures at less than 1% and for malignant disease at less than 10%.

Cement leakage is the most frequent complication and is usually asymptomatic. For osteoporotic fractures, the incidence ranges from 30% to 65% and for malignant disease it is higher, 38%-72.5%. Cortical destruction, presence of a cortical soft tissue mass, highly vascularized lesions, and severe vertebral collapses are likely to increase the rate of complications.

Routes of Cement Leakage

- Epidural space and neural foramina. It can produce radiculopathy and paraplegia as a result of nerve root and cord compression, respectively. Radiculopathy is a minor adverse reaction. It occurs as a result of cement contact with the emergent nerve root and heating of the nerve tissue during polymerization of the cement. If detected at the time of the procedure, a spinal needle should be immediately positioned in the foramina and normal saline injected slowly to cool the nerve root. This radiculopathy may require a brief course of nonsteroidal antiinflammatory agents, oral steroids, or local steroid injection in the affected area. Cord compression is a serious complication and requires urgent neurosurgical decompression to prevent neurologic sequelae.
- Disc space and paravertebral tissue. It is usually of no clinical significance. However, in severe osteoporosis, large disc leaks, especially anterior, could lead to collapse of the adjacent vertebral bodies.

- Perivertebral venous plexus. It can result in pulmonary embolism, which is usually peripheral and asymptomatic, and rarely central causing infarction. Paradoxical cerebral embolization has been reported.

Infection occurs in less than 1%. Strict asepsis should be maintained throughout the procedure. There have been recent reports in literature of postvertebroplasty infection with epidural and soft tissue abscess formation treated with surgery and antibiotics.

Fracture of ribs, posterior elements, or pedicle is rare, with an incidence of less than 1%. It is considered a minor complication.

Risk of collapse of the adjacent vertebral body has a reported incidence of 12.4% and an odds ratio of 2.27.

The risk factors for the development of new compression fractures are older age, multiple levels treated at the initial vertebroplasty, less severe wedge deformity of the treated vertebra, and fractures outside the thoracolumbar junction.

Allergy to the cement is characterized by hypotension and arrhythmias. Anaphylactic reaction to PMMA resulting in death is not an insignificant risk, as has been reported to the U.S. Food and Drug Administration.

Bleeding from the puncture site is associated with localized pain and tenderness, which resolves in 72 hours. It is minimized by 5 minutes of compression once the needle is removed.

Reported complications have usually resulted from poor technique and patient selection, namely due to:
- Injection of cement in its liquid phase resulting in venous intravasation and bony extravasation
- Injection at multiple levels (it is advised not to treat more than five levels at one sitting)
- Incorrect positioning of the needle tip (e.g., in a basivertebral vein or close to the posterior wall)
- Treatment of highly vascular lesions such as metastasis from thyroid and renal cancer
- Poor fluoroscopic image
- Poor radiopacity of cement

Results

Following vertebroplasty for osteoporotic fractures, improvement in pain scores and functional capability is found to be maintained at 1 month and 1 year of follow-up. Ninety percent of patients experience complete pain relief when treated for acute fractures. In patients with chronic osteoporotic fractures more than a year old, results are inferior at 80%. The requirement for analgesic drugs is significantly reduced in 91% of patients and patient satisfaction is 95%-100% for the procedure. Improved mobility is seen following vertebroplasty, being 93% and 50% for acute and chronic osteoporotic fractures, respectively. In patients with malignant disease, pain relief is seen in 60%-80% of patients, while in patients with hemangiomas this ranges between 80% and 90%.

Vertebroplasty has been found to restore vertebral body height. Hiwatashi and colleagues reported a significant 2.2-mm increase in height with a greater than 3-mm fracture reduction in 39 of 85 vertebral fractures treated with vertebroplasty.

In our series, satisfactory results were obtained in 78%, 83%, and 73% of patients with osteoporosis, vertebral tumors, and hemangiomas, respectively.

▬ KYPHOPLASTY

Kyphoplasty, also known as balloon-assisted vertebroplasty, is a technique that was developed in the mid-1990s by Kyphon (Sunnyvale, Calif.). The procedure includes inflation of balloons called *bone tamps* within the vertebral body before cement injection. The procedure aims to restore vertebral body height, reducing kyphosis associated with a vertebral fracture and reducing the complications of cement leakage associated with vertebroplasty.

Indications

In the literature, kyphoplasty has mainly been used for the treatment of osteoporotic vertebral compression fractures. There are few reports of its use in the treatment of malignant vertebral fractures.

In our department, we only use kyphoplasty in the treatment of acute traumatic compression fractures of the vertebral body, Type A1 (Maegryl Classification) in young nonosteoporotic patients. We treat traumatic fractures acutely within the first week, because the fracture is fresh and it is easier to achieve reduction of kyphosis and restore vertebral body height.

We sometimes perform the procedure in conjunction with other surgeons at the time of posterior stabilization of the spine or following posterior stabilization, which converts an unstable fracture into a stable fracture. This avoids an anterior surgical approach, which can be challenging.

Contraindications

In traumatic fractures, the main contraindication is fractures with instability. Other contraindications are the same as those for vertebroplasty.

Preprocedure Imaging

With regard to traumatic fractures, MRI of the spine is mandatory before the procedure. In fact, in all cases of vertebral trauma, spinal MRI is performed to check for cord contusion and epidural and paraspinal hematomas.

Plain radiographs, especially the lateral view, give a global overview of the spine and are useful in quantifying the degree of regional kyphosis induced by the vertebral fracture.

Thin-section CT with multiplanar reconstruction is useful to assess the integrity of the posterior wall and assess the pedicles and the degree of burst component present.

Technique (Fig. 24-14)

The procedure is usually performed with the patient under general anesthesia because inflation of the bone tamps is painful and the hardware used is of much larger caliber compared to percutaneous vertebroplasty.

The procedure can be performed under fluoroscopy alone or with dual image guidance using CT and fluoroscopy.

The patient is positioned prone on the table. Bipedicular access to the vertebral body is gained using the standard transpedicular approach. After insertion of the 8-gauge working cannulas, the high-pressure Silastic balloons are inflated within the vertebral body to achieve reduction of the fracture. This may take up to 30 minutes. Following the creation of the cavity, phosphocalcic cement is injected using bone fillers to fill the cavity in a retrograde fashion. Cement injection is done under continuous lateral fluoroscopic control to allow for early detection of epidural leaks. Due to the creation of the cavity, cement injection is comparatively easy, under low pressure, but the injection of the last milliliters into normal bone may prove difficult and is under high pressure. The cannulas are only withdrawn on completion of cement injection of both sides.

Calcium Phosphate Cements

Calcium phosphate cements are inherently radiopaque but not sufficiently enough for operator comfort, do not produce an exothermic reaction, have been found to be osteoconductive and biocompatible, are more difficult to inject, require more time to cure, and have questionable infiltration into the vertebral body.

Experimental studies have found calcium phosphate cements to be osteoconductive and biocompatible. These biocompatible cements may eliminate concerns about thermal necrosis and

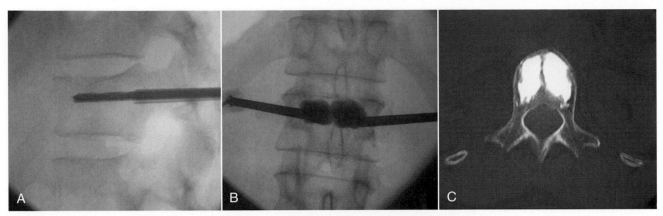

FIGURE 24-14. Kyphoplasty in traumatic compression fracture. **A,** Transpedicular insertion of the 8-gauge working cannulas into the posterior portion of the vertebral body. **B,** Simultaneous inflation of the balloons to achieve fracture reduction, followed by injection of phosphocalcic cement into the created void. **C,** Computed tomography scan.

cytotoxicity. Because they are bioresorbable, these cements are appealing in young patients, because they provide mechanical augmentation immediately and later provide an osteoconductive template for subsequent bone repair and remodeling. Even though inherently radiopaque, these cements are difficult to visualize during injection. The Jectos+ (Kasios, France) cement is a newer generation of cement that has added radiopacity, making it easier to visualize during injection.

Postprocedural Care

Because the procedure is done under general anesthesia, the patient is hospitalized for at least 1 day. Calcium phosphate cement takes a longer time to cure, therefore early mobilization is not advocated. Patients are usually maintained in a recumbent position for 3 days after the procedure to allow the cement to reach maximum strength. Patients can be mobilized earlier but only if a protective brace is used.

Complications

In their review of complications of vertebroplasty and kyphoplasty as reported to the MAUDE database, Nussbaum and colleagues found 33 complications associated with kyphoplasty between 1999 and June 2003, representing approximately 40,000-50,000 total procedures. One patient died. In 20 patients, spinal compression developed, requiring surgical decompression to prevent permanent paralysis. Six patients sustained permanent injury. It is thought that the increased risk of pedicular fractures can lead to spinal compression because of cement leakage or development of an epidural hematoma. The large diameter of the cannula leaves little room for error during insertion through the pedicle and increases the risk of pedicular fracture. Pulmonary cement embolism was noted in one patient and infection in the form of discitis/osteomyelitis was reported in two patients.

On a comparative basis, the number of complications reported with kyphoplasty is much higher than with vertebroplasty, based on the number of cases performed.

Garfin and colleagues reported six major complications in 531 patients (1.1%), four of which were neurologic complications. Majd and colleagues reported a 5.5% complication rate with the procedure.

The incidence of cement extrusion following kyphoplasty has been reported to range from 8.6% to 33%.

Results

Pain relief following kyphoplasty is durable and is seen in 90% of patients.

Box 24-8. Osteoid Osteoma

Ninety percent present before the age of 30 years
Classics symptoms are local pain, worse at night with dramatic improvement after taking aspirin
Brodie abscess and stress fractures should be excluded
Core drill excision, radiofrequency ablation (RFA), alcohol injection, or laser photocoagulation can be used
Nidus must be completely destroyed
Success rates of 91%-100% for laser and 79%-86% for RFA have been reported

---

Outcome for height restoration and improvement of kyphosis is debatable. Liebermann and colleagues reported a height restoration of 35%, which amounts to 2.9 mm; Rhyne and colleagues reported 4.6 mm and Gaitanis and colleagues, 4.3 mm.

With vertebroplasty the amount of height restoration has been reported to range from 2.7 mm to 3 mm.

The mean improvement in kyphosis angle has been reported to range from 3.4 degrees to 8.8 degrees, which was found to be quite similar to that achieved by vertebroplasty (4.3°-6.4°).

Vertebroplasty and kyphoplasty are similar in their clinical outcomes but kyphoplasty is four times more expensive. Hence it is not economically viable to treat all patients with vertebral compression fractures with kyphoplasty.

In our series of 27 patients (mean age 30.8 years) treated with kyphoplasty following acute traumatic fractures, complete pain relief was obtained in 25 patients with significant improvement of kyphosis in 10 patients.

Osteoid Osteoma

Osteoid osteoma is a benign neoplasm of bone, occurring in the first 3 decades of life, with 90% presenting before the age of 30 years and having a distinct male predominance. The classic clinical presentation is local pain that is worse at night and improves dramatically following treatment with aspirin. The characteristic clinical and radiologic findings result in a high level of diagnostic confidence (Box 24-8).

The disease is self-limiting, and pain may be relieved after 5-6 years of conservative medical treatment. However, due to the accompanying severe persistent pain, total removal of the nidus is the treatment of choice.

Surgical removal consists of wide excision of the nidus and curettage. Because the tumor is difficult to localize, a large amount of bone must be resected to ensure complete tumor removal. This

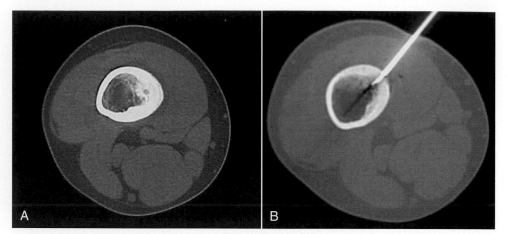

FIGURE 24-15. Femoral osteoid osteoma. **A,** Thin-section computed tomography (CT) scan (1 mm) exquisitely demonstrates the central 5-mm nidus of the osteoid osteoma. **B,** CT-guided placement of the laser fiber in the nidus. The thickened cortex was perforated by a Bonopty needle, through which an 18-gauge spinal needle was coaxially placed in the nidus for passage of the laser fiber.

results in disproportionate bone removal compared to nidus size and results in several weeks of restricted mobility.

Percutaneous minimally invasive techniques such as CT-guided core drill excision, RFA, alcohol injection, or percutaneous laser photocoagulation allow for direct destruction of the nidus without extensive bone excision.

Indication

Patient selection is crucial for effective treatment.

Patients with characteristic findings on CT, MRI, and scintigraphy with consistent and typical clinical findings are the best candidates for treatment.

Brodie abscess and stress fractures need to be excluded because they are the major mimics of osteoid osteoma. Because the nidus is very small, biopsy to establish the histologic diagnosis may be inconclusive.

Contraindications

Lesions within 5 mm of neurologic structures are the main contraindication to treatment.

Patients with bleeding diathesis can be treated following correction of the coagulation disorder.

Technique

The procedure is performed using CT guidance, which allows for accurate positioning of the needle within the nidus, avoiding neurovascular structures. Strict asepsis is maintained throughout the procedure.

The procedure is always performed using general anesthesia or regional nerve bloc anesthesia because nidal transgression is extremely painful.

Interstitial laser photocoagulation (ILP) consists of percutaneous insertion of optical fibers into the tumor. Experimental work has shown that a reproducible area of coagulative necrosis is obtained around the fiber, with good correlation between energy delivered and the lesion size, and with conservation of the biomechanical properties of the bone tissue in the treated area. The size of osteoid osteomas falls within the range that can be effectively coagulated by one or two fibers (Fig. 24-15).

Using CT control, an 18-gauge spinal needle is used to access the nidus. The 400-μm fiber is then inserted coaxially through the needle; the needle is withdrawn about 5 mm so that the tip of the bare fiber lies within the center of the tumor. The diode laser (Diomed 805 nm, Cambridge, UK) is turned on in continuous wave mode, at a power of 2 W for 200-600 seconds, depending on the nidus size (energy delivered, 400-1200 J). For a tumor located away from neurovascular structures, usually a maximum energy of 1200 J

is applied to coagulate the nidus. For a tumor located near neurovascular structures, the amount of energy delivered is calculated according to the formula [(nidus size in mm × 100 J) + 200 J] with a maximum of 1200 J. If the tumor is within 8 mm of neurovascular structures, a cooling solution should be injected continuously into the surrounding region to prevent thermal neural damage. At the end of the procedure, 5-10 mL of naropeine (2 mg/mL) is injected subperiosteally to ease postprocedural local pain.

The technique of RFA is similar to RF neurolysis using thermal technique. The RF electrode is inserted in the nidus and the power is increased progressively to reach 90°C. The nidus is exposed to this temperature for 6-10 minutes. To avoid large necrosis of bone, the cooling system or infusion should not be used in osteoid osteoma. In the case of RFA, the electrode placement should be such that no portion of the tumor is more that 5 mm from the exposed tip. CT control scans are performed during the procedure to detect gas.

Complications

In our experience, CT-guided RFA or ILP of osteoid osteoma is very safe without major complications such as pathologic fractures, neurovascular injury, and infection. Gangi and colleagues reported a single case of reflex sympathetic dystrophy in their series of 114 patients, following treatment of an osteoid osteoma of the lunate. The patient's symptoms completely resolved after 2 months.

Recurrence following percutaneous treatment is very low (6 of 114) and most patients do very well with a repeated ablation or ILP.

Results

In the literature, pain relief after RFA is reported between 79% and 86%, with a complication rate ranging from 0% to 2%. The ILP series has a clinical success ranging from 91% to 100% with a minor complication rate in a range of 4%-33%.

▬ SUGGESTED READINGS

Adam G, Neuerburg J, Vorwerk D, et al. Percutaneous treatment of osteoid osteomas: combination of drill biopsy and subsequent ethanol injection. *Semin Musculoskelet Radiol.* 1997;1:281-284.

Alexandre A, Coro L, Azuelos A, Pellone M. Percutaneous nucleoplasty for discoradicular conflict. *Acta Neurochir Suppl.* 2005;92:83-86.

Aluntas A, Slavin J, Smith PJ, et al. Accuracy of computer tomography guided core needle biopsy of musculoskeletal tumors. *ANZ J Surg.* 2005;75:187-191.

Barr JD, Barr MS, Lemley TJ, et al. Percutaneous vertebroplasty for pain relief and spinal stabilization. *Spine.* 2000;25(8):923-928.

Bernadette Stallemeyer MJ, Zoarski GH, Obuchowski AM. Optimizing patient selection in percutaneous vertebroplasty. *J Vasc Interv Radiol.* 2003;14:683-696.

Bhagia SM, Slipman CW, Nirschl M, et al. Side effects and complications after percutaneous disc decompression using coblation technology. *Am J Phys Med Rehabil.* 2006;85:6-13.

Bosacco SJ, Bosacco DN, Berman AT, et al. Functional results of percutaneous laser discectomy. *Am J Orthop.* 1996;25:825-828.

Brown DB, Gilula LA, Sehgal M, et al. Treatment of chronic symptomatic vertebral compression fractures with percutaneous vertebroplasty. *AJR Am J Radiol.* 2004;182:319-322.

Brunot S, Berge J, Barreau X, et al. Long term clinical follow-up of vertebral haemangiomas treated by percutaneous vertebroplasty. *J Radiol.* 2005;86(1):41-47.

Buy X, Basile A, Bierry G, Cupelli J, Gangi A. Saline-infused bipolar radiofrequency ablation of high-risk spinal and paraspinal neoplasms. *AJR Am J Roentgenol.* 2006;186:S322-S326.

Callstrom MR, Atwell TD, Charboneau JW, et al. Painful metastases involving bone: percutaneous image-guided cryoablation—prospective trial interim analysis. *Radiology.* 2006;241:572-580.

Callstrom MR, Charboneau JW, Goetz MP, et al. Painful metastases involving bone: Feasibility of percutaneous CT- and US-guided radiofrequency ablation. *Radiology.* 2002;224:87-97.

Callstrom MR, William Charboneau J, Goetz MP, et al. Image-guided ablation of painful metastatic bone tumors: a new and effective approach to a difficult problem. *Skeletal Radiol.* 2006;35:1-15.

Carrino JA, Blanco R. Magnetic resonance–guided musculoskeletal interventional radiology. *Semin Musculoskelet Radiol.* 2006;10:159-174.

Casper GD, Hartman VL, Mullins LL. Results of a clinical trial of the holmium:YAG laser in disc decompression utilizing a side-firing fiber: a two-year follow-up. *Lasers Surg Med.* 1996;19:90-96.

Cavanaugh JM, Ozaktay AC, Yamashita HT, et al. Lumbar facet pain: biomechanics, neuroanatomy and neurophysiology. *J Biomech.* 1996;29:1117-1129.

Chen YC, Lee SH, Saenz Y, Lehman NL. Histologic findings of disc, end plate and neural elements after Coblation of nucleus pulposus: an experimental nucleoplasty study. *Spine.* 2003;3:466-470.

Choy DS, Ascher PW, Ranu HS, et al. Percutaneous laser disc decompression. A new therapeutic modality. *Spine.* 1992;17:949-956.

Choy DS, Case RB, Fielding W, et al. Percutaneous laser nucleolysis of lumbar disks. *N Engl J Med.* 1987;317:771-772.

Choy DS. Percutaneous laser disc decompression (PLDD) update: focus on device and procedure advances. *J Clin Laser Med Surg.* 1993;11:181-183.

Choy DS. Percutaneous laser disc decompression: a 17-year experience. *Photomed Laser Surg.* 2004;22:407-410.

Choy DS. Response of extruded intervertebral herniated discs to percutaneous laser disc decompression. *J Clin Laser Med Surg.* 2001;19:15-20.

Cloft HJ, Jensen ME. Kyphoplasty: an assessment of a new technology. *AJNR.* 2007;28:200-203.

Cortet B, Cotton A, Deprez X, et al. Value of vertebroplasty combined with surgical decompression in the treatment of aggressive spinal angioma. *Rev Rhum Ed Fr.* 1994;61:16-22.

Cotten A, Deramond H, Cortet B, et al. Preoperative percutaneous injection of methyl methacrylate and N-butyl cyanoacrylate in vertebral haemangiomas. *Am J Neuroradiol.* 1996;17:137-142.

Cotton A, Boutry N, Cortet B, et al. Percutaneous vertebroplasty: state of the art. *Radiographics.* 1998;18:311-320.

Cotton A, Dewatre F, Cortet B, et al. Percutaneous vertebroplasty for osteolytic metastases and myeloma: Effects of the percentage of lesion filling and the leakage of methyl methacrylate at clinical follow-up. *Radiology.* 1996;200:525-530.

Cyteval C, Fescquet N, Thomas E, et al. Predictive factors of efficacy of periradicular corticosteroid injections for lumbar radiculopathy. *AJNR Am J Neuroradiol.* 2006;27:978-982.

Deramond H, Depriester C, Galibert P, et al. Percutaneous vertebroplasty with polymethylmethacrylate. Technique, indications and results. *Radiol Clin North Am.* 1998;36:533-546.

Dreyfuss P, Halbrook B, Pauza K, et al. Efficacy and validity of radiofrequency neurotomy for chronic lumbar zygapophysial joint pain. *Spine.* 2000;25:1270-1277.

Dupuy DE, Goldberg SN. Image-guided radiofrequency tumor ablation: challenges and opportunities—part II. *J Vasc Interv Radiol.* 2001;12:1135-1148.

Dupuy DE, Rosenberg AE, Punyaratabandhu T, Tan MH, Mankin HJ. Accuracy of CT-guided needle biopsy of musculoskeletal neoplasms. *AJR Am J Roentgenol.* 1998;171:759-762.

Gage AA, Baust JG. Cryosurgery for tumors. *J Am Coll Surg.* 2007;205:342-356.

Gaitanis IN, Hadjipavlou AG, Katonis PG, et al. Balloon kyphoplasty for the treatment of pathological vertebral compressive fractures. *Eur Spine J.* 2005;14:250-260.

Gangi A, Alizadeh H, Wong L, et al. Osteoid osteoma: percutaneous laser ablation and follow-up in 114 patients. *Radiology.* 2007;242:293-301.

Gangi A, Basile A, Buy X, et al. Radiofrequency and laser ablation of spinal lesions. *Semin Ultrasound CT MR.* 2005;26:89-97.

Gangi A, Dietemann JL, Gasser B, et al. Interstitial laser photocoagulation of osteoid osteomas with use of CT guidance. *Radiology.* 1997;203:843-848.

Gangi A, Dietemann JL, Gasser B, et al. Interventional radiology with laser in bone and joints. *Radiol Clin North Am.* 1998;36:547-557.

Gangi A, Dietemann JL, Guth S, et al. Percutaneous laser photocoagulation of spinal osteoid osteomas under CI guidance. *AJNR Am J Neuroradiol.* 1998;19:1955-1958.

Gangi A, Dietemann JL, Ide C, et al. Percutaneous laser disk decompression under CT and fluoroscopic guidance: indications, technique, and clinical experience. *Radiographics.* 1996;16:89-96.

Gangi A, Dietemann JL, Schultz A, et al. Interventional radiologic procedures with CT guidance in cancer pain management. *Radiographics.* 1996;16(6):1289-1304.

Gangi A, Gasser B, Guth S, et al. New trends in interstitial laser photocoagulation of bones. *Semin Musculoskelet Radiol.* 1997;1(2):331-337.

Gangi A, Guth S, Imbert JP, Marin H, Wong LLS. Percutaneous bone tumor management. *Semin Interv Radiol.* 2002;19:279-286.

Gangi A, Kastler BA, Dietman JL. Percutaneous vertebroplasty guided by a combination of CT and fluoroscopy. *Am J Neuroradiology.* 1994;15:83-86.

Gangi A, Sabharwal T, Irani FG, et al. Quality assurance guidelines for percutaneous vertebroplasty. *Cardiovasc Intervent Radiol.* 2006;29(2):173-178.

Gangi A, Wong LLS, Guth S, et al. Percutaneous vertebroplasty: indications, techniques and results. *Semin Interv Radiol.* 2002;19:265-270.

Gardos F, Depriester C, Cayrolle G, et al. Long term observations of vertebral osteoporotic fractures treated by percutaneous vertebroplasty. *Rheumatology.* 2000;39:1410-1414.

Garfin SR, Reilley MA. Minimally invasive treatment of osteoporotic vertebral body compression fractures. *Spine J.* 2002;2:76-80.

Gaugen JR, Jensen ME, Schweickert P, et al. Lack of preoperative spinous process tenderness does not affect clinical success of percutaneous vertebroplasty. *J Vasc Interv Radiol.* 2002;13:1135-1138.

Gerszten PC, Welch WC, King Jr JT. Quality of life assessment in patients undergoing nucleoplasty-based percutaneous discectomy. *J Neurosurg Spine.* 2006;4:36-42.

Gevargez A, Groenemeyer DW, Czerwinski F. CT-guided percutaneous laser disc decompression with Ceralas D, a diode laser with 980-nm wavelength and 200-microm fiber optics. *Eur Radiol.* 2000;10:1239-1241.

Goetz MP, Callstrom MR, Charboneau JW, et al. Percutaneous image guided radiofrequency ablation of painful metastases involving bone: a multicenter study. *J Clin Oncol.* 2004;22:300-306.

Gupta S. New Techniques in Image-guided percutaneous biopsy. *Cardiovasc Intervent Radiol.* 2004;27:91-104.

Hardouin P, Fayada P, Leclet H, Chopin D. Kyphoplasty. *Joint BoneSpine.* 2002;69:256-261.

Hau MA, Kim JI, Kattapuram S, et al. Accuracy of CT-guided biopsies in 359 patients with musculoskeletal lesions. *Skeletal Radiol.* 2002;31:349-353.

Hellinger J. Complications of non-endoscopic percutaneous laser disc decompression and nucleotomy with the neodymium: YAG laser 1064 nm. *Photomed Laser Surg.* 2004;22:418-422.

Hiwatashi A, Moritani T, Numaguchi Y, et al. Increase in vertebral body height after vertebroplasty. *Am J Neuroradiol.* 2003;24:185-189.

Hooten WM, Kinney MO, Huntoon MA. Epidural abscess and meningitis after epidural corticosteroid injection. *Mayo Clin Proc.* 2004;79:682-686.

Hooten WM, Martin DP, Huntoon MA. Radiofrequency neurotomy for low back pain: evidence-based procedural guidelines. *Pain Medicine.* 2005;6(2):129-138.

Houten JK, Errico TJ. Paraplegia after lumbosacral nerve root block: report of three cases. *Spine J.* 2002;2:70-75.

Huntoon MA, Martin DP. Paralysis after transforaminal epidural injection and previous spinal surgery. *Reg Anesth Pain Med.* 2004;29:494-495.

Ide C, Gangi A, Rimmelin A, et al. Vertebral haemangioams with spinal cord compression: the place of preoperative percutaneous vertebroplasty with methyl methacrylate. *Neuroradiology.* 1996;38:585-589.

Jensen ME, Evans AJ, Mathis JM, et al. Percutaneous polymethylmethacrylate vertebroplasty in the treatment of osteoporotic vertebral body compression fractures: technical aspects. *Am J Neuroradiol.* 1997;18:1897-1904.

Kasperk C, Hillmeier J, Noldge G, et al. Treatment of painful vertebral fractures by kyphoplasty in patients with primary osteoporosis: a prospective nonrandomized controlled study. *J Bone Miner Res.* 2005;20:604-612.

Kaufmann TJ, Trout AT, Kallmes DF. The effects of cement volume on clinical outcomes of percutaneous vertebroplasty. *AJNR Am J Neuroradiol.* 2006;27(9):1933-1937.

Kornblum MB, Wesolowski DP, Fischgrund JS, Herkowitz HN. Computed tomography-guided biopsy of the spine. A review of 103 patients. *Spine.* 1998;23(1):81-85.

Laredo JD, Hamaze B. Complications of percutaneous vertebroplasty and their prevention. *Semin Ultrasound CT MRI.* 2005;26:65-80.

Leclaire R, Fortin L, Lambert R, Bergeron YM, Rossignol M. Radiofrequency facet joint denervation in the treatment of low back pain: a placebo-controlled clinical trial to assess efficacy. *Spine.* 2001;26(13):1411-1416.

Lee WS, Sung KH, Jeong HT, et al. Risk factors of developing new symptomatic vertebral compression fractures after percutaneous vertebroplasty in osteoporotic patients. *Eur Spine J.* 2006;15:1777-1783.

Leech JA, Dulberg C, Kellie S, et al. Relationship of lung function to severity of osteoporosis in women. *Am Rev Respir Dis.* 1990;141:68-71.

Lieberman IH, Dudeney S, Reinhardt MK, Bell G. Initial outcome and efficacy of "kyphoplasty" in the treatment of painful osteoporotic vertebral compression fractures. *Spine.* 2001;26:1631-1638.

Lin EP, Ekholm S, Hiwatashi A, et al. Vertebroplasty: cement leakage into the disc increases the risk of new fracture of the adjacent vertebral body. *Am J Neuroradiol.* 2004;25(2):175-180.

Logan PM, Connell DG, Munk PL, Janzen DL. Image-guided percutaneous biopsy of musculoskeletal tumors: an algorithm for selection of specific biopsy techniques. *AJR Am J Roentgenol.* 1996;166:13-141.

Majd ME, Farley S, Holt RT. Preliminary outcomes and efficacy of the first 360 consecutive kyphoplasties for the treatment of painful osteoporotic vertebral compression fractures. *Spine J.* 2005;5:244-255.

Martin JB, Jean B, Sugiu K, et al. Vertebroplasty: clinical experience and follow up results. *Bone.* 1999;25(suppl 2):11S-15S.

Mathis JM, Barr JD, Belkoff SM, et al. Percutaneous vertebroplasty: a developing standard of care for vertebral compression fractures. *AJNR Am J Neuroradiol.* 2001;22:373-381.

Mathis JM, Wong W. Percutaneous vertebroplasty: technical considerations. *J Vasc Interv Radiol.* 2003;14:953-960.

Maynard AS, Jensen ME, Schweickert PA, et al. Value of bone scan imaging in predicting pain relief from percutaneous vertebroplasty in osteoporotic vertebral fractures. *Am J Neuroradiol.* 2000;21:1807-1812.

McGraw JK, Cardella J, Barr JD, et al. Society of Interventional Radiology quality improvement guidelines for percutaneous vertebroplasty. *J Vasc Interv Radiol.* 2003;14:827-831.

McLain RF, Kapural L, Mekhail NA. Epidural steroid therapy for back and leg pain: mechanisms of action and efficacy. *Spine J.* 2005;5:191-201.

Murphy WA, Destouet JM, Gilula LA. Percutaneous skeletal biopsy: a procedure for radiologists—results, review, and recommendations. *Radiology.* 1981;139:545-549.

Nardi PV, Cabezas D, Cesaroni A. Percutaneous cervical nucleoplasty using Coblation technology. Clinical results in fifty consecutive cases. *Acta Neurochir Suppl.* 2005;92:73-78.

Nussbaum DA, Gailloud P, Murphy K. A review of the complications associated with vertebroplasty and kyphoplasty as reported to the Food and Drug Administration Medical Devise related website. *J Vasc Interv Radiol.* 2004;15:1185-1192.

Padovani B, Kasriel O, Brunner P, et al. Pulmonary embolism caused by acrylic cement: A rare complication of percutaneous vertebroplasty. *Am J Neuroradiol.* 1999;20:375-377.

Parlier-Cuau C, Nizard R, Champsaur P, et al. Percutaneous resection of osteoid osteomas. *Semin Musculoskelet Radiol.* 1997;1:257-264.

Parther H, Van Dillen L, Metzler JP, et al. Prospective measurement of function and pain in patients with non-neoplastic compression fractures treated with vertebroplasty. *J Bone Joint Surg Am.* 2006;88(2):334-341.

Peh WCG, Gilula LA, Peck DD. Percutaneous vertebroplasty for severe osteoporotic vertebral body compression fractures. *Radiology.* 2002;223(1):121-126.

Peh WCG, Gilula LA. Percutaneous vertebroplasty: Indications, contraindications and technique. *Br J Radiol.* 2003;76:69-75.

Phillips FM. Minimal invasive treatment of osteoporotic vertebral compression fractures. *Spine.* 2003;28(s):45-53.

Poole KES, Compston JE. Osteoporosis and its management. *Br Med J.* 2006;333:1251-1256.

Puri A, Shingade VU, Agarwal MG, et al. CT-guided percutaneous core needle biopsy in deep seated musculoskeletal lesions: a prospective study of 128 cases. *Skeletal Radiol.* 2006;35:138-143.

Reddy A, Loh S, Cutts J, Rachlin J, Hirsch J. New approach to the management of acute disc herniation. *Pain Physician.* 2005;8:385-389.

Reitman CA, Watters 3rd W. Subdural hematoma after cervical epidural steroid injection. *Spine.* 2002;27:E174-E176.

Rhyne 3rd A, Banit D, Laxer E, et al. Kyphoplasty: report of eighty-two thoracolumbar osteoporotic vertebral fractures. *J Orthop Trauma.* 2004;18:294-299.

Riew KD, Yin Y, Gilula L, et al. The effect of nerve-root injections on the need for operative treatment of lumbar radicular pain. A prospective, randomized, controlled, double-blind study. *J Bone Joint Surg Am.* 2000;82:1589-1593.

Robertson Jr WW, Janssen HF, Pugh JL. The spread of tumor-cell-size particles after bone biopsy. *J Bone Joint Surg Am.* 1984;66(8):1243-1247.

Rosenkranz M, Grzyska U, Niesen W, et al. Anterior spinal artery syndrome following periradicular cervical nerve root therapy. *J Neurol.* 2004;251:229-231.

Rosenthal DI, Alexander A, Rosenberg AE, et al. Ablation of osteoid osteomas with a percutaneously placed electrode: a new procedure. *Radiology.* 1992;183:29-33.

Rosenthal DI, Hornicek FJ, Torriani M. Osteoid osteoma: Percutaneous treatment with radiofrequency energy. *Radiology.* 2003;229:171-175.

Schofferman J, Kine G. Effectiveness of repeated radiofrequency neurotomy for lumbar facet pain. *Spine.* 2004;29(21):2471-2473.

Schubert A, Deogaonkar A, Lotto M, et al. Anesthesia for minimally invasive cranial and spinal surgery. *J Neurosurg Anesthesiol.* 2006;18(1):47-56.

Scroop R, Eskridge J, Britz GW. Paradoxical cerebral arterial embolization of cement during intra-operative vertebroplasty: case report. *AJNR Am J Neuroradiol.* 2002;23:868-870.

Sequeiros RB, Hyvonen P, Sequeiros AB, et al. Osteoid osteoma: MR imaging-guided laser ablation with use of optical instrument guidance at 0.23T. *Eur Radiol.* 2003;13:2309-2314.

Singh V, Piryani C, Liao K, Nieschulz S. Percutaneous disc decompression using Coblation (nucleoplasty) in the treatment of chronic discogenic pain. *Pain Physician.* 2002;5:250-259.

Stoll BA, Parbhoo S, eds. *Bone Metastasis: Monitoring and Treatment.* New York: Raven Press; 1983.

Theodorescu D. Cancer cryotherapy: evolution and biology. *Rev Urol.* 2004;4(suppl 6): S9-S19.

Uppin AA, Hirsch JA, Centenera LV, et al. Occurrence of new vertebral body fracture after percutaneous vertebroplasty in patients with osteoporosis. *Radiology.* 2003;226:119-124.

van Kleef M, Barendse GA, Kessels A, Voets HM, Weber WE, de Lange S. Randomized trial of radiofrequency lumbar facet denervation for chronic low back pain. *Spine.* 1999;24(18):1937-1942.

Voormolen MH, Lohle PN, Lampmann LE, et al. Prospective clinical follow-up after percutaneous vertebroplasty in patients with painful osteoporotic vertebral compression fractures. *J Vasc Interv Radiol.* 2006;17(8):1313-1320.

Watanabe AT, Nishimura E, Garris J. Image-guided epidural steroid injections. *Tech Vasc Interv Radiol.* 2002;5:186-193.

Weill A, Chiras J, Simon JM, et al. Spinal Metastases: Indications for and results of percutaneous injection of acrylic surgical cement. *Radiology.* 1996:241-247.

Witt JD, Hall-Craggs MA, Ripley P, et al. Interstitial laser photocoagulation for the treatment of osteoid osteoma: Results of a prospective study. *J Bone Joint Surg Br.* 2000;82:1125-1128.

Zoarski GH, Snow P, Olan WJ, et al. Percutaneous vertebroplasty for osteoporotic compression fractures: quantitative prospective evaluation of long-term outcomes. *J Vasc Interv Radiol.* 2002;13:139-148.

CHAPTER 25

Image-Guided Tumor Ablation: Basic Principles

Michael D. Beland, MD, and William W. Mayo-Smith, MD, FACR

METHODS OF ABLATION	Interstitial Laser Photocoagulation	IMAGING GUIDANCE
Chemical Ablation	High-Intensity Focused Ultrasound	POSTPROCEDURAL FOLLOW-UP
Radiofrequency Ablation	PERFORMING ABLATION	AND IMAGING
Cryoablation	Patient Preparation	FUTURE DIRECTIONS
Microwave Ablation		

Tumor ablation techniques and applications have received increasing attention, research and experience over the past decade and have become an integral component of the treatment plans of some oncology patients. As techniques of application have become increasingly sophisticated, the patient population who may be considered candidates for thermal ablation has also continued to expand. Many malignancies are poorly responsive to systemic chemotherapy or local radiation therapy. Patients presenting with these tumors often have reduced life expectancy and multiple comorbidities making them poor surgical candidates. Image-guided tumor ablation offers an effective, minimally invasive, less costly approach, often achievable in an outpatient setting.

Chemical ablation will be briefly reviewed but is currently limited in application and has largely been supplanted by the most widely available and most extensively evaluated thermal ablation techniques: radiofrequency ablation (RFA) and cryoablation (Box 25-1). Microwave ablation, interstitial laser photocoagulation, and high-intensity focused ultrasound (HIFU) are also discussed, although these modalities are currently in the early stages of application in the United States. Finally, issues regarding patient preparation, imaging guidance, procedural follow-up, and future directions are discussed.

METHODS OF ABLATION

Chemical Ablation

Chemical ablation is achieved with image-guided instillation of a chemical agent. The most common chemical agent used for tumor ablation is ethanol, although other agents such as acetic acid have been used. Percutaneous ethanol injection (PEI) has been shown to be a safe, inexpensive, and effective treatment for small (3-5 cm) hepatocellular carcinomas (HCCs). Ethanol works by protein denaturation, leading to coagulative necrosis, thrombosis of small vessels, and formation of fibrotic and granulomatous tissue. It is effective for encapsulated tumors, such as HCC, where surrounding tissue is made firm by underlying disease, the cirrhotic liver. Injected alcohol diffuses throughout the tumor but is prevented from diffusing into the liver by the tumor capsule and surrounding cirrhotic parenchyma. PEI is less effective for metastases because they are often firm tumors surrounded by normal tissue. PEI is performed by placing a small (19-gauge) needle or similar sized lateral side-hole needle into the center of the untreated portion of tumor. Absolute ethanol (96%) is injected during continuous sonographic monitoring. Alcohol droplets appear as a hyperechoic cloud.

The volume injected is based on the tumor size, considered as a sphere, using the equation:

$$\text{Injected volume (V)} = 4/3\,\pi\,(r + 0.5)^3$$

Generally, 10-20 mL per injection per lesion is given. Injections are repeated as needed on a weekly basis until the calculated volume is achieved. Multiple needle tracts are to be avoided to decrease the risk of alcohol leaking into the peritoneal cavity, which can be very painful. Although computed tomography (CT) can be used for imaging guidance, ultrasound is the preferred modality for performing PEI in the liver due to the ease of use. Ethanol injection for HCC results in complete tumor necrosis in 70%-80% of cases (Fig. 25-1). Cure rates equal those of surgery in selected patients. Results for metastases are less favorable, with complete necrosis rates closer to 50%. PEI has not gained widespread popularity in the United States, probably because multiple treatments are needed and because it has decreased efficacy in treating colorectal metastasis. As a result, PEI is less effective than other treatments for colorectal metastasis.

Radiofrequency Ablation

RFA works by transforming RF energy into heat, which is deposited into a tumor. An RF generator in the range of 60-250 W is commonly used as the source. After grounding pads are placed on the patient and connected to the power unit, applicators (electrodes) are then placed into the tumor and connected to the RF generator. Alternating current applied to the electrode passes through the patient to the grounding pads. The alternating nature of the current causes ionic agitation of the molecules surrounding the uninsulated electrode tip, ultimately leading to the production of frictional heating. As tissue temperatures increase to the range of 60°C-100°C, irreversible cellular damage referred to as coagulation necrosis occurs instantly. Lower temperatures (50°C-60°C) may induce coagulation in minutes. Temperatures less than 50°C do not reliably induce necrosis. Temperatures greater than 100°C are generally avoided because, as tissues boil, gas is produced, which acts as an insulator and significantly impedes further diffusion of heat energy into the surrounding tumor.

In general, there are three types of RF applicators available: single straight needles, cluster straight needles, and multitined expandable electrodes. The applicator diameters are typically 14-17.5 gauge. The major difference between the different RF applicators is the size of ablation zone possible during a single treatment session. Maximum achievable uniform ablation zone with a single straight electrode is approximately 1.6 cm in vivo. A method has been developed to increase ablation zone size through the use of an internally cooled applicator where chilled perfusate flows through the applicator to decrease temperatures at the tip and allow for a larger ablation zone by preventing the formation of char and vaporization. To further increase ablation zones, other applicator styles have been developed. Cluster electrodes consist of three single electrode needles in one applicator. The diameter of ablation using these devices is approximately 3 cm. The umbrella-style expandable array electrode consists of multiple individual tines that are deployed within the tumor, creating 5- to 6-cm zones of ablation. Some of these electrodes also employ instillation of interstitial saline from the tips of the applicator to spread thermal energy more efficiently while increasing tissue ionicity, which allows for greater flow of current. Finally, the simultaneous use of multiple single probe applicators placed at different locations in the tumor can be used to treat larger neoplasms (Fig. 25-2).

In addition to new applicator technology, new generator designs have allowed more efficient production of larger ablation zones (Box 25-2). Energy pulsing has been developed to augment overall energy transfer while avoiding vaporization and charring. The rapid alternation of low- and high-energy deposition allows preferential cooling of tissue nearest the probe while maintaining continual heating of more distant tissue. Combining energy pulsing with an internally cooled RF applicator synergistically produces greater tissue ablation than either method alone. Connecting multiple probes to a generator (switch box technology) can also be used. The most recent innovation that will likely have a large impact on thermal ablation technology is the development of bipolar RFA, wherein an ablation zone can be created between two electrodes. Bipolar percutaneous RF electrodes are not yet commercially available in the United States.

The length of treatment time to create tissue necrosis varies depending on which type of applicator is used and the size of the tumor being treated. Most single treatments are 10-16 minutes in soft tissue. The goal of treatment is to gain a 5- to 10-mm treatment margin beyond the suspected tumor borders identified on preprocedural imaging. To accomplish this goal, it may be necessary to plan multiple overlapping ablations following intervening applicator repositioning, which can significantly lengthen the total procedure time (Fig. 25-3).

One of the principal advantages of RFA is that it is a minimally invasive outpatient procedure with patients often being treated and discharged on the same day (Table 25-1). In addition to being preferred by patients over a prolonged hospital stay, this leads to significant cost savings to the health care system. There are fewer complications when compared with major surgery and the use of general anesthesia. RFA has an intrinsic cautery effect which may decrease bleeding complications, a major consideration in coagulopathic patients. RFA has also been shown to be synergistic with traditional treatments, such as radiation therapy, which can improve patient survival.

There are two primary factors inherent to RFA which may impede complete tumor necrosis (Box 25-3). Tissue boiling and charring occurs with temperatures greater than 100°C and acts as an electrical insulator, limiting heat conduction to tumor beyond the area of charring. The ability to obtain adequate thermal heating may also be limited by adjacent large blood vessels. This is referred to as the *heat sink effect*, wherein rapidly flowing blood

---

Box 25-1. Solid Tumor Ablation Techniques

CHEMICAL
Percutaneous ethanol injection

THERMAL
Radiofrequency ablation
- Cryoablation
- Microwave ablation
- Interstitial laser photocoagulation
- High-intensity focused ultrasound

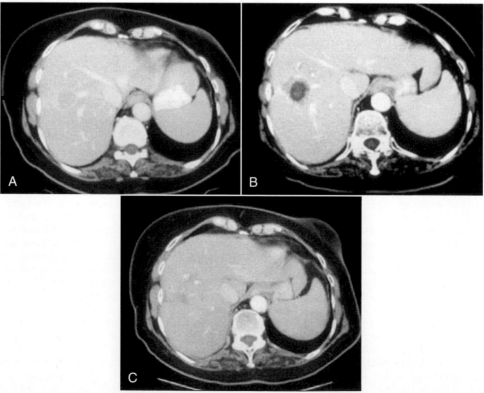

FIGURE 25-1. Contrast-enhanced liver computed tomograph before (**A**), at 3 months (**B**), and at 9 months(**C**) after percutaneous ethanol injection for hepatocellular carcinoma. Note low density in region of alcohol injection in **B**.

carries heat away from the treatment zone. Methods to counteract the heat sink effect have been developed, including preprocedural hepatic artery embolization or temporary occlusion of the hepatic artery and portal vein during the procedure (Pringle maneuver). Other methods showing promise to increase thermal necrosis through synergistic effects include concurrent chemoembolization, external beam radiation, and brachytherapy.

Cryoablation

Cryoablation is the oldest of the applicator-based ablative techniques. It was first described in the liver in 1963. Cryoablation causes tumor necrosis through rapid cell freezing. The

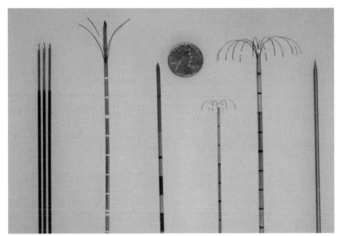

FIGURE 25-2. Various percutaneous ablation probes. Left to right: Cluster radio frequency ablation (RFA), expandable tine RFA with interstitial saline infusion, microwave, small and large umbrella RFA, cryoablation. (Courtesy Damian Dupuy, MD.)

Box 25-2. Strategies to Increase Volume of Coagulation

Necrosis
  Multiple probe or cluster array electrodes
  Cool-tip RFA electrodes
  RF energy pulsing
  Interstitial saline infusion

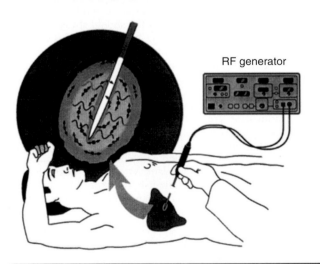

FIGURE 25-3. Schematic representation of radiofrequency ablation procedure. (Courtesy Damian Dupuy, MD.)

mechanisms through which subfreezing temperatures induce cell death are complex and not fully understood but likely occur through multiple mechanisms. Principal contributors to cell death include protein denaturation, cell membrane rupture, cell dehydration, and ischemia secondary to hypoxia.

Recent improvements in cryoablation systems have led to its use as a percutaneous technique. These systems use either a single or mixed refrigerant, such as nitrous oxide or argon gas under high pressure. After the gas flows through the cryoapplicator, it expands at the applicator tip (exploiting the Joule-Thomson effect) causing the temperature to rapidly drop. Temperatures from −80°C to −150°C are possible. Applicators also incorporate helium to cause an active thaw cycle. When the helium expands at the tip, heat is rapidly generated.

Freezing is accomplished by placement of at least one applicator into the tumor, although usually multiple (up to 8) probes are used to treat larger tumors. The length of treatment may vary slightly but is usually a 10-minute freeze followed by an 8-minute thaw cycle. In general, two freeze-thaw cycles are used to treat most solid tumors. Monitoring of the local ablation zone temperature can easily be performed with a thermocouple device to ensure that lethal temperatures are obtained and adequate thawing has occurred, but the zone of ablation (freeze ball) can usually be visualized directly using ultrasound, CT, or magnetic resonance imaging (Fig. 25-4).

Cryoablation offers many of the minimally invasive advantages offered by RFA. In addition, there may be advantages over RFA, including decreased procedure-associated pain in some applications and improved real-time visualization of the treated area. Generally, the attainable zone of ablation is largest with cryoablation for comparable length of treatment given the routine placement of multiple simultaneous applicators. However, the time spent placing multiple applicators may be similar to repositioning RFA electrodes for overlapping ablations.

Microwave Ablation

Microwave ablation (MWA) is a newer technique that uses an electromagnetic device coupled to an applicator to induce tumor necrosis by using frequencies from 900 to 2450 MHz. A rapidly oscillating charge is produced at approximately 2-5 billion times per second. Because water molecules are polar, the oscillating electric charge from microwave radiation interacts with water molecules, causing them to rotate at the microwave's frequency. Microwave radiation is specially tuned to the natural frequency of water molecules to maximize this interaction. The rapid motion of these water molecules causes frictional heating, raising the

TABLE 25-1 Comparison of Thermal Techniques

	Availability	No. of Sessions	Complication Rate	Cost
Radiofrequency Ablation	↑↑↑	↓	↓	↓
Cryoablation	↑↑	↓	↑↑	↑
Microwave	↓↓↓	↓	↑↑	↑↑
Laser	↓↓↓	↑↑	↓	↑↑↑
High-intensity focused ultrasound	↓↓↓	↑↑	↓	↑↑↑

Box 25-3. Strategies to Increase Thermal Injury

↑ Amount or rate of energy deposited
↑ Tissue conduction of heat
↓ Resistance of target tissue to heat

temperature of the local cellular environment. As with RFA, the goal of treatment with MWA is to achieve sustained temperatures greater than 50°C and ideally greater than 60°C.

Because of the different mechanism of action, MWA offers several theoretical advantages over RFA. When compared with RFA, MWA causes a much larger zone of active heating (up to 2 cm surrounding the microwave applicator compared with a few millimeters in RFA) because of a much broader field of power density. This larger heating zone may give a more uniform temperature in the ablation zone, leading to a larger field of cell death. Because of the decreased dependence on thermal conduction, MWA is also less susceptible to the heat sink effect compared with RFA. Given that microwaves are electromagnetic, microwave ablations are not limited by the increased impedance seen with tissue boiling and charring in RFA. This allows for much higher intratumoral temperatures, which translates into considerably larger ablation zones with relatively shorter treatment durations. In addition, current microwave prototypes allow placement of multiple applicators simultaneously to treat larger tumors.

Interstitial Laser Photocoagulation

Interstitial laser photocoagulation (ILP) uses intense pulses of light created by a laser to generate heat. The laser light is conveyed to the tissue by optical fibers passed through 19-gauge needles. The needles are arranged in arrays within the tumor using ultrasound guidance for placement and monitoring of therapy. CT or CT fluoroscopy may aid with difficult tumor localization. Generally 4-8 needles are placed for each 3- to 4-cm lesion. Twelve needles may be required for large or multiple lesions. Complete tumor necrosis in lesions less than 4 cm has been reported in 40%-60% of lesions.

High-Intensity Focused Ultrasound

HIFU was first described in the 1940s as a new method of ablating brain tissue. In HIFU, ultrasound waves generated by piezoelectric elements are focused either through a spherical arrangement, acoustic lens, or paraboloid reflectors. The wave is transmitted between the ultrasound source and the patient's skin through degassed water. Degassed water is used because the acoustic properties are similar to body tissue, which limits the amount of sound absorption and reflection. The sound waves converge at a predetermined focal point, causing a large amount of focused power deposition, which leads to thermonecrosis.

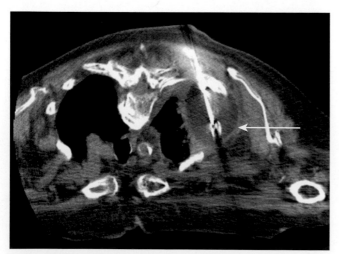

Figure 25-4. Computed tomography–guided cryoablation of a large painful metastasis to the chest wall from non–small cell lung cancer. Note the clearly visible hypodense freeze ball *(arrow)* surrounding one of the cryoprobes.

The size of an ablation zone for a single treatment is very small, approximately 1.5 × 15 mm under normal exposure parameters at 1.7 MHz. The ablation zone is ellipsoidal, with the long axis parallel to the ultrasound beam. It is the confluence of numerous individual ablation zones that make up the overall treatment area. While it only takes 1-3 seconds per treatment, the total time can be substantial depending on tumor size (up to 2 hours or longer for a 2- to 3-cm mass).

The principal advantage of HIFU is the ability to cause tissue necrosis without direct contact between the applicator and the tumor. Tumors that may not be easily accessible by percutaneous methods may be more easily treated. There is also the advantage of very precise control of the ablation zone, especially with MRI guidance. However, bone and air-filled viscera between the transducer and the tumor can lead to complications or incomplete treatments.

PERFORMING ABLATION

Patient Preparation

Because many of the techniques of percutaneous tumor ablation are similar to those of image-guided needle biopsy, patient preparation is also similar. Most busy ablation services function similarly to a surgical practice with a clinic for patient consultations before the procedure and follow-up visits. The goal of the initial patient consultation is to determine whether the patient is a candidate for percutaneous ablation. In most cases this entails reviewing recent cross-sectional imaging examinations. In addition to determining whether the tumor is amenable to treatment, imaging allows evaluation of adjacent structures and is useful for staging the disease. Patients with tumors that can be safely resected for cure should also undergo surgical evaluation. A close relationship with oncologists and oncologic surgeons is imperative. If the lesion is amenable to ablation, histologic sampling to confirm malignancy should be strongly considered. If lesion pathology is unavailable before ablation but imaging is sufficiently characteristic, then percutaneous biopsy may be performed at the time of treatment immediately preceding ablation. If histopathologic diagnosis dictates treatment, this approach mandates on-site pathology personnel for the procedure. Relative contraindications to performing RFA may include excessive tumor burden, untreatable diffuse or distant disease, active signs of infection, uncorrectable coagulopathy, and inability to obtain informed consent. Before treatment, the patient must receive a directed history and physical examination. Anticoagulants (e.g., warfarin, low molecular weight heparin) and antiplatelet agents (e.g., aspirin, clopidogrel, nonsteroidal anti-inflammatories) should be stopped with sufficient time for coagulation status to normalize (or be appropriately substituted with short-acting agents if anticoagulation can be ceased for only a brief window). Preprocedural laboratory studies should always include a coagulation profile and platelet count. Additional studies that may be appropriate include a complete blood count, blood chemistries (tailored to organ system being treated and depending on use of iodinated contrast for imaging), electrocardiogram, baseline appropriate tumor markers, and blood type and match.

On the day of the procedure, interval history and a directed physical examination are performed. Signed informed consent is obtained and intravenous access is initiated. While certain patients may require general anesthesia, many percutaneous ablation procedures are performed with conscious sedation using intravenous fentanyl and midazolam. Vital signs, heart rhythm, and oxygen saturation are continuously monitored by dedicated nursing personnel. Intravenous fluid and oxygen by nasal canula may be administered as necessary.

IMAGING GUIDANCE

Imaging guidance for percutaneous applicator placement and monitoring of treatment can be performed using fluoroscopy, ultrasound, CT, or MRI. The modality used depends on the organ system being treated, the type of ablation being performed, and user preference (Box 25-4).

Fluoroscopy has limited utility for monitoring of probe placement and is not frequently employed given the current wide availability of cross-sectional imaging. However, fluoroscopy may be appropriate in the treatment of osseous lesions, especially when superficial. A major drawback of fluoroscopic guidance is the inability to monitor local tissue changes during the procedure.

Ultrasound allows real-time monitoring of applicator placement without ionizing radiation. If a safe path to the lesion and the lesion itself are well-visualized on ultrasound, then this should be the guidance modality of choice. However, a known lesion is occasionally difficult to demonstrate on ultrasound because of limited soft tissue contrast. Ultrasound visualization may also be hindered by interposed bone, bowel gas, or lung. If local temperatures in RFA or microwave approach 100°C and cavitation occurs, the gas bubbles can obscure visualization of the applicator and the tumor entirely.

CT can provide better intrinsic soft tissue contrast than ultrasound to improve lesion conspicuity depending on the organ system being treated. It also has the advantage of being able to administer intravenous contrast at the time of placement to better assess localization of the lesion. In addition, intravenous contrast can be given following the ablation to immediately check for suspected areas of residual tumor outside of the ablation zone that may need immediate retreatment. The use of CT fluoroscopy allows near real-time visualization of applicator placement. CT also offers excellent visualization of osseous lesions. Disadvantages of CT include limitations in guidance planes (limited by maximum gantry angling) and ionizing radiation exposure to the patient and staff. At many institutions, CT is the imaging guidance of choice for treating lung, renal, and osseous neoplasms (Figs. 25-5 and 25-6).

MRI for imaging guidance increases the complexity of the procedure in that only MR-compatible devices can be used. While

---

Box 25-4. Imaging Guidance for Radiofrequency Ablation

MAGNETIC RESONANCE IMAGING (MRI)
High tumor conspicuity
Multiplanar imaging
Temperature-sensitive sequences
Specialized equipment necessary
Availability limited

COMPUTED TOMOGRAPHY (CT)
Conspicuity between MRI and ultrasound
Ideal when ultrasound is limited (e.g., obese, thorax, gas)
Wide availability
Less operator dependence
Near real-time with CT fluoroscopy

ULTRASOUND
Variable tumor-tissue contrast
Portable/less expensive
Wide availability
Operator/location dependent
Contrast agents can improve conspicuity

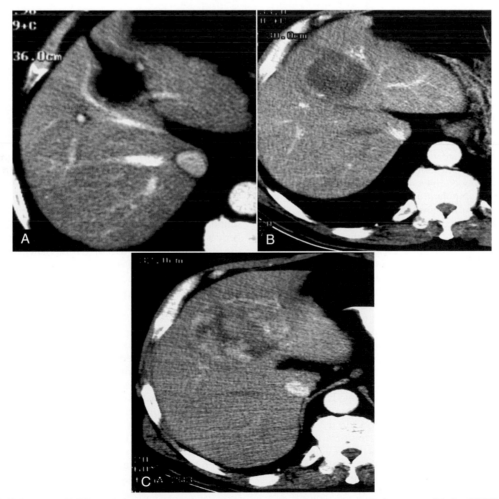

FIGURE 25-5. **A,** Medial segment left hepatic lobe hepatocellular carcinoma. **B,** One month after radiofrequency ablation (RFA). **C,** Ten months after RFA. Note progressive contraction of the nonenhancing ablation zone.

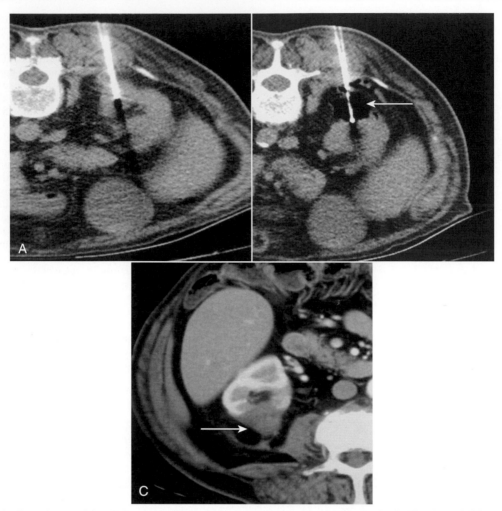

FIGURE 25-6. Renal cell carcinoma with radiofrequency (RF) probe in place **(A)**, gas due to vaporization/boiling *(arrow)* **(B)**, and 3 months after RF ablation with no residual enhancing tumor *(arrow)* **(C)**.

MR-compatible applicators are available, the control unit needs to be kept outside of the MR room. However, specialized temperature-sensitive MR pulse sequences have been devised that allow near real-time monitoring of temperatures in the ablation zone, which is useful to outline treatment margins. An additional disadvantage is the relative high cost compared to other imaging modalities.

Advantages and disadvantages of each modality become especially evident during cryoablation treatment monitoring. On ultrasound, the ice ball is visualized as an echogenic, expanding region during treatment. Ultrasound guidance, however, is limited because only the near edge of frozen tissue is adequately visualized because sound waves do not penetrate frozen tissue and the lesion can become obscured during treatment. This can be partially overcome by probe repositioning, which is easier to accomplish intraoperatively where the probe can be moved into numerous other planes but poses a significant problem for the percutaneous approach. CT guidance offers clear visualization of the entire treatment margin, which becomes very important when treating lesions near vital organs. On CT, the ice ball appears hypodense compared with the adjacent untreated tissue. The margins of the frozen tissue seen on CT do not represent the true margins of tumor necrosis because temperatures at the advancing outer edge of the ice ball are sublethal. Therefore, the visible margin of frozen tissue on imaging is usually extended 5-10 mm beyond the tumor margins seen before the procedure.

Currently, guidance and monitoring of HIFU is performed either by using ultrasound or MRI. When ultrasound is used to guide treatment, a diagnostic transducer is arranged confocally with the therapeutic transducer. The relationship of these two transducers is fixed, allowing reliable positioning of the therapeutic focus based on the diagnostic image. When MRI is used to guide treatments, local temperature elevations can be detected using specialized MR pulse sequences. Initially, low-level ultrasound energy is used to slightly raise the temperature of the target tissue. After this information is used to confirm the position of the ultrasound focus, then higher intensity therapeutic exposures are used for the actual treatment.

▮ POSTPROCEDURAL FOLLOW-UP AND IMAGING

Immediately following the procedure performed with the patient under conscious sedation, patients are generally observed for at least 3-4 hours in a dedicated recovery area and then discharged home. Occasionally, patients may be admitted for overnight observation if there is considerable postprocedure pain or complications. Usually a follow-up phone call is performed 24 hours after the treatment and a clinic visit scheduled around 3-4 weeks after ablation. Appropriate tumor markers can be repeated at that time. If residual or recurrent tumor is suspected at any time due to imaging finding or clinical assessment, reablation or alternative treatment is performed.

Appropriate imaging follow-up depends on the type of tumor being treated, the organ in which the tumor occurs, the confidence of the radiologist that treatment has been effective, and local preferences. Contrast-enhanced CT is probably the most common imaging modality to assess for residual or recurrent tumor. The CT examination protocol is tailored to the type of tumor and its location. MRI is particularly useful in patients with allergies to iodinated contrast agents.

FUTURE DIRECTIONS

The field of thermal ablation has great potential for further investigation, technical improvements, and new applications. While RFA has the most clinical data and is the most widely applied of the available techniques, there continues to be evolution of all ablative techniques. One of the largest questions now being investigated is defining its role amidst currently accepted therapies, such as surgery, chemotherapy, external beam radiation, and brachytherapy. Additional modifications to the way tumor ablation is currently performed are forthcoming.

There are currently multiple researchers investigating ways of gaining more control over the effective ablation zone with all of the percutaneous methods described. One potential method involves injecting solutions with specific thermal properties into the target tissues to enhance cell necrosis of the diseased tissues while preserving the normal tissues from injury.

As the safety and efficacy of thermal ablative techniques continues to be investigated and established, we are likely to see the continued expansion of their indications and application. While these therapies are currently mainly used for treatment of unresectable disease and symptom palliation, their role in curative therapy as a first-line treatment in certain diseases may be established in the future. Continued studies comparing these and possibly newer thermal ablation techniques with current gold standards of treatment, such as surgery, will be needed. New methods of image guidance to improve tumor targeting and minimize collateral damage as well as the use of combination therapies will hopefully lead to improved patient survival and decreased morbidity.

SUGGESTED READINGS

Bilchik AJ, Wood TF, Allegra D, et al. Cryosurgical ablation and radiofrequency ablation for unresectable hepatic malignant neoplasms. *Arch Surg.* 2000;135: 657-664.

Dupuy DE, Goldberg SN. Image-guided radiofrequency tumor ablation: challenges and opportunities-part II. *J Vasc Interv Radiol.* 2001;12:1135-1148.

Gazelle GS, Goldberg SN, Solbiati L, Livraghi T. Tumor ablation with radiofrequency energy. *Radiology.* 2000;217:633-646.

Gervais DA, Arellano RS. Percutaneous tumor ablation for hepatocellular carcinoma. *AJR Am J Roentgenol I.* 2011;197:789-794.

Gervais DA, McGovern FJ, Arellano RS, McDougal WS, Mueller PR. Renal cell carcinoma: clinical experience and technical success with radiofrequency ablation of 42 tumors. *Radiology.* 2003;226(2):417-424.

Giovannini M. Percutaneous alcohol ablation for liver metastasis. *Semin Oncol.* 2002;29:192-195.

Goldberg SN, Charboneau JW, Dodd III GD, et al. For the International Working Group on Image-Guided Tumor Ablation: proposal for standardization of terms and reporting criteria. *Radiology.* 2003;228:335-345.

Goldberg SN, Dupuy DE. Image-guided radiofrequency tumor ablation: challenges and opportunities-part I. *J Vasc Interv Radiol.* 2001;12:1021-1032.

Goldberg SN, Gazelle GS, Mueller PR. Thermal ablation for focal malignancy: a unified approach to underlying principles, techniques and diagnostic imaging guidance. *AJR Am J Roentgenol.* 2000;174:323-331.

Lubner MG, Brace CL, Hinshaw JL, Lee FT. Microwave tumor ablation: mechanism of action, clinical results, and devices. *J Vasc Interv Radiol.* 2010;21(8):S192-S203.

Mayo-Smith WW, Dupuy DE, Parikh PM, Pezzullo JA, Cronan JJ. Image guided percutaneous radiofrequency ablation of solid renal masses: techniques and outcomes of 38 treatments in 32 consecutive patients. *AJR Am J Roentgenol.* 2003;180:1503-1508.

Pavlovich CP, Walther MM, Choyke PL, et al. Percutaneous radio frequency ablation of small renal tumors: initial results. *J Urol.* 2002;167.10-15.

Simon CJ, Dupuy DE, Mayo-Smith WW. Microwave ablation: principles and applications. *Radiographics.* 2005;25:S69-S83.

Thacker PG, Callstrom MR, Curry TB, et al. Original research: palliation of painful metastatic disease involving bone with imaging-guided treatment: comparison of patients' immediate response to radiofrequency ablation and cryoablation. *AJR Am J Roentgenol.* 2011;197:510 515.

Uppot RN, Silverman SG, Zagoria RJ, et al. Imaging-guided percutaneous ablation of renal cell carcinoma: a primer of how we do it. *AJR Am J Roentgenol.* 2009; 192:1558-1570.

Venkatesan AM, Wood BJ, Gervais DA. Percutaneous ablation in the kidney. *Radiology.* 2011;261:375-391.

Welch BT, Atwell TD, Nichols DA, et al. Percutaneous image-guided adrenal cryoablation: procedural considerations and technical success. *Radiology.* 2011;258:301-307.

Wood BJ, Ramkaransingh JR, Fojo T, Walther MM, Libutti SK. Percutaneous tumor ablation with radiofrequency. *Cancer.* 2002;94:443-451.

Zagoria RJ, Traver MA, Werle DM, et al. Oncologic efficacy of CT-guided percutaneous radiofrequency ablation of renal cell carcinomas. *AJR Am J Roentgenol.* 2007;189:429-436.

CHAPTER 26

Image-Guided Ablation of Renal Tumors

Colin P. Cantwell, FRCR, FFR, and Debra A. Gervais, MD

Before the advent of tumor ablation, the curative treatment for primary renal cell cancer (RCC) was to perform laparoscopic or open nephrectomy or partial nephrectomy. Many patients are deemed unsuitable for potentially curative surgical techniques because of limited renal functional reserve, desire to avoid renal replacement therapy, and comorbid conditions.

The development of needle applicators for tumor ablation has provided selected patients who are unsuitable or unwilling to undergo renal surgery with less invasive nephron-sparing treatment options. This chapter focuses on percutaneous ablation procedures.

METHODS OF ABLATION

There are multiple series published of RCC and benign tumor ablation in humans using percutaneous radiofrequency ablation (RFA) and cryoablation (Box 26-1). Medium-term follow-up data exist for microwave ablation in RCC. Reports of in vivo use of laser interstitial thermal therapy and ultrasound ablation exist in normal animal kidney and RCC (Table 26-1). There are first reports of irreversible electroporation in human and animal kidney.

The method of action of each of the ablation techniques is similar in kidney and liver, discussed in Chapter 25.

INDICATIONS AND OUTCOME

Image-Guided Ablation for Renal Cell Cancer

RCC can be ablated for local control in patients who are unsuitable for renal resection, because of comorbidities, limited renal functional reserve, a single kidney, multiple RCCs, or a condition with an increased risk of RCC occurrence in residual renal tissue such as von Hippel-Lindau disease (Box 26-2). Ablation is suitable for RCCs that are predominantly solid or cystic.

Effectiveness and Local Control

At a mean follow-up of less than 2 years, percutaneous computed tomography (CT)-guided RFA achieves successful local control in 93%-100% of patient series for a wide range of tumor sizes. The number of RFAs necessary for complete ablation increases with tumor size (Table 26-2). RCCs smaller than 3 cm are more likely

than larger tumors to be completely ablated in a single session. RCCs that are 3-5 cm in size are completely ablated in one or two ablation sessions. In one series, only 25% of RCCs of 5 cm or larger could be completely ablated by repeated ablation sessions. The upper limits of RCC size suitable for ablation vary among institutions and are not standardized. In general, RCCs that are 4 cm or less (stage T1a) are suitable for RFA, although with newer technology many completely ablated tumors exceed this size. At our institution we have successfully ablated 6- to 8-cm tumors.

Percutaneous CT-guided cryotherapy for primary RCC has a local control rate of 92%-100% in patient series with a wide range of tumor sizes at a mean follow-up of less than 2 years. Overall, 95%-100% of small RCC can be completely ablated in a single ablation session (Box 26-3).

Ultrasound-guided microwave ablation of RCC has achieved 1-, 2-, and 3-year disease-free survival rates of 95.4%, 92.3%, and 92.3%, respectively.

Early data from phase 2 clinical trials regarding ultrasound ablation demonstrate pathologic response in 15%-35% of targeted tissue in resected RCCs treated with extracorporeal high-intensity focused ultrasound.

There are no published data yet regarding the effectiveness and rate of local control of RCC with laser interstitial thermal therapy or irreversible electroporation. Data are available for application in normal animal kidney. Further medium- and long-term follow-up is required to determine the efficacy of all forms of percutaneous ablation.

Quality of Life

A nonrandomized comparison of percutaneous RFA and laparoscopic radical nephrectomy for small renal cell carcinoma demonstrated there was a significant lower baseline quality of life and greater age in those patients who were selected for RFA. This difference in age demographic may reflect indications for RFA in the study which included coexisting morbidities and surgical or anesthetic risk. After treatment, the surgery group demonstrated a significant reduction in quality of life at 1 week, whereas patients who had RFA demonstrated no significant change in quality of life in the first week. There was a tendency toward improvement above baseline for age in quality of life in the RFA group up to 24 weeks after RFA.

TABLE 26-1 Ablation Zone Diameter with Tumor Ablative Techniques

Modality	Mean Ablation Size (cm)	Generator Power (W)	Endpoint Determinant	Tissue Ablated
2-cm multitined expandable electrode (Starburst XL; Rita Medical Systems) with renal collecting system cooling	2.6	NS	Temperature	In vivo pig kidney
2-cm multitined expandable electrode (Starburst XL; Rita Medical Systems) without renal collecting system cooling	2.7	NS	Temperature	In vivo pig kidney
3-cm cooled electrode (Covidien)	2.5	200	12 minutes Impedance control	In vivo pig kidney
2.5-cm cooled cluster electrode (Covidien)	3.1	200	12 minutes Impedance control	In vivo pig kidney
Three 3-cm electrodes placed 1.5 cm apart using switching device (Covidien)	5.0	200	12 minutes Impedance control with switching controller	In vivo pig kidney
Three 3-cm electrodes placed 2 cm apart using switching device (Covidien)	4.4	200	12 minutes Impedance control with switching controller	In vivo pig kidney
Single interstitial laser fiber	1.8	NS	4 minutes	In vivo pig kidney

NS, not stated.

Box 26-1. Renal Tumor Ablative Techniques

Thermal
- Radiofrequency ablation
- Cryoablation
- Microwave ablation
- Laser interstitial thermal therapy
- Ultrasound ablation

Irreversible electroporation

Box 26-2. Indications for Renal Ablation

Patient unsuitable for renal resection
Limited functional renal reserve
Single kidney
Multiple renal cell carcinomas
Von Hippel-Lindau disease

Cost Effectiveness

In an analysis of the relative cost effectiveness of percutaneous RFA and nephron-sparing surgery in patients of 65 years of age with small renal cell carcinoma (<4 cm) performed at our institution in 2007, nephron-sparing surgery yielded a minimally greater average quality-adjusted life expectancy than RFA (2.5 days), but was more expensive (assuming a 10% higher incidence of tumor recurrence after RFA when compared with nephron-sparing surgery). For nephron-sparing surgery to be preferred over RFA, an estimated nephron-sparing surgery cost reduction of $7500, or RFA cost increase of $6229, was necessary. RFA was preferred even if the annual probability of post-RFA local recurrence was up to 48%.

Image-Guided Ablation of Benign Renal Masses

Image-guided ablation has been used for benign tumors such as oncocytomas, angiomyolipomas and renal arteriovenous malformation. Therapy is indicated for angiomyolipomas when there are symptoms such as pain or when the lesion is greater than 4 cm because of a risk of spontaneous hemorrhage; however, angiomyolipomas of this size are typically treated by transcatheter embolization,

and the role of ablation is not well established. Further criteria for treatment of angiomyolipomas include growth of the lesion by 2 cm at annual CT or presentation with acute hemorrhage.

Some institutions consider oncocytomas for ablation as an alternative to imaging follow-up or resection. Case reports describe successful use of tumor ablation in patients with hypertension secondary to oncocytoma.

Image-Guided Ablation for Symptomatic Palliation

Ablation has been used for palliation of gross hematuria in a small group of cases. The rationale for its use stems from the fact that RF technology is modified from electrocautery used in surgery for hemostasis. RFA leads to resolution of gross hematuria in 1-2 days, in most cases. It is an alternative to embolization in patients with renal insufficiency, solitary kidney, or comorbid conditions, or after failed conventional therapies in patients who are not candidates for surgery. However, its utility is limited to targeting small foci responsible for bleeding

ABLATION PLANNING AND PROCEDURE

Preablation Evaluation and Treatment Planning

Like for liver tumor ablation, a clinic visit is an essential component of planning ablation (Box 26-4). A clinic visit involves a general medical review, physical examination, review of imaging, renal function measurement, and discussion of outcome. It may be appropriate to arrange consultation for oncologic or surgical review. In our institution, a percutaneous biopsy is arranged at least 1 week before ablation to allow pathological analysis.

Imaging studies available for renal masses should be current. The choice of multiphase-enhanced magnetic resonance imaging (MRI) or CT scan for evaluation of renal lesions varies among centers. In our center, CT is reserved for patients with a creatinine less than 2 mg/dL. MRI with gadolinium contrast should be avoided in patients with moderate to severe renal impairment (estimated glomerular filtration rate [eGFR] < 30 mL/min/1.73 m^2) and particularly in patients on hemodialysis, because nephrogenic systemic fibrosis (NSF) has been linked with exposure to gadolinium. We do not use positron emission tomography CT for patients with RCC because of the variable avidity of the tumor for fluorodeoxyglucose.

TABLE 26-2 Achievement of Complete Necrosis (Imaging Definition) and Number of Radiofrequency Ablation Sessions to Achieve Complete Necrosis Based on Tumor Size

Tumor size (cm)	% of all Tumors That Will Achieve Complete Necrosis After Multiple Sessions	% of Adequately Treated Tumors That Will Achieve Complete Necrosis After 1 Ablation Session	% of Adequately Treated Tumors That Will Achieve Complete Necrosis After 2 Ablation Sessions	% of Adequately Treated Tumors That Will Achieve Complete Necrosis After 3 Ablation Sessions
<3	100	92	8	NA
3-5	92	53	44	3
>5	25	0	50	50

NA, Not applicable.

BOX 26-3. Local Effectiveness of Ablation

93%-100% for radiofrequency ablation
92%-100% for cryoablation
Renal cell carcinoma (RCC) less than 3 cm can be ablated with single session
RCC between 3 and 5 cm usually requires more than one session
Local control decreases for RCC greater than 5 cm

BOX 26-4. Patient Preparation and Treatment Planning

Clinic visit essential
Current imaging studies required
Imaging checked for extrarenal disease
Guiding modality for treatment chosen
Biopsy performed before ablation

Image studies are also reviewed for the presence of extrarenal disease and the distance from the tumor to the ureter and bowel. Although ablating a margin of "normal" kidney is not as critical as ablation of a liver margin during hepatic ablation, the zone of ablation must cover the entire tumor. In many cases, the zone of ablation extends beyond the tumor. This must be considered when planning the ablation and when considering other structures at risk for injury.

Because RFA is a local treatment, patients with significant extrarenal metastatic disease (renal vein involvement, extension beyond the Gerota fascia, involved lymph nodes, and distant RCC metastases) are not suitable candidates for ablation unless the treatment is for palliation of hematuria or symptoms.

Appropriate imaging guidance for tumor targeting with CT, ultrasound, or MRI is selected based on availability and visibility of the tumor. If ultrasound guidance is planned, it is prudent to perform preprocedure ultrasound to determine the ease of access to the tumor and sonographic visibility of the lesions.

Appropriate coagulation parameters and renal function are checked. A plan for anticoagulation management is put in place if necessary.

Intraprocedural pain control can be achieved with moderate sedation in most cases. General anesthesia is reserved for those with comorbid disease or who fail sedation management of pain during ablation or biopsy. The use of anesthesia or intravenous sedation is generally institution dependent.

Biopsy

A biopsy of the renal lesion is mandatory at the authors' institution before performance of ablation. A coaxial 17-gauge needle is placed in the tumor, and multiple core biopsies and fine-needle

---

BOX 26-5. Ablation Procedure

Contrast material can be used to aid tumor visualization
Applicators placed to "cover" the tumor volume
Pyeloperfusion if tumor less than 1 cm from ureter
Hydrodissection with D_5W, if bowel close
Cryoprobes no more than 2 cm apart

---

aspirates are obtained. However, not all institutions require biopsy before ablation. In the past, focal renal biopsy had a limited role in the management of renal masses because the complication rate and risk of seeding the biopsy tract were overstated and definitive biopsy results were uncommon.

However, histologic techniques have become more reliable and pathologists have become more confident in differentiating oncocytomas, oncocytic cancers, RCC, and fat-poor angiomyolipomas by biopsy.

We know that 12.8% of solid renal masses are found to be benign (25% for masses smaller than 3 cm, 30% for masses smaller than 2 cm, and 44% for masses smaller than 1 cm). Thus, preablation diagnosis can help determine whether treatment is needed. In addition, even when ablation of benign mass is planned, a definitive benign diagnosis has implications for the frequency of postablation imaging, which may not need to be as frequent when disease is benign.

Procedure

Ablation is performed with spinal anesthesia, general anesthesia, or moderate sedation with midazolam, fentanyl citrate, and meperidine hydrochloride (Box 26-5). Antibiotic prophylaxis varies among institutions with most interventional radiologists choosing to administer a single dose before RFA (80 mg gentamicin and 1 g of ampicillin intravenously) only to patients who have retrograde pyeloperfusion catheters placed for protection of the ureter, vesicoureteric reflux, or a refluxing ureteroenteric anastomosis. Ablation in the presence of a urinary tract infection should be deferred until appropriate therapy is completed.

Targeting, Controlling, and Monitoring Therapy

Common to all ablative techniques except ultrasound ablation is the need to place the applicator in the tumor. CT can be used with or without the addition of intravenous contrast to improve tumor visualization. MRI, when available, can target tumors due to the high tissue contrast between tumor and normal kidney.

The patient is positioned ablation side down, prone, with the side for ablation up, or even supine, depending on the position of the lesion, lung, ribs, and transverse processes. For upper pole masses in most cases, placing the ipsilateral side for ablation down displaces the lung superiorly.

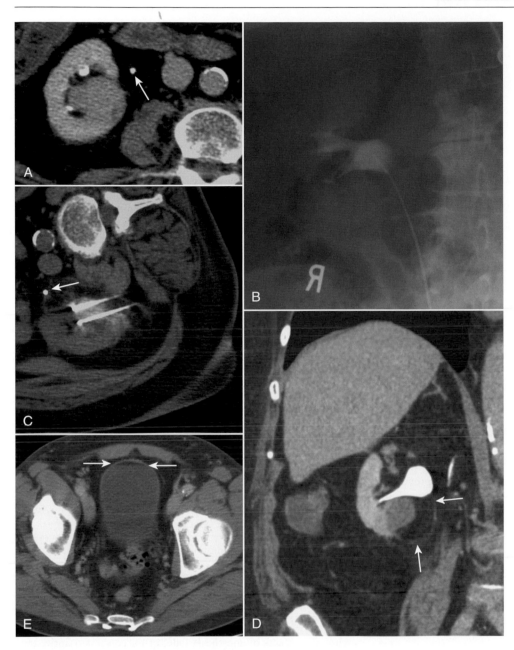

FIGURE 26-1. Radiofrequency ablation (RFA) in a 77-year-old woman with a biopsy-proven right lower pole clear cell renal cell carcinoma (RCC). **A,** Excretory phase postcontrast computed tomography (CT) scan demonstrates a hilar renal mass 9 mm from the ureter *(arrow)*. **B,** Anteroposterior radiograph of a right retrograde pyelogram with the tip of a 5-French FlexTip catheter in the renal pelvis before RFA. **C,** Noncontrast CT scan demonstrates the cluster electrode positioned in the RCC for RFA 9 mm from the ureter *(arrow)*. **D,** Excretory phase coronal CT scan at 3 months demonstrates no hydronephrosis and a halo *(arrows)* of enhancement in the retroperitoneal fat consistent with ablation. **E,** Noncontrast CT scan of the pelvis 3 months after RFA demonstrates a fluid-fat level in the bladder *(arrows)*.

Positioning of the applicator in the tumor is planned using similar techniques as for liver tumor ablation to cover the tumor with the number of placements adjusted for the response of renal tumor to the selected applicator.

Cryoablation usually involves multiple applicator placements depending on lesion size before application of two freeze-thaw cycles. Repositioning applicators can be challenging near the ablation zone after a freeze cycle because of noncompliance of cooled tissues. However, upon thawing, repositioning to an untreated area is possible. Cryoprobes are generally placed no more then 2 cm apart with the peripheral cryoprobes no more than 1 cm from the edge of the tumor.

Size and Geometry of Ablation Zone in Renal Tissue

The geometric shapes of the ablation zones are irregular and ovoid. Edges interfacing with the kidney often are wedge shaped. The transverse diameter of the ablation zone has been studied in vivo for various applicators in normal kidney (see Table 26-1).

Adjunctive Techniques to Protect Organs

A number of techniques have been developed to protect adjacent organs or structures from the zone of ablation. Use of pyeloperfusion with chilled D_5W has been reported during RFA of tumors near the ureter to prevent ureteric stricture. Saline solution is avoided because of its electrical conductivity. Ureteral strictures, which can occur if the ice ball encompasses the ureter during cryoablation, were reported in early cases. Retrograde perfusion of the ureter with room temperature saline has been applied during cryotherapy.

Pyeloperfusion Technique

Perfusion of the ureter with cooled 5% dextrose and water has been described to protect the ureter when within 15 mm of the tumor for RFA. A rigid cystoscope is used by a urologist to advance a 5-French open-ended ureteral catheter (FlexTip, Cook, Bloomington, Ind.) into the renal pelvis/proximal third of the ureter. The catheter tip position is confirmed by contrast injection under fluoroscopy or with a CT scan (Fig. 26-1). A

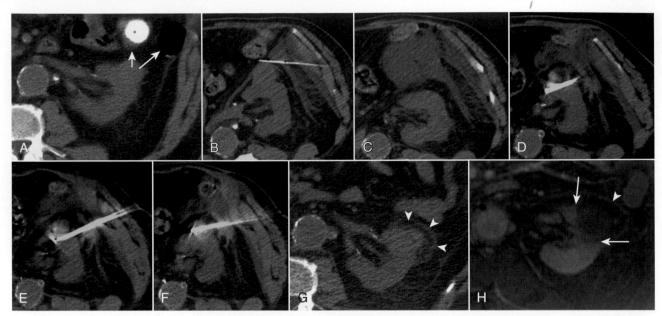

FIGURE 26-2. Radiofrequency ablation in a 67-year-old man with a biopsy-proven left anterior interpolar eosinophilic renal cell carcinoma (RCC). **A,** Axial noncontrast computed tomography (CT) scan of the anterior exophytic RCC positioned posterior to splenic flexure of the colon *(arrows)*. **B,** Axial noncontrast CT of a 20-gauge Chiba needle positioned anterior to the tumor for instillation of D_5W for hydrodissection. **C,** Axial noncontrast CT scan after instillation of 500 mL of D_5W for hydrodissection anterior to the Gerota fascia to separate the transverse colon from the ablation zone. **D, E,** and **F,** Axial noncontrast CT scan before three overlapping ablations. **G,** Noncontrast axial CT scan at 1 month demonstrates a peripheral halo *(arrowheads)* of soft tissue attenuation in the retroperitoneal fat consistent with ablation. **H,** Arterial phase, postcontrast magnetic resonance fat-saturated T1 imaging at 1 month demonstrates no enhancing tumor in the ablation zone (between *arrows*) and a thin peripheral halo *(arrowhead)* of soft tissue signal in the retroperitoneal fat consistent with ablation.

14-16 French Foley catheter is then placed into the bladder, to which the retrograde ureteral catheter is taped to prevent its displacement.

One-liter bags of D_5W are refrigerated overnight at 2°C-6°C. The bags of D_5W are hung from an intravenous pole, 80 cm above patient bed, and connected to the retrograde ureteral catheter using 10-drop IV set (Arrow International Inc, Reading, Pa.). This produces a perfusion pressure of 80 cm H_2O. During the procedure, approximately 1000-1500 mL is perfused into the collecting system. The drip system and Foley catheter output should be frequently monitored during RFA to confirm ongoing perfusion and drainage. The ureteral stent and Foley catheter are removed immediately upon termination of the RFA procedure.

Displacement Techniques

Displacement of adjacent large bowel, duodenum, iliofemoral nerve, and psoas muscle away from the tumor is feasible using carbon dioxide or 250-1000 mL 5% dextrose solution locally injected using a 20-gauge Chiba needle placed adjacent to the tumor (Fig. 26-2). Angioplasty balloons have been used to displace and protect adjacent normal structures from thermal injury during RFA.

Postprocedure Care

Patients can be discharged home on the same day if they are hemodynamically stable, have recovered from sedation in accordance with institutional guidelines, and can tolerate oral intake and pass urine. Additional analgesics may be needed during recovery and in the first 4-7 days after the procedure. Patients should be reassured that, in most cases, a near-normal lifestyle may be resumed within 10 days of the ablation procedure. Some patients may be admitted for observation while coexisting morbidity is managed,

---

> ### Box 26-6. Complications
>
> Radiofrequency ablation has a complication rate of 8%
> Percutaneous cryotherapy has a complication rate of 6%-8%
> Ablative techniques are safer than partial or radical nephrectomy
> In 80% of cases, fever or flulike symptoms (postablation syndrome) develop
> Majority of ablative complications are related to perinephric hematomas and transient hematuria
> Ureteral strictures and large hematomas are rare

while the effects of anesthesia fade, or for continued anticoagulant or analgesia management.

Post–Radiofrequency Ablation Syndrome

Fever or flulike symptoms develop in 80% of patients with RF-ablated renal lesions. Thirty percent of patients with RF-ablated renal lesions have the complete spectrum of post-RFA syndrome: low-grade fever (temperature > 99°F [37°C]) and flulike symptoms. The fever peaks at day 3 and flulike symptoms peak at day 5. Patients with RF-ablated renal lesions experienced less pain and lifestyle interference than patients with RF-ablated liver lesions.

Patients who have persistent or late-onset fever may harbor concurrent infection, including abscess formation or urinary tract infection.

▬ COMPLICATIONS

Percutaneous ablation is safe (Box 26-6). RFA has been associated with complications in 8% of cases, few of which result in long-term morbidity. Percutaneous cryotherapy has a major complication rate of 6%-8%.

Ablation is safer than laparoscopic or open partial or radical nephrectomy. Open radical nephrectomy is associated with postoperative complications in 16%-20% of cases, major complication in 7%, reoperation in 3%, and death within 30 days in 1%-5%. Laparoscopic radical nephrectomy has a postoperative complication rate of 9%-13%.

Partial renal resection techniques have evolved to reduce the invasiveness and preserve renal function. Partial nephrectomy, especially when performed with laparoscopic techniques, is a more complex operation than the traditional radical nephrectomy or open partial nephrectomy, and higher complication rates have been reported. In one study, laparoscopic partial nephrectomy patients had complications in 10%-33% of cases, open conversion in 1%, and reoperation in 2%. Complication rates are higher in larger tumor resections, when tumors are multifocal or bilateral, and when large tumors are resected in a solitary kidney.

The majority of minor complications after RFA consist of small perinephric hematomas and transient gross hematuria, which are considered by many to be normal postprocedure imaging and clinical findings. A hematoma limited by the capsule of the kidney can lead to a Page kidney and hypertension. Rarely, admission for blood transfusion is necessary for a large hematoma. In a single report, central tumors had a 33% risk of bleeding into the urinary system when the RCCs obscured calyces on CT or MRI, but no problems were reported when the tumor merely abutted the calyces.

Cryoablation and RFA have rarely been associated with colorenal fistula formation. In one study of treatment of 100 tumors, RFA of RCC was associated with no complications related to bowel perforation or inflammation, despite tumors being within 1 cm of the bowel in 22 cases.

Ureteral strictures may result from direct thermal injury or perirenal scarring in the inflammatory response to RFA. A safe distance between a proposed RCC ablation and the ureter has not been determined. In one study, strictures of the collecting system developed in 25% (2/8) of tumors within 1 cm of the ureter and in 10% (1/10) of RCCs 1-2 cm away. Stricture did not occur when the ureter was more than 2 cm away from the tumor. Cryoablation is assumed to have a lower rate of ureteric stricture formation but there are case reports of postablation stricture formation in patients treated with cryoablation.

Ablation in the presence of a urinary tract infection has been reported and may result in retroperitoneal abscess formation.

Multisystem injury, disseminated intravascular coagulation, myoglobinuria, and acute lung injury are severe complications associated with large volume hepatic and renal cryoablation, but this complication has not been reported with renal RFA.

Complication rates related to clinical application of microwave, ultrasound, and laser interstitial thermal therapy have not yet been reported.

▬ OUTCOMES AND FOLLOW-UP

Imaging Assessment of Treatment Response

Imaging is critical to response assessment with ablation because tumors are left in situ (Box 26-7). Definitions of residual and local progression of disease remain the same as in liver tumor imaging. In a trial of percutaneous biopsy 1 year or more after RFA of RCC in lesions without CT evidence of local recurrence, there was no evidence of cellular viability. Therefore, CT imaging can reliably monitor treatment efficacy.

While the first scan is performed at 1 month, follow-up unenhanced, parenchymal, and excretory phase contrast-enhanced MRI or CT imaging are performed at 3, 6, and 12 months and

---

Box 26-7. Follow-Up

Contrast-enhanced computed tomography (CT) or magnetic resonance imaging (MRI) can reliably monitor treatment efficacy

First CT or MRI at 1 month

Follow-up CT and MRI at 3, 6, 12 months and then yearly

Ablated lesions checked for enhancement, size change, and metastatic disease

Fat-fluid level in the bladder is common (40%)

Ablation has little effect on renal function

---

then yearly after renal ablation (Fig. 26-3). The intervals between imaging may vary slightly among institutions. The treated tumors are assessed for residual enhancement, size change, and development of new metastatic disease. A thin homogenous rim ("halo") of soft tissue attenuation fibrosis may evolve in the fat peripheral to the tumor in approximately half of patients. CT scan of the pelvis after RFA demonstrates a fluid-fat level in the urinary bladder in 40% of patients (see Fig. 26-1E). The fat-fluid level may resolve and recur. Peripheral nodular enhancement, thick irregular peripheral enhancement, and diffuse tumor enlargement all reflect active tumor. Specific to the renal ablation follow-up, imaging is performed in the excretory phases to detect urine leaks, hydronephrosis, and ureteric injuries. Ablation zone diameters may show significant reduction in size over time. Involution is generally more pronounced after cryoablation than after RFA.

If areas of viable tumor remain amenable to ablation, patients can make additional visits to the radiology department for more ablations. If new tumors develop, then reevaluation can be performed as to whether biopsy and percutaneous ablation is feasible.

Renal Function

There is evidence that RFA of RCC has little effect on renal function in the short term. In a study of 16 patients with a single kidney with an RCC ablated using RFA, one patient who had severe baseline renal insufficiency progressed to end-stage renal disease 2½ years following RFA. Mean glomerular filtration rate (GFR) decreased from 54.2 mL/min/1.73 m^2 preoperatively to 47.5 mL/min/1.73 m^2 at a mean follow-up of 31 months. In a second study, there was no significant change in renal function at 2 years after renal tumor RFA as measured by the serum creatinine level. The mean serum creatinine level was 1.36 ± 0.17 mg/dL before the procedure and 1.6 ± 0.27 mg/dL at the latest follow-up ($P = 0.477$). Similarly, there was no significant difference in the change in the serum creatinine levels when the patients were stratified into two groups: those with a solitary kidney and those with two functioning kidneys.

There is also evidence that ipsilateral radical nephrectomy in the presence of a contralateral normal kidney is associated with significantly more renal insufficiency than partial nephrectomy. Patients who undergo elective surgery for a solitary tumor that is 4 cm or smaller have a 3-year probability that the patient will be free from a new onset eGFR of lower than 60 mL/min per 1.73 m^2 of 35% after radical nephrectomy and 80% after partial nephrectomy.

The need for renal replacement therapy after nephrectomy depends on the demographics and degree of renal disease in patients undergoing surgery, and suffers from selection bias in studies. In one series, 6.5% of patients who had a laparoscopic nephrectomy progressed to end-stage renal disease requiring renal replacement therapy after an average of 8.2 years.

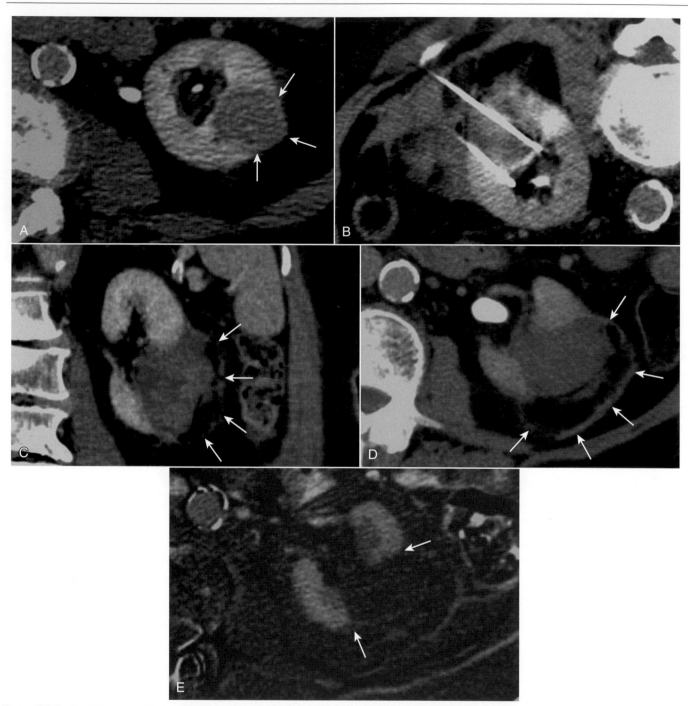

FIGURE 26-3. Radiofrequency ablation (RFA) in a 75-year-old woman with a biopsy-proven left interpolar clear cell renal cell carcinoma (RCC). **A,** Excretory phase contrast-enhanced computed tomography (CT) scan demonstrates a hypoattenuating RCC *(between arrows)*. **B,** Axial postcontrast CT scan with the patient prone demonstrates the RF electrode in the tumor and a small retroperitoneal hematoma. **C,** Postcontrast coronal CT scan at 1 month demonstrates hypodensity of the ablation zone and a peripheral halo *(arrows)* of enhancement in the retroperitoneal fat consistent with ablation. **D,** Postcontrast axial CT scan at 1 month demonstrates hypodensity of the ablation zone and a peripheral halo *(arrows)* of enhancement in the retroperitoneal fat consistent with ablation. **E,** Subtracted arterial phase postcontrast magnetic resonance fat-saturated T1 imaging at 3 months demonstrates no enhancing tumor in the ablation zone (between *arrows*).

■ **SUGGESTED READINGS**

Ahrar K, Matin S, Wood CG, et al. Percutaneous radiofrequency ablation of renal tumors: technique, complications, and outcomes. *J Vasc Interv Radiol.* 2005;16:679-688.

Atwell TD, Farrell MA, Callstrom MR, et al. Percutaneous cryoablation of 40 solid renal tumors with US guidance and CT monitoring: initial experience. *Radiology.* 2007;243:276-283.

Atwell TD, Farrell MA, Leibovich BC, et al. Percutaneous renal cryoablation: experience treating 115 tumors. *J Urol.* 2008;179:2136-2140.

Bretheau D, Lechevallier E, Eghazarian C, et al. Prognostic significance of incidental renal cell carcinoma. *Eur Urol.* 1995;27:319-323.

Cantwell CP, Wah TM, Gervais DA, et al. Protecting the ureter during radiofrequency ablation of renal cell cancer: a pilot study of retrograde pyeloperfusion with cooled dextrose 5% in water. *J Vasc Interv Radiol.* 2008;19:1034-1040.

Chow WH, Devesa SS, Warren JL, Fraumeni Jr JF. Rising incidence of renal cell cancer in the United States. *JAMA.* 1999;281:1628-1631.

Clark PE, Woodruff RD, Zagoria RJ, Hall MC. Microwave ablation of renal parenchymal tumors before nephrectomy: phase I study. *Am J Roentgenol.* 2007;188:1212 1214.

Clark TW, Millward SF, Gervais DA, et al. Reporting standards for percutaneous thermal ablation of renal cell carcinoma. *J Vasc Interv Radiol.* 2006;17: 1563-1570.

Delworth MG, Pisters LL, Fornage BD, von Eschenbach AC. Cryotherapy for renal cell carcinoma and angiomyolipoma. *J Urol.* 1996;155:252-255.

Fielding JR, Aliabadi N, Renshaw AA, Silverman SG. Staging of 119 patients with renal cell carcinoma: the yield and cost-effectiveness of pelvic CT. *AJR Am J Roentgenol.* 1999;172:23-25.

Gervais DA, Arellano RS, McGovern FJ, McDougal WS, Mueller PR. Radiofrequency ablation of renal cell carcinoma: part 2, Lessons learned with ablation of 100 tumors. *AJR Am J Roentgenol.* 2005;185:72-80.

Gervais DA, McGovern FJ, Arellano RS, et al. Renal cell carcinoma: clinical experience and technical success with radiofrequency ablation of 42 tumors. *Radiology.* 2003;226:417-424.

Gervais DA, McGovern FJ, Wood BJ, et al. Radio-frequency ablation of renal cell carcinoma: early clinical experience. *Radiology.* 2000;217:665-672.

Goldberg SN, Charboneau JW, Dodd III GD, et al. Image-guided tumor ablation: proposal for standardization of terms and reporting criteria. *Radiology.* 2003;228:335-345.

Goldberg SN, Hahn PF, Tanabe KK, et al. Percutaneous radiofrequency tissue ablation: does perfusion-mediated tissue cooling limit coagulation necrosis? *J Vasc Interv Radiol.* 1998;9:101-111.

Hafron J, Kaouk JH. Cryosurgical ablation of renal cell carcinoma. *Cancer Control.* 2007;14:211-217.

Jayson M, Sanders H. Increased incidence of serendipitously discovered renal cell carcinoma. *Urology.* 1998;51:203-205.

Kennedy JE. High-intensity focused ultrasound in the treatment of solid tumors. *Nat Rev Cancer.* 2005;5:321-327.

LaGrange CA, Gerber EW, Garrett JE, Lele SM, Strup SE. Interstitial laser ablation of the kidney: acute and chronic porcine study using new-generation diffuser tip fiber. *J Endourol.* 2007;21:1387-1391.

Landman J, Rehman J, Sundaram CP, et al. Renal hypothermia achieved by retrograde intracavitary saline perfusion. *J Endourol.* 2002;16:445-449.

Landman J, Venkatesh R, Lee D, et al. Renal hypothermia achieved by retrograde endoscopic cold saline perfusion: technique and initial clinical application. *Urology.* 2003;61:1023-1025.

Lang K, Danchenko N, Gondek K, Schwartz B, Thompson D. The burden of illness associated with renal cell carcinoma in the United States. *Urol Oncol.* 2007;25:368-375.

Lee SJ, Choyke LT, Locklin JK, Wood BJ. Use of hydrodissection to prevent nerve and muscular damage during radiofrequency ablation of kidney tumors. *J Vasc Interv Radiol.* 2006;17:1967-1969.

Littrup PJ, Ahmed A, Aoun HD, et al. CT-guided percutaneous cryotherapy of renal masses. *J Vasc Interv Radiol.* 2007;18:383-392.

Margulis V, Matsumoto ED, Taylor G, et al. Retrograde renal cooling during radio frequency ablation to protect from renal collecting system injury. *J Urol.* 2005;174:350-352.

Mayo-Smith WW, Dupuy DE, Parikg PM, et al. Imaging-guided percutaneous radiofrequency ablation of solid renal masses: techniques and outcomes of 38 treatment sessions in 32 consecutive patients. *AJR Am J Roentgenol.* 2003;180:1503-1508.

Meraney AM, Gill IS. Financial analysis of open versus laparoscopic radical nephrectomy and nephroureterectomy. *J Urol.* 2002;167:1757-1762.

Neeman Z, Sarin S, Coleman J, Fojo T, Wood BJ. Radiofrequency ablation for tumor-related massive hematuria. *J Vasc Interv Radiol.* 2005;16:417-421.

Onishi T, Nishikawa K, Hasegawa Y, et al. Assessment of health-related quality of life after radiofrequency ablation or laparoscopic surgery for small renal cell carcinoma: a prospective study with medical outcomes Study 36-Item Health Survey (SF-36). *Jpn J Clin Oncol.* 2007;37:750-754.

Pandharipande PV, Gervais DA, Mueller PR, Hur C, Gazelle GS. Radiofrequency ablation versus nephron-sparing surgery for small, unilateral renal cell carcinoma: a cost-effectiveness analysis. *Radiology.* 2008;248:169-178.

Pech M, Janitzky A, Wendler JJ, et al. Irreversible electroporation of renal cell carcinoma: a first in man phase 1 clinical study. *Cardiovasc Intervent Radiol.* 2011;34:132-138.

Raman JD, Stern JM, Zeltser I, Kabbani W, Cadeddu JA. Absence of viable renal carcinoma in biopsies performed more than 1 year following radio frequency ablation confirms reliability of axial imaging. *J Urol.* 2008;179:2142-2145.

Schultze D, Morris CS, Bhave AD, Worgan BA, et al. Radiofrequency ablation of renal transitional cell carcinoma with protective cold saline infusion. *J Vasc Interv Radiol.* 2003;14:489-492.

Silverman SG, Tuncali K, vanSonnenberg E, et al. Renal tumors: MR imaging-guided percutaneous cryotherapy-initial experience in 23 patients. *Radiology.* 2005;236:716-724.

Thomson KR, Cheung W, Ellis SJ, Federman D. Investigation of the safety of irreversible electroporation in humans. *J Vasc Interv Radiol.* 2011;22:611-621.

Wah TM, Arellano RS, Gervais DA, et al. Image-guided percutaneous radiofrequency ablation and incidence of post-radiofrequency ablation syndrome: prospective survey. *Radiology.* 2005;237:1097-1102.

Wah TM, Koenig P, Irving HC, Gervais DA, Mueller PR. Radiofrequency ablation of a central renal tumor: protection of the collecting system with a retrograde cold dextrose pyeloperfusion technique. *J Vasc Interv Radiol.* 2005;16:1551-1555.

Yu J, Liang P, Cheng ZG, et al. US guided percutaneous microwave ablation of renal cell carcinoma: intermediate term results. *Radiology.* 2012;263:900-908.

Zagoria RJ. Imaging-guided radiofrequency ablation of renal masses. *Radiographics.* 2004;24:S59-S71.

Zlotta AR, Schulman CC. Ablation of renal tumors in a rabbit model with interstitial saline-augmented radiofrequency energy. *Urology.* 1999;54:382-383.

CHAPTER 27

Image-Guided Ablation as a Treatment Option for Thoracic Malignancies

Alice M. Kim, MD, and Damian E. Dupuy, MD, FACR

Lung cancer is the leading cause of death in both men and women in the United States. It accounts for approximately 32% of deaths in males and 25% in females. Most patients with primary and secondary lung malignancies are nonsurgical candidates because of poor cardiopulmonary reserve, advanced stage at diagnosis, and severe medical comorbidity. Only about 15% of patients diagnosed with pulmonary malignancies are surgical candidates for open thoracotomy (lobar or sublobar resection). Conventional treatments for patients with lung cancer include external beam radiation therapy with or without systemic chemotherapy. However, chemotherapy and/or radiation therapy is beneficial in only a small percentage of these patients. Many times, no treatment is available and the outcome remains poor. The majority of patients with lung cancer (86%) die of their disease. The overall 5-year survival rate for all clinical stages is dismal at 14%.

Common complications during the course of the disease include pain, dyspnea, cough, hemoptysis, metastases to the musculoskeletal system and central nervous system, obstruction of the superior vena cava, and tracheoesophageal fistula. Therefore palliative care is a crucial part of treatment; however, this is not often successfully achieved. Recent medical literature reports that approximately 50% of patients were dying without adequate pain relief. According to Watson and colleagues, the three main causes of malignancy-related pain are osseous metastatic disease (34%), Pancoast tumor (31%), and chest wall disease (21%). Newer treatment alternatives, such as percutaneous image-guided thermal ablation procedures, may be a viable salvage modality, which will, at minimum, provide symptomatic relief.

Image-guided thermal tumor ablation is a procedure that incorporates direct application of chemicals or thermal therapy to achieve substantial tumor destruction. The advantages of image-guided ablative therapies compared with traditional cancer treatments include reduced morbidity and mortality, in that these procedures are minimally invasive and conserve normal lung tissue, have lower procedural cost, are suitable for real-time imaging guidance, enable the performance of ablations in the outpatient setting, and are synergistic with other cancer treatments. There is also theoretical cytoreduction from thermocoagulation therapy, which allows external beam radiation therapy and/or chemotherapy to be more effective. Grieco and colleagues demonstrated that combined therapy may result in an improved survival over either radiation therapy or radiofrequency ablation (RFA) alone.

Image-guided thermal ablation procedures can be performed on surgically high-risk patients, those who refuse surgery, and those with postoperative recurrence. It is becoming clearer that percutaneous RFA is a safe procedure and technically feasible for unresectable pulmonary malignancies. The goal of thermoablative therapy is to prolong disease-free survival with a reasonable quality of life (Box 27-1).

This chapter discusses the mechanism of image-guided thermal ablation, applications for thermal ablation therapy in the thorax, and the safety and efficacy associated with thermal ablation.

■ RADIOFREQUENCY ABLATION

Patient Evaluation

Patients referred for RFA are initially evaluated in a clinic where the patient's history and pertinent imaging studies are reviewed. During this initial visit, the appropriateness of the RFA procedure, as well as the risks and benefits of the procedure are discussed with the patient and family. All preprocedural studies are ordered. Risks such as bleeding or serious cardiopulmonary issues are addressed, as are the side effects of the RFA, which includes the postablation syndrome. The postablation syndrome is a transient systemic response to the circulating factors such as tumor necrosis factor that results in fever, malaise, and anorexia.

Generally, most patients who are stable enough to undergo computed tomography (CT)-guided needle biopsy are good candidates for pulmonary RFA. Special attention is paid to those patients who only have a single lung remaining and have severe emphysema. Patients with a single lung may need a chest tube after the RFA procedure. Patients with severe emphysema may retain carbon dioxide and lose their respiratory drive. Patients with idiopathic pulmonary fibrosis are considered poor candidates for the pulmonary RFA procedure because exacerbation of the underlying disease may lead to serious respiratory failure and possible death following the RFA procedure.

All patients are told to fast the night before the procedure to limit the risk of sedation-induced nausea and aspiration of gastric contents. Patients with hypertension and cardiac disease are told to take their medications as usual. Insulin-dependent diabetic patients are asked to administer only half of their usual morning insulin dose.

Box 27-1. Rationale for Ablation in Lung Cancer Patients

Most patients with lung cancer are nonsurgical because of advanced stage at diagnosis; only 15% are suitable for surgery

Overall 5-year survival rate for all stages is 14%

Main causes of pain: bone metastasis, Pancoast tumor, and chest wall disease

Goal of ablation is to prolong disease-free survival and improve quality of life

---

Box 27-2. Lung Radiofrequency Ablation Facts

The ideal position for the radiofrequency (RF) probe is along the long axis of the tumor

Normal aerated lung acts as insulation and concentrates RF energy in the tumor

Lung tumor ablation requires less time than similar size liver tumors

Lesions lying close to the visceral pleura are more painful to ablate than deeper lesions

Ablation of lesions near a bronchus may produce a cough response

---

Technique

When the patient arrives at the department, a brief history and physical examination is performed. An intravenous line is placed. Patients are brought to the CT scanner whereby the CT technical staff prepare the patient for the procedure. The appropriate grounding pads are placed on the opposite chest wall from the skin entry site to direct the RF current and prevent damage to adjacent structures in the target area. The site of skin entry is determined using a computer grid after the initial preprocedure images are obtained. The desired skin entry site is matched with the site determined on the computer screen using the horizontal and vertical laser lights in the CT gantry. The skin is prepped and draped in a sterile fashion. A 1% buffered lidocaine hydrochloride solution is used for local anesthesia at the skin and down to the extrapleural soft tissues. Using CT-guided fluoroscopy, the needle tip is identified. A small skin incision is made approximately 1-2 cm into the subcutaneous tissues. The RF electrode is placed through the skin and pleura approximately one-half to two-thirds the distance to the target lesion. The RF electrode angle is corrected as necessary using CT-guided fluoroscopy.

For pleural-based masses, preference is for the shorter RF electrode. Superficial positioning of the electrodes may be difficult from a lateral position due to the protrusion of the electrode in the CT gantry if the gantry is narrow (e.g., 70 cm). A coaxial guiding catheter could also be used in this situation, in which the RF electrode is placed into the mass all at once, after the outer cannula position is confirmed. Central and distal positioning of the RF electrode is adequate for the first ablation for lesions less than 2 cm. The ideal positioning in all RF ablation procedures is along the longitudinal axis so that sequential overlapping tandem ablations can be performed during electrode withdrawal. Lesions larger than 2 cm require larger electrode or several overlapping ablation zones to be performed for adequate thermocoagulation of the target lesion.

The optimal ablative temperature to achieve thermal injury and immediate cell death is 60°-100°C throughout the target volume in a controlled setting. Energy generated during the RFA procedure is accumulated within the lung mass because the normal lung parenchyma acts as an insulator and therefore concentrates the RF energy in the target tissue. There is also a heat sink effect, which dissipates heat away from the normal adjacent tissue and concentrates the energy within the solid component of the target lesion. This same effect may limit successful RFA of larger lesions.

Like for liver tumor ablations, it is best to work around the periphery of larger tumors in the lung to ensure adequate ablation of the soft tissue margins. Large lung tumor ablation procedures require less time and current to achieve adequate thermocoagulation than in liver masses. This may be a result of limited current deposition within small parenchymal masses surrounded by aerated lung. Each ablation should follow the manufacturer's guidelines regarding temperature and/or impedance (Box 27-2).

Conscious sedation is maintained with doses of midazolam (0.5 mg intravenously) and fentanyl (25-50 µg intravenously) during the RF ablation procedure. The nursing staff continuously monitor the patient's vital signs and electrocardiogram throughout the procedure. Generally, pulmonary lesions located away from the visceral pleura require less sedation than painful pleural based lesions. VanSonnenberg and colleagues report using intercostal and paravertebral nerve blocks with long-acting local anesthetic to prevent postprocedural discomfort and pain. RF heating of central lesions near the bronchi may produce a prominent cough response and as a result may require more sedation to prevent patient motion. Vagal nerve stimulation may produce referred pain to the jaw, teeth, chest, or upper extremity similar to pain related to a myocardial ischemic event. If the patient becomes bradycardic, 0.5-mg doses of atropine may be administered. General anesthesia may be necessary for pediatric patients or patients who do not tolerate the RF heating with conscious sedation alone. Dual lumen endotracheal tubes are generally not necessary; given the coagulating effect of the RF current, bleeding related to the RFA procedure is similar to or less than that which occurs with CT-guided biopsies.

Once the target lesion is treated, the RF electrodes are removed and CT-guided fluoroscopy is performed to exclude a pneumothorax. Small asymptomatic pneumothoraces are monitored with immediate and 2-hour postprocedure chest radiographs. These patients are monitored in the recovery room on oxygen for at least 2 hours after the procedure. If the 2-hour postablation chest radiograph demonstrates an increasing pneumothorax or the patient is symptomatic, then a chest catheter is placed and wall suction evacuation is done. If there is interval resolution of the pneumothorax after chest tube placement, the patient is discharged home with a Heimlich valve on the end of the catheter and is told to return in 24 hours for a repeat chest radiograph. Patients are instructed to immediately report any shortness of breath, bloody sputum, or pain. Hospitalization may be required for pain or if the patient is reluctant about outpatient chest tube management. If the pneumothorax is resolved on follow-up, the chest tube is checked for an air leak by having the patient cough with the tube end in a container of sterile water. If no air bubbles are seen, the chest tube is removed with petroleum jelly–based gauze to provide an airtight seal upon removal. Patients with air leaks may require prolonged hospitalization and placement of a surgical chest tube.

Complications

Gillams and colleagues reported that the number of lesions, electrode positions, and anticipated RF electrode trajectory through lung affect the likelihood of pneumothorax development. Therefore careful planning should be performed regarding choice of approach and trajectory of RFA electrode placement. Additionally, Iguchi and colleagues evaluated lung neoplasms close to the heart or aorta for safety and effectiveness. This study looked at 42 patients in two groups: one with tumors 1-9 mm from the heart or aorta (Fig. 27-1) and one with tumors contiguous with the heart or aorta. The overall primary technique effectiveness rate for both

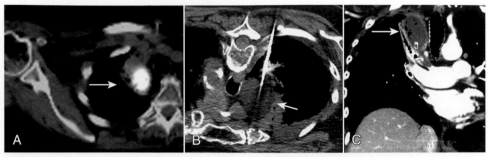

Figure 27-1. An 80-year-old woman with history of bilateral breast cancer status postradiation and chemotherapy in 2000 with fludeoxyglucose (FDG)-avid biopsy-proven metastatic right upper lobe mass abutting the mediastinum and trachea. **A,** Axial positron emission tomography/computed tomography (CT) scan demonstrates an intense focus of FDG uptake in the right lung apex *(arrow)*. **B,** Prone axial nonenhanced CT fluoroscopic image demonstrates the cryoablation probe with ice ball within the mass *(arrow)*. **C,** Coronal contrast-enhanced CT scan demonstrates lack of tumoral enhancement with minimal peripheral enhancement in the ablation site *(arrow)* consistent with adequate treatment 1 month after cryoablation.

groups was 75.8%, 45.9%, and 45.9% at 6, 12, and 24 months, respectively. The local control of tumor was considerably better for the tumors that were close but not contiguous with the heart or aorta. Procedural complications included asymptomatic pleural effusion, pneumothorax, and abscess. No complications related to the specific tumor location occurred. Contraindications to RFA include uncontrollable bleeding diathesis and recent anticoagulation use. According to Skonieczki and colleagues, patients undergoing RFA with implanted cardiac devices such as pacemakers and defibrillators should be cautioned about the possibility of interference with their cardiac devices. The energy in the RF and microwave spectrum (10 RF ablation current [500 KHz] to 10 Hz) can possibly interfere with cardiac devices. According to manufacturers, pacemakers are capable of sensing electrical activity more than 15 cm from the leads and may electrically reset when sensed within 5 cm. Therefore careful positioning of the grounding pads must be performed to direct the flow of the current away from the cardiac device. Microwave ablation (MWA) does not require grounding pads and may be less cumbersome. Coordination with the patient's cardiac electrophysiologists should be done so as to interrogate and program the pacemaker to automatic pacing mode and turn off defibrillators during the RFA procedure. External pacing/defibrillation should be available for emergency use.

The goals of all image-guided thermal ablation procedures are to ablate the tumor and a small margin of normal tissue; avoid injury to blood vessels, central airways, and nerves; and create a large ablation area quickly. Burned tissue and cavitation are limitations of RFA. There is also a theoretical limitation of systemic embolism, including stroke, when small gas bubbles form during burning and "roll-off" impedance. Jin and colleagues reported one case of acute stroke in 200 patients treated. Vaughn and colleagues reported a case of massive hemorrhage in a 70 year-old man undergoing RFA of a lung malignancy. However, the patient was being treated with clopidogrel (Plavix). Other complications include mild-to-moderate intraprocedural pain (usually controlled with adequate analgesics), mild pyrexia (usually self-limiting and lasting up to 1 week), pneumothorax, hemorrhage, hemoptysis, bronchopleural fistulas, acute respiratory distress syndrome, reactive pleural effusion (usually self-limiting), damage to adjacent anatomic structures, skin burns (secondary to inappropriate grounding pad placement), and infection or abscess formation. Sano and colleagues demonstrated in a large single-center study that the overall major complication rate associated with RFA is 17.1%, which included pneumothoraces requiring chest tube placement, pleural effusion requiring drainage, lung abscess, and intrapulmonary hemorrhage. Specifically, the rate of pneumothorax ranges from 9% to 52%. The greater likelihood of pneumothorax development is related to the greater number of pleural punctures, larger needle size, and longer procedure time. Simon and colleagues performed a retrospective study and found the rate of pneumothorax to be 28.4% with a 9.8% chest

Box 27-3. Lung Radiofrequency Complications

Development of pneumothorax is influenced by number of pleural punctures, needle size, and duration of procedure
Tumors contiguous with the heart or aorta have poorer results
Radiofrequency (RF) can interfere with pacemaker devices
Overall, major lung RF ablation complication rate is 17%
Pleural effusions postablation occur in 4%-16%
Pneumothorax rate varies from 9% to 52%

tube insertion rate. Hiraki and colleagues also showed that male patients, as well as patients with no prior history of pulmonary surgery and a greater number of tumors ablated, were at increased risk for pneumothorax. Patients whose tumors were treated in the upper lobes were also at increased risk for chest tube placement for pneumothorax. Pleural effusions occur at a rate of 4%-16% (Box 27-3).

IMAGING FOLLOW-UP

There is no proven imaging modality or time interval for immediate postablation imaging and subsequent imaging to accurately depict success or failure of the initial ablation. Follow-up imaging is used to evaluate interval growth and necessity for repeat ablation. The current follow-up strategy used at our institution is to obtain a 48- to 72-hour postablation imaging study to evaluate the appearance of the ablated lesion. There may be a "cockade phenomenon," which demonstrates concentric rings of varying density.

At 24-48 hours, there is greater than four times the amount of ground-glass opacification in completely RF-ablated lesions (Fig. 27-2). Bojarski and colleagues noted rapid resolution of ground-glass opacity by the end of the first month in 25 of 26 patients. Cavitations may be seen in 25%-31% of the lesions treated and are more commonly seen when the size of the lesion at 1 week exceeds pretreatment size by more than 200% (see Fig. 27-2). Approximately 60% of cavitations decrease in size on follow-up scans. Bubble lucencies may be seen in up to 31% of all cases of RF-ablated lesions (see Fig. 27-2). At 1 week to 1 month after RFA, the lesion can appear as an area of consolidation or nodules with the mean diameter usually larger than the preablative size. Bojarski and colleagues noted pleural thickening in 55% and linear opacification between the treated lesion and adjacent pleura in 64%. Pleural effusions were noted in 15%. At 2-6 months after the ablation, cross-sectional imaging may demonstrate no change or decreased size of the tumor compared to the post-RFA baseline study in patients with complete response (Box 27-4).

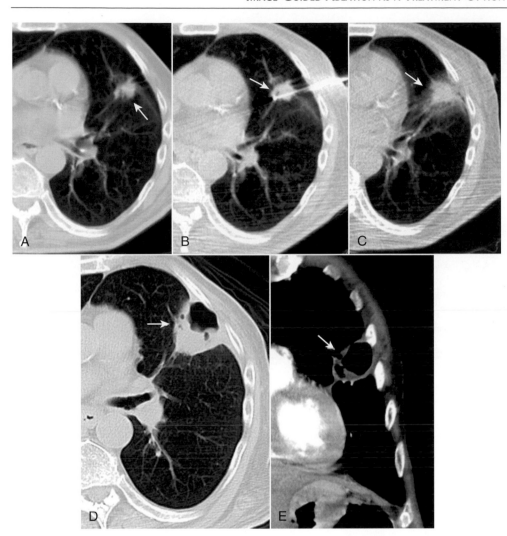

FIGURE 27-2. A 73-year-old man with recurrent disease 7 months after microwave ablation for non–small cell lung cancer. **A,** Axial supine computed tomography (CT) scan before radiofrequency ablation (RFA) demonstrates a 2-cm left lingular nodule *(arrow).* **B,** Fluoroscopic CT image obtained during RFA shows position of the three RF electrodes in the lingular nodule *(arrow).* **C,** Supine CT scan obtained immediately following the RFA procedure and removal of electrode shows increased parenchymal density with peripheral ground-glass opacity surrounding the tumor corresponding to lesion-induced RF heat *(arrow).* No pneumothorax was seen. **D,** CT scan obtained at the same level as in C 3 months later demonstrates a well-circumscribed mass with peripheral cavitation and bubble lucencies internally *(arrow).* **E,** Contrast-enhanced reconstructed coronal CT scan demonstrates no significant peripheral enhancement to suggest recurrent or residual disease at the site of ablation *(arrow).*

Box 27-4. Imaging Features After Lung Radiofrequency Ablation

At 24-48 hours, there is greater than 4 times the amount of ground-glass density (GGO) in ablated lesions
GGO resolves by 1 month
Cavitation is seen in 25%-30% of ablated lesions
Bubble lucencies can be seen in up to 31%
By 2 months, computed tomography may demonstrate no change or decreased size of tumor

---

An enhancing rim of soft tissue around the ablation zone is considered reactive if uniform and less than 5 mm in thickness. A confirmatory positron emission tomography (PET) scan can subsequently be performed. PET scan may be used to follow up post-RFA lesions. A decrease or complete absence of FDG activity (photopenia) is suggestive of necrosis with no residual tumor (Fig. 27-3). If there is residual or recurrent tumor, there is increased FDG uptake within the periphery of the lesion. Akeboshi and colleagues demonstrated that PET was more sensitive than contrast-enhanced CT to detect early tumor progression. Another more recent study by Yoo and colleagues as part of the ACOSOG Z4033 lung cancer RFA trial studied early and 6-month follow-up FDG PET in 26 patients with early stage non–small cell lung cancer. They showed that early PET within 96 hours did not predict treatment outcome but the 6-month follow-up PET did.

Nodule CT densitometry can be performed to evaluate nodule enhancement after contrast administration by assessing the difference in vasculature of benign versus malignant lesions. A study by Suh and colleagues demonstrated significant decrease in mean contrast enhancement at 1-2 months' follow-up (see Fig. 27-3). At 3 months, Suh and colleagues demonstrated a slight interval increase in contrast enhancement, although it was less than the preablation study. Lesion size and degree of enhancement are useful criteria for following post-RFA lesions. One pitfall is that most RFA-treated tumors demonstrate heterogeneous enhancement and may fail to identify tumor activity. There may also be viable areas within a lesion, usually within the periphery of the zone of ablation in a crescentic or nodular shape.

At our institution, the overall increase in size of the soft tissue ablation zone 1.25 times that of the greatest diameter of the baseline CT after ablation, is considered local progression of disease (Figs. 27-4 and 27-5). The presence of soft tissue larger than 9 mm in the maximum dimension with evidence of contrast enhancement (>15 HU) is also indicative of local progression of disease (Box 27-5; see Figs. 27-4 and 27-5).

Radiofrequency Ablation in Primary Versus Secondary Lung Tumors

Primary lung malignancy patients who are nonsurgical candidates may benefit significantly from RFA. This cohort of patients may undergo RFA as a means to cure a small early-stage lung cancer. Others may use it as a palliative measure to achieve tumor

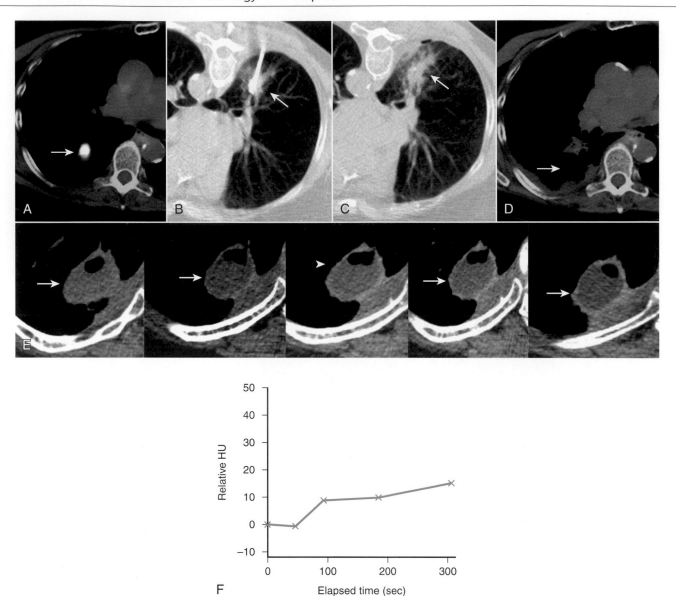

Figure 27-3. An 83-year-old woman with a 2.5-cm biopsy-proven non–small cell lung cancer in the right lower lobe. **A,** Axial positron emission tomography (PET)/computed tomography (CT) image demonstrates increased fludeoxyglucose (FDG) uptake within the right lower lobe pulmonary nodule *(arrow)*. **B,** Axial prone image shows the radiofrequency (RF) electrode within the tumor *(arrow)*. **C,** Axial prone image obtained immediately following the RF ablation demonstrates surrounding ground-glass opacity *(arrow)*. **D,** Axial PET/CT scan 48 hours postablation through the same level as in **A** demonstrates an area of photopenia with mild surrounding increased FDG activity consistent with postablation changes *(arrow)*. **E,** Axial contrast-enhanced images 3 months postablation at 0, 45, 90, 180, and 300 seconds demonstrates no significant enhancement to suggest recurrent or residual tumor. Note benign peritumoral enhancement *(arrow)*. **F,** Relative Hounsfield units versus time demonstrates no significant enhancement (>15 HU) to suggest recurrent tumor within the ablation bed.

reduction before chemotherapy or radiation therapy. Simon and colleagues retrospectively reviewed 153 consecutive patients with 189 primary or metastatic inoperable lung cancers who received RFA and had a median 20.5-month follow-up period. The long-term Kaplan-Meier median 1-, 2-, 3-, 4-, and 5-year survival rates for stage 1 non–small cell lung cancer were 78%, 57%, 36%, 27%, and 27%, respectively, demonstrating a survival benefit especially in nonsurgical candidates. The corresponding survival rates for colorectal pulmonary metastases were 87%, 78%, 57%, 57%, and 57%. However, most of these patients received prior and/or adjuvant chemotherapy; therefore the sole effect of RFA is difficult to evaluate. The 1-, 2-, 3-, 4-, and 5-year local tumor progression-free rates were 83%, 64%, 57%, 47%, and 47%, respectively, for tumors 3 cm or smaller and 45%, 25%, 25%, 25%, and 25% for tumors larger than 3 cm. Tumor size was a statistically significant predictor of local tumor progression.

A large single-center prospective study by de Baère and colleagues followed 60 patients, each with five or fewer tumors with diameters of less than 4 cm. Ninety-seven of 100 targeted tumors were treated; overall survival rate was 71% and lung disease–free survival at 18 months was 34%. At 18 months, the overall survival rates were 76% for primary lung tumors and 71% for metastatic disease (Fig. 27-6). This study also reports a 54% rate of pneumothorax, with chest tube placement in 9% of the procedures. Lencioni and colleagues published their results from a large multicenter study known as the RAPTURE (radiofrequency ablation of pulmonary tumors response evaluation) trial, which included 106 patients. In this study, there were 33 non–small cell lung cancer patients. The 2-year overall survival was 48%. However, most of these high-risk patients died of non–cancer-related causes, as indicated by their 2-year cancer-specific survival, which was much higher at 92%.

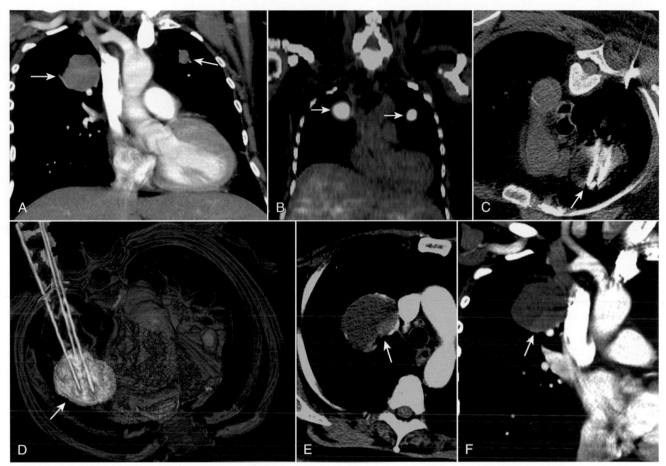

FIGURE 27-4. A 63-year-old woman with metastatic rectal carcinoma to the brain and lungs (bilateral upper lobes). Debulking was performed with microwave ablation before radiation therapy. **A,** Coronal contrast-enhanced computed tomography (CT) scan demonstrates bilateral upper lobe enhancing pulmonary masses (attenuation, 100 HU), which are highly suspicious for metastatic colorectal carcinoma *(arrows)*. **B,** Positron emission tomography/CT scan shows fludeoxyglucose-avid uptake within the bilateral upper lobe masses consistent with biopsy-proven metastatic rectal carcinoma *(arrows)*. **C,** CT-guided fluoroscopy shows the microwave antennae placement within the tumor *(arrow)*. **D,** Three-dimensional reconstructed shaded-surface display image shows three microwave antennae within the right upper lobe mass *(arrow)*. **E,** Axial contrast-enhanced CT scan at the same level as in **F** demonstrates peripheral nodular areas of enhancement posteriorly within the ablation bed, suspicious for residual tumor *(arrow)*. **F,** Coronal contrast-enhanced image through the chest demonstrates nodular enhancing residual tissue inferiorly, suspicious for residual tumor *(arrow)*.

Dupuy and colleagues prospectively studied 24 consecutive medically inoperable patients with stage 1 non–small cell lung carcinoma who were treated with CT-guided RFA followed by radiation therapy (dose of 66 Gy). All tumors were successfully treated with post-RFA temperatures of greater than 60°C and a mean treatment time of 6.8 minutes. The mean follow-up period was 26.7 months and cumulative survival rates at the end of 12, 24, and 60 months were 83%, 50%, and 39%, respectively.

A smaller study by Thanos and colleagues reviewed 27 CT-guided RFA procedures in 22 patients, 14 patients with primary lung cancer and eight with metastatic lung neoplasms. This study demonstrated that RFA is a useful palliative treatment in nonsurgical patients with primary or metastatic lung tumor with a low associated morbidity and mortality. The median progression-free interval for primary lung cancer was 26.2 months and for metastatic tumors was 29.2 months.

In 2004, Lee and colleagues studied 32 patients with early stage non–small cell lung cancer and showed that 100% of tumors less than 3 cm had complete necrosis with no evidence of enhancement at the treatment site, generally with a diameter greater than the preablation diameter. However, larger lesions greater than 3 cm only demonstrated 8% necrosis. The mean survival rate with complete necrosis was higher than in patients with partial necrosis (19.7 vs. 8.7 months). See Box 27-6. Zemlyak and colleagues compared sublobar resection, RFA, and cryoablation in a prospective randomized fashion in 64 patients with non–small cell lung cancer. The probability of 3-year survival for the surgical, RFA, and cryoablation groups was 87.1%, 87.5%, and 77%, respectively, which was not statistically significant. The 3-year cancer-specific and cancer-free survival for the surgical, RFA, and cryoablation groups was 90.6% and 60.8%, 87.5% and 50%, and 90.2% and 45.6%, respectively. The cohort of patients was small and the study was likely underpowered to show statistical significance between the groups.

Metastatic disease is an indication of widespread disease; however, in certain tumors, the metastatic disease process may be isolated to the lungs. In these patients who have a finite number of metastatic lesions in the lung and a tumor with favorable biologic characteristics (e.g., soft tissue sarcoma, renal cell carcinoma, and colorectal carcinoma), resection is a consideration to improve prognosis. Factors that contribute to improved prognosis include nodule size, completeness of resection, and lymph node status. Indications for surgical resection include exclusion of other distant disease, no tumor at the primary site, the likelihood of complete resection, and adequate cardiopulmonary reserve to withstand general anesthesia for an extended period of time. The overall 5-year survival rate after surgical resection of pulmonary metastatic lesions of different tumor types is approximately 36% and mortality approximately less than 2%.

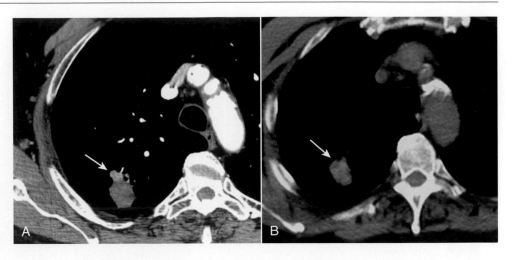

FIGURE 27-5. A 65-year-old man with non–small cell lung cancer after radiofrequency ablation (RFA) with 3-month follow-up computed tomography (CT) scan demonstrating a 7-mm nodular focus of enhancement in the anterior-most aspect of the ablation bed, which demonstrated increased fludeoxyglucose (FDG) uptake consistent with residual tumor. **A,** Axial contrast-enhanced CT-scan obtained 3 months after RF ablation demonstrates a 7-mm focal nodular area of enhancement *(arrow).* **B.** Axial positron emission tomography (PET)/CT scan 6 months after RFA shows focal area of mild FDG uptake (standardized uptake value [SUV] 1.3), which correlates with the nodular area of enhancement seen on CT scan *(arrow).* The current SUV is slightly higher compared to the PET/CT performed immediately 48 hours postablation and is suspicious for residual tumor. The patient underwent repeat ablation of the small residual focus of tumor. **C,** CT-densitometry time density graph of the nodular enhancement shows the intense (60 HU) enhancement within the first 4 minutes after contrast *(arrow).*

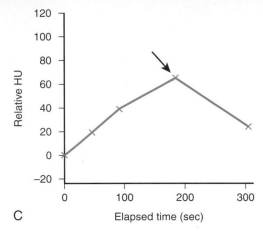

Box 27-5. Imaging Features of Recurrence

A uniform enhancing rim less than 5 mm thick is considered reactive

An increase in size of the ablated lesion more than 1.25 times the size of the original lesion is considered to be local progression

Enhancing soft tissue > 9 mm also suggests local progression

PET is more accurate than contrast enhanced CT for follow-up

There is yet to be a defined size and number of lesions appropriate for thermal ablation therapies. However, the parameters applied for RF ablation of liver tumors (i.e., four or fewer metastatic lesions) are applied to the lung. The maximum size has not been established; however, a study by Kang and colleagues showed that tumors less than 3.5 cm in diameter were relatively well contained. They also demonstrated that lesions less than 3 cm were optimal for the current thermal ablation technology. Another study by Yan and colleagues demonstrated that 70% of patients with lesions greater than 3 cm in size died within 14 months of treatment. The median survival of the entire cohort was 33 months. The exclusion criteria used by Yan and colleagues included more than six lesions per hemithorax, lesions with a diameter greater than 5 cm, international normalized ration greater than 1.5, platelets less than 100×10^9, and extrapulmonary metastatic disease.

A study by Kondo and colleagues demonstrated that metastatic lesions from renal cell carcinoma, sarcoma, and colorectal carcinoma patients will benefit from image-guided thermal ablation procedures. This is critical for patients with renal cell carcinoma because approximately one third of patients will develop pulmonary metastatic lesions and approximately one half of patients who had nephrectomies will develop pulmonary metastases in the future. The biology of metastatic lesions is not optimal for treatment with radiation. Therefore alternative treatments such as thermal ablation can be administered in tandem with many systemic therapies. The survival outcomes of the thermal ablation group with or without adjuvant therapy compare favorably when compared with the surgical cohorts. The presumed theory of RFA palliation is through cytoreduction, destruction of adjacent sensory neural fibers, and decreased neural stimulation by debulking.

■ MICROWAVE ABLATION

MWA is the most recent addition to the field of tumor ablation. It can be performed percutaneously, laparoscopically, or through open surgical access. Electromagnetic microwaves traveling at 9.2×10^8 Hz produce friction and heat by agitating water molecules within the surrounding tissues and causing the molecules to flip. This procedure induces coagulation necrosis and cell death.

The advantages of microwave ablation include consistently higher intratumoral temperatures, larger tumor ablation volumes, fast ablation times, use of multiple applicators, more effective heating of cystic masses, and improved convection profile. The greater diameter of thermocoagulation possible with MWA is likely due to the higher intratumoral temperatures achieved. There is also increased affinity for water-based tissues and decreased heat sink effect.

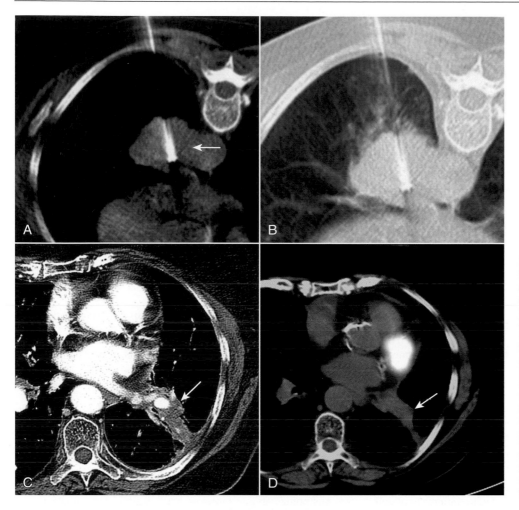

FIGURE 27-6. A 79-year-old man with biopsy-proven non–small cell lung cancer abutting the aorta for radiofrequency ablation (RFA). **A,** Axial prone computed tomography (CT) scan demonstrates 3-cm pulmonary mass abutting the aorta with the RF electrode within the tumor bed *(arrow)*. **B,** Axial prone CT fluoroscopic image at the same level as in **A** in lung windows. **C,** Axial contrast-enhanced CT scan through the level of the pulmonary veins 3 years postablation and radiation therapy shows residual scar, but no evidence of residual enhancing tumor post-RFA *(arrow)*. **D,** Three-year follow-up axial positron emission tomography/CT scan demonstrates mild FDG uptake isointense to mediastinal background in the site of prior RFA with no evidence of residual or recurrent tumor *(arrow)*.

Box 27-6. Lung Radiofrequency Ablation Facts

Primary tumors less than 3 cm in size are associated with a better response to ablation

Primary tumor size is a statistically significant predictor of local tumor progression

A survival benefit has been demonstrated for radiofrequency ablation (RFA) in nonsurgical lung cancer patients

RFA may have a synergistic effect with chemotherapy/radiotherapy by achieving tumor reduction

---

MWA has been successfully used in treatment of hepatic malignancies by several groups. Currently in the United States there are six commercially available microwave systems that use either a 915-MHz (Evident, Covidien, Boulder, Colo.; MicrothermX, BSD Medical, Salt Lake City, Utah; Avecure, Medwaves, San Diego, Calif.) or 2450-MHz (Certus 140, Neuwave, Madison, Wisc.; Amica, Hospital Service, Rome, Italy; Acculis MTA, Microsulis Medical Limited, Hampshire, UK) generator and straight antennae with varying active tips of 0.6-4 cm. Perfusion of the antennae shaft is required in five of the six systems either with room temperature fluid or carbon dioxide to reduce conductive heating of the nonactive portion of the antenna, thus preventing damage to the skin and tissues proximal to the active tip. A single applicator is used with a single generator in four of the systems. Two of the systems have the ability to power up to three antennas with a single generator. Because most of the microwave systems are newly FDA approved, there are no published data yet on their differences in safety or effectiveness. Percutaneous microwave tissue ablation has been FDA approved since 2010. There are at least three MVA devices. The only study in the English literature by Wolf and colleagues using a 915-MHz microwave system studied 50 patients who underwent 66 percutaneous MWAs for 82 intraparenchymal pulmonary masses without chest wall involvement. Patients were followed for a mean period of 10 ± 6.8 months, and during this time, 22% of patients (11/50) were found to have new disease distant from the ablation site. Progressive disease within the treated lobe, but not at the ablation site, was found in 9 of 11 patients, and new metastatic foci in untreated lobes or organs were found in 2 of 11 patients as evidenced by enhancement on routine contrast-enhanced CT or FDG avidity on PET scan. This resulted in a 1-year local control rate of 67% $\pm$ 10% with a mean 16.2 ± 1.3 months to first recurrence distant from the ablation site. Presence of residual enhancing tumor was more commonly found in follow-up of treated tumors greater than 3 cm. Thus index tumor size greater than 3 cm was predictive of residual disease in these patients ($P = 0.01$). However, the presence of residual disease did not correlate with reduced overall survival. The Kaplan-Meier median time to death for all patients (n=50) due to any cause, including the pulmonary malignancy being treated, was 19 ± 1 months. The 1-, 2-, and 3-year actuarial survival rates were 65% $\pm$ 7%, 55% $\pm$ 9%, and 45% $\pm$ 11%, respectively. Analysis of cancer-specific mortality yielded a median time to death of 22 ± 1 month and 1-, 2-, and 3-year survival rates of 83 $\pm$ 6%, 73 $\pm$ 9%, and 61 $\pm$ 13%, respectively.

On initial postablation contrast-enhanced CT, the ablated index tumor was changed in appearance, demonstrating the effects of thermally induced coagulation necrosis. A hazy ground-glass opacification was most commonly observed within and extending from the zone of ablation penetrated by well-defined antennae tracts. At 1-, 3-, and 6-month intervals, ablated tumors (zones of ablation) were measured, and mean maximum postablation diameters were compared with index dimensions. Preliminary data revealed an initial increase in size of 2.4 cm, ($P = 0.02$) with a mean increase in maximum diameter of 0.65 ± 0.27 cm, due to thermal changes in adjacent lung tissue, which was then followed by a persistent reduction in diameter, consistent with consolidation. Cavitary changes were identified in 35 of 82 (43%) treated tumors (26 of 50 patients, 52%); these had a statistically significant inverse relationship to cancer specific mortality ($P = 0.02$). This result may be explained by the fact that cavitary changes occur more frequently when there is more complete tumor kill and the local tissue blood supply has been thermocoagulated.

Like for RFA, percutaneous MWA is usually performed with the patient under conscious sedation (with intravenous midazolam and fentanyl). In certain situations when procedure pain is a problem, general anesthesia is used. Patients are monitored with continuous pulse oximetry and electrocardiography with blood pressure measurements performed every 5 minutes. The standard surgical preparation and draping are performed. Local anesthesia is achieved with 1% buffered lidocaine hydrochloride solution. Using CT or ultrasound guidance, the tumor is localized and the optimal approach is determined. A microwave antenna is then placed within the tumor (see Fig. 27-4). The exposed noninsulated portion of the antenna, which emits the electromagnetic microwave, is placed at the distal margin of the lesion. Because of the inherent properties of the electromagnetic wave, grounding is not necessary with MWA. Intratumoral temperatures can be measured with separately placed thermocouple devices. Unlike in RFA, tissue charring is not a significant limitation of electromagnetic wave propagation used in MWA (Box 27-7).

CRYOABLATION

Percutaneous cryoablation (CA) allows gas in a region of constant temperature to travel through a porous plug of cotton into an area of lower pressure thereby allowing the gas to expand and become cooler. This was first performed by Joule and Thompson (Lord Kelvin) and is therefore known as the Joule-Thompson effect. Argon gas allows expansion from high pressure to low pressure through a constricted orifice (J-T port) within the cryoprobe at ultracold temperatures (approximately −160°C) and forms an ice ball as a marker for identifying the ablative margins (see Fig. 27-1). At the end of the procedure, helium gas is used to warm the probe and facilitate removal. Currently, there are two commercially available percutaneous argon-based cryoablation devices available (Cryohit, Galil Medical, Plymouth Meeting, Pa., and Cryocare, Endocare Inc, Irvine, Calif.). These systems allow the placement of between 1 and 15 individual 1.5- to 2.4-mm diameter cryoprobes. At our institution, each CA treatment consists of a 10-minute freeze, followed by an 8-minute thaw, and then another 10-minute freeze. One advantage of CA is the ability to preserve collagenous and other structural cellular architecture in any frozen tissue. Another advantage is ice ball visualization

under CT allows for direct comparison of the ablative zone in relation to the tumor margins, thus giving the operator greater confidence when treating tumor near critical structures, and allows for measuring the cytotoxic ice margin which lies 3-7 mm within the most peripheral aspect of the ice ball as described by Hinshaw and colleagues.

Kawamura and colleagues performed cryoablation on metastatic pulmonary lesions on 35 tumors in 20 patients showing a 1-year survival rate of 89.4% with local recurrence of seven tumors in seven patients (20%). The primary tumors of the study patients were colorectal (30%), lung cancer (25%), liver cancer (10%), soft tissue sarcomas (10%), head and neck cancer (10%), uterine cancer (10%), and renal cancer (5%). Wang and colleagues studied the feasibility and safety of the procedure for thoracic malignancy and demonstrated that tumor size and location were highly predictive of tumor ice coverage even when controlled for tumor stage and type. A short-term follow-up showed palliative benefits of cryoablation in terms of general health status with increased dietary intake and weight gain.

CONCLUSION

Image-guided thermal ablation procedures are best suited for medically inoperable, high-risk patients with early-stage lung cancers, patients with small, oligonodular and favorably located pulmonary metastatic lesions, and patients who seek palliative measures for tumor-related symptoms or chest recurrences within treatment fields. Image-guided thermal ablation can be repeated and have synergistic effects when combined with other cancer treatments. Further research is being performed to identify the ideal tumor size, cell type, tumor morphology and location. In addition the appropriate imaging follow-up criteria and timing to accurately determine the treatment success has yet to be completely defined. In the future, further delineation of which thermal ablation technique is best for the various clinical scenarios should be performed. Additionally, new advances and emerging technology should be focused on greater ablation volume in shorter time periods with real-time monitoring of the treatment effects.

SUGGESTED READINGS

Akeboshi M, Yamakado K, Nakatsuka A, et al. Percutaneous radiofrequency ablation of lung neoplasms, initial therapeutic response. *JVIR.* 2004;15:463-470.
Bojarski JD, Dupuy DE, Mayo-Smith WW. CT imaging findings of pulmonary neoplasms after treatment with RFA results in 32 tumors. *AJR Am J Roentgenol.* 2005;185:466-471.
de Baère T, Palussière J, Aupèrin A, et al. Midterm local efficacy and survival after radiofrequency ablation of lung tumors with minimum follow up of 1 year: prospective evaluation. *Radiol.* 2006;240(2):587-596.
Dupuy DE, DiPetrillo T, Gandhi S, et al. Radiofrequency ablation followed by conventional radiotherapy for medically inoperable Stage 1 non-small cell lung cancer. *Chest.* 2006;129:738-745.
Dupuy DE, Goldberg NS. Image-guided radiofrequency tumor ablation: challenges and opportunities-part II. *J Vasc Interv Radiol.* 2001;12:1135-1148.
Dupuy DE, Mayo-Smith WW, Abbott GF, et al. Clinical applications of radio-frequency tumor ablation in the thorax. *Radiographics.* 2002;22:259-269.
Dupuy DE, Zagoria RJ, Akerley W, et al. Percutaneous radiofrequency ablation of malignancies in the lung. *AJR Am J Roentgenol.* 2000;174:57-59.
Gadaleta C, Catino A, Ranieri F, et al. Radiofrequency thermal ablation of 69 lung neoplasms. *J Chemother.* 2004;16:86-89.
Ghandi NS, Dupuy DE. Image-guided radiofrequency ablation as a new treatment option for patients with lung cancer. *Semin Roentgenol.* 2005:171-181.
Gillams AR, Lees WR. Analysis of the factors associated with radiofrequency ablation-induced pneumothorax. *Clin Radiol.* 2007;62:639-644.
Goldberg SN, Dupuy DE. Image-guided radiofrequency tumor ablation: challenges and opportunities-part 1. *J Vasc Interv Radiol.* 2001;12:1021-1032.
Goldberg SN, Gazelle GS, Mueller PR. Thermal ablation therapy for focal malignancy: a unified approach to underlying principles, techniques, and diagnostic imaging guidance. *AJR Am J Roentgenol.* 2000;174:323-331.
Griffin JP, Nelson JE, Koch KA, et al. End of life care in patients with lung cancer. *Chest.* 2003;123(suppl 1):312S-331S.
Grieco CA, Simon CJ, Mayo-Smith WW, et al. Percutaneous image-guided thermal ablation and radiation therapy: Outcomes of combined treatment for 41 patients with inoperable stage 1/II non-small cell lung cancer. *J Vasc Int Radiol.* 2006;17:1117-1124.

Hinshaw JL, Sampson L, Lee Jr FT, Laeseke PF, Brace CL. Does selective intubation increase ablation zone size during pulmonary cryoablation? *J Vasc Interv Radiol.* 2008;19:1497-1501.

Hiraki T, Tajiti N, Mimua H, et al. Pneumothorax, pleural effusion and chest tube placement after radiofrequency ablation of lung tumors: Incidence and risk factors. *Radiol.* 2006;241:275-283.

Hoffman PC, Mauer AM, Vokes EE. Lung cancer. *Lancet.* 2000;355:479-485.

Iguchi T, Hiraki T, Gobara H, et al. Percutaneous radiofrequency ablation of lung tumors close to the heart or aorta: evaluation of safety and effectiveness. *J Vasc Interv Radiol.* 2007;18:733-740.

Jain SK, Dupuy DE, Cardarelli GA, et al. Percutaneous radiofrequency ablation of pulmonary malignancies: combined treatment with brachytherapy. *AJR Am J Roentgenol.* 2003;181:711-715.

Jin GY, Lee JM, Lee YC, et al. Primary and secondary lung malignancies treated with percutaneous radiofrequency ablation: evaluation with follow-up CT. *AJR Am J Roentgenol.* 2004;183:1013-1020.

Kang S, Luo R, Liao W, et al. Single group study to evaluate the feasibility and complications of radiofrequency ablation and usefulness of post treatment position emission tomography in lung tumors. *World J Surg Oncol.* 2004;2:30.

Kondo H, Okumura T, Ohde Y, et al. Surgical treatment for metastatic malignancies. Pulmonary metastasis: indications and outcomes. *Int J Clin Oncol.* 2005;10:81-85.

Kvale PA, Simoff M, Prakash UB, American College of Chest Physicians. Lung cancer: palliative care. *Chest.* 2003;123(suppl 1):284S-311S.

Lee JM, Jin GY, Goldberg SN, et al. Percutaneous radiofrequency ablation for inoperable non-small cell lung cancer and metastases: preliminary report. *Radiology.* 2004;230:125-134.

Lencioni RR, Crocetti L, Cioni R, et al. Response to radiofrequency ablation of pulmonary tumours: a prospective, intention-to-treat, multicentre clinical trial (the RAPTURE study). *Lancet Oncol.* 2008;9:621-628.

Licker M, Spiliopoulos A, Frev JG, et al. Risk factors for early mortality and major complications following pneumonectomy for non-small cell lung carcinoma of the lung. *Chest.* 2002;121:1890-1897.

Munden RF, Swisher SS, Stevens CW. Imaging of the patient with non-small cell lung cancer. *Radiology.* 2005:803-818.

Piltz S, Meimarakis G, Wichmann MW, et al. Long-term results after pulmonary resection of renal cell carcinoma metastases. *Ann Thorac Surg.* 2002;73:1082-1087.

Sano Y, Kanazawa S, Gobara H, et al. Feasibility of percutaneous radiofrequency ablation for intrathoracic malignancies: a large single-center experience. *Cancer.* 2007;109:1397-1405.

Skonieczki BD, Wells C, Wasser EJ, Dupuy DE. Radiofrequency and microwave tumor ablation in patients with implanted cardiac devices: is it safe? *Eur J Radiol.* 2011;79:343-346.

Steinke K, King J, Glenn D, Morris DL. Radiologic appearance and complications of percutaneous computed tomography-guided radiofrequency ablated pulmonary metastases from colorectal carcinoma. *J Comput Assist Tomogr.* 2003;27:750-757.

Suh RD, Wallace AB, Sheehan RE, et al. Unresectable pulmonary malignancies: CT guided percutaneous radiofrequency ablation-preliminary results. *Radiology.* 2003;229:821-829.

Thanos L, Mylona S, Pomoni M, et al. Percutaneous radiofrequency thermal ablation of primary and metastatic lung tumors. *Eur J Cardiothorac Surg.* 2006;30:797-800.

Todd TR. The surgical treatment of pulmonary metastases. *Chest.* 1997;112:287S-290.

VanSonnenberg E, Shankar S, Morrison PR, et al. Radiofrequency ablation of thoracic lesions: part 2 initial clinical experience-technical and multidisciplinary considerations in 30 patients. *AJR Am J Roentgenol.* 2005;184:381-390.

Vaughn C, Mychashkiw G, Sewell P. Massive hemorrhage during radiofrequency ablation of a pulmonary neoplasm. *Anesth Analg.* 2002;94:1149-1151.

Watson PN, Evans RJ. Intractable pain with lung cancer. *Pain.* 1987;29:163–173.

Wolf F, DiPetrillo TA, Machan J, Mayo-Smith WW, Dupuy DE. Microwave ablation of lung malignancies: effectiveness, CT findings and safety in 50 patients. *Radiology.* 2008;247:871-879.

Yan T, King J, Sjarif A, et al. Percutaneous radiofrequency ablation of pulmonary metastases from colorectal carcinoma prognostic determinants for survival. *Ann Surg Oncol.* 2006;13:1529-1537.

Yoo DC, Dupuy DE, Hillman SJ, et al. Radiofrequency ablation of medically inoperable stage 1A non-small cell lung cancer: are early posttreatment PET findings predictive of treatment outcome? *AJR.* 2011;11:1529-1537.

Zemlyak A, Moore WH, Bilfinger TV. Comparison of survival after sublobar resections and ablative therapies for stage I non-small cell lung cancer. *J Am Coll Surg.* 2010;211:68-72.

CHAPTER 28

Image-Guided Ablation of Liver Tumors

Colin P. Cantwell, FRCR, FFR, and Debra A. Gervais, MD

Treatment of primary or metastatic hepatic tumors includes surgical resection, hepatic transplantation (for hepatocellular carcinoma), systemic drug therapy, and transarterial chemo and radioembolic therapy. Limited disease may be amenable to surgical resection. However, only 10%-20% of patients with primary hepatocellular carcinoma (HCC) and colorectal metastatic liver tumors are candidates for curative surgical resection. Many patients are deemed unsuitable for potentially curative surgical techniques because of tumor multifocality and size, portal venous tumor invasion, underlying advanced liver cirrhosis, comorbid conditions at the time of selection, tumor growth, development or progression of comorbid conditions, and development of advanced local and/or metastatic disease outside the liver in the period from selection for transplantation and availability of a donor organ.

Even with patient selection, surgical techniques are associated with 2%-5% mortality and 20% morbidity. The development of needle applicators and chemical ablative techniques for tumor ablation has provided less invasive treatment options to selected patients who are otherwise unsuitable for hepatic surgery. This chapter focuses on percutaneous ablation procedures. Other treatments such as transarterial chemoembolization and selective intraarterial radioembolization are discussed elsewhere.

METHODS OF ABLATION

Three groups of image-guided ablation exist: chemical ablation, thermal ablation, and cell membrane perforation with electroporation (Box 28-1). Chemical ablation refers to direct instillation of an agent into a tumor. Thermal ablation uses heat or cold to destroy tissue. Exposure of human tissue and tumor to temperatures in excess of 50°C for 6 minutes leads to cell death, although in practice, even higher temperatures are desirable for an efficient ablation. Wide variability in thermal ablation efficacy is due to underlying tissue characteristics, including cell thermal sensitivity. These parameters have been characterized and mathematically modeled in the form of electrostatic equation coupled to the bio-heat equation, which is simplified to:

Coagulative necrosis = energy deposited × local tissue interactions – heat lost

The majority of heat transfer in thermal ablation is by thermal conduction, and cooling is by blood flow–mediated thermal convection (Fig. 28-1).

Many systems are designed for delivery of cytotoxic thermal ablation (see Chapter 28). The most widely available and most extensively evaluated of these is radiofrequency ablation (RFA). This chapter emphasizes the results of hepatic RFA.

INDICATIONS AND OUTCOMES

Image-Guided Ablation for Hepatocellular Carcinoma

Hepatocellular carcinoma (HCC) can be ablated for local control in a patient who is unsuitable for hepatic resection or transplantation. HCC can be ablated to prolong the period a patient is suitable for liver transplantation by fulfilling the Milan criteria or UCSF criteria. The Milan criteria suggest that patients with a single HCC less than 5 cm or with up to three HCCs all less than 3 cm in diameter have a better outcome after liver transplantation. The UCSF criteria suggest that patients with a single tumor 6.5 cm or smaller, maximum of three tumors with none greater than 4.5 cm, cumulative tumor size 8 cm or less have a better outcome after liver transplantation.

Results of ablation are dependent on tumor size and to a lesser extent on degree of encapsulation. Local control for HCC less than 3 cm, 3-5 cm, and 5.1-9 cm has been reported as 90%, 71%, and 45%, respectively, after RFA. The upper limit of HCC size suitable for ablation varies among institutions and is not standardized. In general, HCCs less than 5 cm are suitable for RFA, although tumors up to 7 cm have been ablated. For multiple tumors, likewise the number of tumors is necessarily limited. Again, no standardized guidelines exist. Some centers ablate up to three tumors while others ablate up to five tumors depending on size, location, and approach.

A randomized controlled trial comparing the effectiveness of RFA and surgical resection as an initial treatment for patients with small HCC found the 1-, 2-, and 3-year local disease control rates were 89%, 82%, and 75%, respectively, in the resection group and 91%, 81%, and 76%, respectively, in the RFA group. The 1-, 2-, and 3-year survival rates were not significantly different at 93%, 85.69%, and 67.26%, respectively, in the resection group and 93%, 82%, and 65%, respectively, in the RFA group.

A further nonrandomized study confirmed survival at 4 years after RFA is equivalent with surgical resection for HCCs of 5 cm or less (96%, 82%, 71%, and 68% at 1, 2, 3, and 4 years).

For RFA as salvage therapy for recurrent HCC that has been previously resected, the 5-year survival rate after RFA of solitary intrahepatic recurrence of HCC is increased when compared with no therapy.

With ethanol ablation, 2-year local recurrence rates among HCCs treated with ethanol instillation with diameters of 2 cm or less, 2-3 cm, and more than 3 cm were 10%, 18%, and 30%, respectively. Elevated baseline α-fetoprotein level, multiple HCCs, and a tumor size larger than 3 cm are predictive of recurrence when using ethanol ablation.

One randomized study comparing ethanol ablation with surgical resection found that alcohol ablation was as effective as surgical resection in the treatment of solitary (≤5 cm) and small HCC. Three-year survival rates of 60%-70% and 5-year survival rates of 30%-50% have been reported. RFA achieves therapeutic efficacy in fewer sessions than ethanol instillation and for this reason has become the preferred ablation modality. The addition of alcohol ablation after RFA improves local control significantly in HCC greater than 3 cm in diameter. A randomized control trial of RFA and microwave had equivalent therapeutic effects, complication rates, and rates of residual foci of untreated disease. However, RF tumor ablation can be achieved with fewer sessions. Survival

rates at 1, 2, and 3 years were 96%, 83%, and 73%, respectively, after microwave ablation.

Microwave ablation has theoretical advantages in comparison to other thermal ablation therapies. The microwave ablation zone may be less affected by proximity to large hepatic vessels.

There is sparse published data as to the rate of local control and long-term survival after cryotherapy and ultrasound ablation. Electroporation remains an experimental technique.

Image-Guided Ablation for Hepatic Colorectal Carcinoma Metastasis

Colorectal carcinoma (CRC) metastasis can be ablated for local control in a patient who is unsuitable for hepatic resection or to make a patient suitable for resection. Hepatic resection in those who are suitable is still the gold standard treatment for hepatic colorectal metastasis.

Local control is achieved in 63%-65% of patients after RFA of CRC metastases but this varies with tumor size. Metastases 3-4 cm or less are more likely than larger tumors to result in a favorable outcome, with local control achieved in up to 98% of small tumors.

Survival data following percutaneous RFA of CRC metastases are not as good as for patients who undergo resection. Reports of cohorts not suitable for surgical resection have shown that survival in those who receive RFA exceeds the historical survival rates with no therapy. Moreover, patients who undergo RFA alone or RFA and resection show better survival than those on chemotherapy alone. Reported ranges of survival after RFA at 1, 3, and 5 years are 91%-93%, 28%-69%, and 25%-46%, respectively.

Magnetic resonance imaging (MRI)-guided laser ablation has been extensively evaluated in Europe and has a reported survival of 94%, 77%, 56%, and 37% at 1, 2, 3, and 5 years, respectively.

A "test-of-time" management approach involves reimaging patients 3-4 months after determination of suitability for resection. Interval development of hepatic metastases prevents patients from undergoing an unnecessary, noncurative surgery. The surgical rationale in these cases is that these new tumors would have developed shortly after surgery, had surgery been immediate, and the patient would not have benefited from a major operation. RFA has been applied in the interval between selection and resection to prevent progression of the existing tumors. Those who develop new metastases can be spared a noncurative operation. Those who demonstrate only local progression of the ablated tumor can still undergo surgery. Those who show no viable tumor have the option of surgery or close surveillance.

Image-Guided Ablation for Other Hepatic Metastases and Tumors

Ablation has been applied to pancreatic, breast, ovarian, sarcomas, ocular melanoma, and neuroendocrine metastases to the liver.

There are limited data on the use of RFA in treating hepatic metastases from breast cancer. Breast cancer is a systemic disease, and systemic therapy remains the primary means of therapy. In 3%-12% of patients, metastases are only in the liver. These patients as well as those who have liver-dominant metastases are those who are likely to benefit the most from ablation. Local control can be achieved in 92% of tumors. Enthusiasm for percutaneous ablation is mitigated by the fact that new metastases develop in 60% of patients.

Neuroendocrine metastases to the liver can be ablated for palliation of hormonal symptoms. However, the extent of disease often makes transcatheter embolization a more effective option.

Standard management of advanced (stages III and IV) ovarian cancer involves surgical resection and chemotherapy. Thermal ablation is effective in achieving local control in selected patients with limited metastasis from ovarian cancer.

Hepatic adenoma has a malignant potential. Image-guided ablation has been used to treat solitary small hepatic adenomas

---

Box 28-1. Tumor Ablative Techniques

Chemical
- Ethanol ablation
- Acetic acid ablation

Thermal
- Radiofrequency ablation
- Microwave ablation
- Cryoablation
- Laser ablation
- Ultrasound ablation

Cell membrane perforation
- Irreversible electroporation

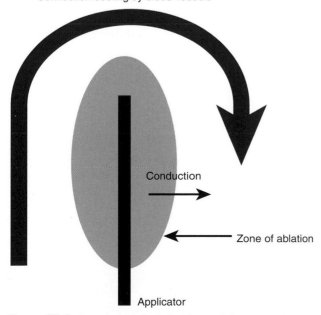

Convection cooling by blood vessels

Conduction

Zone of ablation

Applicator

FIGURE 28-1. Heat loss methods limiting radiofrequency therapy.

that are unsuitable for resection or as an alternative when resection is rejected.

ABLATION PLANNING AND PROCEDURE

Preablation Evaluation and Treatment Planning

The interventional radiologist plays a significant role in the management of patients who undergo ablative therapy. A preablation visit is an essential component of planning ablation.

The components of a preablation clinic visit include a focused history and physical examination. Patients are counseled regarding their diagnosis and given realistic expectations of the potential outcome, complications, postprocedure symptoms, intent of treatment, and course. If not done already, consultation with oncology or for surgical review of the case may be done to determine whether ablation is appropriate and whether timing of chemotherapy coincides with ablation. Informed consent is obtained.

Preprocedure imaging is assessed for adequacy in terms of demonstrating tumor number, location, margins with normal liver, proximity to or invasion of vessels, and proximity to critical structures such as gallbladder, stomach, and colon. Ideally, imaging is performed within 1 month of the ablation. If imaging is not adequate or recent, the imaging should be repeated to ensure that the patient is staged correctly.

The choice of multiphase-enhanced MRI, CT, or PET/CT for evaluation of liver tumors varies among centers; some choose MRI almost exclusively while others use MRI in selected patients because CT is limited to patients with a creatinine less than 2 mg/dL.

Imaging studies are also reviewed for extrahepatic disease burden; for site, size, and number of tumors; and for their relationship to the biliary tree, hepatic veins, portal veins, and hepatic arteries. The ablation of a 0.5- to 1-cm margin beyond the borders of the tumor is considered optimal to achieve complete tumor destruction. Flow in large intrahepatic blood vessels (>3 mm) diminishes RFA-induced coagulation necrosis by cooling tissues. Extrahepatic structures may abut the organ or tumor and may require adjunctive techniques to protect them (Table 28-1). Of note, the gallbladder has proven resilient following ablation of nearby tumors. Chemical cholecystitis can occur when the ablation zone abuts the gallbladder fossa and can be managed conservatively with pain management. Cholecystectomy or cholecystostomy are almost never required.

TABLE 28-1 Protective Techniques

Frequency of Use	Organ	Technique
Common	Bowel	Hydrodissection, carbon dioxide, balloon inflation
Somewhat common	Diaphragm	Hydrodissection, carbon dioxide, balloon inflation
Somewhat common	Lung	Hydrodissection, elective pneumothorax/pleural effusion
Uncommon	Bile duct	Cooled biliary perfusion

Imaging guidance with ultrasound, CT, or MRI is selected based on availability, visibility, and access. If ultrasound guidance is planned, it is prudent to perform preprocedure ultrasound to determine the ease of access to and visibility of the lesions.

Appropriate coagulation parameters, renal function, and tumor marker levels are checked. Oral aspirin, clopidogrel, and Coumadin are stopped 5-7 days before the procedure. If necessary, preprocedure admission for intravenous heparin, direct thrombin inhibitors, or outpatient conversion to subcutaneous low molecular weight heparin are instituted. Mild coagulation abnormalities (international normalized ratio > 1.5) or thrombocytopenia (platelets < 50-70 × 10^3 μL) can be treated with intraprocedural fresh frozen plasma or platelets.

Intraprocedural pain control can be achieved with moderate sedation by the radiologist or by general anesthesia by an anesthesiologist. The use of one or the other is generally institution dependent. If moderate sedation is the default, then in selected patients with significant comorbidities or intolerance of moderate sedation during a prior procedure such as a biopsy, general anesthesia may be needed.

Biopsy

A biopsy of the tumor may be performed on a separate occasion or at the same visit. Whereas many tumors may require biopsy to stage the cancer, imaging is sufficient in some cases. For example, a 1-cm or larger tumor in a cirrhotic liver showing arterial hyperenhancement and portal venous or delayed phase washout on multiphase contrast-enhanced CT/MRI is considered diagnostic for HCC according to the American Association of the Study of Liver Diseases (AASLD) guidelines.

Procedure

Ablation is performed with spinal anesthesia, general anesthesia, or moderate sedation with midazolam (Versed; Roche, Nutley, N.J.), fentanyl citrate (Sublimaze; Jansen, Titusville, N.J.), and meperidine hydrochloride (Demerol, Abbott Laboratories, Ill.). Antibiotic prophylaxis varies among institutions, with most interventional radiologists choosing to administer a single dose to most patients. The authors routinely use 80 mg gentamicin and 1 g of ampicillin intravenously in nonallergic patients. Patients with significant risk factors for abscess formation (biliary stent, previous sphincterotomy, bioenteric anastamosis, or bioenteric fistula) may benefit from a prolonged antibiotic course after RFA.

Targeting, Controlling, and Monitoring Therapy

Common to all the ablative techniques except ultrasound ablation is the need to place the applicator in the tumor (Table 28-2). Tumors can be targeted with ultrasound guidance when they can be seen clearly at ultrasound (Fig. 28-2). CT can be used with or without the addition of intravenous contrast to improve tumor visualization. MRI, when available, can target therapy because there is high tissue contrast between tumor and normal liver.

Based on the size and geometry of the tumor, overlapping ablations are performed if the applicators are insufficient to cover the entire tumor with a single ablation. This can be done

TABLE 28-2 Imaging Response in the Ablation Zone with Tumor Ablative Techniques

Modality	Radiofrequency Ablation	Cryotherapy	Ethanol Ablation
Ultrasound	Hyperechogenicity	Hyperechoic rim and Hypoechogenicity in ice ball	Hyperechogenicity
Computed tomography	Hypodensity and/or Hyperdensity	Hypodensity	Hypodensity
Magnetic resonance imaging	Sequence dependent	Hypointensity	T2 hyperintensity

by repositioning a single applicator or simultaneous activation of multiple applicators to ablate the entire tumor (Fig. 28-3). The operators compare the tumor diameter in the plane of imaging to the expected in vivo ablation diameter of the applicator in use and adjust applicator positions accordingly (Table 28-3). In the orthogonal plane, applicator adjustments are likewise performed based on the expected ablation diameter and tumor size. If the axis of the tumor parallel to the applicator is longer than the expected ablation length, overlap is achieved by pulling the applicator back for the appropriate distance and performing another ablation. The goal is generally to ablate a 5- to 10-mm margin of normal liver parenchyma to minimize the risk of tumor progression.

Thermal ablation using heat produces a transient (30-90 minute) hyperechoic area at ultrasound and mixed hypodensity and hyperdensity on CT, which approximates but does not accurately reflect the zone of coagulative necrosis. The hyperechoic area is due to microbubbles of water vapor and other cellular products forming as a result of tissue vaporization during active heating. The transient hyperechoic zone may prevent tumor visualization and accurate applicator reinsertion.

Noninvasive MRI thermometry makes use of the temperature dependence of some physical property whose spatial distribution can be visualized. Three tissue properties have been used for this purpose: spin-lattice decay time (T1), molecular diffusion of water molecules, and the proton resonance frequency of water molecules.

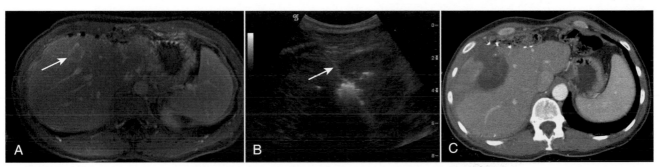

FIGURE 28-2. Radiofrequency ablation in a 42-year-old woman with a segment 8 biopsy-proven hepatocellular cancer (HCC). Previous left lobe resection was performed for HCC. **A,** Portal venous phase, postcontrast magnetic resonance image, fat-saturated T1 image demonstrates a peripherally enhancing tumor *(arrow)*. **B,** Axial oblique ultrasound image demonstrates the radiofrequency electrode *(arrow)* in the tumor with a hyperechoic zone at the time of ablation. **C,** Postcontrast axial computed tomography scan at 1 month demonstrates hypodensity of the ablation zone.

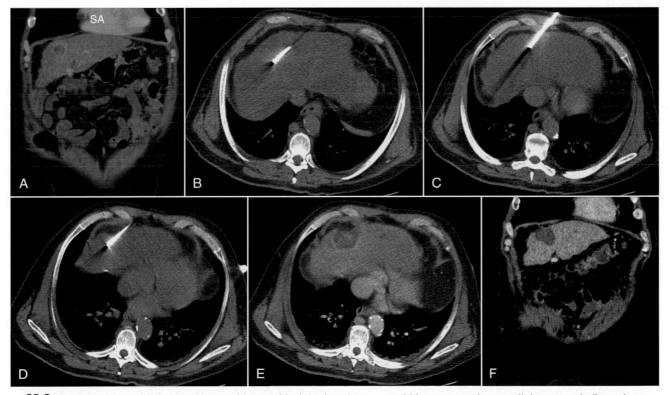

FIGURE 28-3. Radiofrequency ablation in a 63-year-old man with cirrhosis and a segment 8 biopsy-proven hepatocellular cancer. **A,** Coronal reconstruction of a parenchymal phase computed tomography (CT) scan of the abdomen demonstrates a liver lesion in a cirrhotic liver. **B,** Axial noncontrast CT scan of the internally cooled cluster of electrodes positioned in the inferolateral aspect of the tumor and adjacent normal liver parenchyma. **C,** Axial noncontrast CT scan of the internally cooled cluster of electrodes positioned in the anteromedial aspect of the tumor and adjacent normal liver parenchyma. **D,** Axial noncontrast CT scan of the internally cooled cluster of electrodes positioned in the superior aspect of the tumor and adjacent normal liver parenchyma. **E,** Axial parenchymal phase contrast CT scan after completion of four overlapping ablations demonstrates a low-density ablation zone with central high density related to hemorrhage and peripheral benign periablational enhancement. **F,** Coronal reconstruction of a parenchymal phase CT scan of the abdomen performed 3 months after ablation demonstrates a hypodense zone of coagulative necrosis in cirrhotic liver.

TABLE **28-3** Ablation Zone Diameter with Tumor Ablative Techniques

Modality	Axial Ablation Size (cm)	Transverse Ablation Diameter, (Short Axis) (cm)	Generator Power	Endpoint Determinant	Tissue Ablated
2.5-cm single electrode (Valleylab)	3.0	1.8	150 W	Impedance	In vivo pig liver
2.5 cm triple internally cooled cluster electrode (Valleylab)	4.2	3	250 W	Impedance	In vivo pig liver
4-cm LeVeen multitined expandable electrode (Radiotherapeutics)	3.1	3.4	200 W	Impedance double roll off	In vivo pig liver
2-cm LeVeen multitined expandable electrode (Radiotherapeutics)	2.3	2.4	200 W	Impedance single roll off	In vivo pig liver
2-cm LeVeen multitined expandable electrode (Radiotherapeutics)	2.6	2.9	200 W	Impedance double roll off	In vivo pig liver
5-cm multi-tined expandable electrode (Starburst XL; Rita Medical Systems)	3.8	2.7	150 W	Temperature	In vivo pig liver
2.4-mm cryoprobe (PERC-24, Endocare)	NS	0.8	NA	2 cycles: 12- and 8-minute freeze then thawing	In vivo pig liver
2.45-GHz microwave ablation microwave applicator	6.5	5.7	150 W	8 minutes	In vivo pig liver

NA, Not applicable; NS, not stated.

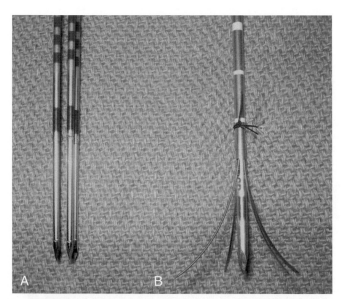

FIGURE **28-4**. Radiofrequency electrode designs. **A,** A cluster electrode with uninsulated distal 2.5 cm. **B,** Multitined expandable electrodes with tines deployed.

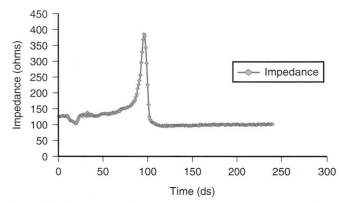

FIGURE **28-5**. Graph of the impedance versus time during impedance control pulsed current delivery in bone. Impedance rises as the temperature of the tissue abutting the electrode rises until it exceeds 30% of the baseline impedance. A low ampere current is instituted for 15 seconds to allow tissue cooling.

Cryotherapy produces acoustic shadowing on ultrasound and can underestimate or overestimate the true extent of the ice ball. CT can detect hypodense changes in the ablation zone. Cryotherapy produces MR signal loss in the ice ball. Cell death occurs approximately 3 mm inside the edge of the ice ball. This clarity allows for monitoring and control of the ablation, minimizes potential complications, and optimizes success.

Chemical ablation produces a hyperechoic area on ultrasound that poorly reflects the extent of treatment. CT can demonstrate a 40-HU drop in attenuation. MRI can demonstrate on diffusion imaging the distribution of alcohol. The injection is stopped and the needle repositioned if filling of a bile duct, portal vein, hepatic vein, hepatic artery, or the gallbladder is seen. The needle can be manipulated into an area of the tumor that has not become echogenic or hypodense, and injection repeated until the tumor becomes completely echogenic or hypodense and/or the target injected volume is reached.

Size and Geometry of Ablation

The geometry of the ablation is determined by the RFA electrode (Fig. 28-4), location of the tumor, tumor consistency, perfusion-mediated cooling effect, and saline distribution for perfusion devices. Primary liver tumors and liver metastases have heterogeneous consistency and impedance. More dense areas of tumor tissue may be partially unaffected by heat, and residual vital tumor cells may remain. Some ablation protocols use applicator cooling with perfusion of the probe with cooled water to stop charring of the applicator and depend on Impedance measurement to guide radiofrequency energy delivery over a treatment period defined in the information for use (Fig. 28-5).

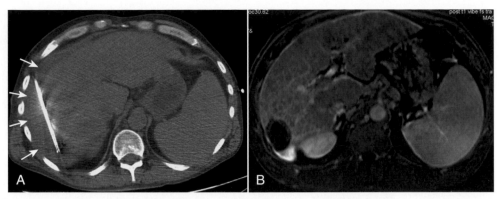

FIGURE 28-6. Radiofrequency ablation in a 50-year-old man with cirrhosis and a segment 7 biopsy-proven hepatocellular cancer. **A,** Hydrodissection with 200 mL of D_5W in the subphrenic space has separated the diaphragm *(white arrows)* and the liver. Axial noncontrast CT confirms that the internally cooled cluster of electrodes is positioned in the tumor by reference to the preprocedure contrast-enhanced axial images. **B,** Parenchymal phase, postcontrast, fat-saturated T1 images at 3 months after ablation demonstrate a low signal ablation zone with no residual tumor enhancement. High signal is seen in Morrison's pouch due to the degradation products of blood.

The relationship of the active length of the electrode to the length of the RFA lesion has been shown to be linear. The diameter of the ablation demonstrates only a small increase from 1 to 2 cm in electrode length and then no difference for an increase in active length greater than 2 cm, although such increases in length would create a longer zone of ablation. The effect of electrode gauge on ablation diameter is minimal; therefore the gauge of the electrode is usually the minimum available to reduce the invasiveness of the procedure.

The single needle electrode, cluster electrode, single microwave antennae, and single cryoprobe produce a coagulation zone that is nearly circular in cross-section and ellipsoid in the coronal plane. A discoid shape is commonly seen with LeVeen multitined expandable electrodes. The Starburst multitined expandable electrode generates a teardrop shape ablation with deformations that correspond to the expandable tines. Perfusion electrodes may produce unpredictable ablation zone shapes due to the spread of the interstitial perfusate.

Multiple cryoprobes or laser fibers produce ablation zones that are dependent upon the number and position of the applicator. Cryoprobes are placed no further than 2 cm apart and produce ablation up to 1 cm from the outer cryoprobes. Chemical ablation produces an unpredictable ablation because it is dependent on diffusion at injection and the degree of tumor encapsulation.

Adjunctive Techniques to Protect Organs

A number of techniques have been developed to protect adjacent organs or structures from the zone of ablation. Hydrodissection using 5% dextrose and water (Fig. 28-6), carbon dioxide, or angioplasty balloons can be used to protect the diaphragm or bowel from thermal injury. Perfusion of the biliary tree has been described to protect the central bile ducts when they are within 6 mm of the ablation zone, but this has not been extensively evaluated.

Adjuvant Therapies

Local therapy combined with transarterial chemoembolization or systemic drug therapy can have additive effects on local tumor control and survival (Box 28-2). Thermal ablation using heat leads to sensitization of the cells to chemotherapeutic agents at the periphery of the tumor which have not undergone coagulative necrosis. Administration of agents such as liposomal doxorubicin have increased efficacy in these heat-sensitized cells.

Combinations of RFA and alcohol ablation have been shown to increase local control rates (Fig. 28-7).

Box 28-2. Strategies to Increase Tumor Ablation

Applicator
- Multitined expandable and cluster radiofrequency (RF) applicators
- Internally cooled RF applicator
- Perfusion applicator: concomitant percutaneous instillation of hypertonic sodium chloride solution

Generator
- High-energy RF generator
- Ramped energy deposition or impedance regulated pulsed energy delivery

Alteration of vascularity
- Preprocedure portal vein or hepatic arterial embolization
- Pringle maneuver or hepatic venous occlusion using an angioplasty balloon placed via the inferior vena cava

Chemotherapy
- Systemic chemotherapy
- Transarterial chemoembolization

Combined ablation techniques
- Thermal and chemical ablation (e.g., RF ablation and ethanol instillation)

Postprocedure Care

After RF ablation, all patients are monitored electronically for blood pressure, heart rate, and oxygen saturation in the radiology recovery area, if they are outpatients, or in the anesthesia recovery area if they received general anesthesia or spinal anesthesia. Patients can be discharged home if they are hemodynamically stable and have recovered from sedation to the point of tolerating oral intake and passing urine 2-4 hours after ablation. Additional analgesics may be needed during recovery and in the first 4-7 days after the procedure. Patients should be reassured that they can resume a near normal lifestyle within 10-14 days of the ablation procedure. Some patients are admitted for observation to manage coexisting morbidity, the effects of anesthesia, or for continued analgesia management.

Five percent of patients are asymptomatic after RFA; 95% suffer a number of symptoms similar to the postembolization syndrome (Table 28-4). Post-RFA syndrome is defined as a combination of flulike symptoms, which includes fever, malaise, pain at the site of ablation, nausea, vomiting, and muscle aches.

Symptoms and fever peak on day 5 and typically resolve by day 10. Symptomatic patients experience significantly greater pain and interference with general and work activities, peaking on day 1. It appears that the number of ablations correlates better with the postablation symptoms than with the maximal diameter of the

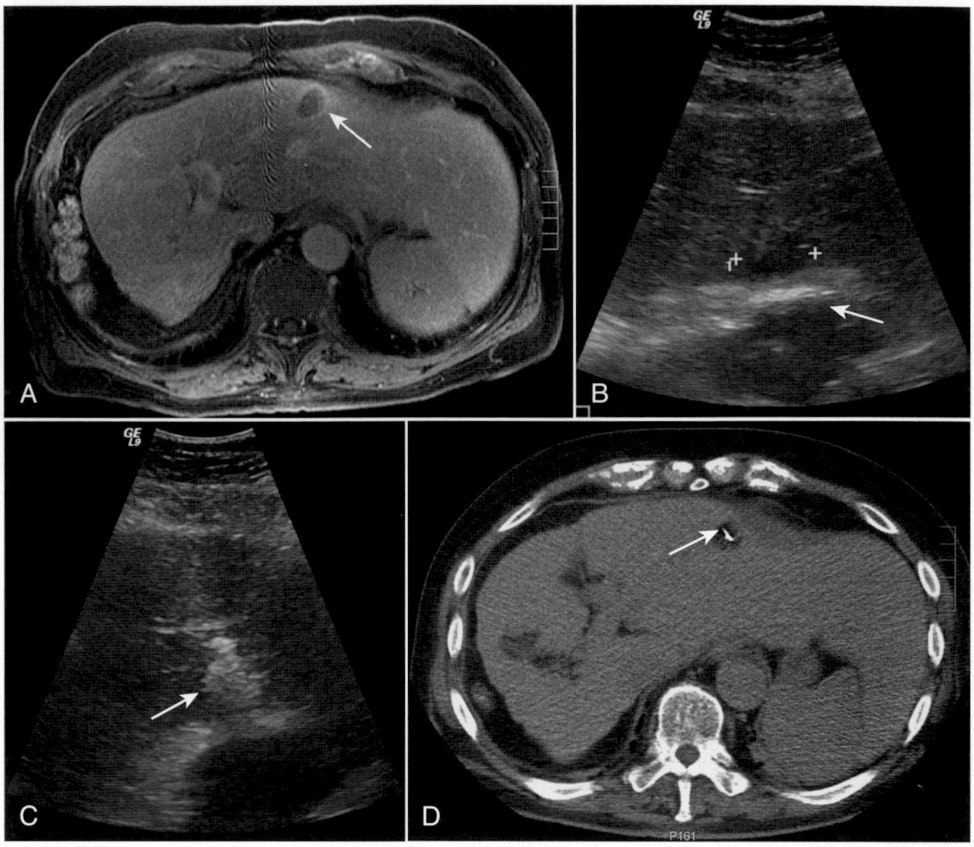

FIGURE 28-7. Radiofrequency ablation in a 75-year-old man with cirrhosis and a segment 3 hepatocellular cancer (HCC) abutting the diaphragm and left ventricle ablated with a combination of alcohol and radiofrequency ablation. **A,** Axial fat-saturated postcontrast T1-weighted magnetic resonance image demonstrates a 2-cm HCC *(arrow)* in segment 3 of the liver with washout. **B,** Ultrasound image of the HCC (between calipers) in close proximity to the left ventricle wall *(arrow).* **C,** Ultrasound image of the hyperechoic HCC *(arrow)* after alcohol ablation. **D,** Noncontrast computed tomography scan after alcohol ablation demonstrates a low-density zone *(arrow)* adjacent to the tip of a radiofrequency electrode that was used to complete the ablation of the inferior margin.

zone of ablation. Patients who have persistent or late onset fever may harbor concurrent infection, including abscess formation.

COMPLICATIONS

In 3554 tumors treated with RFA, six deaths (0.3%) were noted: two caused by multiorgan failure following intestinal perforation, one by septic shock following *Staphylococcus aureus* peritonitis, one by massive hemorrhage following tumor rupture, one by liver failure following stenosis of right bile duct; and one by unknown cause 3 days after the procedure. Fifty (2.2%) patients had additional major complications, including peritoneal hemorrhage, neoplastic seeding, intrahepatic abscesses, and intestinal perforation. The larger the number of RFA-treated tumors, the higher the rate of major complications. Minor complications were observed in less than 5% of patients.

Abscesses tend to occur late in the clinical course, with a reported interval that ranges from 8 days to 5 months. The risk of abscess formation is increased if the patient had recent biliary instrumentation, biliary bypass surgery, bilioenteric fistula, biliary external drainage, or obstruction of the biliary tree.

Conventional ethanol ablation is usually well tolerated, with local pain, transient fever, and intoxication being easily managed. There is a 3.2% major and minor complication rate and 0.1% mortality.

Open cryoablation has been associated with liver fracture, intraperitoneal hemorrhage, and disseminated intravascular coagulation and multiorgan failure (1%). This complication appears to be much rarer with the percutaneous technique and smaller diameter cryoprobes.

Microwave ablation, ultrasound ablation, and RFA have been associated with cutaneous burns at the site of the applicator for all types or at the grounding pad sites in RFA.

Irreversible electroporation uses extremely high voltages. It has been associated with development of arrhythmias and must be performed with general anesthesia and muscle relaxation due

TABLE 28-4 Postablative Syndrome

Symptoms	Incidence
Flulike symptoms and fever	37%
Low-grade fever that ranged from 99° to 102°F (37°C-39°C)	42%
Flulike symptoms: Nausea Vomiting Malaise Myalgia	81%

to muscle stimulation and pain secondary to the high-voltage application.

FOLLOW-UP

Markers

If elevated, tumor specific biological markers including α-fetoprotein, CEA, CA 125, insulin, or urinary catecholamines can be evaluated before therapy so the trend can be monitored for potential recurrence or disease progression.

Imaging Assessment of Treatment Response

Imaging is critical to response assessment with ablation because tumors are left in situ. While the first scan is performed at 1 month, follow-up unenhanced and multiphasic contrast-enhanced MR or CT imaging are performed at 2- to 3-month intervals after ablation. The liver is assessed for residual enhancement in the treated tumor, size of the zone of ablation, and development of new metastatic disease.

Residual disease is defined as persistent enhancement in an area or areas of tumor after ablation, as determined on the 1- or 3-month follow-up study. A thin homogenous rim of peripheral enhancement has been shown to represent evolving granulation tissue and should not be mistaken for residual tumor. Peripheral nodular enhancement, thick irregular peripheral enhancement, or diffuse tumor enlargement all reflect active tumor.

A common interpretive pitfall by those unfamiliar with postablation imaging is to report tumor enlargement on the first postablation scan when in fact what has occurred is development of a zone of ablation larger than the original tumor, a desirable result. Familiarity with the treatment history and postablation imaging findings will help avoid this misinterpretation.

On subsequent follow-up scans, after absence of viable tumor at imaging has been confirmed once, the zone of ablation may stay the same size or slowly decrease in size. Any increase in size of the zone of ablation is generally viable tumor.

Local progression of disease or recurrence is defined as new tumor enhancement after at least one imaging study has demonstrated complete elimination of enhancement. It can also refer to growth of persistent untreated areas on follow-up scans. If areas of viable tumor remain amenable to ablation, patients can make additional visits to the radiology department for more ablations if CT or MRI reveals incomplete treatment on follow-up. If new tumors develop, then reevaluation can be performed as to whether percutaneous ablation and/or other locoregional or systemic therapies are warranted.

▬ SUGGESTED READINGS

Buscarini L, Buscarini E, Di Stasi M, et al. Percutaneous radiofrequency ablation of small hepatocellular carcinoma: long-term results. *Eur Radiol.* 2001;11:914-921.

Chen MH, Yang W, Yan K, et al. Large liver tumors: protocol for radiofrequency ablation and its clinical application in 110 patients—mathematic model, overlapping mode, and electrode placement process. *Radiology.* 2004;232:260-271.

Chen MS, Li JQ, Liang IIII, et al. Comparison of effects of percutaneous radiofrequency ablation and surgical resection on small hepatocellular carcinoma. *Zhonghua Yi Xue Za Zhi.* 2005;85:80-83.

Chen MS, Li JQ, Zheng Y, et al. A prospective randomized trial comparing percutaneous local ablative therapy and partial hepatectomy for small hepatocellular carcinoma. *Ann Surg.* 2006;243:321-328.

Chen MS, Zhang YJ, Li JQ, et al. Randomized clinical trial of percutaneous radiofrequency ablation plus absolute ethanol injection compared with radiofrequency ablation alone for small hepatocellular carcinoma. *Zhonghua Zhong Liu Za Zhi.* 2005;27:623-625.

Cheung TT, Chu FS, Jenkins CR, et al. Tolerance of high intensity focused ultrasound ablation in patients with HCC. *World J Surg.* 2012;36:2420-2427.

Chopra S, Dodd 3rd GD, Chintapalli KN, et al. Tumor recurrence after radiofrequency thermal ablation of hepatic tumors: spectrum of findings on dual-phase contrast-enhanced CT. *Am J Roentgenol.* 2001;177:381-387.

Clark TW, Soulen MC. Chemical ablation of hepatocellular carcinoma. *J Vasc Interv Radiol.* 2002;13:S245-S252.

de Baere T, Bessoud B, Dromain C, et al. Percutaneous radiofrequency ablation of hepatic tumors during temporary venous occlusion. *Am J Roentgenol.* 2002;178:53-59.

de Baere T, Elias D, Dromain C, et al. Radiofrequency ablation of 100 hepatic metastases with a mean follow-up of more than 1 year. *Am J Roentgenol.* 2000;175:1619-1625.

Elias D, Di Pietroantonio D, Gachot B, et al. Liver abscess after radiofrequency ablation of tumors in patients with a biliary tract procedure. *Gastroenterol Clin Biol.* 2006;30:823-827.

Gervais DA, Arellano RS, Mueller PR. Percutaneous radiofrequency ablation of ovarian cancer metastasis to the liver: indications, outcomes, and role in patient management. *Am J Roentgenol.* 2006;187:746-750.

Gervais D, Arellano RS. Percutaneous tumor ablation for hepatocellular carcinoma. *AJR.* 2011;197:789-794.

Gillams AR, Lees WR. Radio-frequency ablation of colorectal liver metastases in 167 patients. *Eur Radiol.* 2004;14:2261-2267.

Giorgio A, Tarantino L, de Stefano G, Coppola C, Ferraioli G. Complications after percutaneous saline-enhanced radiofrequency ablation of liver tumors: 3-year experience with 336 patients at a single center. *Am J Roentgenol.* 2005;184:207-211.

Giorgio A, Tarantino L, de Stefano G, et al. Ultrasound-guided percutaneous ethanol injection under general anesthesia for the treatment of hepatocellular carcinoma on cirrhosis: long-term results in 268 patients. *Eur J Ultrasound.* 2000;12:145-154.

Goldberg SN, Gazelle GS, Compton CC, Mueller PR, Tanabe KK. Treatment of intrahepatic malignancy with radiofrequency ablation: radiologic-pathologic correlation. *Cancer.* 2000;88:2452-2463.

Goldberg SN, Grassi CJ, Cardella JF, et al. Image-guided tumor ablation: standardization of terminology and reporting criteria. *Radiology.* 2005;235:728-739.

Goldberg SN, Solbiati L, Hahn PF, et al. Large-volume tissue ablation with radio frequency by using a clustered, internally cooled electrode technique: laboratory and clinical experience in liver metastases. *Radiology.* 1998;209:371-379.

Gunabushanam G, Sharma S, Thulkar S, et al. Radiofrequency ablation of liver metastases from breast cancer: results in 14 patients. *J Vasc Interv Radiol.* 2007;18:67-72.

Harmon KE, Ryan Jr JA, Biehl TR, Lee FT. Benefits and safety of hepatic resection for colorectal metastases. *Am J Surg.* 1999;177:402-404.

Hori T, Nagata K, Hasuike S, et al. Risk factors for the local recurrence of hepatocellular carcinoma after a single session of percutaneous radiofrequency ablation. *J Gastroenterol.* 2003;38:977-981.

Izumi N, Asahina Y, Noguchi O, et al. Risk factors for distant recurrence of hepatocellular carcinoma in the liver after complete coagulation by microwave or radiofrequency ablation. *Cancer.* 2001;91:949-956.

Jaskolka JD, Asch MR, Kachura JR, et al. Needle tract seeding after radiofrequency ablation of hepatic tumors. *J Vasc Interv Radiol.* 2005;16:485-491.

Jemal A, Murray T, Ward E, et al. Cancer statistics, 2005. *CA Cancer J Clin.* 2005:10-30.

Lawes D, Chopada A, Gillams A, Lees W, Taylor I. Radiofrequency ablation (RFA) as a cytoreductive strategy for hepatic metastasis from breast cancer. *Ann R Coll Surg Engl.* 2006;88:639-642.

Lencioni R, Cioni D, Crocetti L, et al. Early-stage hepatocellular carcinoma in patients with cirrhosis: long-term results of percutaneous image-guided radiofrequency ablation. *Radiology.* 2005;234:961-967.

Lencioni RA, Allgaier HP, Cioni D, et al. Small hepatocellular carcinoma in cirrhosis: randomized comparison of radio-frequency thermal ablation versus percutaneous ethanol injection. *Radiology.* 2003;228:235-240.

Lin SM, Lin CJ, Lin CC, Hsu CW, Chen YC. Radiofrequency ablation improves prognosis compared with ethanol injection for hepatocellular carcinoma <4 cm. *Gastroenterology.* 2004;127:1714-1723.

Livraghi T, Goldberg SN, Lazzaroni S, et al. Hepatocellular carcinoma: radiofrequency ablation of medium and large lesions. *Radiology.* 2000;214:761-768.

Livraghi T, Goldberg SN, Lazzaroni S, et al. Small hepatocellular carcinoma: treatment with radio-frequency ablation versus ethanol injection. *Radiology.* 1999;210:655-661.

Livraghi T, Goldberg SN, Solbiati L, et al. Percutaneous radio-frequency ablation of liver metastases from breast cancer: initial experience in 24 patients. *Radiology.* 2001;220:145-149.

Livraghi T, Lazzaroni S, Meloni F, Solbiati L. Risk of tumour seeding after percutaneous radiofrequency ablation for hepatocellular carcinoma. *Br J Surg.* 2005;92:856-858.

Livraghi T, Lazzaroni S, Meloni F. Radiofrequency thermal ablation of hepatocellular carcinoma. *Eur J Ultrasound.* 2000;13:159-166.

Livraghi T, Solbiati L, Meloni F, et al. Percutaneous radiofrequency ablation of liver metastases in potential candidates for resection the "test-of-time" approach. *Cancer.* 2003;97:3027-3035.

Livraghi T, Solbiati L, Meloni MF, et al. Treatment of focal liver tumors with percutaneous radio-frequency ablation: complications encountered in a multicenter study. *Radiology.* 2003;226:441-451.

Lu DS, Raman SS, Limanond P, et al. Influence of large peritumoral vessels on outcome of radiofrequency ablation of liver tumors. *J Vasc Interv Radiol.* 2003;14:1267-1274.

Lu MD, Chen JW, Xie XY, et al. Hepatocellular carcinoma: US-guided percutaneous microwave coagulation therapy. *Radiology.* 2001;221:167-172.

Mazzaferro V, Regalia E, Doci R, et al. Liver transplantation for the treatment of small hepatocellular carcinomas in patients with cirrhosis. *N Engl J Med.* 1996;334:693-699.

Ohmoto K, Yoshioka N, Tomiyama Y, et al. Thermal ablation therapy for hepatocellular carcinoma: comparison between radiofrequency ablation and percutaneous microwave coagulation therapy. *Hepatogastroenterology.* 2006;53:651-654.

Oshio A, Tamaki K, Shimizu I, et al. Double radiofrequency ablation is more extensive with a spherical zone shape compared to single ablation in a pig liver model. *J Med Invest.* 2007;54:28-34.

Oshowo A, Gillams A, Harrison E, Lees WR, Taylor I. Comparison of resection and radiofrequency ablation for treatment of solitary colorectal liver metastases. *British Journal of Surgery.* 2003;90:1240-1243.

Pereira PL, Trubenbach J, Schenk M, et al. Radiofrequency ablation: in vivo comparison of four commercially available devices in pig livers. *Radiology.* 2004;232:482-490.

Poon RT, Ng KK, Lam CM, et al. Effectiveness of radiofrequency ablation for hepatocellular carcinomas larger than 3 cm in diameter. *Arch Surg.* 2004;139:281-287.

Solbiati L, Livraghi T, Goldberg SN, et al. Percutaneous radio-frequency ablation of hepatic metastases from colorectal cancer: long-term results in 117 patients. *Radiology.* 2001;221:159-166.

Tateishi R, Shiina S, Teratani T, et al. Percutaneous radiofrequency ablation for hepatocellular carcinoma an analysis of 1000 cases. *Cancer.* 2005;103:1201-1209.

Yu HC, Cheng JS, Lai KH, et al. Factors for early tumor recurrence of single small hepatocellular carcinoma after percutaneous radiofrequency ablation therapy. *World J Gastroenterol.* 2005;11:1439-1444.

Index

Page numbers followed by *f* indicate figures; *t*, tables; and *b*, boxes.

Automated spring loaded core biopsy needles, 513, 513f–514f
AVFs. *See* Arteriovenous fistulas (AVFs)
AVMs. *See* Arteriovenous malformations (AVMs)
Axillary artery
  anatomy of, 119
  angiography access and, 44–45, 44f–45f
  angiography of, 123
  occlusion of, 122
Axillary lymph node sampling, 522–523
Axillary vein
  anatomy of, 137, 137f
  pseudolesion, 140f
  thoracic outlet syndrome and, 143–144, 143f
Azygos vein, anatomy of, 138, 138f, 287, 288f–289f

B

Back pain
  disc decompression for, 533–535
  facet joint infiltration for, 530
  nerve root blocks for, 532–533
  rhysolysis for, 531–532
Bacterial infections, 16–17
  sources of, 19t, 20t
  syphilitic aortitis. *See* Syphilitic aortitis
Ballerina sign, 344f
Balloon angioplasty
  for aortic coarctation, 196, 196f
  balloon sizes for, 74, 74t
  burst pressure and, 73, 74f
  catheters for, 75, 75f
  compliant/noncompliant balloons in, 73, 74f
  enhanced balloons for, 75, 75f
  guidelines for, 74–75, 74b, 74f
  "kissing balloon" technique, 212, 212f, 214, 215f
  mechanism of, 73, 73f
  for renal artery stenosis, 273, 274f
  with vascular bifurcation, 76, 76f
  vessel rupture during, 76, 77b, 77f
Balloon dilatation
  of benign biliary strictures, 469–471
    biliary access for, 469, 469f
    indications for, 469
    method of, 469–470, 470f, 471b
    patient preparation for, 469, 469b
    preprocedural evaluation for, 469
    results of, 466t, 471
  of GI tract strictures, 439–441, 439f–440f, 440b
  of ureteric strictures, 506, 507f
Balloon occlusion catheter, 164, 164f
Balloon occlusion hepatic venography, 312–314, 317–318, 317f
Balloon retrograde transrenal obliteration (BRTO) of gastric varices, 325–326
Balloon-expandable stents, 76–77, 78f, 79
  in TIPS procedure, 322, 324f
Balloon-type retention gastrostomy button, 431–432, 431f
Barcelona Clinic liver cancer staging of hepatoma, 249t
Barium studies
  for colorectal cancer, 447–449, 449f
  for colorectal strictures, 441, 442f
  for esophageal strictures, 439, 441, 443f–444f
  for percutaneous gastrostomy, 425–426, 426f
Basilar artery, 99, 102f
Basilic vein
  anatomy of, 136–137, 137f
  for angiographic access, 48–49

Basket devices, 95–96, 96f, 96t
  for stone removal, 472f, 473
Behçet disease
  aortoiliac aneurysms and, 203b
  clinical presentation of, 7t, 8, 9f
Benign prostatic hyperplasia (BPH), 227–228, 227f
Bentson guidewires, 28
β-cell hypertrophy, pancreatic, 245
Betadine, as sclerosing agent, 416, 419f
Bile ducts
  anatomy of, 309–310, 451–452
    variants of, 451, 452f
  gallstones and, 474, 471–473
  injury, in laparoscopic cholecystectomy, 467, 467b
  interventions. *See* Biliary interventions
  obstruction of
    hilar, 457–460
    low CBD, 460
    malignant, 457–467
    tissue diagnosis of, 466–467
Bile leakage treatment, 480
Biliary drainage. *See* Percutaneous biliary drainage (PBD)
Biliary interventions, 451–473
  for benign strictures
    percutaneous balloon dilatation as, 466t, 469–471, 469b, 471b
    stents as, 471
  drainage. *See* Percutaneous biliary drainage (PBD)
  ductal anatomy and, 451–452
  indications for, 453b
  for laparoscopic cholecystectomy complications, 467, 467b
  patient preparation for, 451–452
  percutaneous transhepatic cholangiography, 452–453
  for stent occlusion, 467–469, 468f
  for stones, 471–473
    rendezvous procedure, 471, 471f
    surgery/transhepatic removal, 471–472
    T-tube track removal, 472–473, 472f
Biopsy
  breast, image-guided, 511–521
  gallbladder, 474, 475f
  liver, 390–391
  liver tumor ablation and, 574
  musculoskeletal, 528–529
  percutaneous. *See* Percutaneous image-guided biopsy
  pleural, 419–421
  renal, 556
  transvascular, 97, 97t, 98f
Bipolar RF nucleoplasty, 535–536
BI-RADS categories for breast lesions, 511, 512b
Bird's Nest filter, 297–298, 299f
Bismuth classification of hilar tumors, 457–458, 459f
Bladder
  anatomy of, 487
  embolization of, 226
  empty, 505, 505f
  suprapubic cystostomy of, 506
Bleeding
  abdominal fluid collections and, 417–418, 420f
  of bronchial arteries, 174–176
  gastrointestinal, 239–244, 259
  gynecologic, 225–226
  with pelvic injury, 220–221
  in percutaneous nephrolithotomy, 498
  in portal hypertension, 316–317
  See also Hemorrhage

Bleomycin pleurodesis, 422
Blood pressure
  angiography and, 39, 39t
  high. *See* Hypertension
  low. *See* Hypotension
Blood vessels
  arteries. *See* Arteries
  decreasing flow through, 86–95. *See also* specific interventions
    fundamentals of, 86–87
    techniques/tools for, 87t
  improving lumen, 68–86. *See also* specific interventions
  pathology of. *See* Vascular pathology
  veins. *See* Veins
Blue toe syndrome, 16, 19f, 210, 353–354, 353t, 354f
Blunt trauma
  aortoiliac, 220, 222f
  to cervical vessels, 111–113, 111f
  to inferior vena cava, 303, 303f
  to thoracic aorta, 193, 193f
  to upper extremity arteries, 131–132
Bone biopsy, 528–529
Bone tamps, 542–544
Bone tumors
  benign, 543–544, 543b
  metastatic
    biopsy of, 528–529
    thermal ablation of, 537–539, 537b
    vertebroplasty and, 539–542
Bougienage, 439, 439f
Bovine aortic arch, 178, 180f
Bowels. *See* Intestines
Brachial artery
  anatomy of, 119, 120f
  angiographic access via, 44–45, 44f–45f
  fibromuscular dysplasia of, 134, 134f
  trauma to, 134
Brachial veins, 137, 137f
  for angiographic access, 48–49, 48f
Brachiocephalic artery, 177
Brachiocephalic veins, 137–139, 138f
Branch catheter reforming technique, 30, 30f
Breast biopsy, image-guided, 511–521
  advantages of, 512b
  clip placement, 512, 512b, 512f–513f
  complications with, 511
  contraindications to, 511
  indications for, 511, 512b
  modalities for
    comparison of, 515t
    MRI-guided, 518–521, 520b
    selection of, 514
    stereotactic-guided, 515–517, 516b, 517t, 519b
    ultrasound-guided, 514–515, 515f–516f
  needle selection, 512–513
    automated spring loaded, 513, 513f–514f
    comparisons of, 514t–515t
    vacuum-assisted, 513, 514b
  reports for, 514b
Breast cancer, hepatic metastases from, 573
Breast interventions, image-guided, 511–526
  axillary fine-needle aspiration, 523
  axillary lymph node sampling, 522–523
  biopsy. *See* Breast biopsy, image-guided
  breast lesion excision systems, 521–523
    complications with, 522
    contraindications to, 522
    Intact BLES device, 522
    vacuum-assisted biopsy *vs.*, 522t
  radio-guided occult lesion localization, 526
  wire-guided localization, 523–526, 523b
Bridge grafts, for dialysis access, 151, 151b, 152f
Brödel line, 485